AJN/MOSBY

Nursing
Boards
Review

For the NCLEX-RN Examination

AJN/MOSBY

Nursing Boards Review

For the NCLEX-RN Examination

TENTH EDITION

with 90 illustrations

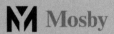

St. Louis Baltimore Boston
Carlsbad Chicago Naples New York Philadelphia Portland
London Madrid Mexico City Singapore Sydney Tokyo Toronto Wiesbaden

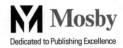

Mosby
Dedicated to Publishing Excellence

A Times Mirror Company

Vice President and Publisher: Nancy L. Coon
Senior Editor: Susan R. Epstein
Senior Developmental Editor: Beverly J. Copland
Associate Developmental Editor: Jerry Schwartz
Project Manager: Dana Peick
Production Editor: Stavra Demetrulias
Designer: Amy Buxton
Manufacturing Supervisor: Linda Ierardi

TENTH EDITION

Printed in the United States of America
Composition by Clarinda Company
Printing/binding by Courier Corporation

Mosby-Year Book, Inc.
11830 Westline Industrial Drive
St. Louis, Missouri 63146

ISBN 0-8151-0080-9

96 97 98 99 00 / 9 8 7 6 5 4 3 2 1

Contributors

COORDINATORS

Patricia Endress Downing, RN, BSN, MN
Clinical Nurse Specialist
Independent Health/Nursing Education Consultant
LaConner, Washington

Susan Droske, RN, MN, CPN
Associate Professor
Texarkana College
Texarkana, Texas

Deborah Antai-Otong, RN, MS, CS
Psychiatric Clinical Specialist; Program Director,
EAP
Department of Veterans Affairs Medical Center
Dallas, Texas

Paulette D. Rollant, RN, MSN, CCRN, PhD
President
Multi-Resources, Inc.
Grantville, Georgia

Marybeth Young, RNC, PhD
Associate Professor
Loyola University—Niehoff School of Nursing
Chicago, Illinois

Contributing Authors

Karen Bernardy, RN, MSN
Conyers, Georgia

Marianne Scharbo-Dehann, RN, BSN, MN, CNM, PhD
Associate Professor
Emory University
Atlanta, Georgia

Gita Dhillon, RN, MA, MS, MEd, CNM
Certified Nurse Midwife
Doctors May-Grant Associates
Lancaster, Pennsylvania

Patricia Endress Downing, RN, BSN, MN
Clinical Nurse Specialist
Independent Health/Nursing Education Consultant
LaConner, Washington

Deborah Ennis, RN, BSN, MSN, CCRN
Professor of Nursing
Harrisburg Area Community College
Harrisburg, Pennsylvania

Sharon Golub, RN, MN
Assistant Professor of Psychiatric Nursing
Mount St. Mary's College
Los Angeles, California

B. Patricia Grace, RN, MSN
Instructor of Nursing
Henry Ford Community College
Dearborn, Michigan

Judith W. Gross, RN, PhD
Assistant Professor
Department of Nursing
Medical University of South Carolina
Charleston, South Carolina

Roberta Kordish, RN, MSN
Principal
Professional Nurse Associates, Inc.
Cleveland, Ohio

Janet Elizabeth Bloomer Kristic, RN, MSN
Assistant Professor, Psychotherapist/Consultant
University of Oklahoma College of Nursing
Oklahoma City, Oklahoma

Alma J. Lubinski, RN, MS, EdD
Chairperson, Professor of Nursing
School of Nursing
North Park College
Chicago, Illinois

Maribeth Moran, RN, BSN, MSN, CPN
Assistant Professor
University of Oklahoma College of Nursing
Oklahoma City, Oklahoma

Judith K. Sands, RN, BS, MS, EdD
Associate Professor, Director of Undergraduate
Students
University of Virginia
Charlottesville, Virginia

Peg Gray-Vickrey, RN(C), BSN, MS, DNS
Assistant Professor
Lycoming College
Williamsport, Pennsylvania

Reviewers

Constance Bobik, RN, BSN, MSN
Assistant Professor
Brevard Community College
Cocoa, Florida

Patricia Castaldi, RN, BSN, MSN
Assistant Dean
Elizabeth General Medical Center School of Nursing
Elizabeth, New Jersey

Alice Day, RN, BS, MS
Health Occupations Teacher
Coffee County High School
Douglas, Georgia

Ralph Matteoli, RN, EdD
Associate Professor
San Francisco State University
San Francisco, California

Anita Norton, RN, MSN
Chairperson, Division of Health Sciences
Jefferson State Community College
Birmingham, Alabama

Susan Speraw, RN, MN, PhD
Associate Professor of Pediatrics
University of Tennessee College of Medicine
Chattanooga, Tennessee

Dorothy Thomas, RN, BSN, MSN
Associate Professor of Nursing
St. Louis Community College at Florissant Valley
St. Louis, Missouri

Debra J. Walden, BA, BSN, MNSc, RNP, CBE
Assistant Professor of Nursing
Arkansas State University
Jonesboro, Arkansas

Introduction

Congratulations! You have passed a big milestone—completing your nursing program. Only one more challenge remains: passing the NCLEX-RN. Your educational program provided a knowledge base to take the boards, but review and study now are essential ingredients to guarantee success on the examination. The *AJN/Mosby Nursing Boards Review* provides a comprehensive review of the essential content you need to pass the NCLEX-RN.

The NCLEX-RN examination focuses on two areas: the nursing process and client needs. It emphasizes the care of both healthy and ill clients. Content areas covered by the test include care of the adult, the child, the child-bearing family, and psychosocial and mental health nursing. Review one clinical area at a time. Start with the one you feel the most comfortable with; this will bolster your confidence to continue. Use a highlighter pen to indicate areas you want to return to for additional study. Make notes in the margins. Use your nursing texts to look up unfamiliar material or to broaden your knowledge base.

The *AJN/Mosby Nursing Boards Review* has three distinct components. Section One introduces you to the format of the computerized NCLEX-RN test and its scoring method including what changes to expect in the new, computerized format. To augment your test-taking skills, this section reviews strategies to increase your competence and confidence. To help you on the day of the examination, it presents techniques to reduce stress. As you study, refer to this section frequently to reinforce principles you will need during the examination.

The second component, contained in Sections Two through Five, covers the four clinical areas. The nursing process provides a consistent framework for organizing client care. Assessment and implementation actions are listed in order of priority. Goals are client centered. Evaluation statements are measurable and reflect the goals. Nursing diagnoses reflect the latest list approved by the North American Nursing Diagnosis Association (NANDA). The content in each section is supplemented by tables, summaries, and illustrations to clarify information and reinforce your knowledge of specific health problems, pharmacology, growth and development, and nutrition. Reprints of articles from the *American Journal of Nursing* and *Maternal/Child Nursing* are provided at the end of each section. These articles have been selected for their relevance to current nursing practice and provide a convenient resource for specific content.

The third component, Section Six, consists of four practice tests of 75 questions each. These sample test questions reflect the stand-alone format of the questions on the NCLEX-RN exam. You may want to use one or two of these as a pretest before you begin your review to identify your strengths and weaknesses. Take the other two practice tests after you have completed your review to see how much you have improved your score.

Answers and rationales are provided for both the correct and incorrect answers for all test questions. The rationales can help clarify faulty thought processes, correct misinformation, and help you learn from your mistakes. Also included is a reference to the section and subsection of this book where relevant content may be found for further review.

Computer disks for both IBM and Macintosh can be found inside the back cover. These disks include the first of the 75 questions, practice tests, and can be used in both a study/review and test format. To reinforce learned information and build confidence, it is recommended that you practice answering questions on a computer to simulate the NCLEX-RN.

Your success with the NCLEX-RN sets you firmly on the road to a professional and challenging career that is full of opportunities. All those responsible for this text—from the staffs at the American Journal of Nursing Company and Mosby to the coordinators and contributing authors who prepared this material—wish you the best of luck on the exam and in your career as a professional nurse.

Contents

3   Nursing Care of the Adult, 108

COORDINATORS   *Patricia E. Downing, RN, BSN, MN*
               Paulette D. Rollant, RN, MSN, CCRN,
               PhD
Contributors   *Patricia E. Downing, RN, BSN, MN*
               Deborah A. Ennis, RN, BSN, MSN,
               CCRN
               Peg Gray-Vickrey, RN (C), BSN, MS,
               DNS
               Alma J. Lubinski, RN, MS, EdD
               Paulette D. Rollant, RN, MSN, CCRN,
               PhD
               Judith K. Sands, RN, BS, MS, EdD

4   Nursing Care of the Childbearing Family, 292

COORDINATOR   *Marybeth Young, RNC, PhD*
Contributors   *Gita Dhillon, RN, MA, MS, Med, CNM*
            B. Patricia Grace, RN, MSN
            Roberta Kordish, RN, MSN
            Marianne Scharbo-DeHann, RN, BSN, MN, CNM, PhD

5 Nursing Care of the Child, 400

COORDINATOR   *Susan Colvert Droske, RN, MN, CPN*

Contributors   *Karen S. Bernardy, RN, MSN*
Susan Colvert Droske, RN, MN, CPN
Judith W. Gross, RN, PhD
Maribeth L. Moran, RN, BSN, CPN

Contents

Chapter *1*

Preparing for the NCLEX-RN

COORDINATOR

Marybeth Young, PhD, MSN, RNC

PRETEST

1. Test items on the NCLEX-RN
   a. describe actual or potential patient health problems.
   b. emphasize knowledge of physiology and safe care.
   c. focus on situations encountered by entry-level nurses.
   d. all of the above choices are correct.
2. The examination requires the graduate nurse to select
   a. one single, best resolution to a problem.
   b. several answers from multiple-choice options.
3. Computer Adaptive Testing (CAT)
   a. requires advanced computer skills.
   b. allows flexibility in changing responses.
   c. individualizes testing by ability level.
   d. penalizes the slow reader.
4. The integrated nursing examination *equally* tests the ability to apply knowledge of
   a. pediatrics, maternity, and medical-surgical nursing.
   b. all five phases of the nursing process.
   c. acute and chronic health problems.
   d. risk factors and measures to promote health.
5. Which of the following test-taking strategies does *not* apply to CAT?
   a. Try to narrow possible responses to two options.
   b. Focus on key words such as *initially* or *least effective*.
   c. Ignore difficult items and return to them later.
   d. Avoid "reading into" the item.

KNOW THE TEST FORMAT

Just as the novice driver needs to know what to expect on the state driving test, each graduate nurse needs a clear idea of the professional licensure exam format. Knowing that you have some questions about the test itself or are unsure of your responses on the pretest, the following brief summary will provide answers.

Success on the national examination is required for entry into professional practice. NCLEX-RN CAT has replaced the paper-and-pencil state boards. This new format reduces the environmental stressors of massive testing rooms by allowing for small-site testing and flexible scheduling.

The framework for the examination continues to follow published guidelines established by the National Council of State Boards of Nursing. Two types of questions are included. The first follows a case study format, in which a situation briefly describing a client's health problems is followed by a multiple-choice question. Each case and subsequent question is discrete; for example, you may need to shift focus from identifying care priorities of an acutely ill adult to teaching an adolescent parent. The second format asks a question that is unrelated to a client case study. Among many possibilities, this type of item may address delegation of care or the responsibilities of a professional nurse.

Graduates may complete the minimum 75 items quickly or continue to test for the maximum of 5 hours or 265 questions. The length of testing is not an indication of performance. The flexibility of CAT tailors each person's exam to a specific ability level.

The test continues to be organized around a broad framework comprised of "Nursing Process" and "Categories of Human Needs." Each part of this plan is summarized briefly; implications for review are suggested.

Nursing Process

The nursing process provides organization for the test as it does for care planning in every clinical setting. Each nursing process phase is equally important in resolving health problems. This consistency is immediately evident to test takers who perceive this equal emphasis. These same graduates are quick to point out that the numbers of items testing maternity and psychiatric nursing are not equal; medical-surgical nursing is heavily emphasized. Table 1-1 suggests a possible test item focus for each phase of the nursing process.

Categories of Human Needs

Concepts that contribute to understanding human needs are another exam focus. Among these are basic human

Table 1-1 Test item focus suggested by the nursing process

Phase	Possible item focus
Assessment	Identifying database
	Selecting appropriate means to gather data
	Gathering information from client/family
	Noting significant observations/data
	Considering environmental factors
	Communicating findings
Analysis	Formulating a nursing diagnosis
	Interpreting data and reporting results of analysis
Planning	Prioritizing nursing diagnoses
	Setting measurable long- and short-term goals
	Involving client/family in planning
	Determining outcome criteria
	Reviewing/modifying plan
Implementation	Carrying out nursing actions safely
	Understanding rationale for care
	Prioritizing care
	Promoting self-care
	Calculating/administering medications safely
	Suggesting diet modifications
	Ensuring safety/comfort
	Preventing infection/injury
	Promoting health
	Responding to emergencies
	Recording/sharing information
	Teaching to client's intellectual level
	Communicating appropriately with client/family/staff
	Supervising/delegating care
Evaluation	Comparing outcomes to goals
	Examining response to therapy
	Seeking more information
	Identifying learning outcomes
	Recognizing risks/problems of therapy
	Communicating evaluation findings
	Evaluating staff learning/caregiving

needs, the teaching-learning process, therapeutic communication, crisis intervention, and developmental theory. Knowledge of anatomy, physiology and pathophysiology, asepsis, nutrition, accountability, the group process, and mental health concepts is basic to the practice of nursing and also is incorporated into many test items. The organization of client needs based on these concepts is identified by the National Council of State Boards of Nursing as "Categories of Human Needs" and is part of the test format. These four categories flow from the ANA Nursing Social Policy Statement and current research on job analysis for entry-level practitioners. The greatest NCLEX-RN exam emphasis is on the categories of physiologic integrity, followed by a focus on health promotion and maintenance. The safe care environment and psychosocial integrity are important, but fewer test items focus on these categories (Tables 1-2 and 1-3). Some overlap is evident as you look at the nursing process framework and the categories of client needs. For example, the nursing process phase of planning addresses both physiologic and psychosocial needs. However, if an individual has a severe fluid volume deficit related to dehydration, emotional needs are attended to *after* setting a goal to resolve life-threatening physiologic problems. Setting priorities is critical to exam success, just as it is in clinical caregiving.

Use your knowledge of the test format to help you identify and review concepts learned throughout your nursing education and to prepare thoughtfully for the examination. However, during the actual NCLEX-RN, do not attempt to identify whether safe, effective care or physiologic integrity is tested in a particular item.

Applied knowledge, rather than mere recall of facts, is measured in most test questions. As you read each question, use the knowledge gained from clinical experience and classroom learning to identify and resolve client problems. Expect to find questions at the beginning of the test fairly easy, followed by increasingly difficult and challenging items. This feature of the CAT allows for individual-

ization of *your* test, and a fit with your ability level. Remember that the NCLEX-RN CAT is a test of competence.

HOW THE TEST IS SCORED

One feature of the CAT is relatively rapid feedback on your PASS/FAIL score. But you must wait several weeks for this information to arrive in the mail. Do not try to keep your own score during the examination; just proceed thoughtfully from one item to the next. If the computer takes a few extra seconds to select an item, remember that it is matching the question difficulty with your ability. Be careful in reading the case study so that you focus on key words. Select the best option thoughtfully. A helpful feature of the CAT is that you are asked to confirm an answer before it registers as your choice. This allows a second opportunity to rethink an answer before moving to another item. Remember, the successful graduate need not be a "computer whiz." Only two keys function during the exam: a space bar and an "enter" key. A brief tutorial will acquaint you with their use. Keep in mind that you will not be able to return to earlier items and change answers as you could on paper-and-pencil tests.

Remember, the NCLEX-RN test plan has been developed to measure critical thinking and nursing competence. Knowing the framework of the exam should dispel some of your fears and help you anticipate and prepare for the test. As you take the test, do not think about the "test plan,"

Table 1-3 Test item focus suggested by categories of human needs

Human needs category	Possible test item focus
Safe, effective care environment	Understanding basic principles
	Using management skills
	Implementing protective measures
	Promoting safety
	Ensuring client/family rights
	Preventing spread of infection
Physiologic integrity	Recognizing altered body function
	Using body mechanics
	Providing comfort measures
	Using equipment safely
	Understanding effects of immobility
	Recognizing untoward responses to therapy/medication/procedures
	Documenting emergency actions
Psychosocial integrity	Identifying mental health concepts
	Recognizing behavior changes
	Referring to resources
	Communicating appropriately
Health promotion/ maintenance	Understanding family systems
	Teaching nutrition
	Promoting wellness
	Strengthening immune responses
	Recognizing adaptive changes to health alterations
	Considering cultural/religious impact on childbearing
	Supporting the dying/family

Table 1-2 Categories of human needs

Categories	Nursing focus
Safe, effective care environment	Coordinating care
	Ensuring quality
	Setting goals
	Promoting safety
	Preparing client for treatments/procedures
	Implementing care
Physiologic integrity	Promoting adaptation
	Identifying/reducing risks
	Fostering mobility
	Ensuring comfort
	Providing basic care
Psychosocial integrity	Promoting adaptation
	Facilitating coping
Health promotion/ maintenance	Promoting growth and development
	Supporting self-care
	Fostering support systems
	Prevention/early treatment of disease

but concentrate on the challenge of each question. Just as the driver attends the road test without wondering, "What is being tested now?" you need only address the problem-solving task.

WHERE SHOULD YOU BEGIN?

When you are familiar with this text and the test format, map out a personal plan for preparation and review. If independent study is planned, set realistic goals within the time available. Ideally, reviewing content over several months is preferable to "cramming" in a few weeks. Studying regularly, over time, helps reinforce knowledge and improves your ability to apply that knowledge.

Begin your review plan by focusing on content that is less familiar to you or about which you feel insecure. Your results on standardized national tests, such as the Assess Test, could serve as a guide, or you may select several case studies from Chapter 6 and answer the questions that follow after reviewing related content. After completing the test items, refer to the correct responses, rationale, and test format classification; then compare your problem-solving abilities to those of content experts. You may find it helpful to return to the review book outline, to a nursing specialty or fundamentals text, or to your class notes to resolve doubts or increase understanding. Look for patterns of test-taking difficulties as you review responses. Becoming aware of your strengths and weaknesses in test taking is an important phase of review and gives more meaningful feedback than counting correct and incorrect responses. By beginning with the greatest challenge and reinforcing understanding, your confidence is renewed as the date of the exam approaches.

COGNITIVE AND AFFECTIVE KEYS TO SUCCESS

Three factors are important in achieving success: *reading,* which affects both reviewing and test taking; being *testwise,* which is defined as the ability to use a test situation to demonstrate learning; and the ability to *control tension* in a major examination, freeing the mind to concentrate on the written questions. Although these factors are interrelated, they are discussed separately. Suggestions and strategies are offered for use during your licensure exam experience (Table 1-4).

Cognitive Strategies to Promote Success

In addition to using this book, other media may meet your needs for review. Audiotapes and videotapes may be helpful in clarifying content or suggesting approaches to test items. You may wish to prepare for the CAT by using one of the many software programs available in schools, libraries, and bookstores.

Reading with concentration is a learned skill that is critical for study, review, and successful examination performance. When preparing for the NCLEX-RN, select an environment that is well lighted and suits your learning style. Avoid reading on a bed—its comfort may induce sleep rather than reinforce knowledge. Gather all materials in advance for the planned study session, including this review book, other appropriate texts, notes, and marker pens to highlight content needing subsequent review.

Skim the review text material, then read for understanding. Look up any unfamiliar terms. Make a note of further questions that come to mind as you review information. Use your knowledge of anatomy, physiology, and pathophysiology to visualize the impact of a specific health alteration. Review the disease process, preventive measures, restoration, and rehabilitation. Refresh your memory of procedures specifically used in treatment. Think about ways in which health might be improved.

While reading test items as practice or in a real situation, be especially observant of *key words.* Notice cues such as *age, risk factors,* and *coping mechanisms.* Clearly identify the question focus (e.g., the concerned parent, the ill child, or the caregiver). Use your knowledge of nursing to think through the question and consider possible responses even before reading all possible options.

Although you must read carefully to understand the questions, avoid reading into the words more than is actually stated. Assume that the health care agency described is ideal and well staffed. If you think that the client's needs would be met by a midnight snack of milk and crackers, do not qualify this with ". . . but it may be impossible to provide this at night."

During the exam, you have no resource for defining vocabulary. Use the sentence context to deduce the meaning of unfamiliar words. Refer to the case study for insight and clarification, and remember to apply your understanding of pathophysiology throughout the exam.

The following examples give you an opportunity to apply several testing strategies to varied questions typical of the NCLEX-RN. Priority setting can be a challenge on an exam. One approach is to view each option as a true/false statement. This is especially helpful if several nursing implementations are correct but you are asked to select a *best* or *initial* action. Ask yourself, "Will the client's health or recovery be affected if one action is *not* carried out initially?"

Consider these test items:

1. Ms. Travis, a 44-year-old kindergarten teacher, was admitted last evening with a medical diagnosis of endocarditis. History includes a cholecystectomy 2 years ago and childhood rheumatic fever. Two days ago her dentist extracted an infected molar after an unsuccessful root canal procedure. Although she usually takes prophylactic penicillin before dental treatment, she forgot to do so. Present temperature is 103°F. IV ampicillin is ordered every 6 hours. She seems uncomfortable and anxious, asking repeatedly if her son has arrived from a distant state. During the initial assessment of Ms. Travis, the nurse notes that 600 ml of 5% dextrose

Table 1-4   Cognitive strategies for success

Prepare	for safe practice
Plan a review	to broaden knowledge
Read carefully	for understanding
Identify key words	to focus attention
Narrow options	by critical thinking
Use an educated guess	not random choice
Set priorities	based on health risk

in 0.225% normal saline has infused in 2 hours. The physician ordered 1000 ml in 10 hours; therefore the *initial action* should be to

① notify the attending physician.
② assess respirations and breath sounds.
③ recalculate the infusion rate.
④ report the problem to the supervisor.

As you would do in a clinical setting, review the assessment data and filter out the information that has less impact on the client's present condition. Identify the actual and potential problems; then read the question and consider each option thoughtfully. As fluid volume is altered, physiologic integrity clearly dictates priority assessments and *immediate* interventions.

In this example say to yourself, "The priority action is to notify the physician. True or false?" Then proceed to the other options. Although responses 1, 2, and 3 are appropriate, the *priority action* is to detect signs of fluid volume excess related to rapid infusion (option 2). Pulmonary edema could further complicate the client's condition. Option 4 is not an initial action, nor should the supervisor be notified until after consulting with the head nurse or unit manager.

2. A physician orders 1000 ml of IV fluids to be infused in 10 hours. The drop factor is 10/ml. The nurse should adjust the rate to

① 2 drops per minute.
② 6 drops per minute.
③ 16 drops per minute.
④ 21 drops per minute.

Calculate the fluid rate using the standard equation. Be sure to label all values such as minutes and milliliters. The correct response is option 3. During the actual exam, use the scrap paper provided to work out the mathematics; never calculate from memory!

3. Mr. Kent had a bronchoscopic examination several hours ago. A topical anesthetic spray was used during the procedure. Because the physician ordered diet as tolerated and the client tolerated sips of water, he was given a general diet for lunch. As he begins to eat, his color turns gray; he appears to have difficulty breathing and then grasps his throat. Select the correct priority action.

① Notify the anesthesiologist.
② Suction secretions from his oral pharynx.
③ Perform a thrust maneuver.
④ Assess for other problems.

The priority action is to ensure a patent airway, option 3. Further reflection may lead you to question if the client's swallowing and gag reflexes were assessed before the meal. In this example, as in many NCLEX-RN test items, one choice suggests the need for further information. Be careful in selecting this response. Although it may be helpful to have more assessment data, this question provides sufficient data to direct quick and safe action.

Communication test items present a special challenge. As in actual practice, nonverbal cues and the environment affect the communication process. When reading questions focusing on nurse/client/family interactions, consider all information carefully. Realize that a reference to an interaction or the presence of quotation marks does not automatically imply therapeutic use of self. Refer to Table 1-5 for suggested ways in which communication test items might vary with *nurse-client* interactions. Apply basic principles and be aware of possible communication blocks. Base choices on a sound rationale, rather than selecting a response that "sounds like" what you actually might say.

4. Ms. Fox, 57, visits the clinic for a Pap smear and describes occasional hot flashes and irregular menstrual periods. She plans to discuss estrogen replacement therapy with her gynecologist. In response to questions about lifestyle, she describes regular activity and rest patterns and a well-balanced diet. A review of her history reveals that two sisters had breast cancer. When asked if she performs breast self-examinations regularly, Ms. Fox appears upset. "I am so afraid of cancer! I'd rather not know if there is a problem! I could not cope with finding a mass." Select an appropriate reply to the client:

① "Fear is no reason to neglect your health."
② "Your risk is very high because of family history."
③ "Tell me more about what you are feeling."
④ "You should not feel afraid; early detection is critical."

This question suggests an initial need for therapeutic communication. Although correct information should be

Table 1-5 Focus of communications test items

Type of interaction	Approach
Interview	Asking purposeful questions
	Identifying risk factors
	Using appropriate vocabulary
	Listening to responses
	Maintaining confidentiality
Information giving	Describing tests/procedures
	Clarifying data
	Explaining treatment to client/family/ staff
Teaching/learning (to client, family, health care providers)	Assessing health, learning needs
	Using developmentally appropriate terms
	Giving instructions to promote safety
	Supporting self-care
	Reinforcing group learning
	Observing a return demonstration
	Involving family in basic care
	Evaluating learning outcomes
Therapeutic use of self	Establishing trust
	Identifying own communication skills
	Developing goal direction
	Listening actively
	Clarifying, reflecting
	Sharing observations
	Anticipating needs
	Reinforcing positive coping styles
	Supporting in loss
	Referring for help

conveyed, risk factors identified, and teaching emphasized, this client needs to express her feelings and concerns. Response 3 indicates the nurse's availability as a listener.

5. A nursing assistant (NA) from the ambulatory care unit is assigned to your acute care setting at a time when several staff have called in sick. He is assigned to work with you. Which of the following tasks could you assign to him?
   ① Changing sterile dressings
   ② Assisting with morning care
   ③ Suctioning tracheostomy tubes
   ④ Monitoring IV fluids

Delegation of care to unlicensed personnel is increasingly the responsibility of professional nurses. Such delegation involves trust and a knowledge of the skills of the assistive worker. In this case, the abilities expected of the NA should include providing for client hygiene, response 2. The other tasks are beyond the ability of an aide without advanced training.

Some questions focusing on Human Needs Categories address potential problems within the environment. Consider the following:

6. During a busy day in the outpatient clinic, the nurse suspects that a young child may have rubella. Of the following clients who were in contact with the child, which individual is at greatest risk?
   ① John Norris, HIV-positive, recovering from tuberculosis
   ② Celia Moran, 8 months pregnant; rubella titer positive
   ③ Lori Ruiz, 1 month old; breast-feeding
   ④ Frances Long, chronic alcoholic with cirrhosis

Rubella exposure is particularly dangerous for any immunosuppressed client (option 1). Although insufficient information is given about the 1-month-old baby's nursing mother and there may be a risk to the client described in option 4, you are asked to identify the individual for whom exposure is *most dangerous*. That client is John Norris.

7. As a nurse makes rounds on a pediatric unit, each of the following is observed. Which situation must be corrected immediately to ensure client well-being?
   ① A school-aged amputee leaves his wheelchair at the bedside.
   ② Several toddlers spread their toys on the playroom floor.
   ③ The stereo volume in the adolescent lounge is too loud.
   ④ The newborn step-down ICU is 68° F.

The low nursery temperature (option 4) is a serious problem and may lead to cold stress. Examine the other options for potential safety problems. The child with a disability should have access to his wheelchair. Although toys should not be left in an area where they create a hazard, risk is minimal in the playroom. The loud music may subsequently affect hearing, but this is typical for adolescents. The question does not mention that other clients are disturbed; therefore there is no need for immediate action.

Some test items ask you to consider potential or actual problems identified in several clients and then decide on an appropriate action. Consider this item:

8. Each of the following assessments is documented by a night nurse on an adult surgical unit. Which observation should be reported *immediately* to the physician?
   ① Jenny Bocci has a temperature of 100° F the night after surgery for a ruptured appendix.
   ② Karen Rosen's knee is hot and swollen 2 days after cartilage repair.
   ③ William Clifford's dressing has purulent drainage shortly after the incision of an abscess.
   ④ George Henderson has blood-tinged urine 12 hours after a transurethral prostatectomy.

In reviewing the data, visualize the operative procedure and expected recovery. Identify problems that may delay healing. The physician should be notified immediately about the orthopedic client's postoperative condition. Option 2 indicates a serious problem that may lead to subsequent bone or systemic infection. All other observations are expected during convalescence for the surgical procedures described.

Affective Strategies for Success

It is difficult to separate cognitive and emotional factors in test performance. There are, however, distinctly separate ways to prepare for the mental and emotional challenges of the examination. Long-range goal setting must include realistic life plans. Anticipate the time that study and review demand; avoid a major life change that increases tension. Because of the increased flexibility of NCLEX-RN CAT, you can schedule your test date so that it does not conflict with a wedding or a 3-week hiking trip.

Realistically evaluate your personal responses to test challenges. Look at past successes and ways you maintain energy and confidence under stress. How have you reacted to past major examinations? What physiologic or psychologic responses to stress are common for you? Many graduates report that tension headaches or gastrointestinal distress occur during the 2 days of testing. Some suggest that lapses of concentration are frequent during a tiring day of problem solving. Expect that your thoughts may "drift" or that you may experience a "failure fantasy," as many other nurses have described. Expect some anger about a specific test item. You may feel that you could have written "better answers than those!"

To use your mind to its fullest and to demonstrate your competence as a nurse, you need to control the effects of anxiety. Several effective ways exist to reduce tension; try one or more of the following:
- Relaxing and contracting muscles progressively from head to toe
- Slow, deep breathing and deliberate calming
- Guided imagery with focus on a peaceful scene
- Meditation, prayer, positive thoughts
- Focusing on a confident self

Select the method of stress reduction that has worked for you in the past, learn new approaches, and practice them during times of tension while studying. For example, to use imagery, see yourself in the setting that is most peaceful for you. Close your eyes and imagine the quiet, the scents, the scenery around you. Feel the warmth and energy. Relax and feel calm. Change the setting as you need to until it is

Table 1-6 Keys to success on the NCLEX-RN

Know the test format
  An integrated exam
  Pass/fail score
  Single-response, multiple-choice items
  Based on measurement of safe nursing behaviors for common
    health problems
Review concepts
  Growth and development
  Pharmacology and pathophysiology
  Effects of culture and nutrition on health
  The nursing process
  Categories of human needs
Where should you begin?
  Consider your strengths and your learning style
How should you prepare?
  Review course notes and texts
  Consider a review program
  Use human resources and support services
Strategies to promote success
  Begin with self-evaluation
  Sharpen test-taking skills
  Learn methods to reduce stress
  Be self-confident
Just before the exam
  Get a good night's rest
  Avoid late cramming
  Eat breakfast
During the NCLEX-RN CAT
  Concentrate on your screen
  Read items carefully
  Draw on your knowledge
  Use relaxation methods

1982, 1988, 1995 Young M, Kopala B.

the perfect relaxing pause. Recall these images during difficult moments in the exam when you need a brief recharge. You will feel your spirits lift and will experience clearer thinking.

Close to the exam date, plan your travel to the testing center. If distance allows, visit the area in advance so that you know the best route and alternates. Consider seasonal problems that may affect travel time. It is critical to arrive at the testing site ahead of time, or you may be refused entry.

Anticipate that even a small test setting may be overwhelming. Plan ways that you can deal with environmental stressors, such as security measures. This is one time in your professional life when *your* needs are a priority. Do what you must to remain calm and confident.

On the exam day, consider your own comfort and nutritional needs. Dress in nonconstricting and attractive clothing that helps you feel good about yourself. It is wise to carry a jacket in anticipation of temperature changes within the testing room. Eat a high-protein breakfast, but avoid excessive caffeine and fluids so that an emergency trip to the restroom is not necessary. Pack fruit, a can of juice, and headache remedies or cough drops so that they are available at the required and optional breaks.

Expect to encounter at least one unfamiliar health problem in the NCLEX-RN CAT. Remain confident that you can use your knowledge of anatomy, physiology, pathophysiology, and nursing to solve the problem. Do not allow anger to destroy your concentration with thoughts such as "Why didn't we learn about that condition in school?" Rather, think to yourself, "I can try to answer these questions." Above all, do not be distracted by the individual who leaves after 1 hour of testing! That person may have a different ability level, or may even be taking a different professional exam.

The keys to success are within you (Table 1-6). Discover your strengths and potential by preparing thoroughly—mentally and emotionally. Study, review, practice test-taking strategies, and learn how to reduce personal tension. The rewards begin with your license to practice as a professional nurse. You are needed in the changing health care field, and you are welcomed as a caregiver and a colleague!

Answer Key for Pretest Questions, p. 2

1. d
2. c
3. d
4. b
5. c

REFERENCES

Changes incorporated into the NCLEX-RN Test Plan, *Issues* 15(4):1, 1994.

Chornick N, Yocom C, Jacobson J: *1992-1993 job analysis study of newly licensed entry-level registered nurses,* Chicago, 1993, National Council of State Boards of Nursing.

Questions and answers on the methodology of the computerized adaptive testing for the NCLEX, Chicago, 1995, National Council of State Boards of Nursing.

Test plan for the national council licensure examination for registered nurses, Chicago, 1995, National Council of State Boards of Nursing.

ACING MULTIPLE-CHOICE TESTS

Just remember confidence, control, content, *and* common sense—*it'll be easier to focus on the questions and answers.*

BY PAULETTE D. ROLLANT

Do multiple-choice exams make your heart race? Do exams on computers challenge your coping skills? Do you have trouble choosing the best answer?

All of the above?

Turn your stress into success! Use the stabilization approach, or what I call the four-point success system.

Houses, cars, chairs, tables, and other useful items are usually based on this system. Each has four points of reference. For example, a car has four tires; if one goes flat, one point of reference is removed. The car can still be driven but not for long. If two tires are damaged, you're out of luck.

Likewise, there are four points of reference to pass exams: the four Cs—*confidence, control, content, and common sense*. If you prepare for multiple-choice exams by using only one or two of these points of reference, you'll lessen your chances of passing. To see how this success system can work for you, let's take a look at each of the points of reference.

CONFIDENCE

You can gain confidence in test taking by learning to read and answer questions precisely. Practice the following easy steps.

Step 1: Be a Detective

Look for clues in the stem, the question, and the responses. Clues include:

Paulette D. Rollant, RN, CCRN, PhD, is president, Multi-Resources, Inc., Atlanta, a firm that develops, presents, and evaluates educational programs.
Modified from AJN: Nursing career guide, Jan. 1994.

Key words: *most, first, initially, immediately, late, toxicity, side effect, toxic effect, complication, usual problem*

Nursing process: assessment, analysis, plan, intervention, evaluation

Time parameters: day one versus day three, preop, postop, during, after

Age group of a patient: the decade determines the developmental need, normal physiologic changes, and will guide an approach for teaching or discharge planning

Absolutes: *always, never, every, none, all, all the time*

Words of essence: *acute, chronic, partial, total,* or diseases that indicate acute or chronic conditions

Locations: outpatient, clinic, hospital, home, postanesthesia unit

Distractors: mystery diseases, absurd situations, content that clashes with your personal beliefs; that is, questions that evoke an emotional response and obscure your thinking

Let's apply these clues to questions.

A patient begins to experience a severe gastrointestinal bleed. The plan of care to meet the patient's fluid needs should include, as a priority, which of the following?

a. accommodating the patient's frequent need for the bedpan or emesis basin

b. monitoring vital signs on an hourly basis

c. maintaining the gastric pH

d. rapidly administering blood and fluid

When questions include key words such as *first* or *priority*, you don't need to look for an incorrect response: All the responses are correct. You must choose the *best response*. Think of us-

ing the ABCs or the nursing process. For the ABCs approach, airway, breathing, and circulation take precedence over any other factors. If the information in the stem defines a situation, try the nursing process. The most likely answer is to do further assessment before an intervention or evaluation. So look for the assessment response. If all the assessment data have been included in the stem, then an intervention response is the likely correct answer.

In the question above, essential words—*priority* and *severe bleed*—guide your selection of the answer. Think ABCs. The only answer that deals with circulation or fluid needs is d. If you are thinking that d is incorrect because at your hospital blood is rarely given, you're reading into the question, as well as letting personal experience influence your answer. Thus, you have answered *a* question rather than answering *the* question asked.

A nurse is caring for a patient with acute myocardial infarction whose recovery is uncomplicated. To prevent complications on the third day, the nurse would do which of the following?

a. Monitor the patient's ability to turn, cough, and deep breathe.

b. Have the patient walk a short distance.

c. Apply antiembolic hose to the patient's legs.

d. Give the patient sublingual nitroglycerin prior to all out-of-bed activity to prevent chest pain.

During a patient's seizure the nurse should

a. suction as needed.

b. ensure safety.

c. elevate head with a pillow.

d. observe the length and aftereffects of the seizure.

The answer to the first question is b. If you read it too quickly, you may have overlooked the time clue of *third day*. If you selected answer c, which is the answer for *a* question about an action on the *first day* post–myocardial infarction, you didn't answer *the* question. By the third day this patient should be walking short distances to prepare for discharge. Answer a might be a good choice for a patient with complications. Response d is incorrect because of the word *all*, an absolute. Not all activity needs preventive medication.

The answer to the second question is b. The key word is *during*. This makes answer d incorrect because it includes information after the seizure. *The* question is asking for general information; select a more general or global response. Response a is too specific, and suctioning is commonly not done during a seizure because the patient's jaws are usually clamped. Elevating the head with a pillow (c) flexes the neck and closes the patient's airway.

The initial content for discharge teaching of a patient, age 26, after the repair of a ruptured appendix with an open incision would be focused on concerns about

a. loss of functional ability.

b. the effects of surgery on intimacy.

c. alterations in body image.

d. fears of not being able to attain life's goals.

The correct answer is c; body image is a major concern of people aged 20 to 29. If the age was changed to 36, b would be correct; if 46, d would be correct; and if 76, a would be correct.

Patients over 60 years of age typically have difficulty with seeing small print, hearing, and manipulating equipment, whereas teenagers may have these abilities but lack the interest or motivation.

A family member of a post–myocardial infarction patient sat in on the discharge teaching session. Which of the following statements indicates the family member understands the steps to successful recovery?

a. "Before we do any activity around the house, a nitroglycerin needs to be taken to avoid chest pains."

b. "We will plan to take a one-hour nap every day."

c. "When we go fishing we'll need to alternate moderate activity with periods of rest."

d. "We have a calendar to mark down the blood pressure and weight in the morning and in the evening."

When a response contains absolutes, it's usually incorrect. Response a is incorrect because of the word *any*. Nitroglycerin should be taken before *strenuous* activity, not just *any activity*. There's no reason for the patient to take a nap every day, so b is incorrect. In response d the activities mentioned are usually done once a day in the morning. The correct response is c.

Ms. Murphy, age 80, who's had diabetes for more than 25 years, visits the clinic for education. She says, "I've cooked the same way for 20 years. I know what I like to eat and I don't plan to change now." At this time, patient teaching for Ms. Murphy should be based on the results of an evaluation of

a. the condition of her feet.

b. her activity level.

c. her serum glucose level.

d. the foods she's eaten.

The correct response is a. Ms. Murphy has a chronic condition and is at the clinic. Her statement indicates that diet education at this time would be ineffective. The clinic nurse would have the most influence on behaviors related to foot care. If the feet were in good condition the nurse could give positive reinforcement. If the feet were in bad condition, the clinic nurse could initiate physical care, then refer Ms. Murphy to a foot specialist. The patient may be more likely to follow up since bad feet are uncomfortable, and this physiologic need commonly supersedes other needs. (Don't forget Maslow's hierarchy of needs.) Response c is incorrect since it's too general—a more specific answer would refer to *when* the glucose was checked (that is, fasting or nonfasting levels). The patient's activity level (b) may be least likely to change due to her age and psychosocial limitations.

The patient with acute disease may be more anxious and have fewer effective coping mechanisms. A patient with a chronic condition, on the other hand, usually has greater coping skills, more available support systems, and a deeper knowledge of the condition to allow for adaptation. These factors will influence your nursing actions in different clinical settings.

Step 2: Read the Stem Systematically

Relax! A tense body results in a tense mind that misses important words and can't think or make decisions. Read the question first. Then read the information above the question. Note any clues in the stem and give all words equal attention. Read the question again. Think of what the answer would be. Then read the given responses.

As you go from question to question, read at an even pace. Avoid spending too much time on a question. Avoid "hangover," which is thinking about prior questions while you're now on a new question.

In the first few seconds of reading a question, avoid the "I know" or "I don't know the content" approach. Remember that your biases from life experiences or emotions may influence how you read the question. For example, if you dislike neuro and had an awful instructor for neuro, when you get to a neuro question this bias automatically kicks into gear. You tense up and can't think. To counter this reaction, for neuro questions tell yourself, "I'm familiar with some part of this situation. I can relate the information. I can make an educated decision." Besides, the question may be asking about something else other than neuro—if you're tense you may not even notice.

After you read the stem, try to act out the situation mentally. Close your eyes, visualize the scenario. Often the correct response will come to mind immediately. For questions about adduction, abduction, flexion, extension, and so forth, you can help yourself choose the right answer by moving your arm or leg in the described manner.

While reading the stem, determine if the background information is important or even related to the question asked. Decide if the question is asking about assessment, planning, intervention, evaluation, or communication content. Or is the question asking about *normal* or *abnormal*? Identifying the focus at this point will help you screen the four responses. Remember that "quotations" don't always indicate a communication or psych question. Be aware that teaching-type questions could be testing correct or incorrect information. For example, questions may be worded "needs additional teaching" or "needs no additional teaching." If you read too quickly or haven't controlled your anxiety, you may overlook small but crucial words like the "no."

Step 3: Read All the Responses, Then Select the Answer

Look for those clues mentioned above in step 1! Concentrate on each word in each response. If possible, narrow your choices to two responses. That will increase your chance of answering the question correctly by 50%. In some cases, you might try to cluster the responses to select the correct answer. That is, categorize the responses: general versus specific, internal/external, immediate/late, drugs/nondrugs, and assessment/intervention. If three of the responses can be grouped, the one outside the category is usually correct.

A patient is constipated and dehydrated. Which intervention would the patient most likely comply with?
  a. drinking Ensure between meals
  b. drinking extra fluids with meals
  c. drinking 8 oz of water every hour between meals
  d. drinking adequate amounts of fluid during the day

The correct answer is c. Note that a, b, and d can be clustered since they are general statements without specific fluid amounts. Or perhaps you found the correct response based on the teaching theory that specific goals more likely result in completion of tasks. (You may want to keep this theory in mind for yourself in preparation for passing those exams.)

With responses that have series of items, read "vertically." For example:

Which set of arterial blood gases should the nurse expect to find in a patient with metabolic acidosis?
  a. pH 7.28, PCO_2 55, HCO_3 26
  b. pH 7.50, PCO_2 30, HCO_3 31
  c. pH 7.48, PCO_2 30, HCO_3 22
  d. pH 7.30, PCO_2 36, HCO_3 18

First, read only the pHs down vertically and look for a lowered pH, acidosis. Using this technique, you can narrow the responses to either a or d. Now look at the HCO_3, since you can recall the rules: for metabolic imbal-

ances the pH and the bicarb move in the same direction and for respiratory imbalances the pH and the CO_2 move in the opposite directions. Note that *the* question is about a metabolic imbalance. Compare the bicarbs in responses a and d. You know the answer is d. By using the vertical technique, you have saved time, energy, and maintained a clearer mind.

If you're stumped by the question, sometimes simply matching similar words or ideas in the stem and response will result in a correct answer. Try these questions.

The patient had his blood pressure taken in lying and standing positions. The nurse explains to him that this is a test for
  a. central nervous system depression.
  b. malignant hypertension.
  c. orthostatic hypotension.
  d. vascular insufficiency.

A patient in acute renal failure develops pulmonary edema. Which of the following interventions would be inappropriate to include in this patient's care?
  a. Administer oxygen.
  b. Encourage coughing and deep breathing.
  c. Place the patient in high Fowler's position.
  d. Replace lost fluids.

In the first question, by matching the idea of *position* in the stem with the associated word *orthostatic,* you choose the correct response, c. In the second question, by matching the concept *edema* in the stem to the word *fluid,* you choose d. (A word of caution: Reserve this technique for when you have no idea what the answer may be.)

When you select an answer, your first hunch is usually correct! Don't change answers unless you're sure that you misread the question or missed some important clues the first time around.

Step 4: Review Practice Questions

When you're preparing for an exam, correct your practice questions. Read all the rationales of all questions if they're available. Rationales frequently include clinical pearls stated in a precise and easy-to-recall manner along with essential factors to consider for the correct response.

Look for patterns of missed questions. For example, you might find

clusters of missed questions at the beginning, middle, or end of the exam. This could reflect periods of fatigue or anxiety. On your next practice test, make a mental note to consciously relax at these times. Take a mental minivacation. Also, if you have the opportunity, review the questions at these patterned intervals to make sure you correctly read the questions before turning in the test. On computer exams you can't go back, so it's best to pause every 15 questions or so for minivacations, deep breathing, or the relaxation exercises that work best for you.

Note the questions for which you have changed answers. Did this help or hinder the number of questions that you got right? If it helped, you have a pattern of changing answers to better your score. Change answers. However, if it didn't help, don't change your answers—no matter what!

Some authorities say that if you have no idea what the answer is, choose "c." The rationale given is that more item writers use "c" as the correct answer. I think that if you would rather choose "a," then do so. In the end it doesn't matter because some research findings report that 25% of any number of multiple-choice questions will be correctly answered by random selection—on a 100-item exam you will get at least 25 questions correct by guessing. Add that to at least 50 questions you will get correct by having studied. You pass the exam.

Review your incorrect responses. For each correct answer you missed, ask yourself: Why did I miss this?

Did I know the content? Make a list of the unfamiliar content. Look it up. Then try to categorize unfamiliar content. Was it cardiac? Renal? If you have time, read parts of the chapter that you think would be most helpful to you.

Ask yourself: What step in the nursing process was more frequently missed? Assessment? Evaluation? The next time you do practice questions pick those types of questions to do. Or be sure when you are doing practice questions to identify these questions, read them more carefully, and try to relax before selecting your response.

Did I misread the questions or responses? Most people fall into this category. Did you overlook a key word in the stem or in one of the responses?

Did you answer *a* question instead of *the* question? When you get your exams back do you say, "I knew that! Why did I choose this"? If you do, you need to sharpen and to more frequently apply confidence skills. Or maybe you need to sharpen and more frequently apply your control skills to lessen your anxiety during exams. Or maybe you need to do both! Your analyses of why you're missing questions will guide you. When you're very nervous, your concentration and perception are below par. You then need to reduce your anxiety through techniques such as deep breathing.

If you practice these strategies for controlling errors in reading test questions, you will certainly boost your confidence in your ability to pass exams. And, as you work on confidence, you can also develop your skills of control.

CONTROL

Control is your ability to maintain a minimum stress level so that your perceptions and decisions are accurate. You're able to read the questions objectively, to think, and to problem-solve. The three most common categories of exam stressors are mental, physical, and psychosocial.

Mental stressors are those messages you play over and over in your mind. Frequently, these messages are negative, draining your confidence, energy, and thinking ability. First, you have to consciously work at becoming aware of these messages. Then you can counter them with positive ones. For example, if you go in to take a test playing the mental message of "I didn't study enough. I know I'll have trouble on this test," counter that thought immediately with something more positive, such as, "I studied as much as I could. I know that content and will use it to figure out related items on the test." Other positive messages might be: "I will slow down and read the questions more carefully." "I will ignore the distractions in the room."

Physical stressors include the environment and your body. The exam room may be too cold, hot, noisy, or crowded, the chairs uncomfortable, and the lighting poor. Plan on the worst. Dress in layers so clothing can be added or removed. You may want to use ear plugs if you find noises distracting. When you do test questions at home, select days when it's hot, cold, or noisy. Practice tuning out the distractions.

To diminish your body's stress, stay away from spicy, fatty, and high-sugar foods, which can make you feel sluggish and heavy, and give you indigestion. Caffeine can make you feel hyper, tense, and anxious, and cause you to make frequent trips to the bathroom. Alcohol depresses the central nervous system as well as dehydrating and depleting important minerals.

Psychosocial stressors result from the behaviors or comments of your colleagues either during study time or right before the exam. Suggest to your group that you have a rule to allow only positive comments during study times or before exams. You may want to distract yourself before testing by listening to music through a headset or by reading something fun or "nonnursing." Also, be aware that a family member's physical problems that are similar to your test material may cause you to answer the question based on your personal experience rather than general theory.

CONTENT

To help you remember content for later application, try this process. Before class on a given topic simply read the introduction and summaries of the chapter that covers the content. Go to class and listen as well as take notes. Every night read over your notes before bedtime. You're more likely to retain content in long-term memory if you study for no longer than an hour and then sleep for at least a few hours. On the following days do some practice questions in that content area, guided by the ones you missed. Refer to your text as much as needed. It's usually students' goal to read all the pages in the text; however, in reality, it's next to impossible. Remember that the content includes facts and the application of facts to clinical situations.

COMMON SENSE

Common sense—don't leave home without it. Pick it up each morning from the kitchen counter and put it in your pocket. Common sense says, "I'll figure this out. I know something. That something will get the answer." Let's practice:

How long does it take to dissolve fibrin?
   a. 1-3 days
   b. 7-10 days
   c. 25-30 days
   d. 60-90 days

If you have no idea what the correct answer is, use common sense plus a little content knowledge. You recall that fibrin has something to do with clotting. So you think of what might be a common situation when a clot forms in the body. You remember that this morning you bumped into the table and bruised your leg. Yes, a bruise is a clot. Then think. You remember that your bruises usually last about a week. Yes! The answer is certainly b.

Another commonsense approach for this question is to look at the numbers in the given responses. Throw out the extremes, the highest and the lowest, answers a and d. Use a conservative approach and select the numbers in b. Try another question.

In the elderly patient sympathetic responsiveness
   a. increases with age.
   b. remains equal to that of a young adult.
   c. decreases with age.
   d. no longer occurs.

As people get older they slow down. Similarly, the sympathetic system most likely does also. The correct answer is c.

The key to becoming a successful test taker? Practice, practice, and more practice in using the four reference points: confidence, control, content, and common sense. Pick up stamina, speed, and steam in thinking and decision making. Remember—that which has your attention determines your direction. Pay attention to these details. I'm sure you'll do well!

Contents

Chapter 2

Nursing Care of the Client with Psychosocial and Mental Health Problems

COORDINATOR

Deborah Antai-Otong, MS, RN, CS

Contributors

Sharon Golub, RN, MN

Janet Kristic, MSN, RN, CS

1. This section reviews content that is general to all nursing—that is, communicating with clients and the nurse-client relationship—as well as content that is specific to psychiatric nursing. The NCLEX-RN examination will test your knowledge of communication and interpersonal relationships in *all* sections of the examination.
2. DSM-IV: The sections in this book are organized in the format of client problem behaviors and the *Diagnostic and Statistical Manual of Mental Disorders,* 4th edition, (American Psychiatric Association, 1994). The DSM-IV categorizes and codes psychiatric diagnoses. These categories and codes are used by physicians, psychiatric nurses, and other mental health care providers to communicate regarding various mental disorders, document clients' records, make diagnoses, compile statistics, refer to nomenclature of diagnostic criteria to strengthen reliability of clinical judgment, apply for grants, and report for third-party payment (insurance). Each diagnosis includes a description of diagnostic criteria. The NCLEX-RN will not ask you to diagnose the client's disorder, but it will use DSM-IV terminology.

PSYCHOSOCIAL CHARACTERISTICS OF THE HEALTHY CLIENT

1. Infant through adolescent
   a. See Table 2-1 and *The Healthy Child,* p. 402
2. Young adult years (20 to 40) (See Table 2-2)
   a. Cognitive development
      1. thinking and learning are problem-centered
      2. thinking is at an abstract level, comparing ideas mentally or verbally with previous memories, knowledge, and experience
      3. learns formally and informally by emphasizing principles and concepts
      4. objective, realistic
   b. Emotional development
      1. sexuality is a powerful determinant
      2. expected to be responsible, have good impulse control
      3. Erikson's task: intimacy versus self-isolation or self-absorption
   c. Moral/religious development
      1. challenges values, principles defined by parents and identifies those to be retained or modified
      2. values become individualized and integrated, and provide basis for future ethical decision making
   d. Body-image development
      1. body image is flexible, subject to constant revision, may not reflect actual body structure
      2. a social and cultural creation
      3. close interdependence between body image and personality, self-concept, and identity; may be altered by illness, injury, disability
   e. Lifestyle options
      1. separates from parents in twenties and develops peer relationships
      2. makes decisions regarding types of relationships to form (marriage, child rearing, communal, homosexual)
      3. settles into career
      4. establishes leisure activities
   f. Developmental tasks
      1. accepts self: stabilizing self-concept and body image
      2. establishes independence
      3. establishes a vocation to make worthwhile contributions
      4. learns to appraise and express love responsibly
      5. establishes intimate bond with another
      6. establishes and manages residence
      7. finds congenial social group
      8. decides on option of a family
      9. formulates philosophy of life
      10. establishes role in community
3. Middle adult years (40-65)
   a. Cognitive development
      1. goal-oriented
      2. enhanced by experiences, motivation
      3. decreased memory functioning
      4. less preserved from verbal information
      5. continued learning emphasized
      6. emphasis on realistic thinking
      7. problem-centered thinking
      8. attitudes may be less flexible
   b. Emotional development
      1. transitional, self-assessment period
      2. channels emotional drives without losing initiative and vigor
      3. masters environment
      4. manages emotional responses
      5. values age and life experiences
      6. Erikson's task: generativity versus self-absorption and stagnation
   c. Moral/religious development
      1. integrates new concepts from wider sources
      2. beliefs are less dogmatic
      3. personal philosophy offers comfort, happiness
   d. Body-image development
      1. adapts to climacteric; changes accepted as part of maturity
      2. reinforces positive self-concept
      3. prefers experiences, insights, values of current age
   e. Lifestyle options
      1. reflects work ethic
      2. increases leisure time
      3. differentiates compulsive work and play from healthy work and play
      4. recognizes self-creativity
      5. increases preparation for retirement
   f. Developmental tasks
      1. develops new satisfaction as a mate; supportive to mate; develops sense of unity with mate
      2. helps offspring become happy, responsible adults
      3. takes pride in accomplishments of self and spouse
      4. balances work with other roles
      5. assists aging parents
      6. achieves social and civic responsibility
      7. maintains active organizational membership
      8. accepts physical changes of middle age
      9. makes an art of friendship

Table 2-1 Life-cycle stages

Common name/age	Freud	Erikson	Sullivan	Tasks
Infancy (Birth-18 months)	Oral Sexual gratification through mouth Dependent drives Pleasure of biting Aggressive drives and body image develop Differentiates self from mother	Trust vs mistrust Exchanges with parents lay basis for trust or mistrust of others in later life	Development of a self-system Others gratify needs and satisfy wishes	Dependent drives Aggressive drive Differentiation from mother/sense of self/trust/security
Toddler (18 months-3 years)	Anal Excretory control learned Concepts of cleanliness, punctuality, self-control, personal independence learned	Autonomy vs shame and doubt Self-control Personal independence and self-worth develop	Acculturation Delay gratification	Shame, disgust Control, cleanliness Punctuality Independence Self-worth
Preschool (3-6 years)	Phallic/oedipal Pleasure through genitals Attachment to parent of opposite sex Competition with parent of same sex Resolves by identifying with parent of same sex Develops sexual identity, guilt	Initiative vs guilt Sharing, competing, self-motivation Learns to control jealousy, rage, envy, guilt	Playmates: forms satisfactory relationships with peers	Guilt, values Establishment of masculine or feminine role Sharing, competing Self-motivation
School age (6-12 years)	Latency Limited sexual image Socialization outside home Intellectual and social growth Friends Control over aggressive, destructive impulses	Industry vs inferiority Skill mastery Work and play in groups Intellectual growth	Chums: relates to friends of same sex	Intellectual and social growth Mastery of skills Establishment of friendships Group work and play Control over aggressive, destructive impulses
Adolescence (12-20 years)	Genital Sexuality focuses on genitals Establishes identity Learns independence from parents, responsibility for self, intimacy with opposite sex	Identity vs role diffusion Sense of self and identity apart from parents	Early: satisfactory relationships with members of opposite sex Late: intimate relationship with member of opposite sex	Independence from parents Responsibility for self Independent identity Acceptance of sexual and peer relationships
Young adult (20-40 years)		Intimacy vs isolation Learns to establish relationship with partner, gratifying social relationships		Establish intimate relationship with partner Gratifying social relationships Work adjustment
Middle age (40-60 years)		Generativity vs self-absorption and stagnation Productivity at home, work, community Child rearing		Productivity at home, work, community Can include reproduction, child rearing
Older adult (60 years-death)		Integrity vs despair views past and remaining life as meaningful whole		Fulfillment Increased dependence Death of spouse, friends, self

Table 2-2 Family developmental tasks

Stage	Task
Early marriage (stage of adjustment)	Psychologic and physical separation from family of origin Establishment of roles Division of tasks/responsibilities Formulation of new rituals Development of new relationships with family of origin and in-laws Establish personal boundaries Form mutually respectful and effective communication patterns Develop a mutually satisfying sexual relationship Decide and plan for children Prepare for childbirth and emerging parental roles
Couple with children	Adjust to parental role and lifestyle changes arising from taking care of infant/child Refine communication patterns with mate and children Reaffirm mutually satisfying sexual relationship with mate Respond to complex demands of family members, including mate, children, and in-laws (e.g., emotional, biologic, social, spiritual, cultural) Prepare children for healthy social relationships in the home, community, and society (e.g., school, college) Encourage healthy separation of children from family system
Middle-aged/older couple	Adjust to midlife biologic, social, and emotional changes (e.g., menopause, children leaving home, retirement) Establish relationship with grandchildren Appraise whether lifelong goals have been established or met Foster generational transmission of cultural/social/ethnic beliefs and values in grandchildren

10. balances leisure with career pursuits
11. develops more depth of personal philosophy by reevaluating values and examining assets
4. Elderly (over 65)
   a. Cognitive development
      1. may decrease as a result of physiologic deterioration
      2. environmental events may affect cognition
         a. loss of self-esteem
         b. isolation
      3. must deal with a will, financial status, and property
   b. Emotional development
      1. reflects on meaningfulness of life, puts success and failure into perspective

2. sense of wisdom, knowledge, and self-reliance, of being able to cope with whatever comes along
3. Erikson's task: integrity versus despair
   c. Moral/religious development
      1. may become more spiritually oriented
      2. value system changes from a material orientation to a more value-oriented outlook
   d. Body-image development
      1. must integrate continued physiologic changes
      2. may see body as less dependable, therefore less desirable
   e. Lifestyle options
      1. may depend on finances, family situation, state of health
      2. increased leisure time after retirement
      3. adjusting to fixed income
      4. developing new hobbies and friends
   f. Developmental tasks
      1. continued self-development (recognizing positive experience of aging)
      2. adapting to family responsibilities
      3. maintaining self-worth, pride, and usefulness
      4. dealing with multiple losses (e.g., mate, friends; changes in lifestyle, body function; upcoming end to life)
5. Sexuality related to the healthy client
   a. Sexuality
      1. an intrinsic attribute of individuals
         a. biologic, sociocultural, psychologic, and ethical components
         b. significant part of Maslow's higher-order needs
         c. integral part of Erikson's task for early adulthood: intimacy versus isolation
      2. definitions
         a. *gender:* internal sense of masculinity or femininity
         b. *sexual role behavior:* all that we do to disclose ourselves as male or female to others
         c. *self-concept/self-esteem:* the perceptions each individual has of self
         d. *body image:* one's opinion of the appearance, function, and separateness of one's own body; a component of self-concept
      3. sexual role dissatisfaction can occur with a wide variety of problems/disease states
         a. common physical problems
            ▪ spinal cord injuries, neuromuscular disease
            ▪ cancer of reproductive organs, genitals
            ▪ diabetes mellitus
            ▪ hypertensive drug regimens
            ▪ cardiac problems (fear)
            ▪ advancing age, menopause
            ▪ colostomy
            ▪ obesity
            ▪ sexually trasmitted diseases
            ▪ infertility
            ▪ endocrine disorders
            ▪ chronic illness (e.g., diabetes, renal failure)
            ▪ rectal, prostate carcinoma

b. common biopsychosocial problems
- disturbances in body image, self-concept
- transvestitism, transsexualism
- orgasmic or erectile dysfunction
- posttraumatic stress disorder

c. drugs that adversely affect sexuality
- alcohol
- antipsychotics or neuroleptics, antidepressants, monoamine oxidase (MAO) inhibitors, sedatives, hypnotics
- antihypertensives
- chemotherapy agents
- hormones and hormone antagonists

4. sexual functioning is multidimensional and influenced by a large number of variables; it is relative to each individual, the individual's lifestyle, quality of relationship with significant others, culture, values, belief system, and choice of love object (e.g., heterosexuality, homosexuality, bisexuality)

5. a critical part of nursing care of the client with respect to sexuality is that the nurse understand his or her own thoughts, feelings, beliefs, and misconceptions about this sensitive area

6. psychosocial counseling with client and significant others includes
   a. verbalizing feelings/concerns/fears/needs
   b. encouraging client to maximize unaltered sexual characteristics
   c. realizing and verbalizing other characteristics that are part of client's individuality, including cultural factors

6. Cultural components related to the healthy client
   a. Culture
      1. definition: *culture* is the organized system of behavior or way of life for an identified social group; it includes knowledge, art, beliefs, morals, laws, customs, and values that are transmitted from one generation to the next
      2. psychosocial support for client and significant others includes
         a. awareness of the components of a cultural orientation
            - social institutions: family, religion, education, economics, politics
            - communication systems
         b. identifying client's specific, culturally related nursing care needs
         c. tailoring interventions to be consistent with cultural practices of client
      3. if culture is mentioned in an NCLEX-RN question, base answer on theory, not past personal experience
      4. the DSM-IV provides an in-depth discussion of *culture-bound syndromes.* This discussion arises from the need to discern whether aberrant behaviors or experiences are culture bound or manifestations of DSM-IV categories. Historically, some of these syndromes have been labeled symptoms of mental disorders rather than unique patterns of specific cultural and ethnic groups. A cultural

assessment is critical to comprehensive diagnosis and care.

7. Spirituality related to the healthy client
   a. Spirituality
      1. defined as an integral aspect of human existence
         a. encompasses values, self-identity, beliefs, and purpose of being
         b. provides understanding of one's relationship to humanity, course and purpose in life, self-worth, and self-concept
         c. an inherent part of love, compassion, faith, hope, caring, warmth, creativity, and insight
         d. significant part of understanding the whole person
         e. a dynamic relationship with and belief in existence of a higher power that is not necessarily part of an established religion
         f. closely tied with psychologic, cultural, and biologic needs; self-integrity; and formation of meaningful relationships
         g. motivates behavior that underlies achievement and meaning of life
         h. provides consolation, hope, healing, comfort, restoration, inner strength, and emotional support, especially during times of stress

ASSESSING AND ADDRESSING THE PSYCHOSOCIAL NEEDS OF CLIENTS IN NONPSYCHIATRIC SETTINGS

1. Role of the nurse
   a. Functions as advocate for client
   b. Actively collaborates with members of the health care team, clients, and families to promote effective treatment outcomes and continuity of care
   c. Gives care that reflects knowledge of client's legal rights as determined by the mental health code of the state in which the nurse practices
   d. Implements nursing care that meets American Nurses Association (ANA) standards as published in *A Statement on Psychiatric–Mental Health Clinical Nursing Practice and Standards of Psychiatric–Mental Health Clinical Nursing Practice.*
   e. Charts in a timely manner both legible and accurate *subjective* client data and *objective* observations, diagnoses and interventions in accordance with accepted nursing practice
   f. Maintains confidentiality of client information
   g. Consults a lawyer when legal clarification is needed
   h. Knows difference between acts of omission and commission
      1. omission: failing to do what should have been done
      2. commission: doing what should not have been done
   i. Ascertains client's understanding of consent to treatment and actively participates in the informed consent process
   j. Provides necessary information at client's level of understanding

   k. Monitors nursing actions relative to client protection to prevent self-harm, assault, or battery
     1. self-harm: self-inflicted behaviors that result in injury or death (e.g., suicide attempt, suicide, self-mutilation)
     2. assault: words or actions that produce genuine belief that action will occur without consent
     3. battery: unconsented touching or restraining of a person without legitimate rationale
   l. Works with or supervises LPN/LVNs, psychiatric or mental health technicians, and various unlicensed assistive personnel
   m. Collaborates with members of the health care team for medical and psychiatric problems
2. Client rights (recent judicial precedents)
   a. Give clients the right to treatment and active participation in treatment
   b. Require institutions to devise individualized plans of client care
   c. Require that plans of treatment be the *least restrictive* of client's liberty considering the individual's condition
   d. Protect civil rights
   e. Maintain confidentiality
   f. Support the client's right to refuse treatment
   g. Support and participate in the informed consent process

SCOPE OF THE PROFESSION

1. Psychiatric nursing is a specialized area of nursing that uses both science and art to provide nursing care to individuals and groups in a wide variety of settings. The nurse-client relationship is the vehicle through which the nurse fulfills independent, interdependent, and dependent roles. Psychiatric/mental health nursing includes promoting mental health and preventing mental illness. It includes the care and rehabilitation of the client with a psychiatric disorder and the psychosocial needs or mental health of the client with a physical condition.
2. Scientific focus: on human behavior
   a. To understand the biopsychosocial principles underlying emotional problems
   b. To be aware of safe and effective treatment measures such as crisis intervention, psychotherapy, medications, electroconvulsive therapy (ECT)
   c. Observe desired and adverse client responses to biopsychosocial interventions and communicate to members of the health care team
   d. Recognize the importance of the research process in evaluating the effectiveness of treatment and in improving the quality of care
3. Purposeful use of self
   a. To apply principles of the nurse-client relationship to all interactions
   b. To be aware of oneself as a principal in the relationship and countertransference issues
   c. To recognize and use one's own feelings and reactions as a guide to increasing empathy and trust and understanding the client
   d. To act as an appropriate behavioral/social role model

   e. Appraise and acknowledge one's cultural and spiritual characteristics and use them as a guide to value these qualities in the client
4. Dependent practice involves implementation and coordination of physician's orders
   a. Know important aspects of each client problem in order to assess, report, and document findings accurately
   b. Apply knowledge and use therapeutic skills in assessment and treatment
   c. Work collaboratively, sharing information about the client's progress
5. Independent practice involves use of the nursing process and development of individualized nursing care plans
6. Interdependent practice involves working with the interdisciplinary team in a variety of settings

INTERPERSONAL RELATIONSHIPS

1. Therapeutic relationships
   a. Relationship between nurse and individual client
     1. initiation, maintenance, and termination of a therapeutic relationship
     2. the nurse collaborates with the client and family to establish outcome criteria (treatment goals) and facilitate positive treatment outcomes
     3. the nurse exhibits appropriate behavior
     4. the nurse treats the client as a unique individual worthy of respect, focusing on the client's symptoms and strengths
     5. the nurse is consistent and reliable, thus increasing the client's trust and security and decreasing defensive acting-out behavior
   b. Group relationship includes
     1. establishing an accepting and trusting environment that facilitates effective communication and behavioral change
     2. helping clients problem solve and manage day-to-day concerns
     3. providing education about major signs and symptoms, causes, and treatment of mental disorders
     4. facilitating adaptive coping behaviors and effective communication
     5. creating a safe environment that facilitates constructive feedback
2. Collaboration with nurses and other health care professionals
   a. Coordinating and formulating a comprehensive continuous plan of care
   b. Sharing implementation of the care plan according to skills needed (e.g., physical therapist, occupational therapist, rehabilitation counselor)
   c. Working interdependently with other health care professionals

ROLES ASSUMED BY THE NURSE

   Nurses are involved directly in the care of the client and may assume diverse, overlapping roles, depending on educational background and clinical expertise. The ANA delineates psychiatric nursing roles as *basic* and *advanced* (minimal education: master's degree) levels, which are discerned by educational background, specific practice, and certification. Promoting and fostering health, providing crisis intervention, milieu therapy, health teaching, and supporting clients as they improve self-care activities are major functions of basic psychiatric nursing practice. In comparison, psychotherapy, prescription of psychoactive agents, clinical supervision or consultation, and consultation-liaison functions lie within the domain of advanced practice psychiatric mental health care nursing. The following is a discussion of specific roles of psychiatric mental health care nurses. Psychotherapy and prescriptive authority are limited to advanced practice psychiatric health nurses; educational preparation, clinical experience, and certification govern the level of care delivered by the nurse in each of the following roles.

1. Counseling: the nurse acts as a counselor.
   a. Counseling may focus on problems of daily living
      1. on a one-to-one basis (nurse-client communication); focus is on problem solving
      2. in groups such as assertiveness groups, stress management, crisis, behavior modification, grooming groups, adolescent groups; focus is on dealing with specific problems, providing emotional support and reality orientation, and increasing social and problem-solving skills and social acceptance
   b. Individual psychotherapy (psychotherapies are limited to advanced practice)
      1. therapist and client meet regularly
      2. because the client re-creates or lives out problems in context of the therapeutic relationship with the nurse, the client is helped to identify own problems and practices new ways of handling them
      3. the client has the opportunity to develop a close relationship with another person (the therapist), practice effective communication skills, grow from the therapeutic experience, gain new insights, and relate adaptive behavior to daily life
   c. Marital/couple therapy
      1. the therapist meets with the couple at established times and encourages them to identify and manage relationship problems
      2. major themes include developing effective communication, conflict resolution, and problem solving skills; appreciating individual and couple needs; and dealing with trust and control issues
   d. Group psychotherapy: nurse may be group leader or co-leader
   e. Family therapy
      1. the therapist meets with the client and the family in various combinations based on subsystems and with a goal of strengthening adaptive or healthy alliances and hierarchy within the family system
      2. family dynamics are stressed, and scapegoating of the "identified client" is decreased
   f. Sociotherapy: within the community mental health care movement, psychiatric nurses provide services aimed at preventing mental illness and reinforcing healthy adaptation; specifically, this is done by teaching, by developing therapeutic relationships, and by recognizing early indications of problems and intervening appropriately
2. Surrogate parent: the nurse is perceived in the role of nurturer, authority figure, or parent as part of therapy with adults and children.
3. Teacher: the nurse provides health teaching regarding biopsychosocial health and developmental needs, mental disorders, coping skills, medications, nutrition, stress reduction, and effective ways of interacting with others.
4. Social agent: the nurse assists the client in using community agencies and social networks and helps people learn about mental health, mental illness, and the prevention of mental illness.
5. Coordinator of client care: the nurse collaborates with mental health and other health care professionals, the client, and family to establish structure; maintain a therapeutic environment; and promote self-care activities. The nurse also administers medications and monitors client's responses to various interventions. Depending on state nurse practice acts and other statutory or federal regulations, the advanced-level nurse may also establish a private practice and be the sole coordinator of client care. This individual may also collaborate with other mental health care professionals for supervision and other activities that promote quality care.
6. Client advocate: the nurse participates in activities (e.g., political, community, state, and national) that promote mental health, decrease social stigma, and increase access to mental health care services.
7. Researcher: the nurse identifies and participates in research activities that promote quality care. The basic-level nurse uses research findings to improve client care; the advanced-level nurse generates research studies to explore, test knowledge, and generate innovative treatment strategies.
8. Administrator: the nurse collaborates with other top management, nurse managers, and staff nurses to determine policies and procedures; resource utilization; standards of practice; continuous quality management; budget management; ethics; hiring, firing, and recruitment practices; and staffing patterns.
9. Supervisor: the nurse works with top management, staff nurses, and other mental health and health care professionals and formulates standards of care and quality management strategies, assesses and provides staff education, analyzes staffing patterns, evaluates staff performance, and oversees the overall quality of care provided to clients by nurses and other health care providers.
10. Case manager: the nurse uses this strategy to collaborate with the client, family members, and other mental health care professionals to coordinate a comprehensive continuous plan of care and effective treatment outcomes. Activities include supportive counseling, crisis intervention, health teaching, and linkage to various community and hospital-based services.

LOCATIONS OF PRACTICE

The role of the nurse is often dictated by the type of mental health care facility.

1. In hospitals the type of involvement the nurse has in client care varies with the theoretical model in use at the individual facility; the nurse may
   a. Participate in the initial and continuous assessment process
   b. Work with psychiatrists, other physicians, and health care professionals, including advanced-practice psychiatric nurses
   c. Formulate comprehensive and continuous plans of care
   d. Observe, support, and listen to clients
   e. Assist clients in developing new adaptive coping behaviors
   f. Provide clients with an environment to try new behaviors
   g. Administer medicines and physical nursing care
   h. Encourage self-care activities
   i. Facilitate individual or group counseling
   j. Provide health teaching regarding signs and symptoms, causes, and treatment of mental disorders; various coping and stress-reducing techniques; and communication and problem-solving skills
   k. Serve as a role model for appropriate behavior and effective communication
   l. Provide crisis intervention to clients and their families
2. In community mental health care centers
   a. The nurse may
      1. participate in the initial assessment and intake process
      2. provide outpatient care using a variety of therapies and based on educational preparation and clinical expertise
      3. enhance primary prevention in the community through
         a. classes designed to fulfill community needs (e.g., parenting classes, stress management, problem solving)
         b. crisis intervention
         c. case management
            ▪ provide counseling
            ▪ health teaching
            ▪ crisis intervention to resolve immediate crisis
            ▪ administer medications and monitor client response
            ▪ coordinate client care with health care team, the client, family, and various hospital and community resources
   b. Frequently there is overlapping of roles as
      1. psychiatrists, psychologists, social workers, basic- and advanced-practice psychiatric nurses, and community mental health care workers collaborate in counseling, home visits, documentation, and medication management
      2. psychiatrists and advanced-practice nurses with prescriptive authority prescribe drugs; nurses administer medications; both make physical and psychosocial assessments
3. In home health settings
   a. The nurse may
      1. collaborate with interdisciplinary team members to facilitate effective client outcomes, provide continuity of care, and engage in continuous assessment of client functioning and evaluation of treatment outcomes
      2. actively engage the family in the decision-making and treatment process
      3. assess and use family strengths to facilitate the client's reentry into the home and community
      4. understand medicare regulations, conditions of major medical insurance, statuary licensing of home health programs, and responsibilities of various members of health care team
      5. employ, orient, manage, and evaluate staff who provide care in home care settings
      6. oversee client care through supervision of licensed and unlicensed assistive personnel
      7. collaborate with the client and family to create an environment conducive to independence, self-care, and responsibility in treatment outcomes
      8. administer medicines and appraise desired and adverse client responses
      9. assess self-care needs and assist in health maintenance activities
      10. provide crisis intervention, appropriate community referrals, and other supportive measures
      11. enlist client and family participation in an ongoing health teaching program
      12. communicate with physician and other health care providers to ensure safe, effective, holistic, continuous, and comprehensive care

LEGAL ASPECTS

The court protects the rights of psychiatric clients using civil and criminal legal procedures. Many individuals are referred to psychiatric services through the courts. Psychiatric expert testimony is used by the courts when a person uses insanity or inability to stand trial as a defense.

1. Civil admission procedures
   a. General information
      1. the Mental Health Systems Act (1980) provides states with a Recommended Bill of Rights for mentally ill clients
      2. each state has its own mental health code determined by the legislature; the code provides guidelines for admission procedures of the mentally ill to hospitals that treat mental illness
      3. state laws differ in legal involuntary admission commitment procedures
   b. Voluntary admission: any legal adult can apply for admission to an institution that treats mental illness
      1. admission implies that the individual agrees to accept treatment and abide by hospital rules
      2. many states require that the client give written notice to the hospital if requesting early discharge
      3. if a physician believes this release to be danger-

ous to the client or others, involuntary admission will be arranged according to state laws

4. in most states a child under the age of 16 may be admitted if the parents sign the required application form

5. in some states the minor has the right to protest admission by parents and petition the court for dismissal

6. clients retain all civil rights with voluntary admission

c. Involuntary admission: application for admission is initiated by someone other than the client and presupposes lack of client consent

1. emergency involuntary admission
   a. person is an immediate danger to self or others
   b. can be initiated by any official or person
   c. client is held temporarily for evaluation and emergency care (usually 3 to 5 days; American Bar Association recommends a maximum of 72 hours for emergency involuntary admission)
   d. hearing usually occurs within 48 hours

2. indefinite involuntary admission
   a. includes initial and indefinite commitments
   b. client is hospitalized for treatment if dangerous to self or others
   c. hearing required by court
   d. client cannot be committed without adequate proof of danger to self or others

3. mandated outpatient treatment
   a. court-ordered
   b. criteria are same as inpatient (i.e., individual is deemed to be a danger to self or others and suffering from a mental disorder)
   c. sometimes used as a preventive measure to decrease further decline in client's mental health and need for involuntary admission

d. Competency hearings: different and separate from admission hearings

1. admission to mental hospital does not mean a person is incompetent to manage own affairs

2. legally, *incompetency* indicates that the person is no longer able to make responsible personal deci-sions, decisions regarding dependents, or deci-sions regarding personal property

3. person declared incompetent has legal status of a minor and cannot
   a. vote
   b. make contracts or wills
   c. manage personal property
   d. drive a car
   e. sue or be sued
   f. hold a professional license

4. a guardian is appointed for the incompetent person and has the power of consent

5. procedure can be instituted by state or family admission

2. Criminal admission procedures

a. *Insanity:* a legal, not psychiatric, term meaning that because of mental illness the accused did not realize the extent or consequences of his or her actions, did not know right from wrong, or had impaired ability to resist wrong and thus is *not criminally responsible* for the unlawful act

1. sanity is determined by jury, based on psychiatric expert testimony

2. the person accused of a crime may stand trial and plead not guilty by reason of insanity
   a. persons found guilty can be sentenced to prison
   b. persons found not guilty are committed to a mental hospital until judged sane by staff
   c. when released, a person who was found not guilty by reason of insanity usually is free and has no legal ruling against self

b. *Inability to stand trial:* a person accused of committing a crime is not mentally responsible at time of trial

1. the person is unfit to stand trial if at that time he or she cannot understand the charge against him or her or is incapable of cooperating with his or her own defense

2. if found unfit to stand trial, the person must be sent to a psychiatric unit until legally determined to be competent for trial

3. once mentally fit, the person must stand trial and serve sentence if convicted

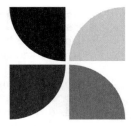

Therapeutic Use of Self

NURSE-CLIENT RELATIONSHIP

1. Purpose: provide counseling, crisis intervention, individual psychotherapy, health teaching
2. Characteristics
   a. Mutually defined relationship
   b. Mutually collaborative
   c. Goal-directed
   d. Interpersonal techniques facilitate trust and open communication
   e. Fosters development of therapeutic relationship
   f. Relationship differs from friendship
      1. specific boundaries established (nurse-client)
      2. purpose, time, and place of interaction are specific
      3. professional demeanor and objectivity maintained
   g. Nurse assists client with problem identification and resolution
   h. Successful relationship leads to mutual growth for client and nurse
3. Facts to remember
   a. It is not a friendship
   b. Its main benefit is to the client
   c. It presents an opportunity for the client to deal with the problems brought to treatment
   d. An accepting and empathetic approach is pivotal to the client's being able to express feelings
   e. Clinical expertise and educational preparation allow the nurse to have more discretion in relating to clients, but inexperienced nurses should use basic communication skills and common sense
4. Therapeutic communication
   a. Interpersonal techniques that facilitate communication
   b. Factors that influence the nurse's response
      1. client's stage of growth and development
      2. stage of the nurse-client relationship
      3. client's level of readiness and motivation to change
      4. goals of the interaction/priorities of care
      5. nurse's level of emotional maturity and stability
      6. countertransference issues of the nurse (both positive and negative responses to the client)
   c. General guidelines: the best responses focus on
      1. actual client behaviors and nursing observations rather than inferences
      2. the here-and-now rather than the past
      3. description rather than judgment, to promote trust
      4. sharing information and exploring alternatives rather than giving advice or solutions
      5. how and what rather than why
      6. orientation and presentation of reality (particularly for confused, disoriented, or sensory-perceptually impaired clients)
      7. degrees of neurobiologic integrity
      8. nursing interventions rather than roles designated to other health care team members
   d. See Table 2-3
5. Phases of the nurse-client relationship: correct response to NCLEX-RN questions may be based on the phase of the relationship
   a. *Initiating or orientating phase:* establishes boundaries
      1. when, duration of meeting, place, number of sessions, how often nurse will meet with client
      2. focus of relationship defined with client
         a. major treatment goals are identified
      3. usually time of anxiety for client and nurse
         a. client may come late to or miss meetings; test boundaries
         b. client may exhibit anxious and tense mannerisms
         c. client may sit silently, hallucinate, or exhibit delusions
         d. nurse may be more likely to use responses that block communication because of own anxiety
      4. preparation for termination begins at this stage
   b. *Working phase:* exhibits reduction of anxiety in both client and nurse
      1. client accepts boundaries of relationship
         a. begins to come to meetings on time
         b. uses the time with nurse as a "working" time
      2. nurse uses interpersonal skills that foster communication
      3. client confronts problems and feelings
      4. client develops insights, learns adaptive coping skills and problem solving
      5. nurse and client see each other as unique people
   c. *Terminating phase:* begins at first session and ends when identified treatment goals have been met; focuses on loss, separation anxiety
      1. client and nurse summarize and evaluate work of relationship
      2. both express thoughts and feelings about termination

Table 2-3 Communication skills in the nurse-client relationship

Therapeutic communication techniques

TECHNIQUE	EXAMPLE
Attending: indicating awareness of what is going on in interaction; includes giving feedback/recognition	Yes (nodding). You have a different haircut.
Encouraging verbalization: promoting continued client verbalization	Um-hmm. And then? Go on.
Verbalization observations: commenting on what nurse has perceived	You sound frustrated. I notice that you're pulling your hair.
Reflecting feelings: verbalizing either stated or implied client feelings	You're feeling anxious. You feel that no one cares about you.
Paraphrasing: restating the content of the message	Client: The doctor said I could go home tomorrow but I'm still having a lot of difficulty focusing. Nurse: You're wondering if you're ready to go home.
Open questioning: promotes freedom of response	What would you like to talk about today? What happens when you feel angry?
Closed questioning: limits freedom of response to short answer or yes/no	Have you ever been hospitalized before? Did you eat dinner?
Giving information: providing factual data	My name is. . . . Lunch is at noon. Visiting hours are 2-8 PM.
Clarifying: promotes understanding of what is unclear	I'm not sure I understand what you are saying.
Validating: checking perception of client verbalization	This is what I heard you say. . . . Let me know if this is how you see it.
Focusing: directing flow of interaction	You were explaining. . . .
Requesting description/comparison: asking client to verbalize perceptions/similarities/differences	Describe how you are feeling now. Tell me when you feel angry. How does this compare with what happened when. . . . ? What other times have you felt this way?
Summarizing: pulling together the salient points of an interaction	Today we have discussed two options for. . . . Last time we talked you were going to. . . .
Presenting reality	I don't hear any voices except yours and mine. Or: Today is Wednesday, September 23, and you're in the emergency room.
Seeking consensual validation: ensuring understanding of client verbalization	Tell me if I understand you correctly. . . .
Decoding or desymbolizing: interpreting meaning of client verbalization	Client: I'm the son of Christ sent to take care of man. Nurse: Do you feel like you want someone to take care of you?
Suggesting collaboration	Let's figure out together what makes you anxious.

BLOCK	EXAMPLE
False assurance	Everything will be all right. Don't worry. You're doing fine.
Giving advice	What you should do is. . . . Why don't you. . . . ?
Giving approval	That's the right attitude. That's the thing to do.
Requesting an explanation	Why are you sad? Why did you do that?
Agreeing with the client	I agree with you. You must be right.
Expressing disapproval	You should stop worrying like this. You shouldn't do that.
Belittling the client's feelings	I know just how you feel. Everyone gets upset at times.
Disagreeing with the client	You're wrong. That's not true. No, it isn't.
Defending	Your doctor is quite capable. This hospital is well equipped. She's a very good nurse. Or: The doctor wouldn't have ordered this for you if it weren't for your own good.
Rejection	I don't think you should be talking about this. . . .
Clichés or stereotypical comments	Look on the bright side. Or: Don't count your chickens before they hatch.
Literal responses	Client: The TV is controlling my mind. Nurse: You need to turn it off then.

THEORETIC KNOWLEDGE OF BASE

1. Theories of behavior: nursing interventions in the realm of human behavior are based on a variety of theories (Table 2-4)
2. Life-cycle stages/family tasks (refer to Tables 2-1 and 2-2, respectively)

   a. Freud: each stage must be negotiated successfully to avoid arrest at any one stage
   b. Erikson: focuses on psychosocial crises and developmental tasks; each crisis must be resolved successfully so the individual will be able to meet subsequent crises

Table 2-4 Theoretic models

Models/proponents	Assumptions	Treatment
Medical-biologic	Emotional disturbance is an illness or defect Illness is located in body or is biochemical Disease entities can be diagnosed, classified, and labeled	Physical/somatic: surgery, electroconvulsive therapy (ECT), chemotherapy Therapists: physicians, others treating under MD's orders
Psychoanalytic (Freud, Erikson)	Emotional disturbance stems from emotionally painful experiences Feelings are repressed Unresolved, unconscious conflicts remain in the mind Symptoms and defense mechanisms develop	Therapy uncovers roots of conflicts through interviews within long-term therapy Therapists: psychoanalysts, usually MDs
Interpersonal (Sullivan, Peplau)	Emotional disturbance results from problematic interpersonal interaction Client is seen as a subsystem of larger systems (e.g., family and community)	Client is approached in a holistic way Intervention includes health promotion/illness prevention and alteration of harmful environments Constructive interpersonal relationship is developed with therapist Therapists: physicians, nurses, or other health professionals

Behavioral-cognitive (Pavlov, Skinner, Wolpe, Beck, Ellis)	Behavior can be modified by operant conditioning
	  Behavior that is reinforced tends to be repeated
	  Behavior that is ignored tends to be eliminated
	Client needs to eliminate faulty thought processes, self-defeating ideas
		Treatment aims at eliminating unwanted behavior by ignoring it and reinforcing wanted behavior
		Response to behavior by therapists must be consistent
		Therapists: physicians, nurses, psychologists, trained assistants, or other mental health professionals

Psychosocial-biologic	Psychosocial factors affect complex biologic processes, such as neuroendocrine and psychoneuroimmune systems Overt biologic responses (e.g., endocrine system) parallel stressful situations One's ability to manage stress effectively is linked with appraisal of stressful situation and available internal and external resources	Biologic interventions such as medications, ECT, vitamins Cognitive therapy can be used to challenge negative self-talk, "all or none" thinking, generalizations Various forms of psychotherapies alone or with other therapies such as chemotherapy Therapists: stress management therapists with prescriptive authority; other psychotherapists; mental health professionals on the treatment team

Social	When stresses and supports are in balance, the individual is socially competent
	Emotional disturbance results from imbalance between stresses and supports (see Table 2-5)
	Too much stress and not enough support lead to social disorientation and disintegration
	Too much support and too little stress lead to social dependence, immobility, regression
		Treatment is aimed at maintaining or restoring balance between stresses and supports
		Levels of prevention of mental illness
		  Primary: promotion of mental health and disease prevention (anticipatory guidance, education, community organization, crisis prevention)
		  Secondary: early treatment to prevent long-term illness (screening, early diagnosis, case finding, brief hospitalization, crisis intervention)
		  Tertiary: treatment of chronic, long-term problems (halfway houses, partial hospitalization, day hospitals)
		Therapists: physicians, nurses, social workers, psychologists, other trained mental health workers

c. Sullivan: focuses on social and environmental factors; a healthy personality develops through meaningful, gratifying interpersonal experiences with others in the environment (Table 2-5)

3. Stress-Appraisal-Coping (Lazarus; Lazarus-Folkman)

The stress-appraisal-coping theory submits that the significance of a potentially stressful circumstance is resolved in terms of whether it threatens one's well-being and that this appraisal governs coping responses. Furthermore, it surmises that stress reactions are determined by a conscious appraisal of harm-loss, threat, or challenge rather than an instinctive reaction. Efforts to manage and assess stressful events are influenced by two forms of appraisal: primary and secondary. *Primary appraisal* is a cognitive evaluative process that determines the meaning or outcome of stressful situations. Factors that influence the outcome of primary appraisal include available resources and options for the situation. In comparison, *secondary appraisal* governs how the situation will be managed.

The Lazarus coping theory is divided three stages of appraisal. During *stage I*, the situation is appraised as either irrelevant to one's well-being, benign (positive) or stressful. When the situation is deemed potentially stressful, the client determines whether it jeopardizes one's well-being,

Table 2-5 Social determinants of mental health and mental illness

Stress	Individual	Support
Social	Genetic information	Social
Poverty	Constitutional traits	Churches and
Poor housing	Developmental traits	synagogues
Unemployment	Coping mechanisms	Schools
Crowding	Ego strength	Social welfare
High rate	Developmental stage	agencies
of mobility	Temperament	Community
Personal	Familial predisposition	resources
Maturational		Personal
Adolescence		Family network
Aging		Friends
Role changes		Clergy
Situational		Bartender
Loss		Hairdresser
Divorce		
Separation		
Illness		

poses imminent harm-loss, or has a potential for positive outcome or challenge. A typical situation involves students taking a pop quiz. The student judges the situation by asking "Am I going to get through this pop quiz or am I going to ace it?" Three types of stress appraisals of this situation exist: harm-loss, threat, and challenge. *Harm-loss* refers to damage that has already occurred—"I do not have a chance of passing this test, it's all over for me." *Threat* refers to anticipation of imminent harm—"If I fail this test I will not graduate." *Challenge* refers to potential for proficiency or achievement and ultimately a positive outcome—"Even though I did not study for this test I know the information and I will do fine."

Stage II is concerned with coping mechanisms arising from the quality of resources and available options. It is also influenced by previous experiences with similar events, perception of self and the world (self-concept), quality of coping skills, and accessible resources. A common predicament emerges when the student regards a stressful situation as either challenging or threatening (harm-loss). In the case of the student who has good study habits, successful test-taking skills, and confidence in passing the test, a pop quiz poses few threats to the student's well-being or graduation. In contrast, the student who has poor study habits, lacks confidence, or does not have positive test-taking experiences will perceive this situation as overwhelming and a threat to the student's well-being and graduation.

Stage III involves reevaluation of the situation and needed revision of coping responses. The first student reviews the situation and determines that it is stressful, but because of good study habits and confidence passes the test and graduates. In comparison, the second student lacks confidence and decides that the situation is hopeless and overwhelming, performs poorly on the test, and fails to graduate.

Coping denotes attempts to mediate environmental and internal demands triggered by the client's response to a po-

tentially stressful appraisal. This complex process is governed by a dynamic interaction among cognitive and behavioral responses, personality traits, early childhood experiences, biologic factors, and other psychosocial issues (see Table 2-5). Furthermore, coping is a repetitive and mutual process between the client and the environment that involves primary and secondary appraisals and reappraisals of a situation. Additionally, coping directs adaptive outcomes by determining the recurrence, degree, and patterns of neurobiologic stress reactions. Possible adaptive outcomes include individual responses that reduce the frequency, severity, and patterns of neuroendocrine responses: problem-focused and emotional-focused coping. *Problem-focused coping* enables the client to eliminate or mediate stress by altering the stressful client-environment interaction. *Emotion-focused coping* enables the client to effectively manage stressful emotions through cognitive appraisal and adaptive behavioral responses that mobilize or alter physiologic responses.

4. Defense mechanisms (Freud)
   a. Psychologic techniques the personality develops to manage anxiety, aggressive impulses, hostilities, resentments, frustrations, and conflicts between the id (pleasure-seeking impulses) and the superego (inhibiting)
   b. Used by both mentally healthy and mentally ill persons
   c. Measure of mental health is determined by the degree that defense mechanisms
      1. distort the personality
      2. dominate behavior
      3. modulate or reduce anxiety
      4. disturb adjustment with others
      5. remain unconscious
   d. Specific defense mechanisms
      1. *suppression:* the conscious, deliberate forgetting of unacceptable or painful thoughts, impulses, feelings, or acts
      2. *repression:* unconscious, involuntary forgetting of unacceptable or painful thoughts, impulses, feelings, or acts
      3. *isolation:* separating thought and affect, allowing only the former to come to consciousness
      4. *dissociation:* walling off certain areas of the personality from consciousness (e.g., trauma)
      5. *denial:* treating obvious reality factors as though they do not exist because they are consciously intolerable
      6. *rationalization:* attempting to justify feelings, behavior, and motives that would otherwise be intolerable by offering a socially acceptable, intellectual, and apparently logical explanation for an act or decision
      7. *symbolization:* using an object or idea as a substitute or to represent some other object or idea
      8. *idealization:* conscious or unconscious overestimation of another's attributes (e.g., hero worship)
      9. *identification:* attaching to oneself certain qualities associated with others; it operates unconsciously and is a significant mechanism in superego development

10. *introjection:* incorporating the traits of others, internalizing feelings toward others
11. *conversion:* the unconscious expression of mental conflict by means of a physical symptom
12. *compensation:* putting forth extra effort to achieve in one area to offset real or imagined deficiencies in another area
13. *substitution:* unconsciously replacing an unobtainable or unacceptable goal with a goal that is more acceptable or obtainable; the process is more direct and less subtle than sublimation
14. *sublimation:* directing energy from unacceptable drives into socially acceptable behavior
15. *reaction formation:* expressing unacceptable wishes or behavior by opposite overt behavior
16. *undoing:* thinking or doing one thing for the purpose of neutralizing something objectionable that was thought or done before
17. *displacement:* transferring unacceptable feelings aroused by one object or situation to a more acceptable substitute
18. *projection:* unconsciously attributing one's own unacceptable qualities and emotions to others
19. *ideas of reference:* believing that one is the object of special and ill-disposed attention by others
20. *fantasy:* satisfying needs by daydreaming
21. *regression:* going back to an earlier level of emotional development and organization
22. *fixation:* never advancing the level of emotional development beyond that in which one feels comfortable
23. *withdrawal:* separating oneself from interpersonal relationships in order to avoid emotional expression or responsiveness

Nursing Process

The format for the NCLEX-RN exam is the nursing process. This means there will be assessment, analysis/nursing diagnosis, planning, implementation, and evaluation questions.

1. Assessment: collecting and organizing data about the client by observation, interview, and examination; identifying strengths and problem areas
   a. Observation (note: appearance, behavior, communication)
   b. Interview
      1. informal data gathering from objective and subjective sources
      2. formal through completion of nursing history
   c. Examination
      1. psychosocial assessment
         a. general appearance and behavior: age, grooming, dress, posture, body movements, eye contact, speech (clarity and rate), affect, mood, gait, attitude and motivation during interview, cultural influences (age, ethnicity, gender, disability, etc.)
         b. thought content: bizarre, obsessions, suicidal ideations, perceptions, delusions, hallucinations, grandiosity, preoccupation, ideas of ref-

erence, illusions; thought process: logical, relevant, coherent, circumstantial, perseveration, flight of ideas, tangential
         c. cognitive functions: orientation, memory, attention and concentration, intellect, judgment, insight, communication, abstract thinking, degree of spontaneous speech
         d. motor functions: presence or absence of tremors and tics, gait, restlessness, pacing, motor coordination, reflexes, grimacing, posture, repetitive or stereotypical movement
         e. social processes: self-concept, interpersonal relations (family, peers, community), activities of daily living (ADL), leisure activities
      2. physical: complete review of systems, growth and development history, diet, exercise, rest, tobacco/drug/alcohol use, body image
2. Analysis/nursing diagnosis: evaluating information gathered during assessment and making nursing diagnoses
3. Planning: developing client goals (outcome criteria) and nursing interventions to meet them
   a. Collaborate with client and family and develop long- and short-term goals.
   b. State goals in behavioral terms.
   c. Specify nursing interventions that will facilitate goal attainment.
   d. Include nursing actions such as setting limits on unacceptable behavior without rejecting the client as a person, increasing or decreasing environmental stimuli, and providing individually appropriate activities.
4. Implementation: carrying out the nursing care plan
   a. Carry out nursing interventions.
   b. Establish a suitable environment for implementation (i.e., therapeutic milieu).
5. Evaluation: appraising client's response to nursing interventions, accomplishing expected outcomes, and modifying the plan as necessary
   a. Appraise client's response to nursing interventions based on their impact on the client's behavior, concerns, and attainment of short-term goals (outcome criteria).
   b. Evaluation is based on input from the individual nurse and members of the health care team.
   c. Continuously assess and modify plan of care as needed.

INTERPERSONAL TREATMENT MODALITIES

1. Psychotherapy
   a. Definition: goal-oriented, restorative emotional experience with a therapist in order to effect behavioral change, including
      1. increased sense of well-being and self-esteem
      2. improved psychologic performance
      3. enhanced social and interpersonal adeptness
      4. expanded biologic function
   b. Length of treatment
      1. less focus on long-term length because of managed care; however, a long-term approach enables the client to gain insight and develop new

coping mechanisms (managed care criteria affect the length of treatment; long-term treatment has to be justified)

2. more likely to be a short-term approach, such as crisis intervention or brief, problem-focused approach (consistent with concepts of managed care model) and time limited

2. Crisis intervention
   a. Definition: a time-limited (approximately 4 to 6 weeks), directive approach to help a client cope with a crisis (a crisis by definition resolves within 6 weeks; whether the outcome or resolution is positive or negative depends on appropriate interventions and quality of coping skills)
      1. person is in crisis when customary methods of coping are not effective
      2. crises resolve within 6 weeks (with or without interventions); however, if the present crisis is ineffectively resolved, the person may have lost some ability to cope with future crises
      3. provides immediate emotional support
      4. person more likely to develop adaptive behavioral changes during crises
   b. Crisis therapy
      1. includes helping an individual or family cope with a present intolerable situation
      2. focuses on here-and-now rather than the past
      3. deals directly and briefly with the individual's present situation to return client to previous level of coping (this level may not be the optimal level, but nonetheless is the goal)
         a. clarifies situation and identifies problem
         b. appraises previous adaptive coping patterns and attempts to adapt to present situation
         c. teaches client new coping skills
         d. identifies current options and mobilizes external and internal resources
      4. expands the client's problem-solving and decision-making skills, thereby promoting growth and adaptation and enhanced ability to manage future crises
      5. minimizes the deleterious effects of present stressors
   c. The process of crisis therapy includes
      1. establishing a nurse-client relationship
      2. providing immediate and ongoing emotional support through the use of self and available resources
      3. helping the client identify viable options for managing the current crisis
      4. emphasizing that the relationship is time limited with a here-and-now focus
      5. establishing a termination date at the beginning of the relationship
      6. actively encouraging the client to express feelings, thoughts, and emotions regarding the crisis situation
      7. facilitating formation of new and adaptive coping skills
      8. having the client take more responsibility in subsequent sessions (if there is more than one)

3. Behavior modification
   a. Definition: refers to a systematic employment of rewards and punishments to modulate or change behavior. Major features:
      1. governed by the premise that behavior is learned and directed by both reward and punishment reinforcers
      2. alterations in consequences result in modified behavior
      3. can be applied in various clinical settings
   b. Process of treatment
      1. identify the behavior to be changed (e.g., adolescent throws temper tantrum when told he or she is grounded)
      2. obtain baseline data regarding the behavior (e.g., frequency)
      3. identify the conditions and reinforcers that promote the behavior (e.g., adolescent allowed to use the telephone [rewarded] to stop temper tantrum)
      4. identify the conditions and reinforcers that will change or eliminate the behavior
   c. Techniques: systematic desensitization, ignoring the behavior, time out, token economy, aversion
   d. Positive reinforcers (rewards) are preferable to aversion techniques

4. Therapeutic milieu
   a. Purposeful use of all interactions to assist client in developing interpersonal and social skills in a conducive physical and emotional environment
   b. Governs (increases or decreases) environmental stimuli to provide limits, protect client, promote optimal functioning
   c. Nurse's role
      1. provide 24-hour milieu management
      2. afford positive role modeling
      3. plan/coordinate care
      4. facilitate formation of adaptive coping behaviors
   d. Activities
      1. government: distributes power, promotes open communications; encourages client-elected officers to run meetings, negotiate with staff, run unit activities (e.g., cleanups, unit parties)
      2. self-care: client required to maintain room, personal hygiene, clothing, nutrition, diversional activities, socialization, and so on to foster independence
      3. occupational therapy: specific programs developed by occupational therapists to encourage nonverbal expressions, increase self-esteem, and expand skills of daily living
      4. activity therapy: art, music, and recreation planned by nurses or activity therapists to increase social skills and self-integrity, decrease regression, and facilitate an optimal level of functioning
      5. health education: focuses on signs and symptoms, causes, and treatment of specific mental disorders; role of client and family in symptom management and relapse prevention

5. Therapeutic groups (psychotherapy): more closely resemble real-life situations than does one-to-one therapy.
   a. Leading these groups requires training beyond basic nursing education.
   b. Beginning nurse may colead a group.
   c. Group may also be led by experienced coleaders.
   d. Group members provide feedback to each other.
   e. Variety of responses and reactions available are exhibited in group settings.
   f. Three stages of development:
      1. group orientation and development of identity
      2. group interaction and observation of dynamics
      3. resolution of dynamics and production of insights
   g. Members may examine patterns of relating to each other and authority figures in supportive atmosphere.
   h. Group therapy more economical than one-to-one therapy; there are usually two therapists and 7 to 12 clients.
   i. The goals and purposes are essentially the same as in one-to-one therapy.
6. Family therapy: focuses on the family rather than on the individual
   a. Major problem:
      1. impaired communication
      2. maladaptive subsystems or family alliances (e.g., unclear boundaries)
      3. inconsistent or unclear family rules
   b. Major objective: to reestablish effective communication between family
      1. family can reassess and recognize dysfunctional alliances
      2. family can resolve to accept individuality of members
      3. family can express feelings and thoughts in an accepting climate
   c. Important difference between family therapy and group therapy
      1. in family therapy, the participants enter therapy with a long-standing system of roles and interactions, which the nurse-therapist must learn
      2. in group therapy, the relationship between participants begins with the first session; they have no history of a relationship
7. Self-help groups: use persons who have themselves surmounted problems. Nurses may serve as consultants/resource persons.
   a. Recovery, Inc.
      1. a consumer-funded group consisting of clients formerly treated for mental illness and persons with emotional problems

2. focus is on the use of willpower in avoiding maladaptive behavior
   b. Other self-help groups
      1. Parents Without Partners
      2. Groups for colostomy clients
      3. Parents whose children have terminal diseases (Candlelighters)
      4. Overeaters Anonymous
      5. Reach for Recovery
      6. Alcoholics Anonymous (see p. 83)
      7. Narcotics Anonymous
      8. Groups for child/wife abusers (Parents Anonymous)
      9. Depressives Anonymous
      10. Alzheimer's Association for a list of support groups and services
      11. Cocaine Anonymous
8. Other therapies
   a. Sex therapy
      1. one must understand one's own sexuality to appreciate the client's sexual concerns
      2. clarifying control issues, self-esteem, body image, cultural influences, and improving communication patterns
      3. improving a person or couple's sexual functioning
      4. active participation in psychotherapy and prescribed experiential learning (e.g., Masters and Johnson's treatment program serves as model for sex therapy)
      5. advanced education and clinical expertise is required
      6. basic-level nurse can provide emotional support and encourage expression of feelings and concerns when sexual dysfunction arises and collaborate with treatment team in making appropriate referrals
   b. Hypnotherapy
      1. may be used for specific symptoms such as anxiety, pain, high blood pressure, smoking, overeating, and phobias
      2. also may be used in conjunction with other therapies to decrease repression
      3. done only by trained professionals
      4. the role of the basic-level nurse is to support client in treatment; communicate with therapist, who may be an advanced-level psychiatric mental health nurse

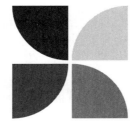

Loss and Death and Dying

LOSS

1. Every human being experiences many losses during a lifetime (e.g., loss of health, loss of a relationship or loved one, change in lifestyle or body image); ideally people deal with loss by grieving and integrating the subsequent changes into their life.
   a. Responses to loss vary greatly depending on several factors: the individual's personality, culture, previous experience with losses, and value of the person or thing lost; available support systems.
   b. Behavior during normal grieving is similar to that seen in a depressed person (e.g., crying, fatigue, feelings of emptiness); unlike grief, depression is a persistent state characterized by low self-esteem; the "depressed mood" is perceived as normal in persons experiencing grief.
   c. People who are dying may experience fear or anticipate feelings of abandonment (e.g., pain, loneliness, meaninglessness).
2. Definitions:
   a. *Loss:* the anticipated or actual removal of something or someone of value to a person.
   b. *Grief:* the normal emotional responses to a loss, which subside after a reasonable time. Duration varies from several months to several years.
   c. *Unresolved grief:* failure to complete the grieving process and cope successfully with the loss because of social and psychologic factors. Circumstances that increase the likelihood of unresolved grief responses include the following:
      1. socially unspeakable loss (e.g., suicide)
      2. uncertainty over loss (e.g., person missing in action)
      3. need to be strong and in control
      4. inability to reach out to others for support
      5. ambivalence over lost object or person
      6. multiple losses
      7. reawakening of an old, unresolved loss or grief
   d. *Mourning:* the expression of sorrow with outward signs of grief as a result of a perceived or threatened loss.
   e. *Grief and mourning process:* the process a person goes through in adapting to a loss; this process is triggered by an *actual* or a *threatened* loss.
3. According to Kübler-Ross (the theorist most often associated with the study of death and dying), there are five stages in the grief and mourning process of the dying person (these stages can be applied to other losses). The stages may overlap, and a person may go back and forth between anger and denial.
   a. Denial: unconscious avoidance that varies from a brief period to the remainder of life; allows a person to mobilize defenses to cope with death.
      1. adaptive responses: crying, verbal denial
      2. maladaptive responses: absence of crying or verbal recognition of loss
   b. Anger: covert or overt expression of realization of loss.
      1. adaptive responses: verbal expression of anger
      2. maladaptive responses: persistent guilt or low self-esteem, aggression, self-destructive ideation or behavior
   c. Bargaining: an attempt to change reality of loss, often done with God.
      1. adaptive responses: bargains for treatment control, expresses wish to be alive for specific events in near future
      2. maladaptive responses: bargains for unrealistic activities or events in distant future
   d. Depression: sadness resulting from actual and anticipated losses.
      1. adaptive responses: crying, social withdrawal
      2. maladaptive responses: self-destructive actions, despair
   e. Acceptance: resolution of feelings about death, resulting in peaceful feelings
      1. adaptive behaviors: may wish to be alone, limit visitors, limit conversation, complete personal and family business
      2. may never reach this stage
4. Child's understanding of and responses to death depend on
   a. Age
      1. preschooler cannot differentiate between death and absence; lacks cognitive understanding of the finality of death and often experiences it as separation from loved one
      2. from 5 to 6 years old, children see death as something others experience; begin to accept death as a fact; believe death is reversible, not final
      3. from 6 to 9 years old, children associate death with injury; personify death (someone bad carries them away); identify death with "old people"
      4. from 9 to 10 years old, children recognize that everyone must die

5. early adolescents understand permanence of death; difficult to see self dying before having a chance to live; may experience resentment, withdrawal, see self as different from others; also concerned about possible different reaction of others (e.g., withdrawal of friends); fantasies of rebirth, re-union, and reincarnation result

6. all ages: underlying fear is of separation and pain, rather than fear of death itself

b. Previous experience with death: relatives, friends, pets, family responses to death

c. Knowledge of what is happening

d. Other influences
1. whether child is hospitalized; staff behavior
2. parents' anxieties and reaction to death and dying
3. reaction of other family members, siblings

Application of the Nursing Process to the Client Experiencing a Loss

ASSESSMENT
1. Current behavior
   a. Stage of grief and mourning
   b. Adaptive or maladaptive
2. Previous losses
3. Support system

ANALYSIS/NURSING DIAGNOSES
1. Safe, effective care environment
   a. High risk for violence: self-directed or directed at others
   b. Sensory-perceptual alterations (visual, auditory, kinesthetic, gustatory, tactile, olfactory)
   c. Altered thought processes
2. Physiologic integrity
   a. High risk for activity intolerance
   b. Pain
   c. Impaired verbal communication
   d. Altered nutrition: high risk for less than body requirements
   e. Sleep-pattern disturbance
3. Psychosocial integrity
   a. Body-image disturbance, identity disturbance, self-esteem disturbance
   b. Anticipatory grieving
   c. Dysfunctional grieving
   d. Social isolation
4. Health promotion/maintenance
   a. Altered family processes
   b. Altered growth and development
   c. Altered health maintenance

GENERAL NURSING PLANNING, IMPLEMENTATION, AND EVALUATION

> **Goal:** Client will identify the stages of grief and resolve it within an acceptable time frame.

Implementation
1. Support the client's method of coping as long as it is not physically or emotionally destructive.
2. Reinforce adaptive behavior; remember that suicidal ideation is not adaptive in any stage.

3. Educate the client and family of the grief stages and normalcy of their feelings and responses to the loss.
4. Help client to express feelings ("You look sad. What are you feeling right now?"); listen attentively and with empathy.
5. Recognize impact of previous losses; help client resolve past and present losses.

Evaluation
Client acknowledges the stages of grief and talks about specific loss; asks questions about future; bargains verbally; expresses anger, sadness.

SELECTED HEALTH PROBLEMS

✷ LOSS (OTHER THAN DEATH AND DYING)

1. Types of loss
   a. Physical losses include loss of
   1. body part (e.g., amputation, mastectomy, enucleation, laryngectomy)
   2. body function (e.g., paralysis of a limb, aphasia)
   3. a valued object (e.g., a house)
   4. economic or role status
   5. youth, beauty, health
   6. a significant other, either through loss of a relationship or through death
   b. Psychologic losses include losses/changes in
   1. meaning in life, beliefs, and values
   2. status, recognition, prestige
   3. meaningful work, creative abilities
   4. self-esteem and self-worth
   5. nurturance and sense of belonging
   6. expected outcome (e.g., a stillborn infant)
   7. role identity, self-concept
   c. Loss may be
   1. threatened loss
   2. perceived loss
   3. actual loss

Nursing Process

ASSESSMENT
1. Specific loss
2. Time of occurrence
3. Meaning of loss to client and family (including cultural factors)
4. Quality and accessibility of support system
5. Previous significant losses

ANALYSIS/NURSING DIAGNOSES (see left)

PLANNING, IMPLEMENTATION, AND EVALUATION

> **Goal:** Client will respond adaptively to the loss.

Implementation
1. Allow client to cry, express anger, or exhibit other adaptive responses to the loss.
2. Provide support for adaptive behavior (e.g., "It must be very difficult for you right now.").
3. Help client to express feelings (e.g., "Other people in

your situation often feel sad or angry. How do you feel?").

4. When client asks questions about living with loss, tell the client only what he or she wants to know at that time (in-depth teaching can be done later when client is ready).
5. Reinforce adaptive behaviors.
6. Expect client to vacillate between behaviors of consecutive stages.

Evaluation
Client asks questions about adapting to the loss; cries, feels sad, plans for future.

✳ DEATH AND DYING

1. Responses to the dying process are highly individualized and may be greatly influenced by the client's physical status and personality; the interaction of client and family will have a strong bearing on the client's healthy progression through the process.
2. Regardless of the age, a life-threatening illness produces a family crisis. Control, fear, and loss issues and grief reactions are examples of the family's emotional response to death and dying.
3. Nurse's responses:
   a. To be effective in helping the dying person, the nurse must explore his or her own beliefs, feelings, and behaviors in regard to death.
   b. The nurse who is unaware of his or her own feelings, fears, and beliefs about death may unintentionally limit client's expression of feelings.
   c. Exploring one's own beliefs about death and how people respond to it enables the nurse to maintain objectivity and facilitate the client's grief work.
4. Establishing priorities:
   a. Priorities may be determined by the client's psychologic and physical status and cultural influences.
      1. at some point, pain or fatigue may demand more attention than psychologic factors
      2. a client who cannot maintain adequate food and fluid intake or remain comfortable requires immediate attention and continuous assessment
   b. The next most important action is helping the client effectively manage the existing stage of grief.
   c. Help the family and client effectively communicate their feelings and thoughts by creating an accepting environment, role modeling, and discussing the normal grief process and death and dying issues.
5. DSM-IV classification: bereavement.

Nursing Process: Adult
ASSESSMENT
1. The impact of the loss on the client's physical and mental status
2. Knowledge of and response to diagnosis; people respond to dying similarly to the way they have responded to other major crises
3. The impact of cultural factors on the client's and family's responses and adaptation to death
4. Stage in dying process: the stage can fluctuate, or client/family may exhibit behaviors of more than one stage at a time

   a. Current response to death and dying
   b. Current affect and feelings expressed
   c. Present and past coping patterns
5. Support from significant others
6. Expectations and resources
7. Spiritual needs and support
8. Cultural needs and support
9. Feelings about treatment setting
10. Family assessment
   a. Perception of diagnosis and prognosis
   b. Stage of loss
   c. Feelings and their influence on client
   d. Communication patterns
   e. Needs and resources
   f. Response to dying person and impact on client
   g. Spiritual needs and support

ANALYSIS/NURSING DIAGNOSES (see p. 30)
PLANNING, IMPLEMENTATION, AND EVALUATION

> **Goal 1:** (Stage 1) Client will begin to cope with the impending death through denial.

Implementation
1. Plan several brief interactions with client each shift or visit (client may try to protect others by being "brave" and perhaps not seek out help and support from others).
2. Teach client that isolation and denial are normal responses when not destructive to the person.
3. Allow denial until client has mobilized other defenses to deal with the impact of diagnosis and prognosis.
4. Be honest when answering the client's questions about life, death, and treatment. Do not be too harsh in your honesty, but do not minimize client's concerns; allow client to maintain hope. Support client's spiritual needs.
5. Do not reinforce or reject client's denial; accept need for denial (e.g., if client says, "I can't believe it! It's not happening," nurse might say, "It must seem a bit unreal to you").
6. Support client in dealing with denial expressed by family and friends.

Evaluation
Client initially denies and then begins to acknowledge the reality of the impending death.

> **Goal 2:** (Stage 2) Client will appropriately express anger about impending death.

Implementation
1. Permit and encourage the verbal expression of anger and other feelings (often the anger is directed toward the nurse). Remember that fear underlies anger; do not take the anger as a personal attack, do not react defensively.
2. Allow expression of guilt (not seeking or following treatment), but help client move away from self-blame.
3. Listen to client's expressions of anger without offering judgment or arguments; help client deal with anger arising from distancing behaviors of relatives and friends.
4. Discuss possible alternative treatment and lifestyle changes introduced by the client; offer clear, factual in-

formation about any alternatives to assist client in making choices.

Evaluation

Client appropriately expresses anger about impending death.

Goal 3: (Stage 3) Client will use bargaining in an attempt to prolong life.

Implementation

1. Permit client to cope by bargaining; client may say things like, "If only . . ." or "Maybe I could . . ."; know that this characteristic "magical thinking" allows client to feel some control.
2. Help client to make amends for past failures or grievances (perceived or real); help client to find meaning and purpose in life by reminiscing and reviewing accomplishments.
3. Discuss importance of what is being bargained for using a sensitive, accepting approach.
4. Allow client to make appropriate decisions and control self-care and ADL when possible (e.g., timing of, intervals between, or lack of interventions) and explore benefits, risks, and possible consequences.

Evaluation

Client continues progress through the grief and mourning process by bargaining.

Goal 4: (Stage 4) Client will verbalize recognition of the inevitable and allow self to feel sadness and depression.

Implementation

1. Provide privacy as needed to express feelings, cry, or raise voice to maintain dignity and humility.
2. Allow client to express sadness by crying, talking, or withdrawing into silence; avoid trying to "cheer" client.
3. Answer questions such as "Am I going to die?" with a response such as "It sounds like you feel you are going to die?" (let client respond) and follow up with, "Tell me what this means to you"; discuss client's responses.
4. Avoid giving false hope.
5. Provide opportunities for client to express feelings about the impending loss of everything known and loved and changes in body image and self-esteem; accept sadness as grieving behavior, not as self-pity.
6. Remind client that sadness is normal; explore the difference that coping with the impending death rather than giving up can make.
7. Help client to focus on the present and to make the most of each day.
8. Use touch judiciously (some clients may welcome touching whereas others do not).

Evaluation

Client verbalizes sad, depressed feelings; begins to talk about own death.

Goal 5: (Stage 5) Client will accept the inevitability of impending death.

Implementation

1. Help client take care of personal and family matters.
2. Continue to allow discussion of the impending death but realize that full acceptance may not be achieved (rather, the client becomes resigned to the situation); do not try to force acceptance.
3. Encourage the client to participate in the decision-making process.
4. Allow client to decide when and if to spend some time alone; allow client to restrict visitors to short periods of time as desired.
5. Promote a peaceful conclusion of the dying process by offering comfort and maintaining dignity, and security measures as necessary.
6. Know that the family may not be at the same level of coping as the client.
   a. Assess the potential disruption the death will have on the family.
   b. Use clear and factual terminology and information when speaking with the family.
   c. Remain calm to avoid increasing family tension. Some families benefit when mutual feelings are shared between nurse and family.
   d. Use family rituals and customs whenever possible.
   e. Spend time with the family discussing their feelings.
   f. Know that families respond to the dying member much as they handled other major crisis situations.
   g. Family's greatest needs may be competent physical care for the ill member and empathy for the difficulty of their situation.
   h. Help family with packing, arrange a comfortable place to sleep, or allow family to call at any time to find out how their ill relative is.

Evaluation

Client moves through the fifth stage of loss at own pace to an acceptable and dignified death; expresses feelings and concerns about impending death; participates in decision making for own ADL for as long as possible; the family or significant other discusses feelings and concerns about death of loved one.

Nursing Process: Child

ASSESSMENT

1. Child's mental status including level of understanding and reaction/feelings about situation; ability to express self
2. Parents' level of understanding and reaction/feelings about situation; parents' strengths and needs; participation in ADL, support systems
3. Child's physical condition (e.g., vital signs, pain, energy level, skin integrity, hydration, eating and sleeping patterns, current medications), ability to perform ADL
4. Staff members' feelings and concerns, need for support
5. Siblings' level of understanding; their responses to the impending death, health changes arising from the child's illness, and separation from ill sibling
6. Family communication and coping patterns
7. History of previous losses and responses
8. Spiritual needs and support
9. Cultural needs and support

ANALYSIS/NURSING DIAGNOSES (see p. 30)
PLANNING, IMPLEMENTATION, AND EVALUATION

Goal 1: Child and family will express feelings, fears, anxieties, and guilt; will verbalize their understanding of the mental and physical health status and the terminal process.

Implementation
1. Determine what the child knows.
2. Encourage parents to take an active role in the child's ADL.
3. Work through own feelings with other staff members.
4. Allow and encourage the parents to express their feelings, and accept those expressions in a nonjudgmental manner.
5. Be available to client and family for frequent interactions.
6. Permit child to express anger and hostility, but at the same time do not be totally permissive regarding unacceptable behavior (child may perceive this permissiveness as total hopelessness and abandonment).
7. Encourage child to draw or play with toys to express feelings.
   a. Draw own body.
   b. Draw a feeling.
   c. Draw family.
   d. Play doctor/nurse and act out feelings, including angry feelings; let nurse be the client.
8. Acknowledge family responses, stages of grieving:
   a. Shock, denial, guilt, bodily distress, anxiety.
   b. Acceptance, belief in God or supreme being.
9. Encourage interaction/involvement of ill child and siblings.
10. Help reduce marital stress by encouraging couple to spend an evening away from the hospital and to call when they feel concerned about their child.
11. Help siblings to express their feelings, use drawing, storytelling, play therapy.
   a. Help parents understand that siblings' perceptions, interpretations, and reactions may not be as intense as parents'.
   b. "Favorite child" angers other siblings; also increased stress experienced by siblings who need a chance to discuss feelings; they, too, may feel they did something to cause sibling to become ill.
12. Refer family to self-help groups or family therapist in community.

Evaluation
Child and family express some degree of awareness of the terminal process; verbalize some feelings associated with grief and mourning.

Goal 2: Child will maintain as much independence as possible in ADL; will have minimal pain and discomfort; will ingest adequate food and fluid to meet body needs.

Implementation
1. Provide pain medication and comfort measures as needed (prn).
2. Ensure adequate fluid and food intake; use supplements when necessary and allow child choice of food if possible.
3. Preserve skin integrity by massage, lotions, sheepskin, water mattress.
4. Encourage child's participation in ADL as long as energy levels are not depleted. Elicit help of parents and encourage active participation in child's ADL.
5. Use passive and active range of motion (ROM).
6. Permit child to have favorite toys, music, and special objects.
7. Explain procedures to parents and child.
8. Ensure continuity of daily life activities by encouraging visits, telephone calls, and letter writing from friends through parents and client.
9. Provide home care through hospice or other home health agencies when requested or appropriate.

Evaluation
Child maintains independence in ADL; has minimal pain and discomfort; ingests food and fluid to meet body needs.

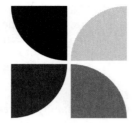

Anxious Behavior

1. Normal anxiety is an innate form of communication, is protective, and is crucial to adaptation and survival. Anxiety is an unpleasant and sometimes distressful phenomenon that consists of biologic and psychosocial components. It is often described as a persistent feeling of dread, apprehension, and impending disaster brought on by a nonspecific threat to self. In milder forms, it is a normal experience that motivates a person to take constructive action in a situation. As anxiety becomes more severe, it can interfere with perception, judgment, and behavior, and it requires outside intervention to help the person to function constructively. Its prominence as a human occurrence makes it one of the most common concerns in psychiatric and psychosocial nursing. Recognition of anxious behaviors and DSM-IV anxiety disorders and the appropriate use of helping interventions are essential nursing skills in any health care setting (Tables 2-6, 2-7, and 2-8).

2. Anticipatory anxiety, anxiety, and fear are all accepted official nursing diagnoses with established defining characteristics.
   a. *Anticipatory anxiety:* an increased level of arousal associated with a perceived *future* threat to the self
   b. *Anxiety:* a generalized feeling of dread and apprehension, which is a subjectively painful warning of a threat to the self or to significant relationships
   c. *Fear:* a feeling of dread related to an *identifiable* source that is perceived as a threat or danger to the self or significant relationships
   d. *Anxious behavior:* refers to a subjective feeling resulting from the experience of anxiety, conflict, fear, or stress; such response ranges from mild to severe and represents a normal human reaction to a sense of threat

3. General causes
   a. A threat to biologic or psychologic integrity
   b. A threat to security of self; anxiety is a warning signal prompting the individual to defend against the threat
   c. Normal coping mechanisms are overtaxed or impaired
   d. An unconscious reaction to danger (defense mechanism)
   e. Genetic predisposition or vulnerability (based on twin and adoption studies)
   f. Neurochemical and neuroanatomic alterations
   g. Distorted cognitions that generate a perceived danger or threat (cognitive theory)

   h. Developmental factors, such as conditioning and reinforcement (learning theory)
   i. Psychosocial factors, including stress and coping patterns

4. Four levels of anxiety: on a continuum from mild to panic, which primarily involves cognitive, psychologic, and neurobiologic (e.g., autonomic nervous system arousal) and level of functioning disturbances
   a. *Mild anxiety:* characteristics
      1. more alert than usual, increased questioning
      2. heightened capacity to deal with perception of impending danger
      3. focus of attention on immediate events
      4. person experiences mild discomfort, restlessness
      5. may be a useful motivating force (e.g., if a person experiences mild anxiety during NCLEX-RN, this may help increase ability to answer questions)
   b. *Moderate anxiety:* characteristics
      1. cognitive disturbances
         a. restricted perception
         b. diminished listening, perceptive, comprehension, and communication capabilities
         c. selective inattention, focus on one specific thing; other information or stimulus is negated or ignored
      2. psychologic disturbances
         a. as tension and discomfort increase and expressed fears of danger emerge
         b. moderate feelings of "doom" or "going crazy"
         c. level of function decreases
      3. neurobiologic disturbances (autonomic nervous system arousal)
         a. muscle tension
         b. restlessness
         c. "keyed up"
         d. dry mouth/throat
         e. hand shakiness
         f. diaphoresis
         g. increased heart rate, breathing, and blood pressure
         h. sleep or eating disturbances
         i. paresthesias (numbness or tingling sensations)
   c. *Severe anxiety:* characteristics
      1. cognitive disturbances:
         a. greatly reduced perception
         b. difficulty attending, understanding, and processing information

Table 2-6 DSM-IV classification of anxiety-related disorders

Anxiety disorders	Somatoform disorders	Dissociative disorders
Panic disorder without agoraphobia	Somatization disorder	Dissociative amnesia
Panic disorder with agoraphobia	Conversion disorder	Dissociative fugue
Agoraphobia without panic disorder	Undifferentiated somatoform disorder	Depersonalization disorder
Specific phobia (e.g., animal, natural environment, situation)	Pain disorder (associated with psychologic disorder; associated with both psychologic factors and a general medical condition)	Dissociative identity disorder (formerly multiple personality disorder)
Social phobia		Dissociative disorder NOS
Obsessive-compulsive disorder	Hypochondriasis	
Posttraumatic stress disorder	Body dysmorphic disorder	
Acute stress disorder	Somatoform disorder NOS	
General anxiety disorder		
Anxiety disorder caused by (indicate the general medical condition)		
Substance-induced anxiety disorder		
Anxiety disorder not otherwise specified (NOS)		

  2. psychologic disturbances
    a. sense of impending doom; dread, horror
  3. neurobiologic disturbances (intense)
    a. increased physical symptoms (e.g., diaphoresis, dizziness, increased muscle tension, pallor, nausea, trembling)
  d. *Panic:* characteristics
    1. altered perceptions of reality
    2. helpless, fearful, panicky feelings
    3. physical symptoms (e.g., tachycardia, hyperventilation)
    4. extreme discomfort; extreme measures to decrease anxiety
    5. feeling of depersonalization (strange or unreal feelings)
    6. severe hyperactivity, loss of control
    7. inability to communicate or function
    8. Frequently unrecognized as panic; clients may think they are having a heart attack or "going crazy"
5. Diagnosis of anxiety: obtained from three kinds of data—neurobiologic changes, psychologic changes (see Table 2-7), and use of coping or defense mechanisms
  a. Neurobiologic changes
    1. involve primarily the arousal of the autonomic nervous system
    2. mild and moderate levels of anxiety tend to arouse neurobiologic processes such as heart rate, breathing patterns, and diaphoresis
    3. level of function is impaired by severe anxiety and panic, resulting in physical paralysis and in prolonged states culminating in death
    4. knowledge of neurobiologic symptoms enables the nurse to intervene before the panic stage
    5. during panic, when the physical symptoms are severe, immediate intervention is imperative
  b. Psychologic changes
    1. psychologic manifestations accelerate as anxiety level increases and can become extremely uncomfortable to the person

Table 2-7 Manifestations of anxiety

Physiologic	Psychologic
Tachycardia	Tension
Palpitations	Nervousness
Excessive perspiration	Apprehension
Dry mouth	Irritability
Cold, clammy, pale skin	Indecisiveness
Urinary frequency	Oversensitivity
Diarrhea	Tearfulness
Muscle tension	Agitation
Tremors	Dread
Narrowing of focus	Horror
	Panic

    2. maladaptive behaviors are mechanisms used to avoid accelerating anxiety to the panic state (e.g., rumination, rituals, compulsivity)
  c. Coping mechanisms: may be a defense mechanism or any means used to resolve, or at least delay, conflict or threats to the self
    1. constructive: client, alerted by warning signal that something is not going as expected, resolves the conflict
    2. destructive or disturbed: client tries to protect self from anxiety without resolving the conflict, which can be expressed in maladaptive or dysfunctional behavior
Major DSM-IV anxiety disorders are listed in Table 2-6.

Application of the Nursing Process to the Client Exhibiting Anxious Behaviors

NOTE: The same nursing process is used with all anxiety-related behaviors regardless of whether they are adaptive or maladaptive.

ASSESSMENT
  1. Level of anxiety (signs and behavior)
  2. Neurobiologic and psychologic signs and symptoms
  3. Causative factors if known

Table 2-8   Stress management

Stress is a generalized, nonspecific response of the body to any demand, change, or perceived threat, whether positive or negative. *Stressors* are the circumstances or events that elicit this response and may be real or anticipated. *Distress* is damaging or unpleasant stress. Altered mental status

SIGNS OF DISTRESS

Accident proneness	Fluctuation in vital signs	Irritability
Alcohol and other drug abuse	Frequent urination	Neck or back pain
Anxiety	Grinding teeth	Perceptual-sensory disturbances
Chronic fatigue	Headache	Nightmares
Decrease or increase of appetite	Impulsive behavior	Sexual problems
Diarrhea or constipation	Inability to concentrate	Stuttering
Emotional instability	Insomnia	Sweating
Emotional tension		

GOAL

The client will maintain homeostasis or optimal adaptive coping by preventing, or recognizing promptly, excessive levels of stress; the client will use effective measures to manage stress by describing a plan to cope with stress in an adaptive way that includes exercise, relaxation, creative problem solving, and sharing feelings and concerns with a significant other.

Stress-reduction techniques	Nursing implications	Stress-reduction techniques	Nursing implications
Identify stressors (e.g., work, relationships, environment, health, age, finances, spiritual/emotional factors)	Have client examine own reaction to life occurrences (e.g., frustration, knot in stomach, loss of control). Discern between positive and negative stressors; explain that stress is unavoidable and can be used to motivate.	Relaxation techniques Progressive relaxation Autogenic training Guided imagery Meditation	Guide patient through a relaxation exercise to experience its usefulness. Begin relaxation with deep breathing. Use guided imagery to induce relaxation (e.g., "Take another deep breath and let all the tension release. With each breath you become more relaxed. Now, imagine yourself in a peaceful, quiet setting [garden, beach, etc]").
Modify or eliminate stressors	Review possibilities for simple and major changes. Discuss alternatives, advantages, and disadvantages of reducing stressors.		
Develop effective coping mechanisms Daily exercise	Suggest methods to reduce stress through exercise (e.g., walking, running, dancing, swimming, gardening, participating in sports, body movement exercises, yoga). Assist in developing a plan of regular activity. Refer to community gyms, health clubs, and YMCAs. Advise consultation with personal physician for contraindications to exercise program.	Diaphragmatic breathing; periodic deep breathing	Refer to cassettes, books, and classes on learning and practicing relaxation techniques. Practice diaphragmatic breathing with client Sit or recline in a comfortable position with legs uncrossed. Place one hand on the chest and the other hand on the diaphragm, approximately 2 inches below the bottom center of the breastbone. Inhale so the diaphragm expands and the hand covering the diaphragm moves out while the other hand remains almost still. As you exhale, the diaphragm relaxes and the hand covering it moves inward.
Develop alternative ways to relax (e.g., drawing, pottery, carpentry, writing, music, photography, reading, watching the sunset, taking a bubble bath)	Review with client activities enjoyed and suggest client devote at least an hour a day to an activity. Refer to recreation departments, adult education programs, community colleges.		

4. Coping mechanisms (adaptive or maladaptive)
5. Problem behavior (e.g., episodes of gastritis indicating moderate anxiety related to demands of nursing school)
6. Level of dangerousness
7. Strengths
8. Support systems and their involvement with client
9. Insight and willingness to change
10. Presence of phobias and ritualistic behaviors

ANALYSIS/NURSING DIAGNOSES

1. Safe, effective care environment
   a. Impaired home maintenance management
   b. High risk for trauma
   c. Knowledge deficit (e.g., effect of anxiety on ability to maintain safety)
2. Physiologic integrity
   a. Impaired verbal communication
   b. Altered nutrition: less/more than body requirements
   c. Sleep-pattern disturbance
   d. Fatigue
3. Psychosocial integrity
   a. Anxiety
   b. Ineffective individual coping
   c. Self-esteem/body-image/personal-identity disturbance
   d. Posttrauma response
   e. Social isolation
4. Health promotion/maintenance
   a. Impaired adjustment
   b. Altered family processes
   c. Altered health maintenance
   d. Self-care deficit (specify)

GENERAL NURSING PLANNING, IMPLEMENTATION, AND EVALUATION

Goal 1: Client will develop an open, trusting relationship with the nurse.

Implementation

1. Approach client in unhurried way and actively listen to concerns and feelings.
2. Encourage client to express feelings and concerns about unmet needs or stressful situation.
3. Be aware of personal feelings and behaviors toward the client's symptoms and their impact on the nurse-client relationship.

Evaluation

Client expresses concerns and unmet needs to the nurse (e.g., concern about failure or rejection or feelings of helplessness).

Goal 2: Client will use anxiety as a motivation for change.

Implementation

1. Create an accepting, attentive, and unhurried environment.
2. Encourage expression of feelings and thoughts about stressful situations, unmet needs.
   a. Invite client to recognize or name the thoughts and feelings being experienced.
   b. Demonstrate genuine interest and concern.

3. Offer reassurance by giving appropriate information, correcting distorted cognitions; repeat the process if necessary because client may have reduced hearing perception; use short, direct, and concise statements.
4. Collaborate with client to identify anxiety-causing situations that can be avoided.
5. Teach client to recognize how client is manifesting anxiety in behavior and biologic responses.
6. Help client identify situations that trigger anxiety.
7. Assist client in using stress-reduction techniques (e.g., biofeedback, visualization/imagery, challenging cognitive distortions, meditation, physical activity or exercise, journaling and homework assignments) to cope with anxiety; refer to Table 2-8.
8. Recognize factors that the nurse and client bring into the relationship.
   a. Anxiety is contagious.
   b. Establish strategies to modulate own anxiety, frustration, or anger.
9. Deter mild anxiety from expanding by realizing nonverbal cues of anxiety (e.g., smiling, restlessness, tense mood) and intervening early, whenever possible.
10. Provide physical care as needed for the severely anxious client

Evaluation

Client expresses feelings; identifies situations that cause anxiety; incorporates at least one stress-reduction technique into daily routine; experiences no more than moderate anxiety.

Goal 3: Client will recognize level of own anxious behavior and gain insight into the cause of maladaptive responses.

Implementation

1. Help client recognize anxiety by exploring the thoughts and feelings that precede anxious behavior.
2. Help client distinguish among thoughts, feelings, and behaviors and their impact on sustaining anxious behaviors.
3. Use the nurse-client relationship to improve the client's insight into the basis of maladaptive behaviors and motivation for change.
4. Provide a new perspective on the situation (i.e., help client "redefine" the problem).
5. Use biofeedback to help client recognize tension levels.
6. Instruct client to evaluate the threat, expectations, or unmet needs and to assess own capabilities realistically.
7. Teach various psychosocial stress-reducing techniques, such as deep-breathing exercises, progressive relaxation, visual imagery, and meditation.

Evaluation

Client identifies own behaviors linked to current anxiety; tells nurse when feelings trigger anxious behaviors; states causes of current anxiety.

Goal 4: Client will demonstrate alternative styles of coping with anxiety.

Implementation

1. Examine client's patterns of coping with anxiety.
2. Reinforce effective and adaptive coping mechanisms.
3. Teach client alternative methods of coping (e.g., visual imagery, relaxation, talking it out, positive self-talk, exercise).
4. Know that the client with mild or moderate anxiety is generally not hospitalized for treatment depending on
   a. Severity of the symptoms
   b. Impact on level of function
   c. Level of dangerousness (e.g., threat to self or others)
   d. Nature of the home environment
   e. Quality of support system
   f. Motivation for change
5. Observe for alterations in mental and physical status and intervene directly as necessary for client's well-being.

Evaluation

Client learns two new coping mechanisms (e.g., verbalizing thoughts and feelings, guided imagery; experiences more control over anxiety).

Goal 5: Client will be able to cope with severe to panic anxiety and reduce anxiety at least one level.

Implementation

1. Understand that a severely anxious client may neglect physical needs, experience alterations in mental status and fatigue, or actually pose a threat to self or others. Provide physical care and emotional support and protection as indicated; maintain safe environment.
2. Remove client from other clients if anxiety increases, and maintain close observation (i.e., do not leave alone).
3. Anticipate mild disturbances and reduce progression into severe or panic stage by identifying early signs and symptoms.
4. Permit client to define stressors that he or she can manage.
5. Recognize that adaptive coping mechanisms modulate anxiety within healthy levels.
6. Maintain a confident and comforting approach.
7. Speak in a calm, reassuring manner and use direct, clear sentences.
8. Use active listening skills.
9. Encourage client to participate in activities that use large muscle groups when appropriate.
10. Avoid challenging the client's coping behaviors.
11. Help client build and use effective, adaptive coping mechanisms.
12. Remove potentially harmful objects from environment and continuously assess the client's level of dangerousness.
13. When antianxiety or anxiolytic agents are prescribed:
    a. Refer to Table 2-9.
    b. Administer anxiolytics or antianxiety drugs to provide symptomatic relief of neurobiologic symptoms and enhance psychosocial interventions.
    c. Assess substance abuse history and realize that these anxiolytics are potentially addictive and should be prescribed for only short periods; drugs may minimize client motivation for change.
    d. Teach client that these drugs should not be taken with alcohol or other central nervous system (CNS) depressants because they potentiate each other.
    e. Teach the client actions and side effects of drugs (a common side effect of anxiolytic agents is drowsiness; therefore persons taking these drugs should avoid operating a vehicle or potentially dangerous equipment).
14. When client's anxiety subsides, negotiate reasonable limits on anxious behavior.
15. Avoid heightening anxiety by giving it excessive attention.
16. Provide physical activity as appropriate to client's condition.

Evaluation

Client reduces anxiety to at least a moderate level; does not injure self or others; manages anxiety using adaptive coping mechanisms (e.g., verbalizing feelings, using relaxation techniques, challenging cognitive distortions).

SELECTED HEALTH PROBLEMS

OBSESSIVE-COMPULSIVE DISORDERS

1. Definition: presence of obsession (uncontrollable, recurring thoughts) or compulsion (a ritualistic act done in an attempt to relieve the anxiety related to the thoughts or to make the thoughts go away); considered to be a complex disorder with multifaceted causes including genetic predisposition, alterations in neurochemical processes and neuroanatomic structures, and psychologic conversion reaction to anxiety.
2. Ego defense mechanisms: displacement and undoing; the person attempts to displace unconscious, hostile, aggressive impulse with unrelated acts (e.g., hand washing); in so doing, the person attempts to undo or negate the unacceptable impulse. NOTE: The person realizes that the obsessions and compulsions are irrational.
3. Signs and symptoms: may include ritualistic behaviors (e.g., compulsive hand washing or cleanliness or habitual responses such as extreme thrift, neatness, or insistence on same daily routine) with panic or bizarre behavior if usual routine is broken.
4. Treatment: individual, family, or group psychotherapy; desensitization; behavior modification; antiobsessional agent (e.g., clomipramine).
5. DSM-IV classification: subclassification of anxiety disorders, obsessive-compulsive disorder: specify with poor insight.

Nursing Process

ASSESSMENT

1. Note patterns of compulsive behaviors, including preceding events, and client's reactions to specific situations and persons.
2. Listen for description of obsessions.
3. Assess level of function and impairment arising from compulsions.

Table 2-9 Antianxiety agents (anxiolytic agents)

Drug	Action	Side effects	Nursing implications
BENZODIAZEPINE DERIVATIVES			

Alprazolam (Xanax)
  0.25-0.5 mg PO tid
  Maximum dosage 4 mg/day in divided doses
Chlorazepate dipotassium (Tranxene)
  15-60 mg/day PO in divided doses for maintenance
Chlordiazepoxide hydrochloride (Librium)
  5-10 mg PO 3-4 x/day (mild-moderate anxiety)
  20-25 mg PO 3-4 x/day (severe anxiety)
  50-100 mg PO for acute alcohol withdrawal
Clonazepam (Klonopin)
  1.5-10 mg per day
Diazepam (Valium)
  2-10 mg PO 2-4 x/day
  10 mg PO 3-4 x first day for acute alcohol withdrawal
	Appears to act on limbic, thalamic, and hypothalamic levels of CNS; produces hypnotic, sedative, anxiolytic, skeletal muscle relaxant, and anticonvulsant effects. Range of CNS depression is from mild sedation to coma.	Hypotension, drowsiness, dizziness, ataxia, lethargy, headache, dry mouth, constipation, urinary retention, changes in libido, paradoxic excitement. Psychologic and physical dependence.	Caution client to avoid potentially hazardous activities because of drowsiness.
			Warn client of danger of concurrent use of alcohol or other CNS depressants.
			Be aware that these drugs may potentiate suicidal tendencies.
			Monitor vital signs.
			Report paradoxic excitement.
			Avoid abrupt withdrawal (may produce reactions).
			Tolerance and psychologic and physical dependence may occur after prolonged use.
			Do not give antacids concurrently.
			In geriatric clients, doses are initiated at lower levels.
			Do not take with meals—slows absorption

Flurazepam (Dalmane)
  15-30 mg PO at bedtime for insomnia
Lorazepam (Ativan)
  2-3 mg PO divided into 2-3 doses/day
Oxazepam (Serax)
  10-15 mg PO 3-4 x/day (mild-moderate anxiety)
  15-30 mg PO 3-4 x/day (severe anxiety)
Temazepam (Restoril)
  15-30 mg total daily dose
	Sedative-hypnotic CNS depressant		

Triazolam (Halcion) 0.25-0.5 mg PO at bedtime for insomnia	Sedative-hypnotic CNS depressant		
PROPANEDIOL			

Meprobamate (Equanil, Miltown)
  1.2-1.6 g daily in 3-4 divided doses
  Maximum dose 2.4 g
	CNS depressant action is similar to barbiturates. Apparently acts on multiple CNS sites—hypothalamus, thalamus, limbic, and spinal cord.	Drowsiness, ataxia, dizziness, vertigo, slurred speech, headache, skin rash, weakness. Psychologic and physical dependence.	Know that meprobamate is highly lethal in overdose; consider the possibility of suicide attempts and take precautions.
			Caution client regarding the concurrent use of alcohol or other CNS depressants.
			Avoid rapid withdrawal (convulsions and death can result).
			Caution client to avoid potentially hazardous activities because of drowsiness.

Continued

Table 2-9   Antianxiety agents (anxiolytic agents)—cont'd

Drug	Action	Side effects	Nursing implications
ANTIHISTAMINES			
Hydroxyzine hydrochloride (Vistaril) Hydroxyzine pamoate (Atarax) 50-100 mg PO qid	Has central cholinergic effect and CNS properties; used for sedative effects as nighttime sleep aid.	Drowsiness, dry mouth, headache.	Caution client to avoid potentially hazardous activities because of drowsiness. Warn client of additive effects with alcohol and other drugs.
BARBITURATES			

The following are sedative doses (hypnotic doses are higher for sleep inducement and preop anxiety)
Amobarbital
  30-50 mg PO bid or tid
Aprobarbital
  40 mg PO tid
Butabarbital sodium
  15-30 mg tid or qid
Mephobarbital
  32-100 mg PO tid or qid
Pentobarbital
  20-40 mg PO bid or tid
Phenobarbital
  30-120 mg PO od
Secobarbital sodium
  100-300 mg od in 3 divided doses (not usually used for sedation; used mostly as a hypnotic)
Talbutal
  30-60 mg PO bid or tid
	Decreases the excitability of both presynaptic and postsynaptic membranes to produce sedative/hypnotic effect. Barbiturates are capable of producing all levels of CNS depression. Used for anxiety, insomnia, alcohol withdrawal syndrome, preoperative sedation, anticonvulsant (only phenobarbital, metharbital, and mephobarbital are effective as oral anticonvulsants).	Tolerance, psychologic and physiologic dependence may occur after prolonged use when used for insomnia; should not be used over 2 weeks; drowsiness.	Warn clients that barbiturates may impair the ability to perform tasks requiring mental alertness (e.g., driving, operating machinery)
			Warn clients not to consume alcohol while taking these drugs.
			Do not withdraw drug abruptly after prolonged use.
			May potentiate side effects of other CNS depressants.
			Dosage in elderly is reduced.
			Obtain blood pressure, pulse, and respiration before administration.
			Watch for paradoxic reactions (e.g., excitement, hyperactivity, confusion, depression).
			Watch for drug interactions (other CNS depressants, anticoagulants, corticosteroids, antidepressants, doxycycline).

ANTIOBSESSIONAL AGENTS			
Clomipramine (Anafranil) (tricyclic) Normal dose: up to 250 mg/day			
Fluvoxamine maleate (Luvox) Normal dose: 100-300 mg/day	SSRI: potent effects on serotonin neurotransmission	Same as other SSRIs	
MISCELLANEOUS			
Buspirone hydrochloride (BuSpar) (20-30 mg PO qd divided)	Anxiolytic; takes 3 weeks for therapeutic effect.	Sleep disturbances, akathisia, tremors, GI disturbances, skin rash, decreased concentration	Observe for EPS; serious drug interactions, particularly MAOIs (e.g., Nardil); teach client to avoid operating potentially dangerous equipment.
Propranolol hydrochloride (Inderal) (10-80 mg PO tid-qid)	Beta-adrenergic blocker used to relieve physical symptoms; attaches to sensors and blocks messages that arouse anxiety states	See Table 3-11.	See Table 3-11.
Imipramine hydrochloride (Tofranil) (30-250 mg PO qd divided)	Antidepressant; regulates brain's reaction to serotonin to prevent panic attacks.	See Table 2-10.	See Table 2-10.

4. Assess client's understanding of impact of disorder on sense of well-being.

ANALYSIS/NURSING DIAGNOSES (see p. 37)

PLANNING, IMPLEMENTATION, AND EVALUATION

Goal: Client will accept limits on repetitive acts and participate in alternative adaptive activities.

Implementation

1. Approach in a calm, accepting, and reassuring manner (appreciate the client's urge to control).
2. Give client a schedule to follow so that ritualistic/repetitive behaviors are *limited, but not prohibited.*
3. Allow client to have choices in schedule and participate in decisions about use of time and energy.
4. Do not abruptly interrupt the repetitive act because it is allaying anxiety; interruption allows the anxiety to break through and can cause panic.
5. Set reasonable limits on repetitive behavior; give the client adequate warning that at a certain time another activity will begin.
6. Engage in alternative activities with client; do not expect the client to proceed in another activity alone.
7. Provide physical protection from repetitive acts; some ritualistic behaviors can cause physical discomfort (e.g., compulsive hand washing).
8. As ritualistic/repetitive behaviors decrease, help client express feelings and concerns in socially acceptable ways.

Evaluation

Client washes hands (or other compulsive act) fewer times a day compared with admission or entry into treatment; begins to participate in constructive activities.

POSTTRAUMATIC STRESS DISORDER

1. Definition: anxiety syndrome resulting from severe external stress that is beyond what is usual or tolerable for most people. This is a complex anxiety disorder arising from cognitive, biologic, and psychosocial factors.
2. Stressors: rape, military combat, natural disasters (e.g., earthquakes), physical accidents involving loss of life of another or loss of body part or its functions (e.g., permanent paralysis after an accident), accidental disasters caused by people (e.g., crashes, fires), intentional disasters (e.g., bombing, torture), victims of criminal assaults (e.g., robbery).
3. Characteristics:
   a. Reexperiencing trauma in at least one of the following ways:
      1. recurrent/intrusive recollections of event
      2. recurrent dreams of event
      3. sudden acting out or feeling as if traumatic event were recurring, because of environmental or thought "triggers" or stimulus
      4. pronounced autonomic arousal arising from recurrent recollection of event
   b. A lack of feelings or numbing responsiveness to or decreased involvement with external world after the trauma:
      1. pronounced apathy in one or more significant activities
      2. social detachment or estrangement from others
      3. constricted affect
   c. At least two of the following symptoms are not present before the trauma:
      1. hyperalertness or exaggerated startle response
      2. sleep disturbance
      3. guilt about surviving or about behavior required for survival
      4. concentration and memory disturbances
      5. avoidance of activities that arouse recollection of traumatic event
      6. heightened symptoms when exposed to events that represent or resemble the traumatic event
4. Related factors:
   a. Physical injury may be present because of the nature of the trauma.
   b. Depression and anxiety are common.
   c. Reaction may be delayed, with symptoms appearing some time after the trauma.
   d. Avoidance behaviors or social isolation may be present.
   e. Risk of self-medication through chemical addiction is increased.
5. Dynamics: loss of self-esteem and loss of control in the traumatic situation have led to the behavior and feelings just described.
6. DSM-IV classification: subclassification of anxiety disorders—posttraumatic stress disorder if symptoms persist more than a month; acute stress reaction if they persist less than a month.

Nursing Process

ASSESSMENT

1. Nature and duration of the traumatic event
2. Duration of symptoms
3. Degree of impairment
4. Preexistence of problems that may complicate situation (e.g., anxiety, depression, unresolved trauma issues, substance misuse)
5. Level of dangerousness toward self and others
6. Presence and degree of symptoms
7. Present and past coping mechanisms
8. Client and family teaching needs
9. Quality of support systems
10. History of previous traumas and treatment
11. Current resources (e.g., financial, career, health insurance)

ANALYSIS/NURSING DIAGNOSES (see p. 37)

PLANNING, IMPLEMENTATION, AND EVALUATION

Goal 1: Client will recall the traumatic event and cope with feelings generated by it.

Implementation

1. Create a safe and accepting treatment environment.
2. Maintain personal space and clear boundaries (e.g., avoid touching without permission).
3. Acknowledge personal reactions that may enhance or impede the treatment process.
4. Support client through process of recounting the event and venting feelings.

5. Acknowledge significance of the traumatic event and the normalcy of client's feelings.
6. If there is a need to return to the scene of the trauma, help the client select appropriate time and supportive accompanying resources.
7. Review goals and plans for crisis intervention (p. 27), depression, rape, and loss (p. 30).
8. Involve client in a recovering group of people with similar problems (e.g., Victims for Victims).

Evaluation
Client describes the event and discusses feelings generated by it (e.g., sadness, anger).

> **Goal 2:** Client will resume involvement in routine daily activities.

Implementation
1. Initiate measures to promote quality social interactions.
2. Remain comfortable during silent periods.
3. Educate client and family about normalcy of feelings
4. Encourage family involvement in treatment, particularly increasing interactions with client.
5. Gradually increase reinvolvement in pretrauma activities.
6. Encourage client to discuss reactions to social involvement.
7. Provide information about social, financial, or health resources.

Evaluation
Client gradually resumes involvement in important life activities.

✖ PSYCHOLOGIC FACTORS AFFECTING MEDICAL CONDITION

1. Definition: Stress-involved physiologic response that exacerbates or intensifies symptoms of a general medical condition on Axis III
2. Reactions: eczema (skin), migraine headaches (neurovascular system), lupus (autoimmune disorder), backaches (musculoskeletal system), gastritis (gastrointestinal disorders), asthma (respiratory disorders), psychogenic pain
3. Occurrence: often seen in medical settings; becomes a psychiatric problem when anxiety escalates in spite of physical disorder
4. Possible secondary characteristics
   a. *Dependence:* a person may manifest abnormal dependency needs resulting from lack of confidence and poor living skills
      1. difficulty in making decisions
      2. extreme lack of confidence
      3. a need for more help in dealing with problems
   b. *Controlling behavior:* attempts to exercise a dominating influence over another person because of perceived helplessness; manipulative techniques include negativism, obstinace, noncompliance, silence, avoidance, talkativeness, crying

Nursing Process
ASSESSMENT (see p. 35)
ANALYSIS/NURSING DIAGNOSES (see p. 37)
PLANNING, IMPLEMENTATION, AND EVALUATION

> **Goal:** Client will express feelings, perceptions, and concerns about symptoms and treatment plan; client will participate in treatment plan.

Implementation
1. Acknowledge and reinforce expression of feelings, concerns, and perceptions.
2. Assess teaching needs and educate client and family about causes, signs and symptoms of anxiety, management of symptoms using medications, and psychosocial interventions.
3. Negotiate areas of self-care and independent activity.
4. Encourage joint exploration of the motivation for client's behavior.
5. Teach alternative anxiety-reducing measures (e.g., talking directly about the concern, asking for help and support, setting limits with others, saying "no" appropriately).
6. Set limits on controlling/manipulative behaviors; state time limits; make expectations clear; do not impose unnecessary controls.
7. Permit the client to retain control when appropriate; avoid power struggles.
8. When manipulative behaviors occur, provide opportunities for staff meetings to vent feelings and coordinate care.
9. Teach effective communication skills (assertiveness training) to assist in getting needs met.

Evaluation
Client accepts limits on controlling/manipulative behaviors; develops alternative coping mechanisms and effective communication skills; participates in self-care.

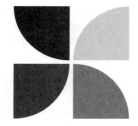

Delirium, Dementia, Amnestic Disorders, and Other Cognitive Disorders

Cognitive disorders can be related to an underlying general medical condition, or they can be substance induced. The DSM-IV delineates four categories of cognitive disorders: delirium, dementia, and amnestic and other cognitive disorders. Cognitive disturbance may be a symptom of a general medical disturbance such as respiratory abnormalities, electrolyte imbalance, infection, biochemical or nutritional imbalances, cerebral vascular disease or destruction, and physical or psychologic trauma. It may be seen in some mental disorders, including severe depression and anxiety disorders, and in acute stress reactions. It also can be substance induced.

Application of the Nursing Process to the Client Exhibiting Confused Behavior

Certain biologic processes and environmental conditions can induce cognitive disturbances. Symptoms of cognitive disturbances may evolve over a rapid period, such as those seen in delirium, or an insidious and progressive period, such as those seen in Alzheimer's disease. Selected health problems will describe various manifestations of cognitive disturbances.

SELECTED HEALTH PROBLEMS

ACUTE COGNITIVE DISORDERS: DELIRIUM

1. Definition: alteration in consciousness with inability to focus or maintain attention.
2. Major manifestations of cognitive disturbances include memory deficits, disorientation, confusion, language difficulties, and perceptual-sensory deficits.
3. The onset of symptoms evolves rapidly (usually hours to days), and symptoms fluctuate throughout the day.
4. Physical examination, history, or laboratory results relate symptoms to a general medical condition (e.g., fluid and electrolyte imbalance, drug interaction, severe anemia, hypoxia, endocrine disorders).
5. Other DSM-IV classifications of delirium: substance-induced delirium (intoxication and withdrawal types); delirium due to multiple etiologies; and delirium not otherwise specified.

PROGRESSIVE COGNITIVE DISORDERS: DEMENTIA

1. Definition: cognitive disturbances arising from degenerative processes in the brain that give rise to symptoms of dementia:
   a. *Alzheimer's type:* memory impairment (inability to learn new information (recent memory) or recall learned information (remote memory); language deficits; motor disturbances; inability to recognize people or objects; severe impairment of abstract thinking, judgment, and organizational mastery. Alzheimer's-type dementia is divided into early onset (before age 65) and late onset (after age 65). Both have subsets of *with delirium, with delusions, with depressed mood, uncomplicated,* and *with behavioral disturbance.* This disorder is an Axis III or medical disorder.
   b. *Vascular dementia:* memory deficits: recent and remote memory deficits; may include one or more of the following: language and motor impairment; difficulty recognizing persons or objects; and impaired abstract thinking, judgment, and organizational skills. Other manifestations include focal neurologic signs, such as hemiparesis and diagnostic findings of multiple cerebral infarctions (cerebral vascular accident) affecting the cerebral cortex. This disorder is also an Axis III disorder and may be classified as *with delirium, with delusions, with depressed mood, uncomplicated,* and *with behavioral disturbance.*
2. Other specific disorders:
   a. Dementia caused by other general medical conditions, such as human immunodeficiency virus (HIV) disease, head trauma, Parkinson's disease, Hunginton's disease, Pick's disease, Cruetzfeldt-Jakob disease, and other conditions.

AMNESTIC DISORDERS

1. Amnestic disorder caused by the general medical condition:
   a. Major symptoms include memory deficits that give rise to a decreased level of function; does not necessarily occur during the course of delirium or dementia; and diagnostic studies link symptoms to an underlying general medical condition such as head trauma. This condition can be classified as transient or chronic (duration more than 1 month). Other DSM-IV classifications include substance-induced

persisting amnestic disorder and amnestic disorder not otherwise specified.

2. Other cognitive disorder not otherwise specified.
3. Varying degrees of cognitive disturbances are noted in cognitive disorders.
4. DSM-IV classification: delirium, dementia, amnestic disorders and other cognitive disorders.

Nursing Process

ASSESSMENT
1. Onset of symptoms history
2. Orientation to person, time, place
3. Problems with cognition: decreased attention, comprehension, abstract thinking, judgment, decision making, calculation
4. Memory: impairment of recent or remote memory; may fabricate experiences or situations in plausible manner to cover memory loss (confabulation)
5. Speech patterns
6. Sensory-perceptual function
7. Self-care abilities
8. Sleep-wake patterns
9. Previous coping mechanisms
10. Personality and affectual (mood) changes
11. Social interaction
12. Feelings and concerns about treatment, impairment
13. Family involvement and perception of client's symptoms
14. Physical problems: respiratory, skin, cardiac, nutrition, rest, activity
15. Current medications, including over-the-counter drugs
16. Alcohol and other drug history use

ANALYSIS/NURSING DIAGNOSES
1. Safe, effective care environment
   a. High risk for injury
   b. Sensory-perceptual alteration (specify)
   c. Knowledge deficit
2. Physical integrity
   a. Activity intolerance
   b. Sleep pattern disturbance
   c. Altered nutrition: less than body requirements
   d. Sensory or perceptual alterations
   e. Altered thought processes
3. Psychosocial integrity
   a. Altered role performance
   b. Social isolation
   c. Personal identity disturbance
   d. Anxiety
4. Health promotion/maintenance
   a. Self-care deficit
   b. Ineffective family coping
   c. Impaired adjustment

PLANNING, IMPLEMENTATION, AND EVALUATION

Goal 1: Client will maintain or improve self-care activities to maintain optimal physiologic functioning.

Implementation
1. Arrange for client to have needed eyeglasses, hearing aid, dentures, and other assistive devices for ADL.

2. Plan ADL schedule based on client's established patterns; allow client to make schedule and activities decisions as appropriate.
3. Give client specific, simple directions for ADL. Provide assistance only if client cannot function alone; allow sufficient time for activities, and give advance notice.
4. Provide ROM exercises at least once daily; assist with ambulation as necessary.
5. Schedule rest periods during the day as needed.
6. Follow client's established bedtime routine; avoid use of sedatives or caffeine products, which may *increase cognitive disturbances.*
7. Offer and encourage nutritionally balanced foods and fluids.
8. Keep skin clean, dry, and free from surface irritants or pressure that impedes circulation.
9. Assist client in maintaining neat, appropriate, attractive appearance.
10. Supervise medication consumption (kind, time, and amount); know side effects of drugs given, and carefully observe and record client responses to all medications and treatments.
11. Record vital signs and fluid intake and output (I&O) daily.

Evaluation
Client performs ADL; attains and maintains ambulation; sleeps sufficient hours to obtain optimal rest; maintains adequate nutritional intake; maintains skin integrity; receives assistance only as required.

Goal 2: Client with dementia will regain an optimal level of contact with reality.

Implementation
1. Establish routine; avoid changes in routine or environment (e.g., assign same staff when possible).
2. Encourage *reminiscence, validation therapy,* and *life review* of positive life experiences to foster positive regard, self-esteem, and integrity. These interventions enable the disoriented client to relive past experiences through memories whether they are correct or not. Restoration of feeling of self-worth, reduction of stress, and reduction of sadness can be attained using these strategies. Because the client with dementia (particularly Alzheimer's disease) can no longer learn new information, traditional methods of reorientation often serve as a reminder of the client's losses and increase agitation and risk of aggression.
3. Enhance orientation by providing family pictures, bold-faced clocks and calendars, signs, and written reminders.
4. Put client's picture and name (big letters) on room door and the bed.
5. Use concrete symbols, such as photographs of client's past, to strengthen sense of continuity.
6. Answer questions as often as needed, using short, simple sentences; demonstrate acceptance nonverbally to reinforce verbal communications; build on the reality-based statements of the client to strengthen con-

versation; talk about familiar subjects; establish eye contact; and face directly when addressing the client.

7. Discover ways to help the client make choices and participate in daily activities and care as often as possible.

8. Provide adequate sensory stimulation, avoiding both sensory deprivation and overload. Structured daily group activities that include music, some form of exercise, or range of motion can help clients maintain adequate sensory stimulation.

9. Use touch: back rub, skin care; hold hands if nurse and client are comfortable doing so.

10. Respect client's privacy, space, time, and possessions.

11. Avoid physical restraints or environmental confinement, which increase helplessness and agitation; assign staff to wandering clients for short times.

12. Administer short-acting anxiolytics (lorazepam) and low-dose neuroleptics (haloperidol) to manage severe agitation and sensory-perceptual disturbances. NOTE: Chronic use of long-acting sedatives and hypnotics may cause toxic or cumulative effects. Major manifestations include delirium, sleep-wake cycle disturbances, daytime drowsiness, further cognitive impairment, loss of equilibrium, and increased risk of falls and fractures.

13. Assess for elder abuse, particularly in the client with numerous dependency needs and self-care deficits.

14. Assess reactions of family and friends to caregiving and its impact on family function. Educate and relate to the family and friends so that they will not withdraw from the client.

   a. Discuss client's behavior and management strategies, memory loss, and confusion; recognize and help them work through their own feelings of helplessness, anger, depression, love, guilt, and grief. Discuss importance of continued interaction for client and significant others.

   b. Help family prepare for client's continuing care by raising questions, exploring alternatives, and deciding on a goal and plan of action that meets their needs as well as the client's.

   c. Refer to an Alzheimer's caregiver's support group.

   d. Provide an environment that facilitates grief work.

   e. Discuss and arrange for respite care.

   f. Assess for signs of depression and make appropriate referrals.

Evaluation

Client has limited orientation to person, time, and place; reminiscences about past successes, interacts with others appropriately; family and friends maintain interaction with client; client and family make reasonable plans for client's continuing care.

Goal 3: Client with delirium will regain and maintain contact with reality.

Implementation

1. Participate in evaluation process to determine underlying medical condition.

2. Approach in a calm and reassuring manner.

3. Keep explanations direct and simple.

4. Arrange for the client not to be left alone; solicit help from family and friends.

5. Continually assess mental and physical status.

6. Orient as needed.

7. Anticipate anxiety and intervene appropriately.

8. Administer short-acting anxiolytics and low-dose neuroleptics to manage severe agitation and sensory-perceptual disturbances sparingly.

Evaluation

Client is oriented to person, place, time; interacts with family and staff appropriately; and maintains contact with reality.

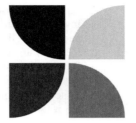

Elated-Depressive Behavior

1. *Affect* is the mood or emotion an individual shows in response to a given situation.
2. Affective disorders comprise a variety of states and syndromes; they include extremes in mood and affect, such as depressive or manic behavior and unresolved grief.
3. Affective states may be viewed as mood states or as full clinical syndromes; for example, the mood state of depression may occur in a normal person who feels sad, in a client with a major depression, or in a client with a medical condition who at intervals may be sad, irritable, anxious, or angry.
4. Biologic research related to affective disorders is rapidly growing and focuses on the role of neurochemical and other neurobiologic processes. There are several hypotheses related to findings that show impairment in the function of biogenic amines, particularly the monoamine neurotransmitters norepinephrine and serotonin. Contemporary research findings show a depletion of these two neurotransmitters in depressed individuals. Other researchers link depression with abnormal cortisol secretion.

    Research also supports the notion that bipolar disorder has a biologic component. Major premises focus on a genetic predisposition and neurochemical causes. Numerous adoption, twin, and family studies support the genetic predisposition of bipolar disorder. A number of studies also show serotonin and norepinephrine disturbances in individuals with bipolar disorders.

    A discussion of biologic component does not negate the psychosocial components of affective disorders. In fact, it supports the premise that these disorders are complex with numerous causes. Stress, loss, pregnancy, abuse of alcohol and other drugs, side effects from prescribed medications, and general medical conditions often play a predominant role in major depressive disorders. Overall, there is less emphasis on the psychodynamic causes of depression and more on biologic and psychosocial influences, which can be affected by stress and loss.
5. Management modalities (treatments) depend on the severity of the symptoms and motivation for change and include psychotherapy, chemotherapy, electroconvulsive therapy (ECT), and milieu therapy in a hospital or ambulatory setting and home health.
    a. Chemotherapy consists of antidepressant drugs (see Table 2-10 and journal reprints at end of chapter).
    b. Psychotherapy focuses on developing insight into the underlying depression and teaching clients about the neurobiologic as well as psychosocial factors involved in depression, thus helping the client and significant other learn how to monitor and manage depressive symptoms.
    c. Therapeutic milieu offers the client safe emotional and physical environments by protecting the client from self-injury, monitoring desired and adverse responses to treatment, and providing problem-solving opportunities in a supportive environment.
    d. Electroconvulsive therapy is a useful and therapeutic biologic alternative in the treatment of depression. The exact therapeutic nature of ECT remains a mystery, but researchers surmise that depressive symptoms are relieved by induced seizures generated by an electrical stimulus that increases the number of neurotransmitters at synaptic sites.
        1. considered effective for
            a. major depressive disorder with psychotic features or severely depressed or suicidal clients who do not respond to antidepressants or psychotherapy
            b. bipolar disorder (acute manic episode)
            c. subgroup of schizophrenia (when illness has short duration and demonstrates concurrent affective symptoms)
            d. positive response to ECT in the past
            e. medical conditions that contraindicate other treatment (e.g., cardiac, pregnancy)
        2. unlikely to be effective for
            a. dysthymic disorder
            b. adjustment disorder with depressed mood
            c. some forms of chronic schizophrenia
        3. electric shock is delivered to brain through unilateral or bilateral electrode placement while the client is under anesthesia
            a. produces immediate unconsciousness
            b. produces a seizure
            c. effective in remission of symptoms
        4. usually given every other day, 3 times a week for a total of up to 20 in a series
        5. Major side effects: transient confusion, amnesia

Allaying client's and family members' fears and misconceptions regarding ECT is a critical intervention for nurses to address when caring for individuals undergoing this procedure. Historically, ECT was primitive, resulting in violent seizures, fractures, and intense fear. Many people con-

Table 2-10 Medications used to treat affective disorders

Name	Usual daily dose (mg)	Action	Side effects	Nursing implications
TRICYCLIC ANTIDEPRESSANTS				
Amitriptyline (Elavil)	100-300	Blocks reuptake of neuro-transmitters at neuronal membrane; effects of norepinephrine and serotonin may be potentiated, resulting in antidepressant effect; strong anticholinergic activity	Dizziness, nausea, excitement, blurred vision, constipation, dry mouth, anorexia, insomnia, drowsiness, excessive perspiration, gynecomastia, skin rash, hypotension	Assess suicide potential Observe side effects and treat symptomatically Do not give with or immediately after treatment with MAO inhibitors Monitor blood pressure Teach client: Avoid alcohol Check with MD before taking over-the-counter medications Ways to avoid problems with orthostatic hypotension Importance of oral hygiene Take with meals to avoid gastric irritation
Amoxapine (Asendin)	150-450			
Imipramine (Tofranil)	100-300			
Doxepin (Sinequan)	100-300			
Combination-clordiaze-poxide/amitriptyline (Limbitrol)	100-300			
Desipramine (Norpramin)	100-300			
Maprotiline (Ludiomil)	100-200			
Nortriptyline (Pamelor)	50-150			
Protriptyline (Vivactil)	15-60			
Trimipramine (Surmontil)	100-300			
TETRACYCLIC ANTIDEPRESSANTS				
Maprotiline hydrochloride (Ludiomil)	75-150	Similar to the tricyclics but do not appear to influence reuptake of serotonin	Same as tricyclics	Institute seizure precautions
Zimelidine (Zelmid)	100-300			
SELECTIVE SEROTONIN REUPTAKE INHIBITORS (SSRIs)				
Fluoxetine hydrochloride (Prozac)	40-80	Inhibition of CNS neuronal uptake of serotonin	Rash, anxiety, nervousness, insomnia, drowsiness, fatigue or asthenia, tremor, sweating, anorexia, nausea, diarrhea, weight loss, headache, dizziness, lightheadedness; may activate mania	Assess suicide potential Observe for mania, side effects. Teach client: Avoid alcohol Avoid driving car or operating heavy machinery until response is determined Check with MD before taking other prescribed medications or over-the-counter medications Notify MD if client becomes pregnant
Paroxetine HCl (Paxil)	20	Blocks reuptake of serotonin at the presynaptic neuronal membrane	Rash, anxiety, nervousness, insomnia, drowsiness, fatigue or asthenia, tremor, sweating, anorexia, nausea, diarrhea, weight loss, headache, dizziness, lightheadedness; may activate mania	Sexual dysfunction (e.g., abnormal ejaculation and orgasm) and sustained increase in BP possible (monitor BP). If a client is taking or has recently taken MAO inhibitors, SSRIs should not be administered for at least 2 weeks after discontinuation because of severe, potentially fatal drug interactions

Continued

Table 2-10 Medications used to treat affective disorders—cont'd

Name	Usual daily dose (mg)	Action	Side effects	Nursing implications
Sertraline hydrochloride (Zoloft)	50-200	Action is presumed to be linked to its inhibition of CNS neuronal uptake of serotonin	Dry mouth, headache, dizziness, nausea, diarrhea, fatigue, insomnia, sexual dysfunction	Do not give with or immediately after treatment with MAO inhibitors Assess suicide potential Teach client to avoid alcohol
Buproprion HCl (Wellbutrin)	150-450	Weakly blocks reuptake of norepinephrine and serotonin, and selectively blocks dopamine	Agitation, dry mouth, insomnia, tremors, headaches, GI disturbances, akathisia, ataxia, seizures	Take precautions against seizures
ATYPICAL ANTIDEPRESSANTS				
Venlafaxine HCl (Effexor)	75-375 in 2-3 divided doses	Serotonin and norepinephrine reuptake inhibitor	Sleep disturbances, sexual dysfunction, dry mouth, nausea, dizziness, constipation, nervousness, sweating, anorexia, possible BP increase	Instruct to take with food Check vital signs; should not be taken in combination with MAO inhibitors or within 14 days of discontinuing treatment because of serious adverse reactions.
MONOAMINE OXIDASE (MAO) INHIBITORS				
Trazodone (Desyrel)	150-300	Multiple effects on serotonin transmission	Dizziness, fainting, cardiac irritability, conduction defects, headache, nausea, priapism	Teach client: Take with food Avoid alcohol, CNS depressants Notify nurse if sexual dysfunction occurs Do not drive
Phenelzine (Nardil) Tranylcypromine (Parnate) Isocarboxazid (Marplan)	15-90 10-30 10-30	Inhibition of monoamine oxidase enzyme (mainly in nerve tissue, liver, and lungs) increases concentration of amines (epinephrine, norepinephrine, dopamine, serotonin), causing an antidepressant effect	Headache, dizziness, dry mouth, blurred vision, postural hypotension, increased appetite, dermatitis, hepatitis, euphoria, activates latent schizophrenia	Potentiates action of narcotics, barbiturates, sedatives, atropine derivatives Avoid tyramine (e.g., aged cheese) and alcohol (may cause severe headaches, hypertension) Teach client food restrictions
LITHIUM				
Lithium carbonate (Eskalith, Lithane)	Dosage determined by blood level and by behavior (typically 900-1800 mg in divided daily doses) Blood level: 0.8-1.5 mEq/L Maintenance level: 0.5-1.2 mEq/L (300 mg/day tid) Toxic level: 2.0 mEq/L or above Acute mania: 1-1.4 mEq/L (20-30 mg/kg/day in 2-3 doses)	Monovalent action that competes with potassium, sodium, calcium, and magnesium at cellular sites; interferes with reuptake of central monoamine neurotransmitters	GI discomfort (nausea, vomiting, stomach, pain, diarrhea), thirst, dazed feeling, drowsiness, hand tremor, tinnitus, blurred vision	Remind client to take medications Assess drug level every 3-4 days Assess suicide potential Monitor salt and fluid intake Teach client importance of administration and blood work schedule to control salt and fluid intake avoid caffeine take with meals Wait 5-14 days for clinical effect

Table 2-10 Medications used to treat affective disorders—cont'd

Name	Usual daily dose (mg)	Action	Side effects	Nursing implications
LITHIUM				
Lithium carbonate (Eskalith, Lithane)	Dosage determined by blood level and by behavior (typically 900-1800 mg in divided daily doses) Blood level: 0.8-1.5 mEq/L Maintenance level: 0.5-1.2 mEq/L (300 mg/day tid) Toxic level: 2.0 mEq/L or above Acute mania: 1-1.4 mEq/L (20-30 mg/kg/day in 2-3 doses)	Monovalent action that competes with potassium, sodium, calcium, and magnesium at cellular sites; interferes with reuptake of central monoamine neurotransmitters	GI discomfort (nausea, vomiting, stomach, pain, diarrhea), thirst, dazed feeling, drowsiness, hand tremor, tinnitus, blurred vision	Remind client to take medications Assess drug level every 3-4 days Assess suicide potential Monitor salt and fluid intake Teach client importance of administration and blood work schedule to control salt and fluid intake avoid caffeine take with meals Wait 5-14 days for clinical effect
OTHERS				
Carbamazepine (Tegretol)	Initial: 200 mg bid Maximum: Adults 1.2 g/day; children 1000 mg/day	Antikindling action resulting in mood stabilization	Drowsiness, dizziness, unsteadiness, nausea, vomiting, dyspnea, rashes, blood dyscrasias	Teach client not to drive until response has been determined avoid alcohol and nonprescription drugs report sore throat, fever, easy bruising, decreased urine output do not stop drug abruptly
Valproic acid (Depakene, Depakote)	15 mg/kg/day to 60 mg/kg/day	Antikindling action resulting in mood stabilization	Drowsiness, nausea, vomiting, indigestion, blood dyscrasias	As above. Both of these drugs are potentially neurotoxic—baseline physical examinations must be done before either of these drugs (or lithium) is begun. NOTE: During the acute stages of bipolar manic episodes, low-dose neuroleptics and anxiolytics are administered to manage symptoms. Antimanic agents are gradually introduced until a therapeutic level or positive client response is achieved.

tinue to harbor this belief. Addressing these myths and fears will reduce anxiety so that clients and families can make a truly informed decision regarding this treatment. NOTE: Other changes regarding ECT include socioeconomic status. For instance, in the 1950s individuals of lower socioeconomic status were more likely to be recipients of ECT. In contrast, recent studies show that people from middle and upper socioeconomic groups are more likely to receive ECT. Moreover, ECT is more likely to take place in private hospitals than in public facilities.

Application of the Nursing Process to the Client with an Affective (Mood) Disorder

ASSESSMENT

1. Affect
   a. Powerlessness, worthlessness
   b. Helplessness
   c. Fear and crying
   d. Anger, hostility (directed inward in depression, outward in elation)
   e. Elation in mania
   f. Sadness in depression
   g. Anxiety
   h. Depression related to guilt and repressed hostility; leads to self-condemnation and punishment
2. Cognition
   a. Limited perception, interests, judgment, and decision-making skills
   b. Impaired concentration and transient memory difficulties
   c. Delusional thinking (e.g., grandiose and persecutory in mania)
   d. Talkative, flight of ideas in elated stage
   e. Distorted cognitions, negative self-talk, overgeneralization in depression
3. Behavior
   a. Decreased (psychomotor retardation) or increased motor activity (agitation or hyperactivity in mania)
   b. Decreased or increased communication
   c. Changes in social interactions: withdrawn in depression and intrusiveness in mania
   d. Self-care deficits
   e. Self-destructiveness (e.g., suicide attempt, substance misuse)
4. Physical: normal patterns and significant changes over the past 6 to 12 months
   a. Appetite and eating patterns
   b. Sleeping patterns
   c. Interest in sex
   d. Weakness, fatigue or increased energy in mania
   e. Constipation/diarrhea
5. Strengths and capabilities
   a. Usual coping strategies
   b. Family and peer relationships
   c. Hobbies and pastimes (often limited in depression)

ANALYSIS/NURSING DIAGNOSES

1. Safe, effective care environment
   a. Impaired home maintenance management
   b. High risk for violence: self-directed
   c. Knowledge deficit
2. Physical integrity
   a. Altered bowel elimination
   b. Altered nutrition: less/more than body requirements
   c. Sleep pattern disturbances
   d. Sexual dysfunction
   e. Fatigue or restlessness
   f. Altered thought processes
3. Psychosocial integrity
   a. Hopelessness
   b. Chronic/situational low self-esteem
   c. Social isolation or intrusiveness in mania
   d. Depression or anxiety

4. Health promotion/maintenance
   a. Impaired adjustment
   b. Altered family processes
   c. Altered health maintenance
   d. Self-care deficit (specify)

GENERAL NURSING PLANNING, IMPLEMENTATION, AND EVALUATION

> **Goal 1:** The depressed client will demonstrate increased ability to cope with feelings by sharing feelings with others.

Implementation

1. Spend time with client at least twice daily; start with 5 to 10 minutes, and increase time as nurse and client can tolerate it; encourage client to identify and verbalize feelings, accept what is said; use silence when appropriate—the presence of a caring person is helpful when learning to cope with painful feelings; *avoid false reassurance, overcheerfulness;* do not attempt to minimize or negate client's feelings.
2. Encourage depressed client to examine distorted cognitions ("I'm a failure because I was laid off"), negative self-talk, overgeneralization, and role in forming and maintaining depressive symptoms.
3. Focus on client's feelings; allow ventilation in ways that are acceptable to the client; help client work through feelings by maintaining a safe, trusting, and accepting attitude.
4. Help client explore meaning of loss, physical symptoms, and significance of feeling. The client may say, "It just isn't worth it anymore." Proper responses might include, "You've had a difficult time lately, and you're learning to deal with your feelings," "You've lost someone you loved, and you're going through grief and mourning," or "Sounds like you remember the positive and negative aspects of this relationship, and you're beginning to be ready to trust again."

Evaluation

Client discusses feelings of sadness and need to cry with nurse and others.

> **Goal 2:** The client will learn techniques that effectively lessen depressive symptoms and the risk of suicide.

Implementation

1. Teach the client major signs and symptoms, causes (e.g., biologic and psychosocial factors), and treatment of depression. This should involve teaching about the role of antidepressants in symptom management.
2. Explore sources of frustration and powerlessness and teach stress-reducing interventions.
3. Apprise client when distorted negative thinking is observed and assist client in assessing reality by challenging negative self-talk, overgeneralizations, and "all-or-none" thinking. Avoid judgmental or patronizing statements.
4. Prevent self-destructive behaviors by removing items

such as sharp objects, matches, glass containers, and cigarettes. When client is in a home health setting, teach family to remove or restrict availability of weapons, alcohol and other drugs, and car keys and report symptoms that need to be evaluated by telephone, office visit, or emergency department (e.g., worsening depression or increased lethality).

5. Encourage client and family to be active participants in treatment.
6. Help client explore ways to cope with feelings through various means such as physical activities, stress management, positive self-talk, journaling, and seeking staff or family rather than socially isolating self.

Evaluation
The client's symptoms decrease, and he or she does not act on suicidal ideations; develops effective coping techniques.

Goal 3: Client will learn how to access available social support and to adapt to environmental demands.

Implementation
1. Client's knowledge of community resources is determined and appropriate referrals are made.
2. Acknowledge client's feelings and thoughts regarding self and others.
3. Help client to express guilt: explore situation and persons with whom the client experiences guilt ("I feel guilty when I . . ."); explore feelings about this. Most situations that involve guilt also involve feelings of anger and resentment; work on these feelings with client. Have client replace the word "guilt" with "resent."
4. Provide positive reinforcement to reality-based behavior and realistic expectations.
5. When appropriate stress the significance of taking antidepressants.
6. Teach strategies that promote sleep, rest, and adequate nutrition.
7. Teach the HALT rule—never get too *H*ungry, *A*ngry, *L*onely, or *T*ired.

Evaluation
Client seeks out support group and complies with medication regimen.

Goal 4: Client will recognize individual signs of relapse and identify actions to obtain assistance from health care providers in managing more severe symptoms.

Implementation
1. Teach symptoms of relapse (e.g., increased isolation, sleep and appetite disturbances, decreased sex drive, increased crying spells, preoccupation with or recurrent substance abuse/dependence).
2. Present client's case during treatment team update and determine needed resources (inpatient and outpatient settings); if in home health care setting, mobilize resources that include family members, support group, sponsor if

client is in a 12-step recovery program, psychotherapist, physician, visiting nurse, and so on.
3. Encourage client to take prescribed medications. If questions or concerns arise contact the nurse case manager.

Evaluation
Client discusses warning signs of relapse and restates available resources.

SELECTED HEALTH PROBLEMS

✳ DEPRESSION

1. Definitions
   a. *Depression* is a multifaceted mood disorder characterized by feelings of dejection, sadness, and hopelessness. Major causes include alterations in neurochemical processes, genetic predisposition, and psychosocial factors.
   b. Psychoanalytic explanation of depression: gratification is received from a love object or representation of environmental relationship that serves as a basis of approval or esteem and basis of success; loss of love object leads to frustration, anxiety, grief, guilt, and hostility. This may result in loss of self-esteem and depression, especially in persons who have a biologic predisposition for decreased levels of serotonin, norepinephrine, and other neurotransmitters associated with depression.
   c. Cognitive theory of depression: activation of three primary cognitive themes that contribute to perception of self and the world. The first consists of prevailing negative feelings toward self; the second is a prominent negative interpretation of personal experiences; and the third is a dismal picture of the future. The first component exists in the majority of persons experiencing depression. Other cognitive themes include feelings of helplessness, hopelessness, and indecisiveness.
2. Precipitating factors
   a. Loss of a loved one through separation or death is the most common precipitant; the loss must be significant to the person.
   b. Threats to self-esteem: disruption in the interpersonal and intrapersonal input of love, respect, and approval results in decreased self-esteem.
   c. Success: paradoxically, one may become depressed on achieving success; this is due to the anticipation of loss of self-esteem if one does not live up to the expectations implied by the success.
   d. Physical illness: depression is often interrelated with many physical illnesses because of real or anticipated loss of function, independence, role of well person (e.g., childbirth); electrolyte disorders; endocrine disorders; stroke; Alzheimer's; multiple sclerosis; and certain medications, such as beta blockers, antihypertensive agents, histamine 2 (H_2) inhibitors, and nonsteroidal antiinflammatory drugs (NSAIDs).
   e. Alterations in self-image: changes in self-image arising from physical, emotional, or lifestyle changes, in-

cluding role changes, body changes, negative self-talk, overgeneralization, all-or-none cognitive distortions.
f. Alterations in neurobiologic processes, particularly neurotransmitter systems (e.g., serotonin, norepinephrine, monoamine oxidase, dopamine).
g. Twin, family, and adoption studies suggest a genetic predisposition and familial history of depression or other mood disorders.
3. States of depression: depression may be felt to some degree by anyone at some point in life; in terms of severity of disruption, there are seven kinds of depression
   a. *Transitory depression*
      1. seldom seen as presenting problem
      2. may be related to psychosocial or physiologic stress
      3. symptoms
         a. affect: quiet, sad, unhappy, helpless, or hopeless
         b. cognition: difficulty making decisions, self-deprecation, feelings of inadequacy, focus on personal problems
         c. behavior: decreased activity, restrained, inhibited, social isolation
         d. physical changes: mild physical discomforts, fatigue, sleep and appetite disturbances
      4. short-lived; person easily resolves
   b. *Grieving*
      1. DSM-IV classification: bereavement
      2. related to precipitating environmental or physiologic stress or personal loss (e.g., death of someone close)
      3. responses follow stages of grief and mourning process (refer to Loss and Death and Dying, p. 29).
      4. symptoms
         a. affect: withdrawn, apathetic, angry, sad, depressed
         b. cognition: personal derogation, suicidal thoughts, preoccupation with loss or stress, self-absorption
         c. behavior: serious impairment of activity, domestic disturbances, social isolation, apathy
         d. physical changes: mild changes, weight loss or gain of less than 10 pounds, feels worse as day progresses, fatigue
      5. complete resolution may take up to 2 years or longer depending on significance of loss, quality of support systems and coping skills, number of losses, and resolution of past grief; grief is normal reactive depression
   c. *Dysthymia*
      1. DSM-IV classification: dysthymic disorder
      2. symptoms usually occur, as indicated by expressed description or observation by family members and others, for at least 2 years in adults and 1 year in children and adolescents
         a. affect: powerlessness, helplessness, anxiety, hostility, anger, fear, crying, hopelessness
         b. cognition: cognitive triad present—negative self-concept, negative view of world, negative expectations of the future; indecisive, self-

blame, impaired concentration and memory, low self-esteem, suicidal ideation
         c. behavior: psychomotor retardation, decreased grooming and self-care, prevailing recurrence of a life experience or regret, decreased social interaction but maintains ability to work, self-criticism
         d. physical changes: weakness, fatigue, somatic preoccupation, poor appetite or overeating, sleep disturbances, decreased sexual interest
         e. a more chronic, less severe form of depression
      3. cognitive changes may be long-standing based on inability to form meaningful relationships and lack of supportive experiences
      4. symptoms of chronic depression emerge in childhood, adolescence, or early adulthood
      5. symptoms are not due to a depressive episode, general medical condition, or psychotic or substance-related disorder
   d. *Major depression*
      1. DSM-IV classification: major depressive disorder
         a. major depressive episode with specifiers
            ▪ psychotic features including severe impairment of reality testing and physiologic disturbances or without psychotic features
            ▪ chronic
            ▪ with catatonic features
            ▪ with melancholic features
            ▪ with atypical features
            ▪ with postpartum onset
      2. depression brought on by severe environmental threats to security; high risk for suicide; may have biochemical/genetic causes; may be associated with chronic general medical condition (diabetes, stroke, myocardial infarction, carcinoma)
      3. symptoms
         a. affect: despondent, little feeling tone, helplessness, worthlessness, emptiness
         b. cognition: delusional thinking in severe depression, cognitive triad present and marked; memory disturbances, thought pattern more lethargic in morning, lifts as day progresses
         c. behavior: greatly depressed or agitated depending on type
            ▪ *agitated depression:* anxious, tense, extreme restlessness; pacing, hand wringing, skin picking, poor eating and sleeping
            ▪ *retarded depression:* general physical and cognitive slowness, inactive, hanging head, looking haggard; indecisive and uncooperative
         d. physical
            ▪ neurovegetative signs: anorexia, weight loss of more than 10 pounds, constipation, decreased libido and concentration, insomnia, amenorrhea/impotence
   e. *Bipolar disorder*
      1. DSM-IV classification: bipolar I disorder, bipolar II disorder (see description of types I and II on p. 56)
         a. episodes of well-defined, self-limiting mania or depression, usually in repeating cycles, with or

without an interval of normalcy; strong evidence of biochemical/genetic predisposition
- person usually recovers completely from both phases, but there is a tendency for recurrence
- may experience only the depressive phase, only the manic phase, or both at different times in life

b. physical changes are the same as for major depression
- insomnia, early-morning awakening
- lack of self-care

f. *Seasonal affective disorder*
1. DSM IV: specifier and refers to the pattern of recurrent major depressive episodes, or bipolar I or II disorder with seasonal pattern
   a. cyclical major depressive disorder that is affected by changes in day length occurring in the fall and winter months (symptoms abate during spring and summer months)
   b. symptoms (appear as the days shorten during winter months)
   - sadness, irritability, and anxiety during depressed periods
   - overeating
   - carbohydrate craving, weight gain
   - sleep duration increases
   - quality of sleep decreases
   - drowsiness during daytime, fatigue
   - difficulties at work, in interpersonal relationships
   c. symptoms may be mediated by the secretion of melatonin, a hormone secreted by the pineal gland that is thought to mediate seasonal behavior and to be affected by day-night rhythms
   d. treatment: studies have shown good results with 20 to 30 minutes of bright light application in the morning or evening hours every day (reverses the depressive changes by extending the photoperiod by 4 to 6 hours); clients respond to treatment after 2 to 4 days

g. *Mood disorder caused by a general medical condition*
1. a persistent mood alteration (either depressed or elated)
2. physical findings suggest that symptoms arise directly from an underlying medical condition (e.g., hypothyroidism, hyperglycemia, certain medications)

Nursing Process

ASSESSMENT

1. Signs and symptoms (refer to States of Depression, p. 52)
   a. Affect
   b. Degree of cognitive change: cognitive triad (negative view of self, world, and the future); unlike other symptoms, the more severe the cognitive triad, the more debilitating the depression
   c. Behavior
   d. Physical changes

2. Severity and level of depression (refer to States of Depression, p. 52)
3. Priorities for care
   a. Safety
   b. Physical needs
   c. Self-esteem
4. Suicide potential
   a. Suicidal risk: persons at high risk for suicide include
      1. adolescents and white males 50 years old and older
      2. single males
      3. persons with psychiatric disorders
      4. young African-American males
      5. persons misusing alcohol and other drugs (refer to journal reprint)
      6. persons with inadequate support systems or distant family ties
      7. police, physicians, dentists
      8. persons experiencing depression
      9. persons hallucinating and responding to voice commands
      10. those with a history of family suicide
      11. persons experiencing a maturational or situational crisis or a chronic or painful illness
      12. previous attempters
      13. persons expressing or experiencing a sense of hopelessness
      14. those with histories of violent or aggressive behavior
      15. persons who are cognitively impaired
      16. those with poor impulse control (e.g., personality disorders, psychosis)
   b. Suicidal plan
      1. method—assess degree of lethality (margin of error)
      2. availability (the more available, the higher the risk)
      3. specificity of plan
   c. Change in behavior (e.g., calmness: may mean person has worked out a plan and no longer feels ambivalent); as depression lifts, client may have energy to carry out plan
   d. Giving away valued possessions: saying goodbye, making amends, asking medical questions
   e. Ambivalent feelings
      1. coexistence of opposing emotions in client (e.g., wants to live/die, experiences love and hate toward deceased or absent person)
      2. inability to express anger and hostility effectively, turns hate and aggression inward, leading to self-destructive thoughts or actions
      3. feelings of ambivalence are common in severely depressed clients, particularly when the depression is related to the loss of a significant other
   f. Significant changes in activities of daily living
      1. sleep patterns
      2. work habits
      3. eating patterns
      4. social interactions
      5. memory or thought process disturbances
      6. impaired decision making and judgement

ANALYSIS/NURSING DIAGNOSES (see p. 50)
PLANNING, IMPLEMENTATION, AND EVALUATION

> **Goal 1:** Client will be able to express self-destructive thoughts rather than act on them.

Implementation

1. Assume responsibility for safety of client; inspect unit for dangerous items such as sharp instruments (e.g., scissors, nail files, glass or metal containers, razor blades), pills; remove from client area. If client is at home, relatives must remove or restrict weapons, drugs, alcohol, and car keys. Provide a 24-hour crisis hotline telephone number; establish a contract for no harm of self and others and identify or designate someone with whom the client feels safe. Refer to appropriate treatment center for depression.
2. Restrict client to observable areas; continuously observe client for suicidal ideations/gestures.
3. Use open questioning about suicidal ideations, plans, and ideas.
4. Set limits on repetition of story of suicidal feelings or gesture.
5. Establish nurse-client relationship that displays the nurse as respectful, competent, knowledgeable, able to assist in problem solving; nurse's attitude should reflect genuine interest and concern, firmness, and confidence.
6. Devise a verbal agreement that the client will not harm self or others and if suicidal thoughts arise that this information will be shared with the nurse or other designated person.
7. Allow client to express feelings.
8. Involve client in challenging activities that ensure success (e.g., attaining small goals in ADL, exercise).
9. Provide realistic reassurance; convey attitude that client will succeed.
10. Assess client's abilities realistically and provide only the help needed; irrational demands should be discussed openly and refused.
11. Stress client's capabilities and strengths.
12. Work with client to prepare list of problems and corresponding solutions; use all resources available, including family and community resources; give client the sense that problems are manageable.
13. Know that suicidal client behavior may generate anger, guilt, or rescue fantasies in the nurse; staff should meet daily for mutual support, planning, and reality testing.
14. Do not withdraw when ambivalence is directed toward nursing staff; continue to listen attentively and maintain socialization.
15. Use emergency methods to counteract suicidal attempts (e.g., lavage, one-to-one observation).
16. If suicide attempt occurs, help client and family to share and work through feelings and concerns.
17. Explore client and family's feelings regarding the unsuccessful attempt. ("That was stupid of me and I am sorry." Or: "I really messed up this time, but next time I will take more pills.")
18. Acknowledge the coexistence of opposing (ambivalent) emotions in the client and family.
19. Communicate and document the presence or absence of suicidal ideations/gestures to members of the health care team, including family members.
20. Observe for change in mood (decreased depression along with increased energy may signal enough energy to act on suicidal ideations and decreased ambivalence).
21. Refer to appropriate treatment for depression.

Evaluation
Client makes no gestures of physical harm; gives all potentially dangerous materials to staff; lists problems, solutions, resources.

> **Goal 2:** Client will meet physical care needs independently.

Implementation
Food and fluid intake:
1. Find acceptable eating pattern based on client's likes, dislikes, and usual eating habits. If client has poor appetite, provide frequent, small meals and snacks of easy foods to eat (leave oatmeal cookies, crackers and cheese, 7-Up, etc. at bedside for small snacks at night or during day). Monitor the food and fluid intake.
2. Weigh weekly (depending on patterns of coping with depression, significant change in weight, either gained or lost, must be assessed).
Sleep/rest:
3. Help client reestablish normal sleeping patterns. If client sleeps continuously during the day and does not rest at night, work with client to maintain schedule of activity and rest during daytime. Recognize that insomnia increases fatigue, and fatigue increases depression. Sedatives are generally ineffective; therefore use other nursing measures (e.g., warm milk, snacks [such as a turkey sandwich], soft music, back rub, warm bath). Discourage use of stimulants before bedtime (e.g., colas, coffee, tea, chocolates, strenuous exercise).
Elimination:
4. Maintain adequate fluid intake.
5. Provide adequate fiber in diet.
6. Monitor elimination.
Grooming and hygiene:
7. Help client reestablish activities of daily living, such as bathing and care of hair, skin, nails, and clothes. If client is unable to initiate self-care, approach in matter-of-fact manner (e.g., "It's time to bathe, Mr. Ekpe"). Convey expectation that client can perform self-care. Give positive reinforcement for any self-care.
Activity:
8. Consider personal preferences and needs; help client do things for self (many depressed clients become dependent on others, but activity usually helps them to feel better).
9. Assign daily responsibility for unit-maintenance to help renew sense of self-worth and purposefulness. Simple tasks (straightening chairs, putting away cards, games, or crafts equipment) with supervision may be appropriate for deeply depressed clients; more diffi-

cult tasks can be gradually introduced paralleling activity tolerance. Assignments should strengthen self-integrity and confidence.

10. Assess previous hobbies and pastimes. Assist with simple crafts that can be finished in one sitting to increase sense of accomplishment; encourage participation in group activities such as singing, poetry reading, painting, or working with clay to help client become more comfortable in groups and to establish community and group socialization. Initially the client may need the nurse's presence to tolerate group activities. Simple exercises and walks may progress to group sports; avoid competitive activities.

11. Plan activity schedule based on client's morning and evening mood variation (i.e., time of day client is most energetic).

Medications:

12. Discuss rationale for medication as client can tolerate and assimilate teaching.

13. Teach desired and side effects, administration, and related drug interactions (see Table 2-10).

14. Discuss causes, major symptoms, and treatment of specific mood disorders.

Evaluation

Client consumes adequate food and fluids; establishes normal sleep and activity patterns; has adequate elimination; dresses and grooms self daily; participates in activities.

Goal 3: Client receiving ECT remains free from preventable injury.

Implementation

1. Participate in informed consent process by explaining procedure thoroughly, and answer client and family questions and concerns.

2. Assess teaching needs and educate the client about ECT. Also provide ample time to identify and dispel myths and allay fears regarding specific treatment.

3. Ensure that consent form is in chart.

4. Arrange for spine x-ray, if required.

5. Gather baseline vital signs.

6. Prepare client as if going to the operating room (OR) (i.e., nothing by mouth [NPO], void, remove dentures, avoid using hairspray).

7. Give medications as ordered: muscle relaxant to reduce tonic/clonic movements; atropine sulfate to dry secretions and prevent bradycardia and asystole; short-acting barbiturate (e.g., Brevital) for sedation.

8. Sit with client before treatment to provide support, and assign staff member to stay with client.

9. After treatment, maintain a patent airway; monitor blood pressure, pulse, respirations, level of consciousness; observe reaction on awakening.

10. Monitor vital signs every 15 minutes for the first hour and hourly for the next 4 hours.

11. Orient client to time and place and to the fact that treatment has been administered (temporary memory loss and confusion are the most distressing side effects of ECT).

12. Stay with client a minimum of 1 hour after ECT; check vital signs; monitor level of consciousness (e.g., confusion); reorient; observe closely for 6 to 8 hours after treatment.

Evaluation

Client recovers from ECT free of injury; is oriented to time, place, and person.

Goal 4: Client will increase interactions with staff, other clients, and family.

Implementation

1. Help client identify, define, and solve difficult problems in social relationships (e.g., client who is hypercritical of self and others can discuss and practice a tactful, more accepting approach).

2. Help client to look at situations in which others are pushed away out of fear of rejection (i.e., reject them before being rejected).

3. Practice social skills; use role-playing and assertiveness training.

4. Observe in group activities, choosing short, simple group activities that client identifies as least threatening (exercise, sports, music).

5. Involve client in activity that provides chance for success (e.g., simple but challenging occupational therapy activities).

6. Refer to Activity, p. 54.

Evaluation

Client spends more time with staff, other clients, and family; identifies problems in relationships; practices new social skills with staff and other clients.

Goal 5: Client will discuss feelings about self and situation. (Refer to General Nursing Goals 1, 2, and 3, p. 50-51.)

Goal 6: Client will increase independent decision making.

Implementation

1. Give positive reinforcement for decisions that are in the patient's best interests.

2. Assist with decision making when client is profoundly depressed.

3. Expect client to make own decisions, with support as depression lifts.

Evaluation

Client participates in planning own activities and schedule.

Goal 7: Family members will maintain supportive relationship with client.

Implementation

1. Provide family members with an opportunity to discuss their feelings of anger, guilt, grief, and inability to help client.

2. Help family understand client's anger, dependency, negativism.

3. Discuss ways family can respond to excessive demands and dependency.
4. Facilitate grief process in family members.
5. Review expectations and goals for family and individual family members; explore alternatives for unrealistic expectations.
6. Provide family members with information that enables them to identify situations that increase stress and incidence of relapse.
7. Educate family about major signs of relapse.

Evaluation

Family members appropriately discuss feelings, expectations, and goals with staff; interact with client by letter, phone, or visit; bring client home when appropriate and assist with recreation and socialization.

✖ MANIA

1. *Mania* is an abnormally and persistently elevated, expansive, or irritable mood that lasts at least 4 days. Additional symptoms: decreased need for sleep, pressured and tangential speech, flight of ideas, delusions (e.g., grandiose and persecutory), irritability, and distractibility. There is a great deal of evidence that this disorder is complex and arises from various neurobiologic causes, such as alterations in the neurotransmitters, and twin and adoption studies suggest a genetic link. Psychosocial theories parallel bipolar disorder with unrealistic family expectations and the need to succeed.
2. Types of mania:
   a. *Mild:* euphoric state of mind, mild exhilaration
      1. happy, unconcerned, uninhibited, expansive, "life-of-the-party" mood
      2. mood can change rapidly to irritability and anger; irritability is expression of anxiety and hostile impulses
      3. very active, but activity is sometimes inappropriate for age and place
      4. relationships are superficial
      5. DSM-IV classification: hypomanic episode
   b. *Acute:* moderate degree of mania
      1. extreme emotional lability ranging from wild euphoria to rage; readily provoked by harmless remarks, seems to forgive and forget
      2. thought disorders: flight of ideas, delusions of grandeur and persecution, short attention span, pressured, tangential, circumstantial, incoherent speech
      3. poor impulse control, poor judgment
      4. little need of sleep, fatigue, uninhibited and actively involved in pleasurable activities such as spending sprees, sexual indiscretions
      5. extremely exaggerated psychomotor activity
      6. often requires hospitalization
      7. client enjoys "high" and is often reluctant to take mood-stabilizing agents, such as antimanic agents
      8. lacks insight into illness
      9. DSM-IV classification: bipolar I disorder, most recent episode manic
   c. *Bipolar disorder with psychotic features:* maximum intensity of reaction
      1. disorganized, seriously delusional (grandiose or persecutory)
      2. disoriented, incoherent, agitated
      3. prone to self-injury, dehydration, and exhaustion
      4. immediate intervention is necessary to meet physical needs
      5. poor judgement and decision-making
      6. DSM-IV classification: bipolar II disorder, severe with psychotic features
   d. *May alternate between manic and depressive phases*
      1. usually hospitalized first for manic episode
      2. may have rapid-cycling manic and depressive phases that succeed each other without a period of remission; DSM-IV classification: bipolar II disorder
      3. may have numerous hypomanic and mild depressive episodes; DSM-IV classification: cyclothymic disorder
3. Prognosis: good, even without treatment, provided that the person does not suffer from complete physical exhaustion in manic phase or commit suicide in depressed phase

Nursing Process
ASSESSMENT
1. Physical needs
   a. Nutrition: decreased appetite or unwillingness to stop activity to eat may lead to weight loss
   b. Hydration
   c. Sleep/rest: activity pattern and insomnia may lead to exhaustion
   d. Elimination: may be incontinent; constipation
   e. May ignore injuries or symptoms of physical illness
   f. Hygiene and grooming: inappropriate dress, excessive makeup; diaphoresis
2. Affect
   a. Degree of euphoria or expansive mood
   b. Lability: rapid mood change from happy to sad without apparent provocation
   c. Anger
   d. Anxiety
   e. Irritability and low tolerance to frustration
3. Cognition
   a. Feelings of worthlessness, loneliness are masked by elation
   b. Flight of ideas
   c. Delusions of grandeur, persecution, or both
   d. Feelings of inadequacy, low self-esteem
   e. Short attention span, easily distracted
   f. Perceptual-sensory disturbances
4. Behavior
   a. Degree and appropriateness of activity
   b. Aggression, manipulation, acting out
   c. Demanding, verbally hostile
   d. Pressured, circumstantial, and tangential speech (talkative)
   e. Easily distracted by extraneous external stimuli
   f. Impulsivity

g. Extreme involvement in pleasurable activities such as exorbitant spending sprees, promiscuity, unwise business ventures
h. Superficial relationships
i. Decreased need for sleep (feels rested after several hours of sleep)
j. Profound intrusiveness

ANALYSIS/NURSING DIAGNOSES (see p. 50)
PLANNING, IMPLEMENTATION, AND EVALUATION

Goal I: Client will meet physical needs independently.

Implementation
Safety:
1. Watch for physical symptoms client may ignore.
2. Maintain safe environment.
3. Monitor dietary and fluid intake.
Food and fluid intake:
4. Nutrition: provide high-calorie finger foods that can be eaten on the run; note amount of food ingested; monitor weight.
5. Hydration: provide fluids at frequent intervals; fluid intake of 2000 ml per day if not contraindicated.
Sleep/rest:
6. Assess client's normal sleeping patterns.
7. Provide medication to promote sleep and rest; provide opportunities for frequent short naps.
8. Reduce environmental stimuli; use soft lighting, low noise level, simple room decorations; quiet or private room if necessary.
9. Restrict caffeine and fluid intake several hours before bedtime.
Elimination:
10. Assess normal elimination patterns, monitor current patterns, maintain fluid intake, establish toileting schedule when indicated.
Hygiene and grooming:
11. Assess self-care needs.
12. Provide flexible schedule for showering and changing clothing; provide loose, comfortable clothing; limit access to clothing if necessary to maintain appropriate dress or decrease frequency of changes; assist with hygiene.
Medications:
13. Administer medications and monitor desired and side effects. Initially administer short-acting anxiolytics (lorazepam) and low-dose neuroleptics (haloperidol) to reduce hallucinations, agitation, delusions and promote rest. Administer lithium and other antimanic medications as ordered (see Table 2-10); observe for side effects, toxic effects, and drug interactions. Teach client and family about lithium therapy.

Evaluation
Client receives adequate sleep and rest; consumes appropriate amounts of food and fluids; maintains hygiene and grooming; remains free from injury; returns to normal thought processes; and verbalizes knowledge of medication regimen.

Goal 2: Client will cope adaptively with hostility and aggression.

Implementation
1. Ignore or respond minimally to hostile behavior that is not destructive to avoid positive reinforcement.
2. Nurse or other staff should not react defensively to criticism or profanity.
3. Set limits on behavior: "I will not allow you to hurt people. You'll have to go to the quiet room for 30 minutes." Be firm, clear, and consistent in limit setting; collaborate with other staff members to establish, implement, and evaluate limit setting.
4. After an explosive or aggressive episode, encourage expression of feelings before, during, and after the episode. Explore self and staff reactions to client's behavior and determine the option of alternative behaviors.
5. Reduce stimuli; use solitary time for hygiene, laundry, and so on.
6. Develop behavioral contract.
7. Approach in an unhurried manner; hurrying will result in more anger and hostility.
8. Use measures to prevent overt aggression (e.g., distraction, reduction of environmental stimuli); avoid competitive games; use large motor skill activities that are not highly structured or confining (e.g., walks, exercise, dance, painting).
9. Using quiet persuasion is most effective.

Evaluation
Client discusses feelings related to hostility and aggression; engages in appropriate physical activities to relieve tension.

Goal 3: Client will demonstrate realistic independence; will develop ability to problem solve, make requests appropriately, and negotiate.

Implementation
1. Do not discuss grandiose ideas or plans.
2. Assess client's abilities.
3. Discuss capabilities calmly with client; reinforce client's self-esteem; convey expectation that client can function independently.
4. Involve client in planning ADL.
5. Assist client PRN.
6. Inform client that staff will not comply with unreasonable demands while conveying acceptance of client.
7. Provide feedback about effects of dependency and demands: "I become irritated when you continually ask me to do things for you that we decided you would do."
8. Help client to identify feelings, needs, means of seeking gratification without manipulation.
9. Assist client in developing decision-making skills; explore possible consequences of decisions and behavior.
10. Help client develop alternative behavior; teach client to use assertion, problem solving, negotiation.

Evaluation
Client makes decisions and takes actions independently, makes requests directly and in a quiet voice, and sets limits on own demanding behavior.

Goal 4: Client will recognize and set limits on own manipulative, acting-out behaviors and impulsivity.

Implementation
1. Avoid impatience and anger if client is manipulative or acts out.
2. Inform client of behaviors expected in short, clear sentences.
3. Set firm, definite limits on client's behavior; consistently enforce limits.
4. Teach client that it is the manipulative behavior that is being rejected, not the client.
5. Avoid arguments or displaying disapproval of vulgarity, profanity, or overt sexual behavior resulting from extreme euphoria.
6. Remove client from public places when this behavior could embarrass the client or family.
7. Protect other clients from sexual advances.
8. Use chemical (anxiolytics, such as lorazepam, and neuroleptics, such as haloperidol) or physical restraints (last alternative) as necessary (e.g., if there is a risk of harm to self or others) to prevent leaving hospital or injuring self or others.

Evaluation
Client's impulsivity and manipulative and acting-out behaviors are less than they were on admission.

Goal 5: Family will recognize indications that client needs treatment for relapse or recurrent symptoms of mania.

Implementation
1. Assess family and client's perception and understanding of present illness.
2. Identify family and client's treatment expectations and their role in outcomes.
3. Explore need for and means of setting limits.
4. Teach family criteria for seeking treatment:
   a. Noncompliance with lithium regimen
   b. Anorexia, weight loss, insomnia
   c. Hyperactivity, excessive spending
   d. Increased use of alcohol and other drugs
   e. Delusions of grandeur or persecution
   f. Sexual impulsivity
   g. Aggressive, demanding, acting-out behavior
   h. Rapid mood changes

Evaluation
Family lists indications of need for treatment.

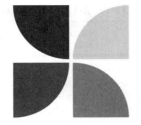

Personality Disorders and Other Maladaptive Behaviors

Personality disorders refer to persistent patterns of internal distress and behaviors that depart from expected social and cultural norms. Primary manifestations of personality disorders include distorted cognitions that affect perceptions of self, others, and circumstances; affect: labile mood, intense feelings, and extreme emotional responses; impaired interpersonal relationships; and poor impulse control.

People with personality disorders normally attribute conflicts to others and the environment and lack insight into their own behavior. Lack of insight, low self-esteem, and difficulty forming and maintaining meaningful interpersonal relationships produce profound distress and global impairment (e.g., social, interpersonal, occupational). Furthermore, inability to modulate frustration, anxiety, and stress tends to generate self-destructive behaviors. Self-destructive behaviors include suicide attempts, abusive relationships, substance misuse, and self-mutilation.

Historically, the basis of personality disorders was linked solely to psychodynamic theories and impaired relationships with primary caregivers. Contemporary studies suggest that the cause of personality disorders is complex and arises from biologic and psychosocial factors. Temperament and genetic predisposition of mood disorders are examples of biologic factors. Psychosocial factors, including early childhood traumas such as sexual, physical, and other forms of abuse, are also believed to play a major role in the formation of borderline and other personality disorders.

Major treatment concerns for persons with personality disorders include their lack of insight into their role in sustaining maladaptive behaviors and the need for treatment. Entry into the health care system parallels the client's inability to manage stress and crises and use of self-destructive behaviors.

Intrafamily violence (child abuse, wife battering, elder abuse, etc.); rape; hostile-aggressive, antisocial, and borderline personality disorders are covered in this section and are examples of other maladaptive behaviors.

Application of the Nursing Process to Clients Exhibiting Socially Maladaptive Behaviors

ASSESSMENT
1. Immediate events that precipitated maladaptive/acting-out behavior: characteristics and frequency
2. Physiologic changes that accompany anger/anxiety
3. Coping behavior that client uses to handle stress and anger: adaptive and maladaptive (e.g., suicide or homicide attempts, drug misuse, antisocial behavior)

4. Defense mechanisms used to cope with anger
5. DSM-IV classification: three clusters (A, B, C)
   a. A: paranoid, schizoid, schizotypal
   b. B: antisocial, borderline, histrionic, narcissistic
   c. C: avoidant, dependent, obsessive-compulsive, personality disorder not otherwise specified (e.g., mixed, passive-aggressive, depressive)

ANALYSIS/NURSING DIAGNOSES
1. Safe, effective care environment
   a. High risk for violence: self-directed or directed at others
   b. High risk for injury
2. Psychosocial integrity
   a. Ineffective individual coping
   b. Self-esteem disturbance, personal identity disturbance
   c. Impaired social interaction
   d. Rape trauma syndrome
   e. Altered patterns of sexuality
   f. Anxiety
3. Health promotion/maintenance
   a. Noncompliance
   b. Ineffective, disabling family coping
   c. Altered family processes

GENERAL NURSING PLANNING, IMPLEMENTATION, AND EVALUATION

Goal 1: The client will exhibit increased adaptive behaviors; uses assertive behaviors as a means of expressing independence and control.

Implementation
1. Provide structure and set limits on behavior that is emotionally and physically destructive to others or the environment.
2. Consistently implement limits. Inconsistent limit setting increases the client's belief that manipulative behavior is productive and increases environmental chaos and tension. It also increases tension and stress and maintains maladaptive behaviors. Consistent limit setting promotes structure and a sense of predictability or security.
3. Examine own nonverbal responses to client; avoid acting defensively or aggressively.
4. Encourage staff to focus interventions that improve maladaptive behaviors rather than criticizing or rejecting the client.

5. Teach client the difference between assertiveness (asking for what one wants without purposely hurting others and standing up for rights) and aggression (getting what one wants at the expense of others).
6. Recognize and point out manipulative behaviors in a nonjudgmental way; do not allow client to manipulate staff or other clients; discuss effect of manipulation on relationships.
7. Reinforce positive (assertive) approaches ("I feel . . ." versus "You make me feel . . .").
8. Discuss consequences of impulsive (maladaptive) actions; help client develop problem-solving skills.
9. Increase self-esteem by supporting strengths and encouraging participation in achievable goals.
10. Teach stress-reduction techniques (e.g., imagery, journaling, relaxation, exercise).
11. Praise efforts of family and significant others as they assist the client in coping.

Evaluation
Client exhibits increased adaptive behaviors; describes the difference between assertion and aggression; demonstrates at least one assertive behavior; uses effective coping mechanisms to handle stress (e.g., relaxation).

SELECTED HEALTH PROBLEMS

✤ VIOLENCE IN THE FAMILY

1. Definitions:
   a. Violence: aggressive drives expressed with the intent or injuring or harming oneself or others
   b. A learned behavior, stemming directly from exposure and imitation or indirectly as seen when an individual using inappropriate measures channels aggressive impulses, such as passive-aggressive behaviors
   c. Has a biologic component (e.g., temperament); often associated with general medical conditions such as delirium, dementia, perceptual-sensory disturbances, and substance-induced intoxication or withdrawal
   d. Family violence and abuse constitute a family crisis
2. Some violent persons feel guilty about their behavior, and others do not. Regardless of the presence or absence of guilt, violent behavior conveys the message that "You are unimportant, irrelevant, and I can demolish you." These messages often underscore numerous mental health problems, including depression, personality disorders, and substance abuse.
3. Victims can include
   a. Children
   b. Siblings
   c. Spouse
   d. Elderly parents or other adults
   e. Children or adults in long-term care settings
4. Potential victims of violence outside the family include homosexuals, and ethnic, religious, or cultural group members.
5. Characteristics of victims and abusers: see Tables 2-11 and 2-12.
6. Multidisciplinary treatment:
   a. Case finding: health care personnel have opportuni-

Table 2-11 Characteristics of abuse

Victim/survivor characteristics	Abuser characteristics
Weaker than abuser	Stronger than victim
Emotionally dependent, compliant, passive	Physically abused as child
Physically dependent	May or may not feel guilt/remorse
Low self-esteem; may feel need for punishment	Defensive about behavior with victim
Ashamed of being abused; quiet	Low self-esteem, self-acceptance
Fearful of retaliation from abuser	Hostility
"Stockholm Response": feeling responsible and sympathy for the abuser	Immaturity
Belief that the abuser will reform	Impulsivity
	Experiences chronic anxiety
	Inadequate knowledge of growth and development
	Seductive behavior toward child
	Aloof, impersonal, dysfunctional attachment
	May have experienced recent crisis—separation; divorce; housing, financial, or personal crisis
	Jealousy
	Perfectionism

Table 2-12 Indications of abuse

Multiple injuries
Injuries that do not fit description of accident
Old, healed fractures; scars, burns
Poor hygiene
Retarded growth or development with no medical explanation
Child has not had immunizations
Child is not properly dressed for weather
Wary of caretaker
Does not seek comfort or affection from caregiver
Young child does not cry when parents leave
Grabbing behavior/lap hunger
Provocative behaviors
Delinquent or runaway behavior
Teenage pregnancy
Bruised or swollen eyes
Bald patches where hair has been pulled out or from prior hematomas
Dislocated joints (especially in the shoulder)
Intraabdominal injuries (especially in pregnant women)
Sexual acting out in young child
Sexually transmitted disease in child
Bruised or edematous genitals

ties to identify high-risk groups and assess children and adults for possible abuse, especially when they are seen for injuries.
   1. be alert for abuse cases, especially in emergency rooms, pediatrics, ambulatory clinics, home health settings

2. carefully document bruises, cuts, and other wounds, as well as their size and location; also document interaction patterns of client and significant others; these may become evidence
3. carefully listen for discrepancies in narrative about how injury occurred—are parent's and child's recollection of events consistent? Is the explanation for injury conceivable? (i.e., a child who "accidentally" got into a bath that was too hot may burn a toe or foot, but would not voluntarily totally immerse in water or remain immersed long enough to sustain third-degree burns on 75% of body)
4. *all suspected child abuse cases must be reported and will be investigated by the state child welfare agency;* in some states elder abuse is also reportable
5. medical personnel are not liable if they report an abuse that does not check out as such
6. offer both abuser and abused referrals for emotional support
   b. Community services: numerous branches of the health care system respond to client abuse situations.
   1. treatment and intervention by child welfare agencies may include alternative living situations for the abused
   2. various community agencies provide classes on parenting, dealing with older parents, problem-solving and conflict resolution skills, and appropriate expression of emotion (e.g., Parents Anonymous—a self-help group for actual or potential child abusers)

Nursing Process

ASSESSMENT

1. Characteristics of survivor and abuser (see Table 2-11)
2. Physical, emotional, behavioral, and psychologic indications of abuse (see Table 2-12)
3. Family communication and interactional patterns
4. Matching history of injury with plausible explanation
5. Client's mental and physical status
6. Parenting, problem-solving, communication, and conflict resolution skills
7. Interactions between parents/marital dyad
8. Substance abuse history of parents, primary caregivers, siblings, adolescent
9. Mental illness
10. Community resources

ANALYSIS/NURSING DIAGNOSES
PLANNING, IMPLEMENTATION, AND EVALUATION

Goal I: The client (abuser) will stop abuse and discuss feelings and needs related to violence openly and honestly.

Implementation
1. Approach the survivor and abuser in a calm, accepting manner.
2. Speak in a calm and confident manner and use direct eye contact to help client regain and maintain control.
3. Acknowledge own feelings about client (abuser) and client (survivor); recognize the needs of both (nurse may feel angry with abuser and sympathetic with survivor); be aware of impact of own feelings on client care.
4. Approach abuser in a nonjudgmental and respectful manner; recognize that the abuser may be a survivor of abuse, may not view own actions as abusive, and may be unable to stop the behavior. Prevailing low self-esteem may require interventions that foster a positive self-regard.
5. Help abuser or caretakers to recognize importance of meeting own needs for affection, belonging, and self-esteem.
6. Delineate appropriate ways to express and meet need.
7. Review expectations regarding psychologic, physical, and emotional needs of survivor.
8. Help client identify events that trigger anger and violence.
9. Teach parenting and stress-reduction skills.
10. Provide the potentially aggressive client with ample physical space.

Evaluation
The client (abuser) talks about feelings, anxieties, and frustrations rather than acting out violently.

Goal 2: The client (survivor) will manage psychologic and physical trauma related to violence.

Implementation
1. Teach and encourage appropriate expression of feelings in both adult and child survivors; provide child/adolescent with sketching materials and dolls to act out feelings when indicated.
2. Discuss adult survivor's strengths, coping abilities, ability to function independently.
3. Attend to physical needs caused by specific trauma (e.g., burns, fractures).
4. Provide physical and emotional comfort (e.g., analgesics, therapeutic use of touch when appropriate, child's personal toy or blanket).
5. Refer to in-hospital support services and community services (e.g., mental health center, crisis intervention hot line, individual and group counseling).
6. Discuss use of support services if violence recurs.
7. If unsafe to return home, contact social service or child/adult protective services for placement.

Evaluation
The client (survivor) expresses feelings; has physical needs met; identifies available support services; verbalizes plan of escape if violence recurs.

Goal 3: The client (abuser) will learn ways to relate to victim without the use of violent behavior.

Implementation
1. Practice open, direct communication and use active listening skills.
2. Document all clinical findings (both objective and subjective data).
3. Help client (abuser) to acknowledge emotional problems when they occur; explore childhood experiences with

violence (some were abused as children and need to learn new ways of handling conflicts).

4. Explore alternative ways of expressing anger (e.g., physical activities, discussion, relaxation).
5. Teach effective problem-solving and conflict resolution skills.
6. Teach parents normal growth and development and realistic expectations of children at various ages; discuss appropriate methods of limit setting and discipline as opposed to emotional or physical use of force.
7. Reinforce positive parenting strategies.
8. Assist in integrating older parent into family home and lifestyle while maintaining independence for all family members.
9. Identify community resources to assist family in managing situation: day/home care agencies to provide respite care from total care for elderly, mental health services, Parents Anonymous to help discuss feelings and problems and share solutions, mental health center for counseling or respite care.

Evaluation
The client (abuser) identifies appropriate alternatives to handle feelings, seeks referral for counseling; attends peer support groups.

▓ HOSTILE AND AGGRESSIVE BEHAVIOR

1. Definitions
   a. Aggression: forceful, goal-directed action that may be verbal, emotional, or physical; the motor counterpart of the affect of rage, anger, and hostility
      1. defensive response to anxiety and loss of self-esteem and power
      2. constructive when it is problem solving and appropriate as a defense against realistic attack, expressed appropriately (e.g., assertiveness)
      3. maladaptive when it is unrealistic, self-destructive, not problem solving, the outcome of unresolved emotional conflict, and results in physical or emotional harm to others
      4. has a biologic component arising from factors noted under Violence in the Family
   b. *Passive-aggressive behavior:* resistance to demands for adequate performance in occupational or social functioning are met by timidity, sullenness, stubbornness, forgetfulness, procrastination, and obstruction
      1. if the behavior is characteristic of the person, it may be considered a personality disorder (e.g., passive-aggressive personality disorder DSM-IV classification)
      2. the person acts out anger in indirect and passive ways (e.g., always late, forgetting to do things that are important to another person); criticizes persons in authority
      3. the anger evoked in another provides the person with attention and release for anger
2. Dynamics
   a. Behavior is a response to a perceived threat.
   b. Feelings of anxiety occur, accompanied by helplessness and frustration.

c. Judgment, reasoning, and cognitive integrity decrease as anxiety increases.
d. Verbal or physical aggression occurs as an attempt to alleviate anxiety.

Nursing Process
ASSESSMENT
1. Refer to Assessment, p. 59
2. Aggressive behaviors
   a. Increase in motor agitation or restlessness
   b. Verbal threat or abusive language
   c. Tense and angry affect
   d. Demanding
   e. Self-directed anger
   f. Manipulative
   g. Uncooperative
   h. Increased tone or rate of speech
   i. Threatening posture, such as clenched fist
3. Level of control
   a. Ability to listen and follow directions
   b. Ability to identify source of anger and verbalize feelings appropriately
   c. Ability to explore alternative ways of expressing anger
4. Nurse's perception of impending violence

ANALYSIS/NURSING DIAGNOSES (see p. 59)
PLANNING, IMPLEMENTATION, AND EVALUATION

> **Goal 1:** Client will increase control and decrease aggressive behavior.

Implementation
1. Refer to General Nursing Plan, p. 59
2. Encourage client to identify source of angry feelings.
3. Explore alternative ways of dealing with anger.
4. Avoid power struggles:
   a. Allow flexibility in decision making as long as it is within safe parameters.
   b. If decision poses risks to self, other clients, or staff, explain reasons the nurse cannot condone them; do not give in.
   c. Establish and apply firm and consistent limits on disruptive behavior.
   d. Develop a plan of action for verbal and physical management of violent or aggressive behavior.
5. Continuously observe for signs of increased loss of control. When determined:
   a. Remove potentially dangerous objects from staff (e.g., jewelry, stethoscope, neckties).
   b. Reduce stimuli; remove objects or persons that agitate client; move client to area with few people and minimal noise, light, or activity.
   c. Designate one staff member to engage in conversation with client and direct the team.
   d. Explain what is happening, that client will be safe; ask whether client has any questions; maintain calm, helpful approach.
   e. If client expresses fear of hurting self or others, initiate steps to avert it; remove weapons or objects that could be used destructively and initiate one-to-one observation.

f. Explain to client that the behavior can be controlled externally if client cannot regain self-control.

g. Offer medication (e.g., anxiolytic, lorazepam) and explain that client is unable to control the behavior voluntarily and will be restrained if medication is refused.

Evaluation

Client's agitation, anxiety, and irritability abate, begins to express feelings appropriately.

Goal 2: Client will be safely restrained to restore control and prevent injury to self and others.

Implementation

1. Be aware of state laws governing use of restraints and parameters of care, and *remember to use as a last resort.*
2. Follow agency's policy and procedure in applying and removing restraints; documenting the subsequent care of client in restraints.
   a. Have sufficient number of staff members (at least four with a fifth person to control the client's head and prevent biting) available to apply restraints. Designate staff positions to control designated areas such as the client's head, legs, trunk, and arms.
   b. Provide an explanation for restraints (e.g., used to help client regain control and prevent injury to self and others) and conditions for removing them (give a few seconds to comply—do not compromise).
   c. Gently raise or turn the client's head to reduce risk of aspiration and feelings of helplessness.
   d. Give ROM exercises for each extremity, and check for full circulation at periodic intervals.
   e. Remove each restraint at specified intervals.
   f. Monitor client in restraints continually and document behavior and care at regular intervals.
   g. Never leave restrained client alone.
   h. Document vital signs and client response to restraints.
   i. Assess and provide ADL.
   j. Continuously assess client's level of dangerousness to self and others; document and report status to members of treatment team.
3. Remove physical restraints when medication takes effect.
4. Explain use of restraints to any other clients who observed episode; encourage discussing fears of loss of control and availability of help. NOTE: Restraints are contraindicated in clients with unstable medical conditions. Agitation arising from dementia and delirium is worsened by restraints.

Evaluation

Client remains free of injury when restrained; released in a timely manner.

❋ SEXUAL AND GENDER IDENTITY DISTURBANCES

1. Definitions (DSM-IV)
   a. *Pedophilia:* includes sex acts with partners who are legally unable to consent (such as children), sex acts with persons who choose not to consent, sex acts ac-

companied by force or violence (rape), and invasion of another person's privacy without that person's knowledge (e.g., voyeurism).
   b. *Voyeurism:* the person observes other people's naked bodies, undressing or engaging in sexual activities without their knowledge or consent in order to obtain sexual gratification.
   c. *Exhibitionism:* a person exposes sexual organs when it is socially unacceptable.
   d. *Sadomasochism:* obtaining sexual pleasure from having pain inflicted on oneself or others; may be part of a rape incident or may be part of other sexual encounter.
   e. *Rape:* legal definitions of rape vary from state to state, but most include sexual intercourse without the consent of the other person; statutory rape is the seduction of a minor, even though the minor consents; victims may be any age; the majority are female, but males can be raped (usually by other males).
2. Characterization of a rapist
   a. Rape is an aggressive sexual act and a crime of violence, power, and control.
   b. Rapists act for the purposes of venting anger and hostility and exercising control, managing their feelings of inadequacy, and power.
   c. Many rapes are planned, and victims may be stalked and brutally tortured and killed.
   d. The majority of rapists are male, and in the case of child victims, usually someone the child knows; acquaintance rape is also a possibility with an adult.
3. Responses to rape
   a. Shame and embarrassment may lead to underreporting.
   b. Common reactions in the survivor include shame, guilt, embarrassment, self-blame, anger; social withdrawal, fears of injury, mutilation, sexually transmitted diseases, and pregnancy; fear of how significant others will react to incident.
   c. The survivor's response varies from expressing feelings through talking or behavioral manifestations (e.g., crying, trembling, agitation) to controlled (outwardly quiet, exerting control over behavior to regain physical and emotional control).
   d. The significant others' reactions to the rape are similar to the survivor's and also vary (e.g., anger, support, isolation).
   e. The psychologic effect of rape may be long lasting, affecting interpersonal relationships with significant others, impairing sexual functioning, and creating feelings of helplessness, anxiety, and depression.
   f. Self-awareness of one's own reaction to rape is imperative to deal therapeutically with the survivor and significant others.

Nursing Process

ASSESSMENT

1. Survivor's perception of incident
2. Survivor's coping ability (both pretrauma and posttrauma)
3. Anxiety level

4. Physical status, including signs of physical trauma (e.g., bruises, scratches)
5. Availability of significant others, support network
6. Impact of rape incident (including cultural factors) on significant others
7. Survivor's immediate concerns (e.g., emotional control, legal information or assistance, physical care, pregnancy, or protection from and information on sexually transmitted diseases

ANALYSIS/NURSING DIAGNOSES (see p. 59)
PLANNING, IMPLEMENTATION, AND EVALUATION

Goal 1: Survivor will return to prerape level of functioning and be amenable to emotional support.

Implementation
1. Provide a private location for interview, examination, and crisis intervention.
2. Document client's perception of incident, physical trauma, psychologic status, coping ability, and physical assessment findings; assist in collecting physical evidence.
3. Use empathetic, nonjudgmental approach; discuss options and guidance to prevent further injury to self or others; be sensitive to survivor's feelings while gathering information and physical evidence; avoid asking for unnecessary repetition of events by client.
4. Maintain clear boundaries and avoid undue touching or invading client's personal space to minimize retraumatization and feelings of helplessness and powerlessness.
5. Encourage verbalization of rape incident; if client is unable to talk about incident, acknowledge difficulty of traumatizing experience; allow immediate use of denial; explain that anger, sadness may occur later.
6. Encourage client to ventilate present feelings about incident; do not dwell on actual sexual act unless client needs to discuss this; allow expression of anger (may be directed at staff).
7. Help client assess present coping ability.
8. Explain common behavioral and emotional responses that may occur.
9. Encourage client to actively problem solve, prioritize concerns, and make decisions (e.g., who to tell, legal recourse, physical care, pregnancy prevention).
10. Explore feelings of guilt or self-blame; reinforce responsibility of rapist, not of survivor, for the act; suggest that whatever client did (either fighting or submitting) was necessary for self-protection.
11. If survivor is child:
    a. Use drawing, play to help child ventilate feelings.
    b. Use calm approach, be aware of own nonverbal communications that may convey anger to child.
    c. Reinforce that child has done nothing wrong and will not be punished.
    d. Explain all procedures thoroughly.
12. Give survivor and significant others information about community resources (e.g., rape trauma group, legal aid, rape crisis center, counseling).
13. Refer for follow-up to crisis counseling; marital or couple's therapy; other psychotherapies.

Evaluation
The survivor (client) verbalizes need for interventions, participates in treatment, and verbalizes willingness to seek referral.

Goal 2: Significant others will verbalize feelings and support survivor.

Implementation
1. Assess significant others' reactions (self-blame or survivor blame are common) and present coping abilities.
2. Reinforce rapist's responsibility for the act and necessity of survivor's actions for self-preservation.
3. Apprise family of expected reactions of survivor and significant others to rape trauma (increased anxiety and fear within 48 hours followed by adjustment; reappearance of anxiety later).
4. Explain how significant others can support client.
    a. Encourage client to ventilate, but do not force discussion of rape.
    b. Help client resume daily activities.
    c. Support survivor's decision for follow-up care, litigation, and so on.
    d. Do not withhold emotional and physical comfort (e.g., touching, holding, stroking).
    e. Avoid overprotection or isolation.
    f. Initiate measures that ensure the client's safety and protection, such as new lock, escort at night.
5. Talk with family away from survivor (client); encourage verbalizing anger to nurse rather than to survivor when appropriate.
6. If survivor is child:
    a. The issue of whether or not the child remains a "virgin" comes up often with families, and when the question arises, it is a source of great anxiety. This is particularly so among families who hold strong religious beliefs about the sanctity of sexual relations, or members of a traditional cultural group in which premarital sex is considered either sinful or damaging in some way. The nurse may be asked whether the child or adolescent is still a virgin. Although there is no ideal answer to this question, the following replies may be helpful to share with families as they try to resolve this issue. First, the hymen can be broken in a number of ways, including nonsexual trauma or by activities such as riding a horse, falling off a bicycle, or using a tampon. Thus the absence of an intact hymen does not necessarily indicate that one's virginity is lost. Moreover, consider other forms of sexual molestation, such as digital penetration, which may not injure the intact hymen. Second, rape or sexual assault is an act of violence and not a consensual sexual act. Hence, although the child is physically violated, there is no intent to "lose virginity"; voluntary consent is frequently the factor deemed wrong or sinful by families. Third, if families continue to struggle with these concerns a referral to a clergy or family therapist may be indicated.
    b. Help parents recognize that the survivor is still a child

and has age-related needs for physical comfort, reassurance, and protection.
   c. Facilitate a return to customary family activities as soon as possible.
   d. Teach parents that child may have a delayed response; issues related to rape may recur.
7. Provide referral to community resources for additional support and assistance.

Evaluation

Significant others discuss traumatic experience and provide adequate support to client (survivor).

ANTISOCIAL PERSONALITY

1. Definition: disorder manifested by persistent pattern of violating the rights of others with a lack of remorse; pattern of lifelong maladaptive behaviors
2. DSM-IV classification: personality disorder
3. Onset in early adolescence
4. Characteristics
   a. Fails to regard the rights of others and conform to social norms and exhibits a history of persistent unlawful acts and arrests since the age of 15
   b. Few close but many superficial relationships
   c. Poor work history and failure to honor fiscal obligations
   d. May engage in sexually deviant behavior
   e. Poor impulse control, chemical addiction, frequent altercations
   f. Articulate communication skills, average to superior intelligence
   g. Able to rationalize or justify behavior
   h. Charming, fabricates stories to impress listener
   i. Manipulative, deceptive, conning, and uses people for personal gratification and gain
   j. Lack of responsibility, unreliable
   k. Lack of insight, decreased tolerance to stress and frustration; does not learn from experience or punishment
   l. Lacks guilt or remorse
5. Rarely experiences real distress; seeking emergency or other services is linked to self-gratification (i.e., drug-seeking or avoiding criminal indictment)
6. Treatment considerations: apply external controls to limit the acting-out behavior
   a. Lacks insight into behavior, subsequently rarely seeks treatment except when forced by law enforcement
   b. Long-term psychotherapy provides limited success, but relatively few clients remain in psychotherapy because of expense, time involved, poor motivation, and lack of insight
   c. Self-help groups have had some success

Nursing Process

ASSESSMENT

1. Reasons for seeking treatment at this time
2. Characteristics of persons with personality disorders
3. Behavior: manipulative, impulsive, self-centered, acts out, is demanding, has need for immediate gratification, has decreased modulation of stress and frustration
4. Substance abuse and dependency history, especially alcoholism
5. Legal history
6. Support systems
7. Psychiatric history
8. Mental and physical status

ANALYSIS/NURSING DIAGNOSES (see p. 59)

PLANNING, IMPLEMENTATION, AND EVALUATION

Goal 1: Client will interact with peers and staff within socially accepted norms; will participate in treatment program.

Implementation

1. Refer to General Nursing Plan, p. 59.
2. Set and apply firm, consistent limits.
3. Call staff conferences to discuss behavior and plans for setting limits and dealing with behavior; document limits on care plans so all staff can follow intervention.
4. Provide client with clear and direct expectations regarding treatment, rules, and routines (e.g., harming self or others, throwing objects is unacceptable behavior); explain consequences if expectations are violated.
5. Recognize manipulative behavior, such as setting up (splitting) staff, playing one staff member against another, and using other clients.
6. Do not make agreements with client before determining what all other staff members have told the client.
7. Confront client in a matter-of-fact way when behavior is not acceptable.
8. Encourage development of positive goals for change.
9. Give positive feedback when client is conforming to socially accepted norms.
10. Explore social relationships and problem areas; role-play social situations; use group therapy to point out problem behaviors.

Evaluation

Client gradually complies with the treatment program; interacts appropriately with others.

BORDERLINE PERSONALITY DISORDER

1. Definition: long-standing pattern of unstable self-image, interpersonal relationships, dysphoria, poor coping patterns, and impulsivity.
2. Dynamics: stems from the early childhood developmental arrest and separation from significant other.
3. Onset: early adolescence.
4. Research *consistently* confirms that persons with borderline personality disorder have extensive histories of early childhood traumas, such as sexual abuse, physical abuse, neglect, and emotional abuse. Biologic factors also play a role in formation of this personality disorder and contribute to depression and other mood and anxiety disorders.
5. Characteristics:
   a. *Splitting:* refers to a defense mechanism that reflects an inability to integrate positive and negative experiences the client has with others. Manifestations of splitting include seeing people as "all good" or "all bad"; leads to idolizing or devaluing people; causes relationships to be intense while idolizing person but short-lived as a result of devaluation.
   b. Often experience inappropriate and intense anger and rage, with extreme and rapid mood changes.

c. Poor judgment and insight.
d. Pervasive feelings of emptiness, loneliness, boredom, and fears of abandonment.
e. Immature and impaired self-concept, identity diffusion.
f. Impulsivity, unpredictability.
g. Increased risk of danger toward self and others (e.g., suicidal attempts, self-mutilation, substance misuse).
h. Poor school and work histories.
i. Unstable or chaotic interpersonal relationships.
j. Tend to evoke intense staff reactions.
k. Brief stress-induced dissociative symptoms or sensory-perceptual disturbances.
6. DSM-IV classification: borderline personality disorder.

Nursing Process
ASSESSMENT
1. Ability to integrate positive and negative qualities in self and others
2. Quality and consistency of relationships with staff, peers, and family
3. Mood
4. Acting-out behaviors
5. Risk of self-injury
6. Ability to accept and express caring
7. Self-concept
8. Judgment and decision making
9. Strengths
10. Chemical addiction history (past and present)
11. Level of function
12. Rape-trauma syndrome
ANALYSIS/NURSING DIAGNOSES (see p. 59)
PLANNING, IMPLEMENTATION, AND EVALUATION

Goal 1: Client will increase socially acceptable behavior.

Implementation
1. Protect client from self-injury (see Depression, Goal 1, p. 59).
2. Establish consistent time and limit setting for interactions with client.
3. Limit impulsive, acting-out behavior in a nonpunitive manner.
4. Discuss meaning and pattern of acting-out behavior.
5. Encourage adaptive expression of feeling (e.g., verbalization, physical activity, relaxation exercises).
6. Develop a behavioral contract (client will write down an-

gry feelings rather than acting out, then discuss feelings with nurse to gain privileges).
7. Role-play behavioral responses to social situations.
Evaluation
Client adheres to behavioral contract, appropriately expresses feelings, and uses effective stress-reducing techniques.

Goal 2: Client will express improved self-esteem.

Implementation
1. Provide opportunities for client to relate to staff and persons in positive manner.
2. Explore client's self-expectations, strengths, and realistic goals.
3. Assist client in developing solitary activities.
4. Reinforce positive behaviors, constructive use of solitary time.
5. Acknowledge and effectively manage staff countertransference reactions.
Evaluation
Client expresses improved self-esteem, realistic self-expectations; lists own strengths; uses solitary time constructively.

Goal 3: Client will improve interpersonal relationships.

Implementation
1. Recognize idolizing or devaluing of staff as part of client's maladaptive interactional patterns; do not act on feelings of hostility or flattery; avoid personalizing client reactions.
2. Be consistent in approach to client; use multidisciplinary conferences to minimize intense transference and countertransference.
3. Examine client's expectations of others.
4. Help client define realistic expectations of others.
5. Help client identify communication problems in interpersonal situations.
6. Role-play social situations and demonstrate effective communication skills.
7. Provide social skills training.
Evaluation
Client establishes and maintains at least one relationship; verbalizes improved ability to evaluate limitations and strengths of others.

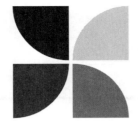

Schizophrenia and Other Psychotic Behaviors

1. Definition: a multifarious mental disorder arising from alterations in neurochemical processes and neuroanatomic structures and influenced by genetic and psychosocial factors. Often described in terms of a retreat from reality that includes affect, motor and sensory-perceptual disturbances, and impaired social, communication, and coping skills.
2. Behavioral continuum:
   a. *Adaptive:* temporarily retreating from a stressful situation and focusing psychic energy internally to think, plan, reflect, and regroup before responding adaptively; a sometimes necessary response
   b. *Maladaptive:* isolating oneself from others and the world to the extent that relationships and the ability to function in society are seriously impaired
      1. may retreat to avoid facing important social situations; social skills are impaired and a cyclical pattern of withdrawal results
      2. examples of maladaptive withdrawal or retreat include
         a. excessive fantasizing that keeps the person from having to deal with day-to-day problems of living
         b. excessive television watching or involvement in only solitary activities to avoid social interactions
      3. schizophrenia is the most severe form of withdrawal; the person's thought patterns, sensory perceptions, communication, and relationships with others prevent functioning in a productive manner
3. Withdrawn behaviors: although withdrawn behaviors occur on a continuum, this section focuses primarily on the most severe form of withdrawal, schizophrenia.
   a. Etiologic factors: exact cause remains unknown; various theories: strong new research points to neurochemical and neuroanatomic causes with genetic predisposition
      1. biologic factors
         a. neurotransmitter alterations: increased levels of dopamine in the limbic system of the brain cause type 1 (positive) symptoms; decreased levels of norepinephrine cause type 2 (negative) symptoms (Table 2-13); neuroleptic medications work toward altering the neurochemical use of dopamine and norepinephrine
         b. neuroanatomic alterations: structural problems in the brain appear to cause decreased cerebral blood flow to frontal areas, altered brain glucose metabolism, changes in ventricular ratios, and decreased gray matter
         c. twin and adoption studies support a genetic predisposition in transmission of schizophrenia
      2. psychologic: internal dynamics in thought process, affect, and behavior cause often profound difficulties in psychologic state
      3. sociologic: Sociologic stresses appear to overload the fragile biochemistry and contribute to severely disrupted family relationships and ability to interact in the community settings; earlier psychoanalytic theories (e.g., mothering styles, double-bind communication) have largely been dismissed
   b. Dynamics: genetic vulnerability and biochemical deficits along with psychologic and sociologic stressors contribute to the client's perception of the world as so threatening that withdrawal from interpersonal relationships, social situations, and reality is the only mode of adapting
   c. Management: long-term management with continuing follow-up is frequently necessary
      1. medications: neuroleptics (antipsychotics) (Table 2-14)
         a. target symptoms: modify intense anxiety, tension, and psychomotor excitement; alleviate delusions, hallucinations, and incoherence
         b. advantages: allow the client to participate in other forms of therapies; increase the level of function, self-care, and self-esteem
         c. side effects: not addictive but do have troublesome, always frightening, sometimes irrevers-

Table 2-13   Positive and negative symptoms of schizophrenia

Positive symptoms (type 1)—few brain structural alterations, more responsive to neuroleptics	Negative symptoms (type 2)—more brain structural alterations, less responsive to neuroleptics
Hallucinations	Blunted affect
Delusions	Loss of interest
Bizarre behaviors	Social withdrawal, apathy
Faster emergence of symptoms	Anhedonia
Few neuroanatomic (brain structure) alterations	Poverty of speech
	Slower emergence of symptoms
	More neuroanatomic (brain) alterations

Table 2-14 Antipsychotic agents (neuroleptics)

Generic name (trade name)	Dosage	Action	Nursing implications
MAJOR PHENOTHIAZINES			
Chlorpromazine (Thorazine)*	100-1000 mg/day	Reduce positive symptoms (e.g. hallucinations, delusions, incoherent thoughts) of schizophrenia by blocking dopamine receptors at pre and postsynaptic neurons in mesolimbic pathways and the extrapyramidal motor system.	For all neuroleptics or antipsychotic agents
Perphenazine (Trilalon)	6-64 mg/day		• Check BP prior to administration; observe for orthostatic hypotension; teach client to rise slowly from sitting or lying position.
Trifluoperazine (Stelazine)	4-10 mg/day: may be slowly increased to 15-20 mg/day		• Monitor periodic liver function tests, blood counts.
Fluphenazine hydrochloride, decanoate or enanthate (Prolixin, Permitil)†	0.5-1. mg po daily, not to exceed 20 mg: 12.5-25 mg q 2wk IM		• Instruct client to notify nurse or physician of complaints of sore throat, nosebleed, rash, fever, or other infections.
Thioridazine hydrochloride (Mellaril)*	20-800 mg/day		• Observe for early signs of pseudo parkinsonism: if present, explain to client and administer antiparkinsonian drug.
Mesoridazine (Serentil)*	initial: 50 mg tid optimal: 100-400 mg/day		
BUTYROPHENONES			
Haloperidol (Haldol, Haldol Decanoate)	Initial 0.05 mg/day gradually increasing over 5-7 days from 0.5 mg-2 mg bid or tid (oral) moderate symptoms; 2-5 mg IM for prompt relieve of acute psychosis/agitation (lower doses in elderly); maintenance with decanoate (Haldol-D) every 4 weeks 50-100 mg initially up to 300 mg deep IM.	Similar to the phenothiazines; more potent dopaminergic effects	• Observe for early warning signs of tardive dyskinesia, such as excessive blinking, muscle rigidity, pill rolling, and tongue-like movements and report.
			• Use abnormal involuntary movement scale (AIMS) to assess for early signs of tardive dyskinesia (TD). (Frequency of tests depend upon facility policies, but usually every 6-12 months or annually).
THIOXANTHENES			• Participate informed process regarding acute and long term side effects of these agents.
Chloroprothixene (Taracian)	100-600mg/day		• Observe for early signs of neuroleptic malignant syndrome (mild rigidity, low grade fever, diaphoresis, change in sensorium).
Thiothixene (Navanc)	6 mg daily, slowly increase to 20-30 mg/day; rarely exceeds 60mg		
*low potency agent: produce significant sedation, anticholinergic effects, and orthostatic hypotension.			Warn client that drowsiness may occur
†high potency agent: high potential for producing extrapyramidal side effects (EPS), such as dystonia, akathisia, and parkinsonian. Injectable agents (decanoale) form lasts 2-4 weeks and increase medication compliancy.			Observe for dryness of mouth, visual or retinal changes, rash, gastric irritation, constipation, difficulty voiding
DIHYDROINDOLONES			
Molindone hydrochloride (Moban)	25-225 mg/day	As per phenothiazines	Do not administer antacids within 1 hour of oral administration of these medications

Table 2-14 Antipsychotic agents (neuroleptics)—cont'd

Generic name (trade name)	Dosage	Action	Nursing implications
DIBENZOXAZEPINES Loxapine hydrochloride (Loxatine C) Loxapine succinate (Loxitane)	25-250 mg/day 25-250 mg/day	Act on ascending reticular activating system	Teach client: • avoid alcohol • consult nurse or physician before taking other medications • appropriate diet and exercise to avoid weight gain • precautions to avoid retina and skin damage from photosensitivity • desired and adverse drug reactions • high-fiber diet, adequate fluids and exercise to prevent constipation
DIBENZODIAZEPINE-DERIVATIVE Clozapine (Clozaril) **BENZISOXAZOR DERIVATIVE** Risperidone (Risperdal)	initial; 25-50 mg/day to reduce the risk of acute hypotension and sedation: increase to 300-450 mg/day at end of 2 weeks; based on clinical response; there is little evidence of benefits in doses >450-600 mg/day. (Should be considered in treatment-resistant clients or when typical neuroleptics are ineffective or produce severe EPS or TD). Normal range 2-8 mg/day (in contrast to clozapine, should be considered with first-episode as well as chronic schizophrenia)	These agents appear to reduce negative (e.g. blunted affect, emotional withdrawal, impoverished thoughts) and positive symptoms of schizophrenia by blocking serotonin 5-HT2 receptors in the frontal cortex and striatal system and adrenergic (norepinephrine) and dopamine receptors: additionally, resperidone is a potent dopamine and histamine antagonist in the basal ganglia and limbic system.	Clozapine: Available only through Patient Management System that ensures weekly white blood count (WBC). Drug supplied only in one-week intervals Contraindicated in clients with compromised bone marrow function, blood dyscrasias or history of bone marrow depression Drug interaction; alcohol, central nervous system depressants and drugs that suppress bone marrow function (e.g. carbanazepine) Monitor vital signs including temperature Teach client: • risk of agranulocytosis (fever, sore throat, malaise) • avoid operating dangerous equipment or driving because of sedation especially during early phases of treatment • encourage to rise slowly from a sitting or supine position • hyper salivation is common Risperidone: Observe for dose-related EPS and early symptoms of TD Teach client: • sleep disturbances are common • to rise slowly from a sitting supine position • avoid operating dangerous equipment of driving during early phase of treatment

ible, and occasionally dangerous side effects such as akathisia, dystonia, tardive dyskinesia, anticholinergic effects, sedation, and sexual dysfunction

   d. nursing role
- administer the medications, observe client response, intervene to prevent complications related to drug side effects (Table 2-15), administer medications to reduce side effects (Table 2-16), and teach client and family about the drug (e.g., action, side effects, and need to take on long-term basis) in efforts to promote medication and treatment compliance; use the abnormal involuntary movement scale (AIMS) to monitor for early signs and symptoms of tardive dyskinesia
- record and report side effects or problems

2. therapeutic milieu: used to increase independence, social skills; see p. 22
3. nurse-client relationship
   a. purpose: helps the client to function as independently as possible and enhance problem-solving skills and manage stress effectively
   b. focuses on development of trust as model for healthy relationships with others
   c. DSM-IV classification: schizophrenia subtypes: disorganized; catatonic; undifferentiated; residual

Application of the Nursing Process to a Client Exhibiting Psychotic Behavior

ASSESSMENT
1. Behavioral manifestations
   a. *Affect* (visible expression of mood)
     1. a specific judgment criterion is the appropriateness of the affect; that is, the degree to which it is in keeping with the situation at hand, both quantitatively and qualitatively. For example, a person

speaking of a sad situation is expected to exhibit a sad or depressed mood (congruency between thought content and affect); however, if the person smiles or exhibits an elated affect (incongruence of mood and thought content), this is probably indicative of an underlying psychosis, particularly in the context of hallucinations and delusions

     2. responses may be excessive, or they may be inappropriately minimal (flat). *Flat* affect is demonstrated by a blunt or dull emotional tone of expression; it is a generalized impoverishment of emotional reactivity
     3. *inappropriate* affect is that which is incongruent with the situation or the content of thought
   b. *Behavior disorganization,* in which the client reacts to stress in an unpredictable or bizarre manner (e.g., pacing, rigid posturing)
   c. *Disregard of hygiene and grooming: self-care deficits* can range from looking unkempt to bizarre clothing and makeup or disregard for bodily care; often severe dermatologic consequences
   d. *Disregard of physical safety: risk of self harm* includes not being concerned about placing self in dangerous situations, such as walking in a busy street or causing self-inflicted wounds; these persons need close observation
   e. *Nutrition deficits* because of poor eating habits, fear of poisoning, and lack of judgment and insight into the need to eat or drink
   f. *Regression,* in which the client returns to behavior patterns exhibited at an earlier stage of development (e.g., thumb sucking, baby talk, fetal position). Unable to cope with the present chaos, behavior regresses
2. Psychologic manifestations
   a. *Autism:* a form of thinking that is completely subjective or self-centered and understood only by the cli-

Table 2-15 Side effects of antipsychotic agents

Parkinsonian-type
  Pseudoparkinsonism
  Dystonia (tonic muscle spasms, especially of eyes, tongue, jaw, and neck)
  Akathisia (restlessness, inability to sit or lie quietly)
Hypotension
Photosensitivity
Anticholinergic effects (blurred vision, dry mouth, constipation, difficulty starting urination)
Agranulocytosis (rare)
Jaundice (rare)
Increased restlessness
Drowsiness
Weight gain
Skin rashes
Amenorrhea with false-positive pregnancy test, galactorrhea
Ejaculation difficulties, gynecomastia
Decreased libido

Table 2-16 Antiparkinsonism medications

Dopaminergics	Anticholinergics
Act by increasing dopamine availability	Act by decreasing acetylcholine availability
Types	Types
Sinemet	Artane
Symmetrel	Cogentin
Parlodel	Akineton
Eldepryl	Parsidol
Side effects	Side effects
Hypotension	Dry mouth
Mydriasis	Nasal congestion
CNS: headaches, dizziness, weakness, confusion, hallucinations, and delusions	Urinary retention
Respiratory: hoarseness, shortness of breath, coughing	Constipation
Gastrointestinal: nausea and vomiting	Mydriasis
	Hypotension
	Sedation
	Decreased sweating

ent. Thoughts emerge in the form of daydreams, delusions, and fantasies.

1. this persistent tendency to withdraw from involvement with the external world and to become preoccupied with ideas and fantasies that are egocentric and illogical causes autistic clients to be unresponsive
2. it is difficult to establish communication with them; they may be mute; their conversations may be irrelevant or lack coherence; they do not respond to affection and fail to attach (bond) normally
3. motor disturbances such as rocking, toe walking, whirling, stereotypic movements

b. *Hallucinations:* a sensory perception that occurs without an external stimulus. Hallucinations function as a protection from the distress of reality.

1. can be auditory, visual, tactile, olfactory, or gustatory
2. usually occurs in psychotic disorders but can occur in both chronic and acute delirium and dementia; visual hallucinations are prominent in underlying general medical condition such as delirium and dementia
3. auditory hallucinations are the most common form occurring in clients with schizophrenia, although visual, tactile, olfactory, and gustatory hallucinations may be experienced; some clients describe the experience as very definite; others describe it with an element of vagueness
4. auditory hallucinations are often threatening, derogatory, and aggressive and commanding; client's response to them may account for acts of violence to self or others
5. when hallucinations occur the client is distracted and unable to interact with real persons in the milieu; such experiences are therefore counterproductive and conducive to further withdrawal from reality; when anxiety and loneliness increase, the client becomes aware that others recognize that client is hallucinating and becomes ashamed and embarrassed; sometimes hallucinations never completely abate, but their severity is reduced by medications and other forms of distractions, such as music or an activity

c. *Delusion:* a false belief or misinterpretation of reality that is unreasonable and distorts judgment. Manifestations of delusions include suspiciousness or intense distrust and paranoia (persecutory) or inflated self-worth (grandiose).

1. delusion of grandeur: false, grandiose, or expansive belief that one is an important or powerful person or entity (e.g., sees self as royalty or as Jesus)
2. delusion of persecution: false belief that one is victim of others' hostility and aggressiveness (e.g., "The FBI is after me" or "My phone is bugged")
3. although delusions represent a withdrawal from reality into fantasy, their function is to secure the client's identity; therefore delusional systems are rigid and inaccessible to reason; any attempt to

correct the client's beliefs strengthens the delusion and portrays the nurse as an enemy.

4. challenging the client's false beliefs only serves to reinforce them
5. best hope for intervention lies in watching for hidden messages in themes of delusion, indicating unmet needs

d. *Depersonalization:* feelings of unreality or strangeness concerning either the environment (derealization), the self, or both.

1. results from the client's poor self-concept
2. client treats self as an object
3. client seems to have resigned not only from the world of reality but also from self; this leads to extreme social isolation

e. *Loose associations:* refers to ideas changing from one unrelated theme to another. Client is unaware that ideas are disorganized or statements are irrelevant or lack significant meaning.

1. the thought process loses its continuity so that thinking and expression become confused, bizarre, incorrect, and abrupt
2. communication is disconnected, follows no logical/orderly sequence, and is confusing to the listener

f. *Ambivalence*

1. occurs normally, from time to time, in all persons and is popularly known as "mixed feelings"
2. Severe disruptive behavior in schizophrenia; client unable to make even the smallest decisions
3. because of the ambivalence, minor difficulties can lead to disruption of relationships with significant others

3. Socialization manifestations

a. Poor social skills: difficulty with conversation and even physical closeness (e.g., aloofness and distant relationships)
b. Retreat from social situations
c. Few or no friends: often has no friends, or relationships are considered to be friendships in spite of minimal contact
d. Often communication disturbances resulting in inability to interact with even closest family member
e. Variable employment history
f. Difficulty maintaining an independent living situation: unable to care for self, will not pay rent regularly or take care of physical needs; some can do the caretaking tasks but tend to isolate themselves (varies among individuals)
g. Self-medication using alcohol and other drugs to manage negative affects and side effects from medications

4. Suicide potential

a. Disordered thinking; aggressive/hostile/command voices; a confused, depressed mood, substance abuse and dependence, poor coping skills, inability to manage anxiety, and low self-esteem increase suicide risk (persons with recent diagnosis of this disorder exhibit high risk for suicide)
b. See Elated-Depressive Behavior, p. 46

ANALYSIS/NURSING DIAGNOSIS
1. Safe, effective care environment
   a. High risk for violence: self-directed or directed at others
   b. Sensory-perceptual alteration (e.g., delusions, visual, auditory)
   c. Impaired home maintenance management
2. Physical integrity
   a. Impaired verbal communication
   b. Sleep pattern disturbance
   c. Altered nutrition: less than body requirements
   d. Self-care deficits
3. Psychosocial integrity
   a. Ineffective individual coping
   b. Chronic low self-esteem
   c. Altered thought processes
   d. Impaired social interaction
   e. Sensory-perceptual alterations (specify)
   f. Anxiety
   g. Self-esteem disturbance
   h. Depression
4. Health promotion/maintenance
   a. Impaired adjustment
   b. Ineffective family coping: compromised
   c. Noncompliance (specify)

GENERAL NURSING PLANNING, IMPLEMENTATION, AND EVALUATION (Table 2-17)

Goal 1: Client will remain free of injury.

Implementation
1. Appraise nature, content, and duration of hallucinations and delusions.
2. Keep harmful objects away from client.
3. Continuously monitor client's behavior and response to interventions.
4. Observe for self-care deficits, such as physical problems (e.g., infection, constipation) that may be outside client's awareness.
5. Administer medications and observe for desired and side effects of drugs. Also provide interventions such as medications to reduce side effects of neuroleptics. (See Table 2-16.)
6. Monitor rest and sleep; use comfort measures such as pillows, snacks, warm baths to induce sleep. Avoid caffeine products in late evening.

Evaluation
Client remains free of injury; experiences desired response to medications and only minimal side effects of drugs; has adequate rest or sleep.

Goal 2: Client will maintain adequate nutrition and fluid and electrolyte balance.

Implementation
1. Observe for signs of dehydration (e.g., dry skin, cracked lips, poor skin turgor); encourage fluids as tolerated.
2. Monitor dietary and fluid intake; if client is not eating, assess the reasons (e.g., delusions about food being poisoned, too agitated to sit for meals, unaware of poor eating habits).
3. Help client find methods to ensure adequate food intake (e.g., permit food from home if client fears hospital food is poisoned; provide finger foods client can eat while walking).
4. Provide positive reinforcement for good eating habits.
5. Teach about nutrition as needed.

Evaluation
Client maintains adequate food and fluid intake; skin turgor is normal.

Goal 3: Client will demonstrate improved hygiene and grooming.

Implementation
1. Identify specific client's self-care needs (e.g., with severe withdrawal, client may need nurse to provide care; client with poor reality orientation or attention span may need assistance; more self-sufficient client may only need encouragement).
2. Use gentle firmness and consistent interest in client's needs.
3. Provide matter-of-fact positive reinforcement for appropriate grooming and cleanliness.
4. Be sure equipment for physical care is available to client.

Evaluation
Client performs own hygienic care (hair, nails, clothing, bathing).

Goal 4: Client will develop a trusting relationship with staff member; will demonstrate increased ability in social interaction.

Implementation
1. Know that staff reactions can be the crucial element negating or facilitating attainment of the therapeutic goal for the client.
   a. Staff members may find themselves withdrawing from the client because the disorder is often chronic, the prognosis is dismal, and client's behavior often provokes feelings of frustration, helplessness, and incompetence.
   b. Withdrawal on the part of the staff reinforces the client's past experiences of rejection and feelings of low self-esteem (mutual withdrawal).
   c. As a protective measure, the client will withdraw further into world of fantasy, negating progress toward therapeutic goals.
   d. The client may test staff involvement by distancing self.
   e. Offer support and encouragement to other staff members; meet regularly to provide support.
   f. Persons with schizophrenia develop relationships slowly and use their ambivalence as a means of distancing; therefore the orientation phase of the relationship is the most difficult.
2. Use consistent, predictable behavior.

Table 2-17 Selected problem behaviors and interventions

Behavior	Interventions
Aggression	Prevention—early recognition of increased excitement. Encourage verbal expression of feelings surrounding behavior. Reduce stimuli. Avoid reinforcement (e.g., competitive games). Provide distraction. Set limits. Protect other clients.
Anger	Acknowledge or name feeling. Explore sources. Encourage to express verbally. Explore appropriate outlets. Avoid arguing.
Anxiousness	Acknowledge or name the behavior or feeling. Explore sources. Encourage appropriate expression. Give reassurance. Recognize that anxiety in nurse increases client's anxiety.
Associative looseness (thought disorder)	Relate in a concrete manner. Focus on immediate situation. Point out reality. Clarify verbalizations that are not understood.
Autism	Accept at stage client is in; do not push. Give ample time for responses. Do not reinforce dependency. Use silence appropriately.
Controlling behavior	Recognize means of controlling: negativism, obstruction, silence, avoidance, insults, yelling, increased chatter, or crying. Do not impose unnecessary controls. Allow client some control. Develop trust, security in giving up control.
Delusions	Avoid arguing. Avoid arousing suspicion. Be honest and reliable. Be consistent. Acknowledge client's feelings. Point out reality: client's beliefs are not shared. Look for themes in content of delusions that may indicate a clue to unmet needs.
Dependence	Assess abilities and capabilities. Provide only help needed. Encourage to solve problems and make decisions. Display attitude of firmness and confidence. Discourage reliance beyond actual need. Encourage successful participation.
Hallucinations	Acknowledge client's fears. Distract client with reality in milieu. Encourage to give up hallucinations. Help to relate with real persons. Do not give attention to content.
Hopelessness, helplessness	Structure small successes. Give encouragement. Exhibit expectation that client will succeed. Encourage identification of strengths.
Hostility	Avoid arguing with the client. Acknowledge and name feelings. Explore the source of hostility with client. Encourage to express hostility verbally rather than resort to physical aggression. Explore appropriate outlets for hostility (e.g., physical activities).
Low self-esteem, feeling worthless	Prevent isolation. Acknowledge client's view. Avoid system of shoulds and should nots and discussions regarding moral judgments. Avoid power struggles. Give minimal tasks, and grade them to manageable size. Prevent self-mutilation.
Manipulation/acting out	Spell out acceptable and unacceptable behavior. Set firm and definite limits. Consistently enforce limits. Avoid involvement in intellectualization (i.e., responsibility for behavior rests with client). Treat infractions with withdrawal of privileges. Ensure that staff is united, firm, and consistent. Maintain sense of authority.
Ritualistic behaviors	Do not interrupt repetitive act: could lead to panic. Set limits on repetitive behavior. Engage in alternative activities with client. Provide physical protection from repetitive acts.
Secondary gain	Understand unconscious motivation of the behavior and differentiate it from malingering. Understand and alleviate primary symptoms. Encourage client to explore the motivation of the behavior. Explore alternatives to the primary symptom for handling anxiety.
Somatic behaviors	Do not focus on physical symptoms. Give appropriate information regarding somatic complaints. Point out reality (i.e., correct misinformation).
Superiority	Suggest solitary activities for client. Put client in charge of things, not people. Give client activities at which client can succeed.

3. Persevere even though client may be unreliable or rejecting.
4. Meet for short intervals at regularly scheduled times to foster trust.
5. Use silence; show willingness to spend time without talking if client so chooses.
6. Afford ample time for response if client is very regressed; use general comments that do not press client for answer.
7. Allow client to set the pace of the relationship.
8. Accept client's particular stage of illness; if communication is to be restored, the nurse must understand that client is frightened and both wants and fears contact from others, makes responses slowly, and needs ample time to trust nurse's sincerity and interest.
9. Listen attentively in a nonjudgmental manner to client's thoughts and feelings.
10. Know that clients experiencing psychosis are extremely sensitive to the feeling tones of others; they pick up negative cues from the nurse, who may be unaware of them.
11. Demonstrate socially appropriate behavior.
12. As client begins to accept the nurse, client may become dependent; a therapeutic goal requires that the nurse maintain contact on a professional level and not reinforce the dependency.

13. Observe verbal and nonverbal behaviors that may indicate any interest in activities; give support to any expression of interest.

Evaluation

Client develops a relationship with one staff member; begins to interact with other clients.

Goal 5: Both the client and family will participate in the health teaching process and accept instruction concerning his or her illness and medications.

Implementation

1. Assess the client's and family's current knowledge and response to present and past treatment.
2. Determine readiness to accept instruction.
3. Focus teaching on causes, signs and symptoms, and treatment of schizophrenia, emphasizing biologic disruptions.
4. Support adaptive coping styles and employ teaching measures that use strengths.
5. Teaching should reflect the actual symptoms the client experiences.
6. Teach early signs of relapse (sleep pattern disturbance, anxiety, recurrent or worsening hallucinations or delusions), and be sure client has access to help. Provide education of situations that increase the risk of relapse (e.g., anger, stress, noncompliance, increased anxiety, substance misuse).

Goal 6: Client will define and test reality; will dismiss internal voices, hallucinations, and delusions.

Implementation

1. Recognize disorientation as manifestation of severe withdrawal related to anxiety and frustration.
2. Be particularly honest and reliable, especially with the suspicious client.
3. Determine content of delusions and hallucinations and their level of dangerousness (e.g., command hallucinations may direct self-harm or harm of others; persecutory delusions may convince the client that the nurse is the enemy, and steps to "protect" self may emerge, posing danger towards others); avoid arguing about content and avoid reinforcing client's perceptions.
4. Acknowledge client's feelings and beliefs; point out that these are not shared.
5. Relate to client in a realistic and concrete manner, focusing on the immediate situation; it is helpful for the nurse to point out reality to the client by saying "I don't understand" and asking for clarification as needed.
6. Help to recognize hallucinations or delusions as a sign of anxiety.
7. Reassure that hallucinations and delusions do go away and can be dismissed as client focuses on real people and situations.
8. Help client relate to real persons.

9. Help client who depersonalizes to discuss feelings of estrangement with trusted individuals:
   a. Initially with familiar nursing staff with whom client has developed a trusting relationship
   b. As client's condition permits, in group therapy sessions or similar groups involving other persons who may recount similar experiences
10. Focus on reality of the client's body and environment during these discussions.

Evaluation

Client dismisses internal voice, hallucinations, and delusions; increases ability to relate to real persons and situations.

Goal 7: Client will increase communication with family members.

Implementation

1. Approach in a calm and accepting manner.
2. Explore present family patterns with client; family assessment and intervention during the client's hospitalization may be needed.
3. Encourage client to describe family interactions.
4. Help client view self as individual with values and beliefs that sometimes differ from family's.
5. Practice social skills to use with family members; use role-playing, assertion techniques.
6. Provide opportunity for family members to talk about the client's illness and treatment to decrease hostility and withdrawal from client; help family explore social resources.

Evaluation

Client effectively communicates with family members.

Goal 8: Client will increase successful decision-making skills.

Implementation

1. Relate in a concrete manner; focus on the immediate situation.
2. Afford decision-making opportunities at level of client's ability; use therapeutic milieu as tolerated by client.
3. Increase complexity of decisions as tolerated.
4. Do not reinforce unneeded dependency.
5. Provide ongoing feedback regarding decision making.

Evaluation

Client increases ability to make decisions.

Goal 9: Client will demonstrate social skills in individual and group settings.

Implementation

1. Role-play appropriate social interactions.
2. Help client develop a relationship with one other client.
3. Encourage client to relate to others during activities.
4. Do not press client beyond present abilities; may need encouragement to begin developing social skills.

5. Help client to relate to others in more complex situations, slowly as tolerated.

Evaluation

Client interacts appropriately in individual and group settings with other clients; demonstrates fewer maladaptive behaviors.

Goal 10: Client will develop ability to be as self-supporting as possible.

Implementation

1. Support client in finding a healthy living situation; may be at home, a halfway house, or in own apartment depending on client's social skills and self-motivation.

2. Support client in finding employment as appropriate; employment history and assessment of skills in occupational therapy can help in developing employment plan.

3. Invite family to discuss feelings about plans for client's living and employment plans; help them evaluate their expectations and role in supporting client in living and employment settings.

4. Connect family with Alliance for the Mentally Ill chapters throughout the country for supportive help in ongoing understanding, crisis management, and learning about disorders, treatment, and medications.

Evaluation

Client finds healthy living situation; develops a plan to be self-sufficient.

Table 2-18   DSM IV Schizophrenia and Other Psychotic Disorders

Type	Characteristics	Additional nursing care
Paranoid	Delusions of persecution/grandeur Hallucinations Ideas of reference Hostility/aggression Superiority	Interventions specific to delusions, hostility, superiority, and aggression
Catatonic	Severe withdrawal, regression Catatonic stupor, waxy flexibility, muteness OR Catatonic excitement, severe agitation, grimacing, bizarre gestures/posturing	Prevent complications of immobility: infection, skin breakdown, urinary and fecal incontinence, constipation
Undifferentiated	Mixed schizophrenic symptoms over long time	See General Nursing Plan, p. 72
Disorganized Incoherent, marked loosening of associations, grossly disorganized behavior Blunt, incongruent, or silly affect *Residual* Longer-term disability. No remaining acute psychotic symptoms, but continuing of blunted affect, social disability, and thought process deficits		
Childhood	Onset in early childhood Withdrawal, impaired relationships, disturbed affect Ritualism Self-mutilation Increased or decreased sensitivity to sensory stimuli *No hallucinations or delusions*	Prevent self-mutilation Behavior modification
Other psychotic disorders • schizophreniform disorders • transient, stress-induced dissociative symptoms or paranoid ideations	Sudden onset Last less than 6 months	See General Nursing Plan, p. 72
Schizoaffective disorder	No prior history of disturbed interpersonal relationships Minimal residual defects	
Atypical psychosis *Induced psychosis disorder:* state in which the psychotic delusion is shared with another person living in close association		

SELECTED HEALTH PROBLEMS

Specific DSM-IV schizophrenia and psychotic disorders include major schizophrenia: paranoid, disorganized, catatonic, undifferentiated, and residual types. Classification of longitudinal course for schizophrenia includes episodic, continuous, single episode, and other or unspecified type. Other disorders in this category include schizophreniform disorder, schizoaffective disorder, delusion disorders, brief psychotic disorder, shared psychotic disorder, psychotic disorder due to a general medical condition, substance-induced psychotic disorder, and psychotic disorder not otherwise specified.

These disorders are characterized by withdrawal from reality because of inability to manage, organize, and respond to incoming stimuli. They may be accompanied by delusions, and all are distinguished by other characteristic behaviors. General Nursing Plans and Evaluations, p. 72 (see also Table 2-17), are used in addition to care specific to the distinguishing characteristics (Table 2-18).

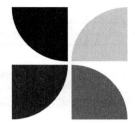

Substance Use Disorders

1. Definitions
   a. Substance use disorder: behavioral changes associated with somewhat regular use of a substance that affects the central nervous system
   b. Polydrug abuse: mixing drugs and alcohol in varying degrees (particularly dangerous because of potentiating and toxic interactions of drugs and alcohol) (Table 2-19)
2. Etiology: not known, but thought to be an interplay of neurobiologic, psychologic, and sociocultural factors
3. Interaction variables
   a. The person
      1. no specific personality type identified even though recent studies suggest a high rate of alcoholism in persons with antisocial personality disorder
      2. most frequently, the person shows signs of immaturity, low tolerance for frustration, low self-esteem, environmental deprivation, conflicts over parental upbringing, and conflict between values and behavior
      3. it is not known if substance abuse fosters development of these characteristics or if the characteristics trigger the abuse
      4. substance-related disorders can coexist with other psychiatric and medical disorders, including schizophrenia, depression, anxiety, and personality disorders; substance abuse may also serve as a form of self-medication in an attempt to cope with psychologic and emotional distress arising from mental disorders, such as depression, schizophrenia, and anxiety and inability to modulate stress and negative feelings
      5. some individuals may be genetically or biologically predisposed to develop an addiction to various substances (e.g., alcoholism and other drugs)
      6. alterations in the brain's reward and neurotransmitter systems are linked with alcoholism and other drug addictions and use
   b. The family: substance abuse may relate to overall anxiety level in family as well as in individual
   c. The environment: social aspects and peer pressure may lead the person into drug culture and antisocial acts
   d. The substance: which substance the person uses depends on the cultural group, availability, costs, and federal regulation of the item (alcohol or drug substances other than alcohol)

4. Three criteria distinguish substance abuse from substance dependence
   a. Pattern of maladaptive use: depending on the substance, client manifests inability to cut down or stop use despite physical problems; needs daily use for adequate functioning; intoxication throughout the day; episodes of a complication of substance intoxication (e.g., alcoholic blackouts)
   b. Impairment of social or occupational functions: legal and economic difficulties because of cost, procurement, or complications of intoxication (e.g., auto accident)
   c. Duration of abuse: disturbance of at least a month
5. Substance dependence
   a. Definition: a more severe form of substance use disorder than substance abuse
   b. Manifestations
      1. a physiologic need for a substance evidenced by withdrawal or tolerance
      2. almost always, a maladaptive use pattern occurs that causes impairment in social or occupational functioning
      3. rarely, manifestations are limited to physical dependence
      4. alcohol or cannabis dependence requires evidence of occupational or social impairment; diagnosis of other substance-dependence categories requires only evidence of withdrawal or tolerance
   c. Length of dependence: regular maladaptive use for over 6 months qualifies as continuous dependence
   d. Social implications: although accessibility, chance, peer pressure, and curiosity play a part in who will ingest a drug and who will not, they do not account for the fact that one person becomes addicted and another does not
   e. Concepts
      1. physical dependence: an altered physical state produced by the repeated administration of the drug, which necessitates its continued administration to prevent a withdrawal syndrome; cross-dependence: dependence on more than one chemical or substance
      2. addiction: the compulsive use of a chemical substance with physical and psychologic dependence
      3. habituation: repeated use of a substance that results in psychologic dependence

Table 2-19 Common drugs of abuse

Drug	Route	Use	Dependency	Overdose	Withdrawal
SEDATIVES/DEPRESSANTS					
Glutethimide (Doriden) Methyprylon (Noludar) Ethchlorvynol (Placidyl) Ethinamate (Valmid) Benzodiazepines Barbiturates Chloral hydrate Methaqualone (Quaalude)	Oral Injection	Relaxation Euphoria	Psychologic Physical	CNS: depression Respiratory: bradypnea CV: decreased BP, P GI: cramps	CNS: marked agitation, insomnia, convulsions, poor muscle coordination GI: nausea/vomiting Psychotic behavior CV: increased BP with postural hypotension
STIMULANTS					
Amphetamines Cocaine Phenmetrazine (Preludin)	Oral Smoking Injection Intranasal	Rush/high Fatigue	Psychologic	CV: increased BP, P; dysrhythmias Respiratory: nasal abnormalities GI: anorexia, dry mouth, vomiting CNS: dilated pupils, hyperactivity, headache Impulsiveness Delusions/hallucinations Poor judgment	Depression Suicide potential Lethargy Somnolence Headache "Crash" paranoia
"Crack" cocaine	Smoking Free-basing	Euphoria	Rapid addiction	CNS: seizures, paranoid psychosis CV: dysrhythmias Respiratory: paralysis	Severe craving Depression Fatigue Hypersomnia Irritability
CANNABINOIDS					
Cannabis (marijuana, hashish, THC) Dronabinol (Marinol)	Smoking Oral	"Dreamy" state Euphoria, hilarity, excitement To control nausea/vomiting of chemotherapy As a bronchodilator	Psychologic	Dropout syndrome Paranoia Confusion Delusions/hallucinations GU; impotence CNS: tremors, poor coordination Red eyes	No clinically significant effects
INHALANTS					
Ether Cleaning fluids Gasoline/kerosene Glue vapor Ethylene oxide Aerosols	Inhalation	Intoxication Exhilaration	Tolerance	Extreme toxicity Airway obstruction Death through damage to liver, kidneys, bone marrow	No clinically significant effects

4. tolerance: greatly increased amounts of the substance are required to achieve the desired effect, or there is a greatly diminished effect with regular use of the same dose
5. withdrawal: a substance-specific syndrome after cessation or reduction of intake
6. lethality: the amount of a substance that constitutes a fatal dose
7. potentiation: two or more substances combined have a greater effect than simple summation (e.g., 1 + 1 = 3)
6. Substance use disorders among health professionals is a serious problem
   a. Narcotic addiction by physicians is estimated at 1% to 2%, or 30 times greater than in the general population
   b. Estimated 40,000 nurses with alcoholism in United States

Table 2-19 Common drugs of abuse—cont'd

Drug	Route	Use	Dependency	Overdose	Withdrawal
PSYCHEDELICS					
PCP LSD Mescaline Psilocybin	Oral Injection Smoking Inhalation	Euphoria Ecstasy but with anxiety	No evidence	Delusions/hallucinations Poor time/space perception Poor memory Multiple individualized effects Depersonalization GI: anorexia, dry mouth, nausea/vomiting CNS: dizziness, dilated pupils CV: increased BP, P, temperature; sweating, chills; dysrhythmias Chromosomal damage Flashbacks Accidents	No clinically significant effects
OPIATE/SYNTHETICS					
Heroin Oxymorphone (Numorphan) Morphine Meperidine (Demerol) Hydromorphone (Dilaudid) Opium alkaloids (Pantopon)	Injection Inhalation Oral	"High" Ecstasy Relaxation Pleasurable feeling	Tolerance Physical	CV: decreased BP GI: anorexia, cramps CNS: grand mal seizures, pinpoint pupils, coma, death Respiratory: slow, shallow breathing GU: urinary retention	*Stage 1* Restlessness Anxiety Craving *Stage 2* Yawning Lacrimation Rhinorrhea Diaphoresis *Stage 3* Dilated pupils Gooseflesh Anorexia Muscle pain *Stage 4* Insomnia Marked agitation Nausea/vomiting Diarrhea

   c. Problems with impaired health professionals' job performance compromise teamwork and result in danger to the clients and the professionals themselves

   d. It is the responsibility of health professionals to report concerns about a colleague to supervisor, and for supervisor to take appropriate actions

   e. Professionals are helping, not harming, a substance-abusing colleague by bringing problems to the attention of someone qualified to help

7. Symptoms of chemically dependent nurses include the following:

   a. Decreased work performance: charting and client care

   b. Sudden mood changes; inappropriate affect; often irritable or suspicious

   c. Absenteeism (before and after days off or payday)

   d. Frequent night-shift work; working all the time

   e. Nurse's clients' consistently complain of inadequate or no relief of pain after medication administration

   f. Frequent errors of judgment and decision making

   g. Problem behavior in handling drugs (offering to give medications for the other nurses, missing drugs, "wasting" of drugs frequently, inaccurate record keeping)

   h. Smell of alcohol on breath

   i. Frequently leaving the unit

   j. Bizarre behavior (paranoia, hallucinations, aggressiveness, elated or depressed mood)

Application of the Nursing Process to a Client with a Substance Use Disorder

ASSESSMENT

1. Substance use history (substance abusers often deny use or seriously understate extent of use; to increase the likelihood of an accurate history, ask questions in a logical, accepting, and nonthreatening manner; family and friends may provide more accurate information or use denial)
   a. History of recent prescription, nonprescription, and illicit drug use
   b. Drugs client has prescribed for self (e.g., nicotine, alcohol, cocaine, marijuana, amphetamine)
   c. Treatment history
2. Psychiatric history: substance users often have a coexistent psychiatric disorder that is often exacerbated by alcohol and other drugs; contributes to noncompliance and impedes sobriety
3. Work performance
   a. Excessive use of sick time
   b. Decreasing productivity or "job shrinkage"
   c. Decreasing ability to meet schedules and deadlines
   d. Disorganized work and reduced productivity
   e. Frequent errors in judgment; in drug-addicted nurses, medication errors, incorrect controlled-drug wastage, or incorrect narcotic counts
4. Physical examinations to rule out underlying medical conditions should include chemistries; renal and liver function tests; test for sexually transmitted diseases, including HIV, reactive plasma reagent (RPR) and venereal disease research laboratory (VDRL) drug (toxicology) screens; electrocardiogram (ECG); complete blood cell count (CBC)
5. Level of consciousness, reality orientation, mental status exam
6. Family history of substance abuse

ANALYSIS/NURSING DIAGNOSES

1. Safe, effective care environment
   a. High risk for injury
   b. Sensory-perceptual alteration: visual, auditory, kinesthetic, gustatory, tactile, olfactory
   c. High risk for violence: self-directed or directed at others
2. Physiologic integrity
   a. Altered nutrition: less than body requirements
   b. Impaired physical mobility
   c. Sleep pattern disturbance
   d. Changes in activity or energy level
   e. Self-care needs
3. Psychosocial integrity
   a. Anxiety
   b. Ineffective individual coping
   c. Chronic low self-esteem
   d. Depression
4. Health promotion/maintenance
   a. Ineffective family coping: compromised
   b. Altered family processes
   c. Noncompliance

GENERAL NURSING PLANNING, IMPLEMENTATION, AND EVALUATION

> **Goal 1:** Client will safely withdraw from substance that is abused or creating dependency.

Implementation

1. It is important *not to do any of the following:*
   a. Lecture, argue, moralize, blame, or threaten
   b. Lose one's temper
   c. Enable person to cover up consequences of actions
   d. Be overly sympathetic or rescuing
   e. Put off facing problem
   f. Personalize derogatory or abusive statements
   g. Approach in judgmental, parental, or demeaning manner
2. Control symptoms with medication (e.g., lorazepam) when required (prn); take vital signs every 2 hours and prn and report elevations or significant changes to physician.
3. Continuously assess the level of dangerousness toward self and others.
4. If client is agitated, confused, assaultive, or belligerent, speak in a calm and firm manner, reorient, stay with client; reduce environmental stimuli, reassure that current symptoms are only the result of body's responding to the abused substance, and that they are temporary; reassure that client will regain control; use restraints *only if necessary* for safety (follow hospital policy carefully).
5. Deal with hallucinations by reinforcing reality; speak slowly in a calm voice; provide a quiet environment; stay with client until the frightening symptoms have decreased.
6. Provide physical care advocated for additional diseases/conditions that client may have.
7. Keep client ambulatory as much as possible; if necessary, walk with client several times a day.

Evaluation

Client safely withdraws from abused substance.

> **Goal 2:** Client will participate in prescribed treatment and learn how to abstain from substance abuse or dependence.

Implementation

1. Meet with client at least twice daily; your presence conveys acceptance and support; be cognizant of your own nonverbal distancing behaviors; establish good eye contact.
2. Do not punish or reprimand client for failures or nonresponse to your suggestions and interventions (punishment serves only to give client fuel for continuing to deal with failure or rejection by drinking or taking drugs); ignore it, but do praise *any positive responses.*
3. Have client make decisions about daily care in hospital and community; involve in some type of occupational therapy or other structured activities, anything in which

client can achieve some measure of success (helps increase self-confidence and self-esteem).

4. Provide opportunities to decrease social isolation and improve social skills (mealtimes, groups, recreation periods, community or occupational activities); calmly and gently point out unacceptable behavior, such as manipulative acts; provide consistent and firm limit setting; reinforce positive social and self-care behaviors (e.g., initiating friendly conversations); and praise all efforts at participation in activities.

Evaluation

Client participates in prescribed treatment.

Goal 3: Client will develop a positive lifestyle that is free from substance use, abuse, or dependence.

Implementation

1. Help the client to gradually become aware of the denial by confronting the denial process; encourage client's assessment of how denial serves client and maintains addiction, including delineation of the self-defeating aspects.
2. Help client look at alternative coping methods and deal with abstinence one day (or one morning, one evening) at a time.
3. Work with client to develop sound discharge planning regarding employment counseling, ongoing support via outpatient counseling, or long-term inpatient treatment.
4. Provide information about other types of therapy and referrals (e.g., stress-reduction programs, medication management for psychiatric and addictive disorders and relapse prevention through employee assistance, 12-step and aftercare programs, psychotherapies, and local mental health clinics or self-help groups).

Evaluation

Client develops a positive lifestyle free of substance abuse or dependence.

Goal 4: Family will explore enabling behaviors.

Implementation

1. Arrange for client and family to attend group counseling sessions, if available in hospital or community settings, to discuss feelings, problems, changing behaviors, coping and communication patterns, pressures, sources of support, and so on.
2. Encourage family to allow time to take care of needs that may have been neglected during years of substance abuse.
3. Teach family new ways to manage frustrations; demonstrate assertion skills.
4. Discuss need for realistic expectations of client behaviors.

Evaluation

Family members participate in group counseling; discuss expectations of client.

SELECTED HEALTH PROBLEMS

✖ ALCOHOL

1. Definitions
   a. *Alcohol* is a mind- and mood-altering substance classified as a central nervous system depressant.
      1. alterations in neurotransmitter systems, such as serotonergic, gamma aminobutyric acid (GABAnergic), dopaminergic, and the brain's reward system play a role in alcoholism and other addictions
      2. twin and adoption studies suggest a strong genetic predisposition
      3. psychosocial and cultural factors also play a role in drinking patterns
   b. *Alcoholism (alcohol dependence):*
      1. no agreement on definition; clinical features: chronicity; preoccupation with drinking; loss of control over drinking; damage to health, relationships, or work; using alcohol as a solution to most problems
      2. the World Health Organization definition: a chronic disease or disorder of behavior characterized by alcohol consumption that exceeds customary use and interferes with the drinker's health, interpersonal relations, or economic functioning
2. Effects
   a. At low levels of consumption, there is little apparent effect on the drinker; moderate levels may produce euphoria; and in large amounts, alcohol acts as a sedative.
   b. Alcohol depresses higher cortical functions, acts as a disinhibitor and tranquilizer, and serves to reduce anxiety rapidly (excessive drinking is often the way a person copes with anxiety).
3. Scope of alcohol abuse and dependence
   a. Estimates
      1. one third of general hospital clients, but these clients are rarely admitted with a diagnosis of alcoholism
      2. about 1 out of 10 Americans who drinks is an alcoholic
      3. about 17 million adults in the United States are alcoholic
      4. about 1 in 10 alcoholics is diagnosed and treated
   b. Occurrence: alcoholism and related problems are widespread among
      1. city residents
      2. various socioeconomic and ethnic populations and cultures
      3. poor men under 25 years of age
      4. persons who have experienced childhood disruptions (e.g., broken homes, childhood traumas, alcoholic parents)
      5. rural or small-town persons who have moved to urban areas
      6. families with a history of alcoholism
4. Characteristics common but not exclusive to persons with alcoholism
   a. Low self-esteem
   b. Feelings of isolation, depression

c. Emotional immaturity and excessive dependence
d. Anger and hostility
e. Highly anxious in interpersonal relationships
f. Inability to express emotions adequately
g. Ambivalence toward authority
h. Grandiosity
i. Compulsiveness, perfectionism
j. Excessive use of denial, projection, rationalization
k. Inability to modulate frustration, stress, and anxiety
l. Poor impulse control and the need for immediate gratification

5. Withdrawal from alcohol and detoxification
   a. Symptoms develop when there is a physiologic dependence and when the intake of alcohol is interrupted or decreased without substitution of other sedation. Symptoms may vary from mild to severe.
   b. Complete cessation of use of alcohol is not necessary for the development of withdrawal symptoms; the beginning of withdrawal can be a reflection of diminished use in those who have developed a high tolerance and physical dependence.
   c. Monitored detoxification for withdrawal is the top-priority need of the client with alcohol dependency.
   d. Withdrawal syndrome has four major manifestations: tremulousness; visual, tactile, and auditory hallucinations; alcohol withdrawal seizures; and delirium tremens. This is a progressive process and involves four stages:
      1. *stage 1;* emerges within 8 hours plus after cessation; symptoms include mild tremors, nausea, intense anxiety and nervousness, tachycardia, increased blood pressure, diaphoresis
      2. *stage 2;* symptoms include profound confusion, gross tremors, nervousness and hyperactivity, insomnia, anorexia, general weakness, disorientation, illusions, nightmares; auditory and visual hallucinations begin
      3. *stage 3;* within 12 to 48 hours after cessation; symptoms include all those of stages 1 and 2, as well as severe hallucinations and grand mal seizures ("rum fits")
      4. *stage 4;* occurs 3 to 5 days after cessation; symptoms include initial and continuing delirium tremens (DTs), which are characterized by confusion, severe autonomic arousal, psychomotor activity, agitation, sleep disturbances, hallucinations, and at onset uncontrolled and unexplained tachycardia; DTs are a medical emergency (fatality rate is 20% even with treatment)

6. Prognosis: motivation and recognition of the problem are necessary for eliminating alcohol use; the person experiences fluctuations of sobriety or recovery, during which acknowledging illness and moving toward a new way of life are challenged by relapse and denial; persons suffering from alcoholism are considered as recovering, not cured

7. Treatment: approaches used in all alcohol treatment models
   a. General measures include vitamin and nutritional therapy, sedatives, tranquilizers, and anticraving agents, such as selective serotonin reuptake inhibi-

tors (SSRIs) (e.g., fluoxetine), naltrexone, and older drugs such as disulfiram (Antabuse); avoid drugs containing alcohol (e.g., elixirs, cough syrups, mouthwashes)
   b. Detoxification: the acute phase of treatment
      1. involves close observation and safety measures to prevent severe reaction while withdrawing from alcohol
      2. fluids are used when dehydration is determined
      3. magnesium sulfate 50% solution and high doses of chlordiazepoxide (Librium) or other benzodiazepines (e.g., lorazepam, especially in the elderly and in individuals with liver damage) are used to prevent alcohol withdrawal seizures and hallucinations
      4. thiamine 50 to 100 mg intramuscularly (IM) to treat malnutrition
      5. education and group process are frequently used after detoxification when client is able to understand instructions
   c. Rehabilitation
      1. aim is to build treatment motivation and overcome denial in clients and significant others
      2. the client with alcoholism has to learn to give up alcohol forever
      3. the person is helped to learn new ways of problem solving and living a satisfying life without alcohol; this is enhanced by a therapeutic relationship that expands the alcoholic's self-confidence, coping skills, feelings of self-worth, and attempts to become more independent
   d. Major models of treatment
      1. chronic disease model
         a. views alcoholism as a primary, physiologic, incurable disease
         b. views psychosocial problems as result of drinking
         c. includes a maintenance program of recovery
         d. emphasis is on self-diagnosis by the person with alcoholism
      2. neurobiologic model
         a. surmises treatment that targets altered neurotransmitter and brain reward systems and includes medications that reduce alcohol craving, such as SSRIs (fluoxetine) and the use of opiate antagonists (naltrexone)
         b. biologic interventions must be supplemented by other psychosocial interventions, including cognitive therapy, 12-step programs, and relapse prevention programs
      3. psychiatric model
         a. varying psychotherapeutic treatment regimen depends on individual
         b. underlying maladaptive issues are assessed and addressed in treatment
      4. family systems model
         a. views family relationships as a contributing factor; chemical dependency is viewed as a family illness
         b. examines childhood development of alcoholic, such as drinking patterns of parents, cultural

and ethnic attitudes, and socialization process regarding drinking behaviors

    c. looks at family roles, communication and problem-solving patterns, family rules, family secrets, and power structure in the family

    d. identifies how present family relations re-create old patterns of avoidance or dependence, which may persist across multiple generations

    e. uses family commitment and caring to promote recovery

    f. integrates recovering alcoholic into revised family structure

  5. neurobiologic theory

    a. numerous studies support the genetic theory of alcoholism (e.g., specific genes have been identified as risk factors of alcoholism)

    b. increased familial vulnerability of alcoholism has also been identified as a risk factor in this disease

e. Alcoholics Anonymous (AA) is a self-help group of recovering persons with alcoholism

  1. a 12-step program enables members to achieve and maintain sobriety at their own pace

  2. run entirely by individuals recovering from alcoholism

  3. requires members to devote themselves completely to mutual help

  4. remarkable success with chronic alcoholism

  5. has member groups for families of alcoholics who themselves suffer from codependency (i.e., dependency on the individual with alcoholism)

    a. Al-Anon is an organization of friends and families of alcoholics

    b. Alateen is an organization of teenagers affected by alcoholism

    c. ACOA is an Al-Anon organization for adult children of alcoholics

    d. the emphasis of Alcoholics Anonymous is on changing oneself to make the most of one's life, develop a healthier lifestyle, education, guidance in relating to the alcoholic family member, the sharing of problems and experiences, and support based on a 12-step program

f. Long-term treatment also may take place in a structured environment, such as a private or public facility or community-based outpatient settings

  1. depending on the particular model used, emphasis varies among group process, education, psychotherapy, family therapy, and AA

  2. AA is the foundation to maintain sobriety; some clients attend daily

8. Preventive measures include helping the client learn to

  a. Cope and effectively modulate psychologic stress and anxiety

  b. Plan ahead for anticipated painful or stressful events (surgery, separation from a loved one, job interview, birth of child)

  c. Reduce social isolation and seek out supportive family and friends

  d. Communicate honestly

  e. Participate in health maintenance activities (e.g., proper nutrition and exercise program)

  f. Use adaptive coping behaviors

9. DSM-IV classifications: alcohol intoxication, alcohol withdrawal, alcohol intoxication delirium, alcohol withdrawal delirium, alcohol-induced persisting dementia, alcohol-induced persisting amnestic disorder, alcohol-induced psychotic disorder, with delusions/with hallucinations, alcohol-induced mood disorder/anxiety disorder/sexual dysfunction/sleep disorder, alcohol-related disorder not otherwise specified, alcohol dependence, alcohol abuse

Nursing Process

ASSESSMENT

1. Physical assessment/history

  a. Skin: spider angiomas, jaundice, acne rosacea, multiple bruises, age of bruises (purple, yellow), mahogany finger stains, "dirty tan," flushed ruddy complexion

  b. Musculoskeletal system: vaguely explained fractures, moderate muscle wasting of proximal muscle groups of lower and upper extremities

  c. Cardiovascular system: a first episode of paroxysmal atrial tachycardia as adult, ventricular premature contractions, paroxysmal atrial fibrillation, erratic hypertensive course (alcohol elevates blood pressure)

  d. Gastrointestinal system: early tooth loss, esophagitis, gastritis, pancreatitis, palpable liver, peptic ulcer, epistaxis, anorexia, weight loss, jaundice, cirrhosis, history of gastrointestinal bleeding, abdominal distention

  e. Neurologic system: tremors that worsen with movement, vertigo and nystagmus that clear during the day, vaguely described memory lapses (blackouts), insomnia, seizures, peripheral neuropathy, hallucinations, cognitive disturbances (e.g., remote and recent memory impairment, confabulation)

  f. Genitourinary system: mild proteinuria, orgasmic/erectile dysfunction; prostatitis

  g. Indications of fluid and electrolyte imbalance

  h. Respiratory system: repeated upper respiratory infections

2. Psychosocial assessment

  a. Suicide potential

  b. Extent of cognitive disturbance

  c. Mental status exam

  d. Occurrence of signs and symptoms related to major psychiatric disorders

  e. Degree of depression or anxiety

  f. Current alcohol type and consumption, age of onset, last drink, and previous history of treatment and sobriety

  g. Perception of use and degree of denial

  h. Quality of support system

3. Other: although not diagnostic themselves, the following raise possibilities and should be explored further

  a. Numerous transient medical symptoms in various organ systems without mention of drinking

  b. Unwarranted complaints and signing out against medical advice (hospitalized clients)

c. Functioning at lower job level than intelligence and education would indicate; changing jobs frequently
d. Alcoholism in close relatives (parental alcoholism increases likelihood fivefold)
e. Child or spouse abuse
f. History of fights or legal problems (e.g., frequent traffic violations)
4. Strengths and stressors, coping mechanisms
5. Beliefs, attitudes, feelings, concerns about alcohol consumption
6. Codependency behaviors in family and friends: enabling behaviors that perpetuate the drinking behaviors; dependence on individuals with alcoholism; overly responsible for others needs and feelings (in children); denial and poor coping; signs of chronic stress
7. Prescription or illicit drug use

ANALYSIS/NURSING DIAGNOSES (see p. 80)
PLANNING, IMPLEMENTATION, AND EVALUATION

Goal 1: Client will withdraw from alcohol and be free of systemic complications.

Implementation
1. Observe for withdrawal symptoms (anxiety, anorexia, insomnia, tremor, agitation, disorientation leading to delirium, tachycardia, hallucinations [prominently visual]) beginning shortly after last drink and lasting 5 to 7 days.
2. Monitor for delirium tremens (severe withdrawal behaviors) beginning 2 to 3 days after cessation of alcohol ingestion and lasting 48 to 72 hours.
3. Administer antianxiety drug, such as lorazepam or diazepam, and monitor for desired and adverse reactions.
4. Institute seizure precautions.
5. Monitor I&O, administer 2500 ml fluid per day as tolerated; avoid caffeinated drinks.
6. Weigh daily to monitor fluid retention.
7. Monitor electrolytes; report abnormalities.
8. Give vitamin/mineral supplements, especially B-complex vitamins.

Evaluation
Client safely withdraws from alcohol without evidence of nutritional imbalance, seizures, fluid and electrolyte imbalances; remains safe during episodes of disorientation, hallucinations.

Goal 2: Client will develop healthier coping mechanisms.

Implementation
1. Express concern for client's situation and confidence in ability to recover.
2. Intervene to decrease denial and manipulative behavior.
3. Share your observations (e.g., client's behaviors) with client, being as direct and genuine as possible; help client relate this behavior to alcohol intake.
4. Deal with angry behavior resulting from confrontation; know that although the anger may be directed at staff,

it may stem from emerging insight into the problems; direct anger into constructive outlets (e.g., exercise, art, journaling, music).
5. Intervene in withdrawal behavior that may result from grieving process and result in relapse; express confidence in client's ability to recover.
6. Discuss drinking pattern with client to identify triggers, cues, "slippery places" (cognitive-emotional-biologic-behavioral responses to stress); talk about what a lifestyle without alcohol would be like.
7. If receiving disulfiram therapy to control impulsive drinking, explain symptoms if alcohol is ingested (headache, severe gastrointestinal distress, tachycardia, hypotension). This form of treatment is enhanced by behavioral contracts.
8. If receiving naltrexone therapy to reduce alcohol craving, explain transient side effects, which include nausea, gastrointestinal distress, musculoskeletal pain, sleep disturbances, and anxiety; this medication has shown success with more severe, chronic post-inpatient forms of alcoholism.
9. Discuss possibilities of continuing psychotherapy, a 12-step program (AA, Al-Anon, Alateen), or a transitional living program; arrange for a referral if client is receptive.
10. Initiate frequent staff conferences to share therapeutic insights and ideas, and air responses to client's manipulative or angry behavior.
11. Collaborate with client and develop a contract for behavior change.

Evaluation
Client practices new coping behaviors; experiences increased self-esteem, social skills; explores group support; initiates insight or behavioral therapy.

Goal 3: Client and family will accept the support of concerned others; will establish a lifestyle without alcohol.

Implementation
1. Involve client in assertiveness training and group therapy to help client recognize the impact of behavior on others.
2. Reinforce contacts with 12-step programs and psychotherapy.
3. Encourage new relationships that do not involve alcohol; be supportive during loss of old relationships.
4. Permit family to express anger regarding client's behavior; help them see their roles as enablers.
5. Help family and staff understand that relapse is a strong possibility but does not mean failure or futility.
6. Know that alcohol-dependent persons are susceptible to adopting other dependencies and developing cross-addictions (e.g., benzodiazepines).

Evaluation
Client and family attend therapy and support groups; client engages in and practices behaviors that decrease social isolation and strengthen new behaviors and drug-free relationships; family recognizes and decreases enabling behaviors.

�֍ DRUGS OTHER THAN ALCOHOL

1. Opiates and opiate derivatives, synthetic opiates (e.g., morphine, Demerol, Dilaudid, codeine, heroin): chronic abuse results in tolerance, physical dependence, habituation, and addiction.
   a. Psychologically, individuals addicted to opiates show a similarity to those using alcohol in some aspects of personality traits (e.g., emotional immaturity; dependent, hostile, and aggressive behavior; and a tendency to take drugs to relieve inner tensions).
   b. Individuals addicted to opiates sometimes differ from alcoholics in that the former handle their feelings passively, by avoidance rather than by acting out; choosing drugs (opiates) seems to suppress these inner tensions.
   c. Availability (abuse may begin after surgery or illness), curiosity, and peer pressure play roles in the use of opiates; social factors, such as urban versus rural differences and social class, may also play a role.
   d. Cultural values regarding the use of opiates may play a role in the rates of addiction.
      1. Asian countries in which opiate addiction has been tolerated have a high rate
      2. Western European countries, where opiate addiction is treated as a medical rather than a legal problem, have low rates
   e. Opiate users may be in a methadone maintenance program as part of treatment and continue to misuse drugs.
2. Barbiturates and other sedative drugs (e.g., meprobamate, glutethimide, chlordiazepoxide, secobarbital, diazepam, alprazolam), if compulsively and chronically abused, cause tolerance, habituation, addiction, and physical dependence.
   a. There is a general, depressant, withdrawal syndrome associated with all of these drugs.
   b. Many users of the sedative drugs began with a physician's prescription; prescription drugs are considered socially acceptable in Western society for the relief of tension and insomnia.
   c. Persons who become chronic and compulsive users of these drugs tend to have a variety of underlying psychologic difficulties:
      1. persistent anxiety or a sense of insecurity
      2. attempts to relieve hostile and aggressive impulses
      3. efforts to reduce tension or escape through the drug's euphoric effect
   d. Gradual withdrawal reduces the incidence of seizures.
3. Amphetamines and cocaine (see also reprint, p. 101) are central nervous system stimulants, and intoxication produces euphoria.
   a. Chronic and compulsive abuse results in tolerance and habituation. NOTE: "Crack" cocaine is the most addictive drug introduced in Western society.
   b. Withdrawal from these drugs results in general fatigue, depression, suicide risk, and changes in sleep electroencephalograph (EEG) patterns; physical dependence is not associated with the abuse of these drugs, and therefore these symptoms are not considered a clinical withdrawal syndrome.
   c. Chronic use or intoxication can produce a substance-induced psychosis, characterized by vivid hallucinations, agitation, autonomic nervous system arousal (increased blood pressure and heart rate, dilated pupils, sweating), and persecutory delusions.
   d. Social, cultural, neurobiologic, and psychologic factors have all been cited as causative: family history of alcoholism and maladaptive behaviors, availability, peer pressure, curiosity, and misuse or prolonged use of prescriptive drugs. The use of these drugs for obesity or depression is more socially acceptable than their illicit use.
   e. Individuals addicted to amphetamines or cocaine tend to use other drugs, such as barbiturates, alcohol, or opiates.
4. Hallucinogens (e.g., lysergic acid diethylamide [LSD], mescaline, "angel dust" [PCP], STP, 3,4-methylenedioxymethamphetamine [MDMA] [Ecstasy, Adam, XTC, X] produce tolerance and in some persons habituation.
   a. These agents do not produce physical dependence with its concomitant withdrawal syndrome or addiction.
   b. May produce acute panic and anxiety states and substance-induced psychosis, characterized by hallucinations, agitation, persecutory delusions, and in extreme cases self-mutilation.
   c. Historically, these drugs have played a major role in religious practices of Native Americans and Mexican Indians.
   d. Recently they have been used by persons, particularly adolescents, who wish to explore their feelings in altered states of drug-induced intoxication.
   e. Persons who abuse these drugs are thought to be psychologically insecure, dependent, hostile, and immature.
   f. Social class seems to be a factor in the use of hallucinogens, with well-educated, middle or upper class persons being more frequent users.
   g. The potency of these agents is less (20 to 80 μg per dose) compared with 100 to 200 μg per dose in the 1960s.
5. DSM-IV classification: substance dependence, substance abuse (or diagnoses that include a specific drug, such as cocaine dependence, amphetamine dependence, opioid dependence, phencyclidine [PCP] dependence, sedative dependence, hypnotic dependence, anxiolytic dependence, etc.).

Nursing Process
ASSESSMENT
1. Physical status/examination: respiratory, circulatory, neurologic problems associated with withdrawal (priority); see Table 2-19
2. After emergency treatment, assess for problems arising from
   a. Consequences of drugs
      1. nasal septum erosion (cocaine)
      2. potential seizures (cocaine, barbiturate withdrawal)
      3. tolerance

4. stroke secondary to cerebral aneurysm (cocaine)
5. sudden death or myocardial infarction (cocaine)
   b. Sepsis associated with drug injection
      1. abscesses of skin and subcutaneous fat deposits
      2. hepatitis
      3. septicemia
      4. endocarditis
   c. Neglect of nutritional needs
      1. malnutrition
      2. loss of teeth, dental caries
      3. respiratory infections
   d. Increased risk of sexually transmitted disease (e.g., HIV) through contaminated needles or unsafe sex practice secondary to disinhibition
3. Behavior problems
   a. Denial or underreporting of use
   b. Somatic complaints
   c. Blaming others
   d. Anger, hostility, self-pity, mistrust
   e. Family, social, employment, and financial problems
   f. Inability to modulate stress and frustration effectively
   g. Criminal or antisocial activities (e.g., theft, stealing, murder)
   h. Grandiosity
   i. High dependency needs
   j. Violence toward self and others
   k. Suicidal attempts
4. Pattern of drug use, family problems

ANALYSIS/NURSING DIAGNOSES (see p. 80)
PLANNING, IMPLEMENTATION, AND EVALUATION

Goal 1: Client will safely withdraw from drug, remain free from respiratory failure, shock, substance-induced psychosis.

Implementation
1. Approach in a calm, reassuring, and nonjudgmental manner.
2. Intervene in respiratory failure: maintain a patent airway, give oxygen, administer naloxone hydrochloride (Narcan).
3. Administer intravenous fluids for shock or dehydration.
4. Observe the level of consciousness or changes in sensorium.
5. Administer drugs to minimize deleterious effects of withdrawal or substance-induced psychosis.
6. Give antibiotics when indicated.
7. Assess need for restraints and use as last resort for safety.

Evaluation
Client safely withdraws from drug and is free of major complications.

Goal 2: Client will decrease purposeful drug-seeking, manipulative, and acting-out behaviors.

Implementation
1. Set firm and consistent limits.
2. Clearly define acceptable and unacceptable behavior and consequences.

3. Know that the client often will complain that a nurse who does not cooperate lacks trust.
4. Be aware that the client may plead, cry, ask for money, steal, simulate drug withdrawal syndrome to obtain drugs.
5. Have entire staff employ consistent approach to client's behavior.

Evaluation
Client decreases purposeful drug-seeking, manipulative, and acting-out behaviors; accepts limits of treatment setting.

Goal 3: Client will decrease intellectualization; will focus on problem solving and activities of daily living.

Implementation
1. Know that client may exhibit dependency behaviors, blame parents, society, world conditions for drug-taking behaviors; be aware that the client may try to involve the nurse in intellectual discussion about these issues, but the nurse should avoid discussing these subjects with the client.
2. Keep focus on client's responsibility for own behavior; do not plead or exhort.
3. Focus on problems in ADL and possible solutions.

Evaluation
Client effectively discusses living problems and develops some solutions.

Goal 4: Client will minimize denial and superficiality; explore alternative coping mechanisms; verbalize some consequences of own actions.

Implementation
1. Confront the client face-to-face with facts about self that client attempts to avoid; use only after foundation of trust and acceptance has been laid or when group relationship is cohesive.
2. Limit discussions of "why" client abuses drugs.
3. Avoid pressuring client to promise total rehabilitation; realistic approach to possibilities of success must be taken.
4. Know that 90% of drug abusers relapse (this is part of the recovery process).
   a. The most effective treatment to date has been that given by former abusers (e.g., Narcotics Anonymous); having been in the situation, these persons are familiar with the demanding behaviors, manipulations, rationalizations, intellectualizations, and denial of drug abusers, and are able to consistently set firm limits using a supportive approach; clients are less likely to manipulate them.
   b. Do not make moral judgments.
   c. Avoid "rescuing" or enabling the client, assess the meaning of intense feelings of anger or hostility toward the client, and use informal peer support groups to address these issues.

Evaluation

Client decreases use of denial; begins to explore alternative coping behaviors; visits postdischarge treatment facility; decreases number and frequency of drug-misuse incidents.

> **Goal 5:** Family will recognize roles as codependents or enablers.

Implementation

1. Recognize that 50% of families in the United States have problems with substance abuse/dependence.
2. Avoid power struggles with client or family; focus on analyzing and restructuring relationships; teach how to avoid enabling behaviors.
3. Assess health teaching needs and initiate individualized teaching regarding various substances, short- and long-term effects of drugs, and behaviors that maintain addiction and trigger drug use.
4. Refer to self-help groups and 12-step programs as adjuncts to family therapy.
5. Collaborate with client and family and develop strategies that increase adaptive coping behaviors.
6. Recognize the possibility of relapse; be supportive while encouraging positive lifestyle changes during relapse.
7. Explore judicious use of confrontation strategies and therapeutic and supportive interventions.

Evaluation

Family discusses healthier lifestyle behavior; confronts client about unhealthy behaviors.

✴ ANOREXIA NERVOSA

1. Definition: a symptom complex with compulsive resistance to eating and maintaining body weight; intense fear of becoming obese, yet obsessed with food; loss of weight in excess of 15% of recommended body weight with no known physical illness to account for weight loss; body-image disturbance (feel fat when thin and emaciated); in females, absence of at least three consecutive menstrual periods
2. Onset: usually 12 to 18 years of age
3. Possible etiologies: biologic factors arising from complex neurochemical processes in the hypothalamic region; often linked with atypical affective disorder; phobic avoidance of adulthood; control of one's identity; disturbance in family relationships, especially with mother; societal demands for perfection and control; ambivalent feelings toward mother and independence
4. Prevalence reported in 12- to 18-year-old girls ranges from 1 in 100 to 1 in 800; 90% to 95% of all anorexics are females
5. Prognosis: reports that up to 21% die from malnutrition, intercurrent infection, or other physical problems; 17% to 77% recover
6. DSM-IV classification: other disorders include feeding and eating disorders of infancy and early childhood, which include pica (craving unnatural foods such as plaster from walls, dirt, clay) and rumination disorder, childhood, adolescent, and adult eating disorders include anorexia nervosa (specify type: binge-eating/purging type); bulimia (specify type: purging/nonpurging type); and eating disorder not otherwise specified.
7. Complications: metabolic abnormalities, muscle wasting, weakness, fatigue, bradycardia, orthostasis, decreased systolic blood pressure, body temperature below 36° C
8. Treatment: bed rest, hospitalization for intravenous or oral feedings to restore electrolyte and nutritional balance, psychotherapy, behavior modification, family therapy, pharmacotherapy (tricyclics, cyproheptadine [Periactin] with caution)

Nursing Process

ASSESSMENT

1. Weight and percentage of normal body weight lost
2. Eating patterns and duration of symptoms (time, amount, and types of foods taken)
3. Vomiting after eating or if food is forced
4. Anemia, hypotension
5. Amenorrhea (menstrual cycle)
6. Hair loss or thinning
7. Physical activities
8. Sleep
9. Relationships and interactions with parents, friends, staff, other clients
10. Feelings about eating, body image, self
11. Age at onset of altered eating patterns
12. Positive coping mechanisms, strengths, interests
13. Family history of anorexia or bulimia
14. Fluid/electrolyte balance
15. Dental erosion, oral hygiene
16. Vital signs
17. Mental status exam; level of dangerousness (e.g., suicide risk, self-mutilation)
18. Medication history, particularly misuse of laxatives, diuretics, or enemas
19. Psychiatric and medical treatment history
20. Substance misuse history, including over-the-counter and prescription medications (e.g., laxatives, diuretics, caffeine)

ANALYSIS/NURSING DIAGNOSES (see p. 80)

PLANNING, IMPLEMENTATION, AND EVALUATION

> **Goal 1:** Client will regain/maintain fluid and electrolyte balance and have adequate nutrition for growth and development.

Implementation

1. Approach in a calm and accepting manner; establish rapport.
2. Avoid threats, pleas, lectures, and health advice.
3. Keep accurate intake and output record; observe amounts and types of food eaten.
4. Observe for 2 hours after eating to prevent vomiting/regurgitation.
5. Administer tube feedings/intravenous feedings when indicated.
6. Provide positive reinforcement for weight gain rather than amount of food eaten.

7. Use the same scales to weigh client daily to three times a week.
8. Inspect the client's clothing for hidden objects that may inaccurately increase weight.
9. Explore client's feelings regarding increased weight gain.
10. Assist client in identifying "triggers" or high-risk situations or feelings that contribute to binging and purging.

Evaluation

Client regains/maintains fluid and electrolyte balance and has adequate nutrition for growth and development.

> **Goal 2:** Client will express feelings and concerns about self and treatment plan; will improve self-concept, will participate in treatment plan.

Implementation

1. Provide opportunities for decision making in treatment plan and ADL (e.g., time of meal, type of food to be eaten, hygiene, exercise, leisure activities).
2. Know that control issues are important dynamics; client must accept responsibility for self without guilt or ambivalence. Set and maintain firm limits; be clear about limits and consistent with treatment plan.
3. Provide opportunities for staff to meet to vent feelings about manipulative and self-destructive behavior.
4. Afford opportunities for challenging successful endeavors and positive reinforcement for adaptive behaviors.

Evaluation

Client expresses feelings and concerns about self and treatment plan; participates in treatment plan (e.g., makes decisions about schedule and activities).

BULIMIA

1. Definition: syndrome characterized by recurrent binge eating with lack of control (average of two binge episodes per week for 3 months), regular self-induced vomiting, use of laxatives or diuretics, dieting/fasting, vigorous exercise to prevent weight gain, overconcern with weight and body shape; usually maintains normal weight and appears healthy
2. Onset: adolescence or early adulthood (17 to 23 years of age)
3. Prevalence: reports of 1% to 4.5% of women affected, 0.4% of men
4. Etiology: same as anorexia
5. Prognosis: good if identified early; tends to be episodic with remissions and relapses
6. Complications (usually result of vomiting and laxative abuse): callus formation on back of hand caused by trauma from teeth while stimulating gag reflex; dental erosions and cavities; Mallory-Weiss tears resulting in bloody vomitus and blood loss; acid-base changes, especially hypokalemia; ipecac toxicity; hyperactivity; depression/suicide attempts
7. Treatment: psychotherapy, family therapy, behavioral therapy, hospitalization, outpatient treatment, pharmacotherapy (tricyclic antidepressants and MAO inhibitors), diet therapy, restoration of normal fluid/electrolyte balance
8. DSM-IV classification: listed with other eating disorders of adolescence

Nursing Process

See Assessment and Planning, Implementation, and Evaluation for anorexia, p. 87.

PSYCHOLOGIC FACTORS AFFECTING MEDICAL CONDITION (SPECIFY MEDICAL CONDITION)

1. Definition: psychologically meaningful environmental stimuli are temporarily related to the initiation or exacerbation of a physical condition with demonstrable general medical condition or known disease process
2. Sometimes confused with hypochondriasis (exaggerated concern with one's physical health); no association with an underlying general medical or physical condition
3. Reactions: eczema (skin), migraine headaches (cardiovascular system), backaches (musculoskeletal system), gastrointestinal and respiratory disorders, psychogenic pain
4. Ego defense mechanism used is repression: emotional tension is unconsciously channeled through organs
5. Occurrence: often seen in medical settings and becomes a psychiatric problem when anxiety escalates because of physical disorder
6. Possible secondary characteristics
   a. *Dependence:* a person may manifest abnormal dependency needs resulting from lack of confidence and poor living skills
      1. difficulty in making decisions
      2. extreme lack of confidence
      3. a need for more help in dealing with problems
   b. *Controlling behavior:* attempts to exercise a dominating influence over another person because of helpless feelings; manipulative techniques include negativism, obstinacy, silence, avoidance, talkativeness, crying
   c. Self-centeredness (narcissism)
      1. excessive self-attention because of low self-esteem
      2. DSM-IV: classified under psychologic factors affecting physical condition and the physical condition specified

Nursing Process

ASSESSMENT (see p. 80)

ANALYSIS/NURSING DIAGNOSES (see p. 80)

PLANNING, IMPLEMENTATION, AND EVALUATION

> **Goal 1:** Client will express feelings, perceptions, and concerns about symptom and treatment plan; client will participate in treatment plan.

Implementation

1. Verbally recognize and reinforce authentic communication of feelings, concerns, and perceptions.

2. Give appropriate information about medications and treatment.
3. Negotiate areas of self-care and independent activity.
4. Focus intervention on understanding and alleviation of primary symptoms.
5. Facilitate mutual exploration of the motivation for client's behavior.
6. Explore alternatives to the primary symptom for handling anxiety (e.g., talking directly about the concern, asking for help and support, setting limits with others, saying "no" appropriately).
7. Set clear and consistent limits on controlling/manipulative behaviors; state time limits; ensure consistency among staff; do not impose unnecessary controls.
8. Permit the client to retain control when appropriate; avoid power struggles with client/family
9. When manipulative behaviors occur, provide opportunities for staff meetings to air feelings and coordinate care.

Evaluation

Client accepts limits on controlling/manipulative behaviors; develops alternative coping mechanisms; participates in self-care.

BIBLIOGRAPHY

General

American Nurses Association: *Statement on psychiatric–mental health clinical nursing practice and standards of psychiatric–mental health clinical nursing practice,* Washington, DC, 1994, American Nurses Publishing.

American Psychiatric Association: *The diagnostic and statistical manual of mental disorders,* ed 4, Washington, DC, 1994, American Psychiatric Association.

Antai-Otong D: *Psychiatric nursing: biological and behavioral concepts,* Philadelphia, 1995, Saunders.

Baumann A, Johnston NE, Antai-Otong D: *Decision-making in psychiatric and psychosocial nursing,* 1990, St Louis, Mosby.

Beck C, Rawlins M, Williams S: *Mental health–psychiatric nursing: a holistic life-cycle approach,* ed 3, St Louis, 1992, Mosby.

Carpenito LJ: *Nursing diagnosis: application to practice,* Philadelphia, 1995, Lippincott.

Colorado Society of Clinical Specialists in Psychiatric Nursing: client's rights, *J Psychosoc Nurs Ment Health Serv* 28(2):38, 1990.

Colorado Society of Clinical Specialists in Psychiatric Nursing: Ethical guidelines for confidentiality, *J Psychosoc Nurs Ment Health Serv* 28(3):43, 1990.

Jost KE: Psychosocial care: document it, *Am J Nurs* 95(7):56, 1995.

Krupnick SLW, Wade AJ: *Psychiatric care planning,* Springhouse, Penn, 1993, Springhouse.

Rawlins R, Heacock P: *Clinical manual of psychiatric nursing,* St Louis, 1992, Mosby.

Sandler RL: Clinical snapshot: restraining devices, *Am J Nurs* 95(7):34, 1995.

Stuart G, Sundeen S: *Principles and practice of psychiatric nursing,* ed 5, St Louis, 1994, Mosby.

Varcarolis E: *Foundations of psychiatric nursing,* ed 2, Philadelphia, 1994, Saunders.

Loss and death and dying

Douville LM: The power of hope, *Am J Nurs* 94(12):34, 1994.
Nelson L: When a child dies, *Am J Nurs* 95(3):61, 1995.
Sanders TM: The good soldier, *Am J Nurs* 95(3):23, 1995.

Anxious behavior

Antai-Otong D: The client experiencing an anxiety disorder. In Antai-Otong D, editor: *Psychiatric nursing: biological and behavioral concepts,* Philadelphia, 1995, Saunders.

Badger JM: Calming the anxious patient, *Am J Nurs* 94(5):46, 1994.

Breakwell H: Are you stressed out? *Am J Nurs* 90(8):31, 1990.

Grainger R: Dealing with feelings: anxiety interrupters, *Am J Nurs* 90(2):14, 1990.

Hayes G, Goodwin T, Miars B: After disaster: a crisis support team at work, *Am J Nurs* 90(2):61, 1990.

Stolley JM: When your patient has Alzheimer's disease, *Am J Nurs* 94(8):34, 1994.

Stolley JM: Freeing your patients from restraints, *Am J Nurs* 95(2):31, 1995.

Townsend M: *Drug guide for psychiatric nursing,* St Louis, Mosby.

Elated-depressive behavior

Badger JM: Reaching out to the suicidal patient, *Am J Nurs* 95(3):24, 1995.

Cardell R, Horton-Deutsch S: A model for assessment of inpatient suicide potential, *Arch Psychiatr Nurs* 8(6):366, 1994.

Valente SM: Recognizing depression in elderly patients, *Am J Nurs* 94(12):18, 1994.

Personality disorders and other maladaptive behaviors

Chez N: Helping the victim of domestic violence, *Am J Nurs* 94(7):32, 1994.

Kinkle SL: Violence in the ED: how to stop it before it starts, *Am J Nurs* 93(7):22, 1993.

Whiting S: The client with a personality disorder. In Antai-Otong D, editor: *Psychiatric nursing: biological and behavioral concepts,* Philadelphia, 1995, Saunders.

Schizophrenia and other psychotic behaviors

Perry K, Antai-Otong D: The client with altered sensory perception: schizophrenia and other psychotic disorders. In Antai-Otong D, editor: *Psychiatric nursing: biological and behavioral concepts,* Philadelphia, 1995, Saunders.

Substance use disorders

Antai-Otong D: Helping the alcoholic patient recover, *Am J Nurs* 95(8):22, 1995.

Bennett EG, Woolf D: *Substance abuse: pharmacologic, developmental and clinical perspectives,* ed 2, Albany, NY, 1991, Delmar.

Hughes TL, Smith LL: Is your colleague chemically dependent? *Am J Nurs* 94(9):31, 1994.

Jansen E: A self psychological approach to treating the mentally ill, chemical abusing and addicted patient (MICAA), *Arch Psychiatr Nurs* 8(6):381, 1994.

Kinney J: *Clinical manual of substance abuse,* St Louis, 1991, Mosby.

Navarro T: Enabling behavior: the tender trap, *Am J Nurs* 95(1):50, 1995.

Plumlee AA: The client with addictive behaviors. In Antai-Otong D, editor: *Psychiatric nursing: biological and behavioral concepts,* Philadelphia, 1995, Saunders.

HELPING THE VICTIM OF DOMESTIC VIOLENCE

When your patient is one of the millions of women battered by a spouse or significant other each year, your instinct is to rescue her—but that's exactly what you can't *do.*

BY NANCY CHEZ, RN, MA

When I first met Ms. Blake, I was disturbed by the bruise around her eye and the overwhelming sadness of her expression. She'd been admitted by her family physician because of recurring headaches.

"How long have you had the headaches?" I asked.

"About a month," she said, "and I think they've gotten worse. This is the first chance I've had to see my doctor and he thought I should go into the hospital."

"The bruise around your eye," I continued, "how did you get that?"

"I bumped into something," she replied. "I've been very accident-prone lately."

An anxious look flickered across her face. She leaned toward me and whispered, "Listen, you really should ask my husband. He'll be here any minute. He can tell you whatever you want to know."

Something was wrong with this picture. Why the black eye? Why did she wait so long to get help? Why was she so eager to have her husband give her history instead of answering the questions herself?

I suspected Ms. Blake was being physically abused by someone at home. Though her admitting diagnosis of "R/O migraine" would be the primary focus of her care, the violence in her home was probably the real and more dangerous problem.

EVERY 15 SECONDS

An act of adult domestic violence occurs in the United States every 15 seconds—more frequently than any other crime. The great majority of its victims are women.

Broadly, the term "domestic violence" refers to a pattern of regularly occurring abuse and violence, or the threat of violence, in an intimate (though not necessarily cohabiting) relationship. Whether the abuse is physical, sexual, psychological, or economic, the heart of the problem is always an imbalance of power. The abuser learns that coercion "works," that it's effective in controlling the relationship and in reinforcing the power imbalance. In fact, control and domination can, in themselves, be forms of abuse. (See *The Five Forms of Domestic Abuse* on page 37.)

In the absence of physical injuries, one of the first indications of an abusive relationship can be—paradoxically—the husband's solicitousness toward his wife. When Mr. Blake arrived, I was struck by his persistence in wanting to see the doctor immediately. He seemed so devoted and concerned that his wife receive the very best care. "Why do we have to wait so long?" he protested. "My wife has a bad headache. Did she tell you how she got the black eye? Did she tell you that she's been really clumsy lately? That's my Jane," he said, smiling, "always bumping into something."

I suggested we use the time to finish Ms. Blake's history. But no matter how I phrased my questions and directed them toward Ms. Blake, her husband continued to answer for her. I asked if he'd like to sit in the lounge while I did my physical assessment. He refused outright. "I'm staying right here, in case my Jane needs me," he said.

SIGNS OF ABUSE TO LOOK FOR

Of course, in this case Ms. Blake did have physical evidence of abuse: her bruised eye. Though this wasn't absolute proof, it was a clue and needed to be investigated, especially because her story was so implausible. How could someone accidentally "bump into something" with enough force to produce the bruising and swelling that usually occurs with a black eye? What's more, her physical injury was in a central area of her body, making it unlikely that an accident was the cause.

Physical signs that a person may have been abused include:

• Injuries on unusual parts of the body, on several different surfaces, or in central areas—for example, the face, neck, throat, chest, abdomen, or genitals.

• Fractures that require significant force or that rarely occur by accident—for example, a spiral fracture, the result of a twisting motion.

• Multiple injuries at various stages of healing.

• Patterns left by whatever was used to inflict injury, such as teeth, ropes, hands, or utensils.

Nancy Chez is the clinical instructor in the emergency department at The New York Hospital in Manhattan. This article is based on the firsthand experiences, as well as the writings, of various domestic violence experts nationwide. The author wishes to acknowledge in particular the New York State Coalition on Domestic Violence and the New Jersey Coalition for Battered Women.
Modified from AJN, July 1994.

• Telltale burns such as those shaped like a cigarette tip or curling iron, or resembling a glove or sock because the extremity was immersed in scalding water.

• Injuries to a pregnant woman.

Behavioral indicators are subtle and may have no physical clues to confirm them. Recall that Ms. Blake described herself as "accident-prone" and put off seeing a physician for a month after the onset of symptoms. These are important clues. Many victims behave this way—ascribing their injuries to random accidents, avoiding medical attention—because they're too embarrassed, or feel responsible, or deny the abusive situation even exists. Some seek medical attention belatedly because they've been forbidden to leave the house.

The behavioral indicators of abuse that you may see include:

• Perhaps most important, recurrent episodes of injury attributed to being "accident-prone."

• Repeated visits to health care facilities.

• Complaints of pain without tissue injury.

• Thoughts about or attempts at suicide.

• Depression.

• Substantial delay between onset of injury and presentation for treatment.

Sometimes, patients report nonspecific complaints that result from abuse or the stress of an abusive situation. The health care team may not see these complaints as serious because there's no physical evidence. Instead, they may view the patient as having psychosomatic problems or as being hypochondriacal. As a result, the surface complaint is evaluated and the real and more dangerous problem is never discussed. What's worse, the patient is sent back to the environment where that problem still exists.

Be alert to these nonspecific complaints as possible indicators of abuse: headaches, musculoskeletal complaints (such as neckaches or backaches), malaise or fatigue, insomnia, chest pain or palpitations, hyperventilation, GI disorders, chronic pain, and anxiety.

FIRST, WHAT *NOT* TO DO

Once you've recognized that your patient is a victim of abuse, what should you do? First, beware of per-

BEYOND THE MYTHS: RECOGNIZING ABUSE VICTIMS

Our culture has supported various myths about domestic violence that may hinder your ability to recognize it. Here's a look at some of the more stubborn myths and the corresponding realities.

Myth: Family violence is most prevalent among the lower class.
Reality: Family violence occurs at all levels of society and without regard to age, race, culture, status, education, or religion. It may be less evident among the affluent because they can find and afford private physicians, attorneys, counselors, and shelters. In contrast, individuals with less financial resources must turn to more public agencies for help.

Myth: Violence rarely occurs between dating partners.
Reality: Estimates vary depending on which studies you read, but violence occurs in a large percentage of dating relationships.

Myth: Abused spouses can end the violence by divorcing their abuser.
Reality: According to the U.S. Department of Justice, about 75% of all spousal attacks occur between people who are separated or divorced. In many cases, the separation process brings on an increased level of harassment and violence.

Myth: The victim can learn to stop doing those things that provoke the violence.
Reality: In a battering relationship, the abuser needs no provocation to become violent. Violence is the abuser's pattern of behavior and the victim can't learn how to control it. Even so, many victims blame themselves for the abuse, feeling guilty—even responsible—for doing or saying something that triggers the abuser's behavior. Friends, family, and service providers reinforce this by laying the blame and the need to change on the shoulders of the victim.

Myth: Alcohol, stress, and mental illness are major causes of physical and verbal abuse.
Reality: Abusive people—and even their victims—frequently use those conditions to excuse or minimize the abuse. But abuse is a learned behavior, not an uncontrollable reaction. People are abusive because they've acquired the belief that violence and aggression are acceptable and effective responses to real or imagined threats.

Fortunately, since violence is a learned behavior, abusers can benefit from counseling and professional help to alter their behavior. But dealing only with the perceived problem (for example, the alcohol, the stress, or the mental illness) won't change the abusive tendencies.

Myth: Violence only occurs between heterosexual partners.
Reality: Increasing evidence suggests that gay and lesbian partners experience violence for varied but similar reasons as heterosexual partners do.

Myth: Being pregnant protects a woman from battering.
Reality: Battering frequently begins or escalates during pregnancy. According to one theory, the abuser who already has low self-esteem views his wife as his property. As a result, he resents the intrusion of the fetus as well as the extra attention his wife gets from friends, family, and health care providers.

Myth: Abused women tacitly accept the abuse by trying to conceal it, by not reporting it, or by failing to seek help.
Reality: Many women, when they do try to disclose their situation, are met with denial or disbelief. This only discourages them from persevering.

This information was adapted from the Domestic Violence Training Curriculum produced by the New York State Governor's Commission on Domestic Violence.

petuating the myth that something is wrong with *her*. The idea that a person could be so vulnerable that she would feel forced to continue living in a threatening, dangerous, and destructive environment is almost impossible for many people to accept. Often, well-meaning family members, friends, and health care professionals will say things like: "Why don't you just leave?" or "I would never let that happen to me!" or "What did you do to make him angry?"

Think of the effect those words can have on the victim. It's as if the other person were saying: "There must be something wrong with you." The implication is that the victim is inferior or weak for staying in the relationship and that she's knowingly and willingly tolerating the abuse. But assigning responsibility to the victim instead of the abuser only intensifies the victim's self-doubt and feelings of low self-esteem. As a result, she remains isolated, afraid to ask for help, and ultimately afraid to try to escape.

If you had a patient you knew or suspected was being abused, your first inclination would probably be to assure her safety after she's discharged. Commendable though that may be, you're not the person to do it. The person most qualified to determine whether the domestic abuse victim will be safe upon leaving the hospital is the victim herself.

That may sound like harsh advice, but it's important for three reasons. First, she has the right; the law views adults as responsible for their own care and as capable of making their own decisions. Second, only the victim can judge the safest time to leave without endangering lives, including her own. Third, victims of abuse have had their self-esteem attacked and every aspect of their lives controlled. Making decisions for them not only isn't helpful, it reinforces the loss of control that the victim is already feeling.

EMPOWERING THE VICTIM

The primary goal of intervention is empowerment. By sharing your observations, by agreeing that what's happening is wrong, just by listening in a warm and accepting way, you give the victim strength and determination. Many victims are relieved at the opportunity to tell the truth instead of constantly covering up. You may learn that you're the first person to confirm that the feelings of hurt and anger, the desire for support and change, are normal. Perhaps most important, you will have supported the patient's independence and autonomy as a decision-maker and helped her to recognize her strengths and resources as a survivor.

To facilitate this exchange, conduct the interview in a quiet, private environment where confidentiality is assured. Pick a time when you won't be interrupted, since your patient may interpret an interruption as rejection or lack of interest. (If you can't be sure of uninterrupted time, see if she'd be willing to talk with a chaplain or social worker.) If others are present, have them leave "until the patient is examined."

Ask the patient direct, nonthreatening questions in an empathetic manner. Examples of such questions are:

"Many patients tell me they've been hurt by someone close to them. Could this be happening to you? Are you being beaten?"

"You seem frightened when your husband is present. Does he frighten you? Why?"

"Are you in a relationship where you're being hurt physically or emotionally?"

If the patient confirms your observations, be ready to listen. As you do, look for opportunities to reassure her that nothing she could have done deserves this type of treatment. Emphasize that no one has the right to abuse another person, that it's in fact illegal, and that she has the right to personal

safety. Let her know that you're concerned about her physical safety and emotional well-being.

As you interact with the patient, be attentive to possible signs of a serious mental health problem such as depression, posttraumatic stress disorder, or suicide risk. Your patient may be clinically depressed if she's unable to sleep or having nightmares, isn't eating, is neglecting her physical needs, can't cope with social situations, experiences constant feelings of anxiety, or has thoughts of harming herself. Research suggests that victims of domestic abuse respond to their stress much like anyone who is subject to life-threatening situations over a period of time and that some of their behavior may reflect adaptation to chronic victimization and battering. In these instances, assessment should be followed through by a qualified mental health professional who is familiar with the field of domestic violence.

'DID SOMEONE HIT YOU?'

I decided to speak to Ms. Blake after the 10 AM medications and before visiting hours. Naturally, I had some doubts about how to raise this painful subject, but a straightforward approach seemed best. "Ms. Blake, I'm concerned about you," I said. "I've noticed the bruises on your face and that you seemed fearful when I asked how you got them. I'm also concerned because you waited so long to get help for yourself. Are you in a relationship that's hurting you physically or emotionally? Did someone hit you?"

At first she seemed reluctant to answer. She was just upset about her headaches, she said. But as she realized her explanation of the black eye wasn't believable, she began talking about the fight she had with her husband that led to the injury.

Eventually, Ms. Blake told me of frequent arguments, physical battering, and not being allowed to leave the house for weeks at a time. She also saw no escape from her husband's assaults because "he's all I've got." I told her that many patients tell me they've been hurt by someone close to them. I assured her that she still had the right to personal safety.

I avoided suggesting she should leave her husband and any implication that would make her feel guilty for

---

HOTLINE NUMBERS FOR VICTIMS OF ABUSE

National Organization for Victim Assistance (NOVA): 1-800-TRY-NOVA (for community information and referrals); (202) 232-6682
National Coalition Against Domestic Violence: (202) 638-6388; (303) 839-1852

IS THERE A TYPICAL ABUSER?

No one can say for sure why one person would habitually abuse another. But certain common traits do turn up in abusive or violent persons. Frequently, they were abused as children, or they witnessed someone else being abused. From this they learned that it's acceptable, even effective, to manage an intimate relationship by responding abusively or violently when they're feeling emotions such as stress, anger, and frustration. In short, they learned that violence is normal and that loving and hurting aren't incompatible. Also, abusive persons usually have low self-esteem, extreme possessiveness, and strong jealousy. They use these feelings to minimize the seriousness of the violence or to blame it on the victim's provocation.

FOR YOUR INFORMATION. . .

Domestic Violence, a two-part video program hosted by author Nancy Chez, is available from the American Journal of Nursing Company. Approved for 1.5 contact hours of CE credit, the program covers characteristics of abusers, forms of abuse, legal issues, and nursing responsibilities. For more information, call 1-800-CALL-AJN.

THE FIVE FORMS OF DOMESTIC ABUSE

Here are some illustrations of abusive behaviors that reflect domestic struggles for power and control.

Physical
- *Inflicting or attempting to inflict physical injury and/or illness*—for example, grabbing, pinching, shoving, slapping, hitting, hair-pulling, biting, arm-twisting, kicking, punching, hitting with blunt objects, stabbing, shooting.
- *Withholding access to resources necessary to maintain health*—for example, medication, medical care, wheelchair, food or fluids, sleep, hygienic assistance.
- *Forcing alcohol or other drug use.*

Sexual
- *Coercing or attempting to coerce any sexual contact without consent*—for example, marital rape, acquaintance rape, forced sex after physical beating, attacks on the sexual parts of the body, bestiality, forced prostitution, unprotected sex, fondling, sodomy, sex with others, use of pornography.
- *Attempting to undermine the victim's sexuality*—for example, treating her or him in a sexually derogatory manner, criticizing sexual performance and desirability. Also, accusations of infidelity, withholding sex.

Psychological
- *Instilling or attempting to instill fear*—for example, intimidation, threatening physical harm to self, victim, and/or others, threatening to harm and/or kidnap children, menacing, blackmail, harassment, destruction of pets and property, mind games.
- *Isolating or attempting to isolate victim from friends, family, school, and/or work*—for example, withholding access to phone and/or transportation, undermining victim's personal relationships, harassing others, constant "checking up," constant accompaniment, use of unfounded accusations, forced imprisonment.

Emotional
- *Undermining or attempting to undermine victim's sense of self-worth*—for example, constant criticism, belittling victim's abilities and competency, name calling, insults, put-downs, silent treatment, manipulating victim's feelings and emotions to induce guilt, subverting a partner's relationship with the children, repeatedly making and breaking promises.

Economic
- *Making or attempting to make the victim financially dependent*—for example, maintaining total control over financial resources including victim's earned income or resources received through public assistance or social security, withholding money and/or access to money, forbidding attendance at school, forbidding employment, on-the-job harassment, requiring accountability and justification for all money spent, forced welfare fraud, withholding information about family finances, running up bills for which the victim is responsible for payment.

Source: New York State Office for the Prevention of Domestic Violence

---

not getting out of an abusive and dangerous situation, or blaming her for its continuation. Instead, I let her know that I was concerned for her safety and wanted to offer her information about where help was available. I suggested that when she was ready, *she* would decide to use the available resources.

Fortunately, Ms. Blake was childless. Of the men who batter their wives, nearly three-quarters also batter their children. In fact, spouse abuse is one of the most identifiable risk factors for predicting child abuse—which affects millions of children each year as victims or witnesses.

ADDITIONAL STRATEGIES FOR HELP

The best resources I could give Ms. Blake were the local 24-hour toll-free hotline numbers for domestic violence and victims' service. (These numbers are available in all telephone books.) I assured her that the counselors who answer the phones have the experience and resources to provide information and emotional support to hundreds of victims. To give her some encouragement, I told her about some of the community resources I thought the counselors might suggest. They included:

• Emergency shelters that offer safe, temporary living space, food, clothing, transportation, advocacy to court, welfare, and health care systems, child care, and assistance with other alternative housing options.

• Appropriate counseling referrals, based on the caller's needs.

• Legal recourse if it's necessary to prevent continued harm and facilitate change. I explained that judges and police are becoming more sensitive to the needs of victims of domestic violence, but I also stressed that involving the police had to be *her* choice.

I offered her some brochures that I'd obtained from local victim support agencies and my hospital's social work department. She shook her head. "My husband would find them," she explained. I congratulated her on having the courage to make that decision, even though she might have felt obligated because I was trying to be helpful.

Since Ms. Blake had visible trauma, I asked if she'd agree to signing a consent form that would let me take an instant photograph of her face. I assured her I'd keep the photograph with her chart in case it needed to be reviewed from a legal standpoint at a later time. I marked the photo with her name and medical record numbers, and documented this interaction in my nurse's notes.

WHY SO MANY WOMEN STAY

As Ms. Blake intimated, many abused women don't believe they have any alternatives. The reasons are many. Some stay because they're afraid, don't have any money, have no other place to live, or don't think they can get a job. Others fear that family members will shun them, or that they'll lose custody of their children. Still others stay because of ties to the abuser, religious or cultural taboos, traditional or stereotypical ideas about marriage, or the desire to maintain a cohesive family for the children.

If your patient decides to return to her abusive husband, try to remain nonjudgmental. Assure her that you respect her judgment and recognize that this is a difficult time for her. Avoid the need to take control, "rescue" her, or limit her choices. Encourage her to take steps to protect her safety.

Offer your help in developing an action plan in case violence recurs. If she accepts, suggest that she have the following readily available:

• Access to documents that validate identification and eligibility for assistance—for example, birth certificate, social security number, income tax forms

  • Access to transportation
  • Extra set of keys
  • Emergency money
  • Emergency phone numbers
  • A safe place to go for the night
  • A packed suitcase, perhaps kept at a neighbor's
  • If she has children, whatever she'll need to take them along.

Ms. Blake chose to return home after three days of hospitalization. Natu-rally, I was concerned about her. But I hoped I had made some impact by letting her know that there were people who cared and that there would be resources available to her when she was ready. If nothing else, I felt I had at least planted a seed of hope.

SELECTED REFERENCES

Burge, S.K. Violence against women as a health care issue. *Fam. Med.* 21:368-373, Sept.-Oct. 1989.

Chez, R.A. If you suspect a patient is a victim of abuse. *Contemp. Ob/Gyn* 132-147, June 1987.

The Governor's Commission on Domestic Violence, New York (State) Department of Social Services and New York (State) Department of Health [now the New York State Office for the Prevention of Domestic Violence]. *Domestic Violence, A Curriculum for Hospital Emergency Departments.* Albany, NY, 1987.

Randall, T. Domestic violence intervention, call for more than treating injuries. [News] *JAMA* 264:939-944, Aug. 22-29, 1990.

Sabatino, F. Hospitals cope with America's new 'family value.' *Hospitals* 66:24-30, Nov. 5, 1992.

Schechter, S. Empowering interventions with battered women. In *Guidelines for Mental Health Professionals.* Washington, DC, National Coalition Against Domestic Violence, 1987, pp. 9-13.

THE POWER OF HOPE

How do you remain optimistic when the odds against your patient's recovery seem insurmountable? This nurse shares what she learned from her patient's remarkable response to an experimental form of cancer treatment.

BY LINDA M. DOUVILLE, RN, BSN

Jim Browning, 26, and his wife Margaret had been married two weeks when I first interviewed him to assess his eligibility for our adoptive immunotherapy program. I recall despairing at the destruction the metastatic malignant melanoma had caused in his body. CT scans revealed an 8- × 5-cm right renal mass, making his right kidney nonfunctional, and extensive retroperitoneal and mediastinal lymphadenopathy. His liver function was also deteriorating.

I could tell Jim was gravely ill just be looking at him. His pallor was striking, and he reported that he'd lost 25 pounds in the past four months. He walked slowly and carefully because of the pain in his right flank, mid-lower back, and right pelvic area. He also complained of intermittent shortness of breath at night.

As I mentally recorded his 19 sites of metastasis, I doubted Jim's chances of recovery and became skeptical about his participation, even though he met all the criteria for eligibility. To be considered for the program, a person must be between ages 18 and 75, and have either metastatic or renal cell carcinoma that is evaluable by observation or diagnostic imaging. He must also have a life expectancy of at least 12 weeks and be able to carry out all self-care activities. Even if a person has met these criteria, though, he may be ineligible if he has major systemic dysfunctions or has undergone prior treatment with interleukin-2 (IL-2).

All the conventional forms of cancer therapy had failed to help Jim. Im-

munotherapy seemed to be his last chance for life, and he and Margaret wanted desperately to try it. He was accepted into the program.

During the 10 weeks between our initial meeting and Jim's admission to the hospital for treatment, the optimism that he and Margaret displayed gradually transformed my uneasiness. I began to share their enthusiasm. My greatest fear, however, was that he wouldn't become a member of our 30% responder group, which includes patients who've experienced a complete response (total disease regression) or a partial response (at least 50% tumor reduction).

HOW IMMUNOTHERAPY WORKS

Jim wanted to learn more about immunotherapy, which has been in use for over 10 years. The treatment, I explained, is based on the fact that the surfaces of some types of cancer cells—melanoma being one of them—have structures, or molecules, that differ from the surface characteristics of noncancerous cells. When the body recognizes these tumor-associated antigens (TAA), it activates an immune response.

If that's true, Jim wondered, why didn't his body develop an initial immunity to the cancer cells and fight them off? I explained that the malignant cells in his body do elicit an immune response, but it isn't strong enough to kill them. And as the tumor cells grow and multiply, they become more aggressive, making the immune response even less effective.

Adoptive immunotherapy restores this imbalance by maximizing the body's existing immune response. In short, T lymphocytes—a type of immune cell that can successfully destroy

tumor cells—are isolated from the patient, expanded to greater numbers outside the body, and then reinfused into the patient to activate the immune response.

Jim was scheduled for surgery and a tumor tissue sample was taken from diseased retroperitoneal lymph nodes, since the T lymphocytes found on or near a tumor—called tumor-infiltrating lymphocytes (TIL)—are most effective against it. In the laboratory, the cells of the specimen were processed to disconnect them from each other in order to isolate the TIL. The TIL were then activated with a monoclonal antibody against the CD3 molecule, a structure that's found on all T lymphocytes. It plays an important role in inducing T cell proliferation, activating their destructive mechanism, and producing cytokines, which are crucial for activating other immune cells, such as natural killer (NK), lymphokine-activated killer (LAK), and B cells, involved in the rejection of tumor cells.

Finally, the TIL were expanded in IL-2, a T cell growth factor. When Jim's TIL culture had grown to therapeutic numbers—500 billion lymphocytes—we'd be able to start infusing him with doses of TIL and low-dose IL-2, which would activate the TIL in his body.

DECLINING RENAL FUNCTION

After six weeks, the culture had multiplied enough for us to begin treatment. Jim and Margaret were eager to start. Pretreatment CT scans of the chest, abdomen, and pelvis and a bone scan confirmed rapid disease progression. Jim's renal function continued to decline. It became clear that unless therapy was started soon, his elevated creatinine and blood urea nitrogen lev-

Linda M. Douville is clinical coordinator, Biologic Cancer Therapy Program, Brigham and Women's Hospital, Boston, MA.
Modified from AJN, December 1994.

els would soon render him ineligible for our protocol, since IL-2 tends to further impair renal function.

Jim was admitted on a Sunday and received three infusions of TIL that Monday, Wednesday, and Friday. Intravenous boluses of IL-2 were administered through a central venous line every eight hours, for a total of 28 days. After each TIL infusion was completed, Jim assured me that the lymphocytes had "gone to do their thing"—attacking the cancerous melanotic cells. He used visualization and described the "little Pac-Men" that were invading his cancer.

Not once did Jim or Margaret speak of the possibility of failure; their faith in the therapy's success, unlike my own, never wavered. They spent each day of the 10-day regimen planning their future together, dreaming of the honeymoon that Jim's diagnosis had interrupted and planning the family they wanted.

MEETING EACH NEW CHALLENGE

There were days when Jim had to fight off the desire to give up—though he didn't let on at the time. He later confided that he'd hung onto Margaret's strength "like threads," praying they wouldn't break.

Jim capitalized on the mind-body connection to combat his illness and keep his spirit strong. He'd been using visualization techniques successfully, and I searched the literature for concrete examples of the beneficial effects of support, prayer, and a positive attitude to reinforce their use.

Jim's increasing nausea, vomiting, diarrhea, and mucositis continually tested their resolve. He also experienced severe fluid retention from the expected capillary leak syndrome and gained about 25 pounds despite the gastrointestinal fluid loss. But somehow Jim and Margaret met the challenge of managing each new toxic symptom. With the nursing staff's assistance, they patiently sketched out a plan that would somehow make each of these adverse effects tolerable.

To successfully tolerate the IL-2, for example, Jim needed adequate hydration. To combat his nausea and vomiting, the nursing staff designed a schedule for administering antiemetics to improve his oral intake of fluids. About 40 minutes after each IL-2 dose, Jim would begin drinking large volumes of fluids in an attempt to maintain his urinary output at greater than 10 mL/hour. Administration of antidiarrheals was similarly timed to decrease the frequency of his liquid stools.

The oral mucositis that Jim developed during the second week of treatment inhibited his fluid intake. He tried gargling with viscous xylocaine 15 minutes before eating and drinking, and that relieved the pain enough so that he could swallow. By trial and error a medication regimen was devised that optimized his nutritional intake. Jim experienced nasal congestion and dry, painful nasal mucosa, which were alleviated by using a saline nasal spray. He also developed a dry, pruritic rash that worsened during the course of his therapy. We used Eucerin cream to alleviate the cracking and peeling and hydroxyzine to control the itch.

Jim also had trouble tolerating the TIL infusions, so before each subsequent dose we administer meperidine 25 to 50 mg IV. This helped prevent the adverse effects and relieved some of the discomfort the therapy had been causing him.

SIGNS OF IMPROVEMENT

Toward the end of treatment, blood work revealed that Jim's renal function appeared to be improving. This is unusual for patients undergoing IL-2 therapy, whose renal function typically diminishes during therapy but then returns to normal when the therapy is stopped. Jim's hepatic function improved too, which was also surprising. It was still too early for celebration, though. I informed Jim and Margaret that the most definite indicator of response would be CT scans taken four to six weeks post-treatment showing tumor regression.

At the end of his discharge interview, Jim gave me a beautiful flowering primrose in a ceramic pot. The accompanying note, which I'll hold dear forever, read: "Thank you so much for all your special care and commitment to my progress. Margaret and I can't begin to tell you how much it's meant to us."

Still, I'd never seen someone with such gross disease have such a complete response, and my initial skepticism was revived. I once again feared that Jim wouldn't make it into the responder group.

During the next few weeks I was busy treating other cancer patients and their families, and the waiting period for Jim's results passed swiftly. One morning the call came from Jim's oncologist. When I heard him say, "Jim's disease has regressed more than 90%," I screamed with delight.

After the oncologist shared the good news with Jim, he consulted with Jim's surgeon to see if he'd consider resection of both the kidney and remaining liver disease to render Jim disease-free. The surgeon agreed that surgery was indicated, and Jim's admission was scheduled for the following week.

The surgery was successful, and once again Jim and Margaret started planning their honeymoon. They were elated that the diseased kidney and portions of the liver were removed; they'd been blessed with a reprieve from the cancer.

Jim was discharged from the hospital only four days postoperatively. He was eager to learn if residual disease would be discovered histologically and asked me to call him as soon as I received the pathology report. When it came in seven days later, it indicated that Jim had had a complete response from the therapy. The kidney and resected liver tissue revealed only necrotic melanotic cells; no viable tumor cells were seen. Jim's postop CT scans also revealed no evidence of metastatic disease.

In all my years of nursing, I've never experienced greater joy for a patient than I did for Jim at that moment. Together, he and Margaret had beaten the odds. They scheduled a honeymoon cruise to St. John's, St. Thomas, and Martinique.

UNCHARTED TERRITORY

Almost two and a half years have passed since Jim's treatment, and his follow-up course of CT scans every four to six months remains uneventful. Although I'm hesitant whenever I answer the phone and hear his voice—for fear his disease might have recurred—I often think back to the day I met Jim and Margaret. I can recall vividly my feelings of doubt and recognize how much I learned from Jim while participating in his care.

Many nurses find it difficult to remain optimistic in the face of terminal illness. In coping with our own feelings of sadness and helplessness, we may struggle prematurely with a patient's fate (or what we feel is the patient's fate), as I did in caring for Jim. My involvement with cancer care research has taught me that nothing is impossible.

Although only a small percentage of the patients with such extensive metastasis respond as dramatically as Jim to adoptive immunotherapy treatment, I'm now able to remain hopeful yet realistic through the course of my patients' therapy. Experimental treatments of terminal illnesses are consistently appearing, and we may all be involved in caring for patients whose course may be less familiar than with conventional methods.

Incidentally, Jim and Margaret have recently purchased their first home and are planning a family. They continue to look forward to a long and full life together.

SELECTED REFERENCES

Eberlein, T.J., et al. CD3 activation of tumor-infiltrating lymphocytes. In *Immunotherapy of Cancer with Sensitized Lymphocytes,* ed. by Alfred E. Chang and Suyu Shu, Chicago, R.G. Landes Co., 1994, pp. 15-31.

Pennebaker, J.W. *Opening Up: The Healing Power of Confiding in Others.* New York, Avon, 1990.

Rosenberg, S.A. Adoptive immunotherapy for cancer. *Scientific Amer.* 262:62-69, May 1990.

Temoshok, L., and Dreher, H. *The Type C Connection.* New York, Random House, 1992.

AFTER DISASTER

A crisis support team at work

BY GLENYS HAYES/TRENA GOODWIN/BECKY MIARS

Ring-g-g.

Barely awake, I reached for the phone that Sunday morning back in May 1988.

"Trena? It's Glenys Hayes. We've got a disaster on our hands. A school bus crash. At least 12 children are dead and many more are injured. Can you go?"

Minutes earlier, Glenys had received a similar call from the Cincinnati Red Cross. We were asked to be part of a crisis-intervention team at the crash scene—about 55 miles away near Carrollton, Kentucky.

Glenys told me to report to the National Guard Armory in Carrollton, where a temporary morgue had been set up—and where I'd find Barb Hamond and Becky Miars, both experienced disaster nurses and members of the Red Cross Crisis Support Nursing Team (CSNT).

I dressed quickly, grabbed my Red Cross badge, and headed for Carrollton. On the way, I heard the news report on the radio. A church youth group from Kentucky was returning from an outing at an amusement park just north of Cincinnati. About 11 PM, a pickup truck hit the bus head-on, causing the bus to burst into flames. I tried to steel myself for what I'd find in Carrollton.

I arrived at the armory and met with the rest of the team to plan our work. We were told that 24 children and three adults had died and that many of the survivors had been taken to area hospitals. Since none of the bodies had yet been identified, we could not tell the families when they arrived whether their children were among the dead.

While Becky met the first family to arrive on the scene, I attended to the rescue workers in the morgue. Several were showing signs of exhaustion; one was crying. I suggested to their supervisor that they break for rest and food away from the scene. As I talked with the workers and with some of the church youth group's officials, I continued to plan how we could best help the families involved.

Meanwhile, Barb was arranging a reception area for the families. We needed a private area away from media and onlookers for the families and for the Red Cross staff. We also needed several motel rooms and additional phone lines. A nearby Holiday Inn and other local businesses provided everything we needed.

The loss of so many children had stunned the community; many felt a deep need to help in any way possible. All those who assisted with the disaster relief operation, especially those from the Kentucky State Police and the Kentucky Coroner's Office, did so with compassion and strength.

As we talked with each family, we felt a part of their pain. Parents asked, "Why?" and "How can we go on?" and "Can we see our child?" Some were hopeful that their children would be found alive. Others asked about making funeral arrangements.

Some of the families had been waiting all night long at the children's church for the ill-fated bus to return. Most of them were exhausted and had eaten nothing. They were beginning to feel the physical effects of their emotional strain. Some seemed to be in a state of shock; we provided them a place to lie down and blankets to keep them warm.

They needed privacy, a place where they were sheltered from questions of curious onlookers and the media. We comforted the families of missing children, helped them fill out missing-person forms, and generally provided a safe, nurturing environment similar to the one suggested by William James Black, Jr., which he called the "libidinal cocoon."[1]

Most of the parents expressed some degree of denial. They needed to hear the details of the accident to help them comprehend its reality. We asked them to tell us what their children looked like and what they were wearing—anything that might help the disaster workers locate them. As is the case with most disasters, we found it incredible to see so many lives altered forever.

HELPING THE VICTIMS

The Carrollton bus crash was just one of the many disasters the Cincinnati Red Cross Crisis Support Nurse Team has attended over the past two years. Most often, the nurses help the victims themselves, either at the scene or in the days that follow, when they need to be linked with the appropriate community services. A few recent incidents best illustrate what the CSNT does.

A CSNT volunteer went to the scene of an apartment fire where a single mother had lost two of her three children. The nurse stayed with the distraught mother, who, by the way, had

Glenys Hayes, RN, MSN, a volunteer coordinator for the Cincinnati Red Cross Crisis Support Nurse Team (CSNT), is a psychiatric staff nurse at University of Cincinnati (OH) Hospital. Trena Goodwin, RN, MSN, is a licensed professional clinical counselor, volunteer training coordinator for the CSNT, an adjunct assistant professor of psychiatry at the University of Cincinnati College of Medicine and a clinical specialist at the Central Psychiatric Clinic, Cincinnati. Becky Miars, RN, BSN, is director of the Deaconess Home Health Care Program in Cincinnati and chairs the Cincinnati Red Cross nursing and health committee.

Modified from AJN, February 1990.

[1]Black, J.W. Jr. *The libidinal cocoon: a nurturing retreat for the families of plane crash victims.* Hosp. Community Psychiatry 38:1322-1326, Dec. 1987.

a history of suicide attempts, to help her through the initial stages of shock and grief.

The woman vacillated between overwhelming grief and unresponsiveness. Her grief was compounded by feelings of guilt over not responding faster to her children's cries. It seems she'd thought that, as was often the case, the children were bickering. At times, she imagined that her children were still alive and that she had to get home to get her five-year-old ready for his graduation from kindergarten, schedule to take place later that same morning.

The nurse attempted, physically and verbally, to keep the woman oriented to reality. She tried to focus the mother's attention on the needs of her surviving 11-year-old developmentally disabled son. She also evaluated the amount of support family members and friends could provide. She asked neighbors to arrange that the door to the burned apartment be padlocked to keep the woman and her son from entering—something their degree of denial made it seem likely they'd attempt. And finally, the nurse made living arrangements for the woman and persuaded her to agree to emergency medical and psychiatric evaluation.

After another fire at a multiple dwelling, a CSNT volunteer shepherded a 10-year-old survivor through the aftermath of losing her entire immediate family and a close friend. The nurse comforted the girl and encouraged her to talk about what had happened. Additional members of the team worked with other bereaved relatives, later helping the families contact available community resources. Since several of the children who died in the fire had attended the same school, a CSNT volunteer discussed with the school's principal the classmates' reactions to the tragedy and how the school's staff could help them work through their grief.

Another time, at the request of a concerned Red Cross Social Services caseworker, a CSNT nurse visited a couple who, hours earlier, had lost their three-year-old and their home in a fire set by their four-year-old. The nurse found the couple distraught and unable to talk with one another. The nurse helped the couple talk about their feelings of anger and grief individually and

TRAINING PSYCHIATRIC NURSE VOLUNTEERS

Psychiatric nurses who volunteer their services to the Cincinnati Red Cross become well versed in crisis intervention strategies. The Red Cross CSNT training sessions focus on the psychological reactions of disaster victims and their families, the needs of special groups such as the severely mentally disabled, rescue-worker stress, disaster injuries, and debriefing.

Nursing process is effective in crises: one assesses needs and plans to meet them. Nurses, who find ready acceptance by victims and families, can watch for physical effects, the exacerbation of existing health problems, and for signs that the person is succumbing to the emotional trauma.

At disaster sites, inexperienced crisis nurses are paired with seasoned colleagues who provide on-site supervision and support. The Red Cross also stages disaster drills periodically to help prepare crisis-support nurses to respond to emergencies.

Because the CSNT is a volunteer group, close monitoring of the training process is essential; poorly prepared volunteers would not only be counterproductive at the scene, they'd soon feel overwhelmed and perhaps leave the volunteer service.

HOW THE CRISIS TEAM GOT ITS START

The very specific emotional needs of crisis victims became painfully apparent when the Cincinnati area suffered two disasters six years apart. The first was the 1977 fire that killed 161 people at a local supper club; the second was the fire that killed 23 people on board an airplane making an emergency landing.

Later, Glenys Hayes, an RN with a master's degree in psychiatric nursing, attended a workshop on disaster health services given at the Cincinnati Chapter of the Red Cross.

Red Cross staff nurse Jean Ellsworth recognized the psychological needs of disaster victims, families and friends of the victims, and rescue workers. So, with Red Cross nursing staff, Ellsworth, and several other nurses who'd had graduate-level psychiatric training, Hayes organized a volunteer program to address those needs: the Crisis Support Nurse Team (CSNT).

The CSNT consists of a coordinator, two assistant coordinators, a telephone chairperson, a training coordinator, and several psychiatric nurses. When a tornado, flood, plane crash, fire, or any other disaster occurs, the Red Cross responds. Most often, the Red Cross asks the CSNT to respond to disasters that involve loss of life.

then to each other. The nurse also helped them plan temporary housing and convinced them to keep their surviving four-year-old child with them rather than sending him to live with other relatives as they had planned.

Besides emotional support and appropriate referral, disaster victims and relatives also need personal care. After a tragedy, some survivors needed help getting their regular prescribed medicines. Many tend to consume alcohol and coffee in dangerous quantities, smoke cigarettes incessantly, and lose sight of their personal needs. CSNT volunteers gently remind them that mood-altering chemicals can only

worsen their anxiety—and might even precipitate other problems. The nurses also help survivors with their most basic needs, reminding them to eat, to drink enough fluids, and to bathe.

During disasters that involve many people, the Red Cross is often called upon to open and maintain a shelter—for a few hours or even for a week or more. The CSNT has developed a list of supplies to have on hand at such shelters, specifically for meeting the mental-health needs that arise. Crossword puzzles, card games, drawing materials, and toys, for example, are used for diversionary, recreational, and therapeutic purposes.

HELPING THE HELPERS

Disaster workers rarely notice how stressed they become during a crisis. Ideally, any one worker should not remain on the scene for more than eight hours at a time; in reality, such is not always the case.[2]

Besides encouraging workers to take breaks, the CSNT volunteers move among them, offering gentle encouragement and support. The nurses, too, need to be aware of their own levels of stress and take time out when they need to regroup.

---

[2]*Mitchell, J., and Resnick, H.L.* Emergency Response to Crisis. *Bowie, MD, Robert J. Brady Co., 1981, pp. 183-195.*

The Red Cross encourages all disaster workers, including the nurses, to go through a debriefing process immediately after their on-site work has been completed and again when the entire disaster operation ends. Debriefing is a process that focuses on feelings. It is designed to help rescue workers recognize the impact of a disaster on themselves and on others. Depending on the magnitude of the disaster, the formal debriefing may consist of one session or of several sessions conducted over time.

The program has had gratifying results on different levels. Nursing's support for a community in a time of crisis brings out the community's own strength. Nursing also achieves greater recognition of its skills. And individually, every nurse involved in the effort has expressed an enormous personal satisfaction.

For professionals who work with those who have chronic mental health problems and whose treatment is long term, immediate, positive results aren't often seen. For the crisis support nurse, however, who comes as a stranger to grieving families, shares their sorrow, and guides them through a horrible period in their lives, immediate gratification becomes a lasting reward.

IS YOUR COLLEAGUE CHEMICALLY DEPENDENT

Don't shrug off signs of possible impairment—the problem is more common than you might think. Knowing how to recognize and report it can literally make the difference between life and death.

BY TONDA L. HUGHES, RN, PhD, AND LINDA L. SMITH, RN, MN, CAP

"I thought she was just having a bad day."

That's what a distraught staff nurse at a major metropolitan hospital said about the day when colleague Luisa Velez (not her real name) died. Luisa had been found in her car shortly after her shift ended the day before. Syringes and broken vials—the debris of a lethal dose of Demerol—lay beside her, along with a half-empty whiskey bottle.

Most of Luisa's co-workers were just as shocked. At a critical incident debriefing session, several said they'd noticed unusual behavior, but thought Luisa was probably having personal problems. One had noticed Luisa's eyes were glassy and her hands trembled, that she seemed hurried and out of sorts. Another said Luisa's speech sounded slurred one day when she'd called in sick. But they hadn't been trained to look more closely and to intervene appropriately when signs like these appear. Their observations were never documented or reported,

Modified from AJN, September 1994.
Tonda L. Hughes is assistant professor of psychiatric nursing and postdoctoral fellow at the Prevention Research Center of the University of Illinois at Chicago School of Public Health. Linda L. Smith is executive director of the Intervention Project for Nurses in Jacksonville, FL, a statewide program to assist nurses whose practice may be impaired due to substance abuse or psychological or physical conditions.

and nothing that could have helped Luisa was done.

Could there be a Luisa working on your unit? Don't dismiss the question lightly: Chemical dependency is more common among nurses than you might think, and it isn't always obvious. Fortunately, you're in an excellent position to spot a chemical dependency problem in a co-worker. Few professional relationships, after all, are as intimate as those between nurses who work together. Here we'll describe the overt characteristics of chemical dependency and how to distinguish them from a "bad day." We'll outline what steps to take—and what not to do—in reporting a colleague's problem. And we'll look at how the chemically dependent nurse can be helped.

A HARSH REALITY

The American Nurses Association has estimated that 6% to 8% of nurses use alcohol or other drugs to an extent sufficient to impair their professional performance. And, it's clear that Luisa's wasn't an isolated case. A Texas researcher found that nearly two-thirds of chemically dependent nurses studied had seriously considered taking their own lives, compared to fewer than one in five nondependent nurses.

Denial is a defining feature of addiction, and the chemically dependent nurse is often the last to see that she has a life-threatening illness. But, as in Luisa's case, the nurse's colleagues also may be slow to recognize or acknowledge the problem.

Partly, that's due to most nurses' lack of knowledge about addiction. Nursing school courses generally focus on the physiologic effects of alcohol and other drugs, and deal little with the psychological process of addiction and even less with chemical dependency in nurses. Consequently, nurses may hold stereotypical views of alcoholics and drug addicts as "skid row bums" or inner city "junkies"—not people who hold important positions, and certainly not those responsible for the lives of others.

Many of us are also blinded by fear of what will happen to the nurse or to us if her problem is discovered. In Luisa's case, one nurse explained, "I've heard of nurses losing their jobs and licenses because of problems like this." Although her concern about Luisa was understandable, it may have prevented Luisa from getting the help she badly needed. And as long as Luisa was willing to accept help, she might have kept both her license and her job.

Another nurse wondered, "What would happen if I were wrong? Could I be sued?" She could, of course, but most nurse practice laws contain some protection for the nurse who reports in good faith a colleague who appears to be impaired. Many health care facilities' policies also address this issue.

Nurses also worry about being labeled a "whistle blower" or "not a team player," even though they know that duty to patients who could be in jeopardy is a higher imperative than loyalty to institution or co-workers.

Then there's our own denial. Because of the stigma attached to chemical dependency, we may be reluctant to acknowledge to ourselves or others that a member of the profession, a colleague, and perhaps a friend has a problem.

Still, nurses have both an ethical and a legal responsibility to report chemical dependency in a co-worker. An ethical duty to report is implied by the American Nurses Association's *Code of Nurses,* which states that a nurse will act to safeguard patients and the public when health care is affected by incompetent, unethical, or illegal practice. And in about 25 states, nurses are legally required to report any colleague who uses alcohol or drugs at work or who they suspect is chemically dependent. It's a good idea to know the law in your state and your legal responsibilities. Accordingly, your hospital policy may require nurses and other employees to report signs and symptoms that could indicate substance abuse by a co-worker.

ALCOHOL ABUSE MOST PREVALENT

The signs of chemical dependency vary with the substance involved and the amount used. An alcoholic nurse, whose drug supply is outside the workplace, will exhibit a different behavior pattern at work (absenteeism, abuse of lunch and other break periods) from that of a nurse dependent on the hospital's supply of meperidine (working extra shifts, "hanging around"). A nurse who is abusing marijuana or cocaine, like the nurse who is alcoholic, may also present with a pattern of absenteeism and deteriorating work performance.

Although the use of controlled substances, particularly those taken from narcotics cabinets, tends to get the most attention in the professional literature and popular media, alcohol abuse is much more prevalent. Of drugs other than alcohol, especially those obtained at work, meperidine is by far the most commonly used by nurses.

Signs of chemical dependency fall into three general categories: decline in job performance and professional image, personality and mental status changes, and behavior suggesting drug diversion (see *Warning Signs of Chemical Dependency,* opposite, for some of the most common signs).

One or a few of these signs in isolation don't necessarily mean a co-worker has a substance abuse problem. It's the rare nurse who doesn't make a charting error now and then. Lack of sleep or stress on the job may lead to an occasional memory lapse or even emotional irritability. But when a pattern begins to emerge of behavioral and work performance changes—inappropriate emotional responses, mistakes in patient care, inaccuracies in charting and communication—it may indicate that your co-worker is having more than a bad day or a passing personal crisis.

If you've witnessed several of these signs with increasing regularity over a period of weeks or months, or more than one serious error or problem over one or a few days, it's time to act. When in doubt, it's better to document and discuss your concerns with your supervisor than to make assumptions about potential causes of the problem.

Phillip Chang had always been a good nurse who got along with everyone, so his colleague, Samantha Johnson, was surprised that he became defensive when she asked about an error in his narcotics counts from the previous day. Later that week, Samantha noticed that Phillip volunteered to give pain medications to two other nurses' patients even though he was quite busy himself.

The next day, one of Phillip's patients complained that she hadn't received her pain medication. When Samantha tried to find Phillip, he was missing from the unit. Although he apologized and gave an explanation for his disappearance, something didn't feel quite right to Samantha. After that, she began to pay more attention, and noticed that Phillip made more trips to the bathroom than usual and that his charts indicated that he routinely gave his patients their full dosage of pain medication when nurses on other shifts were giving the same patients lower dosages.

WHEN AND HOW TO REPORT

When you begin to discern a pattern such as Samantha saw, take private notes of your observations. In your notes, stick to the facts and include dates and times. You might record, for example, "Today, September 8, Faye Martin was absent from the unit between 2:00 and 2:45 PM, and didn't explain her absence." Don't draw conclusions, such as "I think Faye left the unit to have a drink."

If you observe unmistakable signs of chemical impairment—breath that smells of alcohol, slurred speech, shakiness, hand tremors—report your observations to your supervisor *immediately.* If Luisa's co-worker had told the supervisor of Luisa's glassy eyes and trembling hands, her problem might have been recognized.

When to report a constellation of more subtle signs is a more difficult question. However, if the signs you've seen persist or worsen over days or weeks (depending on their seriousness), don't delay sharing your observations with your supervisor.

You may feel that without sufficient documentation you'll be wrongly "accusing" the colleague. But the worst mistake you can make isn't to express concerns that may later prove unfounded, but to do nothing. Keep in mind that your goal isn't to diagnose chemical dependency, but to make sure a problem is recognized before a patient or the nurse herself is harmed. Too often, chemical dependency has reached a serious stage by the time signs of impairment are discernible in the workplace. Early action provides the best chance for successful intervention and recovery.

Also remember that your co-workers may be reporting their own observations. While you may not be sure you see a pattern, your supervisor may recognize one from several individuals' reports. Had Luisa's colleagues each reported their few observations, her supervisor might have spotted a pattern in her behavior.

In speaking with your supervisor, again, don't offer conclusions or judgments, but focus on specific concerns about job performance, including patient care and interpersonal communication. Refer to the notes you've taken of incidents, dates, and times.

Your supervisor should treat your report confidentially. There's no need to share your observations with other co-workers, which could lead to rumors that hinder dealing with the problem constructively.

For many of the reasons we mentioned earlier, your supervisor may be reluctant to follow up on your report. If this occurs, continue to document your observations and apprise her of them. If she still doesn't respond, be prepared to discuss your concerns with her manager. Remember, if patients'

WARNING SIGNS OF CHEMICAL DEPENDENCY

Job Performance
- Excessive use of sick time, especially following days off. (This is most common in alcohol dependency.)
- Absence without notice or last-minute requests for time off.
- Long breaks or lunch hours.
- Frequent or unexplained disappearances from the unit.
- "Job shrinkage." The nurse increasingly does the minimum work necessary for the job.
- Increasing difficulty meeting schedules or deadlines.
- Sloppy or illogical charting.
- An excessive number of mistakes—frequent medication errors or errors of judgment in patient care.
- Smell of alcohol on breath.
- Excessive use of breath mints, chewing gum, or mouthwash.
- Elaborate, implausible excuses for behavior.

Personality and Mental Status
- Emotional lability. The nurse becomes unusually quiet or irritable or has frequent mood swings.
- Inappropriate verbal or emotional responses such as snapping at colleagues, uncontrolled anger, or crying.

- Diminished alertness (perhaps appearing dazed or preoccupied), confusion, or frequent memory lapses.
- The nurse increasingly isolates herself from co-workers. She eats alone, avoids informal staff get-togethers, or requests transfer to the night shift.

Diversion
- Consistently volunteering to be the "medications nurse."
- Often signing out more controlled drugs than co-workers.
- Frequently reporting medication spills or other waste.
- Failing to obtain co-signatures.
- Reports reflecting excessive use of PRN medications.
- Discrepancies in end-of-shift medication counts.
- Evidence of tampering of vials or other drug containers.
- Waiting until alone to open the narcotics box or cabinet, or disappearing into the bathroom after opening it.
- An increase in patients' complaints of unrelieved pain.
- Defensiveness when questioned about medication errors.
- Consistently coming to work early and staying late.
- Volunteering to work with patients who receive regular or large amounts of pain medication.

safety is at risk, immediate action is called for.

There are several things you *shouldn't* do. Some nurses, meaning to help an impaired colleague, will cover for her errors and inconsistencies ("The unit was so crazy today, it's no wonder Laraine didn't get a chance to chart Mr. Smith's meds"). Or they'll make excuses for her behavior to co-workers or her supervisor ("She must be having family problems"). But this only prevents the nurse from getting the help she needs and may endanger patients as well.

As a concerned co-worker you may be tempted to assume the role of counselor to the nurse, but you shouldn't try to do more than call her attention to resources ("I'm concerned about you—you seem to be having problems. Maybe you should go talk to Sarah, the counselor with the hospital's employee assistance program"). Taking on a primary counseling role and getting involved with a chemically dependent nurse's personal life requires a tremendous amount of energy—maybe even interfering with your own performance—and can actually do harm by enabling her to avoid the specialized treatment that chemical dependency requires.

WHAT WILL HAPPEN?

It's not possible to describe in much detail how a nurse's chemical dependency problem will be handled; it depends on the individual circumstances of the case and on the institution's culture and policies. Formal measures are sure to be taken, both to protect patients and to help the nurse obtain needed assistance, if the supervisor determines there's been a serious decline in the nurse's job performance. Someone experienced in formal intervention, such as a counselor from the institution's employee assistance program (EAP) or a consultant with the state nurse assistance program, should be involved or at least consulted. Ideally, a plan is developed according to hospital policy and is carried out by nursing administration in consultation with employee health, the EAP, or the state program. (We'll discuss these programs more later.)

Many hospitals have specific policies on the use of alcohol or other drugs while on duty (such as "Fitness for Duty" policies). These outline what's to be done if an employee's performance falls below acceptable levels and what tests are to be performed to determine the employee's health status and ability to practice safely. Fitness-for-duty evaluations are usually performed by an employee health physician or EAP specialist, and many include a physical and mental status examination, blood and urine drug screening, and, if necessary, arrangements for transporting the

employee to an appropriate treatment facility.

Although not legally required to do so, employers should conduct these investigations and interventions in a nondiscriminatory manner that respects the nurse's civil and professional rights. For example, the nurse has a right to engage legal counsel and to have a family member or other supportive person present during questioning. Employers should refrain from trying to elicit a "confession" or self-incriminating evidence, which can later become the basis for legal charges. That runs counter to the goal of motivating the nurse to seek treatment and rehabilitation.

The American Hospital Association encourages all health care facilities to implement clear written policies that comply with Title I of the Americans with Disabilities Act (ADA). The ADA generally prohibits employers from discriminating against a qualified individual with a disability in job application procedures, hiring, advancement, discharge, compensation and training, as well as other terms, conditions, and privileges of employment. It doesn't, however, protect an employee or applicant who's currently using drugs illegally.

A growing number of hospitals and other employers of nurses are developing return-to-work procedures to structure and ease reentry into the work-

WHERE TO TURN FOR HELP

American Nurses Association
600 Maryland Avenue SW
Washington, DC 20024-2571
(202) 554-4444
Can provide information on state nursing association programs.

Drug and Alcohol Nursing Association (DANA)
660 Lonely Cottage Drive
Upper Black Eddy, PA 18972-9313
(610) 847-5396
National association of chemical dependency nurses providing education and resource information.

Employee Assistance Professionals Association (EAPA)
2101 Wilson Boulevard, Suite 500
Arlington, VA 22201
(703) 522-6272
Can provide a national listing of all EAP services available and also provides training on issues such as addressing impairment in the workplace.

National Consortium of Chemical Dependency Nurses (NCCDN)
1720 Willow Creek Circle, Suite 519
Eugene, OR 97402
1-800-876-2236
National association of chemical dependency nurses providing education and resource information.

National Council of State Boards of Nursing, Inc.
676 North St. Clair Street, Suite 550
Chicago, IL 60611-2921
(312) 787-6555
Can provide information and listings of all formal diversion programs and also has model program information.

National Nurses Society on Addictions (NNSA)
4101 Lake Boone Trail, Suite 201
Raleigh, NC 27607
(919) 783-5871
National association of chemical dependency nurses providing education and resource information.

place. These procedures are carried out in conjunction with the nurse's drug treatment and her "aftercare plan," the ongoing support that's been arranged to keep her recovery on course.

CONFIDENTIAL ASSISTANCE AVAILABLE

When available, employee health services or EAPs provide a wide range of confidential assistance to employees on various personal problems, including chemical dependency. This typically includes consultation, assessment of problem areas and need for intervention, short-term counseling, and referral to community agencies such as substance abuse treatment centers, mental health facilities, rape crisis centers, or financial counselors. EAPs also often monitor employees following treatment for chemical dependency. The programs are usually staffed by certified, licensed clinicians. In hospitals or other institutions without EAPs, the employee health or human resources department may provide some of these services.

Many states now have formal programs that serve as alternatives to the usual disciplinary processes for nurses whose practice is impaired by chemical dependency or emotional or psychological problems. These confidential programs are designed to help the nurse obtain appropriate counseling and treatment. The chemically dependent nurse, usually referred by her employer, refrains from practice until she completes an agreed-upon course of treatment, then is permitted to go back to work with the understanding that her performance will be monitored.

In addition, the nurse is required to participate in an ongoing 12-step or nurse support program. These requirements vary in length from two to five years. As long as she complies with the treatment and recovery program, no formal disciplinary action is taken and the employer isn't compelled to report her to the licensing board. Your state's licensing board can tell you whether your state offers these programs.

Many state nurses' associations have "peer assistance" programs that can help nurses who have problems such as chemical dependency. These vary considerably in the services offered. Some provide mainly consultation-referral and educational services. Others with more comprehensive service also sponsor support groups for chemically dependent nurses and offer assistance in monitoring during the nurse's return to the workplace.

Other organizations can also provide information on your legal responsibilities, planning a successful intervention, and referral to treatment (see *Where to Turn for Help* on page 34).

PAIN BEFORE HEALING

Certainly, confronting chemical dependency in a colleague is never easy and often painful. The nurse who hasn't yet come to terms with her problem may feel that she's been betrayed by those she suspects reported her, and may express this to co-workers. But our duty to protect patients' health and safety obligates us to act.

It's important to keep in mind that recovery from chemical dependency is possible. It doesn't necessarily spell the loss of a job or the end of a career. A chemically dependent colleague who's been helped because you cared enough to intervene may someday say, "Thanks for saving my life."

SELECTED REFERENCES

American Nurses Association. Impaired nursing practice. *ANA News Release,* Mar. 1987.

Bissell, L., and Haberman, P.W. *Alcoholism in the Professions.* New York, Oxford University Press, 1984.

Hughes, T.L. *Chief Nurse Executives' Responses to Chemically Dependent Nurses.* Chicago, University of Illinois, 1989. (Unpublished doctoral dissertation)

Hughes, T.L., and Solari-Twadell, A. Response to chemical impairment: policy and program initiatives. In *Addiction in the Nursing Profession: Approaches to Intervention and Recovery,* ed. by M.R. Haack and T.L. Hughes, New York, Springer Publishing Co., 1989.

McMahon, J.M. *Characteristics of Chemically Dependent Nurses in a Large Metropolitan Area in the State of Texas.* Houston, University of Houston, 1986. (Unpublished doctoral dissertation)

Naegle, M.A. Creative management of impaired nursing practice. *Nurs. Adm. Q.* 9:16-26, Spring 1985.

Valentine, N. *Stress, Alcohol, and Psychoactive Drug Use Among Nurses in Massachusetts.* Boston, Brandeis University, 1991. (Unpublished doctoral dissertation)

WHEN A CHILD DIES

Practical, sensitive advice for helping parents through their worst nightmare.

BY LUCY NELSON, RN, BSN

The phone on your busy pediatric ICU rings. A five-year-old boy, Justin Christopher, has been brought to the ED after being struck by a car. He has severe head and abdominal trauma, and the prognosis is poor.

The staff rushes to prepare for the patient. In the blur of high-tech clinical activity, it's easy to forget that there's a real child on the way—a child who's part of a family. But eventually you'll have to speak to Justin's parents. What will you say to them?

There's no script to follow in breaking the bad news to parents or supporting them as they grieve over their loss. But there are some simple steps you can take, a few kind words and gestures you can offer, to help them through this difficult time.

HELP THE PARENTS FOCUS ON THE CHILD

As Justin's parents arrive on the unit, help them tune out the beeps and alarms of the ICU and focus on their child. First, introduce yourself. Be sure to make eye contact. Explain clearly that you're the nurse responsible for Justin's care on the unit. Ask them how they'd like to be referred to. I've had some parents say they were offended by being called "mom" or "dad." Other parents find "Mr.," "Ms.," or "Mrs." impersonal. Use the names the parents prefer as you introduce them to other caregivers.

Take the parents' emotional temperature. Ask how they're doing, and note their facial expressions and whether they're crying. If they're emotionally out of control, do your best to

Lucy Nelson is a West Chicago, Illinois-based grief consultant with 12 years of pediatric and pediatric ICU nursing experience.
Modified from AJN, March 1995.

calm them. One way is speak to them in mild, even tones. Most parents will eventually match your tone and emotional pitch.

When you meet the Christophers, they may already be deep in a flood of "what ifs"—imagined scenarios that may or may not come true. Ask them what they know about the accident and Justin's condition. It's essential that you do this before you tell them very much. Most likely, you won't be the first to talk to the parents; rather, you'll be reinforcing and clarifying what the physician has already told them. But parents often won't completely grasp or retain what the physician has said. Now's the time to correct any mistaken assumptions or misunderstandings. Of course, it helps to be present when the physician speaks with the family, but this isn't always possible.

The next step is to prepare the parents for what they'll see. Try to determine what they want to know. You can say, "I can tell you about the equipment attached to Justin" or ask, "Do you want to know how we can tell how Justin is doing?" Some families want to know the function of every piece of equipment and the meaning of every electronic beep or squiggle; others only want the basics. Tailor what you say to meet their needs. Be sure to use language they can understand. Simple sentences are best. you might explain, "We've taken Justin's clothing off so we can see him better, but we're using a lamp to keep him warm," or "There's a machine breathing for him, and we've given him medicine for pain." If the parents don't understand English, wait for an interpreter.

Frequently ask the parents how they're doing. Let them know they can ask questions as they arise. I always stress to parents that we don't expect them to remember everything. Parents

will often forget things and ask the same questions repeatedly. This is a defense mechanism that protects them from having to deal with painful facts before they're ready to. Unfortunately, it can be very frustrating to the staff and even lead to conflict with parents—unless you're sensitive to it.

SILENCE: YOUR ALLY AT THE BEDSIDE

Once you bring the Christophers to the bedside, anything can happen. Let silence be your ally. Give them time to get used to their surroundings. Be present in case they need you, but don't intrude. Watch for subtle signs. For example, when the parents make frequent eye contact with you without saying anything, they may have questions they're hesitating to ask.

Observe whether the Christophers are keeping a distance away from Justin. Most parents need permission to touch their child. They rarely feel comfortable enough to approach the bed on their own. Help the Christophers find a spot that allows the care team access to Justin without asking them to move. Encourage them to touch and speak to Justin. If it seems appropriate, help them to focus on positive or unchanged aspects of the child's appearance. Again, simplicity is the key. Phrases like, "He looks so peaceful," "She has such pretty hair," "You must love him very much," said sincerely, often help.

Reinforce the parent's role as primary caregiver. Remind them that the decisions about Justin's treatment are theirs to make. Involve them in simple care measures, such as bathing or oral suctioning. I've asked parents to bring in photos of the child or his favorite stuffed animal to keep at the bedside.

Acknowledge that the situation "must be terribly difficult" for them. But don't say or imply that you know how they feel, even if you've had a similar experience. You may come across as trying to devalue their pain.

GIVE THE PARENTS SOME TIME ALONE

Limit the parents' first encounter at the bedside to no more than 10 minutes, if possible. After that, suggest that they take care of phone calls, paperwork, or other tasks that will distract them. Allow them some time alone to sort out their thoughts and feelings.

Provide the Christophers with privacy during their time away from the bedside by showing them to an empty conference room or office. Allow them the choice of having other family members, such as grandparents, with them, but offer yourself as the gatekeeper to screen visitors. This takes the pressure off the family and gives them some time alone if they want it. Now's a good time to give the parents whatever written material you have, such as lists of phone numbers, visiting information, the names of the care team members, and those of the chaplain, social worker, and other resources. Most people won't remember this information if it's not in writing. Hospitals usually require parents to fill out a form about the child. This is a good time to have them do it.

WHEN DEATH COMES

Despite the efforts of the team, Justin dies the morning after his admission. There's no need to deny or hide your emotions as you speak to his parents. Don't be afraid to express grief or even to cry. But take care not to shift the focus from the family's grief by speaking of your own past losses. Also, try to avoid euphemisms like "passed away," "went to be with the angels," or "no longer with us." By using the word "died," you'll encourage Justin's parents to acknowledge his death, which is the first step toward acceptance. And you'll leave no room for misunderstanding.

You'll probably have to inform and direct the parents on arrangements for transferring the body. Know your social workers and chaplain. They're usually familiar with the arrangements and paperwork required for funerals and disposition of the body. They may also have the time to spend with the family while you attend to other responsibilities.

Provide a private space for the Christophers at this time. Check first to see if they need something to drink or to use the rest room, and check in again periodically. Offer to call relatives, friends, or community clergy they may want on hand. You might suggest that they ask someone to notify extended family for them so they can have some time undisturbed.

Also keep in mind the following dos and don'ts in supporting the grieving family:

• *Always call the child by name.* The family may interpret references to their child as "your son" or "the patient" or even as "him" or "her" as cold and objectifying. Calling the child by name shows respect for the person the child was and that you sincerely cared about him.

• *Don't offer platitudes.* Rote phrases such as "It's God's will" or "She's at peace now" may be interpreted by family members to mean they should stop talking. Many family members ask questions like "Why my child?" or "How could this happen?" These questions are rhetorical, and you shouldn't try to answer them. Silence is very powerful during these moments.

• *Don't automatically offer tissues.* Make sure they're on hand, but offer them only when someone asks. Offering tissues to grieving parents interrupts the flow of thoughts and emotions. And it may seen to them like a cue to stop crying and control themselves.

• *Listen attentively.* Many patients will need to relive memories of their child. If you don't have time to stay, say so honestly and find someone else—the nurse manager, chaplain, or social worker, or a hospital volunteer. Minimize interruptions and distractions. Turn off the phone and make sure tissues and a pitcher of water are in the room. If the parents or other family members begin to ramble on about unrelated matters, try to direct them back to pleasant, happy memories of the child.

• *Allow parents, siblings, and other family members time alone with the child.* After you've cleaned the body and removed medical equipment, invite the parents into the room. Suggest that they hold their child or lie in bed with him. Let them know they have as much time as they need and that you'll be right outside. Then leave and close the door, but stay close by.

Let the parents choose which family members to allow in. But encourage them to let their other children say good-bye too. Though parents often want to protect them from the reality of death, children older than three benefit from a final contact with their sibling. The child should be carefully prepared and accompanied into the room by an adult who can provide support and answer questions. Parents may not be able to do this; if not, a grandparent or other adult relative may be. If you've developed a relationship with the child, it may help for you to be present. Be sure to emphasize that you'll answer the child's questions in keeping with the family's faith or belief system.

SOMETHING TO REMEMBER THE CHILD BY

If the Christophers are like most parents, they haven't collected mementos of their son since he was a baby. In just a few minutes you can create and preserve memories of Justin. These are gifts you can give to a family that will otherwise go home empty-handed. (Don't collect these mementos, however, unless the child has already died.)

One simply keepsake is a record of the child's weight and height (or length). Once a child is past infancy, these measurements are noted much less frequently, so the parents may not have them. Record the measurements on a clean sheet of paper or certificate (if available) with the child's full name, date of birth, and date of death.

Another memento is a handprint or footprint. A plaster cast handprint is better than an ink print, but isn't always possible to obtain. If you experience deaths with any frequency on your unit, it helps to keep ink pads and plaster and disposable pie tins for casts readily available. If deaths are rare, you may just want to note where you can get these items and keep this information with your death records.

A lock of hair has long been treasured as a remembrance of a loved one. But always ask the parents before cutting the child's hair; some religions and cultures, such as certain Native

American cultures, proscribe it. If the family accepts your offer, take the hair from the back of the head and place it in a sealable plastic bag.

Finally, offer a blanket or pajamas or other clothing that the child has worn recently. Seal the item in a plastic bag. The smell of the child will be preserved. Through this may sound morbid, it can be very comforting to parents. The child's scent will linger for a long time.

The parents may not accept some of these things at the time of death. But keep them at the hospital for at least six months, preferably a year, after the child's death, in case the parents change their minds.

COPING WITH YOUR OWN FEELINGS

Even if a child was in your care for just a few hours, it's hard not to be moved emotionally by his death. Along with grief and empathy for the parents, you may have feelings of helplessness. And if you, too, are a parent, you may be haunted by thoughts that "this could have been my child."

Those of us who frequently care for dying children develop ways to cope with these feelings. One way is to keep busy; caring for others can often keep your emotions from overwhelming you before you have the chance to work through them. Another is to share your feelings with your co-workers or with a chaplain; many pediatric ICUs and other units have formal programs, such as support groups, to encourage this.

But carrying out the steps outlined in this article can also help. Whether you witness a child's death once a week or once in a lifetime, supporting parents in their moment of loss can foster your emotional healing as well as theirs.

Contents

Chapter *3*

Nursing Care of the Adult

COORDINATORS

Patricia E. Downing, RN, BSN, MN

Paulette D. Rollant, RN, MSN, CCRN, PhD

Contributors

Patricia E. Downing, RN, BSN, MN

Deborah A. Ennis, RN, BSN, MSN, CCRN

Peg Gray-Vickrey, RN (C), BSN, MS, DNS

Alma J. Lubinski, RN, MS, EdD

Paulette D. Rollant, RN, MSN, CCRN, PhD

Judith K. Sands, RN, BS, MS, EdD

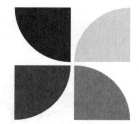

The Healthy Adult

HEALTH

1. Definitions
   a. No universally accepted definition
   b. World Health Organization (WHO), 1946: "state of complete physical, mental, and social well-being and not merely the absence of disease or infirmity . . . fundamental right of every human being."
   c. American Nurses' Association (ANA Social Policy Statement), 1980: "dynamic state of being in which the developmental and behavioral potential of an individual is realized to the fullest extent possible."
2. Characteristics
   a. Dynamic state, dependent on individual's ability to adapt continually to changing internal and external environments
   b. Continuum, extending from obvious disease through absence of discernible disease to state of optimal functioning
   c. Determinants
      1. biologic and genetic factors
      2. macroenvironmental and microenvironmental factors
      3. psychosocial factors
   d. Aspects: physical, emotional, and social
   e. Norms change with age
3. Life expectancy (LE)
   a. Statistically determined number of years an individual of a given age can expect to live
   b. Used as an indicator of a nation's health
   c. Increases with advances in disease control
   d. Born in United States in 1900: 47 years; born in United States in 1992: 75.8 years
4. Levels of health promotion
   a. Primary: health promotion and disease prevention
   b. Secondary: early diagnosis, prompt treatment, and disability limitation
   c. Tertiary: restoration and rehabilitation

Characteristics of the Healthy Young and Middle-Aged Adult (20 to 65 years)

1. Physiologic characteristics
   a. General
      1. growth and development appropriate for age
      2. symmetric body
      3. no pain
      4. balanced sleep pattern
   b. Integument
      1. skin
         a. clean, intact, smooth, warm, dry
         b. normal turgor and texture; elastic
         c. odorless
         d. no lesions
         e. normal color (e.g., no jaundice, cyanosis)
      2. mucous membranes
         a. pink, intact, hydrated
         b. no lesions
      3. hair
         a. normal distribution and amount
         b. normal texture
         c. no dandruff, no scales
      4. nails
         a. semitransparent; smooth, convex surface
         b. pink nail beds
         c. normal capillary filling of nail beds (within 5 seconds after compression); contralateral side equal
   c. Neck
      1. symmetric
      2. trachea in midline
      3. no masses
   d. Eyes
      1. symmetric placement
      2. white sclera
      3. pink conjunctiva
      4. normal lacrimation
      5. pupils equal, round, react to light and accommodation (PERRLA)
      6. eye movements coordinated and parallel
      7. visual acuity 20/20 without or with correction
   e. Ears
      1. symmetric placement
      2. auditory acuity normal (e.g., can distinguish softly whispered words at 1 to 2 feet)
      3. no drainage from external auditory canal
      4. equilibrium maintained (no vertigo)
   f. Thorax and lungs
      1. open, unobstructed airway
      2. respirations (eupneic)
         a. rate: 12 to 20 per minute at rest
         b. rhythmic, normal depth
         c. effortless, noiseless
         d. odorless
         e. excursion of diaphragm: bilateral and equal

3. thorax: symmetric, normal anteroposterior (AP) diameter (i.e., AP diameter less than lateral-to-lateral diameter)
4. normal breath sounds: tracheobronchial, bronchovesicular, vesicular (no adventitious sounds)
5. resonant (no dullness) on percussion
6. no cough or sputum

g. Cardiovascular
1. normal sinus rhythm (NSR)
2. heart rate: 60-80 beats per minute at rest
3. normal heart sounds, no extra sounds or murmurs
4. blood pressure (BP): systolic pressure <130 mm Hg and diastolic pressure <85 mm Hg at rest
5. no chest pain
6. no palpitations
7. palpable peripheral arterial pulses (radial, brachial, femoral, popliteal, posterior tibial, dorsalis pedis)
8. normal skin color and temperature (e.g., no cyanosis or pigmentation)
9. no peripheral edema
10. no varicosities or ulcerations of extremities

h. Abdomen
1. soft, nontender
2. flat, no distention
3. normal, active bowel sounds
4. no palpable organomegaly, masses, or hernias

i. Gastrointestinal/nutrition
1. normal weight for height
2. normal appetite
3. normal digestion (e.g., no food intolerance or indigestion)
4. well nourished
5. teeth present, in good repair
6. normal mastication (i.e., no difficulty or pain with chewing)
7. no dysphagia
8. regular bowel habits; stools brown and formed

j. Musculoskeletal
1. good posture and body alignment
2. body movements coordinated (no tremors or involuntary movements)
3. muscles firm, symmetric, strong, normal tone (no spasms, contractures, weakness, atrophy, or paralysis)
4. normal heel-to-toe gait (foot strikes heel to toe, normal base of support, arms swing in coordination with leg movements)
5. joints
   a. full, unimpaired range of motion
   b. no deformities
   c. nontender, nonswollen, no crepitation

k. Neurologic
1. mental and cognitive function
   a. oriented to person, place, time
   b. alert, conscious
   c. appropriate response to visual, auditory, tactile, and painful stimuli
   d. short-term and long-term memory intact
   e. capable of abstract thinking
   f. able to articulate without difficulty
   g. appropriate behavior and mood (no excessive aggression, violence, withdrawal, or depression)
2. sensory perception
   a. pain perception intact
   b. light touch, pressure, and vibration perception intact
   c. temperature perception intact
   d. sight, hearing, taste, and smell perception intact
3. motor (see also Musculoskeletal, this page)
   a. coordinated, balanced movement
   b. reflexes intact and normal (including deep tendon reflexes)
   c. proprioception (awareness of body position)

l. Genitourinary
1. genitals
   a. normal pubic hair distribution
   b. normal appearance/structure
   c. no lesions or abnormal discharge
2. breasts
   a. symmetric size and placement
   b. no masses
   c. no discharge from nipples
3. sexual function viewed by individual as satisfying, rewarding, and adequate
4. micturition (urination)
   a. painless
   b. voluntary control
   c. normal stream
   d. no frequency or urgency
   e. bladder empty after voiding
   f. approximately 300 ml per voiding; 1000 to 1500 ml per day
   g. urine: yellow to amber, specific gravity 1.010 to 1.025, pH 4.6 to 8.0; no protein or glucose; no microscopic red blood cells (RBCs), white blood cells (WBCs), or bacteria

2. Psychosocial characteristics (see Chapter 2, Psychosocial Characteristics of the Healthy Client, p. 14.)

Characteristics of the Healthy Elderly Adult (Over 65 Years)

1. Aging
   a. A normal progressive process, not a disease
   b. Norms: normal physiologic changes vs. abnormal pathologic changes not completely identified
2. Physiologic characteristics
   a. General changes
      1. general tissue desiccation and slowed cell division
      2. slowed, weakened speed of response to stimuli
      3. slowed rate of tissue repair
      4. decreased metabolism
      5. less rapid and less efficient mechanisms of homeostasis
      6. decreased immunocompetence
      7. rate of aging is individual, influenced by such factors as heredity and stress
      8. high incidence of health problems (e.g., congestive heart failure [CHF], osteoporosis, cataracts)

b. Integument
  1. skin
    a. dry, wrinkled, loss of elasticity
    b. decreased perspiration and sebum
    c. fragile, easily injured
    d. decreased subcutaneous tissue
    e. decreased skin turgor
    f. increased sensitivity to cold
  2. hair
    a. decreased number of hair follicles, generalized loss
    b. scant, fine, graying
    c. hirsutism (female)
    d. possible hereditary baldness
  3. nails
    a. dry
    b. thick
    c. brittle
c. Eyes
  1. decreased visual acuity
    a. farsightedness because of slow lens accommodation (presbyopia)
    b. narrowed field of vision (tunnel vision)
  2. slowed accommodation to light
  3. decreased lacrimal secretions
d. Ears
  1. decreased auditory acuity
  2. sensorineural hearing deficit (presbycusis): gradual decreased sensitivity to high-frequency tones
e. Thorax and lungs
  1. decreased lung capacity
  2. decreased elasticity of tissue
  3. increased AP diameter of thorax
f. Cardiovascular
  1. decreased vascular elasticity
  2. increased systolic and diastolic BP
  3. decreased cardiac output
  4. less tolerance to position change (e.g., orthostatic hypotension)
g. Gastrointestinal/nutrition
  1. decreased metabolism: caloric requirement approximately 1000 calories per day
  2. slowed digestion; increased food intolerances
  3. redistribution of body fat: increased fat in trunk, especially in the abdomen
  4. teeth and gum problems common
  5. atonia constipation common
h. Musculoskeletal
  1. easily tired, less stamina
  2. symmetric decrease in muscle bulk
  3. decreased muscle strength and tone
  4. impaired range of motion resulting from stiff joints
  5. generalized loss of 6 to 10 cm in stature because of
    a. flexion of knee and hip joints
    b. narrowing of intervertebral disks
  6. body takes on bony, angular appearance
  7. osteoporosis common, especially in women
  8. osteoarthritis common
i. Neurologic
  1. general
    a. slowed speed of impulse transmission

b. progressive decrease in number of functioning neurons in central nervous system (CNS) and sense organs
    c. normal neurologic functioning possible because of tremendous reserve of numbers of neurons
  2. mental and cognitive function
    a. altered capacity to retain new information and learn new tasks
    b. some impairment of memory and mental endurance
  3. sensory (see also Eyes, Ears, this page)
    a. some impairment of sensory perception (hearing, smell, sight, taste, touch, temperature, pain)
    b. gradual decrease of visual and auditory acuity
  4. motor (see also Musculoskeletal, this page)
    a. slowed reaction to stimuli; lengthening of reaction time
    b. decreased coordination and balance
j. Genitourinary
  1. genital
    a. female: menopause secondary to decreased estrogen (see Nursing Care of the Childbearing Family, p. 301)
    b. male: decreased testosterone, spermatogenesis, and size of testes; increase in size of prostate
    c. ability to function sexually may continue well into older years
  2. urinary
    a. decreased number of nephrons, renal plasma flow (RPF), glomerular filtration rate (GFR), and tubular function resulting in decreased kidney function
    b. decreased renal capacity to concentrate urine at night, resulting in nocturia
k. Immunity
  1. decline in cell-mediated immunity, decreased antibody response
  2. increased susceptibility to infections (e.g., pneumonia, influenza)
3. Psychosocial characteristics (see Chapter 2, Psychosocial Characteristics of the Elderly Healthy Client, p. 16)

APPLICATION OF THE NURSING PROCESS TO THE HEALTHY ADULT
ASSESSMENT
1. Health history
  a. Usual health status
  b. Present health status
  c. Family history
  d. Previous illness
  e. Immunization status
  f. Allergies (allergen and reaction)
  g. Psychosocial
    1. age, sex, race, marital status
    2. role in family
    3. cultural heritage
    4. language
    5. education
    6. economic status
    7. occupation
    8. housing
    9. religious practices

10. recreational/social activities
11. personal habits (e.g., tobacco, alcohol)
   h. Physical
      1. personal hygiene habits/practices
      2. eating habits/patterns
      3. dental history
      4. bowel and bladder habits
      5. sleep and rest habits
      6. activity level
      7. work habits
      8. sexual habits
2. Physical exam
   a. Methods
      1. inspection: looking, observing
      2. auscultation: listening
      3. palpation: feeling, touching, pressing
      4. percussion: tapping
   b. Head-to-toe appraisal (see Physiologic Characteristics of the Young, Middle-aged, and Elderly Adult, pp. 110-112)

ANALYSIS/NURSING DIAGNOSIS

1. Safe, effective care environment
   a. Knowledge deficit (specify)
   b. Risk for injury
   c. Sensory or perceptual alteration (specify)
2. Physiologic integrity
   a. Altered growth and development
   b. Altered nutrition: more/less than body requirements
   c. Risk for activity intolerance
3. Psychosocial integrity
   a. Self-esteem disturbance
   b. Spiritual distress (distress of the human spirit)
   c. Altered sexuality patterns
4. Health promotion/maintenance
   a. Knowledge deficit (specify)
   b. Health-seeking behaviors (specify)
   c. Altered health maintenance

GENERAL NURSING PLANNING, IMPLEMENTATION, AND EVALUATION

Goal 1 Adult individual will use health practices that promote optimal health.

Implementation
1. Promote personal health habits as necessary that help individual to
   a. Maintain personal hygiene.

b. Maintain good nutrition:
   1. eat a nutritionally adequate, well-balanced diet (Fig. 3-1; Tables 3-1 and 4-8)
   2. eat a variety of foods
   3. choose foods low in fat, saturated fat, cholesterol, and simple sugars (Table 3-12)
   4. eat foods with adequate starch and fiber
   5. use salt and sodium in moderation (Table 3-13)
c. Maintain desirable body weight.
d. Exercise regularly.
e. Obtain adequate rest and sleep.
f. Reduce stress.
g. Avoid tobacco use.
h. Limit alcohol use (no more than two drinks per day).
i. Avoid prolonged sun exposure.

Evaluation
Individual maintains healthful lifestyle.

Goal 2 Adult individual will experience safe environment; will be free from accidental injury.

Implementation
1. Teach as necessary to ensure that individual
   a. Has safe home (e.g., fire alarms, ample lighting).
   b. Works in safe environment (e.g., safety devices, no toxic material exposure).
   c. Travels safely (e.g., automobile seat belts).
   d. Recreates safely (e.g., no diving in shallow water).

Evaluation
Individual is free from serious accidents.

Goal 3 Adult individual will undergo routine health exams.

Implementation
1. Recommend and help schedule as necessary
   a. Annual physical exam
   b. Routine dental visits
   c. Attendance at screening clinics (e.g., hypertension, glaucoma, diabetes)
2. Teach guidelines for early detection of cancer (see Table 3-66)

Evaluation
Individual has dental exam every 6 months and physical exam every year.

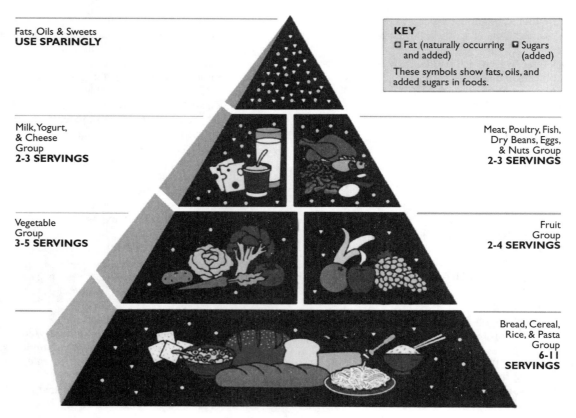

Fig. 3-1   Food guide pyramid; a guide to daily food choices. (From U.S. Department of Agriculture: *USDA's food guide pyramid*, USDA Human Nutrition Information Pub. No. 249, Washington, D.C., 1992, U.S. Government Printing Office.)

Table 3-1   U.S. recommended daily nutrition for an average healthy adult (23-50 years)

	Women	Men
	120 lb (55 kg)	154 lb (70 kg)
	64 in (163 cm)	70 in (178 cm)
Calories	2000 kcal	2700 kcal
Protein*	44 g	56 g
	(176 kcal)	(224 kcal)
Fat†	66 g	90 g
	(594 kcal)	(810 kcal)
Carbohydrate‡	285 g (1140 kcal)	383 g (1532 kcal)
Cholesterol	300 mg	300 mg
Sodium	1100-3300 mg	1100-3300 mg
Calcium	800 mg	800 mg
Iron	18 mg	10 mg
Fluids	1500 ml	1500 ml

From *Recommended Daily Allowances* (RDA), National Research Council. Daily Goals for the United States, U.S. Senate Select Committee on Nutrition and Human Needs, American Heart Association.
*8%-12% of total calories; 0.8 g/kg of ideal body weight.
†30% of total calories (10% saturated fat and 20% from polysaturated or monosaturated fat).
‡58% of total calories (48% complex carbohydrate, 10% simple sugar).

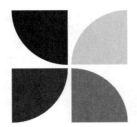

The Adult Client Undergoing Surgery

OVERVIEW OF PHYSIOLOGY

1. Surgery is a stressful event.
2. Close monitoring of cardiovascular, respiratory, and renal systems is needed particularly throughout the perioperative period.
3. The most common problems during the immediate postanesthetic phase are airway obstruction, hypoventilation, hypotension, cardiac dysrhythmias, and pain.
4. The most common types of complications in the postoperative period:
   a. Respiratory
      1. atelectasis: the incomplete expansion of a lung or portion of it, partly because of the absence of periodic deep breaths
      2. hypostatic pneumonia
   b. Circulatory
      1. thrombophlebitis and phlebothrombosis (see Peripheral Vascular Problems, p. 138)
      2. shock; volume depletion (refer to Shock, p. 129)
   c. Wound
      1. hemorrhage
      2. infection
      3. dehiscence: separation of wound edges
      4. evisceration: separation of wound edges with protrusion of viscera through incision
   d. Urinary
      1. retention
      2. oliguria
   e. Gastrointestinal
      1. paralytic ileus: neurogenic disruption of intestine often related to hypokalemia or decreased autonomic innervation
      2. singultus (hiccoughs)
   f. Negative nitrogen balance: greater nitrogen excretion than amount ingested
5. Factors affecting client's response to surgery and development of complications:
   a. Age: very old and very young are less able to tolerate stress of surgery.
   b. Nutritional status:
      1. malnutrition: increases risk of infection and poor wound healing
      2. obesity: increases risk of poor wound healing, infection, respiratory complications, and thrombophlebitis

   a. Presence of other chronic illnesses:
      1. chronic obstructive pulmonary disease (COPD) increases risk of pulmonary problems
      2. cardiovascular disease decreases ability to deal with stress of surgery
      3. renal disease increases risk of fluid and electrolyte problems, particularly hyperkalemia and fluid overload
      4. diabetes mellitus increases risk of poor wound healing
      5. chronic glucocorticoid therapy increases risk of fluid and electrolyte problems, poor wound healing
   b. Prolonged immobility after surgery increases risk of thrombophlebitis, abdominal distention, urinary retention, and pulmonary complications.
   c. Type of operation: some operations are more frequently associated with complications (e.g., atelectasis after open gallbladder surgery).
1. Each institution has basic admission, preoperative, intraoperative, and postoperative routines. The following content emphasizes general principles of care that apply to all situations.

APPLICATION OF THE NURSING PROCESS TO THE ADULT CLIENT UNDERGOING SURGERY

1. Preoperative care may need to be completed within 1 or 2 hours in an emergency or day surgery situation, or it may be given over a longer period for elective surgery.
2. Immediate postoperative care may be given in the recovery room, the intensive care unit (ICU), or on the general floor.
3. Adequate physiologic and psychologic preparation and care are extremely important to the client's successful recovery.
4. For day surgery clients: Many procedures are now performed in ambulatory surgery or day surgery settings. These persons need the same care as that required by inpatients. Diagnostic tests are usually done on an outpatient basis the week before surgery. The client may see the anesthesiologist, sign consent forms, and receive some preoperative teaching at this time. Postoperatively, a time and place must be provided to instruct the client and family about diet, fluids, activity, care of wounds, medications, and what to expect regarding discomfort, nausea and vomiting, and returning to work. Clients need

someone to help them get home from the hospital if they receive a general anesthetic.
5. Discharge planning starts at admission.

Nursing Process

ASSESSMENT
1. Total health status of the client and activities of daily living (ADL) preoperatively
2. General physical exam preoperatively as described for the healthy adult (if time is limited, focus on cardiovascular, pulmonary, neurologic, and renal exams)
3. Psychologic readiness: anxiety, fears
4. Learning needs; expectations of surgery and how pain will be managed
5. For day surgery clients: ability to get home, do care at home, support persons at home
6. Diagnostic tests (preoperative)
   a. Every client
      1. hematocrit/hemoglobin
      2. urinalysis
   b. Specific clients
      1. white blood cell count (WBC) (e.g., when infection suspected, after radiation, with immunosuppressive or steroid therapy, with collagen-vascular diseases)
      2. electrolytes (client over age 60, diabetes, use of diuretics, dysrhythmias, renal disease)
      3. electrocardiogram (ECG) (males over 40, women over 45, suspected or known cardiac disease)
      4. chest x-ray (when pulmonary condition is known or suspected)
      5. type and crossmatch blood (as necessary)
      6. prothrombin time (PT), partial thromboplastin time (PTT), bleeding time or clotting time
         a. underlying bleeding or coagulation problem
         b. receiving anticoagulants or to receive anticoagulants during surgery
         c. liver problems or presence of jaundice
      7. blood gases and pulmonary function tests (if pulmonary problem is present or pulmonary-cardiovascular surgery is planned)
7. Diagnostic tests (postoperative) will vary with type of surgery
8. Postoperative assessment focuses on systems affected by surgery and on potential complications
9. Discharge assessment
   a. Client's ability to perform self-care
   b. Significant others available to help
   c. Home situation

ANALYSIS/NURSING DIAGNOSIS
1. Safe, effective care environment
   a. Knowledge deficit (preoperative)
   b. Risk for injury (intraoperative)
   c. Risk for injury: perioperative positioning
   d. Risk for infection (postoperative)
2. Physiologic integrity
   a. Ineffective breathing pattern, risk for ineffective airway clearance (intraoperative, postoperative)
   b. Risk for decreased cardiac output (intraoperative, postoperative)
   c. Urinary retention (postoperative)
   d. Pain (postoperative)
   e. Risk for altered nutrition: less than body requirements (postoperative)
3. Psychosocial integrity
   a. Anxiety (preoperative)
   b. Fear (preoperative)
   c. Body-image disturbance (postoperative)
   d. Acute confusion (postoperative)
4. Health promotion/maintenance
   a. Self-care deficit (specify) (postoperative)
   b. Knowledge deficit (postoperative)
   c. Altered health maintenance (postoperative)

PLANNING, IMPLEMENTATION, AND EVALUATION

> **Goal 1** Client and significant others will be prepared for surgery.

Implementation
Day before or immediately before surgery (for emergency or day surgery clients):
1. Allay anxiety/fears as much as possible. (Refer to Anxious Behavior, Nursing Care of the Client with Psychosocial and Mental Health Problems, p. 34.)
2. Explain surgical procedure; provide sensory information.
3. Clarify expectations of surgery.
4. Explain preoperative procedures, postoperative routine to client and significant others.
5. Obtain informed surgical consent.
6. Ensure that diagnostic tests are completed, results acceptable.
7. Evaluate nutritional status.
8. Instruct client to take nothing by mouth (NPO) after midnight if required.
9. Prep bowel if required.
10. Ensure that client receives adequate rest the night before surgery; sedate as required.
Day of surgery:
11. Monitor vital signs and report immediately if different from previous baseline vital signs.
12. Validate NPO status if ordered.
13. Have client shower if ordered.
14. Remove hairpins, jewelry, and medals to avoid loss or injury.
15. Remove prosthetic devices (e.g., contact lenses, partial dentures). When possible permit client to wear eyeglasses, hearing aids, and dentures to operating room. Removal enhances feelings of helplessness and makes communication with client difficult. Make their presence known to operating room (OR) staff, who can remove and protect them before or after induction of anesthesia.
16. Apply antiembolic stockings as ordered.
17. Have client void immediately before administering any premedications.
18. Premedicate as ordered (not used as frequently as in the past).
19. Put side rails up after premedication.
20. Provide quiet environment.

Evaluation

Client and significant others explain surgery and postoperative routine accurately; client demonstrates deep breathing, coughing, and turning correctly.

> **Goal 2** Client will experience a safe environment in the operating room.

Implementation

1. Prepare skin as appropriate.
2. Maintain sterility of equipment and operating team.
3. Prevent electrical dangers.
4. Position client appropriately.
5. Maintain contact with client during induction of general anesthesia (Table 3-2).

Table 3-2 Stages of general anesthesia

Stage	Duration	Manifestations
I	Beginning of induction to loss of consciousness	Loss of judgment Hearing acute
II	Loss of consciousness to loss of eyelid reflex	Cerebral or voluntary control lost Hypersensitive to incoming impulses Hearing acute
III	Extends from loss of eyelid reflex to cessation of respiratory effort; surgery performed in this stage; reflexes absent and muscles relaxed	Functions of medulla retained
IV		Respiratory paralysis Cardiac failure Death

6. Assist in monitoring for potential complications of anesthetic agents (Table 3-3).
7. Promote hemostasis and have appropriate equipment, supplies available.
8. Perform counting procedures (e.g., sponges).
9. Estimate blood loss.

Evaluation

Client experiences no injuries from improper positioning; client's BP, pulse, rhythm, and oxygenation are maintained at normal levels during the induction of anesthesia and during surgery; client is free from signs of shock or cardiac dysrhythmias during surgery.

> **Goal 3** Immediately postoperatively, client's respiratory, circulatory, fluid, electrolyte, and neurologic status will be optimal.

Implementation

1. Monitor respiratory rate and character, other vital signs, intake and output (I&O), intravenous (IV) infusion, electrolytes, drainage tubes, neurologic status, and surgical wound dressing.
2. Report changes to physician.
3. Begin turning, coughing, and deep-breathing exercises every hour (qh) after airway tube is removed.
4. Suction nasopharyngeal secretions as needed.
5. Administer respiratory-assistance drugs as ordered.
6. Use inspiratory spirometer as indicated.
7. Give IV therapy and drugs as ordered (Table 3-4).
8. Use voiding-inducement techniques as necessary.
9. Start oral fluids and food when appropriate (Table 3-5).
10. Keep side rails up until client's neurologic status is normal.
11. Use restraints as necessary.
12. Care for surgical wound using aseptic technique.

Table 3-3 General points regarding anesthetic agents

Type	Definition	Major complications
General		Cardiac dysfunction (dysrhythmias, arrest)
Inhalation	Gases and vapors administered through mask or endotracheal (ET) tube; block pathways to brain and render client unconscious; used for major operations of thorax, abdomen, head, and neck.	Respiratory dysfunction (bronchospasms and laryngospasms, aspiration, failure) Cardiovascular dysfunction (shock, hypotension) Neurologic complications (convulsions, cerebrovascular accident [CVA]) Others (renal and liver problems, malignant hyperthermia)
Intravenous	Drugs given directly into vein; used for induction and as adjuncts to inhalation agents; do not abolish all pain reflexes.	Respiratory dysfunction (arrest, bronchospasm and laryngospasms) Cardiac and cardiovascular dysfunction (hypotension, depression) Neurologic dysfunction (convulsions), nuchal rigidity
Regional	Drugs injected into nerve track/endings to block selected fibers; may be given topically or locally (spinal, epidural, etc.); do not decrease anxiety, fear; must have a cooperative client.	Hypotension, anaphylactic shock Respiratory paralysis can occur with spinal anesthesia Headache
Local	Drugs applied topically or infiltrated into tissue; results in loss of sensation in the immediate area of application.	If sufficient amount of drug is absorbed, systemic toxicity may occur

Table 3-4 Calculating IV rates

$$\frac{\text{Amount of IV fluid (ml)}}{\text{Time to infuse (min)}} \times \text{Drip factor (gtt/ml)} = \text{IV rate (gtt/min)}$$

Example: The order is for 1000 ml D_5W to run for 10 hours. The drip factor is 15 gtt/ml.

$$\frac{1000 \text{ ml}}{600 \text{ min}} \times \frac{15 \text{ gtt}}{1 \text{ ml}} = \text{IV rate of 25 gtt/min}$$

$$(60 \text{ min} \times 10 \text{ hr}) = 600 \text{ min}$$

Table 3-5 Postoperative diet modifications

Diet	Foods allowed	Comments
Clear liquids	Tea, gelatin, broth, strained juices	Provides liquids but inadequate calories and nutrients
Full liquids	Soups, milk, unstrained juices, ice cream, custards, pudding	Provides more calories and nutrients; if selected carefully, can meet many nutritional needs

Evaluation

Client takes deep breaths and coughs well; breath sounds are clear; BP remains stable; fluid intake and urinary output are adequate; skin is warm and dry; nail beds blanch briskly; surgical dressing is dry and intact; client responds appropriately to commands.

> **Goal 4** Client will be free from discomfort during the postoperative period.

Implementation

1. Assess pain: every 2 hours during first postoperative day; more often if pain is poorly managed or if interventions are changed.
    a. Presence of pain: *single most reliable* indicator of pain and its severity is client's report
    b. Source
    c. Location, character, and duration
    d. Intensity: use self-report measurement scales (e.g., numerical or adjective rating and scales)
    e. Level of anxiety
    f. Factors that intensify of decrease discomfort
    g. Client's cultural background
    h. Type of surgery
    i. Type of anesthesia
  Consult *Acute Pain Management in Adult: Operative Procedures* (Acute pain management clinical practice guideline), U.S. Dept of Health and Human Service, Public Health Service, Agency of Health Care Policy and Research.
2. Give analgesics as appropriate; may use patient-controlled analgesia (PCA) (Table 3-6).
    a. Check vital signs before and after administering analgesic.
    b. Assess and document effectiveness.

Table 3-6 Classes of analgesics

OPIOID AGONIST

Morphine
Codeine
Fentanyl transdermal system (Duragesic)
Hydromorphone (Dilaudid)
Hydrocodone (in Lorcet, Lortab, Vicodin)
Methadone (Dolophine)
Levorphanol (Levo-Dromoran)
Oxycodone (in Percocet, Percodan)
Oxymorphone (Numorphan)
Meperidine (Demerol)

OPIOID AGONIST-ANTAGONIST AND PARTIAL AGONIST

Buprenorphine (Buprenex)
Pentazocine (Talwin)
Nalbuphine (Nubain)
Butorphanol (Stadol)

NONSTEROIDAL ANTIINFLAMMATORY DRUGS (NSAIDs)

Aspirin
Acetaminophen
Ibuprofen (Motrin)
Fenoprofen (Nalfon)
Diflunisal (Dolobid)
Naproxen (Naprosyn)
Ketorolac (Toradol)

3. Use nonpharmacologic management to supplement, not replace, pharmacologic interventions.
    a. Cognitive-behavioral intervention (e.g., relaxation, distraction, imagery)
    b. Physical interventions (e.g., positioning, heat, cold, massage)
    c. Assess and document effectiveness
4. Prevent immobility.
    a. Turn every 2 hours.
    b. Begin range-of-motion (ROM) exercise as appropriate.
    c. Ambulate as appropriate to prevent abdominal distention.
5. Prevent nausea and vomiting.
    a. Determine cause (e.g., type of anesthesia or surgery).
    b. Give antiemetics as ordered.
    c. Give frequent oral hygiene.

Evaluation

Client's pain is relieved; offers no complaints of nausea.

Goal 5 Client and significant others are prepared for client's discharge.

Implementation

1. Begin discharge planning at first encounter with client.
2. Determine discharge date by consulting with physician.
3. Give *written* discharge instructions to client and significant others; allow time for them to read and discuss instructions.
4. Give client and significant others appropriate information about medications, return appointments, treatments, activity level, diet, and dressings.
5. Instruct client and significant others to report signs of complications to physician immediately (e.g., fever, reddened incision, chest congestion).
6. Refer to appropriate community health agency as needed.

Evaluation

Client states time of return appointment, activity allowed; lists medicines and how to take them; demonstrates correctly how to do prescribed treatments.

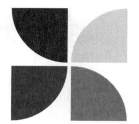

Oxygenation

OVERVIEW OF PHYSIOLOGY

1. The cardinal purpose of the cardiovascular and respiratory systems is to provide adequate oxygenation to the entire body.
   a. Respiratory system: responsible for the intake of oxygen (O_2) and elimination of carbon dioxide (CO_2); plays a major role in maintaining acid-base balance
   b. Cardiovascular system: responsible for the transport of O_2, CO_2, nutrients, and waste products
2. The heart is enclosed and protected in a fibrous sac known as the pericardium; between the pericardium and epicardium there is a small space that contains a few drops of fluid that lubricate the heart surface.
3. The heart wall is composed of three layers:
   a. Epicardium: outer layer
   b. Myocardium: middle layer; responsible for contraction of the heart
   c. Endocardium: inner layer; lines inner chambers, valves, chordae tendineae, and papillary muscles
4. The heart is a high-energy, four-chamber pump that forcefully ejects blood with enough pressure to perfuse the pulmonary and systemic circulatory systems.
5. The heart is innervated by the autonomic nervous system.
   a. Sympathetic stimulation increases the heart rate.
   b. Parasympathetic (vagal) stimulation decreases the heart rate.
6. The cardiac cycle consists of
   a. systole, the period of contraction during which the chambers eject blood
   b. diastole, the period of relaxation during which the chambers fill with blood
7. Preload is the volume of blood distending the ventricle at the end of diastole. Afterload is the resistance against which the left ventricle must eject blood into the aorta.
8. The cardiac impulse originates automatically in the sinoatrial (SA) node, travels to the right and left atria → atria contract. Then the impulse reaches the atrioventricular (AV) node; accelerates through the bundle of His, bundle branches, and Purkinje's fibers; and is distributed rapidly and evenly over the ventricles → ventricles contract.
9. Flow of blood through the heart: Deoxygenated blood via superior and inferior vena cava enters the right atrium → tricuspid valve → right ventricle → pulmonic valve → pulmonary arteries → lungs. Oxygenated blood from lungs via pulmonary veins enters left atrium → bicuspid (mitral) valve → left ventricle → aortic valve → aorta → systemic circulation (Fig. 3-2).
10. The blood supply to the heart itself is furnished by the right and left coronary arteries (Fig. 3-3).
11. The vascular system is a continuous network of tubes that carry blood throughout the body. The arterial system, made up of arteries, arterioles, and capillaries, delivers oxygenated blood from the heart to body organs and tissues. In the microscopic capillary bed, oxygen, nutrients, and metabolic waste products are exchanged between blood and tissue cells. The venous system, made up of venules and veins, collects blood from the capillary bed and returns it to the heart.
12. Mean arterial pressure = cardiac output × total peripheral resistance; cardiac output = stroke volume (amount of blood ejected/beat) × heart rate. Arterial pressure can be increased by increasing cardiac output (either stroke volume, heart rate, or both), or by increasing total peripheral resistance. Both cardiac output and total peripheral resistance are influenced by a variety of factors, particularly the autonomic nervous system. Stimulation of the sympathetic nervous system increases heart rate, stroke volume, and total peripheral resistance.
13. Blood pressure varies throughout circulation: greatest in the arterial system; lowest in the venous portion. Central venous pressure (CVP) is the pressure within the right atrium (normal = 4 to 10 cm H_2O [2 to 7 mm Hg]).
14. The respiratory system is composed of upper and lower airway structures:
   a. Upper airway: nose and nasopharynx, mouth, oropharynx, and larynx
   b. Lower airway: trachea, main stem of bronchi, bronchioles, alveolar ducts, and alveoli
   c. Airways filter, warm, and humidify inspired air
15. The lungs lie in and are protected by the airtight thoracic cavity. The bony cage is composed of the sternum and ribs anteriorly and the ribs, scapulae, and vertebral column posteriorly. The thoracic cavity is lined with a serous membrane, the pleura; one surface of the pleura lines the inside of the rib cage (parietal pleura), and the other covers the lungs (visceral pleura). The pleural space (really a potential space) exists between the surfaces of the two pleurae. Subatmospheric pressure in the pleural space is responsible for the continued expansion of the lungs.

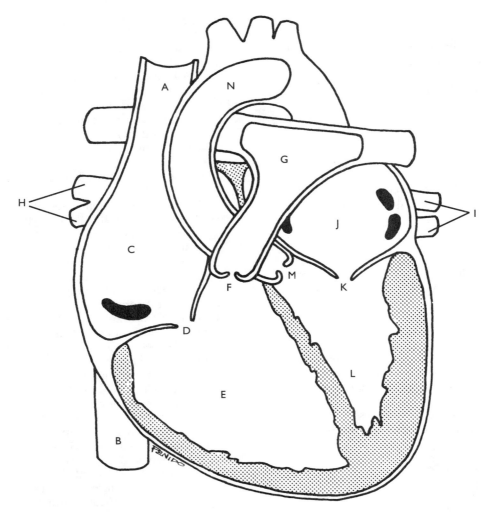

Fig. 3-2 The normal heart. *a*, Superior vena cava; *b*, inferior vena cava; *c*, right atrium; *d*, tricuspid valve; *e*, right ventricle; *f*, pulmonic valve; *g*, pulmonary artery; *h*, right pulmonary veins; *i*, left pulmonary veins; *j*, left atrium; *k*, bicuspid (mitral) valve; *l*, left ventricle; *m*, aortic valve; *n*, aorta.

16. The basic gas-exchange unit of the respiratory system is the alveolus. Pulmonary capillaries lie adjacent to each alveolus; O_2 and CO_2 are exchanged across the alveolar-capillary membrane by the process of diffusion.

17. The neural control of respirations is located in the medulla. Under normal conditions, this center is stimulated directly or reflexly by the concentration of CO_2 in the blood (Pco_2). Also, chemoreceptors located in the carotid arteries and aortic arch respond primarily to hypoxemia (reduced Po_2). These chemoreceptors also stimulate the medulla.

18. The rhythmic breathing pattern is dependent on the cyclical excitation of the respiratory muscles by the phrenic nerve (to the diaphragm) and the intercostal nerves (to the intercostal muscles).

19. Blood is the fluid that circulates through the cardiovascular system.
   a. Composition:
      1. cells: RBCs, WBCs, platelets
      2. plasma: water, protein, electrolytes, and various organic constituents
   b. Functions:
      1. RBCs (hemoglobin): carry O_2 from the lungs to tissue and CO_2 from tissue to lungs
      2. WBCs: defend against microbial invasion
      3. platelets: hemostasis
   c. total volume: approximately 5000 ml

20. The major steps of clot formation are thromboplastin $\rightarrow$ prothrombin $\rightarrow$ thrombin $\rightarrow$ fibrinogen $\rightarrow$ fibrin (clot).

APPLICATION OF THE NURSING PROCESS TO THE CLIENT WITH OXYGENATION PROBLEMS

ASSESSMENT
1. Health history
   a. Dyspnea or chest pain/discomfort
      1. when (e.g., rest, activity)
      2. relieved by what

b. Cough
1. when
2. nonproductive or productive; if productive, character and amount of sputum
c. Smoking
1. type, quantity, duration
2. if stopped, duration
d. Allergies
1. allergen
2. allergic reaction
e. Orthopnea or paroxysmal nocturnal dyspnea (PND)
1. when
2. relieved by what (e.g., number of pillows, rest)
f. Edema, syncope, dizziness, or headache
1. when
2. relieved by what
g. Fatigue or weakness
1. when
2. relieved by what
3. compare with client's normal level of exercise
h. Changes in lifestyle
1. ADL
2. work
3. leisure
i. Diet (have client describe previous 24-hour intake)
1. restrictions (e.g., sodium, cholesterol)
2. difficulties complying with prescribed diet
3. alcohol intake
4. food preferences and intolerances
5. who shops for food and prepares meals

j. Medications (prescription and nonprescription)
1. dosage
2. side effects
3. effectiveness
k. Personal or family history
1. cardiac problems (e.g., angina, myocardial infarction, hypertension)
2. pulmonary problems (e.g., tuberculosis, pneumonia, asthma)
2. Physical examination
a. Vital signs
1. blood pressure: lying, sitting, standing, in both arms
2. pulse: rate, rhythm, and volume
3. respirations: rate, depth, rhythm, and effort
4. temperature
b. Inspection of chest
1. use of accessory muscles
2. presence of retraction
3. degree of excursion
4. chest deformity
c. Palpation of chest
1. areas of pain or tenderness
2. presence of carotid thrills, atypical pulsation
3. change in tactile fremitus
4. point of maximal impulse (PMI): slight pulsation palpable at apex area (Fig. 3-4)
d. Percussion of chest
1. resonance = normal air
2. hyperresonance = trapped air
3. dullness = fluid or consolidation
e. Auscultation of the lungs
1. normal breath sounds
a. vesicular: heard over most of lungs
b. bronchovesicular: heard over main stem of bronchi
c. bronchial: heard over trachea and main stem of bronchi
2. adventitious breath sounds
a. rales or crackles
▪ high-pitched crackling

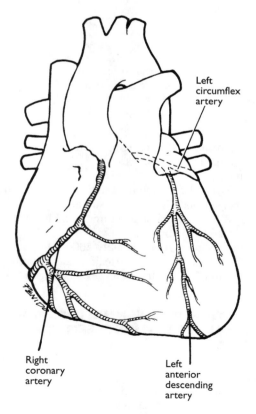

Fig. 3-3 Coronary blood supply.

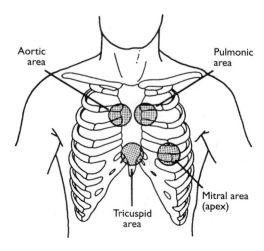

Fig. 3-4 Areas of auscultation of heart valves.

- predominantly inspiratory
- caused by air passing through abnormal secretions in alveoli

b. rhonchi or gurgles
  - loud, coarse gurgling
  - predominantly expiratory
  - caused by air passing through abnormal secretions in bronchi

c. wheezing
  - high-pitched whistling
  - caused by air passing through narrowed bronchi

d. bronchial (tubular) breath sounds audible over peripheral lung
  - expiratory and inspiratory
  - indicates consolidation (e.g., pneumonia)

e. Auscultation of the heart

3. anatomic landmarks: aortic, pulmonic, tricuspid, and mitral area correspond to where valve closing is heard the loudest (Fig. 3-4)

a. aortic: second intercostal space to the right of the sternum

b. pulmonic: second intercostal space to the left of the sternum

c. tricuspid: fourth and fifth intercostal space slightly left of the sternum

d. mitral: at the apex of the heart in the fifth intercostal space in the midclavicular line

4. apical pulse
  a. Auscultated best at apex area (Fig. 3-4)
  b. rate and rhythm
  c. pulse deficit = apical minus radial pulse (NOTE: the two pulses must be taken at the same time by *two* practitioners)

5. normal heart sounds
  a. S_1 (lub)
    - closing of mitral and tricuspid valves
    - at onset of ventricular systole
  b. S_2 (dub)
    - closing of aortic and pulmonary valves
    - at onset of ventricular diastole

6. extra heart sounds
  a. S_3, S_4
    - abnormal in adults
    - sometimes normal in children and young adults
  b. murmurs: caused by turbulent blood flow

f. Capillary filling time of nail beds (normal is less than 5 seconds)

g. Inspection of neck veins (jugular)

h. Auscultation of carotid and femoral arteries for bruits

i. Palpation of peripheral pulses
  1. rate
  2. rhythm
  3. strength (absent → bounding)
  4. equality relative to contralateral artery
  5. compressibility of vessel wall (elastic → rigid)

j. Inspection of skin
  1. color
  2. temperature
  3. texture
  4. pigmentation
  5. pain/tenderness
  6. paresthesia
  7. hair distribution
  8. nails
  9. lower extremities
    a. ulceration
    b. varicosities
    c. edema

3. Diagnostic tests
  a. Pulmonary function tests: the direct or indirect measurement of various lung volumes to assess lung function (Fig. 3-5)
    1. *tidal volume* (TV): volume of gas inspired and expired with a quiet, normal breath (500 ml)
    2. *inspiratory reserve volume* (IRV): maximal volume that can be inspired at the end of a normal inspiration (3100 ml)
    3. *expiratory reserve volume* (ERV): maximal volume that can be forcefully exhaled after a normal expiration (1200 ml)

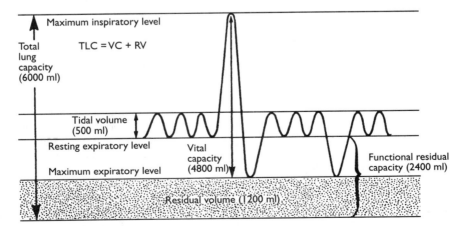

Fig. 3-5 Pulmonary volumes and capacities of an adult; values vary with age, sex, weight, and height. (From Kersten L: *Comprehensive respiratory nursing: a decision making approach,* Philadelphia, 1989, Saunders.)

4. *residual volume* (RV): volume of gas left in lung after maximal expiration (1200 ml)
5. *minute volume* (MV): volume of gas inspired and expired in 1 minute of normal breathing (6 L/min)
6. *vital capacity* (VC): maximal amount of air that can be expired after a maximal inspiration (TV + IRV + ERV) (4800 ml)
7. *forced expiratory volume* (FEV): volume of air that can be forcefully expelled after maximal inspiration; FEV_1: FEV in first second

b. Sputum specimens
   1. examinations
      a. smear: acid-fast bacilli (AFB)
      b. culture and sensitivity (C&S)
      c. cytology
   2. nursing care
      a. collect specimen in morning
      b. have client cough after three deep breaths and expectorate into sterile specimen container
      c. collect at least 5 ml sputum, not nasal/oral mucus or saliva

c. Chest x-rays or tomograms

d. Lung scan: after injection of radioactive material, lung is scanned for presence of obstruction or areas that are poorly perfused

e. Bronchoscopy
   1. insertion of a rigid or flexible fiberoptic bronchoscope through the oral cavity into the bronchus in order to view the area; bronchial brushing, biopsy, or bronchogram may be done during the procedure
   2. nursing care: preparation
      a. explain procedure
      b. NPO 6 to 12 hours
      c. oral hygiene
      d. remove dentures
      e. premedicate
   3. nursing care: postprocedure
      a. NPO until gag reflex returns
      b. observe respirations
      c. observe hoarseness, dysphagia
      d. observe for subcutaneous emphysema (crackling under the skin when pressed, caused by air from perforated airway)
      e. bloody sputum normal after biopsy

f. Electrocardiogram (ECG)
   1. graphic recording of the electrical activity of the heart (Fig. 3-6); used primarily to identify cardiac dysrhythmias and myocardial damage
   2. types
      a. resting
         ▪ standard 12 lead
         ▪ continuous-monitor 1 or 2 lead
      b. exercise (stress test)
         ▪ treadmill or bicycle
         ▪ abnormalities may show only during exercise
      c. ambulatory continuous
         ▪ Holter monitor
         ▪ abnormalities may show only during daily activities

g. Myocardial scan: after injection of radioactive thallium, heart is scanned to evaluate myocardial perfusion

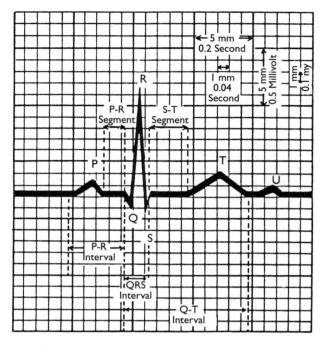

Fig. 3-6 Components of a normal electrocardiogram. The P wave represents atrial depolarization; the P-R segment, atrial depolarization and transmission of the cardiac impulse through the AV node. The QRS complex presents ventricular depolarization; the ST segment, the refractory period of the ventricular muscle. The T wave represents ventricular repolarization. The U wave may not be present.

h. Echocardiogram: movement of heart structures is viewed by ultrasound
i. Cardiac catheterization or angiography (see also Table 5-19)
   1. insertion of a radiopaque catheter into the heart via a peripheral vein (right heart catheterization) or artery (left heart catheterization). Injection of radiopaque dye permits viewing of heart chambers, valves, and vessels. Pressures and oxygen concentrations are also measured
   2. preparation
      a. explain procedure
      b. NPO 6 to 12 hours
      c. take and record all peripheral pulses
      d. check for allergy to iodine or shellfish
   3. nursing care: after procedure
      a. monitor vital signs
      b. monitor pulse and temperature in area distal to arterial puncture site (spasms or emboli can cause these to diminish or disappear); embolus formation requires immediate intervention
      c. Maintain hemostasis at insertion site; use pressure dressing
      d. prevent stress on incision line (e.g., no bending of affected limb, no ambulation for 12 to 24 hours if femoral site)
j. Pulse oximetry: noninvasive measurement of arterial O_2 saturation (normal 95% to 100%)

k. Hematologic studies
1. arterial blood gases (ABGs)
   a. tests of arterial blood to assess oxygenation, ventilation, and acid-base status
   b. normal values
      - pH: 7.35 to 7.45
      - Po_2: 80 to 100 mm Hg
      - Pco_2: 35 to 45 mm Hg
      - O_2 saturation: 95% to 100%
2. complete blood cell count (CBC)
   a. WBC: 5000 to 10,000 per mm^3
   b. RBC:
      - men: 4.7 million to 6.1 million per mm^3
      - women: 4.2 million to 5.4 million per mm^3
   c. hemoglobin (Hgb)
      - men: 14 to 18 g/dl
      - women: 12 to 16 g/dl
   d. hematocrit (Hct)
      - men: 42% to 52%
      - women: 37% to 47%
   e. platelets: 150,000 to 400,000 per mm^3
3. electrolytes
   a. sodium: 136 to 145 mEq/L
   b. potassium: 3.5 to 5.0 mEq/L
   c. chloride: 90 to 110 mEq/L
4. lipids
   a. cholesterol: 150 to 200 mg/dl
   b. triglycerides: 40 to 150 mg/dl

ANALYSIS/NURSING DIAGNOSIS

1. Safe, effective care environment
   a. Risk for injury
   b. Knowledge deficit (specify)
   c. Risk for infection
2. Physiologic integrity
   a. Decreased cardiac output
   b. Impaired gas exchange
   c. Activity intolerance
3. Psychosocial integrity
   a. Ineffective individual coping
   b. Anxiety
   c. Body image disturbance
4. Health promotion/maintenance
   a. Impaired adjustment
   b. Health-seeking behaviors (specify)
   c. Noncompliance (specify)

GENERAL NURSING PLANNING, IMPLEMENTATION, AND EVALUATION

Goal 1 Client will maintain patent airway and adequate oxygenation.

Implementation
1. Monitor respiratory status (e.g., vital signs, breath sounds, skin color, ABGs, pulse oximetry).
2. Reduce anxiety.
3. Limit or space activities to decrease O_2 need.
4. Turn frequently if on bed rest.
5. Place in Fowler's position to increase air exchange.
6. Humidify air.
7. Administer O_2 as needed.
8. Encourage to cough and deep breathe frequently.

9. Avoid sedatives that depress respirations and cough reflex (e.g., narcotics).
10. Force fluids to liquefy bronchial secretions.
11. Suction as needed; provide hyperoxygenation before and after suctioning to decrease chances of hypoxia.
12. Carry out postural drainage to promote drainage of lung and bronchi by gravity, if needed.
    a. Give humidified air or bronchodilators 10 to 15 minutes before.
    b. Do no longer than 15 minutes at one time.
    c. Clapping or vibrating helps loosen secretions.
    d. Avoid clapping or vibrating over sternum, over breast tissue, below ribs.
    e. Follow with coughing to be effective; do not allow client to cough in head-down position.

Evaluation
Client is well-oxygenated (Po_2 is greater than 80 mm Hg).

Goal 2 Client's cardiac workload will be decreased.

Implementation
1. Monitor cardiovascular status (e.g., vital signs, pulse deficit, skin color).
2. Limit activity to decrease O_2 need.
3. Promote rest.
4. Administer O_2 as needed.
5. Monitor I&O of fluids to detect circulatory overload.
6. Give antihypertensives and diuretics as ordered to reduce preload and afterload (Table 3-7).
7. Prevent constipation (e.g., use stool softeners).
8. Reduce anxiety.

Evaluation
Client's cardiac workload is decreased; pulse decreases from 100 to 84.

Goal 3 Client will remain free from the hazards of immobility.

Implementation
1. Turn frequently.
2. Encourage to deep breathe and cough as needed.
3. Provide passive ROM exercises as needed.
4. Teach client ankle flexion exercises.
5. Give good back care.
6. Apply antiembolic hose.
7. Give anticoagulants if ordered (Table 3-8).

Evaluation
Client remains free from thrombophlebitis, pressure ulcers, pulmonary consolidation.

SELECTED HEALTH PROBLEMS RESULTING IN INTERFERENCE WITH CARDIAC FUNCTION

✠ CARDIOPULMONARY ARREST

1. Definition: sudden cessation of adequate cardiac and pulmonary function
2. Classification: medical emergency

Table 3-7   Antihypertensive drugs

Name	Action	Side effects	Nursing implications
DIURETIC AGENTS			
Thiazide diuretics Chlorothiazide (Diuril) Hydrochlorothiazide (Oretic, HydroDIURIL, Esdrix) Chlorthalidone (Hygroton)	Increases sodium chloride and water excretion by inhibiting renal reabsorption between the ascending loop and distal tubules. Enhances potassium excretion.	*Hypokalemia* *Hyponatremia* *Hyperuricemia* (usually asymptomatic; can cause gouty arthritis) *Hyperglycemia* (usually asymptomatic)	Monitor I&O, BP, weight, serum electrolytes. Modify dietary sodium and potassium as needed. Administer potassium supplement as ordered.
Loop diuretics Bumetanide (Bumex) Ethacrynic acid (Edecrin) Furosemide (Lasix)	Primarily inhibits reabsorption of sodium chloride and water in loop of Henle.	Same as thiazides plus hypochloremia and GI upset	Same as thiazides.
Potassium-sparing diuretics Spironolactone (Aldactone)	Increases sodium chloride and water excretion and decreases potassium excretion by blocking aldosterone.	*Hyperkalemia* *Hyponatremia*	Weak diuretic. Monitor for hyperkalemia.
ANTIADRENERGIC AGENTS			
Reserpine (Serpasil, Reserpoid, Sandril, Rau-Sed) Methyldopa (Aldomet) Guanethidine (Ismelin) Propranolol (Inderal)* Clonidine (Catapres) Metoprolol (Lopressor) Prazosin (Minipress)	Acts by various complex mechanisms to inhibit synthesis, storage, and transport of norepinephrine, thereby depressing sympathetic nerve activity—as a result, cardiac output and peripheral vascular resistance are decreased. Reserpine and methyldopa also have central depressant effects.	Depression, fatigue and drowsiness, vivid dreams, dry mouth, impotence, bradycardia (except prazosin)	Monitor BP, P, weight. Teach importance of compliance. Advise hard candy for dry mouth. Instruct to rise and change position slowly.
VASODILATING AGENTS			
Hydralazine (Apresoline) Minoxidil (Loniten) Nitroprusside (Nipride) injection	Acts directly on vascular smooth muscle to decrease peripheral resistance.	Headache, tachycardia, palpitation, angina, GI disturbances, lupuslike syndrome (especially long-term administration with high doses), sodium and fluid retention, postural hypotension	Monitor BP, P, weight. Teach importance of compliance. Instruct to rise and change position slowly.
ANGIOTENSIN-CONVERTING ENZYME (ACE) INHIBITORS			
Captopril (Capoten) Enalapril (Vasotec) Lisinopril (Prinivil, Zestril)	Inhibits angiotensin II formation; decreases aldosterone secretion; reduces peripheral resistance.	Vertigo, cough, anorexia, dysrhythmias, proteinuria, rash, impotence	Monitor BP, heart rate. Check renal function. Contraindicated with renal artery disease.
CALCIUM CHANNEL BLOCKERS*			
Nifedipine (Procardia) Diltiazem (Cardizem) Verapamil (Calan)	Reduces tone of blood vessels; causes arterial dilation.		

*See also Table 3-9.

Table 3-8 Anticoagulant and thrombolytic drugs

Name	Action	Side effects	Nursing implications
ANTICOAGULANT AGENTS			
Heparin sodium	Prolongs clotting. Prevents formation of thrombin from prothrombin. Onset almost immediate. Lasts 4 hours. No effects on existing thrombi.	Hemorrhage epistaxis, hematuria, melena, ecchymosis, bleeding gums	Parenteral: IV or subcutaneous. Monitor partial thromboplastin time (PTT). PTT maintained at 1½-2 times normal (normal = 30-40 seconds). Discontinue if there is evidence of bleeding or if the PTT is overly prolonged. ANTIDOTE: Protamine sulfate. Use bleeding precautions (e.g., soft toothbrush, electric razor).
Bishydroxycoumarin (Dicumarol)	Prolongs clotting. Inhibits synthesis of prothrombin and other vitamin K–dependent clotting factors. Slow onset (2-3 days). Lasts up to 9 days after last dose. No effect on existing thrombi.	Hemorrhage epistaxis, hematuria, melena, ecchymosis, bleeding gums. GI disturbances: diarrhea, vomiting, anorexia. INTERACTION: Salicylates *increase* anticoagulant effect.	Oral. Monitor prothrombin time (PT). PT maintained at 1½-2 times normal (normal = 11.0-12.5 seconds). Discontinue Dicumarol or Coumadin if the PT is overly prolonged or if bleeding occurs. No aspirin. ANTIDOTE: Vitamin K (AquaMEPHYTON). Use bleeding precautions as above. Carry ID stating that anticoagulants are being taken.
Warfarin sodium (Coumadin)	Same as Dicumarol. Onset occurs within 18-24 hours. Cumulative effect lasts up to 7 days.	Same as Dicumarol.	Same as Dicumarol.
THROMBOLYTIC AGENTS			
Streptokinase (Streptase)	Activates plasminogen and converts it to plasmin, which degrades fibrin clots. Immediate onset; residual effects last up to 12 hours after infusion.	Hemorrhage, oozing at site of puncture, incision, or cut; fever, allergic reaction, reperfusion dysrhythmias.	Parenteral: IV. Monitor PT, PTT, and thrombin time. Monitor for hemorrhage. Maintain bleeding precautions. Start heparin before streptokinase is discontinued. Solu-Cortef frequently given before infusion to prevent allergic reaction. Administer all drugs through preexisting IV lines, by mouth, or by NG tube while streptokinase is infusing. Monitor cardiac rhythm for reperfusion dysrhythmias. No true antidote.
Tissue Plasminogen Activator (t-PA) (Activase)	Converts plasminogen to plasmin at fibrin surface; is more clot specific than streptokinase. Immediate onset; action lasts approximately 10 minutes.	Hemorrhage, oozing at site of puncture, incision, or cut; reperfusion dysrhythmias.	Parenteral: IV. Monitor PT, PTT, and thrombin time. Monitor for hemorrhage. Maintain bleeding precautions. Start heparin before t-PA is discontinued. Administer all drugs through preexisting IV lines, by mouth, or by NG tube while streptokinase is infusing. Monitor cardiac rhythm for reperfusion dysrhythmias.

Nursing Process

ASSESSMENT

1. Responsiveness
   a. Tap or gently shake victim.
   b. Shout "Are you OK?"
2. A——airway: determine airway patency
3. B—breathing
   a. Determine breathlessness in 3 to 5 seconds
   b. *Look* for chest to rise and fall.
   c. *Listen* for air escaping during exhalation.
   d. *Feel* for flow of air.
4. C—circulation
   a. Determine pulselessness in 3 to 10 seconds.
   b. Check carotid pulse.

ANALYSIS/NURSING DIAGNOSIS (see p. 125)

PLANNING, IMPLEMENTATION, AND EVALUATION

Goal 1 Unresponsive victim will be recognized promptly and receive emergency medical services (EMS) intervention as soon as possible.

Implementation

1. Determine unresponsiveness quickly.
2. If unresponsive:
   a. Activate EMS system *immediately,* before beginning cardiopulmonary resuscitation (CPR) (i.e., phone 911 or equivalent emergency number).
   b. Call for defibrillator.

Evaluation

Unresponsive victim receives EMS intervention within 10 minutes of collapse.

Goal 2 Breathless, unresponsive victim will have an open airway and receive adequate ventilation.

Implementation

1. Place victim in supine position on flat, firm surface.
2. Assume rescuer position at victim's side.
3. Clear airway of foreign matter if present (finger sweep).
4. Open airway by head tilt–chin lift maneuver (lifts tongue away from back of throat).
5. Watch for breathing.
6. If spontaneous breathing is obvious, roll unresponsive victim without cervical trauma onto his or her side (recovery position) and maintain open airway.
7. If no breathing, ventilate mouth-to-mouth.
8. Give two initial slow breaths of 1½ to 2 seconds each.
   a. Maintain open airway with head tilt–chin lift maneuver.
   b. Pinch nose closed with thumb and index finger.
   c. Seal lips around victim's lips to create airtight seal.
9. If unable to ventilate:
   a. Reposition head.
   b. Ventilate.
10. If still unable to ventilate, use Heimlich maneuver (subdiaphragmatic abdominal thrust) to clear airway of foreign body.
11. Watch for breathing.

12. Continue mouth-to-mouth ventilation, if no breathing but pulse is present, at rate of 10 to 12 breaths per minute.
13. Take a breath after each ventilation.
14. If available:
    a. Use barrier devices (e.g., latex gloves).
    b. Use ventilatory devices.
    c. Administer 100% oxygen.

Evaluation

Victim is adequately ventilated; i.e., chest rises with each ventilation, air escape is heard and felt during exhalation.

Goal 3 Breathless, pulseless, unresponsive victim will circulate adequately oxygenated blood.

Implementation

1. Check carotid pulse.
2. If carotid pulse is absent, begin external chest compression after initial two breaths.
3. Maintain victim in horizontal supine position on firm flat surface.
4. Assume rescuer position at victim's side.
   a. Arms straight, elbows locked
   b. Shoulders directly over hands and victim's sternum
5. Locate lower half of victim's sternum.
6. Locate proper hand position.
   a. Place heel of one hand on lower half of sternum.
   b. Place other hand on top of hand on sternum so hands are parallel.
   c. Have long axis of hand heel over long axis of sternum.
   d. Have fingers extended or interlocked, but off chest.
7. Depress sternum approximately 1½ to 2 inches at rate of 80 to 100 compressions per minute.
8. After each compression, release pressure completely without lifting hands from chest and allow chest to return to its normal position.
9. One rescuer: give 15 compressions per 2 ventilations. Two rescuers: give 5 compressions per 1 ventilation.
10. Determine if victim has resumed spontaneous breathing and circulation by reassessing breathlessness and pulselessness at about the end of first minute and every few minutes thereafter.
11. Continue CPR until spontaneous respirations and pulse return.
12. If available:
    a. Monitor ECG.
    b. Defibrillate as soon as possible for ventricular fibrillation.

Evaluation

Victim has carotid pulsation with each compression; maintains systolic arterial blood pressure of 60 to 80 mm Hg.

Goal 4 Breathless, pulseless, unresponsive victim will receive appropriate emergency drugs.

Implementation

1. Start IV for drug administration.
2. Administer emergency drugs as ordered (Table 3-9).

Table 3-9 Emergency drugs*

Name	Indications
FIRST-LINE DRUGS	
Adenosine (Adenocard)	Complex tachycardias
Atropine sulfate	Bradycardia, asystole
Epinephrine	Asystole and ventricular fibrillation; to increase heart rate, cardiac output, and BP
Lidocaine hydrochloride (Xylocaine)	Ventricular dysrhythmias
SECOND-LINE DRUGS	
Bretylium tosylate (Bretylol)	Ventricular dysrhythmias unresponsive to lidocaine
Dopamine hydrochloride (Intropin)	To increase BP and cardiac contractility; in small doses improves renal perfusion
Procainamide hydrochloride (Pronestyl)	Ventricular dysrhythmias when lidocaine is not effective
Verapamil (Calan)	Paroxysmal supraventricular tachycardia (PSVT)
Sodium bicarbonate	Not recommended routinely during cardiac arrest

*Drugs that should be readily available for all cardiac emergencies; recommended by American Heart Association.

Evaluation

Victim receives appropriate doses of ordered drugs; victim's heart resumes normal sinus rhythm

SHOCK

1. Definition: state in which tissue perfusion is inadequate to sustain life
2. Etiologic classification
   a. Hypovolemic (decreased volume)
   b. Cardiogenic (inadequate pump)
   c. Vasogenic (pooling caused by vasodilation)
      1. neurogenic
      2. septic
      3. anaphylactic
3. Precipitating factors
   a. Hemorrhage
   b. Gastrointestinal (GI) loss of fluid and electrolytes
   c. Burns
   d. Myocardial infarction
   e. Dysrhythmias
   f. Spinal cord trauma
   g. Spinal anesthesia
   h. Infections, particularly gram-negative bacteria
   i. Allergic reactions
4. Body's response to shock
   a. Stimulation of the adrenal medulla by the sympathetic nervous system
      1. tachycardia
      2. tachypnea
      3. vasoconstriction
      4. redistribution of blood
      5. cool, clammy skin; oliguria; decreased bowel sounds
   b. Stimulation of renin-angiotensin-aldosterone system and antidiuretic hormone (ADH)
      1. thirst
      2. decreased urine volume
      3. increased concentration of urine
   c. Stimulation of cortisol and growth hormone secretion
      1. increased glucose metabolism
      2. increased fat mobilization

Nursing Process

ASSESSMENT

1. Identify high-risk client
2. Vital signs: tachycardia, tachypnea; early BP may be normal because of compensatory mechanisms but will decrease later
3. Mental status: restless, early increased alertness; as hypoxia occurs, alertness decreases, lethargy and coma follow
4. Skin changes
   a. Pale, cool, clammy skin (hypovolemic and cardiogenic shock)
   b. Flushed, cool if vasodilation present (vasogenic shock)
5. Fluid status: check skin turgor, I&O, urine specific gravity, central venous pressure (CVP)
   a. CVP increased in cardiogenic shock
   b. CVP decreased in hypovolemic and vasogenic shock

ANALYSIS/NURSING DIAGNOSIS (see p. 125)

PLANNING, IMPLEMENTATION, AND EVALUATION

Goal 1 High-risk client will remain free from undetected change in cellular perfusion.

Implementation (high-risk client)

1. Assess vital signs q4h, more frequently if unstable.
2. Measure I&O at least q8h, qh if unstable.
3. Note skin turgor, temperature, and color q8h.
4. Monitor ECG if dysrhythmias are present.
5. Obtain blood work as appropriate (CBC, electrolytes, blood urea nitrogen [BUN], creatinine, blood gases).

Evaluation

Client maintains stable vital signs, fluid balance; has no signs of impending shock.

Goal 2 Client will have adequate perfusion.

Implementation

1. Monitor blood pressure (mean should be at least 80), pulse, and respiration.
2. Note and report dysrhythmias.
3. Monitor CVP (normal = 4 to 10 cm H_2O); measure the same way each time.
4. Maintain urine output of at least 30 ml/hr and proportional to intake.
5. Monitor mental status.
6. Monitor GI function.
7. Administer fluids as ordered: blood, colloid fluids, or electrolyte solutions as necessary (until CVP = 6 to 10 cm H_2O).
8. Administer drugs only after circulating volume has returned to normal.
   a. Adrenergic agonists (e.g., epinephrine, dopamine, dobutamine, norepinephrine [Levophed], isoproterenol [Isuprel]) are used to increase cardiac output by increasing heart contractility and rate.
      1. administer with a controlled-volume regulator
      2. monitor BP every 15 minutes continually
      3. wean off drugs as soon as possible
      4. know that some of these drugs cause severe vasoconstriction and can worsen organ damage (renal failure, hepatic failure)
      5. watch for extravasation of vasopressors (if norepinephrine or dopamine extravasates, infiltrate around area with phentolamine [Regitine])
      6. titrate drug infusion to keep BP at a mean of 80, or as ordered.
   b. Vasodilators (nitroprusside [Nipride]) may be used to decrease cardiac work in cardiogenic shock.
   c. When using adrenergic stimulants and vasodilators together:
      1. if BP drops, decrease vasodilator first; then increase adrenergic stimulant
      2. if BP increases, decrease adrenergic agonists and then increase vasodilator
   d. Administer other drugs as ordered (e.g., cardiac glycosides to enhance cardiac contractility) (Table 3-10).
9. Place in modified Trendelenburg's position (feet up 45 degrees and head flat).

Evaluation

Client's BP is maintained at a mean of 80 mm Hg.

Goal 3 Client will have adequate O_2 and CO_2 levels.

Implementation

1. See General Nursing Goals 1 and 2, p. 125.
2. Provide comfort measures. (NOTE: If giving pain medications, do not use intramuscular (IM) or subcutaneous (SQ) route because medications may accumulate and not be absorbed; when perfusion improves, client may get overdose.)
3. Keep client warm, not hot or cold (heat causes sweating; cold causes shivering).

Evaluation

Client is well oxygenated (Po_2 is greater than 80 mm Hg; no air hunger or cyanosis).

Goal 4 Client will be protected from injury and complications.

Implementation

1. Keep bed's side rails up; if client is confused, watch carefully and avoid using restraints.
2. Apply antiembolic stockings to prevent venous stasis.
3. Turn frequently to prevent pressure ulcers, pulmonary problems.
4. Use sterile technique with all procedures (e.g., changing IVs) because client has decreased resistance to infection.

Evaluation

Client is free from preventable complications (e.g., falls, infections).

❖ ANGINA PECTORIS

1. Definitions
   a. Atherosclerosis: fatty plaque deposits in the intima of the artery
   b. Arteriosclerosis: calcium deposits in the media of the artery
   c. Angina pectoris: chest pain caused by temporary ischemia of the myocardium; usually caused by atherosclerosis, arteriosclerosis, thrombus, or coronary artery spasm

---

Table 3-10 Cardiac glycoside drugs

Name	Action	Side effects	Nursing implications
Digitoxin (Crystodigin) Digoxin (Lanoxin) oral and injection	Increase strength of myocardial contraction. Cardiac output is increased. Decreases heart rate. Promotes diuresis.	GI upset, visual disturbances, supraventricular dysrhythmias, heart block. Hypokalemia potentiates digitalis action.	Take pulse before administration: if below 60, hold medication and notify MD. Monitor serum K, Mg. High-potassium diet as needed. Monitor serum drug levels. (Therapeutic levels; Digoxin 0.5-2.0 ng/ml; Digitoxin 25-35 ng/ml)

2. Coronary artery disease (CAD) risk factors
   a. Modifiable
      1. hypertension
      2. hyperlipidemia
      3. smoking
      4. obesity
      5. diabetes
      6. stress
      7. sedentary lifestyle
   b. Nonmodifiable
      1. age
      2. sex: male
      3. family history
3. Precipitating factors (immediate)
   a. Five *E*s
      1. *e*xercise
      2. *e*xertion: arteries able to provide blood to myocardium at rest, but increased demand on coronary circulation cannot be met temporarily
      3. *e*motions: stimulation of sympathetic nervous system leads to increased demand on heart
      4. *e*ating a heavy meal: increased perfusion of the gastrointestinal tract for digestion; pressure from full stomach against diaphragm
      5. *e*xposure to cold
   b. Smoking

Nursing Process
ASSESSMENT
1. Precipitating factors
2. Pain
   a. Pattern varies with each individual but is usually the same for a specific person
   b. Usually retrosternal
   c. Tends to radiate into neck, jaw, shoulder, and down inner aspect of left arm (see Fig. 3-7).
   d. Short duration (1 to 3 minutes)
   e. Usually relieved by rest and nitroglycerin
3. ECG changes (if any) are not permanent
ANALYSIS/NURSING DIAGNOSIS (see p. 125)
PLANNING, IMPLEMENTATION, AND EVALUATION

> **Goal I** Client will have improved perfusion of the myocardium.

Implementation
1. Give antianginal drugs as ordered (Table 3-11).
2. Know actions and side effects of these drugs.
Evaluation
Client performs daily activities without anginal pain.

Table 3-11 Antianginal drugs

Name	Action	Side effects	Nursing implications
NITRATES			
Nitroglycerin (Nitrostat)	Rapid generalized vasodilation Oxygen consumption and demand on myocardium are decreased	Pounding headache, flushing, tachycardia, dizziness, orthostatic hypotension	Usually taken sublingually. Take at pain onset; repeat in 5 min × 2; if no pain relief, go to ER. Also taken prophylactically before pain onset.
Nitroglycerin ointment (Nitro-Bid) Nitroglycerin disk (Transderm Nitro, Nitro-Dur)	Slowly absorbed through skin; long-acting vasodilation	Same as nitroglycerin	Topical; disk applied to intact, hairless skin. Rotate sites. Use dermal patches intermittently (tolerance develops with use).
Erythrityl tetranitrate (Cardilate) Isosorbide dinitrate (Isordil, Sorbitrate)	Long-acting vasodilation	Same as nitroglycerin; can cause gastric irritation, nausea, vomiting	Sublingual or oral
Pentaerythritol tetranitrate (Peritrate)	Possible long-acting vasodilation	Same as nitroglycerin	Take on empty stomach.
CALCIUM CHANNEL BLOCKERS			
Nifedipine (Procardia) Diltiazem (Cardizem) Verapamil (Calan)	Coronary artery spasm is inhibited Oxygen consumption of myocardium is decreased	Fatigue, headache, transient hypotension, nausea, constipation	
BETA-ADRENERGIC BLOCKERS			
Propranolol (Inderal)	Heart rate, cardiac contractility, cardiac output, and BP are reduced; oxygen consumption of myocardium is decreased	Fatigue, bradycardia, postural hypotension, nausea, vomiting, diarrhea, bronchospasm	Heart rate must be 50 or more before the drug is administered.

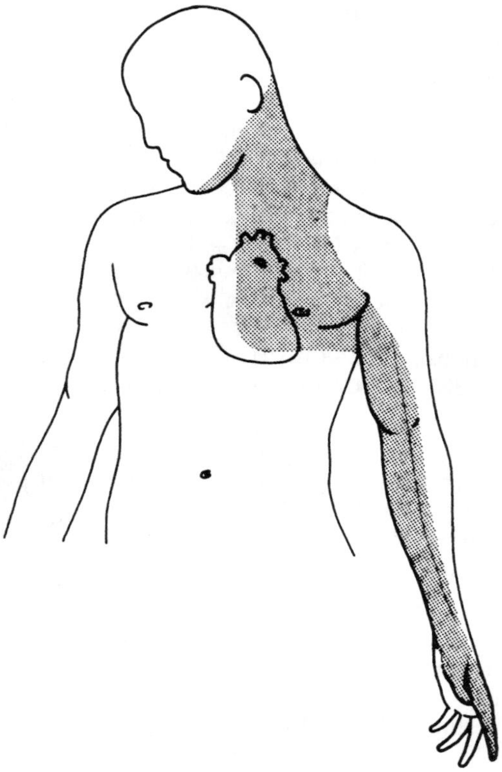

Fig. 3-7 Distribution of typical angina pain.

Goal 2 Client will learn methods to prevent attacks.

Implementation
1. Teach client
   a. To recognize symptoms.
   b. To take medications and cope with any side effects.
   c. When to take medications (e.g., before activity).
   d. To avoid precipitating factors if possible.
   e. To decrease risk factors (e.g., quit smoking, control hypertension).
   f. To reduce dietary cholesterol, fat, and saturated fat to prevent further atherosclerosis (Table 3-12).
2. Define activity level: space activities, eliminate those that might precipitate angina (e.g., mowing grass, shoveling snow).

Evaluation
Client performs daily activities without anginal pain by spacing activities and by taking a nitroglycerin tablet before bathing, eating, or taking daily walk.

Goal 3 Client will be able to state what to do if symptoms change.

Implementation
1. Teach client to identify own pain pattern and to recognize change in pain.
2. Instruct client to notify physician of change.

Table 3-12 Cholesterol and saturated fat content in selected items*

Food items	Serving	Cholesterol (mg)	Saturated fat (g)
DAIRY PRODUCTS			
Milk, skim	8 oz	0	0
Yogurt, low fat	8 oz	11	1.8
American cheese	1 oz	27	5.6
Butter	1 tbs	31	7.1
Milk, whole	8 oz	33	5.1
Ice cream	8 oz	59	8.9
FISH AND SHELLFISH			
Clams	3 oz	50	0.4
Fish, lean	3 oz	59	0.3
Shrimp	3 oz	126	0.5
MEATS AND POULTRY			
Beef liver	3 oz	372	2.5
Egg	1 whole	213	1.7
Beef, lean	3 oz	56	2.4
Chicken breast	3 oz	63	1.3
FRUITS AND VEGETABLES			
All fruits All vegetables	No cholesterol and generally no saturated fats (vegetable oils in italics below are two exceptions)		
VEGETABLE OILS			
Coconut oil	1 tbs	0	11.8
Palm oil	1 tbs	0	6.7
Olive oil	1 tbs	0	1.8
Corn oil	1 tbs	0	1.7
Safflower oil	1 tbs	0	1.2

*Exact amount of cholesterol and saturated fat varies with brand of food item.

Evaluation
Client correctly explains ways of dealing with a change in anginal pain.

MYOCARDIAL INFARCTION (MI)

1. Definition: occlusion of one or more coronary arteries causing an area of necrosis in the myocardium (infarct); see Figs. 3-3 and 3-8
2. Incidence
   a. Leading cause of death in the United States
   b. More common in men; rate in women rises after menopause
3. Risk factors (see coronary artery disease risk factors, p. 131)

Nursing Process

ASSESSMENT
1. Chest pain
   a. Intense, crushing, substernal
   b. Not relieved by rest or nitroglycerin
2. ECG changes: ST elevation or depression; T-wave inversion; pathologic Q waves
3. Serial serum enzymes (Table 3-13)

ANALYSIS/NURSING DIAGNOSIS (see p. 125)
PLANNING, IMPLEMENTATION, AND EVALUATION

> **Goal** Client will undergo pacemaker implantation free from preventable complications.

Implementation
1. Postprocedure
   a. Monitor for changes in pulse rate and rhythm.
   b. Monitor insertion site for bleeding or infection.
   c. Maintain strict asepsis at insertion site.
   d. Monitor for temperature elevation.
2. Teach client to
   a. Modify activity level as needed.
   b. Take own pulse daily.
   c. Monitor for signs and symptoms of pacemaker failure: vertigo, syncope, palpitations, hiccoughs, bradycardia.
   d. Avoid improperly grounded electric appliances (e.g., some power tools).
   e. Avoid sources of high-frequency signals (e.g., radio towers).
   f. Avoid magnetic resonance imaging (MRI) procedures.
   g. Have battery replaced per recommended schedule.
   h. Carry identification card.
   i. Continue medical follow-up care.

Evaluation
Client maintains a regular, normal heart rate after pacemaker implantation.

CONGESTIVE HEART FAILURE (CHF)
1. Definition: state in which cardiac output is inadequate to meet the metabolic needs of the body; characterized by circulatory congestion
2. Etiology: one or more of the following:
   a. Inflow of blood to heart greatly increased (e.g., excessive IV fluids or sodium and water retention)
   b. Outflow of blood from heart obstructed (e.g., damaged valves, narrowed arteries)
   c. Functional capacity of myocardium decreased (e.g., myocardial infarction, dysrhythmias)
   d. Metabolic needs of body accelerated (e.g., fever, pregnancy)
3. Cardiac compensation
   a. Mechanisms
      1. *tachycardia:* increases cardiac output
      2. *ventricular dilation:* increases volume of chambers
      3. *myocardial hypertrophy:* fibers of myocardium increase in length and diameter; heart contracts more forcibly
   b. Terminology
      1. *compensated CHF:* compensatory changes maintain adequate cardiac output
      2. *decompensated CHF:* compensatory changes unable to maintain adequate cardiac output; CHF becomes symptomatic
4. Left-sided congestive heart failure: left ventricle cannot accept all blood from pulmonary bed
   a. Etiology
      1. hypertension
      2. mitral or aortic valvular disease
      3. ischemic heart disease: damage or infarction of the left ventricle
   b. Pathophysiology: blood backs up in the *pulmonary* bed (Table 3-16)
5. Right-sided congestive heart failure: right ventricle cannot eject all blood from right atrium; therefore right atrium cannot accept all blood from systemic circulation
   a. Etiology
      1. left-sided CHF
      2. pulmonary disease
      3. tricuspid and pulmonic valvular disease
      4. ischemic heart disease: damage or infarction of the myocardium of the right ventricle
   b. Pathophysiology: blood backs up in *systemic* circulation (Table 3-16)

Nursing Process
ASSESSMENT
1. Left-sided CHF
   a. Dyspnea
   b. Abnormal breath sounds (e.g., rales)
   c. Abnormal heart sounds (e.g., S_3)

Table 3-16 Congestive heart failure

Results	Signs and symptoms
PATHOPHYSIOLOGY OF LEFT-SIDED HEART FAILURE: Blood backs up from left ventricle to *pulmonary* bed.	
Pulmonary congestion	Dyspnea, orthopnea, rales, paraoxysmal nocturnal dyspnea
Pulmonary edema	(PND), decreased vital capacity, cyanosis
Cerebral anoxia	Irritability, restlessness, confusion
Decreased O_2 to cells	Extreme weakness, fatigue, oliguria
PATHOPHYSIOLOGY OF RIGHT-SIDED HEART FAILURE: Blood backs up from right ventricle to *systemic* circulation.	
Increased hydrostatic pressure in systemic circulation	Peripheral pitting edema, dependent edema: sacrum, ankles
Elevated venous pressure	Distended neck veins
Congestion in kidneys, retention of sodium	Oliguria
Venous congestion in extremities	Cool and cyanotic legs
Congestion in GI tract	Anorexia, nausea, bloating

d. Decreased O_2 saturation (i.e., <95%)

e. Decreased Po_2 (i.e., <80 mm Hg)

2. Right-sided CHF
   a. Elevated central venous pressure
   b. Distended neck veins
   c. Hepatomegaly
   d. Abnormal liver function (hepatic congestion)
   e. Peripheral pitting edema
3. Both right-sided and left-sided CHF
   a. Cardiomegaly; displacement of point of maximal impulse (PMI)
   b. Oliguria
   c. Weight gain
   d. Tachycardia

ANALYSIS/NURSING DIAGNOSIS (see p. 125)

PLANNING, IMPLEMENTATION, AND EVALUATION

Goal 1 Client will experience improved ventricular function.

Implementation

1. Administer cardiac glycoside as ordered to strengthen myocardial contractility (inotropic effect) (see Table 3-15).
2. Administer vasodilator as ordered to decrease afterload by reducing vascular resistance to ventricular outflow (e.g., angiotensin converting enzyme [ACE] inhibitors) (see Table 3-7).
3. Monitor vital signs closely.

Evaluation

Client's resting heart rate is decreased from 88 to 72.

Goal 2 Client will eliminate excess fluid.

Implementation

1. Give diuretics as ordered (see Tables 3-7).
2. Give ACE inhibitors as ordered to promote diuresis by decreasing aldosterone secretion (see Table 3-7).
3. Keep accurate I&O.
4. Weigh daily.
5. Restrict sodium intake.

Evaluation

Client's weight decreases to pre-CHF level.

Goal 3 See General Nursing Goal 2, p. 125.

Goal 4 See General Nursing Goal 3, p. 125.

Goal 5 Client will remain free from pulmonary edema.

Implementation

1. Monitor closely for symptoms of fluid in aveolar and interstitial tissue of the lung.
   a. Severe dyspnea, tachypnea
   b. Audible rales
   c. Cough, frothy, blood-tinged sputum

Table 3-17 Bronchodilator drugs*

Name	Action	Side effects	Nursing implications
ADRENERGIC AGENTS			
Epinephrine (Adrenalin) Ephedrine	Stimulates alpha- and beta-adrenergic receptors of sympathetic nervous system. Alpha: peripheral vasoconstriction, increased BP. Beta: bronchodilation, increased cardiac irritability, increased heart rate.	Nervousness, tremors, headache, palpitation, tachycardia, dysrhythmias	Monitor BP, pulse. Use cautiously for clients with hypertension and coronary insufficiency.
Isoproterenol (Isuprel)	Stimulates beta-adrenergic receptors of sympathetic nervous system: relaxes bronchioles, stimulates heart.	Similar to epinephrine	
Terbutaline (Brethine) Albuterol (Proventil, Ventolin) Metaproterenol (Alupent)	Selective beta-2 agonists.	Similar to epinephrine and isoproterenol, with fewer cardiovascular effects.	
XANTHINE COMPOUNDS			
Aminophylline Theophylline	Relaxes smooth muscle of bronchial airway and blood vessels. Also has diuretic effect. Acts synergistically with adrenergic bronchodilators.	Dizziness, hypotension, restlessness, dysrhythmias, GI irritation (oral), cardiac stimulation	Monitor BP; observe for hypotension. Give oral preparations with food.

*See also Table 5-18.

d. Extreme anxiety
e. Cyanosis
f. Diaphoresis
2. Institute therapy *immediately if pulmonary edema develops.*
   a. Place in high Fowler's position.
   b. Give O_2 by positive pressure if available (increases O_2 and helps push fluid from alveolar space).
   c. Give morphine sulfate IV (relieves anxiety, slows respirations, reduces venous return)
   d. Give diuretic as ordered (e.g., furosemide [Lasix]). (see Table 3-7.)
   e. Give bronchodilator (aminophylline IV) (see Table 3-17.)
   f. Administer cardiac glycoside as ordered (see Table 3-10.)
   g. Apply rotating tourniquets (Fig. 3-9) to reduce circulating blood volume by obstructing *venous* flow in three extremities.
      1. rotate one tourniquet every 15 minutes in *one* direction.
      2. remove one at a time when edema is controlled.
   h. Monitor closely:
      1. vital signs
      2. urinary output
      3. skin color
      4. level of consciousness
      5. arterial O_2 saturation
         a. pulse oximetry
         b. ABGs

Evaluation
Client has normal respiratory rate (e.g., 16 per minute); client's lung fields are clear on auscultation.

> **Goal 6** Client and significant others will be able to explain need for care after discharge.

Implementation
1. Teach
   a. Level of activity, balance between activity and rest
   b. Sodium-restricted diet (see Table 3-14), high potassium diet as necessary (see Table 3-15)
   c. Medication administration, schedule, side effects
   d. Application of antiembolic hose
2. Instruct client: weigh daily to monitor fluid balance.

Evaluation
Client correctly describes care needed for home (e.g., drug therapy, how to take own pulse).

✖ HYPERTENSION

1. Definition: a chronic elevation of systemic arterial BP in which the systolic pressure at rest is *consistently over 140 mm Hg and the diastolic pressure at rest is 90 mm Hg or higher*
2. Incidence
   a. Affects all age groups
   b. Prevalence increases with age
   c. One of the major causes of illness and death in the United States
3. Chief risk factor for CVA

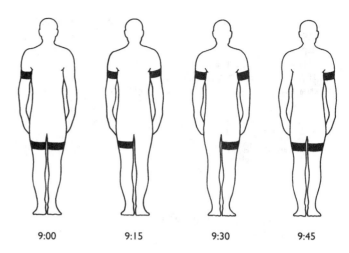

Fig. 3-9 Pattern for rotating tourniquets. Rotate one tourniquet every 15 minutes in the same direction.

4. Major risk factor for MI
5. Blood pressure physiology
   a. Determinants
      1. cardiac output
      2. total peripheral resistance
   b. Regulation
      1. neural stimulation: autonomic nervous system
      2. humoral stimulation (e.g., catecholamines, aldosterone, angiotensin)
6. Pathophysiology
   a. No obvious early pathologic changes in blood vessels and organs
   b. Large vessels (aorta, coronary arteries, basilar artery to brain, peripheral vessels in limbs) eventually become sclerosed and tortuous
   c. Vessel lumens narrow, resulting in decreased blood flow to heart, brain, and lower extremities
   d. Vessels become completely occluded or rupture, resulting in hemorrhage
   e. Damage to the intima of small vessels causes local edema and intravascular clotting
   f. Decreased blood supply to tissues of heart, brain, kidneys, and eyes causes dysfunction of these target organs
7. Types
   a. *Primary* (essential): approximately 90% of all cases: etiology unknown; types include
      1. *benign:* slowly progressive
      2. *malignant:* rapidly accelerating
   b. *Secondary:* approximately 10% to 15% of all cases; caused by an identifiable primary disease (e.g., pheochromocytoma)
8. Predisposing factors
   a. Stress
   b. Familial history
   c. Obesity

Nursing Process
ASSESSMENT
1. BP elevated on at least three different occasions
2. Headache

3. Change in vision (hemorrhages in retina, blurred vision)
4. Epistaxis
5. Personality change: forgetful and irritable

ANALYSIS/NURSING DIAGNOSIS (see p. 125)
PLANNING, IMPLEMENTATION, AND EVALUATION

Goal I Client's BP will decrease to safe level and permanent damage will be prevented.

Implementation
1. Monitor BP.
2. Modify lifestyle to reduce stress.
3. Lose weight if obese.
4. Modify diet.
   a. Sodium restricted (see Table 3-14).
   b. Fat and cholesterol restricted (see Table 3-12)
   c. Calories reduced if needed.
   d. High potassium if needed (see Table 3-15).
5. Exercise in a regular, planned program.
6. Avoid smoking.
7. Administer antihypertensive medications as ordered (see Table 3-7).

Evaluation
Client's elevated blood pressure is reduced and maintained at 140/90.

Goal 2 Client will carry out self-care activities after discharge.

Implementation
1. Teach client to
   a. Take and record own BP.
   b. Modify lifestyle as needed.
   c. Institute exercise program.
   d. Modify diet as needed.
   e. Modify smoking and alcohol habits as needed.
   f. Understand medications (see Table 3-7).
      1. administration
      2. schedule
      3. side effects
      4. importance of compliance
2. Emphasize importance of follow-up care.

Evaluation
Client lists all components of therapeutic regimen; keeps appointment for return visit.

✣ PERIPHERAL VASCULAR PROBLEMS

1. Definition: problems caused by changes in arterial and venous blood vessels peripheral to the heart
2. Common examples of arterial problems
   a. *Arteriosclerosis obliterans:* atherosclerotic plaque formation that involves arteries of lower extremities; occurs in men aged 50 to 70 and women after menopause
   b. *Raynaud's disease:* intermittent constricting spasms

of arterioles of digits and extremities, resulting in pain and cyanosis
   c. *Buerger's disease* (thromboangiitis obliterans): diffuse, inflammatory, proliferative changes in arteries and veins of extremities
3. Common examples of venous problems
   a. *Varicose veins:* dilated, tortuous superficial veins; incompetent valves cause dilation; increased pressure causes tortuosity; increased capillary pressure causes edema
   b. *Varicose ulcers:* ulcers resulting from circulatory insufficiency
   c. *Thrombophlebitis:* inflammation of vein with thrombus formation
   d. *Phlebothrombosis:* thrombus formation in a vein without inflammation

Nursing Process: Arterial Problems

ASSESSMENT
Signs and symptoms of impaired peripheral arterial circulation (Fig. 3-10).
ANALYSIS/NURSING DIAGNOSIS (see p. 125)
PLANNING, IMPLEMENTATION, AND EVALUATION

Goal I Client will have adequate arterial blood flow to extremities.

Implementation
1. Teach client to eliminate or avoid
   a. Tobacco
   b. Exposure to temperature extremes
   c. Trauma: tissue injury and infections
   d. Excessive exercise
   e. Vasospastic drugs (e.g., epinephrine)
   f. Constrictive clothing
2. Maintain good foot care.
3. Walk to tolerance to promote collateral circulation.
4. Modify diet
   a. Low cholesterol
   b. Moderate fat
   c. Reduced calories if client is obese
5. Give thrombolytics or anticoagulants as ordered (see Table 3-9).

Evaluation
Client's extremities are warm; peripheral pulses are strong and equal.

Goal 2 Client will have minimal discomfort.

Implementation
1. Have client rest when pain occurs.
2. Administer peripheral vasodilator adrenergic medications as ordered (e.g., isoxsuprine [Vasodilan]).

Evaluation
Client develops schedule of activities that keeps pain under control.

Chronic venous insufficiency
(advanced)

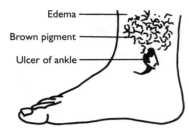

Edema

Brown pigment

Ulcer of ankle

Chronic arterial insufficiency
(advanced)

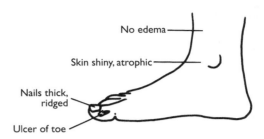

No edema

Skin shiny, atrophic

Nails thick,
ridged

Ulcer of toe

	Venous Conditions	Arterial Conditions
Pathophysiology	Impaired/occluded peripheral *venous* circulation	Impaired/occluded peripheral *arterial* circulation
Involved areas	Lower extremities	Upper and lower extremities
Signs and symptoms		
Pain	None or aching tiredness, positive Homan's sign (thrombophlebitis)	Severe ischemic (e.g., intermittent claudication) Late: pain on rest
Edema	Pronounced	Usually none
Peripheral pulses	Present, difficult to palpate with edema	Diminished or absent
Skin	Thickened Stasis dermatitis	Trophic changes: shiny, hairless, tightly drawn, dry, scaly skin; thick ridged nails
Color	Brawny pigmentation of ankle and lower leg Cyanosis with dependency	Pallor/cyanosis Rubor with dependency
Temperature	Warm	Cool or cold
Ulcers	May develop; nonpainful	May develop; painful
Gangrene	Not present	Present with occlusion
Effect of position		
Elevation	Improves symptoms	Aggravates symptoms
Dependency	Aggravates symptoms	Improves symptoms
Common conditions	Varicose veins Varicose ulcers Thrombophlebitis	Arteriosclerosis obliterans Raynaud's disease Buerger's disease

Fig. 3-10 Common manifestations of chronic arterial and venous peripheral vascular problems.

Goal 3 Client will be able to explain when surgery might be used; will be free from preventable complications.

Implementation
1. Know that bypass surgery with graft may be used for localized arterial occlusion; that sympathectomy may be used to relieve vasospasm; that amputation is the treatment for gangrene; that embolectomy is advisable for acute arterial occlusion.
2. Provide postoperative care after graft: avoid strain on incision (do not bend joint over which graft passes), moni-

tor for hemorrhage resulting from disruption or occlusion of graft, administer anticoagulants as ordered (see Table 3-8).
3. See Amputation, p. 253.

Evaluation
Client explains the type of surgery that he or she may receive; is free from complications postoperatively (e.g., no split incision or frank hemorrhage).

Nursing Process: Venous Problems
ASSESSMENT
Signs and symptoms of impaired venous circulation (see Fig. 3-10).

ANALYSIS/NURSING DIAGNOSIS (see p. 125)
PLANNING, IMPLEMENTATION, AND EVALUATION

Goal 1 Client will have adequate venous blood flow from extremities.

Implementation
1. Teach client to eliminate or avoid
   a. Tobacco
   b. Injury and infections
   c. Constrictive clothing (e.g., garters)
   d. Standing or sitting for long periods
   e. Crossing legs at knee
   f. Oral contraceptives
2. Teach client to
   a. Wear antiembolic hose
   b. Elevate legs
   c. Do ankle push-ups when standing (promotes venous return)
   d. Walk daily to tolerance

Evaluation
Client's lower extremities are warm and free from edema.

Goal 2 Client with thrombophlebitis will be protected from dislodgement of thrombus.

Implementation
1. Maintain bed rest 7 to 10 days.
2. Prevent Valsalva's maneuver (forced expiration against a closed glottis).
3. Elevate legs.
4. Apply antiembolic hose.
5. Apply warm, moist packs to involved site (prevent burns).
6. Do not rub legs.
7. Give thrombolytics or anticoagulants as ordered (see Table 3-8).

Evaluation
Client is free from any signs or symptoms of pulmonary embolism.

Goal 3 Client's leg ulcers will heal.

Implementation
1. Maintain bed rest with leg elevated when ulcer is acute.
2. Monitor for signs of cellulitis and report immediately.
3. Give antibiotics as ordered if infected.
4. Know and inform client that skin grafting may be necessary.
5. Explain the long-term nature of treatment to client.

Evaluation
Client's ulcer remains clean and uninfected; heals well.

SELECTED HEALTH PROBLEMS RESULTING IN INTERFERENCE WITH FORMED ELEMENTS OF THE BLOOD

Refer to Nursing Care of the Child, pp. 458-461.

SELECTED HEALTH PROBLEMS RESULTING IN INTERFERENCE WITH PULMONARY FUNCTION

✖ CHRONIC OBSTRUCTIVE PULMONARY DISEASE (COPD) OR CHRONIC OBSTRUCTIVE LUNG DISEASE (COLD)

1. Definition: group of chronic respiratory disorders that involve a persistent obstruction of bronchial airflow
2. Incidence
   a. Fastest-growing cause of death in the United States
   b. Occurs in adults and children
3. Predisposing factors
   a. Smoking
   b. Environmental factors: smoke, coal, hay, asbestos, air pollution
   c. Allergic factors
   d. Chronic, recurrent respiratory infections
   e. Genetic factors (possibly)
4. Pathophysiology
   a. Thoracic excursion is reduced because of bronchial obstruction, air trapping, and thoracic overdistention; possible inflammatory reaction in airways causes bronchial spasm and increased secretions
   b. Tidal volume, vital capacity, expiratory volume, and inspiratory reserve necessary for effective coughing are decreased
   c. Accessory muscles of respiration used to facilitate breathing; pursed lips used to maintain open bronchioles with expiration
   d. Bronchial obstruction and air trapping lead to destruction of lung, permanently reduced alveolar ventilation, and CO_2 retention
   e. Decreased resistance and stasis of secretions increase susceptibility to respiratory infections (e.g., pneumonia)
   f. Respiratory acidosis (compensated) commonly occurs secondary to chronic CO_2 retention
5. Hypoxemia
   a. Definition: deficient oxygenation of the blood
   b. Frequently chronic, possibly acute
   c. Characterized by
      1. restlessness, agitation, headache, drowsiness, and confusion (because of less O_2 to the brain and stimulation of the sympathetic nervous system)
      2. tachycardia and hyperventilation early; possibly followed by bradycardia and hypoventilation
      3. hypertension caused by sympathetic nervous system stimulation may be present early
      4. decreased PO_2 (<80 mm Hg)
      5. late: cyanosis
6. Hypercapnia
   a. Definition: excess of CO_2 in the blood
   b. Can occur with hypoxemia; may be chronic or acute
   c. Characterized by
      1. CNS depression: drowsiness, inability to concentrate, progressive loss of consciousness
      2. early behavioral changes: irritability; inability to get along with others; inability to sleep
      3. headache

4. rubor
5. tremors, dizziness, cardiac dysrhythmias
6. increased P_{CO_2} (>45 mm Hg)
7. Common examples of COPD
   a. *Bronchial asthma*
      1. chronic lung disease characterized by
         a. airway hyperresponsiveness to a variety of stimuli
         b. airway inflammation
         c. usually reversible airway obstruction
      2. refer to Nursing Care of the Child, p. 449
   b. *Chronic bronchitis*
      1. definition: chronic inflammation of the bronchi with production of copious amount of sputum that causes bronchial obstruction
      2. etiology and pathophysiology: air pollution or smoking causes inflammation of bronchial mucosa with resulting edema and copious production of mucus; reduced ciliary motility in the bronchi causes predisposition to recurrent respiratory infections
   c. *Emphysema*
      1. definition: chronic lung condition characterized by overdistention and destruction of alveoli
      2. etiology: exact cause not identified; 80% associated with smoking
      3. pathophysiology: air trapped behind partially obstructed bronchioles produces overdistention and destruction of alveoli; loss of elastic recoil of lungs reduces respiratory flow; residual volume increases; barrel chest develops

Nursing Process
ASSESSMENT
1. Respiratory distress (dyspnea on exertion progressing to dyspnea at rest)
2. Apprehension
3. Cough (productive)
4. Lethargy (results from hypoxemia)
5. Use of accessory (intercostal and abdominal) muscles
6. Increased anterior-posterior (AP) diameter of chest (emphysema)
7. Abnormal breath sounds (rales, rhonchi, wheezing, decreased breath sounds)
8. Weight loss
9. Skin color
   a. Cyanosis (hypoxemia)
   b. Flushed (hypercapnia)
10. Abnormal pulmonary function tests (e.g., decreased expiratory and vital capacity volumes)
11. Blood gases
    a. P_{O_2} decreased only with activity at first, then decreased continuously
    b. P_{CO_2} increases as disease worsens
12. Respiratory acidosis, compensated (from chronic CO_2 retention) (Table 3-18)
13. Hematocrit, sometimes elevated
14. Frequent respiratory infections (decreased resistance)
ANALYSIS/NURSING DIAGNOSIS (see p. 125)
PLANNING, IMPLEMENTATION, AND EVALUATION

Goal 1 Client will maintain a P_{O_2} of at least 60 mm Hg; airway will be clear, sputum will be thin and clear.

Implementation
1. See General Nursing Goal 1, p. 125.
2. Administer bronchodilators as ordered (see Table 3-17).
3. Administer expectorants as ordered (see Table 3-19).
4. Administer nebulizer as ordered.
   a. Bronchodilators (see Table 3-17)
   b. Mucolytics (see Table 3-19)
   c. Corticosteroids (Table 3-20, see Table 5-18)
5. Teach relaxation techniques and breathing exercises (e.g., pursed-lip breathing).
6. Administer low concentrations of humidified O_2 (1 to 2 L/min); CAUTION: high O_2 flow may precipitate respiratory failure in presence of hypercapnia and hypoxia.
7. Encourage activity to tolerance.
8. If client must be confined to bed for any period (usually infection or asthma attack)
   a. Use semi-Fowler's or Fowler's position.
   b. Turn frequently.
   c. Encourage to take frequent deep breaths and to breathe out slowly and completely.
   d. Perform active ROM exercises (passive if client too weak to do active exercises).
   e. Employ diversional activities to avoid napping during the day to prevent insomnia and nocturnal restlessness.
   NOTE: *Avoid bed rest if at all possible to prevent hypoventilation, stasis of secretions, weakened ventilatory muscles, weakness of other muscles, and decreased cough reflex.*
9. Give diet as tolerated (e.g., small amounts of soft food 4 to 5 times per day); increase fluids unless contraindicated.
Evaluation
Client's P_{O_2} remains greater than 60 mm Hg; pH remains between 7.35 and 7.45; sputum is clear and thin.

Goal 2 Client will be protected from any injuries.

Implementation
1. Know that with hypoxia, hypercapnia, or uncompensated respiratory acidosis, client may be lethargic, confused, or comatose.
2. Use bed's side rails, pad if necessary.
3. Keep bed low to floor.
4. Avoid restraints, sedatives, or tranquilizers.
5. If client is confused, have someone stay with client.
6. Maintain quiet environment.
7. Speak in low, calm, soothing tone.
Evaluation
Client is free from injury.

Goal 3 Client will be protected from CO_2 narcosis.

Table 3-18   Acid-base imbalance

Problem	Etiology	Assessment	Compensating mechanisms	Nursing implications
RESPIRATORY ACIDOSIS				
pH < 7.35 Pco_2 > 45 Hco_3 normal	Hypoventilation Acute causes Respiratory infections CNS depressant over-dose Paralysis of respiratory muscles Atelectasis Brain damage Postoperative abdominal distention Chronic causes Obesity Ascites Pregnancy	Hypoventilation; tachycardia, irregular pulse; decreased chest excursion; headache, dizziness; cyanosis; drowsiness leading to coma	Kidneys retain and manufacture more bicarbonate leading to pH 7.4 Pco_2 > 45 Hco_3 > 28	Turn, cough, and deep breathe qh. Suction as needed. Monitor vital signs. Give respiratory stimulants as ordered. Give bronchodilators. Give O_2 cautiously to prevent CO_2 narcosis.
RESPIRATORY ALKALOSIS				
pH > 7.45 Pco_2 < 35 Hco_3 normal	Hyperventilation Emotions, hysteria O_2 lack Fever Salicylate poisoning CNS stimulation by drugs/disease	Hyperventilation Light-headedness Tingling of hands and face (tetany) Convulsions, diaphoresis, low serum K^+	Kidneys excrete large amounts of bicarbonate leading to pH 7.4 Pco_2 < 35 Hco_3 < 22	Calm client. Slow the rate of ventilation. Use rebreather mask to increase Pco_2. Administer O_2 as needed.
METABOLIC ACIDOSIS				
pH < 7.35 Pco_2 normal Hco_3 < 22	Bicarbonate loss Diarrhea GI fistula Acid gain Diabetic ketoacidosis Lactic acidosis Renal failure Salicylate intoxication K^+ excess	Headache, dizziness; Kussmaul's respiration; fruity breath odor; disoriented; coma; nausea/vomiting; high serum K^+	Lungs hyperventilate to blow off CO_2 and reduce plasma carbonic acid content leading to pH 7.4 Pco_2 < 35 Hco_3 < 22	Administer sodium bicarbonate as ordered. Give insulin as ordered. Monitor I&O, vital signs. Support client.
METABOLIC ALKALOSIS				
pH > 7.45 Pco_2 normal Hco_3 > 26	Acid loss Vomiting or GI suction Steroid therapy Thiazide diuretics Bicarbonate retention Excess use of bicarbonate (baking soda) as antacid Excess infusion of Ringer's lactate Citrated blood	Headache, numbness and tingling leading to tetany and convulsions, hypoventilation, confusion and agitation, low serum K^+	Lungs hypoventilate to retain CO_2 and increase plasma carbonic acid content leading to pH 7.4 Pco_2 > 45 Hco_3 > 26	Give IV ammonium chloride as ordered. Maintain K^+ level with diet or drugs. Teach client high K^+ diet if taking thiazide diuretics. Give acetazolamide (Diamox) as ordered. Maintain calm, quiet environment.

Table 3-21   **Antibiotic drugs**

Name	Action	Side effects	Nursing implications

			All antibiotics:
			    Take culture if ordered *before* starting antibiotic.
			    Instruct client to take *entire* prescription.
			    Assess allergy and toxic effect history before administering.

PENICILLINS			

Natural penicillins
Penicillin G
    Aqueous crystalline IV or IM
    Procaine (Wycillin) IM only
    Benazathine (Bicillin) IM only
    Penicillin V (Pen-Vee) Oral
	Bactericidal (inhibits cell-wall synthesis); effective against numerous gram-positive cocci, spirochetes, actinomycetes, and some gram-negative organisms.	Hypersensitivity (rash, urticaria, anaphylaxis); GI disturbance (oral); superinfection	Observe for hypersensitivity.

Penicillinase-resistant penicillins Methicillin (Staphcillin) Oxacillin (Prostaphilin) Nafcillin (Unipen)	Semisynthetic penicillin; effective against penicillin-resistant organisms such as *S. aureus*.	Same as Penicillin G and V	Same as Penicillin G and V.

Extended-spectrum penicillins
Aminopenicillins
    Ampicillin (Polycillin)
Carboxypenicillins
    Carbenicillin (Geopen)
    Ticarcillin (Ticar)
Ureidopenicillins and Piperazine penicillin
    Mezlocillin (Mezlin)
    Azlocillin (Azlin)
    Piperacillin (Pipracil)
	Semisynthetic penicillin; effective against many gram-positive and gram-negative organisms.	Same as Penicillin G and V	Same as Penicillin G and V.

Penicillin/beta-lactamase inhibitor combinations Amoxicillin-clavulanic acid (Augmentin) Ticarcillin-clavulanic acid (Timentin) Ampicillin-sulbactam (Unasyn)	Semisynthetic penicillin combined with beta-lactamase inhibitor; increases the activity of penicillin against resistant beta-lactamase–producing bacteria such as *S. aureus*	Same as Penicillin G and V	Same as Penicillin G and V.
MACROLIDES Erythromycin (E-Mycin) Erythromycin ethylsuccinate (E.E.S.) Erythromycin estolate (Ilosone) Erythromycin stearate (Erythrocin)	Bacteriostatic (inhibits protein synthesis); antimicrobial spectrum similar to penicillin G	GI disturbance, hypersensitivity (urticaria, pruritus), superinfection, hepatotoxicity with some forms No cross-sensitivity to penicillin	Used as penicillin substitute for allergic client.
CEPHALOSPORINS Cephalothin (Keflin) Cephalexin (Keflex) Cefaclor (Ceclor) Cefadroxil (Duricef) Cefotetan (Cefotan) Cefoxitin (Mefoxin) Cefixine (Suprax) Ceftazidime (Fortaz)	Bactericidal (inhibits cell wall synthesis, similar to penicillin); broad-spectrum activity against most gram-positive cocci and many gram-negative bacilli	Hypersensitivity (rash, urticaria, pruritus), GI disturbance, cross-sensitivity to penicillin (but anaphylaxis rare)	Check for history of allergy to penicillin.

Continued

Table 3-21 Antibiotic drugs—cont'd

Name	Action	Side effects	Nursing implications
TETRACYCLINES			
Tetracycline* (Achromycin) Minocycline (Minocin) Oxytetracycline (Terramycin) Demeclocycline (Declomycin) Doxycycline (Vibramycin)	Bacteriostatic (inhibits protein synthesis); effective against a broad spectrum of gram-positive and gram-negative organisms, rickettsiae, chlamydia, trophozoite forms of amebae, and actinomycetes.	GI disturbance; hypersensitivity (rash, urticaria); photosensitivity; superinfection; permanent tooth discoloration during development	Do not give with milk, food, or antacids. Avoid sun exposure. Do not administer to pregnant women or children under 8 years.
AMINOGLYCOSIDES			
Neomycin* Gentamicin (Garamycin) Kanamycin (Kantrex) Streptomycin† Tobramycin	Bactericidal (inhibits protein synthesis); effective against a wide range of gram-positive and gram-negative organisms and mycobacteria.	Significant toxicity Ototoxicity Nephrotoxicity Neuromuscular blockade	Monitor hearing function. Monitor renal function. Do not administer to client with neuromuscular disorder
POLYPEPTIDES			
Bacitracin*	Bactericidal (hinders cell-wall synthesis); effective against most gram-positive organisms.	Significant toxicity: Nephrotoxicity	Used primarily as topical agent because of its nephrotoxicity.
Polymyxins* Polymyxin B (Aerosporin) Colistin (Coly-Mycin)	Bactericidal (hinders cell-wall synthesis); effective against nearly all gram-negative organisms, except the *Proteus* group.	Neurotoxicity Nephrotoxicity Neuromuscular blockade	Used topically. Use parenterally with caution. Parenteral: monitor renal function; use cautiously for clients with respiratory insufficiency.

SULFONAMIDES See Table 3-43, p. 189

*See also Table 3-60.
†See also Table 3-22.

3. malnutrition
4. debilitating diseases
5. immunosuppressive condition
   b. Virulence of organism
   c. Length of exposure
5. Transmission
   a. Usually by inhalation of airborne particles (droplet nuclei) that contain *Mycobacterium tuberculosis* from person with infectious TB
   b. Communicable as long as tubercle bacilli are present in sputum
6. Pathophysiology
   a. Most common site of organism implantation is alveolar surface of lung parenchyma.
   b. Induces hypersensitivity response in host.
   c. Inflammation occurs; localized pneumonitis develops.
   d. Characteristic tubercle (caseous nodule) is formed around organism.
   e. If host response is adequate, organism is walled off within tubercle (becomes a healed calcified mass). With reduced host resistance, organism can become active again (reactivation process).
   f. If host response is inadequate, organism spreads, multiple fibrotic tubercles are formed throughout the lungs; total amount of functional pulmonary tissue is reduced.
   g. Disease may also spread systemically through lymph and blood vascular systems (miliary tuberculosis).
   h. If medical therapy fails, surgical resection of one or more lobes may be advised.

Nursing Process
ASSESSMENT
1. History of TB exposure
2. Productive cough
3. Low-grade fever, especially in afternoon
4. Night sweats
5. Weight loss
6. Anorexia
7. Fatigue
8. Dyspnea
9. Pleuritic pain
10. Rales
11. Hemoptysis (late symptom)
12. Mantoux tuberculin skin test
    a. TB screening test
    b. *Intradermal* injection of purified protein derivative (PPD) on volar surface of forearm

Implementation
1. Encourage ambulation unless contraindicated.
2. Perform active and passive range of motion.
3. Apply antiembolic stockings.
4. Maintain adequate hydration, steady IV rates.
5. Avoid strain, Valsalva's maneuver (straining against a closed glottis).
6. Turn, cough, deep breathe every 2 hours.
7. Administer prophylactic low-dose heparin as ordered.

Evaluation
Client is free from signs and symptoms of respiratory difficulty.

Goal 2 Client's pulmonary perfusion and ventilation will improve.

Implementation
1. Observe for signs and symptoms of hypoxia.
2. Monitor respiratory rate and rhythm.
3. Turn every 2 hours.
4. Administer O_2 at prescribed concentrations.
5. Administer thrombolytics or anticoagulants as ordered (Table 3-8).

Evaluation
Client exhibits no respiratory distress; has pink nailbeds, normal skin and mucous membrane color.

Goal 3 Client will maintain adequate cardiac output.

Implementation
1. Monitor for signs and symptoms of acute right ventricular heart failure.
2. Measure CVP as ordered.
3. Auscultate heart sounds.
4. Monitor cardiac rhythm.
5. Monitor I&O.
6. Administer pulmonary bronchodilator (e.g., aminophylline) as ordered (see Table 3-17).
7. Administer diuretics (e.g., furosemide) (see Table 3-18).

Evaluation
Client has normal heart rate and rhythm; BP, urine output within normal limits.

Goal 4 Client will experience reduced apprehension, fear, and anxiety.

Implementation
1. Administer sedation as ordered.
2. Provide a quiet, nonstimulating environment.
3. Provide calm reassurance.
4. Explain all procedures thoroughly.
5. Stay with client during episode of severe dyspnea or chest pain.

Evaluation
Client appears calm; verbalizes reduction in anxiety.

Goal 5 Client will remain free from recurrence of thrombus formation and pulmonary embolus.

Implementation
1. Teach
   a. Methods to prevent venous stasis
   b. Anticoagulant medication dosages and side effects (Table 3-8)

Evaluation
Client develops no recurrent thrombi.

CHEST TUBES AND CHEST SURGERY

1. Clients who experience open-chest injuries or surgery require similar care because of the opening of the thoracic cavity and the subsequent use of chest tubes.
2. Lung expansion is supported by subatmospheric pressure of pleural space.
3. Causes of disruption of airtight thoracic cavity:
   a. Spontaneous pneumothorax
   b. Stab wound
   c. Bullet wound
   d. Tear of pleura by fractured rib
   e. Thoracotomy
4. Tension pneumothorax:
   a. Cause: closed chest wound; air is unable to escape from pleural space on expiration; lung collapses; mediastinal contents shift to *unaffected* side of thorax as intrathoracic tension increases.
   b. Emergency treatment: chest tube if available; otherwise, insert a needle to allow air to escape.
5. Chest tube drainage:
   a. Definition: one or two catheters (tubes) inserted through chest wall into pleural space for drainage of air or fluid. Drainage end of tube *must* be submerged in water (acts as one-way valve) so that air and fluid travel down tube but atmospheric air is prevented from traveling up into chest.
   b. Purpose: used after thoracotomy and lung collapse
      1. to remove air or for drainage from pleural space
      2. to help reexpand the lung
      3. to prevent tension pneumothorax
      4. not used after pneumonectomy
   c. Placement of tubes:
      1. anterior, upper thoracic area for air removal
      2. posterior (if required), lower thoracic area for drainage
   d. Forms (Figs. 3-11 and 3-12):
      1. one-bottle system
      2. two-bottle system
      3. three-bottle, or Pleur-Evac, system
   e. Application of suction
      1. uncontrolled suction: suction control bottle controls amount of suction
      2. controlled suction: intermittent positive pressure is used to facilitate drainage and lung reexpansion

Nursing Process
ASSESSMENT
1. Client: breathing (rate, regularity, depth, ease, breath sounds), anxiety, chest discomfort, level of understanding

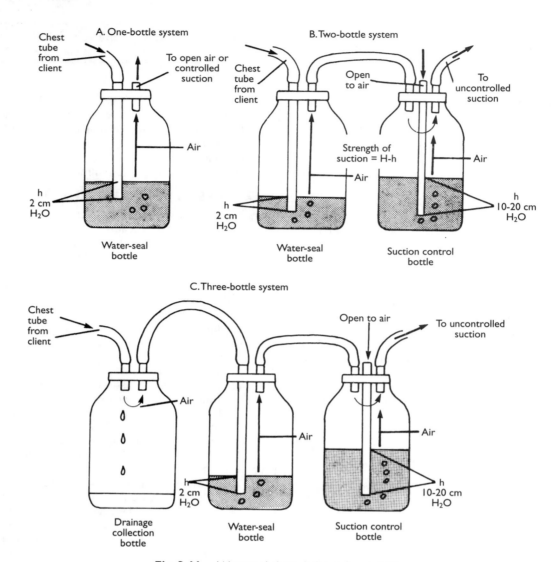

Fig. 3-11 Water-seal chest drainage (*h* = height).

2. Entry site: dressing, drainage, subcutaneous emphysema
3. Tubing: tight, taped connections; no kinks, compressions or dependent loops
4. Bottles (Fig. 3-11)
   a. Bottles kept below chest level.
   b. *Water-seal bottle:* chamber filled and tube submerged to ordered level (usually 2 cm); vent open to air, controlled suction, or suction control bottle. Column of fluid in submerged tube fluctuates with respiration *(up with inspiration, down with exhalation);* air bubbles *intermittently* from submerged tube with exhalation, coughing, or sneezing (no fluctuation or intermittent bubbling may indicate reexpansion of lung or blockage [e.g., kinking] of chest tube); *continuous* bubbling from submerged tube indicates air leak.
   c. *Suction control bottle:* chamber filled and tube submerged to ordered level (usually 20 cm); submerged tube open to air; one vent to water seal bottle, other vent to uncontrolled suction; air bubbles gently and

continuously from submerged tube. (NOTE: *The amount of suction applied is determined by the depth the tubes in the suction control and water-seal bottles are submerged in water, not by the amount of suction applied to the system. Excess suction merely draws air in through the vent of the submerged tube of the suction control bottle. This is what produces the continuous gentle bubbling in this bottle.*)
   d. *Drainage collection bottle:* used only in three-bottle system; volume, type, and rate of drainage monitored.
5. Suction source
   a. No control bottle: suction set at ordered level
   b. Control bottle: suction set so that gentle, continuous bubbling occurs

ANALYSIS/NURSING DIAGNOSIS (see p. 125)
PLANNING, IMPLEMENTATION, AND EVALUATION

Goal I Client will experience well-functioning water-seal system.

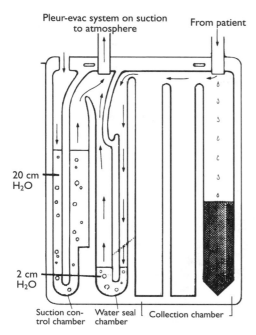

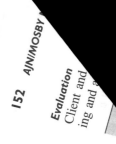

152 AJN/MOSBY

Evaluation
Client and a...
ing and a...

Pleur-evac system on suction
to atmosphere — From patient

20 cm
H₂O

2 cm
H₂O

Suction con-
trol chamber | Water seal
chamber | Collection chamber

Fig. 3-12   Pleur-Evac system. A Pleur-Evac unit consists of three chambers comparable to a three-bottle water-seal drainage system. The suction control chamber is equivalent to bottle no. 3—the suction control bottle. The water-seal chamber is equivalent to bottle no. 2—the water-seal bottle. The collection chamber corresponds to bottle no. 1—the drainage collection bottle.

Implementation
1. Check functioning of system.
2. Check that tubes are submerged at appropriate level or that water levels in Pleur-Evac are correct.
3. Tape all connectors.
4. Know what to do if system breaks: have tube clamps at bedside and use clamps appropriately.

Evaluation
Client's water-seal drainage remains intact; client remains free from respiratory distress.

> **Goal 2** Client will have tube patency maintained.

Implementation
1. Position chest tubes correctly; ensure that they are not kinked.
2. Attach chest tube to bed linens to prevent it from falling over side and pulling at insertion sites.
3. Check for fluctuation of fluid in tube of water-seal bottle *(up with inhalation or cough, down with expiration)*.

Evaluation
Client has adequate air and fluid drainage through patent tubes.

> **Goal 3** Client will experience adequate lung reexpansion.

Implementation
1. Help with daily chest x-ra·
2. Measure amount of draina·
   and time of measuremen·
   ml/hr for the first few·
   creases to 10 to 20 ml/·
3. Monitor for respiratory·
4. Cough and deep breat·
5. Provide comfort mea·
   as ordered (see Table 3-6).
6. Position the client to ensure optimal lunₓ
   a. Pneumonectomy: lie either on *affected* side ...
      back.
   b. All other thoracotomies: lie on *unaffected* side or
      back.
7. Help with removal of tube:
   a. Equipment needed: gauze sponges, tape, and scissors
      to cut suture holding the tube.
   b. Instruct client to exhale or inhale and hold breath.
   c. Apply airtight dressing (Telfa or petrolatum gauze).

Evaluation
X-ray shows adequate lung reexpansion; client breathes easily; has normal skin color.

✴ CANCER OF THE LUNG

1. Incidence
   a. Leading cause of cancer death in men and women; peaks in middle age
   b. Increasing in frequency, especially among women
2. Mortality rate is 20 times higher for those who smoke two or more packs of cigarettes daily
3. Medical treatment
   a. Surgical intervention
      1. pneumonectomy
      2. lobectomy
   b. Medical intervention
      1. radiation
      2. chemotherapy

Nursing Process
ASSESSMENT
1. No early signs
2. Cough: chronic, persistent
3. Abnormal chest x-ray
4. Positive findings from sputum cytology
5. Positive biopsy results
6. Hemoptysis, weakness, anorexia, weight loss, dyspnea, chest pain: symptoms of advanced disease
7. Pleural effusion (peripheral tumors)
ANALYSIS/NURSING DIAGNOSIS (see p. 125)
PLANNING, IMPLEMENTATION, AND EVALUATION

> **Goal 1** Client and significant others will be able to explain diagnostic tests and procedure care.

Implementation
1. Assess level of knowledge of client and significant others.
2. Explain procedures (e.g., bronchoscopy, sputum exams; see p. 124).

significant others describe what to expect during... fter procedures.

Goal 2 Client and significant others will be able to explain planned medical treatment.

Implementation
1. Know that radiation therapy and chemotherapy are often given if surgery is not possible, or preoperatively in conjunction with surgery.
2. Prepare client and significant others for radiation and chemotherapy (see Cellular Aberration, p. 257).

Evaluation
Client describes expected actions and side effects of planned medical therapy.

Goal 3 Client and significant others will be able to explain preoperative care, postoperative needs, operating room, postanesthesia care unit, surgical intensive care unit (OR-PACU-SICU) environment, and purpose of chest tubes.

Implementation
1. Refer to Perioperative Period, p. 115; Cellular Aberration, General Nursing Goal 3, p. 260; and chest tube care, p. 149.
2. Tour ICU.

Evaluation
Client demonstrates adequate coughing and deep breathing; correctly describes ICU environment.

Goal 4 Postoperatively, client will have adequate respiratory function, stable cardiac function, and adequate pain control.

Implementation
1. Refer to Perioperative Period, p. 115.
2. Monitor chest tubes; position appropriately for lung expansion (see Chest Tube Care, p. 149).

Evaluation
Client remains free from postoperative complications (breathes easily, has adequate I&O, experiences good pain control).

Goal 5 Client and significant others will discuss fears and concerns.

Implementation
1. Assess level of anxiety.
2. Give emotional support and help relieve anxiety.
3. Maintain hope.
4. Refer to appropriate support groups.

Evaluation
Client and significant others discuss fears and ask questions concerning diagnosis.

Goal 6 Client and significant others will be prepared for discharge.

Implementation
1. Teach
   a. Levels of activity and rest.
   b. How to prevent respiratory infections (e.g., avoid crowds).
2. Encourage client to stop smoking.
3. Arrange follow-up appointment.

Evaluation
Client knows date for return appointment with physician; states a willingness to comply with restrictions.

✖ CANCER OF THE LARYNX

1. Incidence: most common malignancy of upper respiratory tract
2. Risk factors
   a. Irritants to mucous membranes (e.g., chemicals, allergens)
   b. Smoking
   c. Excessive alcohol intake
   d. Familial predisposition
   e. Chronic laryngitis
   f. Voice abuse
3. Medical treatment
   a. Surgical intervention
      1. laryngectomy
      2. laryngectomy with modified, radical neck dissection
   b. Medical intervention
      1. radiation therapy
      2. chemotherapy *not* used

Nursing Process
ASSESSMENT
1. Persistent hoarseness (early symptom)
2. Dysphagia, burning with hot liquids
3. Persistent sore throat
4. Pain in laryngeal prominence
5. Feeling that something is in throat
6. Swelling of the neck
7. Diagnostic tests: abnormal results of laryngoscopy and biopsy

ANALYSIS/NURSING DIAGNOSIS (see p. 125)
PLANNING, IMPLEMENTATION, AND EVALUATION

Goal I Client and significant others will be able to explain planned medical treatment.

Implementation
1. Know that radiation is often used as adjuvant therapy to surgery.
2. Prepare client and significant others for radiation (see Cellular Aberration, p. 257).

Evaluation
Client describes expected actions and side effects of radiation therapy.

Goal 2 Client and significant others will be able to explain preoperative care, postoperative needs, and the OR-PACU environment.

Implementation

1. Refer to Perioperative Period, p. 115, and Cellular Aberration, General Nursing Goal 3, p. 260.
2. Give frequent oral care.
3. Advise no smoking or drinking alcohol.
4. Teach about postoperative procedures.
   a. Presence of drains and HemoVac
   b. Tracheostomy care and suctioning
   c. Breathing through tracheostomy tube and inhalation treatments
   d. Possible IVs or tube feedings
5. Discuss communication problems that will result.
6. Determine methods of postoperative communication (e.g., writing pad, picture board, call bell, magic slate, hand signals).

Evaluation

Client explains tracheostomy care; client, significant others, and nurse have plan for postoperative communication.

Goal 3 Postoperatively, client will have adequate respiratory function.

Implementation

1. Refer to Perioperative Period, p. 115.
2. Assess frequently:
   a. Patency of airway
   b. Breath sounds, respiratory rate and depth
3. Elevate head of bed 30 to 45 degrees (promotes drainage and facilitates respirations).
4. Support head and neck.
5. Administer humidified oxygen.
6. Suction tracheostomy frequently.
   a. Use sterile suction equipment.
   b. Hyperoxygenate client (suctioning can lower Po_2 10 to 30 mm Hg).
   c. Lubricate catheter (with H_2O-soluble lubricant) and insert catheter with suction *off* until obstruction is met.
   d. Withdraw catheter 1 cm (away from mucosa).
   e. Withdraw catheter while rotating and applying suction.
   f. Limit suctioning to 10 to 15 seconds at a time.
   g. Hyperoxygenate client.
   h. Repeat procedure, allowing client to rest and be hyperoxygenated between suctionings.
   i. Observe cardiac monitor if in use; if bradycardia or dysrhythmias occur, terminate suctioning immediately and hyperoxygenate client.
   j. If client has inflated endotracheal or tracheostomy tube in place and cuff must be deflated, use the following procedure:
      1. suction trachea secretions through tube as outlined above
      2. suction oropharynx and nasopharynx
      3. open new sterile setup, then deflate cuff and apply suction through tube immediately
      4. reinflate cuff only until air can no longer be heard, being careful not to overinflate cuff
7. Give laryngeal-tube care; clean tube at least q8h.
8. Suction nasopharyngeal secretions and tracheostomy using separate sterile catheters (or apply suction to tracheostomy first and nasopharynx second with same catheter).
9. Give frequent oral hygiene.
10. Check neck drains and HemoVac for drainage.

Evaluation

Client remains free from respiratory distress; has stable vital signs; rests comfortably.

Goal 4 Client will have satisfactory communication with staff and significant others postoperatively.

Implementation

1. Use communication measures decided on preoperatively.
2. Stay with client as often as possible.
3. Explain to client how to summon nurse; respond promptly when called.
4. Have significant others remain with client.

Evaluation

Client communicates needs effectively.

Goal 5 Client will receive adequate nutrition postoperatively.

Implementation

1. Give IV therapy as ordered.
2. Give nasogastric (NG) tube feedings as ordered.
3. Give vitamin supplements as ordered.
4. Supervise first oral intake; know that aspiration is not possible unless a fistula has formed.
5. Check skin turgor to monitor adequate hydration of tissues.
6. Monitor I&O.

Evaluation

Client's weight remains stable; fluid output approximates intake.

Goal 6 Client will cope with change in body image.

Implementation

1. See Loss and Death and Dying, p. 29.
2. Enlist help of role models such as rehabilitated laryngectomy clients.

Evaluation

Client's grooming and attitude demonstrate a positive self-concept.

Goal 7 Client and significant others will be prepared for discharge.

Implementation

1. Teach importance of
   a. Tube care
   b. Stoma care
   c. Proper clothing
   d. Diet
   e. Activity and recreation
   f. Bathing
   g. Oral hygiene
   h. Medic Alert bracelet (neck breather)
2. Refer to community support group (e.g., Laryngectomee Club of American Cancer Society).
3. Refer to speech therapist.
4. Arrange follow-up appointment.

Evaluation

Client correctly explains care of tube and stoma. Client knows when and where to return for follow up care.

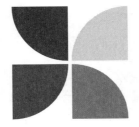

Nutrition and Metabolism: The Digestive Tract

OVERVIEW OF PHYSIOLOGY

1. Function: to transfer food and water from the external to the internal environment of the body and transform these substances into a form suitable for distribution to the cells by way of the circulatory system
2. Anatomy (Fig. 3-13)
   a. Upper gastrointestinal (GI) tract
      1. mouth, teeth, and salivary glands
      2. esophagus
      3. stomach
   b. Lower gastrointestinal tract
      1. small bowel
      2. large bowel
      3. rectum
      4. anus
   c. Accessory organs of digestion
      1. liver
      2. gallbladder
      3. pancreas
3. Processes
   a. Digestion: the process of breaking down proteins, polysaccharides, and fat; accomplished by the action of acid and enzymes secreted into the GI tract
   b. Secretion: the process of elaborating a specific product as a result of glandular activity (Table 3-23)
      1. saliva (mouth): contains salivary amylase (ptyalin), which hydrolyzes starch into maltase
      2. gastric secretions
         a. mucus: lubricates and protects stomach lining and content
         b. hydrochloric acid (HCl): essential to provide the acid medium necessary for the function of pepsin
         c. pepsin: breaks down proteins to polypeptides
         d. gastric lipase (small amounts): digests butterfat
         e. gastrin: regulates secretion of HCl
      3. small bowel secretions
         a. peptidases: split polypeptides into amino acids
         b. sucrase, maltase, isomaltase, and lactase: split disaccharides into monosaccharides
         c. intestinal lipase: splits fats into glycerol and fatty acids
         d. secretin, cholecystokinin-pancreozymin: stimulate the pancreas and gallbladder
      4. pancreatic secretions
         a. trypsin, chymotrypsin, nucleases, carboxypeptidase, pancreatic lipase, and pancreatic amylase: break down protein, fats, and carbohydrates
         b. bicarbonate-rich isoosmotic electrolyte solution
      5. gallbladder secretions
         a. bile: emulsifies fat
   c. Absorption: the process by which the small molecules that are the result of digestion cross cell membranes of the intestine and enter the blood and lymph
      1. carbohydrates and proteins are absorbed by active transport along with sodium
      2. fatty acids are absorbed by diffusion
      3. water and electrolytes are absorbed in the small and large intestines
      4. synthesis and absorption of vitamin K, thiamin, riboflavin, vitamin B_{12}, folic acid, biotin, and nicotinic acid take place in the large intestine as a result of bacterial activity, primarily *E. coli*
   d. Motility: the process by which contractions of the smooth muscle lining the walls of the GI tract produce movement of substances through the GI tract while digestion and absorption occur
      1. GI tract contains an intrinsic nerve supply that controls tone and peristaltic action
      2. nerve fibers from both the sympathetic and parasympathetic branches of the autonomic nervous system supply the intestinal tract and interact with intrinsic nerve supply
      3. the vagus nerve (the major autonomic nerve supplying the GI tract) is composed of motor parasympathetic fibers and many sensory fibers; parasympathetic stimulation *increases* motility and secretion; sympathetic stimulation *decreases* motility and secretion
   e. Metabolism
      1. all of the changes or body processes that take place in order to sustain life; the chemical changes that occur allow chemical energy to be changed to other forms of energy so that cellular functions can be maintained
      2. intermediary metabolism includes all the cellular functions in the body's internal environment; this phase of metabolism begins after the ingestion and digestion of foodstuff from the external environment

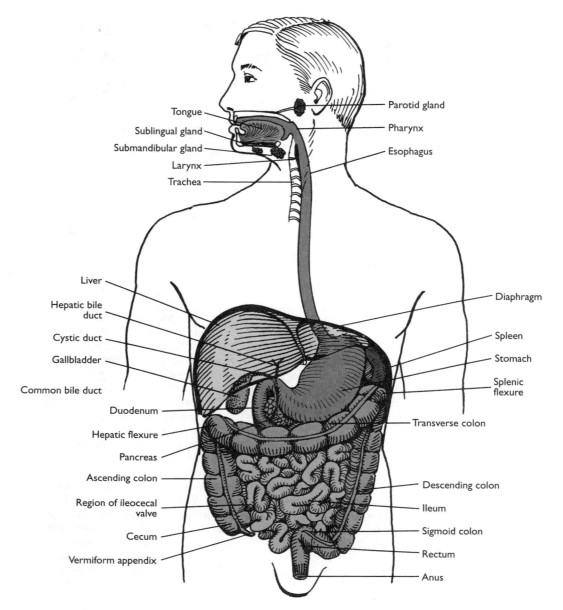

Fig. 3-13 The primary and accessory organs of digestion. (From Long BC, Phipps WJ: *Medical-surgical nursing: a nursing process approach,* ed 3, St Louis, 1993, Mosby.)

3. two-part process
   a. anabolism: the process of synthesis of smaller molecules to larger molecules; energy is saved
      - building process: proteins from amino acids, fats from fatty acids, and polysaccharides from monosaccharides
      - increased during growth, pregnancy, recovery states, or times of increased intake
   b. catabolism: the breaking down of larger molecules into smaller molecules
      - protein, fats, and carbohydrates are broken down into units that can be used by the cells
      - excesses in catabolism are seen in starvation, illness, and trauma

   - breakdown involves the release of CO_2, water, and urea with amino acid metabolism
4. adenosine triphosphate (ATP) is the high-energy phosphate that is the major source of energy for cellular function
5. adenosine diphosphate (ADP) is one of the end products released when energy is used and ATP is broken down
6. metabolic balance remains intact unless a change in the internal or external environment produces imbalances (for the balance to be maintained, the rate of catabolism must equal anabolism)
7. variances in metabolic rate occur with differences in sex, age, hormonal environment, seasonal and

Table 3-23 Digestive enzymes

Enzymes that digest	Source	Selected action and products
CARBOHYDRATES		
Amylase	Parotid and submaxillary glands	Hydrolyzes starch to maltose.
Sucrase, maltase, isomaltase, lactase	Intestinal fluids	Split diaccharides into monosaccharides.
Pancreatic amylase	Pancreas	Splits starches into maltose and isomaltose.
FATS		
Gastric lipase	Gastric mucosa	Digests butterfat.
Intestinal lipase	Intestinal fluids	Splits fats into glycerol and fatty acids.
PROTEIN		
Pepsin	Gastric mucosa	Breaks down dietary protein into proteoses, peptones, and polypeptides.
Peptidases	Intestinal glands	Splits polypeptides into amino acids.
Trypsin	Pancreas	Splits proteins into peptide and amino acids.
Chymotrypsin	Pancreas	Splits proteins into polypeptides.
Carboxypeptidase	Pancreas	Splits polypeptides into smaller peptides.
OTHER		
Enterokinase	Duodenal mucosa	Activates trypsin.
Nucleases	Pancreas	Splits nucleic acids.

environmental temperature changes, culture, activity levels, and ingestion of drugs (e.g., caffeine, nicotine, epinephrine)

8. materials needed for metabolism
   a. nutrients to supply energy and build tissue: glucose, glycerol, fatty acids, and amino acids
   b. minerals, electrolytes
   c. materials (primarily proteins) to promote synthesis of enzymes and hormones
   d. vitamins that function as coenzymes
   e. enzymes and hormones to function as organic cellular catalysts
9. metabolism governs the activities of muscle contraction, nerve impulse transmission, glandular secretion, absorption, and elimination

APPLICATION OF THE NURSING PROCESS TO THE CLIENT WITH DIGESTIVE TRACT PROBLEMS

ASSESSMENT

1. Health history
   a. Normal dietary pattern: changes in appetite
   b. Normal weight: changes in weight (how much, time period, planned vs. unplanned)
   c. Change in energy level: weakness, fatigue, general malaise
   d. Stool: changes in frequency, color, character
   e. Urine: dark, orange or clear color, frequency
   f. Indigestion or heartburn: pattern, frequency, drugs used, effectiveness
   g. Difficulty in swallowing: dysphagia with onset by solids or liquids
   h. Eructation or regurgitation: frequency
   i. Difficulty tolerating certain foods: allergies
   j. Vomiting or nausea: character of vomitus; amount,

characteristics, pattern of nausea; relationship to intake, other events
   k. Abdominal pain: presence, location, character, or pattern
   l. Abdominal distention, flatus, excess fullness
   m. History of abdominal surgery or trauma
   n. Bleeding: onset, duration, and extent
   o. Alcohol habits
   p. Family history, lifestyle patterns
2. Physical examination
   a. Inspection
      1. oral assessment: lips, gums, tongue, teeth, and mucous membranes; NOTE: gloves should be worn during this examination
      2. skin characteristics: turgor, scars, striae, engorged veins, spider angiomas, bruising, and jaundice
      3. abdominal structure: visible peristalsis, pulsations, or masses
      4. abdominal contour: rounded, protuberant, concave, or asymmetric; abdominal girth
   b. Auscultation: listen to all four quadrants of abdomen
      1. bowel sounds: location, frequency (normally 8 to 20 per minute in each quadrant), characteristics
         a. normal: succession of high-pitched clicks and gurgles
         b. abnormal
            ▪ hyperperistalsis: prolonged, loud, multiple gurgles; the term *borborygmi* may be used for exaggerated waves of peristalsis that can indicate the attempt to push fluid and air against an obstruction
            ▪ paralytic ileus: absent or infrequent sounds (listen for at least 1 minute in each quadrant)
   c. Percussion
      1. stomach (tympany normal—clear, hollow sound)

2. liver size (liver area is normally dull to percussion)
3. large intestinal areas: check for gaseous distention; a tympany reflects gas
   d. Palpation (NOTE: *performed last to avoid stimulating bowel sounds*)
   1. pain, tenderness, organ size and position
   2. masses, especially liver enlargement
3. Diagnostic tests
   a. Hematologic studies: normal values will vary slightly from laboratory to laboratory
      1. general function
         a. electrolytes
            ▪ sodium: 136 to 145 mEq/L
            ▪ potassium: 3.5 to 5.0 mEq/L
            ▪ chloride: 90 to 110 mEq/L
         b. CBC (see Oxygenation, p. 120)
      2. liver function
         a. aspartate aminotransferase (AST) (formerly SGOT): 5 to 40 U/ml (Frankel)
         b. alanine aminotransferase (ALT) (formerly SGPT): 5 to 35 U/ml (Frankel)
         c. alkaline phosphatase (ALP): 30 to 85 U/L
         d. ammonia: 15 to 45 μg/dl
         e. albumin: 3.2 to 4.5 g/dl
         f. globulin: 2.3 to 3.5 g/dl
         g. total bilirubin: 0.1 to 1 mg/dl
         h. cholesterol: 150 to 250 mg/dl
         i. prothrombin time: 11 to 12.5 seconds; NOTE: may be expressed as international normalized ratio (INR)
      3. GI function: gastrin 40 to 150 pg/ml
      4. pancreatic function
         a. glucose levels
            ▪ glucose: 70 to 115 mg/dl (fasting)
            ▪ postprandial: less than 140 mg/dl
         b. lipase: 20 to 180 IU/L
         c. amylase: 56 to 190 IU/L
   b. Urine tests
      1. glucose, acetone
      2. urobilinogen
   c. Stool tests
      1. ova and parasites (stool must be warm)
      2. occult blood (guaiac)
      3. fecal fat (sent to lab after a 72-hour collection)
      4. culture
   d. Radiographic studies
      1. flat plate of abdomen
      2. GI series (barium swallow)
         a. definition: x-ray of esophagus, stomach, and duodenum after oral intake of 16 to 20 ounces of contrast medium (barium)
         b. nursing care pretest: keep NPO for 8 hours before test
         c. nursing care posttest
            ▪ give laxatives, force fluids to remove barium
            ▪ encourage mobility to stimulate peristalsis
      3. cholecystography
         a. definition: x-ray visualization of gallbladder and biliary tract after oral ingestion of iodine

dye (isopanoic acid tablets); use of this test has largely been replaced by ulrasonography
      b. nursing care pretest
         ▪ check for allergies to iodine, shellfish, contrast dyes
         ▪ administer tablets (dose based on patient's body weight) one at a time with specified amount of water at 5-minute intervals 2 to 3 hours after a low-fat evening meal and 12 hours before test
         ▪ assess for side effects of tablets: diarrhea, nausea, vomiting, or abdominal cramps; report to physician or radiologist
         ▪ keep NPO for 8 hours before test
      4. IV cholangiography
         a. definition: x-ray visualization of gallbladder and biliary tract after injection of radiopaque dye; NOTE: test may also be performed via T-tube or during surgery
         b. nursing care pretest
            ▪ check for iodine or shellfish allergies
            ▪ keep NPO for 8 hours before test
            ▪ ensure that signed consent form is on chart if needed
            ▪ give laxative or enema if ordered before exam
         c. nursing care posttest: force fluids (x-ray dye acts as a diuretic)
      5. abdominal computed tomography (CT) scan: with or without contrast medium
      6. percutaneous transhepatic cholangiography (PTHC)
         a. definition: passing a needle through the liver into a dilated intrahepatic bile duct and directly injecting iodinated dye; used with clients who have elevated bilirubin and jaundice
         b. nursing care pretest: refer to IV cholangiography
         c. nursing care posttest
            ▪ assess for signs and symptoms of peritonitis, bleeding, sepsis
            ▪ keep client NPO and on bed rest as ordered
            ▪ assess vital signs according to postprocedure routine
   e. Endoscopy
      1. definition: direct visualization of a part or parts of the GI tract through a lighted scope; may be used as a treatment modality (e.g., polypectomy, removal of foreign objects, cauterization of GI bleeding sites)
      2. types
         a. esophagogastroduodenoscopy
         b. peritoneoscopy (liver, gallbladder, and mesentery)
         c. endoscopic retrograde cholangiopancreatography (ERCP) (pancreas and biliary tree)
         d. colonoscopy (entire colon)
         e. proctoscopy (rectum), sigmoidoscopy (rectum and sigmoid colon)
      3. nursing care pretest
         a. keep NPO for 8 hours before test

b. administer bowel prep for lower GI endoscopy
c. ensure that a signed consent form is on the chart
d. give pretest sedation as ordered
4. nursing care posttest
a. check vital signs frequently the first 24 hours
b. feed when gag reflex returns after upper GI endoscopy
c. observe for bleeding (indicated by frequent swallowing and bloody emesis after exam of the upper GI system or bloody stools after exam of lower GI system), sharp pain in the abdomen (indicates perforation)
d. force fluids as needed

f. Ultrasonography
1. definition: use of high-frequency sound waves to evaluate organ size, shape, and structure; painless, safe procedure
2. nursing care pretest
a. if client has had prior barium contrast studies, laxatives and cathartics may be given the evening before
b. gallbladder: keep NPO for 8 hours before test, low-fat evening meal before test
c. pelvic: have client drink 6 to 8 glasses of water just before test and not void until test is over, or clamp Foley catheter (full bladder acts as a landmark)
d. all other organs: no food or fluid restrictions
3. nursing care posttest: no special concerns

g. Analytic studies
1. gastric analysis
a. definition: to determine amount of gastric secretion with and without stimulation; may be done with nasogastric (NG) insertion or administration of Diagnex blue tablets by mouth
b. nursing care (with NG tube)
▪ keep NPO for 8 hours
▪ insert NG tube
▪ collect fasting specimen and a specimen after stimulation by food or drugs (Histalog)
c. nursing care (without NG tube)
▪ keep NPO for 8 hours
▪ have client empty bladder, discard urine
▪ administer caffeine to stimulate gastric secretions
▪ administer Diagnex blue tablet
▪ collect urine after 2 hours and check color (if gastric secretion has a pH of 3 or less, the dye will be absorbed and excreted in urine)
2. Schilling test
a. definition: to identify the reason for vitamin B_{12} deficits—either a lack of intrinsic factor (pernicious anemia) or a defect in absorption
b. nursing care
▪ keep NPO 8 to 12 hours before exam
▪ after administration of radioactive oral vitamin B_{12} usually by nuclear medicine personnel, administer vitamin B_{12} IM as directed (usually 1 to 2 hours after oral dose)
▪ start 24-hour urine specimen collection after IM injection to assess levels of radioactive B_{12} excreted (normal is 8% to 40% excretion of injected material within 24 hours)
▪ allow client to resume eating after IM injection

h. Biopsies
1. excisional
a. intestinal (done at time of sigmoidoscopy or colonoscopy)
b. gastric (done at time of gastroscopy)
2. needle (percutaneous liver biopsy)
a. definition: a blind needle biopsy of liver tissue to establish a microscopic picture of the liver
b. nursing care pretest
▪ ensure that informed consent is on chart
▪ check prothrombin time (if less than 40%, test will not be done)
▪ check platelet count (test may not be done if count is less than 100,000)
▪ instruct client to exhale and hold breath for 1 to 2 seconds while biopsy is being done and not to move during procedure; client may be in a supine position with the right arm under the head during the procedure
c. nursing care posttest
▪ have client lie on right side with pillow or sandbag over the insertion point under costal margin for 1 to 2 hours, bed rest for 24 hours
▪ take frequent vital signs the first 24 hours
▪ assess for pain or respiratory difficulty (pneumothorax or hemothorax)

ANALYSIS/NURSING DIAGNOSIS
1. Safe, effective care environment
a. Knowledge deficit
b. Risk for infection
2. Physiologic integrity
a. Pain
b. Constipation or diarrhea
c. Nutrition, altered: less than body requirements
3. Psychosocial integrity
a. Ineffective individual coping
b. Situational low self-esteem
4. Health promotion/maintenance
a. Health-seeking behaviors
b. Management of therapeutic regimen (individual or family), ineffective

GENERAL NURSING PLANNING, IMPLEMENTATION, AND EVALUATION

Goal I Client will eat a diet that conforms to prescribed restrictions yet contains all needed nutrients.

Implementation
1. Increase or decrease dietary nutrients as ordered.
2. Teach client the rationale for dietary restrictions.
3. Help client identify factors in lifestyle that may interfere with adherence.
4. Provide needed support and encouragement; involve family if possible.

Evaluation
Client selects appropriate diet from sample menus; verbalizes rationale for restrictions; expresses positive attitude toward diet changes.

Goal 2 Client will be as comfortable and with as little discomfort as possible.

Implementation
1. Administer pain medications as appropriate.
2. Use noninvasive comfort techniques such as positioning, massage, and distraction.
3. Teach client and significant others about measures that will minimize pain when client is discharged (e.g., dietary regimen, medications).

Evaluation
Client states that pain is either minimal or absent; verbalizes measures to control pain after discharge.

Goal 3 Client's fluid and electrolyte balance will return to normal.

Implementation
1. Institute replacement therapy or restrictions as ordered.
2. Keep accurate I&O.
3. Monitor daily weight.

Evaluation
Client's fluid and electrolyte levels are within normal limits.

Goal 4 Client will be knowledgeable about disease process, medications, and the prevention of complications.

Implementation
1. Explain disease process.
2. Discuss rationale for ordered treatment regimen.
3. Provide information regarding the administration and side effects of all medications.
4. Help client and significant others identify factors that might trigger complications of the disease.

Evaluation
Client lists medications; describes the prevention of complications.

Table 3-24 Related problems in ingestion and digestion

Disorders	Description	Medical management	Nursing management
Gastroesophageal reflux	Reflux of stomach contents into esophagus causing heartburn and regurgitation; in severe cases it may progress to painful or difficult swallowing, ulceration, or stricture	Prn use of antacids, H_2 receptor antagonists (Cimetidine/Ranitidine), or metoclopramide (Reglan) to increase lower esophageal sphincter (LES) pressure; avoid anticholinergic agents	Diet—smaller, more frequent meals; high-protein, low-fat diet; avoid caffeine, alcohol, and chocolate Position—remain upright after eating; elevate head of bed 6-12 inches (blocks or foam wedge) Activity—avoid activity that increases intraabdominal pressure (e.g., lifting, tight clothes, bending over)
Hiatal hernia	Herniation of a portion of stomach through enlarged esophageal opening in diaphragm; common problem in middle age that is usually asymptomatic but may be accompanied by chronic reflux and heartburn	(See above regimen) If reflux is severe, surgical repair (fundoplication of stomach around esophagus) may be performed	(See above regimen) Surgical care involves meticulous respiratory management; small feedings because of reduced stomach capacity
Acute gastritis	Transient severe inflammation of the gastric mucosa, with possible hemorrhage and erosion; associated with excess aspirin ingestion, extreme physical stress, alcohol abuse, infection, radiation treatment and chemical poisoning; symptoms vary with severity but may include nausea, vomiting, pain, eructation, and bleeding	Condition is usually self-limited; treatment may necessitate fluids, antiemetics, antacids, or antibiotics; vitamin B_{12} may be needed in chronic cases	NPO or liquid diet; comfort measures; monitor I&O and electrolyte status; NG lavage to neutralize substance if ordered

Table 3-25   A comparison of gastric and duodenal ulcers

	Predisposing factors	Pathophysiology	Clinical manifestations
Gastric ulcers	Excessive use of salicylates, nonsteroidal antiinflammatory drugs (NSAIDs) Genetic predisposition Severe physiologic stress *H. pylori* infection	Acid secretion rate is usually normal or reduced. *H. pylori* infection damages the mucosa, impairs bicarbonate secretion, and impairs the quality of the mucus	Epigastric pain—often severe. Not related to food intake and may not respond to antacids. Anorexia, nausea and vomiting, bloating and weight loss. Hemorrhage is common.

Duodenal ulcers	Acid oversecretion related to:
	    Excess parietal cell mass
	    Increased postprandial gastrin release
	    Increased gastrin sensitivity
	    Genetic predisposition
	    H. pylori infection
		Gastrin stimulates acid secretion, which overwhelms the mucosal integrity. Gastric emptying also may be accelerated, causing acid load to exceed the buffering capacity.	Pain similar to gastric but episodic and rhythmic—relieved by food or antacid. Nighttime pain is common. Bleeding is more likely to be chronic, and perforation is more common.

SELECTED HEALTH PROBLEMS RESULTING IN PROBLEMS WITH DIGESTION

✠ GASTROESOPHAGEAL REFLUX; HIATAL HERNIA; ACUTE GASTRITIS

Refer to General Nursing Planning, Implementation, and Evaluation, p. 159. Specific nursing care can be found in Table 3-24.

✠ PEPTIC ULCER DISEASE

1. Definition: sharply defined break in mucosa, which may involve the submucosa and muscular layers of the esophagus, stomach, duodenum, and jejunum
2. Incidence: estimated to affect 1% of the total adult population, although most of those affected are asymptomatic; varies widely by age, sex, and site; increases sharply with age
   a. Duodenal: most common form; peak occurrence from age 40 to 50; men most commonly affected
   b. Gastric: risk higher in elderly; peak occurrence after age 50; incidence highest in females
3. Predisposing factors (Table 3-25)
4. Pathophysiology (Table 3-25)
5. Diagnostic aids
   a. Fiberoptic endoscopy with biopsy to rule out malignancy
   b. Barium swallow
   c. Stool exams for occult blood
   d. *H. pylori* sampling
6. Complications
   a. Bleeding: occurs in 15% to 20%; may involve coffee-ground emesis, tarry stools (melena) with slower rates of bleeding, or the passage of bright-red blood rectally (hematochezia) with profuse upper GI tract hemorrhage
   b. Hemorrhage: occurs when ulcer erodes a blood vessel; treatment of shock and emergency surgery may be necessary
   c. Perforation: ulcer penetrates entire stomach or duodenal wall, releasing stomach contents, which results in a chemical burn and peritonitis
   d. Obstruction: repeated cycles of ulceration and healing in the pyloric region may cause scar tissue buildup around the sphincter
7. Medical treatment
   a. Drugs (Table 3-26)
      1. histamine$_2$ receptor antagonists, proton pump inhibitors
      2. antacids and mucosal healing agents
      3. antibiotics for inflammation
      4. anticholinergics (rarely used)
   b. Diet modification
   c. Rest
   d. Surgical intervention (used primarily for intractable ulcers and to manage acute complications)
      1. Billroth I: removal of part of stomach, anastomosis of remaining portion to duodenum
      2. Billroth II: resection of distal two thirds of the stomach; anastomosis of jejunal loop to remaining portion with remaining duodenal stump sutured shut
      3. vagotomy: severing of vagus nerve to decrease acid-secreting stimulus to gastric cells—can be truncal or affect only selective portions of the nerve
      4. pyloroplasty: revision of passage between pyloric region and duodenum to enhance emptying; usually performed in conjunction with vagotomy

Nursing Process
ASSESSMENT
1. Pain: type; severity; location; duration; response to food, liquids, or antacids; ulcers are frequently asymptomatic
2. Anorexia, nausea, or vomiting
3. Weight loss
4. Alcohol and smoking histories
5. Melena or occult blood in stool
6. Hematemesis
7. Complications of peptic ulcers
   a. GI hemorrhage
   b. Perforation or peritonitis
      1. sudden onset of severe abdominal pain

Table 3-26 Peptic ulcer drug therapy

Generic name (trade name)	Action	Use	Side effects
ANTACIDS			
Aluminum hydroxide (Alterna-GEL, Amphojel) Dried form (Alu-Cap)	Nonsystemic; works by neutralization	To treat gastric and duodenal ulcers; manage phosphate stone formation and high phosphate levels in renal failure	Constipation, phosphorus deficiency, intestinal obstruction
Basic aluminum carbonate (Basaljel)	As with Amphojel	As with Amphojel	Constipation
Calcium carbonate (Alka-2, Tums, Rolaids)	Rapid onset; high neutralizing capacity	Peptic ulcers	Constipation, hypercalcemia, rebound hyperactivity
Magnesium hydroxide (Milk of Magnesia)	Neutralizes HCl, demulcent effect	Antacid Laxative	Diarrhea, abdominal pain, nausea
Sodium bicarbonate	Systemic and local alkalizer	Antacid	Acid rebound, systemic alkalosis
ANTIFLATULENT			
Simethicone (Mylicon)	Decreases surface tension of gas bubbles; prevents formation of mucus-surrounded gas bubbles	Antiflatulent	None
COMBINATION MIXTURES			
Magaldrate (Riopan)	Combination of aluminum and magnesium hydroxide; nonsystemic neutralizing substance	Antacid	Mild constipation or diarrhea Hypermagnesemia in renal failure
Aluminum and magnesium hydroxide (Maalox; Maalox 1, 2, and Concentrate)	As above	Antacid	As above
Aluminum and magnesium hydroxide and simethicone (Mylanta, Mylanta II, Maalox Plus)	As above	Antacid Antiflatulent	
INHIBITORS OF GASTRIC ACID SECRETION			
Cimetidine (Tagamet)	Inhibits release of HCl by occupying histamine receptors in gastric mucosa	Duodenal ulcers; gastric hypersecretory states; prevent recurrent ulcers	Mild diarrhea, mental confusion, dizziness, gynecomastia Not recommended when drug interactions are of concern
Ranitidine (Zantac)	As above; greater reduction of acid secretion, longer duration of action	As above	As above, but side effects are fewer; no gynecomastia or confusion
Famotidine (Pepcid)	As above	As above	Dizziness, headache, constipation
Nizatidine (Axid)	As above	As above	As above
Proton pump inhibitor Omeprazole (Losec, Prilosec)	Profoundly inhibits gastric acid secretion for a prolonged period	Peptic ulcers	Headache, dizziness, GI distress, constipation or diarrhea
MUCOSAL HEALING AGENTS			
Sucralfate (Carafate)	Action unclear; may stimulate synthesis of gastric prostaglandins or adhere to protein in ulcer base	Peptic ulcers	Constipation; do not take with antacids
Misoprostol (Cytotec)	Enhances mucosal defenses by replacing gastric prostaglandins; has some antisecretory activity	Used for prevention of gastric ulcers for clients taking NSAIDs.	Crampy abdominal pain or diarrhea

Table 3-26 Peptic ulcer drug therapy—cont'd

Generic name (trade name)	Action	Use	Side effects
H. PYLORI DRUG TREATMENT			
Regimens are experimental but commonly include Bismuth compounds (Pepto Bismol) Amoxicillin or Tetracycline Metronidazole (Flagyl, Protostat)	Eradicate *H. pylori* infection	When chronic gastritis complicates ulcer healing and relapses are common	Nausea, diarrhea, and abdominal pain are common
ANTICHOLINERGICS (RARELY USED)			
Propantheline (Pro-Banthine)	Decreases quantity of GI secretions by inhibiting action of acetylcholine	Adjunct to ulcer treatment	Dry mouth, constipation, drowsiness

  2. diffuse abdominal tenderness
  3. diminished bowel sounds
  4. boardlike abdomen with diffuse distention
 c. Obstruction
  1. fullness, nausea
  2. profuse vomiting of undigested food

ANALYSIS/NURSING DIAGNOSIS (see p. 159)
PLANNING, IMPLEMENTATION, AND EVALUATION

Goal 1 Client will be free from pain.

Implementation
1. Give 30 ml antacid drugs 1 to 3 hours after meals, at bedtime, and prn but not within 30 minutes of histamine receptor antagonists or sucralfate ingestion.
2. Give histamine receptor antagonists as ordered with meals or at bedtime.
3. Teach client to eliminate or reduce intake of foods that cause increased pain.
   a. Try small, frequent meals; avoid eating at bedtime.
   b. Avoid common stimulants of gastric acid secretion during the healing process (e.g., caffeine, beer, alcohol, and spicy foods).
4. Provide for increased rest; promote a calm, peaceful environment.
5. Assist client to stop smoking, if possible.

Evaluation
Client can tolerate diet without discomfort; states or institutes measures that decrease or prevent pain.

Goal 2 Client will identify activities to prevent ulcer recurrence.

Implementation
1. Help client plan to balance work, play, and rest.
2. Clarify dietary modifications. Avoid overeating and bedtime snacking. Encourage a high-fiber, low-saturated-fat diet.

3. Encourage reduction or elimination of smoking, alcohol, caffeine intake.
4. Encourage follow-up health care as recommended for *H. pylori* infection management.
5. Teach regarding medications, side effects; time and method of administration; avoid medications that irritate ulcer (e.g., acetylsalicylic acid (ASA), NSAIDs, steroids).

Evaluation
Client states measures that will reduce the chances of recurrence; follows prescribed diet; takes medication correctly; has a balanced activity schedule; stops or decreases smoking or alcohol ingestion.

Goal 3 Client will recover from GI hemorrhage or ulcer perforation with minimal complications.

Implementation
1. Monitor vital signs every 5 to 15 minutes; record I&O.
2. Establish large-bore IV line for fluid replacement.
3. Institute measures to control bleeding if ordered. NOTE: it is estimated that ulcer bleeding will stop spontaneously in 85% of cases.
   a. Insert gastric lavage tube; irrigate stomach with 250 ml of room-temperature tap water or saline until clear; allow to dwell for approximately 2 minutes before removing; repeat as needed. Connect to low suction.
   b. Position client with head of bed (HOB) elevated at least 45 degrees to prevent aspiration. Turn on side if tolerated.
   c. Give cimetidine (Tagamet) after acute bleeding has stopped. Administer antacids if ordered.
   d. Administer IV fluids; type and crossmatch client's blood in order to replace blood loss as ordered.
   e. Offer emotional support and remain calm.
4. Minimize consequences of perforation.
   a. Give antibiotics and analgesics as ordered.
   b. Insert NG tube and administer IV fluids as ordered.

c. Keep client in Fowler's position to localize gastric contents to one area of peritoneum.

d. Monitor vital signs frequently, and prepare client for surgery if needed.

Evaluation

Client experiences control of gastric bleeding; maintains vital signs within normal limits. Client with perforation is stable and prepared for surgery.

Goal 4 Client undergoing gastric surgery will recover free from complications.

Implementation

1. Provide standard postoperative care; encourage deep breathing to promote lung expansion; refer to Perioperative Period, p. 115.

2. Keep client NPO for 5 to 7 days to allow incision to heal; monitor for return of peristalsis; progress from clear liquids to a diet as tolerated.

3. Keep client in semi-Fowler's position.

4. Maintain NG tube to suction.
   a. Do not routinely irrigate or reposition NG tube unless ordered. Only sterile saline should be used for irrigation.
   b. Record all NG drainage as output.
   c. Observe color of drainage: should progress from bloody drainage to old blood to gastric secretions (greenish) within 24 hours.

Evaluation

Client recovers from surgery free from respiratory complications, infection, and hemorrhage.

Goal 5 Client will recover from gastric surgery with minimal anemia.

Implementation

1. Know that 20% to 50% of clients will experience anemia for 1 to 2 years after significant gastric resection.
   a. Vitamin B_{12} deficiency (pernicious anemia) may develop if parietal cells of the stomach were removed (loss of intrinsic factor).
   b. Iron deficiency from blood loss and poor absorption may occur.

2. Give dietary supplements as ordered.

Evaluation

Client recovers; is free from anemia; if anemic, seeks follow-up care.

Goal 6 Client will exhibit an understanding of dumping syndrome and ways to control it.

---

1. Teach client
   a. Causes of dumping syndrome (following subtotal or total gastrectomy)
      1. food enters duodenum rapidly
      2. hyperosmolarity of intestinal contents pulls H_2O from vascular bed and stimulates a neuroendocrine response

3. blood glucose levels rise rapidly after a meal containing simple sugars and triggers a reactive hypoglycemia several hours after the meal
   b. Symptoms of dumping syndrome
      1. symptoms occurs within *30 minutes* of eating and may continue for 1 hour
      2. client feels dizzy, weak, nauseated, and diaphoretic
      3. tachycardia, orthostatic hypotension, faintness are more common
      4. skin becomes cool, clammy
      5. diarrhea may occur
   c. Prevention techniques
      1. eat six small meals that are dry and contain moderate protein and fat and limited simple carbohydrates; avoid refined sugars
      2. drink liquids between meals only
      3. rest or lie down on left side for 20 to 30 minutes after meals if possible to slow gastric emptying
   d. Control of diarrhea or steatorrhea if present; have client:
      1. eliminate lactose and fluids during meals; limit glutens; limit fat intake
      2. use antimotility medications as needed
      3. report incidence of weight loss
      4. supplement vitamins and minerals as needed
      5. verbalize that there is decrease in severity in first year

2. Know that if conservative measures do not relieve the problem, surgical intervention with pyloroplasty may be necessary to narrow the opening between stomach and intestine.

3. For some clients, dumping syndrome and subsequent malabsorption become chronic, unrelieved problems.

Evaluation

Client states symptoms of and methods to prevent dumping syndrome; selects appropriate foods from diet list.

✖ CHOLECYSTITIS WITH CHOLELITHIASIS

1. Definition: inflammation of the gallbladder usually caused by presence of stones (composed of cholesterol, bile pigment, or calcium)

2. Incidence: common health problem affecting 15% of the U.S. population; higher in women

3. Predisposing factors
   a. Two times more common in women, particularly Caucasian, Mexican American, and American Indian
   b. Obesity
   c. Middle age
   d. Multiparity, use of birth control pills, estrogen replacement

4. Medical treatment
   a. Medical intervention
      1. low-fat diet can decrease the severity of symptoms but does not prevent the development of stones (Table 3-27)
      2. dissolution therapy (chenodeoxycholic acid

[CDCA]) by percutaneous transhepatic catheter; used experimentally for selected patients

3. shock wave lithotripsy; used experimentally for selected patients

b. Surgical intervention
1. cholecystectomy (removal of gallbladder and cystic duct); still necessary when stones are found in the common bile duct; Jackson-Pratt or Penrose drain may be placed in gallbladder bed
   a. removal of stones from common bile duct usually necessitates placement of T-tube to maintain duct patency during healing (Fig. 3-14)
2. Laparoscopic cholecystectomy: laser dissection of gallbladder by the insertion of a laparoscope through an umbilical incision. Technique reduces pain and recovery time (see Box 3-1 for Home Care after Laser Cholecystectomy)

Nursing Process

ASSESSMENT
1. Abdominal pain and acute tenderness in the right upper quadrant; may radiate to back or scapula; onset of pain follows ingestion of a large or rich meal
2. Fullness, eructation, dyspepsia following fat ingestion
3. Nausea and vomiting (distention of bile duct initiates stimulation of vomiting center)
4. Low-grade fever
5. Abnormal ultrasound
6. Signs of obstructed bile flow (less than 10% of patients)
   a. Mild jaundice
   b. Clay-colored stools, dark-amber urine

ANALYSIS (see p. 159)
PLANNING, IMPLEMENTATION, AND EVALUATION

Goal 1 Client with an acute attack of cholecystitis will be comfortable with relief of symptoms.

Implementation
1. Relieve pain with analgesics as ordered; meperidine (Demerol) is usually ordered because morphine causes spasms of bile ducts.
2. Relieve reflex spasms with antispasmodic drugs prn as ordered.
3. Relieve vomiting and decrease gastric stimulation with NG tube to suction.
4. Give broad-spectrum antibiotics as ordered. Monitor fever.

Table 3-27   Principles of a low-fat diet

Trim all visible fat from foods.
Use only lean meats; remove skin from poultry.
Restrict use of eggs.
Do not use fat for food preparation; no frying.
Use skim milk and low-fat cottage cheese.
Avoid use of sauces, gravies, and rich desserts.
Increase use of fish and seafood.

Evaluation
Client is pain free without nausea, vomiting, or fever.

Goal 2 Client will recover from abdominal cholecystectomy without complications (refer to General Nursing Plans, p. 159.)

Implementation
1. Provide liberal pain medication (postoperative pain is severe and persistent).
2. Place in low to semi-Fowler's position; encourage frequent coughing and deep breathing to prevent atelectasis.
3. Change dressings as needed (bile with a pH of 7.6 to 7.8 is extremely irritating to skin).
4. Care for T-tube if present.
   a. Avoid tension and obstruction of tubing.
   b. Measure amount of drainage carefully; record as output (drainage will be 200 to 1000 ml per day for first several days; continuing large amounts indicate obstruction).
   c. Clamp as ordered in 3 to 4 days before meals to allow bile to drain into duodenum; assess tolerance (absence of nausea or vomiting); client may need discharge teaching for care of tube because it is common for clients to go home with a T-tube. Stool will regain its brown color as bile begins to flow into the duodenum.
   d. Usually removed 10 to 12 days postoperatively after T-tube cholangiogram to determine status of duct.
5. Advance from clear liquids to low-fat diet as tolerated when ordered.

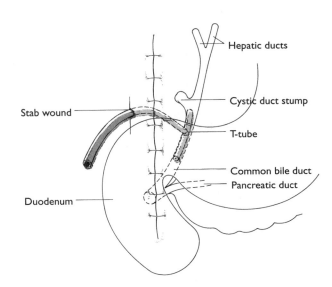

Fig. 3-14   The T-tube. The crossbar of the T-tube lies in the common bile duct. The long end is brought out through a stab sound in the abdomen and connected to gravity drainage. (From Beare P, Myers J: *Principles and practice of adult health nursing*, ed 2, St Louis, 1994, Mosby.)

Box 3-1

HOME CARE AFTER LASER CHOLECYSTECTOMY

1. Take NSAID or prescription pain medication as needed for adequate pain relief.
   a. Pain often radiates to the shoulder area.
   b. A heating pad may increase comfort.
2. Report the development of any severe pain or tenderness in the right upper quadrant, increase in abdominal girth, or drainage from the puncture sites promptly to the physician.
3. Monitor response to oral fluids and food.
4. Ambulate for short distances at least 4 times a day and take 10 deep breaths in the standing position. Ensure adequate rest and avoid fatigue.

Evaluation

Client recovers from surgery free from skin irritation, diet intolerance, and biliary tract complications; ambulates without difficulty.

✂ PANCREATITIS

1. Definition: acute or chronic inflammation of the pancreas
2. Pathophysiology: stimulation of the pancreas triggers digestive enzyme release; movement is blocked by edema or stones in the duct resulting in
   a. Duct rupture and enzyme escape
   b. Autodigestion within the pancreas
   c. Interstitial hemorrhage, tissue necrosis, or development of pseudocysts
   d. Chronic pancreatitis: destruction of parenchyma with fibrosis formation
3. Risk factors
   a. Gallbladder disease (40%)
   b. Alcohol abuse (40%)
   c. Abdominal trauma or surgery
   d. Infections (especially viral)
   e. Idiopathic causes (15%)
4. Medical treatment:
   a. Generally conservative
   b. Control pain
   c. Rest pancreas
   d. Support nutrition and hydration

Nursing Process

ASSESSMENT

1. Abdominal pain, usually epigastric or left upper quadrant; constant, ranges in severity from mild to extremely severe
2. Nausea and vomiting
3. Abdominal distention and severe tenderness
4. Low-grade fever
5. Signs of fluid deficits
6. Elevated serum amylase and lipase
7. Elevated urinary amylase
8. Shock (kinin is a vasodilator activated by trypsin secretion), tachycardia, hypotension

9. Chronic steatorrhea
10. Hyperglycemia

ANALYSIS/NURSING DIAGNOSIS (see p. 159)

PLANNING, IMPLEMENTATION, AND EVALUATION

> **Goal 1** Client will be free from pain or have minimal pain.

Implementation

1. Keep NPO until inflammation subsides and serum amylase levels fall.
2. Know that meperidine (Demerol) is the narcotic of choice; morphine may cause spasm of the sphincter of Oddi.
3. NG tube to suction if vomiting is severe or ileus is present.
4. Histamine receptor antagonists, anticholinergics, and antacids may be used in selected situations.
5. Be alert to signs of alcohol withdrawal.

Evaluation

Client states that pain is subsiding.

> **Goal 2** Client will be free from shock in the acute phase (refer to Shock, p. 129).

> **Goal 3** Client will maintain adequate nutrition.

Implementation

1. Maintain NPO during acute phase; NG suctioning may be used. Carry out specific mouth care orders.
2. Monitor I&O balance, daily weight, and abdominal girth to monitor fluid shifts.
3. Administer total parenteral nutrition (TPN) (Table 3-28) as ordered if inflammation persists; gradually progress to a bland, low-fat diet after inflammation subsides. A regular diet is gradually resumed.
4. Teach client to avoid stimulants, and alcohol.
5. Monitor blood glucose, urine glucose, and acetone levels (short-term prn insulin may be necessary).
6. Know that pancreatic enzymes may be given with meals to aid fat digestion in chronic pancreatitis if damage is severe.

Evaluation

Client is free from nutritional deficiencies and digestive problems; ingests and tolerates the prescribed diet; has no weight loss; chooses bland, low-fat foods from the diet menu.

> **Goal 4** Client will institute measures to prevent chronic pancreatitis.

Implementation

1. Discuss with client ways to eliminate the underlying cause when possible.
2. Instruct client to avoid alcohol and caffeine.

3. Suggest alcohol rehabilitation programs if indicated.
4. Implement orders to treat biliary disease if present.
Evaluation
Client experiences no recurrences of inflammation; avoids alcohol use.

Table 3-28   Total parenteral nutrition (TPN)

DEFINITION

TPN is a method for nutritionally sustaining clients who cannot or should not ingest, digest, or absorb nutrients. TPN solutions consist of an individually calculated combination of amino acids, glucose, minerals, vitamins, and trace elements. Lipid emulsions are frequently added to make the feedings complete.

ADMINISTRATION

TPN may be delivered through either a peripheral or central vein. Peripheral delivery necessitates excellent venous access, and glucose concentrations are restricted to 10%. Solutions of 15%-35% glucose may be administered centrally. TPN is associated with significant potential risks of infection and metabolic imbalance and necessitates careful monitoring.

NURSING INTERVENTIONS

Monitor insertion site; provide site care and dressing changes according to institution policy.
Administer TPN solutions through inline filters; lipids do not require filters.
Weigh client daily and maintain records.
Assess for fluid overload.
Monitor laboratory values daily.
Avoid drawing blood or administering other fluids and medications through TPN catheter or port.
Monitor blood glucose levels throughout therapy; provide sliding-scale insulin coverage with short-acting insulins as needed.
Encourage active exercise as tolerated to support the production of muscle rather than fat cells.
Monitor respiratory rate; excess carbohydrates increase CO_2 production and may cause tachypnea.
Instruct client to use Valsalva's maneuver and then clamp I.V. tube during tubing changes to prevent air emboli.
Carefully monitor infusion times but do not increase rate to catch up if behind. Rate changes of no more than 10% are usually the rule of thumb.

✴ HEPATITIS

1. Definition: acute inflammatory disease of the liver caused by virus (most common), bacteria, toxic or chemical injury.
2. Major types (Table 3-29): hepatitis D occurs as a coinfection or superinfection with hepatitis B; hepatitis E resembles hepatitis B in most respects
3. Pathophysiology
   a. Virus invades portal tracts and lobules of liver, causing inflammation and destruction of parenchymal cells
   b. Hyperplasia of Kupffer cells, tissue inflammation, impaired bilirubin metabolism
   c. Activation of complement system and formation of immune complexes
   d. Damaged cells are gradually phagocytized and cell regeneration occurs
4. Medical treatment
   a. Rest, symptomatic support
   b. Interventions to minimize transmission

Nursing Process
ASSESSMENT
Preicteric:
1. Flulike symptoms: malaise, fever, and chills
2. Dull pain and tenderness in right upper quadrant (RUQ) of abdomen; liver enlargement
3. Anorexia, nausea and vomiting
Icteric (2 to 6 weeks):
4. Jaundice
5. Clay-colored stools, dark-amber urine
6. Pruritus
7. Anthralgia
8. Severe fatigue, weakness, anorexia, abdominal tenderness
9. Abnormal liver function tests: elevated bilirubin, AST, and ALT
Posticteric (2 to 6 months):
10. Resolving jaundice
11. Gradual return of appetite and energy
ANALYSIS (see p. 159)
PLANNING, IMPLEMENTATION, AND EVALUATION

Table 3-29   Major forms of hepatitis

Factor	Hepatitis A	Hepatitis B	Hepatitis C (non-A, non-B hepatitis)
Primary route of infection	Oral, fecal, parenteral	Parenteral, direct and sexual contact, secretions and breast milk	Parenteral, sexual contact
Primary sources of infection	Contaminated food and water	Contaminated blood, blood products, and instruments	Contaminated blood, instruments, and dialysis
Incubation	15-50 days	50-150 days	14-182 days
Age group primarily affected	Children and young adults	Any age	Any age
Severity	Usually mild	Severe	
Vaccine	Hepatitis A vaccine (Havrix)	Hepatitis B vaccine (Hepatavax)	
Treatment for exposure	Immune globulin may be given	Same as Hepatitis C	Hepatitis B immune globulin (HBIG) may be given, but repeated infections are possible.

Goal 1 Client will have reduced metabolic demand on liver.

Implementation
1. Place on bed rest; explain reason to client.
   a. Limit activities until symptoms have subsided.
   b. Provide environment for adequate rest.
   c. Provide diversionary activities as needed.
2. Monitor liver function tests throughout care for a decreased level.
3. Avoid administering drugs toxic to the liver; use sedatives and opiates with caution.
4. Provide general comfort measures and interventions to control pruritus (e.g., baths, fresh linens, light clothing, diversion, cool room temperatures, short nails, and antihistamines).

Evaluation
Client rests most of the day; sleeps throughout the night; skin remains intact.

Goal 2 Client will have adequate nutrition.

Implementation
1. Encourage well-balanced diet with adequate nutrients and calories; restrict fats if poorly tolerated; encourage fluids during febrile period.
2. Use mild antiemetics if needed before meals; offer small, frequent meals.
3. Know that good nutrition is hard to maintain because of anorexia and nausea.
4. Have food available at client's bedside (e.g., hard candy).

Evaluation
Client's nutritional status remains adequate: minimal weight loss, intake equals output, and gradual return to normal energy level.

Goal 3 Significant others and staff will be protected from the client's infection.

Implementation
1. Follow guidelines for standard precautions.
2. Reinforce importance of scrupulous personal hygiene and good hand washing.

Hepatitis A:
3. Recommend disposable eating utensils and dishes.
4. Follow hospital protocol for handling and disposal of linens.
5. Provide immune globulin to close household and sexual contacts.
6. Recommend Havrix vaccine (one injection) for persons at risk such as food preparation workers.

Hepatitis B; non-A, non-B hepatitis:
7. Provide hepatitis B immune globulin to exposed persons.
8. Strongly recommend hepatitis B (three spaced injections) vaccine for all health care workers. Repeat titers and vaccine every 5 years as needed.
9. Follow hospital protocol for handling and disposal of linens.

Evaluation
Staff members and client's significant others remain free from disease.

Goal 4 Client will remain free from reinfection.

Implementation
1. Provide health teaching and information about preventive measures.
   a. Encourage optimal sanitation and hygiene.
   b. Instruct not to share personal care items.
   c. Instruct to wash clothing separately in hot water.
   d. Instruct to avoid sexual activity until blood values normalize.
   e. Encourage to refrain from alcohol use.
   f. Instruct not to donate blood.

Evaluation
Client states methods to prevent transmission and recurrence.

CIRRHOSIS
1. Definition: chronic degenerative disease of the liver causing diffuse inflammation and fibrosis, destruction, fibrotic regeneration, and hepatic insufficiency
2. Incidence: twice as common in men as in women; higher in people 40 to 60 years old, but can occur at any age
3. Predisposing/precipitating factors
   a. Malnutrition
   b. Effects of long-term, severe alcohol or drug abuse
   c. Necrosis from hepatotoxins or viral hepatitis
   d. Chronic congestive heart failure
4. Pathophysiology
   a. Fatty infiltration of the liver is the first step. Liver cell damage results in inflammation and hepatomegaly followed by fibrosis.
   b. Fibrotic changes gradually produce a small, nodular liver.
   c. Hepatic function is slowly impaired.
   d. Obstruction of venous and sinusoid channels blocks hepatic blood flow and causes portal hypertension.
5. Medical treatment
   a. Eliminate or relieve causative factors.
   b. Provide rest, nutritional and fluid support.
   c. Liver transplant is only the definitive treatment.

Nursing Process

ASSESSMENT
1. Early signs
   a. Anorexia, nausea, indigestion
   b. Aching or heaviness in right upper quadrant
   c. Weakness, fatigue, malaise
   d. Weight loss masked initially by fluid retention
2. Later signs
   a. Abnormal liver function tests: elevated bilirubin, AST, ALT, alkaline phosphatase
   b. Intermittent jaundice and pruritus
   c. Edema and ascites, prominent abdominal wall veins
   d. Prolonged prothrombin time, decreased platelet count, decreased serum albumin
   e. Anemia: folic acid deficiency, decreased RBC production, increased RBC destruction in spleen

f. Hormonal abnormalities, elevated estrogen levels
   1. palmar erythema, spider angiomas
   2. testicular atrophy, impotence, gynecomastia, amenorrhea

ANALYSIS/NURSING DIAGNOSIS (see p. 159)
PLANNING, IMPLEMENTATION, AND EVALUATION

> **Goal 1** Client will have reduced metabolic demands on liver.

Implementation
1. Provide bed rest during periods of acute malfunction.
2. Have client rest before and between activities if anemia becomes worse.
3. Eliminate ingestion of all substances toxic to liver, including sedatives, opiates, alcohol, and acetaminophen.

Evaluation
Client rests comfortably; spaces activities throughout the day; sleeps through the night.

> **Goal 2** Client will have adequate nutrition and hydration.

Implementation
1. Give a well-balanced, moderate-protein, high-carbohydrate, high-calorie (over 2000) diet.
2. Restrict fluids and sodium intake if there is edema or ascites present.
3. Plan small, frequent meals.
4. Administer multiple-vitamin therapy as ordered (higher doses of thiamin and fat-soluble vitamins if there is deficient fat absorption).
5. Monitor I&O and daily weights.
6. Monitor serum potassium, and offer supplementation if indicated.

Evaluation
Client eats prescribed diet; is adequately hydrated; maintains a stable body weight.

> **Goal 3** Client will not experience bleeding problems.

Implementation
1. Monitor urine, stool, gums, and skin for signs of bleeding or bruising.
2. Avoid injections; apply pressure to venipuncture sites for at least 5 minutes.
3. Monitor for increased prothrombin time, PTT; decreased platelet count, WBCs.
4. Teach client to use soft toothbrush for oral care.
5. Handle client gently and prevent skin damage from scratching.
6. Administer vitamin K as ordered.
7. Instruct client not to strain at stool.

Evaluation
Client remains free of bleeding.

COMPLICATIONS OF LIVER DISEASE

✥ ESOPHAGEAL VARICES

1. Definition: dilation of collateral veins that bypass a scarred liver to carry portal blood to vena cava; may occur in esophagus and stomach.
2. Pathophysiology:
   a. As liver becomes increasingly cirrhotic, portal hypertension increases.
   b. Collateral circulation in the esophagus develops in vessels that are weaker than normal vessels.
   c. As pressure in collateral vessels increases, vessels become overdistended and can rupture and bleed.
3. Usually asymptomatic until the varices rupture.
4. Mortality rate associated with hemorrhage is as high as 50%.
5. Treatment:
   a. Medical intervention includes gastric lavage with Sengstaken-Blakemore tube; vasopressin infusion.
   b. Endoscopic sclerotherapy, ligation and shunting procedures.
   c. Surgical intervention: portacaval shunt (anastomosis between the portal vein and inferior vena cava [has a high mortality rate]).

Nursing Process
ASSESSMENT
1. Abrupt, active bleeding after
   a. Increased abdominal pressure (physical exertion, Valsalva's maneuver, sustained coughing)
   b. Mechanical trauma (abrasions from swallowing poorly chewed food)
   c. Esophageal irritation by HCl acid, pepsin
2. Hematemesis

ANALYSIS/NURSING DIAGNOSIS (see p. 159)
PLANNING, IMPLEMENTATION, AND EVALUATION

> **Goal** Client will have esophageal bleeding effectively controlled.

Implementation
1. Assist with insertion of Sengstaken-Blakemore tube (Fig. 3-15).
   a. Ensure balloon patency and accurate labeling of all ports before insertion.
   b. Monitor balloon pressure frequently (at least qh); deflate balloons to relieve tissue pressure as ordered.
   c. Help client expectorate secretions, or gently suction secretions from oral cavity (*client cannot swallow around tube*).
   d. Monitor airway (*danger of airway obstruction if tube moves*); elevate head of bed 30 to 45 degrees.
   e. Provide comfort measures such as mouth and nasal care and positioning (esophageal balloon may be left inflated for up to 48 hours).
   f. Administer lavage fluids or antacids as ordered.
2. Monitor and treat client for shock as needed (see Shock, p. 129).
   a. Establish adequate venous access.

b. Administer blood transfusions as ordered.
c. Administer vitamin K for clotting problems.
3. Administer gastric lavage, saline cathartics, lactulose, and enemas as ordered to reduce ammonia formation and possibility of hepatic coma.
4. Give intestinal antimicrobials (e.g., neomycin) as ordered to decrease intestinal bacterial action on blood in GI tract.

Evaluation

Client's esophageal bleeding is promptly identified and controlled; condition remains stable.

ASCITES

1. Definition: an abnormal intraperitoneal accumulation of watery fluid containing small amounts of protein
2. Pathophysiology: results from a complex series of factors
   a. Decreased colloid osmotic pressure from decreased liver albumin production
   b. Increased capillary hydrostatic pressure from portal hypertension
   c. Increased levels of aldosterone
3. Medical treatment (depends on severity of ascites)
   a. Sodium (200 to 1000 mg) restriction; fluid restriction of 1.0 to 1.5 L per 24 hours may be ordered
   b. Diuretic therapy: spironolactone (Aldactone), an aldosterone antagonist, is often first drug used; a thiazide or loop diuretic may be added
   c. Salt-poor albumin to restore plasma volume
   d. Placement of LeVeen or Denver peritoneal shunt (catheter to move ascitic fluid from peritoneum to vena cava)
   e. Paracentesis
      1. used only for diagnosis or when fluid volume compromises comfort and respiration
      2. fluid tends to reaccumulate rapidly

Nursing Process

ASSESSMENT

1. Enlarged abdominal girth, protruding umbilicus
2. Increased weight
3. Fatigue
4. Fluid status: general dehydration
5. Abdominal discomfort, respiratory difficulty

ANALYSIS/NURSING DIAGNOSIS (see p. 159)

PLANNING, IMPLEMENTATION, AND EVALUATION

Goal Client will experience a reduction of ascites and an increase in comfort.

Implementation

1. Maintain bed rest or restricted activity.
2. Provide a sodium-restricted diet.
3. Monitor fluid and electrolyte balance, I&O, and daily weight.
4. Measure abdominal girth at umbilicus at least every shift.
5. Maintain high-Fowler's position for maximum respiratory effectiveness and comfort. Encourage deep breathing and use of incentive spirometer.
6. Support abdomen with pillows.
7. Administer diuretics as ordered.
8. Administer salt-poor albumin IV as ordered; during the

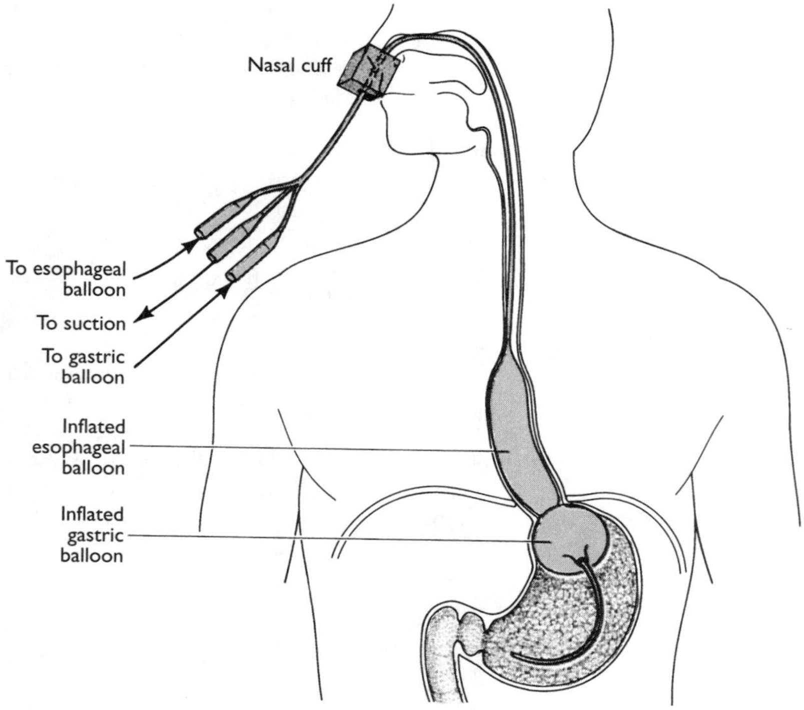

Fig. 3-15 The Sengstaken-Blakemore tube. (From Beare P, Myers J: *Principles and practice of adult health nursing,* ed 2, St Louis, 1994, Mosby.)

infusion monitor carefully for signs of CHF, pulmonary edema, dehydration, and electrolyte imbalance.

9. Assist with paracentesis if performed.
   a. Get a permit signed if appropriate.
   b. Have client void before the procedure.
   c. Prepare the client for a sitting or high-Fowler's position during the procedure.
   d. Monitor vital signs during and after the procedure. Watch for hypovolemia and electrolyte imbalance.
   e. Observe puncture wound for leakage, signs of infection.

Evaluation

Client is comfortable; experiences a reduction in abdominal girth and respiratory distress.

PORTAL SYSTEMIC ENCEPHALOPATHY (HEPATIC COMA)

1. Definition: cerebral dysfunction associated with severe liver disease
2. Pathophysiology: inability of the liver to metabolize substances that can be toxic to the brain, such as ammonia, which is produced by the breakdown of protein
3. Medical treatment (depends on severity)
   a. Restriction or elimination of dietary protein (NOTE: the effectiveness of this traditional intervention is now being questioned)
   b. Lactulose or neomycin to inhibit protein breakdown, decrease bacterial ammonia production, cleanse bowel of bacteria and protein

Nursing Process

ASSESSMENT

1. Mental status, level of consciousness: lethargy progressing to coma
   a. Dullness, slurred speech, confusion
   b. Behavioral changes, lack of interest in grooming or appearance, apathy
2. Neurologic exam: decreased reflexes, muscle twitching, muscular incoordination, asterixis (a flapping tremor)
3. Elevated serum ammonia level
4. Abnormal electroencephalogram (EEG)

ANALYSIS (see p. 159)

PLANNING, IMPLEMENTATION, AND EVALUATION

Goal 1 Client will have decreased ammonia production.

Implementation

1. Reduce dietary protein to 20 to 40 g per day (Table 3-30); maintain adequate calories to prevent catabolism.
2. Decrease ammonia formation in the intestine:
   a. Give laxatives, enemas as ordered.
   b. Administer lactulose (Cephulac) and neomycin (oral or rectal) as ordered. Two to four soft stools daily, not diarrhea, are the goal.

Evaluation

Client's serum ammonia level returns to normal limits; client tolerates a low-protein diet.

Goal 2 Client will remain free from injury.

Implementation

1. Perform general nursing measures for the unconscious client (refer to Sensation and Perception, p. 219).
2. Assess mental status frequently.

Evaluation

Client regains consciousness; is free from injury.

Goal 3 Client and significant others will learn to prevent future episodes of encephalopathy.

Implementation

1. Counsel client regarding low-protein diet and prescribed medications.
2. Ensure that client and family understand how to avoid and treat constipation.
3. Teach family early signs of encephalopathy: restlessness, slurred speech, decreased attention span.

Evaluation

Client states measures to ensure proper bowel functioning; states principles of a low-protein diet and planned rest periods.

Table 3-30 Low-protein diet sample menu

	Serving	Protein (g)
BREAKFAST		
Orange juice	½ glass	1
Farina	½ cup	1
Margarine	1 tbsp	trace
Sugar	1 tbsp	—
Low-protein bread	1 slice	1
Jelly	1 tbsp	—
Milk	½ cup	3.5
Coffee		—
LUNCH		
Fruit salad:		
Peaches (canned)	1	trace
Pears (canned)	1	trace
Apple (fresh)	1	trace
Low-protein bread, toasted	1 slice	1
Margarine	1 tbsp	trace
Jelly	1 tbsp	—
Sherbet	½	1
Ginger ale with added sugar	1 glass	—
Tea		—
DINNER		
Omelette	2 eggs	13
Aspargus	½ cup	trace
Carrots	⅔ cup	1
Baked potato	1	3
Margarine	1 tbsp	trace
Ginger ale with added sugar	1 glass	—
Coffee	—	—
Cantaloupe	¼	½
	TOTAL	26 g*

*Usual protein intake: 40-60 g.

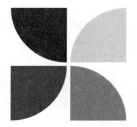

Nutrition and Metabolism: The Endocrine System

OVERVIEW OF PHYSIOLOGY

1. The endocrine system is a chemical system that functions together with the nervous system as the body's communication network.
   a. Endocrine glands synthesize and secrete chemical substances (hormones) that control and integrate body functions (Table 3-31).
      1. secreted in minute amounts
      2. circulated in the blood
      3. regulated by
         a. negative feedback systems
         b. changes in the plasma concentration of specific substances
         c. direct autonomic nervous system activity
         d. circadian rhythms
      4. actions alter specific physiologic responses
         a. growth and development
         b. reproduction
         c. metabolism
         d. responses to stress and injury
   b. Health problems involving the endocrine system result from hormone imbalances.
      1. primary problems: involvement of the target gland of the hormone
      2. secondary problems: involvement of the primary gland of secretion (e.g., pituitary or hypothalamus)
2. Glands:
   a. Pituitary:
      1. anatomy
         a. lies in the sella turcica above the sphenoid bone at the base of the brain
         b. consists of two lobes connected by the hypothalamus
      2. functions (see Table 3-31 for hormones and actions)
         a. regulates the function of the other endocrine glands through the stimulation of target organs
         b. controlled through the action of releasing and inhibiting factors from the hypothalamus
   b. Thyroid gland:
      1. anatomy
         a. located at or below the cricoid cartilage in the neck, anterior to the trachea
         b. consists of two highly vascular lobes
      2. functions (see Table 3-31 for hormones and actions)
         a. controls the rate of body metabolism

   c. Parathyroid glands:
      1. anatomy: four small glands located near or imbedded in the thyroid gland
      2. functions: control calcium and phosphorus metabolism in the body
   d. Adrenal glands:
      1. anatomy: two small glands lying in the retroperitoneal region, capping each kidney
      2. functions (see Table 3-31 for hormones and actions)
         a. adrenal cortex (outer capsule)
            ▪ secretes the adrenocortical steroids, mineralocorticoids, and androgens
         b. adrenal medulla (inner parenchyma of gland)
            ▪ secretes catecholamines
   e. Pancreas:
      1. anatomy
         a. long, soft gland that lies retroperitoneally
         b. head of the gland is in the duodenal cavity and the tail lies against the spleen
      2. functions
         a. exocrine function to produce digestive enzymes
            amylase: aids CHO digestion
            lipase: aids fat digestion
            trypsin: aids protein digestion
         b. endocrine function to control carbohydrate metabolism

APPLICATION OF THE NURSING PROCESS TO THE CLIENT WITH ENDOCRINE SYSTEM PROBLEMS

ASSESSMENT

Hormones have diverse systemic effects. Hypofunction or hyperfunction can result in dysfunction in a wide variety of organs and organ systems.

1. Health history
   a. Current symptoms
      1. change in client's energy level or stamina
      2. change in body characteristics or personal appearance
         a. size of head, hands, or feet
         b. weight, skin, or hair
         c. secondary sex characteristics
      3. increased sympathetic nervous system activity
      4. change in alertness or personality
      5. change in sexual functioning
   b. Past or family history

Table 3-31 Endocrine Glands, and Hormones with Actions

Gland	Hormone	Action
Hypothalamus	Releasing hormones	Stimulates release of hormones from pituitary gland.
	Inhibiting hormones	Inhibits release of hormones from pituitary gland.
Pituitary, anterior lobe	Growth hormone (GH)	Acts directly on bones and other tissues to stimulate growth.
	Prolactin (PRL)	Stimulates development of mammary tissue and lactation.
	Thyrotropic hormone (TSH)	Controls all functions of the thyroid gland.
	Adrenocorticotropic hormone (ACTH)	Controls release of glucocorticoids and adrenal androgens.
	Melanocyte-stimulating hormone (MSH)	Stimulates darkening of the skin.
	Luteinizing hormone (LH)	Initiates ovulation and formation of corpus luteum.
	Follicle-stimulating hormone (FSH)	*Women:* stimulates ovarian development of graafian follicle.
		Men: maintains spermatogenesis.
Pituitary, posterior lobe	Antidiuretic hormone (ADH, also called vasopressin)(produced in hypothalamus and stored in pituitary)	Facilitates reabsorption of H_2O in the kidneys, vasoconstriction in arterioles.
		Major regulator of osmolality and body water volume.
	Oxytocin (also produced in hypothalamus)	Initiates expression of breast milk; stimulates uterine contractions at delivery.
Thyroid	Triiodothyronine (T_3)	Control and influence: body metabolism physical and mental
	Thyroxine (T_4)	growth; nervous system activity; protein, fat, carbohydrate metabolism; reproduction.
	Calcitonin	Lowers serum calcium levels; inhibits bone resorption.
Parathyroid	Parathormone (PTH)	Regulates calcium and phosphorus metabolism.
Pancreas	*Endocrine function*	
	Insulin (from beta cells)	Enables glucose to freely enter cells; helps muscle and tissue oxidation of glucose; promotes storage of glycogen.
	Glucagon (from alpha cells)	Increases gluconeogenesis in liver.
Adrenal cortex	Glucocorticoid: cortisol (hydrocortisone)	Decreases protein synthesis; regulates serum glucose by increasing rate of gluconeogenesis; suppresses the inflammatory and immune response; increases fat mobilization; supports adaptation during stressful situations.
	Mineralocorticoid: aldosterone	Facilitates reabsorption of NA^+ and elimination of K^+.
	Adrenal androgens	Responsible for development of secondary sex characteristics.
Adrenal medulla	Catecholamines:	
	Epinephrine	Initiates stress response.
	Norepinephrine	Causes vasoconstriction.
Ovaries	Estrogen	Responsible for secondary sex characteristics, mammary duct system, growth of graafian follicle in women.
	Progesterone	Prepares corpus luteum; maintains pregnancy.
Testes	Testosterone	Responsible for secondary sex characteristics and normal reproductive function in men.

1. abnormal progression in growth and development
2. family history of diabetes, hypertension, infertility, mental illness
2. Physical exam
   a. Inspection: subtle or dramatic deviations from normal in body size, muscle tone, skin, hair, voice, and sexual characteristics
   b. Palpation: limited to the thyroid gland
3. Diagnostic tests (multiple tests available for each gland; see specific disorders)
   a. Interrelationships between hypothalamus, anterior pituitary gland, and target glands
   b. Measurement of the amounts of hormones present in serum or urine
   c. Fluctuations in daily pattern of hormone secretion cause random specimens to have limited value
4. Medical treatment

   a. Medical intervention: hormone replacement therapy, diet adjustment
   b. Surgical intervention: partial or total gland removal

ANALYSIS
1. Safe, effective care environment
   a. Knowledge deficit
   b. Risk for injury
2. Physiologic integrity
   a. Activity intolerance
   b. Risk for fluid volume deficit
   c. Nutrition: more or less than body requirements
3. Psychosocial integrity
   a. Anxiety
   b. Impaired individual coping
   c. Body-image disturbance
4. Health promotion/maintenance
   a. Impaired adjustment

b. Management of therapeutic regimen, ineffective (individual or family)
c. Health-seeking behaviors

GENERAL NURSING PLANNING, IMPLEMENTATION, AND EVALUATION

Refer to General Nursing Goals 1, 3, and 4 for digestive tract problems, pp. 159-160.

> **Goal** Client will successfully adapt to changes in body image.

Implementation
1. Assess client's perceptions of body.
2. Encourage client to verbalize concerns.

3. Provide client with accurate information about the degree of symptom reversibility.

Evaluation

Client expresses self-acceptance; engages in usual social activities.

SELECTED HEALTH PROBLEMS

✖ DISORDERS OF THE PITUITARY GLAND
See Tables 3-32 and 3-33.

✖ HYPERTHYROIDISM
1. Definition: oversecretion of the thyroid gland; second to diabetes in incidence; also called thyrotoxicosis

Table 3-32 Pituitary disorders

Disorder	Description	Symptoms	Medical management
HYPERPITUITARISM			
Anterior pituitary (acromegaly or prolactin hypersecretion)	Excess prolactin or growth hormone secretion. Usually caused by a benign adenoma or ectopic stimulation. More common in women.	Acromegaly: coarse facial features; protruding, enlarged jaw and nose; enlarged hands and feet; voice changes	Options include Transsphenoidal hypophysectomy (Table 3-33) or adenectomy Radiotherapy Drugs to suppress release of hormone
		Prolactin excess: Galactorrhea and menstrual disturbance (female) Gynecomastia and decreased libido (male) Visual defects, fatigue and lethargy, headache	Hypopituitarism is a risk with all treatments.
Posterior pituitary (syndrome of inappropriate secretion of ADH [SIADH])	Disorder is characterized by the inappropriate continued release of ADH, which can result in water intoxication, water excess, and hyponatremia. Disorder may be triggered by neoplasms, trauma, surgery, and drugs.	Depend on severity and rapidity of development. Weight gain, falling urine output, anorexia and nausea, confusion and lethargy. Seizures and coma may accompany very low sodium levels.	Fluid restriction to 500 ml will usually reverse the disorder. Drug therapy may inhibit renal ADH response; 3%-5% IV saline administration may be needed.
HYPOPITUITARISM			
Anterior pituitary (deficiency in childhood results in dwarfism): deficiency in growth hormone (GH)	Rare disorder that usually involves partial or complete deficiency of hormone secretion and results in multiple deficiencies. May be triggered by neoplasms, infection, or hereditary conditions.	Symptoms are variable and depend on the specific deficiencies. Most result from hypogonadism. They include menstrual irregularities, impotence, lethargy and fatigue, decreased stress response.	Options include hormone replacement (corticosteroids, levothyroxine, estrogen or testosterone), transsphenoidal surgery, or radiotherapy.
Posterior pituitary (diabetes insipidus): deficiency in antidiuretic hormone (ADH)	Condition of impaired renal water conservation resulting from a deficiency in ADH. It may develop idiopathically or result from trauma, surgery, tumors, infections, or in response to drugs.	The syndrome causes abrupt onset of extreme thirst with polyuria and polydipsia. Urine volume may reach 4-20 L/day with frequent urination. Dehydration may develop rapidly.	Treatment involves fluid replacement and drug therapy, usually with intranasal or injectable vasopressin.

a. Graves' disease (most common form)—a recurrent syndrome of autoimmune glandular oversecretion that may be precipitated by stress, infection, or trauma.

b. Toxic nodular goiter—thyroid hyperplasia related to elevated TSH stimulation possibly related to iodine deficiency. Nodules form that function autonomously. The disease is generally milder than Grave's disease.

c. Both common forms occur primarily in women 30 to 50 years of age.

2. Diagnosis
   a. Classic clinical picture (See following assessment)
   b. Elevated serum T_3, T_4, TSH assays and radioactive iodine uptake (RAIU) (test for thyroid antibodies)
   c. Abnormal findings from thyroid scan

3. Complications
   a. Cardiovascular disease (hypertension, angina, CHF)
   b. Thyroid storm or crisis: life-threatening hypermetabolism with excessive adrenergic response

4. Medical treatment
   a. Medications
      1. propylthiouracil (PTU): antithyroid drug that depresses the synthesis of thyroid hormone; takes about 3 months to be completely effective
      2. propranolol (Inderal) or other adrenergic blockers: relieve the adrenergic effects of excess thyroid hormone (e.g., sweating, tachycardia, tremors)
      3. iodine preparations (saturated solution of potassium iodide [SSKI], Lugol's solution): decrease the size and vascularity of the gland (short-term use) usually as preparation for surgery
   b. Radioactive iodine: limits the secretion of hormone by damaging or destroying thyroid tissue; treatment of choice for most adults (Table 3-34)
   c. Surgical intervention (performed only when client is in a euthyroid state)
      1. subtotal thyroidectomy (for large goiters)
      2. total thyroidectomy (if carcinoma present)

Nursing Process

ASSESSMENT

1. Cardiovascular: elevated BP, bounding pulse, tachycardia, palpitations
2. Nutrition: weight loss, increased appetite, frequent stools

Table 3-33 Nursing care associated with transphenoidal hypophysectomy

Refer to Intracranial Surgery (p. 227).

Monitor for increases in intracranial pressure.

Monitor for CSF leak through muscle plug in nose. Assess for positive glucose test on drainage, which is a halo ring on dressing, frequent swallowing, or complaints of postnasal drip. Change nasal drip pad (moustache dressing) as needed.

Provide frequent gentle oral care with rinses and tooth sponges. Do not brush teeth.

Assess for patency of gingival suture line.

Monitor for signs of diabetes insipidus (Table 3-32).

Administer Vasopressin IM or by nasal spray as ordered.

Teach client about the need for lifelong hormone replacement therapy and regular medical follow-up.

3. Integument: flushed, moist skin; heat intolerance
4. Musculoskeletal: fatigue, muscle weakness and wasting, fine tremors
5. Psychologic: anxiety, restlessness, insomnia, mood swings, personality changes
6. Other: menstrual irregularities, change in libido
7. Exophthalmos (protruding eyes from fat and fluid deposits in retroocular tissue—occurs only with Graves' disease)

ANALYSIS/NURSING DIAGNOSIS (see p. 173)

PLANNING, IMPLEMENTATION, AND EVALUATION

Goal I Client will return to a euthyroid state.

Implementation

1. Assess vital signs. Instruct client to report incidence of palpitations or chest pain.
2. Provide calm, restful physical environment with low levels of sensory stimulation.
   a. Ensure physical comfort; cool environmental temperature.
   b. Provide adequate rest; avoid muscle fatigue.
   c. Assist client to cope with anxiety and emotional lability.
3. Provide adequate nutrients.
   a. High-calorie (4000 to 5000/day), balanced diet during hypermetabolic state.
   b. Increased fluid intake.
   c. Small, frequent meals if hypermotility is present. Avoid stimulants.
   d. Monitor body weight.
4. Provide eye care if exophthalmos present.
   a. Eye drops, dark glasses, eye patches if necessary.
   b. Elevate head of bed for sleep. Avoid sleeping in the prone position.
   c. Assess visual acuity and adequacy of lid closure.
   d. Restrict dietary sodium.

Table 3-34 Care associated with administration of radioactive iodine*

Client should be euthyroid before treatment but drug free for 3-5 days to maximize absorption of iodine.

Dose is administered orally with client remaining in outpatient department for 4 hours to ensure tolerance.

At discharge client is taught to:

Avoid close contact with children or pregnant women for 24 hours.

Increase fluid intake and empty bladder frequently to avoid concentrations of isotope in urine. Flush toilet 2-3 times after each use.

Use separate utensils for 24 hours if the radiation dose is high.

Report symptoms of hypothyroidism (common long-term complication of treatment)

Follow up with physician for specified checks.

*[131]I therapy is the treatment of choice for middle-aged adults with moderate disease. It is safe and effective and associated with minimal or mild treatment effects.

Evaluation

Client enjoys restful sleep; verbalizes decreased discomfort and fatigue; maintains or increases body weight; is free from corneal damage.

> **Goal 2** Client undergoing thyroidectomy will be free from postoperative complications.

Implementation

1. Ensure prompt access to O_2, suction, tracheostomy set, and calcium gluconate or calcium chloride in the early postoperative period.
2. Monitor for signs of bleeding or excessive edema.
   a. Elevate head of bed 30 to 45 degrees.
   b. Check dressings frequently; assess for constriction. Loosen dressings if needed.
   c. Check behind the neck for bleeding.
3. Assess for signs of respiratory distress, stridor, hoarseness. (Laryngeal damage is possible, but worsening hoarseness is usually the result of edema.)
4. Be alert for the possibility of
   a. Tetany (owing to hypocalcemia caused by disruption of parathyroid glands): assess for numbness, tingling, or muscle twitching.
   b. Thyroid storm: sharply increased temperature and pulse with increasing restlessness and agitation.
5. Administer food and fluid with care (dysphagia is common). Begin with fluids and a soft diet.
6. Encourage client to gradually increase range of motion of neck. Support head and neck in position changes.
7. Answer call light promptly. Immediately postop and for about 24 hours the client may only be able to softly whisper.

Evaluation

Client maintains normal vital signs; experiences no excessive bleeding or respiratory distress; supports head and neck during movement.

> **Goal 3** Client will establish normal levels of thyroid hormone.

Implementation

1. Provide client with information about prescribed medications (i.e., name, dosage, side effects) and the importance of ongoing medical supervision.
   a. Total thyroidectomy necessitates lifelong replacement medication.
   b. Subtotal thyroidectomy necessitates careful monitoring for the return of thyroid function.
   c. Teach client receiving radioactive iodine treatment symptoms of thyroid deficiency (hypothyroidism is common within 2 to 5 years).

Evaluation

Client follows prescribed medication regimen; is euthyroid.

✵ HYPOTHYROIDISM

1. Definitions: underactive state of the thyroid gland resulting in diminished secretion of thyroid hormone
   a. Creates a diffuse clinical syndrome

   b. Most common in women in their middle years
   c. Effects may be overt or extremely subtle, especially in the elderly
2. Diagnosis
   a. Decreased T_3 and T_4
   b. Elevated TSH and cholesterol
3. Complications
   a. Cretinism: severe physical and mental retardation resulting from severe deficiency in infancy or childhood
   b. Myxedema: rare syndrome that may occur from prolonged untreated disease in adults
      1. accelerated development of coronary artery disease
      2. severely depressed core temperature and basal metabolism
      3. myxedema coma: rapid development of impaired consciousness and suppression of vital functions, usually in response to a major stressor such as surgery, trauma, or infection
4. Medical treatment: thyroid replacement
   a. Levothyroxine (Synthroid) is the drug of choice, introduced slowly to prevent excessive strain on the heart.
   b. Other preparations may be used for clients with allergic histories or special problems.

Nursing Process
ASSESSMENT

1. Fatigue, weight gain, constipation
2. Thickened, dry skin, cold intolerance
3. Coarse, thinning hair
4. Mental sluggishness, apathy
5. Thick tongue, slurred speech
6. Menstrual irregularities, infertility, decreased libido
7. Extreme sensitivity to narcotics, barbiturates, anesthetics—can trigger myxedema coma

ANALYSIS/NURSING DIAGNOSIS (see p. 173)
PLANNING, IMPLEMENTATION, AND EVALUATION

> **Goal** Client will return to a euthyroid state.

Implementation

1. Provide a warm environment conducive to rest.
2. Avoid use of all sedatives until condition improves.
3. Assist client in choosing low-calorie diet.
4. Increase intake of fluid and roughage to relieve constipation.
5. Increase physical activity and sensory stimulation gradually as condition improves.
6. Monitor cardiovascular response to increased hormone levels carefully.
7. Provide information about prescribed medication (i.e., name, dosage, side effects) and the importance of lifelong medical supervision.

Evaluation

Client follows prescribed medication regimen; loses weight gradually; experiences increased activity tolerance and alertness.

✺ DISORDERS OF THE PARATHYROID GLAND

See Table 3-35.

✺ HYPERFUNCTION OF THE ADRENAL GLANDS

1. Definition: oversecretion of hormones from either the adrenal cortex or adrenal medulla
   a. Adrenal cortex
      1. Cushing's syndrome: excessive secretion of glucocorticoid and possibly androgens from the adrenal cortex
      2. hyperaldosteronism: excessive secretion of aldosterone from the adrenal cortex because of a tumor, adenoma, or a secondary response to chronic sodium loss (Table 3-36)
   b. Adrenal medulla
      1. pheochromocytoma: catecholamine-producing tumor of the adrenal medulla (Table 3-36)
2. Incidence
   a. Cushing's syndrome
      1. true Cushing's syndrome is relatively rare but occurs most frequently in women aged 20 to 60
         a. primary disease typically results from adrenal tumors

Table 3-35 Parathyroid gland disorders

Disorder	Description	Symptoms	Client management
Hyperparathyroidism	Disorder of calcium, phosphate, and bone metabolism characterized by hypersecretion of parathyroid hormone (PTH) from increased gland mass. May be caused by benign adenomas or secondary responses to hypocalcemic states. Incidence rises sharply after age 50.	Usually detected on routine chemistry profiles because most clients are asymptomatic. Symptoms are related to excess calcium and include hypertension, renal stones, muscle weakness, GI distress, constipation, and bone pain.	Surgical removal of affected gland; increased fluids and calcium-blocking agents (used short term).
Hypoparathyroidism	May be produced by a variety of disease states associated with impaired secretion of parathyroid hormone (PTH) and surgical damage during anterior neck surgery. May be idiopathic.	Symptoms are variable and primarily related to the severity and rapidity of the deficiency. Calcium deficiency is primary aspect with muscle tetany, abdominal cramping. Cardiac depression and seizures may occur.	Medications to replace calcium and vitamin D and control phosphate levels.

Table 3-36 Other adrenal gland disorders

Disorder	Description	Symptoms	Client management
Pheochromocytoma	A rare disorder that may occur in middle age in either sex and appears to have some familial patterns. They are highly vascular tumors that produce, store, and secrete catecholamines. Diagnosed through elevated metanephrine and catecholamine levels and urinary vanillylmandelic acid (VMA).	Paniclike hypermetabolic state. Sustained or paroxysmal hypertensive attacks associated with headache, palpitations, sweating, and anxiety. MI and CVA are significant risks.	Surgical adrenalectomy is treatment of choice after control of catecholamine release and blood pressure has been established.
Hyperaldosteronism	The primary disorder affects mainly women in middle age and usually involves a benign adenoma, adrenal hyperplasia, or tumor. Secondary disease results from the activation of the renin angiotensin system by a nonadrenal stimulus such as sodium loss, renal arteriolar narrowing, nephrosclerosis, and cirrhosis.	Usually asymptomatic but may have hypertension, headache, fatigue, and hypokalemia.	Options include surgical adrenalectomy and medications to control blood pressure and restore potassium levels.

b. secondary disease occurs from excessive pituitary secretion of ACTH or an ectopic source of ACTH secretion in the body (e.g., oat cell lung cancer)

c. iatrogenic disease is a frequent result of the chronic use of exogenous steroids for any purpose

2. hyperaldosteronism is usually the result of a benign adenoma or adrenal tumor (see Table 3-36)

3. pheochromocytoma is a rare disorder resulting from a highly vascular tumor (see Table 3-36).

3. Diagnosis: increased serum cortisol, elevated urinary 17-hydroxysteroids and 17-ketosteroids; abnormal electrolytes—decreased potassium, increased calcium, and elevated blood glucose

4. Complications
   a. Cardiac problems (e.g., CHF or hypertension)
   b. Skeletal fractures
   c. Opportunistic infections

5. Medical treatment
   a. Surgical adrenalectomy if tumor is present
   b. Hypophysectomy for tumor of pituitary (see Table 3-33)
   c. Drug therapy with cortisol inhibitors
   d. Alteration in exogenous steroid dose if possible

Nursing Process
ASSESSMENT

1. Cushing's syndrome
   a. Abnormal fat distribution
      1. weight gain, increased appetite, thick trunk, thin legs
      2. moon face, buffalo hump (cervical dorsal fat pad)
   b. Skin changes
      1. thin fragile skin, red cheeks, easy bruising
      2. purple striae (stretch marks)
      3. body hirsutism, acne
   c. Cardiovascular
      1. sodium and water retention, hypokalemia
      2. hypertension
      3. fluid overload, CHF
   d. Musculoskeletal
      1. muscle weakness, decreased muscle mass, fatigue
      2. osteoporosis, bone pain, fractures
   e. Increased susceptibility to infection
   f. Decreased resistance to stress
   g. Increased secretion of pepsin and HCl
   h. Hyperglycemia
   i. Mental changes and mood swings
   j. Changes in secondary sex characteristics, menstrual irregularities, amenorrhea

ANALYSIS/NURSING DIAGNOSIS (see p. 173)
PLANNING, IMPLEMENTATION, AND EVALUATION

Goal I Client with Cushing's syndrome will manage disease symptoms effectively.

Implementation

1. Provide diet low in calories and sodium but high in protein, potassium, and calcium.

a. Offer diet in small, frequent feedings.
   b. Monitor for signs of hyperglycemia, GI bleeding.

2. Protect client from unnecessary exposure to infection.
   a. Monitor vital signs regularly.
   b. Use strict hygiene and asepsis.
   c. Institute reverse isolation if needed.

3. Provide atmosphere conducive to rest; space activities and help with care as needed.

4. Observe for signs of CHF.

5. Monitor daily weight, I&O, blood and urine glucose measurements.

6. Assess mental status regularly. Offer needed support in dealing with changes in body image and labile moods.

Evaluation

Client maintains or loses weight; experiences increased strength and stamina; is free from infection, accidental injury, or peptic ulceration; refers to self in a positive way.

Goal 2 Client treated with adrenalectomy will be free from complications.

Implementation

1. Measure urine output accurately and frequently.
2. Monitor vital signs frequently.
3. Watch for signs of adrenal crisis; have IV fluids, pressor drugs, corticosteroids readily available.
4. Minimize physiologic and psychologic stress.
5. Prevent thrombotic and respiratory problems.
6. Monitor wound healing carefully.
7. Teach regarding postdischarge self-care (e.g., diet, medications, activity level, and follow-up care).

Evaluation

Client maintains stable vital signs, adequate urine output and respiratory gas exchange postoperatively; states self-care needs to expect after discharge.

✺ HYPOSECRETION OF THE ADRENAL GLANDS

1. Definition: cortisol insufficiency (Addison's disease)—insufficient secretion of glucocorticoid, mineralocorticoid, and possibly androgens from the adrenal cortex

2. Incidence
   a. Rare disease occurring in 1 in 100,000; affects both sexes and usually occurs in middle age
   b. True Addison's disease is usually caused by autoimmune adrenalitis, but cortisol insufficiency can occur after bilateral surgical removal of the adrenal glands or withdrawal of exogenous steroids after long-term suppression

3. Diagnosis
   a. Low serum cortisol levels
   b. Low serum sodium and glucose
   c. Elevated serum potassium
   d. ACTH stimulation tests (increased ACTH levels but low plasma cortisol response)

4. Complications: adrenal crisis—acute adrenal insufficiency with sudden, marked deprivation of adrenocortical hormones producing severe hypovolemia, vascular collapse, coma, and possibly death

5. Medical intervention: steroid replacement maintained throughout life
   a. Glucocorticoid
      1. hydrocortisone usually given for maintenance
      2. dose will need to be increased at any time of increased stress, including illness or surgery
   b. Mineralocorticoid: fludrocortisone (Florinef) 0.05 to 0.2 mg daily (if more needed, long-acting preparation may be given)
   c. Periodic testosterone injections to support protein anabolism

Nursing Process

ASSESSMENT
NOTE: The clinical picture from the history and symptoms is often vague.
1. Lethargy, apathy, depression
2. Muscle weakness and fatigue
3. Gastrointestinal symptoms: anorexia, nausea, weight loss, abdominal pain
4. Increased pigmentation of skin and mucous membranes; bronzing
5. Hypotension, fluid deficit
6. Hypoglycemia, hyponatremia, hyperkalemia
7. Adrenal crisis
   a. Hypovolemia, hypotension, or shock
   b. Confusion, restlessness, or coma
   c. Fever
   d. Nausea, diarrhea, and abdominal pain
   e. Severe headache

ANALYSIS/NURSING DIAGNOSIS (see p. 173)
PLANNING, IMPLEMENTATION, AND EVALUATION

Goal 1 Client will recover from an adrenal crisis.

Implementation
1. Give large dose of glucocorticoids and vasopressors by IV infusion.
2. Encourage complete bed rest; prevent physical activity and emotional stress.
3. Monitor vital signs (especially BP for hypotension), fluid and electrolyte balance, and glucose levels frequently until condition stabilizes.

Evaluation
Client maintains vital signs within normal limits; exercises and returns to normal activity levels gradually.

Goal 2 Client will maintain normal hormonal balance.

Implementation
1. Provide information about prescribed medications (i.e., name, dosage, or side effects) and the importance of ongoing medical supervision.
2. Teach to balance activity and rest, maintain a regular activity pattern.
3. Promote good nutrition; monitor weight, fluid status, and I&O.

4. Help client to deal effectively with stress.
5. Teach client the signs and symptoms of underdose or overdose of medications and conditions that will require dosage adjustments (see Table 3-20).

Evaluation
Client is asymptomatic; takes and adjusts medications as indicated; maintains ongoing medical care.

HYPOFUNCTION OF THE PANCREAS: DIABETES MELLITUS

1. Definition: a chronic, systemic disease producing disorders in carbohydrate, protein, and fat metabolism; results from disturbances in the production, action, or use of insulin; eventually produces destructive changes in a wide variety of organs and tissues; insulin deficiency may be relative or absolute
2. Incidence
   a. Most common endocrine disorder; more than 10 million diabetics in the United States
   b. Diabetes and its complications are among the leading causes of death and disability in the United States
3. Etiology
   a. Basic etiology remains unknown
   b. Considered to be a group of syndromes whose development is influenced by genetic factors, viruses, autoimmunity, and environmental factors such as stress and obesity
4. Types
   a. Insulin-dependent diabetes mellitus (IDDM; type I): results from destruction of the beta cells of the pancreas resulting in little or no insulin production; requires daily insulin administration; most common in children under 20—peak incidence at 11 to 12 years
   b. Non–insulin-dependent diabetes mellitis (NIDDM; type II): probably results from a disturbance in insulin reception in the cells or loss of beta cell responsiveness to glucose; most common in middle-aged, overweight adults; 80% of all cases
5. Pathophysiology: IDDM (type I)
   a. Normally blood-glucose levels are maintained in the homeostatic range of 60 to 100 mg/dl by a series of feedback mechanisms
   b. In the absence of insulin, glucose accumulates in blood and urine leading to
      1. hyperglycemia
      2. glycosuria
   c. Glucose is hypertonic and depletes the body of large amounts of water (from extracellular fluid) as it is excreted by the kidneys causing
      1. polyuria
      2. polydipsia
      3. loss of sodium and potassium
   d. Glucose is then not available for cellular nutrition, and this causes polyphagia
   e. Fat and protein stores are broken down and used for energy; fatty acid and triglyceride accumulation cause ketone buildup with
      1. ketoacidosis
      2. ketonuria
      3. weakness

f. Other metabolic effects
1. microcirculatory and macrocirculatory changes producing atherosclerosis and arteriosclerosis (e.g., coronary artery disease, peripheral vascular disease, retinal and kidney damage)
2. alteration in immune and inflammatory response
   a. glucose concentration in the skin creates an excellent medium for infection
   b. glucose inhibits the phagocytic action of leukocytes, leading to decreased resistance
3. alterations in perception and coordination caused by developing neuropathies (a common complication, the cause of which is not well understood)
6. Pathophysiology: NIDDM (type II)
   a. Serum-insulin level may be low, normal, or elevated
   b. Pathology thought to be a combination of
   1. slowed response in insulin release
   2. reduced number of insulin receptors
   3. peripheral resistance to insulin
   4. reduced beta-cell responsiveness to glucose
7. Medical treatment
   a. Drug therapy (Table 3-37)
   1. insulin: short-, intermediate-, and long-acting forms
   2. oral hypoglycemic agents

b. Diet: individually planned regimens based on the client's age, sex, weight, and usual lifestyle (Table 3-38)
1. diet is manipulated to distribute the nutrient intake appropriately over a 24-hour period
2. diet is planned using the American Diabetic Association's (ADA) exchange method of meal planning
3. diet is used to correct obesity when necessary
c. Exercise

Nursing Process

ASSESSMENT
1. IDDM: initial symptoms
   a. Polyphagia, polyuria, polydipsia, weight loss
   b. Hyperglycemia, glycosuria, ketonuria
   c. Weakness, fatigue
2. NIDDM: initial symptoms
   a. May not have any classic IDDM signs
   b. Often diagnosed with development of complications (e.g., neurologic, vascular, infection)
   c. Weakness, chronic fatigue
   d. Hyperglycemia, glycosuria
3. Fasting glucose greater than 140 mg/dl or random glu-

Table 3-37   Hypoglycemic agents

Description	Drugs that act to either stimulate the islet cells in the pancreas to secrete more insulin (oral) or act as insulin replacement when pancreatic function ceases (parenteral)
Uses	Treatment of diabetes mellitus
Side effects	Hypoglycemic reactions, GI distress, neurologic symptoms, alcohol intolerance (oral preparations), allergic reactions
Nursing implications	Know onset and duration of action for each agent and teach to client; monitor for and teach client to monitor for hypoglycemic reaction; stress compliance with total diabetic regimen: exercise, diet, medications; check for beef or pork allergy (insulin preparations); see Goals 2 and 3 on pp. 181-182. Check for Sulfa allergies before administration of oral agents

Type of examples	Peak (hours)	Duration (hours)
ORAL AGENTS		
First generation		
Acetohexamide (Dymelor)	8-12	18
Chlorpropamide (Diabenese)	3-6	24-60
Tolbutamide (Orinase)	4-6	up to 24
Tolazamide (Tolinase)	4-8	6-12
Second generation		
Glipizide (Glucotrol)	1-3	12-24
Glyburide (Diabeta, Micronase)	4-8	12-24
INSULIN (USUALLY ARE STANDARD PURITY)		
Rapid acting (onset ½-1 hr)		
Regular	2-4	4-6
Regular Iletin	2-4	5-8
Regular human (Humulin-R, Novolin-R)	1-3	3-5
Intermediate acting (onset 4 hr)		
NPH Iletin	4-12	
Lente Iletin	8-12	10-14
NPH human insulin isophane (Humulin-N, Novolin-N)	8-12	12-16+
		12-16+
Long acting (onset 4-6 hr)		
Insulin zinc suspension extended (Ultralente)	16-24	>36
Ultralente human (Ultralente Humulin)	18	24-36

cose greater than 200 mg/dl on at least two occasions accompanied by symptoms

4. Abnormal glucose tolerance test, the definitive test

ANALYSIS/NURSING DIAGNOSIS (see p. 173)

PLANNING, IMPLEMENTATION, AND EVALUATION

> **Goal 1** Client will demonstrate knowledge of the principles of diet control.

Implementation

1. Assess client's knowledge of a diabetic diet.
2. Reinforce teaching of the dietitian as needed.
3. Encourage client to use the individualized meal plan.
4. Reinforce the importance of not skipping meals; the need to measure foods accurately and not estimate them.
5. Discuss with client the diet modifications needed to compensate for changes in lifestyle or illness.
6. Assist client with NIDDM to lose weight as indicated.

Evaluation

Client makes appropriate selections from sample menus; maintains normal body weight; maintains fasting blood-glucose levels within normal ranges.

> **Goal 2** Client will correctly administer insulin or other hypoglycemic agent as indicated.

Implementation

1. Assess client's knowledge of hypoglycemic agents.
2. Teach client preparation of injection, storage of insulin, and the principles of site rotation.
   a. Insulin in current use may be stored at room temperature for up to 30 days, all others in refrigerator or cool area. Do not freeze.
   b. Insulin must be at room temperature before administration.
   c. Roll insulin to mix; double-check label concentration.
   d. If client mixes insulin, do so in same sequence each day; e.g., always draw up regular or shorter-acting insulin first followed by longer-acting preparations (i.e., clear to cloudy).
   e. Rotate sites so that no individual site is used more frequently than once every 4 to 6 weeks; sites should be at least 1½ inches apart, and all sites in one area should be used before moving on to another area.
   f. Know that switching from separate injections to a mixture of insulins in one injection may alter local response.
   g. Inject at 45-degree or 90-degree angle depending on subcutaneous tissue layer thickness.
   h. Press (do not rub) the site after injection.
   i. Avoid smoking for 30 minutes after injection (cigarette smoking decreases absorption). Active exercise of injected extremity increases rate of absorption.

Table 3-38 Diabetic meal planning

NUTRIENT BALANCE (PERCENT OF TOTAL CALORIES)

Carbohydrate	55%-60%	Fiber	up to 40 gms/day
Fat	less than 30%	Alcohol	<1-2 equivalents 1-2 times per week
Protein	12%-20%		1 equivalent = 1.5 oz alcohol, 4 oz wine, 12 oz beer

EXAMPLES OF FOODS IN EXCHANGE LISTS

Free foods	List 1 Milk exchanges (quantity 1 cup)	List 2 Vegetable exchanges (quantity ½ cup)	List 3 Fruit exchanges (quantity approx. ½ cup)	List 4 Bread/starch exchanges (quantity 1 slice, ½ cup)	List 5 Meat exchanges (quantity 1 oz)	List 6 Fat exchanges (quantity 1 tsp or 1 tbs)
Coffee, tea	Whole milk (omit 2	Asparagus	Apple	Bread	Meat and poultry	Butter or margarine
Clear broth	fat exchanges)	Beets	Applesauce	Cereals	Fish	Bacon (crisp)
Gelatin (unsweet-	Skim milk	Broccoli	Banana	Spaghetti, noodles	Shellfish	Cream
ened)	Buttermilk made	Cabbage	Strawberries	Crackers	Eggs	Mayonnaise
Pepper and other	with skim milk	Cauliflower	Cantaloupe	Beans and peas	Cheese: cheddar,	Nuts
spices	Yogurt	Cucumbers	Cherries	(dried and	cottage	Olives
		Chard	Grapefruit	cooked)	Peanut butter	
		Collards	Orange juice	Corn	Cold cuts	
		Mushrooms	Pear	Potatoes		
		Onions	Pineapple	Rice		
		Tomatoes	Prunes, dried			
		Turnips	Watermelon			
		Raw vegetables				

GENERAL RULES (FOR ALL CLIENTS TO KNOW AND FOLLOW CAREFULLY)

1. Eat all meals about the same time daily. Do not skip meals.
2. Eat foods in the amount given only on the diet list.
3. Do not eat between meals unless it is part of the dietary plan; unless it is replacing food not eaten at a previous meal, or unless an insulin reaction is "coming on."

3. Provide opportunities for multiple return demonstrations.
4. Teach at least one family member to administer insulin.
5. Teach client factors that influence the body's need for insulin.
    a. Increased need: trauma, infection, fever, severe psychologic or physiologic stress.
    b. Decreased need: active exercise.

Evaluation
Client properly administers own insulin; shows no signs of lipodystrophy.

Goal 3 Client will monitor diabetic status regularly and correctly through the use of blood glucose monitoring, urine testing, or both.

Implementation
1. Assess client's knowledge of glucose and urine ketone monitoring.
2. Teach client proper technique for finger sticks.
    a. Follow product guide carefully for timing results.
    b. Use sides of fingertips or earlobes.
3. Teach client principles of urine ketone testing.
    a. Ketones are tested whenever blood glucose exceeds 250 mg/dl, especially during periods of illness, infection, or high stress.
    b. Consistent use of one product.
    c. Test before meals and at bedtime using a fresh urine sample.
    d. Record results in percentages, not pluses.
4. Keep accurate date and time records for both urine and finger-stick testing.
5. Teach client to notify physician if urine ketones or finger-stick results are greater than the physician-specified limit.

Evaluation
Client demonstrates accurate urine testing and blood glucose measurements; correctly interprets the results; maintains consistent, accurate records of the results; knows when to contact physician.

Goal 4 Client will implement a pattern of regular exercise.

Implementation
1. Assess client's knowledge of the relationship between exercise and diabetes.
2. Individualize exercise plan for each client; focus on aerobic exercise of light intensity; instruct the client with NIDDM to have a cardiovascular evaluation before beginning an exercise program.
3. Tell client to perform exercise 1 to 3 hours after meals to ensure an adequate level of blood glucose.
    a. Teach client with IDDM to carry a rapid-acting source of glucose, and take extra carbohydrates if vigorous exercise exceeds 30 minutes.
    b. Teach client that excessive or unplanned exercise may trigger hypoglycemia.
    c. Teach client to take daily insulin dose before active

exercise but to avoid injection into an exercising limb.

Evaluation
Client engages in planned regular exercise, 5 to 6 days per week at approximately the same time, without experiencing difficulties with hypoglycemia.

Goal 5 Client will practice good personal hygiene and positive health promotion to avoid diabetic complications.

Implementation
1. Assess client's knowledge of health promotion and complications.
2. Teach client diabetic foot care.
    a. Perform daily gentle cleansing and inspection.
    b. Wear properly fitting shoes.
    c. Use lanolin cream or oil to prevent dryness and cracking of feet and heels.
    d. Avoid going barefoot.
    e. Wear socks with shoes.
    f. Visit a podiatrist as needed for care of nails, calluses, and corns. Cut nails straight across.
    g. Test the temperature of bath water and avoid the use of heating pads or hot water bottles on the extremities.
3. Teach client interventions to prevent peripheral vascular disease (refer to Peripheral Vascular Problems, p. 138).
4. Teach client the adjustments that must be made in the event of minor illness (e.g., colds, flu).
    a. Continue taking insulin or oral hypoglycemic agent regularly (infection increases the body's need for insulin).
    b. Maintain fluid intake; replace diet with liquids if unable to eat solid food.
    c. Increase the frequency of blood/ketone testing.
    d. Contact physician if necessary.
5. Help client identify stressful situations in lifestyle that might interfere with good diabetic control.
6. Encourage good daily hygiene and regular checkups by dentist and ophthalmologist.
7. Teach prompt and thorough care for minor skin cuts and abrasions; avoid clothing and activities that cause chafing and irritation.

Evaluation
Client maintains teeth and gums in good repair; maintains soft, intact skin; states adjustments that are to be made to maintain control during periods of minor illness.

Goal 6 Client will recognize the signs of hypoglycemia and ketoacidosis and, if present, take appropriate actions.

Implementation
1. Assess client's knowledge about hypoglycemia and ketoacidosis.

Table 3-39 Differentiating hypoglycemia from ketoacidosis (hyperglycemia)

	Hypoglycemia (insulin reaction)	Ketoacidosis (diabetic coma)
Causes	Delayed or missed meals, excess insulin, excess exercise (glucose less than 50 mg/dl)	Inadequate insulin, too much food, infection, injury, physical or emotional stress (glucose greater than 350 mg/dl).
Symptoms	Anxiety, weakness, sweating, hunger, tremor, nausea, shallow, rapid respirations (severe: headache, confusion, unconsciousness); moist, cool skin	Thirst, increased urination, weakness, nausea, abdominal pain (classic: acetone breath odor, Kussmaul's (deep, rapid) respirations, decreased consciousness); hot, dry skin.

Treatment	5 to 15 g of carbohydrate:
	    4 oz soft drink (regular, not diet)
	    4 oz orange or other fruit juice
	    6-8 Life Savers
	    1-1½ Tbs honey, jam
	    4 cubes or 2 packets of sugar
	    2 squares of graham crackers
	Administer glucagon if unable to swallow
	Give some complex carbohydrate from meal plan within 1 hr after initial treatment
		Correct volume depletion with IV fluids (isotonic saline)
		Administer regular insulin by infusion.
		Replace electrolytes as volume restored.
		Monitor vital signs, I&O, blood glucose, and level of consciousness.

2. Teach signs of hypoglycemia and the situations that may trigger it (Table 3-39).
   a. Too much insulin or too little food
   b. Strenuous, unplanned exercise
3. Teach client to reverse hypoglycemia if possible with 5 to 15 g of a simple oral carbohydrate.
4. Teach client signs of ketoacidosis and situations that may trigger it (Table 3-39).
   a. Failure to take insulin
   b. Episode of illness, infection, stress, or trauma
5. Teach client that development of ketoacidosis requires immediate transport to a health care facility.
   a. Correct dehydration by administering IV fluids.
   b. Correct blood glucose with administration of regular insulin (usually low-dose infusion).
   c. Record I&O accurately (Foley catheter may be necessary if client is unconscious).
   d. Assess level of consciousness (LOC) and cardiopulmonary status at frequent intervals. Monitor for signs of hypokalemia as treatment progresses.
   e. Monitor urine ketones and blood glucose at frequent intervals.
   f. Replace electrolytes as ordered.
6. Tell client to wear a diabetic alert bracelet or tag at all times.
7. Be alert to the development of hyperosmolar nonketotic coma (HNKC) in elderly clients (Table 3-40).

Evaluation
Client lists the symptoms of hypoglycemia and ketoacidosis; states appropriate actions to take for each; wears a diabetic alert tag.

Table 3-40 Hyperosmolar nonketotic coma

A life-threatening condition characterized by severe elevation of blood glucose, dehydration, and stupor or coma. It occurs primarily in elderly NIDDM or previously undiagnosed diabetics. It has a 15%-20% mortality rate.

PATHOPHYSIOLOGY

The crisis is frequently caused by an infection or stressor that causes an outpouring of steroids and raises the blood glucose. Enough insulin is produced to prevent ketosis, but hyperglycemia and dehydration become life threatening, especially if the client cannot take oral fluids.

SYMPTOMS

Severe dehydration
Hypothermia, hypotension
Severe weakness and lethargy
Depressed mental status to coma
Blood glucose greater than 600 mg/dl
Elevated serum sodium
Serum osmolality above 350 mOsm/L
Absence of ketones in urine

TREATMENT

IV fluid replacement
Low-dose IV insulin
Careful monitoring for complications (e.g., CHF, pulmonary edema, electrolyte imbalance, seizures)

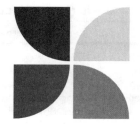

Elimination: The Kidneys

OVERVIEW OF PHYSIOLOGY

1. Kidneys
   a. Location: paired organs that lie in the retroperitoneum at the costovertebral angle (CVA)
      1. upper border: T12
      2. lower border: L3
   b. Size: 120 to 170 g (4 to 6 oz) each
   c. Regions (Fig. 3-16)
      1. cortex
         a. outer layer
         b. contains glomeruli, proximal and distal tubules
      2. medulla
         a. middle layer
         b. composed of 6 to 10 renal pyramids, formed by collecting ducts and tubules
         c. deepest part of loop of Henle
      3. pelvis
         a. innermost layer
         b. hollow collection area composed of calyces
         c. papillae move urine into ureter by peristaltic action
   d. Nephron (Fig. 3-17)
      1. functional unit of kidney
      2. one million nephrons in each kidney
      3. composition
         a. glomerulus
         b. tubule
            ▪ Bowman's capsule
            ▪ proximal convoluted tubule
            ▪ loop of Henle
               • descending limb
               • ascending limb
            ▪ distal convoluted tubule
            ▪ collecting duct
      4. action: all elements to be excreted or conserved are acted on in the nephron by the processes of filtration, concentration, reabsorption, or secretion
2. Ureters
   a. Join with renal pelvis; distal end implanted in bladder
   b. Composed of smooth muscles that have peristaltic action
   c. Narrow at ureteropelvic junction, bifurcation of iliac vessels and join with bladder
3. Bladder
   a. Stores urine until eliminated
   b. Muscular organ (detrusor muscle)
4. Urethra
   a. Passageway for urine during excretion
   b. Surrounded by prostate gland in men
5. Functions of the kidney
   a. Fluid and electrolyte balance (Tables 3-41 and 3-42)
      1. control of sodium balance
         a. intake in normal diet is usually greater than needed
         b. filtered by glomeruli
         c. reabsorption in tubules is controlled by active and passive processes and by the renin-angiotensin-aldosterone system; presence of aldosterone causes reabsorption of sodium
      2. control of chloride balance follows sodium
         a. intake in normal diet is usually greater than needed
         b. filtered by the glomeruli
         c. actively transported out of the ascending loop of Henle
      3. control of potassium balance
         a. intake adequate in normal diet
         b. filtered by glomeruli
         c. almost all filtered potassium is reabsorbed in proximal tubules
         d. secreted into distal tubules and into distal ducts where there is selective secretion or reabsorption
         e. dependent on hormonal influence
            ▪ increase of aldosterone causes increased potassium secretion into distal tubules
            ▪ decrease of aldosterone causes decreased potassium secretion into distal tubules
         f. potassium also lost through GI tract
      4. control of H_2O balance
         a. intake controlled by social habits and thirst
         b. reabsorption controlled by ADH concentration in the renal tubules
   b. Control of acid-base balance (see Table 3-18)
      1. excretion of organic acids
         a. HPO_4 buffer system; $H + HPO_4 \rightarrow H_2PO_4$
         b. NH_3 buffer system
            ▪ $NH_3 + H \rightarrow NH_4$
            ▪ $NH_4 + NaCl \rightarrow NH_4Cl + Na$
         c. liberation of free hydrogen ions
      2. conservation of bicarbonate
   c. Excretion of waste products (primarily products of protein metabolism: urea and creatinine)

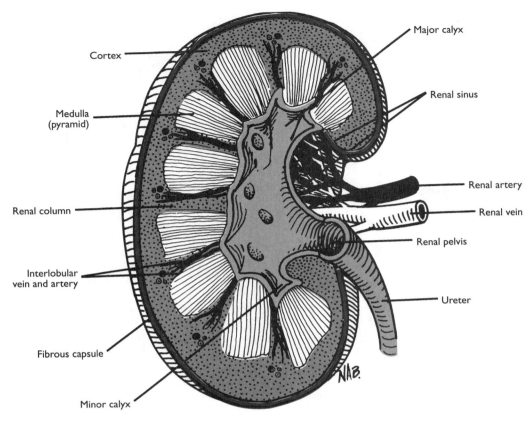

Fig. 3-16 Frontal section of kidney. (From Long BC, Phipps WJ: *Medical-surgical nursing: a nursing process approach,* ed 3, St Louis, 1993, Mosby.)

d. Production and secretion of erythropoietin in response to hypoxemia, an abnormal deficiency of oxygen in the arterial blood (erythropoietin stimulates bone marrow to produce erythrocytes)

e. Manufacture and activation of vitamin D (plays a role in calcium metabolism: active form of vitamin D must be available for parathormone to work)

f. Regulation of arterial blood pressure: renin and aldosterone
   1. kidneys secrete an enzyme called renin, which acts on plasma protein to cause the release of angiotensin (a vasoconstricting substance)
   2. angiotensin increases total peripheral resistance, leading to increased aldosterone secretion by adrenal cortex
   3. increased aldosterone stimulates increased sodium reabsorption
   4. increased sodium reabsorption leads to increased water retention and plasma volume, which increases arterial BP

APPLICATION OF THE NURSING PROCESS TO THE CLIENT WITH KIDNEY PROBLEMS

ASSESSMENT

1. Health history
   a. Urinary retention, stasis (e.g., associated with pregnancy, neurogenic bladder, immobility, diabetes)
   b. Bladder infections: caused by contamination from large intestine (especially young girls)
   c. Intrusive procedures (e.g., catheterization, cystoscopy, coitus)
   d. Bone demineralization
   e. Metabolic disease
   f. Changes in color of urine (e.g., hematuria)
   g. Changes in volume of urine
      1. polyuria: greater than 2500 ml per day
      2. oliguria: less than 400 ml per day
      3. anuria: less than 100 ml per day
   h. Changes in voiding pattern
      1. nocturia
      2. frequency
      3. hesitancy
      4. urgency
      5. change in urinary stream
      6. incontinence
         a. amount
         b. frequency of occurrence
         c. dribbling
   i. Medications
      1. diuretics
      2. antibiotics
      3. nephrotoxic agents: aspirin (ASA), acetaminophen, mercaptomerin sodium, phenylbutazone, sulfonamides, gentamicin, other aminoglycosides
      4. cholinergics, anticholinergics

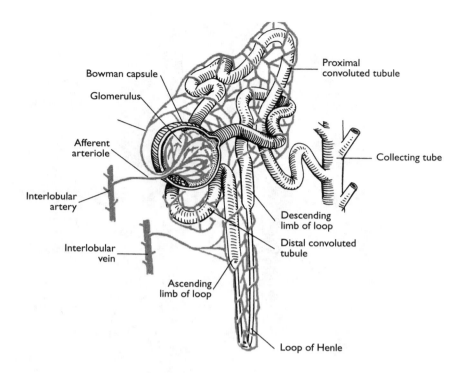

Part of nephron	Function	Substance
Glomeruli	Filtration	H_2O and solute, electrolytes (Na, K, PO_4, Ca, Cl, Mg), urea, creatinine, uric acid, glucose, amino acids
Proximal tubules	Reabsorption, secretion	H_2O, electrolytes (Na, K, Mg, Ca, Cl, HCO_3), glucose, amino acids
Loop of Henle	Reabsorption	H_2O, electrolytes (Na, K)
Distal tubule	Acid-base balance, secretion	Hydrogen ions (H), Na
Collecting tubule	Concentration	H_2O

Fig. 3-17 Nephron. (From Long BC, Phipps WJ: *Medical-surgical nursing: a nursing process approach,* ed 3, St Louis, 1993, Mosby.)

2. Physical examination
   a. Inspection of genitals
   b. Palpation of kidneys
   c. Palpation of prostate
   d. Pain
      1. back
      2. flank
      3. CVA tenderness
3. Diagnostic tests (Table 3-43)
   a. Urine (visual inspection)
      1. color: pale to deep amber; changes with medication, food, or disease
      2. volume: 30 ml or more each hour
      3. appearance: clear
      4. odor: normally aromatic; strong ammonia after stored for a period of time

   b. Urinalysis: microscopic exam for color, appearance, pH, protein, glucose, ketones, RBCs, WBCs, and casts
      1. specific gravity: 1.015 to 1.025 (random samples)
         a. reflects concentrating ability of kidneys
         b. increases (greater than 1.035) with glucosuria, proteinuria, and dehydration
         c. decreases (less than 1.002) with distal renal tubular disease, endocrine disorders associated with insufficiency of ADH, and overhydration
         d. fixed (1.010) with glomerulonephritis
      2. pH: 4.8 to 8.0
         a. reflects the acid-base balance
         b. greater than 8.0: alkaline; occurs with metabolic alkalosis, overuse of alkalizing medica-

Table 3-41   Fluid imbalances

Etiology	Assessment	Nursing implications
OVERHYDRATION		
Renal failure Excessive fluid intake Excess IVs Water intoxication (GU irrigation with hypotonic fluids) Hypernatremia	Level of consciousness, vital signs, weight (increases), peripheral edema, venous pressure (increases), pulmonary edema, symptoms of CHF or increased intracranial pressure	*Prevention* Monitor IV fluids closely. Monitor urine output, I&O, weight. *Treatment* Reduce edema (e.g., positioning). Give diuretics as ordered. Limit intake. Maintain low sodium intake.
DEHYDRATION		
Nausea and vomiting Increased urinary output Diuretics Insufficient intake (because of age, immobility, etc.) Inadequate replacement following excess fluid loss (diaphoresis, diarrhea)	Level of consciousness, vital signs, weight (may be decreased), skin turgor (poor), thirst, urine output increased dry mucous membranes	*Prevention* Monitor I&O. Replace lost fluids. Client teaching about excess perspiration. *Treatment* Replace fluids carefully. Monitor I&O and weight.

tions, in presence of urinary tract infection (UTI)

c. less than 4.8: acidic; occurs with metabolic acidosis, uncontrolled diabetes, some medications (e.g., ammonium chloride, high doses of vitamin C)

3. glucose
   a. normally not present
   b. may occur after heavy meal, emotional stress, or with infusion of glucose
   c. occurs abnormally with diabetes mellitus, pancreatic disorders, impaired reabsorption in the proximal tubules

4. ketones
   a. normally not present
   b. occur with uncontrolled diabetes, fasting, severe infections accompanied by nausea and vomiting

5. protein
   a. normally not present
   b. occurs with serious kidney or proximal tubular disorders, nephrotic syndrome, toxemia
   c. may occur after heavy protein meal, strenuous exercise, or prolonged standing

6. red blood cells
   a. normally 0 to 3 per high-power field
   b. increase with kidney malfunction, trauma to urinary tract, tumor, or infection in urinary tract

7. white blood cells
   a. normally 0 to 4 per high-power field
   b. increase with infection within urinary tract system

8. hyaline casts
   a. normally not present
   b. indicate acute glomerulonephritis or pyelonephritis, chronic renal disease, or renal calculi

9. granular casts
   a. normally not present
   b. indicates acute renal rejection (transplant), pyelonephritis, or chronic lead poisoning

c. Urine culture and sensitivity
   1. voided specimen (clean catch): bacterial count over 100,000 organisms per milliliter (if infection is present)
   2. sterile, catheterized specimen: over 10,000 organisms per milliliter

d. Tests of filtration function
   1. creatinine clearance (the most important test of kidney function)
      a. amount of creatinine filtered by glomeruli (because creatinine is not reabsorbed and is only minimally secreted, this test is a measure of glomerular filtration rate)
      b. determined by 24-hour urine specimen
      c. normal values
         - 115 ± 20 ml/min
         - serum creatinine: 0.7 to 1.5 mg/dl
      d. as glomerular filtration rate falls, serum creatinine rises and 24-hour urine creatinine decreases
      e. advantage of serum creatinine: independent of protein metabolism
   2. BUN
      a. normal: 5 to 20 mg/dl
      b. urea: end product of protein metabolism
      c. increases with decrease in glomerular filtration
      d. less reliable measure than serum creatinine because
         - after being filtered, urea is reabsorbed back into renal tubular cells
         - urea production varies according to the state of the liver function and protein intake and breakdown

Table 3-42 Electrolyte imbalances

Problem	Etiology	Assessment	Nursing implications
SODIUM			
Hypernatremia Na$^+$ > 145 mEq/L	*Hyperosmolar* Sodium increased in relation to water, water loss without sodium loss, dehydration	Increased hemoglobin, signs of dehydration, thirst, decreased BP, concentrated urine with high specific gravity	Offer sodium-restricted diet and fluids. Maintain strict I&O. Prevent shock. Maintain adequate urine output. Monitor serum Na.
	Sodium excess Both sodium and water increased, renal failure, cirrhosis, steroid therapy, aldosterone excess	Edema, weight gain, hypertension, symptoms of fluid outload	Offer low-sodium diet, water restriction. Maintain strict I&O. Monitor signs of CHF or increased intracranial pressure. Measure daily weight Administer diuretics (Na wasting) as ordered.
Hyponatremia Na$^+$ < 136 mEq/L	*Hypoosmolar or "dilutional"* Water increased in relation to sodium, water intoxication, exercise, IVs without NaCl, sodium-restricted diet	Fluid volume excess, increased urine output with low specific gravity, no thirst, nausea/vomiting, weakness/cerebral dysfunction	Restrict water. Monitor I&O, serum Na. Watch for circulatory overload. Replace Na carefully. Give high-Na diet.
	Sodium deficit Both sodium and water decreased, diuretics, GI losses, burns	Decreased BP, poor skin turgor, dehydration/shock, oliguria	Monitor for shock. Provide good skin care. Give isotonic fluids. Monitor I&O, serum Na.
POTASSIUM			
Hyperkalemia K$^+$ > 5.0 mEq/L	Severe burns, crush injuries, Addison's disease, renal failure, acidosis, excessive K intake (oral or IV)	ECG changes (high T wave), skeletal muscle weakness, bradycardia, cardiac arrest, oliguria, intestinal colic, diarrhea	Monitor cardiac function, serum K, neurologic signs. Limit K intake. Give D$_{50}$ plus insulin as ordered. Give exchange resins (sodium polystyrene sulfonate [Kayexalate] PO or enemas) as ordered. Give bicarbonate to correct acidosis. Dialysis (renal/peritoneal).
Hypokalemia K$^+$ < 3.5 mEq/L	Diuretic therapy (thiazides), poor intake, GI loss, ulcerative colitis, Cushing's syndrome, alkalosis	Digitalis toxicity, muscle weakness and decreased reflexes, flaccid paralysis, paralytic ileus, CNS depression, lethargy, hypotension, anorexia, ECG changes (flattened T wave)	Administer K slowly IV. Monitor ECG. Teach adequate K replacement when taking diuretics. Administer PO K drugs/diet.
CALCIUM			
Hypercalcemia Ca^{++} > 10.5 mg	Immobility, hyperparathyroidism, bone metastasis, excess vitamin D intake, parathyroid tumor, osteoporosis, decreased renal excretion	Skeletal muscle weakness; bone pain; renal calculi; pathologic fractures; CNS depression, altered level of consciousness (LOC); GI (constipation, nausea, vomiting, anorexia); decreased serum phosphorus	Limit intake. Client teaching. Prevent fractures. Give phosphorus. Maintain adequate I&O. Monitor neurologic signs.

Table 3-42   Electrolyte imbalances—cont'd

Problem	Etiology	Assessment	Nursing implications
CALCIUM—cont'd			
Hypercalcemia Ca^{++} > 10.5 mg	Immobility, hyperparathyroidism, bone metastasis, excess vitamin D intake, parathyroid tumor, osteoporosis, decreased renal excretion	Skeletal muscle weakness; bone pain; renal calculi; pathologic fractures; CNS depression, altered level of consciousness (LOC); GI (constipation, nausea, vomiting, anorexia); decreased serum phosphorus	Limit intake. Client teaching. Prevent fractures. Give phosphorus. Maintain adequate I&O. Monitor neurologic signs.
Hypocalcemia Ca^{++} < 9 mg	Hypoparathyroidism, low vitamin D in diet, parathyroidectomy, pregnancy and lactation, postthyroidectomy, rickets, renal disease	Tetany, tingling, paresthesias of fingers and around mouth, muscle twitching, cramps; positive Chvostek's and Trousseau's signs; laryngospasm; increased phosphorus	Give Ca as needed. Monitor for early muscle spasms, neurologic signs. Monitor those at risk. Give phosphate-binding antacids. Monitor serum Ca.
MAGNESIUM			
Hypermagnesemia Mg^{++} > 3.0 mEq/L	Renal insufficiency, diabetic ketoacidosis, excess Mg intake (antacids), dehydration	CNS and neuromuscular depression, hypotension, sedation, or arrest	Monitor replacement carefully. Support respiration. Teach client correct antacid intake. Monitor neurologic signs.
Hypomagnesemia Mg^{++} < 1.6 mEq/L	Alcoholism, malnutrition, loss (GI, diuresis), low intake, hypercalcemia, diabetes, toxemia, renal disease	Tremors and neuromuscular irritability, disorientation, positive Chvostek's and Trousseau's signs, convulsions	Give Mg cautiously as ordered. Monitor closely for Mg excess. Teach adequate intake. Monitor neurologic signs.

Table 3-43   Laboratory tests used to evaluate renal function

Test	Normal range	Usual range in renal disease	What it measures
Hemoglobin	12-18 g/dl	Lowered	Formation of red blood cells, influenced by renal erythropoetin
Blood urea nitrogen (BUN)	5-20 mg/dl	Elevated	Renal excretory function
Electrolytes			
Sodium	136-145 mEq/L	Elevated or lowered; depends on water retention or loss	Fluid and electrolyte balance
Potassium	3.5-5 mEq/L	Elevated	Electrolyte balance
Chloride	90-110 mEq/L	Elevated or lowered; has partnership with sodium	Fluid and electrolyte balance
Serum creatinine	0.7-1.5 mg/dl	Elevated	Renal excretory function
Serum osmolality	275-300 mOsm/kg	Elevated or lowered	Dissolved particles in the blood
Glucose	70-115 mg/dl	Slight hyperglycemia	Renal function
Blood pH	7.35-7.45	Usually lowered	Acidity vs. alkalinity of blood
Calcium	9.0-10.5 mg/dl	Usually lowered	Renal excretory function
Phosphorus	2.5-4.5 mg/dl	Elevated	Renal excretory function
Albumin	3.2-4.5 g/dl	Usually lowered	Albumin (helps maintain blood's osmotic pressure), renal function

e. Radiologic tests
  1. KUB: kidney, ureters, bladder
    a. simple x-ray without contrast medium
    b. results indicate size, position, and any radiopaque calcifications
  2. tomography
    a. x-ray at different angles: no contrast medium
    b. useful for clear picture when colon and other organs block kidney
    c. can distinguish solid tumors from cysts
  3. intravenous pyelogram (IVP) (excretory urogram)
    a. injection of contrast medium that is excreted by kidneys

  b. allows visualization of kidneys, ureters, and bladder

  c. used to diagnose masses, cysts, obstructions, renal trauma, bladder dysfunction

  d. contraindicated in severe renal disease or dehydration and individuals allergic to shellfish or iodine

  e. nursing care pretest
- check for iodine or shellfish allergies
- ensure that informed written consent is on the chart
- tell client that a dye is injected and x-rays are taken at 2-, 5-, 10-, 15-, 20-, 30-, and 60-minute intervals
- administer strong cathartic, enemas night before
- NPO after midnight
- have client void immediately before test

  f. nursing care posttest: check for signs and symptoms of allergic reaction to dye and signs of acute renal failure

4. nephrotomogram

  a. techniques of tomography with IVP

  b. provides a clearer visualization

5. retrograde pyelogram

  a. catheter is passed through urethra, urinary bladder, and into right or left ureter, where contrast medium is injected

  b. allows more detailed visualization of the urinary collecting system independent of the status of renal function

  c. disadvantages: increased chances of trauma from catheter manipulation and infection

  d. nursing care pretest
- check for iodine allergies
- ensure that informed written consent is on the chart
- teach client about the procedure
- administer cathartics, enemas evening before
- keep NPO after midnight

  e. nursing care posttest
- observe amount of urine
- watch for hematuria
- watch for signs of urinary sepsis
- check for signs and symptoms of allergic reaction to dye

6. renal angiography, arteriography

  a. catheter is introduced through the femoral artery to the renal artery

  b. contrast medium is injected and 2 or 3 x-rays are taken at 2-second intervals

  c. allows visualization of renal arteries, capillaries, and venous system

  d. used to diagnose renal artery stenosis, renal masses, trauma, thrombosis, and obstructive uropathy

  e. risks: bleeding, thrombosis, damage to vessels, allergic reaction

  f. nursing care pretest
- check for iodine allergies

- ensure that informed written consent is on the chart
- administer cathartics, enemas the evening before
- ensure that chart contains the hematologic evaluation
- have client void immediately before test

  g. nursing care posttest
- maintain bed rest 12 to 24 hours; flat, no sitting
- check insertion site for hematoma formation
- check pressure dressing on insertion site
- monitor postoperative vital signs
- check peripheral pulses distal to insertion site
- measure urine output; observe for a decrease; may have an increase for about 24 hours from the diuretic effect of the x-ray dye

7. cystography

  a. a flexible metal tube is inserted into the bladder and a dye is injected; x-rays are taken at 30-minute intervals

  b. assesses bladder function and explores the possible presence of stones in the bladder

  c. nursing care: same as retrograde pyelogram

8. cystoscopy

  a. a cystoscope is inserted into bladder through the urethra

  b. direct inspection of bladder to biopsy and resect tumors, remove stones, cauterize bleeding areas, dilate ureters, and implant radium seeds

  c. nursing care pretest
- ensure that written informed consent is on the chart
- administer prep as ordered
- teach client about procedure (e.g., position [lithotomy], darkened room)
- keep NPO if general anesthesia will be used
- administer preoperative medications as ordered

  d. nursing care posttest
- monitor urine output for a decrease
- monitor urine color; blood-tinged urine is common
- provide comfort measures (back pain, bladder spasms, feeling of fullness are common) such as sitz baths and analgesics (e.g., belladonna and opium [B&O] suppository as ordered)
- check temperature and urine for signs of infection
- encourage increased fluid intake unless contraindicated

9. renal biopsy

  a. a specially designed needle is inserted percutaneously to obtain sample of kidney tissue

  b. determines histology of glomeruli and tubules

  c. contraindications: a single functioning kidney; infection; tumors; hydronephrosis; coagulation disorders; client who is uncooperative

SELECTED HEALTH PROBLEMS RESULTING IN ALTERATION IN URINARY ELIMINATION

✖ CYSTITIS/PYELONEPHRITIS

1. Definitions
   a. *Cystitis:* inflammation of the bladder wall
   b. *Pyelonephritis:* inflammation of the kidney caused by bacterial infection
      1. acute (short course): organisms gain access to the kidney by ascending from the lower urinary tract or via bloodstream; no permanent renal impairment
      2. chronic (slowly progressive): multiple, recurrent, acute attacks that scar the renal parenchyma, damaging tubules, vessels, glomeruli
2. Incidence: both more common in women
3. Risks/predisposing factors
   a. Cystitis
      1. prostatic hypertrophy with urinary retention (men)
      2. contamination from large intestine (women)
      3. intrusive procedures: catheterization, cystoscopy
      4. coitus (women)
      5. atonic bladder (spinal cord injury)
      6. chronic disease (e.g., diabetes)
      7. pregnancy (because of pressure of uterus on bladder and urethra)
      8. chronic stasis (e.g., atonic bladder, immobility, and infrequent voiding)
   b. Pyelonephritis
      1. anomalies of the kidney
      2. pregnancy
      3. calculi
      4. diabetes mellitus
      5. neurogenic bladder
      6. instrumentation (i.e., procedures)
      7. bacterial infection elsewhere in the body

Nursing Process
ASSESSMENT
1. Cystitis (often asymptomatic)
   a. Burning
   b. Frequency
   c. Urgency
   d. Suprapubic pain
   e. Slight hematuria
2. Pyelonephritis
   a. Symptoms of cystitis may or may not be present
   b. Severe flank pain, CVA tenderness
   c. Hematuria, pyuria
   d. Fever
   e. Chills
3. Diagnostic tests
   a. Urinalysis, urine culture and sensitivity (C&S): midstream urine specimen for evaluation of bacterial content
   b. CBC: leukocytosis

ANALYSIS/NURSING DIAGNOSIS (see p. 191)
PLANNING, IMPLEMENTATION, AND EVALUATION
Refer to General Nursing Goals 1, 2, and 3, p. 191.

✖ URINARY CALCULI

1. Types of stones
   a. Calcium oxalate: hard, small; alkaline urine
   b. Calcium phosphate: large, soft; alkaline urine
   c. Cystine: metabolic, familial; acid urine
   d. Uric acid: may be accompanied by gout; acid urine
   e. Struvite: large, soft; associated with urinary tract infections, alkaline urine
2. Incidence: can occur at any age
3. Locations
   a. Bladder
   b. Ureter (especially at narrow points)
   c. Pelvis of the kidney
4. Risk factors
   a. Supersaturation of urine with poorly soluble crystalloids (calcium, uric acid, cystine)
   b. Infection: alkaline urine leads to precipitation of calcium and struvite
   c. Increased concentration of urine
   d. Stasis
   e. Bone demineralization leading to increased calcium phosphate in serum and urine
   f. Metabolic diseases (e.g., gout [increased uric acid])
   g. Certain medications (e.g., corticosteroids, vitamin D [hypervitaminosis D])
5. Medical treatment
   a. Medical interventions
      1. ambulation to increase the likelihood of passing the stone
      2. fluids to decrease the concentration of substances involved in stone formation, to promote passage of the stone, and to prevent infection
   b. Surgical intervention (Fig. 3-18)
      1. *ureterolithotomy:* incision into ureter through an abdominal or flank excision to extract stones from the ureter
         a. ureteral catheter is inserted to act as splint; ureter not sutured to avoid stricture; catheter is never irrigated to maintain patency
         b. Penrose drain inserted around ureter to collect any extra drainage
      2. *pyelolithotomy:* removal of a stone from renal pelvis through a flank incision; Penrose drain inserted outside renal pelvis
      3. *nephrolithotomy:* parenchyma of kidney is cut and stone extracted through a flank incision
         a. nephrostomy tube placed to divert urine and drain pelvis to allow kidney to heal; never irrigated unless specifically ordered
         b. Penrose drain inserted
      4. lithotripsy
         a. percutaneous lithotripsy: percutaneous nephrostomy tract made through a small incision over the kidney; an endoscope is passed through this tract, and a basket is used to remove the calculi; if unable to remove the stone, ultrasonic lithotripsy is used to disintegrate the calculi
         b. transcutaneous shock wave lithotripsy: client is submerged in a large tub of water; ultrasonic

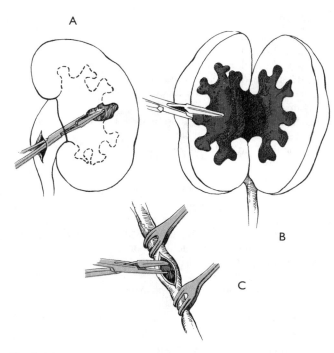

Fig. 3-18 Location and methods of removing renal calculi from upper urinary tract. **A,** Pyelolithotomy, removal of stone through renal pelvis. **B,** Nephrolithotomy, removal of staghorn calculus from renal parenchyma (kidney split). **C,** Ureterolithotomy, removal of stone from ureter. (From Long BC, Phipps WJ: *Medical-surgical nursing: a nursing process approach,* ed 3, St Louis, 1993, Mosby.)

    shock waves are fired at the area of the calculi; results in disintegration of the calculi
  5. *nephrectomy:* removal of kidney through a flank incision
    a. may be needed if stone and infection have caused extensive damage to kidney parenchyma
    b. Penrose drain inserted into renal bed

Nursing Process

ASSESSMENT
1. Pain
    a. Renal colic: sudden, sharp, severe; located in deep lumbar region; radiating to side
    b. Ureteral colic: same type pain radiating to genitalia and thigh
2. Renointestinal reflex: nausea and vomiting, diarrhea, constipation
3. Hematuria, frequency, altered pH of urine
4. Increased WBC
5. Fever, chills
6. Signs of paralytic ileus with right-sided renal colic
7. If stone is formed in renal pelvis, may be asymptomatic for years until signs of infection occur
8. IVP results
9. Urine tested for mineral precipitate
10. Blood levels of uric acid, calcium, and phosphorus if metabolic problems suspected

ANALYSIS/NURSING DIAGNOSIS (see p. 191)
PLANNING, IMPLEMENTATION, AND EVALUATION

> **Goal 1** Client will be free from pain.

Implementation
1. Administer analgesics as ordered (often morphine is necessary because of severity of pain).
2. Administer anticholinergics, propantheline (Pro-Banthine) as ordered, to relax smooth muscles.
3. Encourage client to ambulate.

Evaluation
Client is free from discomfort.

> **Goal 2** Client will be free from infection leading to urinary calculi (refer to General Nursing Goal 1, p. 191).

> **Goal 3** Client will decrease risk of stone formation.

Implementation
1. Teach client importance of maintaining adequate fluid intake (3000 ml per day).
2. Teach client about medications and reason for prescription (e.g., to maintain recommended urinary pH).
3. Teach client about any medication ordered to decrease levels of minerals (e.g., aluminum hydroxide [Amphojel] + $PO_3 \rightarrow AlPO_3$, eliminated through the GI tract).
4. Teach client how to measure urine pH.
5. Assess diet for excess intake of substances that contribute to stone formation.
6. Teach client about dietary restrictions.
7. Explain advantages of regular exercise and voiding at least every 2 hours (e.g., to prevent stasis calculi).

Evaluation
Client states importance of maintaining high urine output; lists actions and need for medication to maintain recommended pH; demonstrates ability to monitor urinary pH; demonstrates adherence to dietary restrictions.

> **Goal 4** Client will be free from postoperative complications.

Implementation
1. Refer to Perioperative Period, p. 115.
2. Note urine: amount, color, and specific gravity.
3. Maintain adequate respiratory function after a flank incision. Client may be reluctant to deep breathe and cough because of incisional pain close to rib cage.
4. Encourage early ambulation.
5. Monitor for
    a. Hypostatic pneumonia.
    b. Hemorrhage.
    c. Paralytic ileus (from reflex paralysis).
    d. Severe pain.
    e. Urinary tract infection.

f. Redness or bruising at site of lithotripsy shock waves.

g. Renal colic pain 3 or more days after lithotripsy and report to physician.

h. Weight gain after lithotripsy (may indicate urinary retention).

6. Give urinary antiseptics and antiinfectives as ordered (see Table 3-44).

Evaluation

Client rests comfortably; is free from signs of UTI (e.g., no leukocytosis, urine culture less than 100,000 organisms per milliliter), complications of surgery.

> **Goal 5** Client will verbalize interventions for home care.

Implementation

1. Refer to General Nursing Goal 3, p. 191.

2. Teach client how and why to avoid upper respiratory tract infection.

3. Tell client to avoid heavy lifting for 4 to 8 weeks after surgery.

Evaluation

Client lists home care measures.

CANCER OF THE BLADDER

1. Characteristics
   a. More than 66% of cases occur in men
   b. Most tumors start as benign papillomas or as leukoplakia
   c. Multiple tumors frequent
   d. Tumors often recur

2. Risk factors: probably a disease of multiple etiologies, not yet specifically identified; industrial carcinogens, smoking, aniline dyes, benzene, asbestos, and alcohol have been implicated

3. Medical treatment
   a. Surgical intervention
      1. transurethral bladder resection if tumors are of the trigone or posterior bladder wall (85%)
      2. complete cystectomy when cure highly probable with urinary diversion
         a. *ileal conduit:* a portion of the ileum becomes a conduit; the ureters are transplanted into one end and the other end becomes an external stoma
         b. *cutaneous ureterostomy:* dissection of one or both ureters, bringing them to the skin, forming one or two stomas (for inoperable tumors)
         c. *continent internal ileal reservoir:* created from a segment of ileum that is isolated; the ureters are implanted into the side of the reservoir; a special nipple valve connects the reservoir to the exterior of the skin and also prevents reflux of urine into the renal pelvis; patients will catheterize the reservoir and have urinary continence
   b. Radiation therapy
      1. preoperative irradiation improves survival in clients with high-grade tumors
      2. external or internal radiation therapy for nonoperable tumors or clients who refuse surgery

Nursing Process

ASSESSMENT

1. Painless hematuria
2. Abnormal cystometric examination
3. Abnormal blood and urine studies
4. Cystoscopy, biopsy results

ANALYSIS/NURSING DIAGNOSIS (see p. 191)

PLANNING, IMPLEMENTATION, AND EVALUATION

> **Goal 1** Client will be prepared for surgery.

Implementation

1. Refer to Perioperative Period, p. 115.
2. Give or arrange for sexual counseling regarding impotence (in men).
3. Give bowel prep as ordered.
4. Arrange for introduction to enterostomal therapist.
   a. Diversionary appliance demonstrated to client
   b. Ensure that stoma site (right lower quadrant) is marked.

Evaluation

Client is able to discuss planned surgery and its implications; inspects diversionary appliance.

> **Goal 2** Client will remain free from postoperative complications.

Implementation

1. Refer to Perioperative Period, p. 115.
2. Check ureteral splints for patency, output, and color of urine qh.
3. Monitor stoma for normal color (pink or red; dark purplish color indicates vascular compromise).
4. Record I&O for at least 3 days; encourage up to 3000 ml fluid intake per day.
5. Offer psychologic support as needed.

Evaluation

Client maintains intake of 3000 ml per day; shows no signs of shock or hemorrhage (e.g., tachycardia, hypotension, apprehension, cold clammy skin, decreased BP, increased pulse).

> **Goal 3** Client will exhibit behaviors for care of urinary diversion appliance and adjustment to alteration in body image.

Implementation

1. Have enterostomal therapist orient client to appliance and its care.
2. Reinforce all teaching regarding skin care, cleanliness, and odor control.
3. Allow client an opportunity to express feelings and concerns regarding changed body image.
4. Encourage client to assume full care of appliance as soon as possible.

Evaluation

Client begins to adapt to body-image change (e.g., discusses change, cares for appliance); achieves self-care management of appliance with successful odor control.

✖ ACUTE RENAL FAILURE

1. Definition: a sudden and potentially reversible loss of kidney function
2. Categories and causes of renal failure
   a. *Prerenal* (outside kidney): poor perfusion, decrease in circulating volume
   b. *Renal:* structural damage to kidney resulting from acute tubular necrosis
   c. *Postrenal:* obstruction within urinary tract
3. Risk/predisposing factors
   a. Prerenal
      1. reduction in blood volume (shock)
      2. trauma
      3. septic shock
      4. dehydration
      5. cardiac failure
   b. Renal
      1. hypersensitivity (allergic disorders)
      2. obstruction of renal vessels (embolism, thrombosis)
      3. nephrotoxic agents (bacterial toxins and drugs)
      4. mismatched blood transfusion
      5. glomerulonephritis
   c. Postrenal
      1. kidney stones or tumors
      2. benign prostatic hypertrophy or obstruction

Nursing Process

ASSESSMENT

1. Oliguric phase (urine volume less than 400 ml per day)
   a. Decreased serum sodium and increased potassium; decreased calcium and bicarbonate
   b. Increased BUN, creatinine maintaining a 10:1 ratio (normally 20:1 ratio)
   c. Increased specific gravity
   d. Hypervolemia, hypertension
   e. Usually lasts 8 days to 3 weeks

2. Diuretic phase (urine volume greater than 3000 ml per day)
   a. Serum sodium and potassium may return to normal, stay elevated, or decrease
   b. Increased BUN and serum creatinine
   c. Decreased specific gravity of urine
   d. Hypovolemia
   e. Weight loss
   f. Usually lasts several days to 1 week
3. Recovery phase: gradual return of normal function over period of 3 to 12 months

ANALYSIS/NURSING DIAGNOSIS (see p. 191)
PLANNING, IMPLEMENTATION, AND EVALUATION

Goal 1 (if prerenal failure) Client will experience increased renal blood flow through an increased circulating blood volume.

Implementation

1. Monitor vital signs as ordered, especially BP and pulse.
2. Maintain strict I&O; monitor urinary output hourly.
3. Administer IV fluids as ordered.
4. Treat shock if present.
5. Administer prescribed medications to increase renal flow (e.g., dopamine 2 to 5 µg/kg/min).
6. Administer prescribed diuretics to increase production of urine (e.g., mannitol, furosemide) if client still has output (Tables 3-7 and 3-45).

Evaluation

Client has adequate renal blood flow as evidenced by urine output greater than 30 ml per hour.

Goal 2 Client will maintain fluid, electrolyte, and nitrogen balance.

Implementation (oliguric phase)

1. Weigh client daily.
2. Measure I&O carefully.
3. Administer only enough fluid to replace losses.

Table 3-45   Osmotic diuretics

Name	Action	Side effects	Nursing implications
OSMOTIC DIURETICS			
Mannitol (Osmitrol)	Draws water from the cells and extracellular spaces into the intravascular. Used to treat or prevent oliguric phase of acute renal failure. Reduces intraocular and cerebrospinal fluid.	Transient circulatory overload and edema, headache, confusion, blurred vision, thirst, nausea, vomiting, fluid/electrolyte imbalance, water intoxication, cellular dehydration	Monitor I&O. Check for electrolyte imbalance, water intoxication, cellular dehydration. Be aware of renal and cardiovascular function. Give frequent mouth care to relieve thirst.

THIAZIDE DIURETICS (see Table 3-7, p. 126)
POTENT DIURETICS (see Table 3-7, p. 126)
POTASSIUM-SPARING DIURETICS (see Table 3-7, p. 126)

4. Include insensible losses in measurement of output.
   a. 500 ml per day if less than 5000 feet above sea level.
   b. 1000 ml per day if more than 5000 feet above sea level.
5. Observe for edema and electrolyte imbalance.
6. Monitor serum lab test results.
7. Administer 50% dextrose with 5 to 10 units regular insulin as ordered, to drive potassium into cells.
8. Administer ion-exchange resin Kayexalate enema as ordered, to lower high potassium levels.
9. Reduce potassium, sodium, and phosphorus in diet.
10. Administer IV sodium bicarbonate for acidosis.
11. Administer phosphate binders such as aluminum hydroxide (Amphojel) or aluminum carbonate (Basaljel) for hyperphosphatemia.
12. Reduce protein in diet and teach client rationale; provide high-biologic-value protein for diet.

Implementation (diuretic phase)
1. Prevent dehydration; balance I&O; daily weights.
2. Increase dietary sodium and potassium to normal levels.
3. Maintain positive nitrogen balance and sufficient calories to prevent body protein from being metabolized.
4. Prevent infection.

Evaluation
Client maintains approximately equal intake and output and stable weight; remains free from signs of electrolyte imbalance, edema, and dehydration; selects foods on a low-potassium, low-protein diet.

> **Goal 3** Client will be free from infection and further damage to kidneys (refer to General Nursing Goal 1, p. 191).

✳ CHRONIC RENAL FAILURE

1. Definition: a progressive, irreversible deterioration of renal function that ends in fatal uremia unless kidney transplant or dialysis is performed
2. Risk/predisposing factors
   a. Urinary tract obstruction and infection
   b. Infectious diseases that cause hypertension and increased catabolism with retention of metabolites (glomerulonephritis)
   c. Metabolic disease (diabetes)
   d. Nephrotoxic agents (bacterial toxins, drugs)
   e. Acute renal failure
3. Pathophysiology
   a. Initially some nephrons destroyed; some remain intact
   b. Intact nephrons hypertrophy to maintain kidney function
   c. As more nephrons are destroyed, oliguria occurs with retention of waste products
   d. End products of protein metabolism accumulate in blood (BUN, creatinine)

Nursing Process

ASSESSMENT
1. Urine output: oliguria, anuria
2. Metabolic indicators
   a. Elevated BUN, creatinine (azotemia)
   b. Hyperphosphatemia
   c. Hyperkalemia
   d. Hypocalcemia
   e. Metabolic acidosis
   f. Elevated, normal, or decreased serum sodium depending on water retention
3. Cardiovascular indicators
   a. Hypervolemia, hypertension, tachycardia
   b. Congestive heart failure
   c. Pericarditis
4. Hematologic indicators
   a. Anemia (decreased renal production of erythropoietin)
   b. Alteration of platelet function leading to bleeding tendencies
   c. Susceptibility to infection (changes in leukocyte function)
5. Respiratory indicators
   a. Pulmonary edema
   b. Uremic pneumonitis
   c. Uremic pleurisy
6. Gastrointestinal indicators
   a. Mucosal irritation in GI tract
   b. Ammonia on breath (uremic fetor)
   c. Anorexia, nausea, vomiting, hiccoughs
7. Central nervous system indicators
   a. Early: mild deficit in mental functioning
   b. Late: altered sensorium, slurred speech, generalized seizures, encephalopathy with toxic psychosis, coma
8. Peripheral nervous system indicators
   a. Peripheral neuropathy involving all extremities
   b. Burning, painful paresthesias
9. Musculoskeletal indicators
   a. Renal osteodystrophy
   b. Bone pain in feet and legs when walking and standing, pathologic fractures
10. Dermatologic indicators
    a. Pruritus
    b. Dry skin: caused by atrophy of sweat glands
    c. Easy bruising, petechiae, and purpura
    d. Pallor related to anemia
    e. Sallow, yellow-tan color to skin
    f. Brittle, dry hair
    g. Dry and ridged nails
    h. Uremic frost: crystallization of urea on skin (late sign)
11. Endocrine indicators
    a. Hypothyroidism
    b. Decreased T_4 level
12. Reproductive indicators
    a. Infertility
    b. Loss of libido
    c. Amenorrhea in women
    d. Decreased testosterone and sperm count in men

ANALYSIS/NURSING DIAGNOSIS (see p. 191)
PLANNING, IMPLEMENTATION, AND EVALUATION

> **Goal 1** Client will maintain fluid and electrolyte balance (refer to Acute Renal Failure Goals 1 and 2, p. 196).

> **Goal 2** Client will remain free from infection (refer to General Nursing Goal 1, p. 191).

Goal 3 Client will maintain adequate caloric intake to prevent muscle wasting and prevent own body stores from being metabolized.

Implementation
1. Initiate daily calorie count.
2. Give medication to control nausea and vomiting before meals.
3. Adjust level of protein in diet to client's serum levels of BUN and creatinine.
4. Encourage protein of high biologic value (containing all essential amino acids), such as milk, meat, fish, and eggs.
5. Serve food attractively and at appropriate temperature.

Evaluation
Client maintains a calorie intake of 35 to 40 calories per kilogram, which will maintain BUN and creatinine at a stable level.

Goal 4 Client will be protected from self-injury during period of altered sensorium.

Implementation
1. Restrain if necessary.
2. Institute seizure precautions.
3. Perform neurologic checks frequently.
4. Monitor BUN and creatinine closely.
5. Teach significant others about cause of altered sensorium.

Evaluation
Client is free from injury during periods of confusion; significant others state awareness of relationship between disease process and altered sensorium.

Goal 5 Client will be relieved of itching and maintain skin integrity.

Implementation
1. Avoid soap.
2. Use soft cloth.
3. Add oil to tepid bath water (baking soda in water may help).

Evaluation
Client's itching is relieved; skin remains intact.

Goal 6 Client and significant others will be supported emotionally (refer to General Nursing Goal 4, p. 191, and Table 2-4).

Goal 7 Client will adapt to altered sexual functioning.

Implementation
1. Teach client and significant other about alterations in sexual functioning.
2. Provide or arrange for sexual counseling if necessary.
3. Encourage client and significant other to discuss the problem.

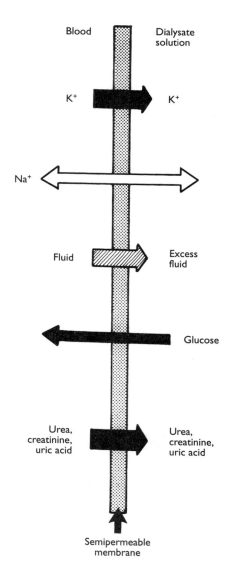

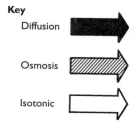

Fig. 3-19 Schematic representation of dialysis.

Evaluation
Client and significant other discuss change and alteration in sexual expression.

✴ DIALYSIS
Dialysis is the passage of particles (ions) from an area of high concentration to an area of low concentration (diffusion) across a semipermeable membrane; simultaneously, water moves (osmosis) toward the solution in which the sol-

Table 3-46 Comparison of peritoneal dialysis and continuous ambulatory peritoneal dialysis (CAPD)

	Peritoneal dialysis	CAPD
Type of catheter	Tenckhoff	Tenckhoff
Number of exchanges per day	Average of 24	3 during day 1 at night
Dwell time	20-30 min per exchange	Day: 4-5 hr Night: 8 hr
Amount of dialysate	1500-2000 ml per exchange	Average 2000 ml per exchange
Type of dialysate	1.5%, 2.5%, 4.25% (4.25% is most concentrated and will remove most fluid)	Day: 1.5%, 2.5% Night: 4.25%
Activity of client	Usually bed rest—may turn from side to side	Ambulatory as desired
Diet of client	Increase protein to 1 g/kg/day 40 kilocalories/kg/day Restrict fluids to 400-500 ml/day Restrict sodium to 1-2 g/day Restrict potassium to 1500-2000 mg/day Limit phosphorus Take daily water-soluble vitamin supplement	Increase protein to 1.2-1.5 g/kg/day Limit phosphorus Include liberal potassium Include liberal fluids Avoid fats and sweets to control cholesterol level and high-density lipoprotein levels

From Williams SR: *Nutrition and diet therapy,* ed 7, St Louis, 1993, Mosby.

ute concentration is greater. When dialysis is used as a substitute for kidney function, the semipermeable membrane used is either the peritoneum (peritoneal dialysis) or an artificial membrane (hemodialysis). The principle of exchange is the same with both methods. The pores in the membrane are large enough to allow the passage of urea, electrolytes, and creatinine but are too small to allow the passage of blood cells and other protein molecules (Fig. 3-19).

Peritoneal Dialysis

1. Definition: placement of catheter through abdominal wall into peritoneal space
2. Procedure: body or room temperature dialysate is allowed to flow into the peritoneal cavity by gravity; the solution remains in the abdomen for exchange to occur and then is drained from the peritoneal cavity by gravity; it carries with it waste products and excess electrolytes; can last from 12 to 24 hours
3. Number of cycles: varies according to the client's problems, tolerance, response, and type of solution
4. Types (Table 3-46)
   a. Intermittent manual
   b. Intermittent automatic
   c. Continuous ambulatory (CAPD)
      1. dialysate remains in peritoneum 24 hours per day with several dialysate exchanges each day
      2. advantages
         a. lower BP (9 out of 10 clients can discontinue BP medications)
         b. increased Hct and Hgb
         c. less expensive
         d. greater freedom for client
         e. weight gain from glucose absorbed from dialysate (later can become a disadvantage)
      3. disadvantages and risks
         a. peritonitis
         b. infection at catheter exit site

   c. dialysate leakage
   d. hypotension
   e. hypoalbuminemia (caused by increased loss of protein from repeated peritonitis and large pores in peritoneum)
5. Peritoneal access (e.g., Tenckhoff peritoneal catheter extends access to the peritoneal cavity for weeks to months)

Nursing Process

ASSESSMENT
1. Temperature, pulse, respirations, and blood pressure
2. Blood chemistries (electrolytes, albumin, BUN, creatinine, glucose)
3. Daily I&O
4. Daily weight (after fluid is drained from cavity)
5. Catheter site for signs of infection or leakage (redness, tenderness, pain, or exudate)

ANALYSIS/NURSING DIAGNOSIS (see p. 191)
PLANNING, IMPLEMENTATION, AND EVALUATION

> **Goal 1** Client will be protected from peritonitis.

Implementation
1. Use scrupulous aseptic technique throughout dialysis.
2. Check dialysate for cloudiness (sign of infection).
3. Notify physician immediately if peritonitis is suspected (cloudy peritoneal fluid, fever, chills).
4. Obtain peritoneal fluid sample for fluid analysis, culture, and sensitivity.
5. Initiate antibiotic therapy as ordered (cephalosporins or aminoglycosides either systemically or instilled into dialysate).
6. Take temperature q4h.
7. Change catheter site dressing at least daily; cleanse with iodine solution and apply topical antibiotic ointment.

Evaluation

Client's peritoneal fluid remains clear; temperature remains within normal limits.

Goal 2 Client will experience successful intermittent dialysis evaluated by maintaining optimal concentrations of blood chemistries.

Implementation

1. Weigh client daily before dialysis.
2. Have client empty bladder and bowel before paracentesis.
3. Place client in comfortable supine position.
4. Warm dialysate to body temperature using warming pads before instilling.
5. Permit 2 L of dialysate to flow unrestricted into peritoneal cavity (inflow).
6. Leave fluid in peritoneal cavity for 20 to 30 minutes so that solution can equilibrate (dwell time).
7. Drain equilibrated fluid from peritoneal cavity.
8. Record amount of fluid loss or gain; outflow should be approximately 100 to 200 ml more than inflow; have client turn on sides to localize fluid and promote drainage; if retention continues after three consecutive exchanges, stop the dialysis and notify physician.
9. Repeat cycle as ordered.
10. Perform blood chemistries as ordered.
11. Maintain client comfort during dialysis.

Evaluation

Client has a stable BUN and creatinine; normal electrolyte levels.

Goal 3 Client will be free from hypertension.

Implementation

1. Monitor BP standing and sitting.
2. Monitor BP during dialysis (should decrease as fluid volume is reduced).
3. Use a more hypertonic dialysate if hypertension persists.
4. Restrict fluid and sodium intake.
5. Give antihypertensive medications as ordered.
6. Notify physician if symptoms of hypotension occur during procedure; it is usually treated during hemodialysis by administering normal saline directly into the arterial or venous line and slowing the dialyzing procedures.

Evaluation

Client's BP remains within predetermined guidelines.

Goal 4 Client will be successful with CAPD at home if client's condition requires chronic dialysis.

Implementation

1. Educate client and significant others in the principles, process, and techniques of CAPD.
   a. Instill 2 L of room-temperature dialysate.

b. Leave in peritoneal cavity 4 to 8 hours.
c. Go about daily activities.
d. Drain fluid and discard.
e. Replace with 2 L of fresh dialysate.
f. Repeat procedure 4 times per day.
g. Leave dialysate in peritoneal cavity overnight.
2. Educate about the use of sterile technique and its importance in preventing peritonitis.
3. Have client keep a written record of daily weight and BP with physician-recommended guidelines of when to notify physician of changes in BP and weight.
4. Provide diet instruction to replace lost protein; liberalize protein, potassium, salt, and water intake.
5. Teach the importance of regular medical and nursing follow-up for lab work, catheter change, evaluation of dialysis technique, monitoring of weight and BP, and any other problems.

Evaluation

Client uses CAPD at home free from any problems; explains proper diet and the importance of follow-up.

Goal 5 Client will accept assistance to cope psychologically with ongoing dialysis treatments (refer to Hemodialysis Goal 3, p. 202).

Hemodialysis

1. Definition: passage of heparinized blood from client through a tube consisting of a semipermeable membrane immersed in a dialysate bath composed of all important electrolytes in their ideal concentration. Diffusion and ultrafiltration occur between the client's blood and the dialysate. Protamine sulfate may be used to counteract the heparin effects.
2. Procedure: fresh dialysate is used continuously until the client's electrolyte and fluid balances are within safe levels.
3. Schedule varies with clinical condition and type of dialyzer.
   a. Up to 3 times per week.
   b. 4 to 6 hours per day is possible for coil and hollow-fiber dialyzers; 10 to 12 hours per day is necessary for plate-type dialyzers.
4. Access to client's circulation (Fig. 3-20):
   a. Arteriovenous (AV) shunt
      1. external device
         a. composed of two nonthrombogenic Silastic rubber tubes or cannulas with Teflon tips, one sutured in artery, the other in vein
         b. between dialysis, the two tubes are joined by Teflon connector
         c. most commonly used vessels are the radial artery and cephalic vein of forearm
   b. Arteriovenous fistula: access of choice for hemodialysis
      1. internal access
         a. created by side-to-side or end-to-end anastomosis between adjacent vein and artery (often radial artery and cephalic vein)
         b. creates enlarged superficial vein with easy access for venipuncture

2. Donor
   a. Live
   b. Cadaver
3. Rejection of the grafted kidney is a significant problem
   a. Attempts to minimize: tissue typing before transplantation (must indicate high degree of histocompatibility)
   b. Types of rejection
      1. *hyperacute:* occurs on the operating room table
      2. *acute:* first episode can occur 5 to 7 days after transplant; subsequent episodes can occur within the first year
      3. *chronic:* rejection continues despite repeated attempts at immunosuppression
      4. rejection rates
         a. 20% to 25% of cadaver grafts
         b. 5% to 10% of live donor grafts
         c. greatly increased by the presence of diabetes
4. Immunosuppressive drugs are given to all transplant recipients; see Table 3-47.

Nursing Process

ASSESSMENT
1. Metabolic state
2. Tissue histocompatibility
3. Immunologic defense status
4. Psychologic and emotional status
5. Potential sources of postoperative infection (carious teeth, infected donor kidneys) because client will be immunosuppressed
6. Age; desires of the client regarding this risk-filled procedure

ANALYSIS/NURSING DIAGNOSIS (see p. 191)

PLANNING, IMPLEMENTATION, AND EVALUATION

Goal I Client will be adequately prepared preoperatively to maximize the chances of a successful outcome.

Table 3-47 Immunosuppressive drugs

Generic name (trade name)	Action	Side effects	Nursing implications
Azathioprine (Imuran)	Inhibits RNA and DNA synthesis. Inhibits lymphoid tissue (where cells divide rapidly during the rejection process) thereby diminishing the rejection process.	Skin rash, alopecia, nausea, vomiting, leukopenia, thrombocytopenia	Begin drug 1-5 days before surgery and continue afterward. Monitor hematologic status. Institute reverse isolation if needed. Monitor for fever, chills, unusual bleeding, bruising, and sore throat.
Cyclosporine (Sandimmune)	Strongly inhibits the antibody production that leads to graft rejection. Use should be accompanied by adjunct steroid administration.	Nephrotoxicity, hypertension, tremor, gum hyperplasia, hepatotoxicity, hirsutism	Monitor kidney and liver function. Dilute oral solution with milk or orange juice and give at room temperature. Observe for anaphylaxis for at least 30 minutes after start of IV infusion of drug.
Lymphocyte immune globulin (Atgam)	Inhibits cell-mediated immune response.	Hypotension, chest pain, nausea, vomiting, anaphylaxis	Monitor for signs and symptoms of infection. Refrigerate drug. Do not use drug if more than 12 hours old. Skin test before first dose. Do not give if allergic to equine products.
Muromonab-CD3 (Orthoclone OKT3)	Restores function of allograft and reverses rejection; decreases T-lymphocytes	Chest pain, nausea, vomiting, fever, chills, tremors, dyspnea	Use only one time (an antibody preparation). Obtain chest x-ray before treatment (risk of pulmonary edema). Give antipyretics before a dose to decrease incidence of fever or chills.

Corticosteroids (see Table 3-20)

Implementation

1. Refer to Perioperative Period, p. 115.
2. Maintain accurate I&O; adhere to fluid restriction; daily weights.
3. Know that the client may need to undergo preoperative hemodialysis to achieve an optimal metabolic state.
4. Protect client from possible sources of infection per Centers for Disease Control and Prevention (CDC) guidelines for immunocompromised clients.

Evaluation

Client will be physiologically prepared for surgery as evidenced by lack of signs of infection, appropriate fluid and electrolyte balance.

> **Goal 2** Client will be psychologically prepared for the surgery.

Implementation

1. Refer to Perioperative Period, p. 115.
2. Allow client the opportunity to discuss feelings and concerns regarding the surgery and its chances of success.
3. Answer client's questions as honestly and completely as possible.
4. Allow client an opportunity to discuss any ambivalent feelings about the donor (may be a close relative).
5. Know that significant others also need support and information.

Evaluation

Client experiences only a moderate level of anxiety preoperatively; expresses realistic hope regarding outcome of transplant.

> **Goal 3** Client will be free from postoperative complications.

Implementation

1. Refer to Perioperative Period, p. 115.
2. Assess fluid and electrolyte balance carefully.
   a. Measure urine output (may range from massive diuresis [live donor] to aneuresis [cadaver donor]).
   b. May require hemodialysis.
3. Protect client from infection.
   a. Give urinary catheter care.
   b. May be in category *specific isolation: immunocompromised.*
   c. Monitor temperature.
4. Observe for signs of acute rejection of transplant.
   a. Oliguria, anuria
   b. Fever (temperature greater than 37.7°C)
   c. Increased blood pressure
   d. Swollen, tender kidney
   e. Flulike symptoms
5. Maintain integrity of venous access.

Evaluation

Client has vital signs within normal limits; output equivalent to fluid intake; remains free from infection.

> **Goal 4** Client will take medications correctly.

Implementation

1. Teach client that immunosuppressive drugs are the main defense against transplant rejection.
2. Teach side effects and complications of these drugs and that withdrawal (if it is ever appropriate) must be done gradually.
3. Tell client that he or she is more susceptible to infection while taking these drugs and to notify physician at the first sign of a cold or infection.
4. Teach client how to avoid or at least decrease exposure to sources of infection.

Evaluation

Client lists side effects of all drugs; states when to call physician regarding drug-related problems; states an awareness of administration schedule and importance of maintaining it.

✖ BENIGN PROSTATIC HYPERTROPHY (BPH)

1. Incidence: more than 50% of all men over age 50
2. Predisposing factors: unknown
3. Medical treatment
   a. Surgical intervention
      1. transurethral resection of prostate (TURP) is most common
      2. suprapubic and retropubic approaches also used
   b. Medical intervention
      1. Finasteride (Proscar)—lowers levels of dihydrotestosterone (high levels cause hypertrophy of prostate); may take 6 months to see results; client may still require surgery at a later date

Nursing Process

ASSESSMENT

1. Urinary dysfunction: retention, dysuria, nocturia, urgency
2. Symmetric, smooth enlargement of prostate
3. Signs and symptoms of hydronephrosis followed by renal failure (late)

ANALYSIS/NURSING DIAGNOSIS (see p. 191)

PLANNING, IMPLEMENTATION, AND EVALUATION

> **Goal 1** Client will have adequate urinary flow preoperatively (Fig. 3-21).

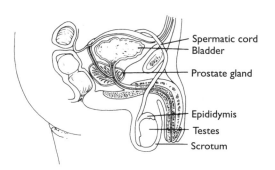

Fig. 3-21 Normal male anatomy.

Implementation

1. Insert urinary catheter.
   a. On initial insertion: prevent bladder collapse by clamping draining tube after 1000 ml urine is drained.
   b. Unclamp tube after 1 hour and repeat protocol.
2. Measure I&O.
3. Know that a suprapubic catheter may be necessary if obstruction is large.

Evaluation

Client's urine output is 30 ml or more per hour.

> **Goal 2** Client will be able to describe surgical approach and postoperative care (Table 3-48; Fig. 3-22).

Implementation

1. Teach client that postoperatively the client will have a catheter with a large diameter and large balloon. This will cause an urge to void that is normal, and the discomfort can be controlled with medication.

2. Client may have a continuous irrigation solution infusing into catheter to keep the catheter free of obstruction.

Evaluation

Client describes a TURP; knows what to expect postoperatively (e.g., pain and discomfort, ambulation).

> **Goal 3** Client will have normal urinary drainage, clear to lightly pink tinged in color; will be without hemorrhage.

Implementation

1. Know that a three-way urinary catheter with 30 ml balloon will be inserted postoperatively.
2. Ensure that urinary catheter is patent.
3. Maintain traction on the urinary catheter for 24 hours (puts pressure on prostatic bed).
4. Maintain constant bladder irrigation (CBI).
5. Increase speed of irrigation if increased blood seen; notify physician if this is not effective.
6. Measure I&O each shift.

Table 3-48 Prostatectomies

Type	Surgical approach	Common problems	Nursing implications
Transurethral resection (TUR)	Client in lithotomy position Gland removed through resecting cystoscope	Not all of gland removed Constant bladder irrigation to decrease bleeding	Explain that benign prostatic hypertrophy can recur. Ensure catheter patency. Run irrigant at rate to keep urine light pink; use only isotonic solution to prevent water intoxication.
	Most common approach	May damage internal sphincter leading to incontinence or bladder-neck strictures	Teach perineal exercises to be done q 2-4 hours.
		May or may not cause sterility	Reassure client that potency is *not* affected.
Suprapubic	Abdominal approach Bladder is opened Allows abdominal exploration	Suprapubic catheter or drain with urinary drainage Hemorrhage common; large-balloon urinary catheter with traction is used to stop bleeding Bladder spasms common	Do frequent dressing changes; Prevent infection or irritation. Watch closely for bleeding; check catheter patency; irrigate with saline prn to prevent clots. Reposition client; give propantheline bromide (Pro-Banthine).
		Causes sterility	Reassure client potency *not* affected.
Retropubic	Low abdominal incision; no bladder incision Allows complete, direct removal of gland with less bleeding	Can be done for cancer or BPH Causes sterility Less chance of bleeding; sometimes constant bladder irrigation is ordered for 24 hours	Reassure client potency *not* affected. Watch for bleeding.
		Few spasms	Medicate prn.
Perineal, radical (for cancer)	Incision in perineum between scrotum and rectum Client in lithotomy position	Causes impotence, sterility, and some incontinence Large perineal wound with risk of infection and bleeding Straining or rectal trauma may increase bleeding May be done for castration if carcinoma	Allow expression of feelings. Teach perineal exercises. Clean well; check and change dressing prn Avoid rectal temperature or tubes. Give stool softeners. Talk to client about concerns or feelings. Explain changes.

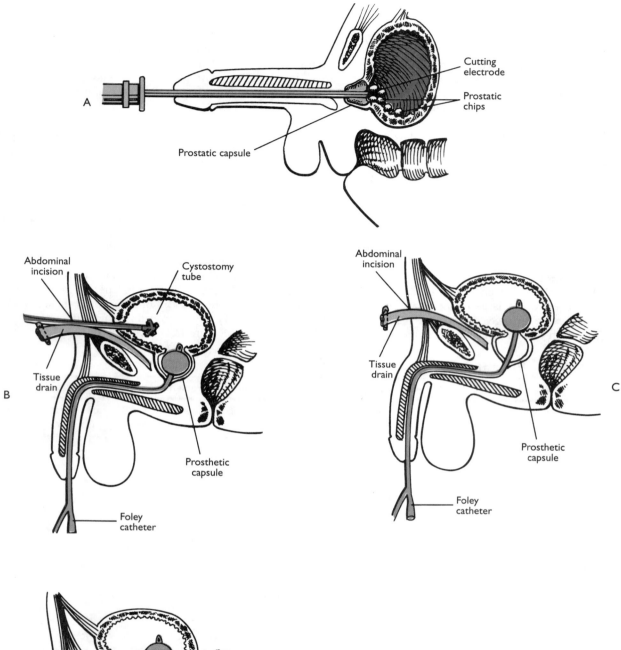
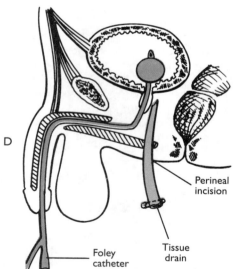

Fig. 3-22   Types of prostatectomies. **A,** Transurethral prostatectomy. **B,** Suprapubic prostatectomy. **C,** Retropubic prostatectomy. **D,** Radical perineal prostatectomy. (From Long BC, Phipps WJ: *Medical-surgical nursing: a nursing process approach,* ed 3, St Louis, 1993, Mosby.)

7. Monitor urinary output after urinary catheter is removed (2 to 3 days).
8. Care for dressing around suprapubic catheter if suprapubic prostatectomy done.

Evaluation

Client's urine remains clear and pink to amber colored without hemorrhage.

Goal 4 Client will have minimal discomfort from bladder spasms and minimal postoperative complications.

Implementation

1. Know that a large balloon on the urinary catheter can stimulate spasms (more likely to be used with TURP).
2. Administer narcotics plus anticholinergic drugs as ordered.
3. Administer belladonna and opium suppositories as ordered.
4. Institute strategies to prevent thrombophlebitis.
5. Know that incisional infection is more frequent with suprapubic prostatectomy.
6. Observe for signs of epididymitis (swelling, pain of scrotum, testes).
7. For epididymitis place ice pack under testes and scrotum.

Evaluation

Client states that discomfort has resolved; is free of postoperative infections or epididymitis.

Goal 5 Client will understand activities allowed after discharge.

Implementation

1. Teach client
   a. To refrain from postoperative sexual activity, heavy lifting, and straining for approximately 3 weeks.
   b. To avoid driving car for approximately 2 weeks.
   c. To monitor urine, which should be continually clear.
   d. To increase fluid intake (i.e., 1 glass of liquid qh).
   e. To avoid alcohol for 6 weeks.
   f. That dribbling may occur after removal of catheter and that perineal exercises can help increase sphincter tone.

Evaluation

Client describes activity restrictions; states intent to monitor urine at home.

✠ CANCER OF THE PROSTATE

1. Incidence
   a. Increasing
   b. Most common cancer in men
   c. Most frequent in 50-plus age group
2. Predisposing factors
   a. Family tendency
   b. Environmental risks and oncogenic virus suspected
3. Other information
   a. Usually starts in posterior lobe
   b. Most commonly adenocarcinoma
   c. Usually palpable on rectal exam

4. Medical treatment: surgical intervention
   a. Radical retropubic prostatectomy (preferred)
   b. Radical perineal prostatectomy
   c. TURP for palliation followed by hormonal manipulation (diethylstilbestrol) or bilateral orchiectomy

Nursing Process

ASSESSMENT

Findings depend on size of tumor.

1. Prostatic specific antigen (PSA) elevated for early detection
2. Rectal exam: if small tumor, hard nodule on prostate
3. Transrectal ultrasound to locate nonpalpable tumors
4. Positive biopsy of prostate
5. BPH resulting from large tumor
6. Signs of metastasis (usually spine): low back and leg pain
7. Increased acid phosphatase with spread beyond capsule
8. Increased alkaline phosphatase with bone metastasis

ANALYSIS/NURSING DIAGNOSIS (see p. 191).

PLANNING, IMPLEMENTATION, AND EVALUATION

Goal 1 Client will exhibit an understanding of the planned surgery and what to expect postoperatively.

Implementation

1. Refer to Perioperative Period, p. 115.
2. Counsel client regarding impotence and available penile prosthetic devices.
3. Include significant others in preoperative discussion.

Evaluation

Client describes planned surgery in own words.

Goal 2 Client's incision will have a clean and intact incision.

Implementation

1. Do not take rectal temperatures or insert rectal tubes.
2. Use brief-type underwear to hold dressing after a perineal approach.
3. When food allowed, follow a low-residue diet until wound healing is advanced.
4. Maintain patency of urinary catheter (may be in place for 2 to 3 weeks).

Evaluation

Client's incision heals without complication.

Goal 3 Client will remain free from postoperative complications.

Implementation

1. Refer to Perioperative Period, p. 115.
2. Monitor for lymphedema if pelvic lymph nodes removed.

Evaluation

Client is afebrile; maintains clear lung sounds; is free from leg edema.

Goal 4 Client will regain perineal muscle tone and urinary continence.

Implementation

1. Teach perineal exercises.
2. Institute exercises 48 hours postoperatively; have client do them qh in the first few weeks after surgery.
3. Reassure client that some urinary control can be obtained.

Evaluation

Client demonstrates perineal exercises; expresses a positive attitude about regaining continence.

Goal 5 Client will be able to explain alternative methods of sexual expression.

Implementation

1. Encourage client to discuss concerns and fears.
2. Encourage client to discuss sexuality with significant other; have them explore different ways to satisfy each other sexually.

Evaluation

Client shows a willingness to discuss sexual concerns and alternatives.

Goal 6 Client and significant other will understand the therapy for advanced disease.

Implementation

1. Explain hormonal manipulation and side effects of female hormones.
2. Prepare client for bilateral orchiectomy if indicated. Answer questions concerning prosthetic devices or inguinal incision.
3. Prepare client for TURP if cancer is causing obstruction but is not surgically treatable.

Evaluation

Client is able to describe treatment modalities for advanced disease.

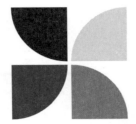

Elimination: The Large Bowel

OVERVIEW OF PHYSIOLOGY

1. The large intestine extends from the ileocecal valve to the anus (cecum, ascending colon, transverse colon, descending colon, sigmoid colon, rectum, and anal canal).
2. The major functions of the colon are the absorption of water and electrolytes in the proximal half of the large intestine and storage of feces in the distal half until defecation occurs.
3. Bacterial action in the large bowel not only provides gases to increase the bulk of and propel the feces but also facilitates synthesis of vitamin K, thiamin, riboflavin, vitamin B_{12}, folic acid, biotin, and nicotinic acid.

APPLICATION OF THE NURSING PROCESS TO THE CLIENT WITH LARGE BOWEL PROBLEMS

ASSESSMENT

1. Health history
   a. Bowel habits: frequency and character of stool patterns
   b. Changes in bowel habits: decrease or increase in frequency, change in consistency (more liquid leads to diarrhea; less liquid leads to constipation)
   c. Presence of blood or change in color of stool
   d. Use of laxatives or other methods that affect elimination
   e. Effect of dietary habits on elimination
   f. Presence of abdominal or rectal pain
   g. Altered weight
2. Physical examination
   a. Inspection
      1. abdomen
         a. scars, striae, wounds, fistulas, ostomy
         b. engorged veins
         c. skin characteristics
         d. visible peristalsis and pulsations
         e. visible masses and altered contour
      2. anus
         a. presence of dilated veins
         b. constipation
         c. breaks in skin, fissures
   b. Auscultation
      1. bowel sounds
      2. bruit
      3. hum and friction rub
   c. Percussion
      1. liver size
      2. presence of fluid or excessive air
   d. Palpation
      1. masses
      2. rigidity of abdominal muscles
      3. pain/tenderness
      4. fluid waves
3. Diagnostic tests
   a. Stool examinations
      1. odor, consistency, color
      2. presence or absence of mucus
      3. occult blood (by guaiac exam)
      4. ova and parasites
      5. fecal fat
   b. Barium enema
      1. definition: barium is instilled in the rectum through a rectal catheter
         a. permits x-ray visualization of large intestine
         b. used to detect polyps, tumors, diverticula, positional abnormalities (e.g., malrotation)
      2. nursing care pretest
         a. explain procedure
         b. administer cathartics as ordered the day before procedure
         c. administer a suppository if ordered on the day of the procedure
         d. may restrict diet to clear liquids for 24 hours before exam
         e. keep NPO after midnight
      3. nursing care posttest
         a. administer laxatives after procedure as ordered to prevent impaction
         b. instruct client that stool will remain light clay colored from the barium for 24 to 72 hours
   c. Proctoscopy, sigmoidoscopy, colonoscopy
      1. definition: visualization of inside of entire colon (colonoscopy), sigmoid colon (sigmoidoscopy), or rectum (proctoscopy) through a lighted scope
         a. proctoscopy: rigid scope
         b. colonoscopy: flexible scope
         c. sigmoidoscopy: rigid or flexible scope
      2. nursing care pretest
         a. explain procedure
         b. give clear liquids 24 to 48 hours before exam
         c. prepare bowel with laxatives, enemas, or suppositories as ordered
      3. nursing care posttest
         a. observe for hemorrhage, abdominal distention, pain

Table 3-49   Antidiarrheal and laxative drugs

Drug	Action	Use	Side effects	Nursing implications
ANTIDIARRHEALS				
Local acting Kaolin and pectin (Ka-opectate) Bismuth subsalicylate (Pepto-Bismol)	Reduce liquidity of feces Act within the bowel to soothe the intestinal tract and increase the absorption of water, electrolytes, and nutrients	Treat acute and chronic diarrhea	Constipation Intestinal obstruction in chronic use Drug absorbs nutrients	Advise clients to stop the medication and notify physician if drug is not effective in 48 hours. Advise to maintain fluid intake during diarrhea. Instruct to shake well before taking a liquid drug. Hold drug and call physician if abdomen becomes distended, if bowel sounds diminish or are absent, or if impaction is suspected.
Systemic acting Diphenoxylate hydrochloride with atropine sulfate (Lomotil) Loperamide (Imodium) Camphorated tincture of opium (Paragoric)	Act systemically to inhibit the peristaltic reflex and reduce GI motility	Same as above	CNS: drowsiness, headache, sedation, dizziness CV: tachycardia GU: urinary retention GI: dry mouth, nausea or vomiting, constipation	Check for presence of glaucoma; if present do not give medications containing atropine.
LAXATIVES				
Bulk formers Psyllium (Metamucil) Methylcellulose (Citrucel) Bran	Produce soft stool by retaining fluid Working time: 1-3 days	Prophylaxis and treatment of functional constipation	GI: abdominal cramps, diarrhea, nausea or vomiting; intestinal obstruction if taken dry or chewed	Discontinue drug if abdominal pain occurs Advise to take 1 hour apart from other oral medications to prevent absorption of drugs by laxative. Give with 8 oz fluids
Emollients Docusate sodium (Co-lace) Docusate calcium (Surfak) Docusate potassium (Dialose)	Docusate salts act as detergents in the intestine, reduce surface tension of interfacing liquids, thus promoting incorporation of fat and additional liquid, softening the stool	For clients who must avoid straining at stool	Increased absorption if used with mineral oil Throat irritation if liquid used Mild abdominal cramping	Advise loss of effectiveness with long-term use. Dilute liquid, but not the syrup preparations, to improve taste. Discontinue if severe abdominal cramping occurs.
Irritants Cascara (Cas-Evac) Senna (Senokot) Castor oil (Alphamul) Bisacodyl (Dulcolax)	Stimulates intestine, promotes peristalsis Working time: 1-3 hours	Preoperative cleansing, diagnostic studies; treat constipation unresponsive to other agents	Abdominal cramps, diarrhea In excessive use: electrolyte imbalance Constipation after catharsis Laxative dependence	Advise cascara may color urine reddish-pink or brown depending on urine pH. Monitor for electrolyte imbalance or laxative dependence.

Continued

Table 3-49   Antidiarrheal and laxative drugs—cont'd

Drug	Action	Use	Side effects	Nursing implications
Lubricant				
Mineral oil	Acts in the colon, lubricates the intestine, and retards colonic fluid absorption Working time: 6-8 hours	Cleansing enema, preparation for bowel studies, constipation	Impaired absorption of fat-soluble vitamins, digitalis glycosides, sulfonamides, anticoagulants, oral contraceptives Potential toxic absorption levels of mineral oil if taken with stool softeners. Nausea, vomiting	Prevent aspiration by not allowing the client to lie flat during or after drug administration. Monitor clients for impaired absorption of medications or vitamins. Obtain detailed history if client takes mineral oil as a regular laxative.
Saline/osmotics				
Milk of magnesia Magnesium sulfate Magnesium citrate (Epsom salt) Lactulose (Cephulac)	Produce watery stools that distend the bowel; promotes peristalsis and bowel evacuation Working time: 1-6 hours	Preprocedure cleansing, constipation	Abdominal cramps Flatulence Diarrhea with dehydration and loss of electrolytes	Monitor for fluid and electrolyte balance and dehydration.
For all laxatives	1. Teach clients the importance of exercise, proper fluid intake, and high-fiber diet to promote regular bowel elimination patterns. 2. Do not use any laxative if obstruction is suspected. 3. Avoid routine use of laxatives.			

b. check for return of normal bowel function after procedure

d. Biopsy
   1. definition: removal of polyps or biopsy specimens through a specialized piece of equipment inserted during endoscopy
   2. nursing care pretest and posttest
      a. same as for proctoscopy

ANALYSIS/NURSING DIAGNOSIS
1. Safe, effective care environment
   a. Risk for infection
   b. Knowledge deficit
2. Physiologic integrity
   a. Constipation, diarrhea, bowel incontinence
   b. Altered nutrition: less than body requirements
3. Psychosocial integrity
   a. Anxiety
   b. Body-image disturbance
   c. Altered pattern of sexuality
4. Health promotion/maintenance
   a. Altered health maintenance
   b. Knowledge deficit
   c. Impaired adjustment

GENERAL NURSING PLANNING, IMPLEMENTATION, AND EVALUATION

Goal 1 Client's bowel elimination will follow a normal pattern.

Implementation
   1. Instruct client how to promote proper bowel function; adjust teaching if client has an ileostomy or colostomy.
   2. Teach client to respond to defecation reflex because holding feces can contribute to constipation.
   3. Instruct client on the use of foods high in bulk and roughage: skin and fibers of fruits and vegetables.
   4. Increase fluid intake if allowed.
   5. Encourage regular exercise to aid in elimination of waste.
   6. Teach about the relationship of stress to altered bowel function.
   7. Prevent diarrhea through proper sanitation and hygiene.
   8. Restrict fruit juices and raw fruits and vegetables that contribute to diarrhea.
   9. Observe client with diarrhea for signs of fluid and electrolyte imbalance.
   10. Administer antidiarrheals (Table 3-49).
   11. Encourage intake of electrolyte-containing drinks (e.g., Gatorade).

Evaluation
Client establishes a normal pattern of bowel elimination; lists and consumes foods that promote bowel evacuation; establishes a pattern of regular exercise; passes stool of normal consistency.

Goal 2 Client's dietary intake will follow prescribed restrictions yet provide all needed nutrients.

Implementation
   1. Increase or decrease dietary nutrients as ordered.
   2. Teach client rationale for restrictions.
   3. Explore with client means of fostering compliance.
   4. Provide needed support and encouragement.

Evaluation

Client selects appropriate diet from sample menus; verbalizes rationale for restrictions; expresses a positive attitude toward diet alteration.

Goal 3 Client will be knowledgeable about disease process, medications, and the prevention of complications.

Implementation

1. Explain disease process and its relationship to medications.
2. Discuss rationale for ordered treatment regimen.
3. Provide data concerning the administration and side effects of all medications.
4. Help client identify potential stressors in lifestyle that might trigger complications of the disease; discuss appropriate client actions.

Evaluation

Client takes medications as ordered, returns for follow-up care; remains free from preventable complications.

SELECTED HEALTH PROBLEMS RESULTING IN ALTERATION IN LARGE BOWEL ELIMINATION

✖ ALTERATION IN NORMAL BOWEL EVACUATION

1. Definitions
   a. *Constipation:* difficult or infrequent defecation with passage of unduly hard and dry fecal material
   b. *Diarrhea:* frequent passage of abnormally watery bowel movements
   c. Normal bowel evacuation: 2 to 3 movements per day to 2 per week; varies in healthy individuals
2. Precipitating factors
   a. Constipation: worry, anxiety, fear, improper diet, intestinal obstruction, tumors, excessive use of laxatives, use of certain drugs, atony or spasticity of intestinal musculature
   b. Diarrhea: diet, inflammation or irritation of intestinal mucosa, GI infections, use of certain drugs, psychogenic factors

Nursing Process
ASSESSMENT
1. Stool consistency, appearance
2. Acute or chronic pain, rebound tenderness
3. Weight loss, malnutrition
4. Dehydration
5. Nausea, vomiting; projectile vomiting
6. Electrolyte imbalance, especially sodium, potassium, chloride
7. Aggravation by certain foods and milk products
8. Drug history
9. Malabsorption of foods

10. Mass in abdomen
11. Low-grade fever
12. Anemia
13. Anorexia
14. Presence of bowel sounds: increased or decreased
15. Abdominal distention
16. Decreased flatus

ANALYSIS/NURSING DIAGNOSIS (see p. 211)
PLANNING, IMPLEMENTATION, AND EVALUATION
Refer to General Nursing Goal 1, p. 211.

✖ CHRONIC INFLAMMATORY BOWEL DISEASE (REGIONAL ENTERITIS, ULCERATIVE COLITIS)

1. Definition
   a. *Regional enteritis* (Crohn's disease) is a small-bowel, segmental, transmural inflammatory process that may involve any part of the alimentary tract; the ileum is the principal site (Table 3-50)
   b. *Ulcerative colitis* is a large-bowel, continuous inflammatory process of the mucosa, primarily of the colon and rectum (Table 3-50)
2. Incidence: young people between 20 and 40 years of age
3. Etiology: unknown: possibly result of infection, stress, or autoimmunity; familial tendency
4. Pathophysiology
   a. Regional enteritis symptoms include pronounced thickening of the submucosa with lymphedema, hyperplasia, granulomas, ulcerations, and fissures; the longitudinal ulcers and transverse fissures produce a cobblestone effect; in the later stages, full-thickness penetration of the intestinal wall results in the formation of fistulas and abscesses
   b. Ulcerative colitis symptoms include congestion, edema, multiple superficial ulcerations, and crypt abscesses in the rectum and distal colon and spread upward; characterized by profuse watery diarrhea containing blood, mucus, and pus
5. Diagnostic test
   a. Stool for blood, fat, and culture
   b. Barium enema (cathartics are contraindicated as a prep)
   c. Proctosigmoidoscopy, colonoscopy with biopsy (not routinely done because of need for vigorous bowel preparation)

Nursing Process
ASSESSMENT
1. Rectal bleeding
2. Diarrhea: frequent liquid stools with tenesmus; may contain blood, mucus, or pus
3. Abdominal cramps before bowel movement; colicky cramping with urgency to defecate
4. Pain, usually located in the left lower quadrant, with ulcerative colitis
5. Anorexia, nausea, vomiting
6. Dehydration
7. Electrolyte imbalance (e.g., decreased potassium and sodium, metabolic acidosis)
8. Weight loss

Table 3-50   Comparison of ulcerative colitis and regional enteritis (Crohn's disease)

	Ulcerative colitis	Crohn's disease
Usual area affected	Left colon, rectum	Distal ileum, right colon
Extent of involvement	Diffuse areas, contiguous	Segmental areas, noncontiguous
Inflammation	Mostly mucosal	Transmural
Mucosal appearance	Ulcerations	Cobblestone effect, granulomas
Character of stools	Blood present	No blood present
	No fat	Steatorrhea
	Frequent liquid stools	Three to five semisoft stools per day
Abdominal pain	May occur, mild	Right lower quadrant pain, cramping
Abdominal mass	No	Common in right lower quadrant
Complications	Toxic megacolon	Fistulas
	Pseudopolyps	Perianal disease
	Hemorrhoids	Strictures
	Hemorrhage	Abscesses
		Perforation
Extraintestinal manifestations	Anemia	Anemia
	Erythema nodosum	Malabsorption of fat and fat-soluble vitamins
	Pyoderma gangrenosa	Arthritis
	Arthritis	Hepatobiliary disease
	Liver disease	Iritis, conjunctivitis
	Irritis, conjunctivitis	Renal stones, obstructive uropathy
	Stomatitis	
	Thrombophlebitis	
Reasons for surgery	Poor response to medical therapy	Presence of complications
	Complications	
Response to surgery	Curative	Noncurrative, high recurrence rate

From Phipps WJ, et al: *Medical surgical nursing concepts and clinical practice,* ed 5, St Louis, 1975, Mosby.

9. Weakness, debilitation, malnutrition
10. Anemia
11. Fever
12. Emotional concerns, immature and dependent personality
13. Dietary habits

ANALYSIS/NURSING DIAGNOSIS (see p. 211)
PLANNING, IMPLEMENTATION, AND EVALUATION

Goal 1 Client will be well nourished and hydrated.

Implementation
1. Weigh client daily.
2. Keep NPO in acute stage; give parenteral fluids with vitamins and minerals as ordered.
3. Administer total parenteral nutrition (TPN) as ordered.
4. Initiate high-protein, high-calorie, bland, low-residue diet as tolerated (Table 3-51).
5. Avoid gas-producing or irritating foods and milk products.
6. Offer small feedings as necessary.
7. Replace deficiency of fat-soluble vitamins (A, D, E, and K).
8. Record caloric intake.
9. Avoid too hot or too cold foods.
10. Urge up to 3000 ml fluid intake per day (if not contraindicated); keep I&O (include measurement of liquid stools).

Table 3-51   Foods to be *avoided* on low-residue diets

Types of food	Foods to be avoided
Beverages	Milk in excess of 2 cups
Breads and cereals	Whole grain or bran
Desserts	Any containing fruits and nuts
Fruits	Any with seeds or skins, raw fruits except bananas
Meats, fish, poultry, cheese, and eggs	Tough meats, pork, fried or highly seasoned meats, fish, cheese
Vegetables	Raw vegetables

11. Involve client and significant others with dietitian for proper diet instructions.

Evaluation
Client maintains weight; states meal plan using high-protein, low-residue, high-calorie, bland diet; maintains at least 2500 ml fluid intake daily.

Goal 2 Client will experience reduced physical and psychologic stress.

Implementation
1. Enforce bed rest to decrease intestinal motility in acute stage.

2. Maintain quiet, comfortable, nonstressful environment.
3. Keep room odor free.
4. Empty bedpan promptly and have within easy reach of client during acute episodes.
5. Keep perianal area clean and dry, applying lubricant or ointments as necessary.
6. Administer pain medications as ordered.
7. Give sitz baths at least 3 times per day or as needed.

Evaluation
Client states relief of pain; rests comfortably.

Goal 3 Client will be free from infection.

Implementation
1. Prevent and treat secondary infection through use of sulfonamides (e.g., sulfasalazine [Azulfidine]) as ordered (see Table 3-44).
2. Help and teach client to turn, cough, and deep breathe q2-4h (during acute stage).
3. Check temperature q4h; avoid taking rectal temperature if anus is excoriated.
4. Administer oral hygiene as necessary.
5. Provide good skin care.

Evaluation
Client remains free from signs of infection (e.g., increased temperature, infiltrate in lungs, or secondary infection in mucous membranes of mouth, skin, or colon).

Goal 4 Client will have fewer bowel movements than when admitted.

Implementation
1. Administer antidiarrheal medications as ordered (see Table 3-49).
   a. Opium alkaloids (Paregoric)
   b. Diphenoxylate (Lomotil)
   c. Anticholinergic drugs (tincture of belladonna, Donnatal)
   d. Kaolin and pectin (Kaopectate)
2. Reduce inflammation by administration of
   a. Azathioprine (Imuran) (immunosuppressive agent)
   b. 6-mercaptopurine (see Table 5-25)
   c. Corticosteroids (see Table 3-20)
3. Check bowel sounds q2-4h; report increase or decrease to physician.
4. Note frequency, color, and amount of stools.
5. Report increase in abdominal distention to physician.
6. Reduce emotional stress (direct influence on course of illness).

Evaluation
Client has a decrease in frequency and amount of stools; has no increase in abdominal distention.

Goal 5 Client will maintain a balance of adequate rest and exercise.

Implementation
1. Encourage rest after meals.
2. Do not confine to bed unless very weak.

3. Provide calm, reassuring environment.
4. Give sedation as necessary to provide adequate night's sleep.
5. Initiate ambulation at short, frequent intervals.
6. Allow for frequent rest periods.

Evaluation
Client verbalizes feeling rested; sleeps through the night; increases periods of ambulation as strength returns.

Goal 6 Client will accept alteration of lifestyle imposed by chronic illness.

Implementation
1. Provide teaching regarding
   a. How to live with chronic disease.
   b. Factors in environment that aggravate colitis (emotional stress, dietary indiscretion, ingestion of irritants, overfatigue, infections, or pregnancy).
   c. How to maintain nutrition.
   d. Importance of medical management of the disease.
   e. Need for biannual sigmoidoscopy and barium enema (increased incidence of carcinoma of large intestines).
2. Provide emotional counseling and support as needed.
3. Encourage verbalization of anxieties.
4. Provide diversional activities.

Evaluation
Client verbalizes acceptance of disease; lists lifestyle modifications to be initiated.

✖ TOTAL COLECTOMY WITH ILEOSTOMY

1. Definition: surgical removal of the entire colon, rectum, and anus with the construction of permanent ileostomy to provide for passage of feces
2. Indications: when medical management fails and constant relapses with intractability occur; occurrence of complications (e.g., perforation, hemorrhage, obstruction, toxic megacolon, abscess, and fistula); more effective as treatment for ulcerative colitis

Nursing Process
ASSESSMENT
1. Physical status
2. Emotional status
3. Acceptance of ostomy
4. Understanding of ostomy function
5. Ability to verbalize feelings

ANALYSIS/NURSING DIAGNOSIS (see p. 211)

PLANNING, IMPLEMENTATION, AND EVALUATION

Goal I Client will be physically and psychologically prepared for surgery.

Implementation
1. Refer to Perioperative Period, p. 115.
2. Give TPN as ordered to improve preoperative nutritional status.
3. Prepare bowel for surgery: low-residue diet, clear liquids, oral antibiotics, cathartics, enema.
4. Obtain help of an enterostomal therapist, if available, to

plan site of stoma placement and to introduce client to appliance.

5. Encourage client to express fears and concerns regarding change in body image.
6. Introduce client to concept of ostomy support groups; obtain volunteer if desired.

Evaluation
Client is prepared physically and psychologically for surgery.

Goal 2 Client will remain free from infection and complications postoperatively.

Implementation
1. Refer to Perioperative Period, p. 115.
2. Observe stoma size, color.

Evaluation
Client remains free from any signs of postoperative infection or complications (e.g., has normal temperature, clear lungs).

Goal 3 Client will maintain normal fluid and electrolyte balance.

Implementation
1. Monitor I&O, weigh daily, NG tube drainage.
2. Monitor state of hydration (skin turgor and condition of mucous membranes), urine output.
3. Monitor serum electrolyte and H & H levels.
4. Monitor ileal output; postoperative drainage begins immediately; the effluent is liquid.
5. Administer IV fluids as ordered, until client can take oral nourishment.

Evaluation
Client has I&O and electrolytes within normal limits.

Goal 4 Client will verbalize dietary restrictions.

Implementation
1. Teach client that food ingested will pass through the ileostomy within 4 to 6 hours.
2. Teach client that each individual has different food tolerances.
3. Provide diet information: most ostomy clients are discharged on a low-residue, high-protein, high-carbohydrate diet rich in high-potassium foods and low in gas-producing, highly seasoned, or fried foods.
4. Know that vitamin supplements A, D, E, K, and B_{12} may be necessary.
5. Prepare client for possible weight gain resulting from increased food tolerance postoperatively.
6. Refer to dietitian as necessary.

Evaluation
Client states dietary changes; verbalizes intent to work out a diet plan within the limits of the individual variations.

Goal 5 Client will achieve self-care management.

Implementation
1. Instruct client (step by step) and receive return demonstration on stoma care, including
   a. Equipment: type, how to use, and where to purchase.
   b. Skin care: ileostomy drainage is erosive and continuous.
   c. Application of appliance.
   d. Odor control.
2. Use services of enterostomal therapist if available.
3. Refer to home care nurses for home follow-up or continue follow up by enterostomal therapist.

Evaluation
Client successfully manages self-care of ileostomy.

Goal 6 Client will successfully cope with altered body image.

Implementation
1. Encourage verbalization of concerns.
2. Assure client that major change in lifestyle is not necessary.
3. Encourage involvement in ostomy club.
4. Provide emotional support to the significant other in adjusting to ostomy.
5. Obtain sexual counseling for client, if needed.

Evaluation
Client discusses altered body image; shows evidence of coping with change and resumption of normal activity.

✖ MECHANICAL OBSTRUCTION OF THE COLON

1. Pathophysiology
   a. Obstruction can be partial or complete
   b. Emergency situation if blood supply is compromised
   c. If blood supply is not compromised, fluid and electrolyte deficiency becomes the major problem
   d. Absorption decreases and fluids and electrolytes accumulate in GI tract
   e. Fluid will either stay in GI tract or be lost through vomiting
   f. Subsequent decrease in extracellular fluid volume (dehydration)
   g. Metabolic acidosis results
2. Risk/causative factors
   a. Small intestine: adhesions, hernia, volvulus
   b. Large intestine: neoplasm, stricture, diverticulitis
3. Medical treatment
   a. Medical intervention
      1. decompression with intestinal tubes; for a small-bowel obstruction
         a. Cantor tube: permanent mercury-weighted tip
         b. Miller-Abbott tube: has port for injection of mercury
         c. length to be passed is determined by physician
      2. fluid and electrolyte replacement
         a. Surgical intervention
      1. colon resection with end-to-end anastomosis or temporary or permanent colostomy
      2. abdominoperineal resection with permanent colostomy

Nursing Process

ASSESSMENT

1. Abdomen distended; altered bowel habits; most common with large intestine obstruction
2. Projectile vomiting and severe pain, most common with small-intestine obstruction
3. Decreased or increased bowel sounds

ANALYSIS/NURSING DIAGNOSIS (see p. 211)
PLANNING, IMPLEMENTATION, AND EVALUATION

> **Goals 1 through 4** Refer to Total Colectomy with Ileostomy, p. 214.

> **Goal 5** The client will have appropriate bowel decompression or preparation for surgery.

Implementation

1. Attach NG tube to intermittent suction.
2. Care for intestinal tube if ordered.
   a. After the tube is passed, tell client to lie 2 hours in each of the following positions in order: right side, back, left side; this will facilitate passage of the tube into the intestine (usually passes at a rate of 2 to 3 inches per hour).
   b. Do not allow tube to pass rapidly because twisting and knotting may result.
   c. Monitor for correct tube placement by testing for pH of aspiration contents (>7 = tube is in small intestine; <7 = tube is in stomach).
   d. Do *not* tape tube until it has passed into the small intestine.
   e. If massive stomach content loss occurs, monitor for metabolic alkalosis (see Table 3-18); if massive intestinal loss, monitor for acidosis.
   f. Remove slowly when ordered to prevent twisting the intestine.

3. Know that the client additionally will undergo preoperative bowel preparation that will include
   a. Clear liquids several days preoperatively; then NPO
   b. Bowel sterilization routine as ordered with neomycin and sulfonamides
   c. Several enemas and cathartics
4. Monitor I&O, urine specific gravity, and gastric output.
5. Give narcotics sparingly (may mask symptoms); avoid morphine (decreases intestinal motility).

Evalution

Client's bowel is decompressed, clean, and prepared for surgery.

> **Goal 6** Client will cope successfully with altered body image.

Implementation

1. See Total Colectomy with Ileostomy Goal 6, p. 216.
2. Instruct client about irrigation and dietary management for regulation of colostomy (Fig. 3-23).
   a. Most physicians advocate colostomy regulation with diet.
   b. If irrigation is required
      1. allow 1 hour for the process
      2. remove old pouch and clean skin around stoma
      3. apply irrigation assembly and sleeve
      4. use 500 to 1000 ml of warm water; hang bag no higher than shoulder level, 18 to 24 inches above stoma
      5. insert irrigating cone into stoma (use of cone is safer than inserting tube)
      6. let water run in slowly
      7. remove cone and allow solution to drain
      8. remove irrigation assembly and sleeve; clean around stoma
      9. apply clean pouch and barrier

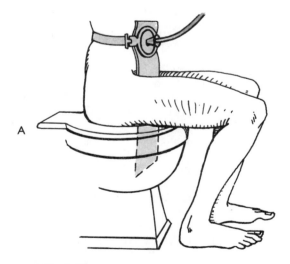
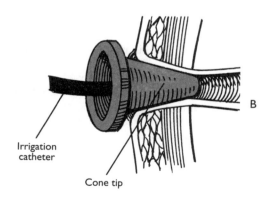

Irrigation catheter

Cone tip

Fig. 3-23 Colostomy irrigation. **A,** Colostomy irrigation with person sitting on toilet: irrigating sleeve drains into toilet. **B,** Cone irrigating tip inserted in stoma. (From Long BC, Phipps WJ: *Medical-surgical nursing: a nursing process approach,* ed 3, St Louis, 1993, Mosby.)

3. If the colostomy is to be closed at a future date, encourage client to look forward to that day. At the same time reinforce the importance of good daily care and adjustment to a temporarily changed body image.

Evaluation

Client discusses altered body image; expresses a willingness to adjust and to maintain colostomy, until closure can be accomplished if indicated with a temporary colostomy.

✚ CANCER OF THE COLON

1. Definition: malignant neoplasm of the large bowel; 70% of cases occur in the rectosigmoid area
2. Incidence
   a. Second most common malignancy in adults
   b. Equal in both sexes
   c. Occurs after fourth decade; peaks in the seventh decade
   d. Most are adenocarcinoma
3. Risk factors
   a. Family history
   b. History of ulcerative colitis, polyps
   c. Possibly related to increased fat in diet, food additives, low-fiber diet, or chronic constipation
4. Diagnostic tests
   a. Rectal exam (almost 50% of these tumors are palpable on digital exam)
   b. Sigmoidoscopy, colonoscopy
   c. Barium enema
   d. Stool exam for occult blood
   e. Alkaline phosphatase and serum glutamic-oxaloacetic transaminase (SGOT): metastasis to liver
   f. Carcinoembryonic antigen (CEA) level: elevated in advanced adenocarcinoma
6. Medical treatment
   a. Surgical intervention: colon resection
      1. colectomy with anastomosis of the remaining colon or colostomy
      2. abdominal-perineal resection (removal of anus and rectum) with a permanent colostomy
   b. Medical intervention
      1. radiation therapy
      2. chemotherapy

Nursing Process

ASSESSMENT

1. Change in bowel habits; blood in stool (more likely with left colon and rectal involvement)
2. Vague, dull pain (more likely with ascending-colon involvement)
3. Anorexia, weight loss, weakness, and anemia
4. Signs of obstruction
5. Hemorrhage
6. Perforation with peritonitis, abscess, and fistula formation

ANALYSIS/NURSING DIAGNOSIS (see p. 211)
PLANNING, IMPLEMENTATION, AND EVALUATION

Refer to Total Colectomy with Ileostomy, p. 214, and Mechanical Obstruction of the Colon, p. 215. Refer to Cellular Aberration for information and goals pertinent to chemotherapy and radiation therapy.

✚ DIVERTICULOSIS/DIVERTICULITIS

1. Definitions
   a. Diverticulum: outpouching of the musculature of the intestine
   b. Diverticulosis: the condition of being afflicted with diverticula
   c. Diverticulitis: inflammation of the diverticula
   d. Fiber and roughage: plants or foodstuff not digested by the body
   e. Residue: that part of foodstuff left after digestion, eventually collected in the large intestine
2. Most common in the sigmoid colon
3. Risk factors
   a. Diet low in fiber and high in refined and processed foods
   b. Age (frequently over 40 years of age)
   c. Chronic constipation
4. Medical treatment
   a. Medical intervention
      1. acute episodes: NPO, antibiotics, IV fluids; if eating a low-fiber, low-roughage, low-residue diet
      2. ongoing care: high-fiber, high-roughage diet, high or low in residue (physician's choice), bulk laxatives, antispasmodics
   b. Surgical intervention: bowel resection with or without a temporary colostomy

Nursing Process

ASSESSMENT

1. Diverticulosis is usually asymptomatic
2. Diverticulitis
   a. Crampy pain in left lower quadrant
   b. Constipation, possibly alternating with diarrhea
   c. Fever and leukocytosis

ANALYSIS/NURSING DIAGNOSIS (see p. 211)
PLANNING, IMPLEMENTATION, AND EVALUATION

> **Goal I** Client will recover from an acute episode without complications.

Implementation

1. Give antibiotics, IV fluids, monitor electrolytes as ordered.
2. Keep client NPO until pain subsides, then advance to liquid diet.
3. Keep on bed rest to decrease intestinal motility.
4. Observe for complications of perforation or peritonitis.

Evaluation

Client remains free from pain and complications; has normal bowel function; tolerates diet.

> **Goal 2** Client will recover from any necessary surgery (e.g., bowel resection, colostomy) without complications. Refer to Total Colectomy, p. 214.

> **Goal 3** Client will take measures to control diverticulosis.

Implementation

1. Teach client
   a. To eat a high-fiber, high-roughage diet (Table 3-52).
   b. To take bulk laxatives (e.g., psyllium hydrophilic [Metamucil]) as ordered.
   c. About use of ordered antispasmodics (e.g., propantheline [Pro-Banthine], oxyphencyclimine [Daricon]).
   d. Ways to decrease stress in life and lifestyle.
   e. To increase daily fluid intake.
   f. To avoid activities that increase intraabdominal pressure.
   g. To avoid all nuts or fruits and vegetables with seeds to prevent the seeds from lodging in the intestinal pouches and causing infection.

Evaluation

Client remains free from symptoms of diverticulitis; tolerates high-fiber, high-roughage diet; decreases stress.

✸ HEMORRHOIDS OR ANAL FISSURE

1. Definitions
   a. *Hemorrhoids:* dilated veins under the mucous membranes in the anal area; may be either internal or external
   b. *Anal fissure:* linear ulceration on the margin of the anus
2. Predisposing factors
   a. Straining at stool
   b. Pregnancy
   c. Portal hypertension
   d. Congestive heart failure
3. Complications
   a. Bleeding
   b. Thrombosis
   c. Strangulation
   d. Infection
4. Medical treatment
   a. Medical intervention
      1. high-roughage diet and 6 to 8 glasses of fluid per day
      2. stool softeners
      3. ointments or suppositories to shrink hemorrhoids
      4. warm sitz bath
      5. injection of a sclerosing substance into the tissues at the base of the vein
      6. rubber-band ligation
   b. Surgical intervention
      1. hemorrhoidectomy: excision of dilated veins
      2. fissurectomy: excision of fissure

Nursing Process

ASSESSMENT

1. Pain and pruritus around anus
2. Character and amount of rectal drainage
3. Usual bowel habits
4. Abdominal distention
5. Urinary retention
6. Anemia caused by chronic bleeding

ANALYSIS/NURSING DIAGNOSIS (see p. 211)

PLANNING, IMPLEMENTATION, AND EVALUATION

Goal 1 Client will remain free from postoperative complications.

Table 3-52 High-fiber, high-roughage diet

Food groups	Recommended foods
Fruits	Fresh fruits with skin
Vegetables	Raw vegetables
Breads	Whole wheat and whole grain
	Bran-type cereals
Grains and flour	Wheat germ, cornmeal, rice, buckwheat
Protein substitutes	Legumes

Implementation

1. Refer to Perioperative Period, p. 115.
2. Have client avoid sitting for prolonged periods; while sitting, use flotation pad.
3. Prevent infection.
   a. Initiate procedures as ordered for thorough preoperative bowel cleansing.
   b. Do *not* take rectal temperature.
   c. Administer perineal care with antiseptic solution after each stool.
   d. Administer sitz baths as necessary to clean incision.

Evaluation

Client remains free from complications (e.g., infection).

Goal 2 Client will experience relief of pain.

Implementation

1. Give analgesics as ordered.
2. Avoid supine position; if supine position is unavoidable, use flotation pad under buttocks.
3. Apply ice packs or warm, moist compresses if ordered.
4. Do *not* use rubber rings to sit on for long periods.
5. Administer topical anesthetic as ordered.

Evaluation

Client states that pain is controlled; is comfortable in all positions.

Goal 3 Client's bowel function will return to normal.

Implementation

1. Give low-residue, soft diet as tolerated for first week postoperatively; then advance diet to include roughage and fresh fruits.
2. Force fluids to 2500 to 3000 ml per day unless contraindicated.
3. Administer stool softener/lubricant or laxative as ordered (see Table 3-49).
4. Provide support during initial bowel movement, noting presence of blood in stool; be alert for vertigo; and administer analgesic as necessary before bowel movement.
5. Teach client how to avoid constipation after discharge.
6. Watch for and teach client symptoms of anal stricture (and report to physician).
   a. Increased pain with bowel movement
   b. Difficulty passing stool

Evaluation

Client passes soft, brown, formed stool on third postoperative day with minimal discomfort; lists ways to prevent constipation; states signs of anal stricture.

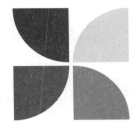

Sensation and Perception

OVERVIEW OF PHYSIOLOGY

1. Nervous system: like an electrical conduction system; coordinates and controls all activities of the body
   a. Receives stimuli or information from internal and external environments over varied sensory pathways
   b. Communicates information between distant parts of body (peripheral and central nervous systems)
   c. Computes or processes information received at various reflex (spinal cord) and conscious (higher brain) levels to determine responses appropriate to existing situations
   d. Transmits information rapidly over varied motor pathways to effector organs for body-action control or modification
2. Central nervous system
   a. Brain
      1. cerebrum or cerebral cortex
         a. hemispheres: right and left; speech is function of left hemisphere for all right-handed and most left-handed people
         b. frontal lobe: functions
            ▪ personality
            ▪ higher intellectual functions (e.g., learning, problem solving)
            ▪ ethical, social, and moral behavior
            ▪ posterior edge of frontal lobe: center for initiation of motor function
         c. parietal lobe: responsible for interpretation of sensory input
         d. temporal lobe: center for hearing, taste, and smell
         e. occipital lobe: visual center
         f. structure
            ▪ skull
            ▪ meninges: three membranes covering brain and spinal cord
               • dura mater
               • arachnoid
               • pia mater
            ▪ brain tissue
      2. brainstem: contains midbrain, pons, and medulla oblongata
         a. relays impulses from spinal cord to cerebrum
         b. controls basic body functions (cardiac, respiratory, and vasomotor centers [medulla])
      3. cerebellum
         a. orientation of body in space (equilibrium)
         b. coordination and inhibition of movement
         c. control of antigravity muscles
         d. coordination of muscle tone
   b. Spinal cord
      1. 31 segments (do not correspond in name to the vertebral segments)
         a. 8 cervical: supply neck and upper extremities, diaphragm, and intercostals
         b. 12 thoracic: supply thoracic and abdominal areas
         c. 5 lumbar: supply lower extremities
         d. 5 sacral: supply lower extremities; urinary tract and bowel control
         e. 1 coccygeal
      2. anterior portion of cord carries *motor* information (descending tracts)
      3. posterior section of cord carries *sensory* information (ascending tracts)
      4. lateral columns contain preganglionic fibers for autonomic nervous system
3. Peripheral nervous system
   a. Cranial nerves (12 pairs); numbered according to the order in which they arise from the brain, and named according to their function or distribution (Table 3-53)
   b. Spinal nerves (31 pairs); named and numbered according to the level of the vertebral column at which they emerge from the spinal cord
4. Autonomic nervous system: concerned with the control of involuntary bodily functions; divided into parasympathetic (craniosacral) and sympathetic (thoracolumbar) divisions (Table 3-54)
   a. Divisions
      1. parasympathetic or craniosacral division controls normal body functioning
      2. sympathetic or thoracolumbar division prepares body for fight or flight
   b. Most effector organs receive innervation from both sympathetic and parasympathetic fibers
   c. Vascular supply of skeletal muscle receives only sympathetic innervation
5. Vision
   a. Major function of eyes is to produce vision: light waves→cornea→lens→retina→optic nerve (II)→occipital lobe of brain
   b. Cranial nerves of the eye
      1. optic (II): vision
      2. oculomotor (III), trochlear (IV), abducent (VI): external muscles of the eye
      3. oculomotor (III) also controls pupil size

c. Exterior of eye
  1. tears secreted by lacrimal glands to lubricate lids and keep corneas moist; excess tears drain through lacrimal ducts into nasal cavity

Table 3-53   Cranial nerves

Number	Name	Type
I	Olfactory	Sensory
II	Optic	Sensory
III	Oculomotor	Motor, parasympathetic
IV	Trochlear	Motor
V	Trigeminal	Sensory, motor
VI	Abducent	Motor
VII	Facial	Sensory, motor parasympathetic
VIII	Acoustic or auditory	Sensory
IX	Glossopharyngeal	Sensory, motor, parasympathetic
X	Vagus	Sensory, motor parasympathetic
XI	Accessory	Motor
XII	Hypoglossal	Motor

2. six extrinsic eye muscles produce movements of eyeball
3. outer layer of eye
   a. cornea: nonvascular transparent fibrous covering of eye
   b. sclera: white, dense connective tissue covering all of eye except cornea
   c. canal of Schlemm: venous sinus at the junction of the sclera and cornea
d. Interior of eye (Fig. 3-24)
   1. iris: circular muscle that constricts or dilates pupil
   2. lens: focuses image accurately on retina
   3. aqueous humor and vitreous humor: liquids act along with lens as refracting media
   4. aqueous humor production: secreted continuously by ciliary process of ciliary body behind iris into posterior chamber→through pupil→anterior chamber→drained off into canal of Schlemm→bloodstream
   5. choroid: black, inner surface of eye that prevents scattering of light rays
   6. retina: light-sensitive layer of eye; sensations of vision result from retina's focused response to image
   7. optic disc: entrance of optic nerve into eyeball

Table 3-54   Parasympathetic and sympathetic effects of the autonomic nervous system

Site	Parasympathetic effects	Sympathetic effects
Eye	Pupils constricted	Pupils dilated
	Far-vision accommodation	Near-vision accommodation
Lungs	Bronchoconstriction	Bronchodilation
	Cardiac rate slowed	Cardiac rate increased
	Contraction force decreased	Contraction force increased
	Coronary vessels constrict	Coronary vessels dilate
Liver	Hepatic glycogenesis	Hepatic glycogenolysis and lipolysis
Stomach and intestine	Secretion and peristalsis stimulated	Secretion and peristalsis inhibited
Urinary bladder	Bladder contracted	Bladder relaxed
	Sphincter open	Sphincter closed
Adrenal medulla		Epinephrine and norepinephrine secretion
Penis	Erection	Ejaculation

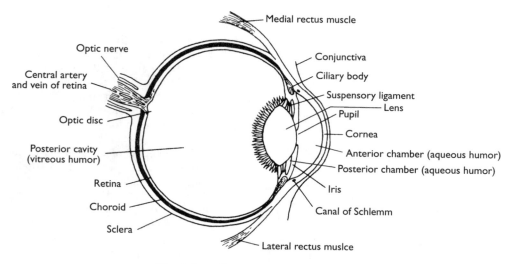

Fig. 3-24   The eye (horizontal section).

8. optic pathway: transmits visual data to occipital lobe of the cerebrum (Fig. 3-25)
6. Hearing
   a. The major functions of the ears are balance and hearing; hearing pathway: sound waves→pinna→external ear canal→tympanic membrane→ossicles in middle ear→cochlea→auditory nerve (VIII)→auditory cortex in temporal lobe
   b. External ear
      1. pinna: external flap of cartilage covered with skin that gathers and concentrates sound waves
      2. external ear canal cavity in skull lined with skin; ceruminous glands produce cerumen (wax) to assist in protecting the canal from small foreign particles; conveys sound waves from pinna to tympanic membrane
      3. tympanic membrane: flexible membrane that closes distal end of external auditory canal; membrane vibrates in response to sound, transmitting vibrations to middle ear
   c. Middle ear
      1. ossicles: malleus, incus, and stapes
      2. set into motion by sound waves from tympanic membrane
      3. amplifies sound waves and transmits them to inner ear
      4. connected with nasopharynx by eustachian tube
   d. Inner ear
      1. cochlea: organ of sound perception
      2. innervated by the auditory nerve VIII
         a. cochlear branch: transmits auditory impulses from the cochlea to auditory cortex of brain
         b. vestibular branch: controls balance
   e. Auditory portion of cerebral cortex interprets auditory information (temporal lobe) (Fig. 3-25)
7. Nose
   a. Air passageway
   b. Contains sensory receptors for smell
   c. Lined with mucosa, hair
      1. secretes mucus
      2. filters, warms, and humidifies inspired air
   d. Paranasal sinuses drain into nasal cavity

APPLICATION OF THE NURSING PROCESS TO THE CLIENT WITH PROBLEMS OF SENSATION AND PERCEPTION

ASSESSMENT
1. Health history
   a. Family history
   b. History of problem: date of onset, precipitating factors, extent, duration or frequency, interventions that have been effective, location, any changes in description
   c. Headaches
   d. Seizures
   e. Medications: prescription and nonprescription
   f. Recent change in behavior or personality
2. Physical examination
   a. Neurologic examination
      1. cognitive function
         a. general behavior, emotional status

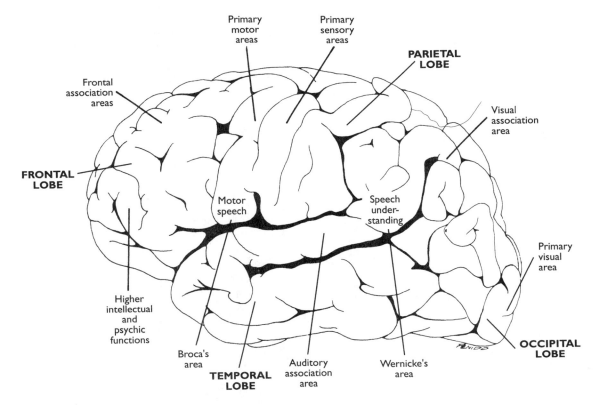

Fig. 3-25 Functional areas of the cerebrum.

b. level of consciousness (LOC): major index of client's neurologic status
c. attention span
d. ability to follow commands
e. memory: short- and long-term
f. arithmetic ability
g. abstract thinking
h. language/speech
  ▪ *motor aphasia* (expressive): inability to speak or write words
  ▪ *sensory aphasia* (receptive): inability to comprehend written words (visual) or spoken words (auditory)
  ▪ *dysarthria*: difficult speech caused by paralysis of muscles
2. cerebellar function
  a. balance
  b. coordination
3. motor function
  a. muscle size, tone, and strength
  b. involuntary movements (e.g., tremors)
  c. coordination and accuracy of movement
  d. motor integration
  e. bowel and bladder function
4. sensory function
  a. superficial sensation: touch and pressure
  b. superficial pain
  c. sensitivity to temperature and vibration
  d. deep pressure, pain
  e. motion and position sense
  f. vision
    ▪ amount of sight with or without glasses or contact lenses
    ▪ distortion
      • halos around lights
      • difficulty adjusting to dark room
      • diplopia
      • floaters
  g. hearing
    ▪ hearing acuity
      • use of hearing aid
      • tinnitus or other noises
    ▪ *conductive deafness* (common causes: otosclerosis, otitis media)
      • impairment of outer- and middle-ear conduction of sound waves
      • causes problems of perception of volume, not discrimination of sounds
      • can benefit from amplification of sound by a hearing aid
    ▪ *sensorineural deafness* (common causes: aging [presbycusis] noise, drug toxicity)
      • impairment of inner-ear nerve conduction
      • diminishes ability to hear high-frequency sounds (consonants)
      • hearing aid not as beneficial as for conductive deafness
    ▪ general speech pattern
    ▪ indications of hearing loss
      • says "huh" frequently
      • asks you to repeat what you said

• does not respond to questions or conversation
• responds inappropriately to questions or comments
5. reflexes: superficial and deep tendon
6. cranial nerves (see Table 3-53)
  b. Neurologic check
    1. LOC
      a. most reliable indicator of neurologic status
      b. Glascow Coma scale (GCS): quantitative assessment of LOC (Table 3-55)
    2. vital signs
    3. pupils: size and reaction to light
    4. motor function
      a. move all extremities
      b. muscle strength (grip)
    5. sensory function: response to touch or painful stimuli
    6. seizures
    7. blood or cerebrospinal fluid (CSF) leakage from nose or ears
    8. posturing (pathologic motor responses)
      a. *decorticate posture* (corticospinal tract): rigid flexion of arms, wrists, and fingers with adduction of upper extremities, and extension with internal rotation of legs (Fig. 3-26)
      b. *decerebrate posture* (midbrain and pons): rigid extension of neck, back, arms, and legs, with hyperpronation of arms and plantar flexion of feet (Fig. 3-27); prognosis grave
3. Diagnostic tests
  a. Lumbar puncture (LP)
    1. description

Table 3-55 Glasgow Coma Scale

	Score
Eyes open	
Spontaneously	4
To speech	3
To pain	2
No response	1
Motor response (to painful stimuli)	
Obeys verbal command	6
Localizes pain	5
Flexion withdrawal	4
Flexion abnormal	3
Extension abnormal	2
No response	1
Verbal response	
Oriented	5
Conversation confused	4
Inappropriate speech	3
Incomprehensible sounds	2
No response	1

Best (highest) response is recorded.
Eye, motor, and verbal scores are totaled.
Range: 3-15.
Poor prognosis (low score <3-4); good prognosis (score >8).

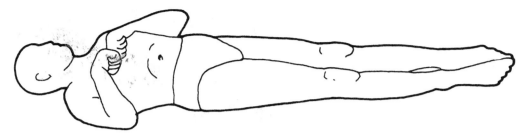

Fig. 3-26   Decorticate posturing.

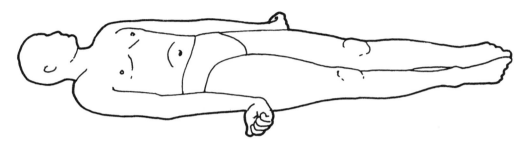

Fig. 3-27   Decerebrate posturing.

a. collection of CSF, measurement of pressure and characteristics of spinal fluid
b. Queckenstedt's test can be done during LP: with manometer still in place, compress jugular veins for 10 seconds
  ▪ normal response: rise in spinal fluid pressure of approximately 100 mm H_2O within 10 seconds, and return to normal within 30 seconds after compression is removed
  ▪ abnormal response: drop in spinal fluid pressure or no rise in pressure; indicates complete obstruction of flow of spinal fluid
2. nursing care
  a. explain procedure carefully to client before procedure
  b. position client on side with legs flexed onto abdomen and head bent down
  c. keep client flat in bed up to 24 hours after test to avoid a headache caused by fluid-tension change
  d. observe CSF characteristics
  e. force fluids to replace loss and restore fluid balance
  f. observe for headache
b. Radiologic exams
  1. x-rays of skull and spine
  2. computerized tomography (CT) scanning
    a. description: 360-degree photographed view of brain in 1-degree angles; provides data on integrity of intracranial structures and precise location of abnormalities; used with or without contrast medium
    b. nursing care
      ▪ explain procedure to client beforehand
      ▪ know client needs to lie still on table for 30-60 minutes

3. magnetic resonance imaging (MRI)
  a. description: noninvasive scan by which body structures are imaged by use of a magnetic field
  b. contraindications
    ▪ obesity
    ▪ pregnancy
    ▪ claustrophobia, confusion, agitation
    ▪ implanted metal devices (e.g., pacemaker, aneurysm clips, inner ear implants)
  c. nursing care
    ▪ explain procedure to client
    ▪ instruct client to expect loud machine noise (ear plugs or earphones may be offered)
    ▪ remove all metal (e.g., watches, jewelry)
4. myelogram (see Mobility, p. 246)
5. brain scan
  a. description: after administration of oral or IV radiopharmaceutical, the head is scanned and uptake of the material is recorded
  b. nursing care
    ▪ explain procedure to client
    ▪ reassure about temporary radioactivity
6. cerebral arteriogram
  a. description: injection of a radiopaque dye through a catheter inserted into femoral, carotid, or vertebral artery; aortic arch; or brachial vessels to study cerebral circulation
  b. nursing care
    ▪ explain procedure and posttest routine to client before test
    ▪ ensure that pretest baseline neurologic status is documented
    ▪ check for allergies to iodine and report if present
    ▪ remove hairpins and dentures as ordered

- bed rest 8 to 24 hours after test, with head of bed elevated 30 degrees
- check incision for hemorrhage, hematoma
- maintain pressure dressing to incision site if femoral or brachial artery used; apply ice bag to reduce swelling
- watch for symptoms of sensitivity to dye (urticaria, pallor, respiratory difficulty) and report immediately
- watch for neurologic changes that indicate emboli in cerebrovascular system (limb weakness or paralysis, facial paralysis, speech difficulty, disorientation, change in level of consciousness); report changes immediately
- observe and record vital signs and neurologic signs according to protocol (usually q15min until stable, then qh for several hours, then q4h)

c. EEG
  1. description: study of electrical activity of brain
  2. nursing care
     a. give information to client to allay fear of being electrocuted
     b. clean client's hair before the test
     c. have client remain on anticonvulsant
     d. have client eat meal before test (fasting affects electric pattern) but avoid stimulants (e.g., coffee, tea, cola, cocoa)
     e. tell client to remain calm and quiet during the test
     f. remove EEG paste from hair after test
d. Electromyogram (see Mobility, p. 247)
e. Eye tests
  1. Snellen test (eye chart) (see Nursing Care of the Child, p. 409)
  2. ophthalmoscopic exam
  3. intraocular pressure (normal: 12 to 20 mm Hg)
f. Ear/hearing tests
  1. otoscopic exam
  2. whisper test for gross hearing: cover the ear not being tested and whisper words into the other ear or hold a ticking watch near the ear
  3. audiogram
     a. client wears earphones in soundproof room and signals when tone is heard, when tone disappears, and in which ear the tone is heard
     b. hearing is measured in *intensity* (dB = decibels) and *frequency* (cps = cycles per second or Hz = hertz)
  4. Weber and Rinne tests (see Nursing Care of the Child, p. 410)
g. Nose/sense of smell tests: provide various scents for client to identify with eyes closed (e.g., alcohol, chocolate, tobacco)
h. Mouth and throat/sense of taste tests: provide various things for client to taste with eyes closed (e.g., chocolate, peppermint)

ANALYSIS/NURSING DIAGNOSIS
1. Safe, effective care environment
   a. Risk for injury
   b. Knowledge deficit
   c. Sensory-perceptual alteration (specify)
   d. Decreased adaptive capacity intracranial
2. Physiologic integrity
   a. Risk for activity intolerance
   b. Risk for aspiration
   c. Pain
   d. Impaired physical mobility
   e. Ineffective breathing pattern
   f. Impaired verbal communication
   g. Hyperthermia
3. Psychosocial integrity
   a. Fear
   b. Altered thought processes
   c. Social isolation
4. Health promotion/maintenance
   a. Altered family process
   b. Altered health maintenance
   c. Knowledge deficit (specify)
   d. Self-care deficit

GENERAL NURSING PLANNING, IMPLEMENTATION, AND EVALUATION

Goal I Client will be free from increased intracranial pressure.

Implementation
1. Monitor for early signs of increased intracranial pressure (ICP)
   a. Decreasing level of consciousness
   b. Vital signs changes
      1. BP: widening of pulse pressure (systolic increases, diastolic remains the same)
      2. rise in temperature with failing thermoregulator
      3. bradycardia
      4. slow, deep, irregular respirations
   c. Pupils: unequal, progressing to fixed and dilated.
   d. Other clinical signs and symptoms (classic triad)
      1. headache (generalized)
      2. projectile vomiting
      3. papilledema
2. Assess at least q15min.
3. Administer osmotic diuretics (e.g., mannitol) as ordered (see Table 3-45), then monitor urine output qh.
4. Keep client slightly dehydrated to reduce or prevent cerebral edema.
5. Administer corticosteroid therapy, if ordered.
6. Prevent transient increases in intracranial pressure.
   a. Elevate head of bed 15 to 30 degrees.
   b. Avoid neck flexion.
   c. Maintain calm environment.
   d. Avoid Valsalva's maneuver (straining).
   e. Administer stool softeners, and teach client not to strain with bowel evacuation.
   f. Avoid bending over, coughing, sneezing, or vomiting.
   g. Avoid isometric contraction of muscles (e.g., pushing up in bed on elbows, pressing feet against a footboard).

Evaluation

Client's intracranial pressure remains within normal limits (5 to 10 mm Hg).

Goal 2 Client will remain free from complications of unconsciousness.

Implementation

1. See General Nursing Goal 4, Mobility, p. 247.
2. Prevent contractures and immobile joints (e.g., use range-of-motion exercises).
3. Keep skin clean, dry, and intact.
4. Keep mucous membranes clean, moist, and intact.
5. Maintain adequate bowel and bladder function.
6. Ensure normal respiratory function (e.g., turn client frequently).
7. Provide safe environment (e.g., bed side rails).
8. Insert NG tube and administer tube feedings as ordered.
    a. Place client in high-Fowler's position for tube insertion.
    b. Check to be sure tube is in stomach and not lungs. (Aspirate gastric contents and test aspirant for acidity with litmus paper; inject 10 ml of air into tube while listening with stethoscope over gastric area for swishing sound.)
    c. Know that client will probably be given no more than 2 L per day of liquid feeding with a concentration of 0.5-1 kcal/ml.
    d. Give feeding at room temperature.
    e. Give feeding at slow rate.
    f. Observe for regurgitation during and after feeding.
    g. Observe for gastric retention.
    h. Irrigate tube with water after each feeding if feedings are intermittent.
9. Administer TPN as ordered (see Table 3-28).
10. Check tissue hydration.
11. Monitor fluid and electrolyte balance.
12. Prevent corneal damage (e.g., use eye patches as needed).
13. Maintain communication with client.

Evaluation

Client is free from contractures, immobile joints, pressure sores, fecal impactions, respiratory distress, injuries, malnutrition, and fluid and electrolyte imbalances.

Goal 3 Client with aphasia will maximize ability to use and understand written and spoken words.

Implementation

1. Determine client's level of understanding.
2. Determine client's use of speech or communication skills.
3. Use gestures if client understands that method best.
4. Use aids to increase and improve communication: word cards, pictures, slate boards, and audiotapes.
5. Talk slowly using natural tone (do not abbreviate; reducing sentences to a shorter, incomplete form does not help comprehension).
6. Use simple words and phrases.

7. Allow client time to respond; be patient.
8. Listen and watch carefully when the client attempts to communicate.
9. Keep distractions to a minimum.
10. Maintain a calm, accepting manner.
11. Sit level with client and maintain eye contact.
12. Arrange for referral to speech therapist as needed.

Evaluation

Client attempts to communicate using written and spoken words.

Goal 4 Disabled client will function as independently as possible.

Implementation

1. Determine client's strengths and deficits.
2. Establish realistic, long-range goals with client and significant other.
3. Devise measures with client to achieve goals.
    a. Institute measures for gaining bowel and bladder control if necessary.
    b. Arrange for physical therapy.
    c. Arrange for occupational therapy and recreational therapy.
    d. Give client and significant others emotional support (e.g., adapting to altered body image; see Loss and Death and Dying, p. 29).
    e. Refer to appropriate community agency.

Evaluation

Client performs ADL, to extent possible, without assistance.

Goal 5 Client will adapt to visual deficits.

Implementation

1. Call client by name when approaching.
2. Identify yourself when approaching client.
3. Communicate in usual manner.
4. Ambulate with client.
5. Teach client
    a. How to summon staff.
    b. Where possessions are.
    c. Physical layout of room.
    d. Placement of food on tray.
    e. Arrangement of food on plate.
    f. Use of cane to aid in walking.
6. Provide meaningful sensory input.
    a. Interaction with staff and significant others
    b. Radio, records, and TV
    c. Physical exercise
7. Provide safe environment (e.g., remove unnecessary equipment).
8. Encourage and reinforce client's independence.
9. Refer to appropriate community agency.

Evaluation

Client functions in hospital environment without difficulty.

Goal 6 Client will adapt to hearing loss.

Implementation

1. Face client when speaking.
2. Keep light on speaker's mouth so client can watch mouth of speaker.
3. Speak with normal speech pattern.
4. Supplement speech with gestures.
5. Speak slowly; allow more time than usual for communication.
6. Remove background noise (e.g., turn down TV sound).
7. Help client obtain hearing aid, if appropriate.

Evaluation

Client responds to spoken directions appropriately.

SELECTED HEALTH PROBLEMS RESULTING IN AN INTERFERENCE WITH NEUROLOGIC FUNCTION

✷ ACUTE HEAD INJURY

1. Clients with acute head trauma need close scrutiny immediately after trauma; shock is rarely seen
2. Common types
   a. *Concussion:* no structural alteration, but immediate and transitory impairment of neurologic function resulting from mechanical force and release of enzymes
   b. *Contusion:* structural alteration (bruised cortex) characterized by extravasation of blood
   c. *Laceration:* a tear in brain tissue or blood vessel
   d. *Hemorrhage*
      1. extradural or epidural: arterial blood collects between skull and dura rapidly; usually results from a tear in an artery
         a. may lose consciousness and regain it temporarily
         b. within a few hours, rapid deterioration: lethargy, coma, hemiplegia
      2. subdural: venous bleeding (hematoma) below dura accompanied by manifestations of increased ICP
         a. acute: develops within few days after injury; surgical intervention needed
         b. subacute: develops between few days to 3 weeks; surgical intervention follows
         c. chronic: develops weeks to months after injury

Nursing Process

ASSESSMENT (refer to Neurologic Exam, p. 221)
ANALYSIS/NURSING DIAGNOSIS (see p. 224)
PLANNING, IMPLEMENTATION, AND EVALUATION

Goal 1 Client will have an open airway at all times.

Implementation

1. Establish and maintain airway.
2. Position client for optimum ventilation.
3. Maintain adequate O_2 level through use of respiratory aids as necessary.

Evaluation

Client's airway remains unobstructed; color is normal; arterial blood gases are within normal limits.

Goal 2 Client will be protected from increasing intracranial pressure.

Implementation

1. Refer to General Nursing Goal 1, p. 224.

Evaluation

Client is free from papilledema; maintains normal vital signs and stable LOC.

Goal 3 Client will maintain optimal fluid and electrolyte status.

Implementation

1. Monitor and record I&O.
2. Administer IV fluids as ordered (fluids are usually restricted because of fear of increased intracranial pressure).
3. Give osmotic diuretics (e.g., mannitol) as ordered (see Table 3-45).
4. Monitor: serum electrolytes (hyponatremia or hypernatremia [see Table 3-42]); syndrome of inappropriate antidiuretic hormone [(SIADH); see Table 3-32]; elevated plasma cortisol.

Evaluation

Client's output remains greater than intake.

Goal 4 Client will have any CSF or blood draining from nose or ears detected.

Implementation

1. Observe and record at least qh any leak of blood or clear fluid from nose or ears.
2. Do not pack nose or ears; have fluid drain onto sterile towel or dressing.
3. Report to physician immediately if any drainage is found.

Evaluation

Client remains free from CSF or blood leakage from nose and ears.

Goal 5 Client will be free from infection or injuries.

Implementation

1. Protect from chilling.
2. Take seizure precautions: use bed with padded side rails, have a nonmetal airway and suction apparatus at bedside. (See Seizure Disorders, p. 441.)
3. Employ aseptic technique during all invasive procedures.
4. Do not permit visitors with respiratory infections.

Evaluation

Client remains afebrile; has skin and mucous membranes free from cuts, ecchymosis, and abrasions.

✠ INTRACRANIAL SURGERY

1. Definition: surgery performed inside the cranial cavity
   a. *Craniotomy:* any operation on the cranium
      1. tentorium: fold of dura mater between cerebellum and occipital lobes
      2. supratentorial: above the cerebellum (e.g., cerebrum, anterior two thirds of brain)
      3. infratentorial: posterior cranial fossa (e.g., cerebellum, brainstem, posterior third of brain)
   b. *Cranioplasty:* repair of cranial defect by inserting a bone graft or a plate made of a synthetic substance; protects the brain from trauma
2. Reasons for surgery
   a. To debride or repair any trauma to the skull and underlying structures
   b. To control intracranial hemorrhage (e.g., aneurysms)
   c. To remove space-occupying lesions (e.g., scar tissue, abscess, tumor)
   d. Intracranial neoplasms
      1. all potentially fatal unless treated because of lack of space within skull
      2. more than 50% are malignant
      3. types
         a. gliomas (within brain substance)
         b. meningiomas (external to brain substance)

Nursing Process

ASSESSMENT
1. Establish baseline data preoperatively (refer to Neurologic Exam, p. 221)
2. Client and significant others' knowledge of procedure and expected outcome

ANALYSIS/NURSING DIAGNOSIS (see p. 224)

PLANNING, IMPLEMENTATION, AND EVALUATION

Goal 1 Client and significant others will be able to explain preoperative and postoperative care, and OR-PACU-ICU environment and care.

Implementation
1. Refer to Perioperative Period, p. 115.
2. Prepare client for the likelihood of postoperative periocular edema and photophobia.

Evaluation
Client and significant others describe planned procedure and postoperative routine.

Goal 2 Client will be physically prepared for surgery.

Implementation
1. Refer to Perioperative Period, p. 115.
2. Know that narcotics are contraindicated preoperatively.
3. Prepare scalp.
   a. Wash hair.
   b. Cut hair (save according to agency policy); shave scalp.
   c. Wash head and cover with clean towel.
4. Ensure that baseline neurologic status is measured and documented.

5. Carry out any special order (e.g., insert indwelling Foley catheter, give enemas slowly to avoid straining and increased intracranial pressure).

Evaluation
Client is physically prepared for surgery correctly.

Goal 3 Client will remain free from respiratory, circulatory, renal, neurologic, or psychologic complications or any infections postoperatively.

Implementation
1. Refer to Perioperative Period, p. 115.
2. Perform frequent neurologic checks; compare with preoperative baseline (refer to neurologic exam, p. 221).
3. Observe for seizures.
4. Monitor breathing; client must not cough.
5. Support head when turning client.
6. Position properly and frequently.
   a. Supratentorial craniotomy: do not position on operative site if large tumor was excised; elevate head 45 degrees.
   b. Infratentorial craniotomy: keep head of bed flat and client's head aligned with vertebral column at all times; position on either side for first 24 hours, not on back; avoid flexion of neck (danger of brainstem compression).
7. Do not suction through nose.
8. Do not use central nervous system depressants (e.g., opiates, sedatives).
9. Check ears, nose, and dressing for drainage (blood or CSF leakage).
10. Change dressings only when ordered; reinforce as needed.
11. Use strict aseptic technique for all dressings and other procedures.
12. Assess periocular edema; relieve with ice packs.
13. Administer steroids (e.g., dexamethasone sodium [Decadron]) as ordered to prevent or relieve cerebral edema (see Table 3-20).
14. Do not take oral temperatures.
15. Give passive ROM exercises q8h.

Evaluation
Client remains free from complications in the postoperative period.

Goal 4 Client and significant others will accept lengthy rehabilitation period.

Implementation
1. See General Nursing Goal 4, p. 225.
2. Inform client of residual effects that may be temporary (e.g., diplopia) or permanent (e.g., aphasia, paralysis).
3. Inform client of cosmetic aids available when indicated (e.g., hairpiece.)
4. Prevent client from striking or bumping head.

Evaluation
Client and significant others express willingness to participate in rehabilitation program; verbalize understanding of the need for patience and persistence.

✠ CEREBROVASCULAR ACCIDENT (CVA)

1. Definition: sudden development of neurologic deficits caused by an abrupt, severe decrease in cerebral circulation by either a thrombus, embolus, or hemorrhage that causes a cerebral infarct; also called a stroke
2. Types
   a. Hemorrhagic (20%)
      1. intracranial
      2. subarachnoid
   b. Ischemic (80%)
      1. thrombus
      2. embolus
3. Incidence
   a. Third leading cause of death in the United States
   b. Leading cause of serious disability in the United States
   c. Age
      1. 20 to 60 years, ruptured aneurysm most common
      2. 60 to 69 years, thrombosis most common
4. Symptoms depend on
   a. Location of the infarct (see Fig. 3-25)
   b. Amount of collateral circulation to affected area of the brain
   c. Type of pathophysiology involved
5. Risk factors
   a. Hypertension—chief risk factor of CVA
   b. Arteriosclerosis/atherosclerosis
   c. Intracranial aneurysms
   d. Diabetes mellitus
   e. Peripheral vascular disease
6. Etiology
   a. Rupture of the wall of a cerebral artery (aneurysm)
   b. Trauma to a cerebral artery
   c. Severe spasm of a cerebral artery
   d. Embolus or thrombus blocking a cerebral artery

Nursing Process

ASSESSMENT
1. Refer to Neurologic Exam, p. 221, and areas of the brain that control certain motor and sensory functions (see Fig. 3-25)
2. Hemiplegia (paralysis) or hemiparesis (muscular weakness)
3. Aphasia (most common with left cerebral infarct)
4. Ataxia (staggering gait)
5. Nuchal rigidity (with hemorrhage)
6. Perceptual deficit
7. Emotional lability
8. Emotional needs of clients and significant others
9. Results of diagnostic studies
   a. CT scan
   b. MRI
   c. Cerebral arteriogram (angiogram)
   d. Digital subtraction angiography (DSA) used in selected cases
   e. Lumbar puncture

ANALYSIS/NURSING DIAGNOSIS (see p. 224)
PLANNING, IMPLEMENTATION, AND EVALUATION

Goal 1 Client will be free from any additional cerebral damage.

Implementation
1. Monitor neurologic status frequently until stable.
2. Do not stimulate cough.
3. Give passive ROM.
4. If thrombus is cause of CVA administer vasodilators and anticoagulants as ordered (see Tables 3-7 and 3-8).
5. If hemorrhage is cause of CVA
   a. Elevate head of bed 30 to 45 degrees (to improve venous drainage).
   b. Turn *gently* to *unaffected* side.
   c. Decrease environmental stimuli (e.g., keep room in semidarkness).
   d. Maintain complete bed rest until bleeding has been controlled and client's condition is stable.

Evaluation
Client remains stable, free from additional cerebral damage.

Goal 2 Client will ingest adequate fluids and food.

Implementation
1. Help client feed self as needed.
2. Provide adequate fluids to maintain skin turgor and sufficient output.
3. Give small, frequent feedings as indicated (more easily tolerated than three large meals).
4. Administer tube feedings if client is unable to take food and fluids orally (see General Nursing Goal 2, p. 225).
5. Monitor electrolyte levels.

Evaluation
Client's weight remains stable; skin turgor is normal; urinary output is greater than 30 ml/hr; urine is clear, straw colored, free from pus and blood.

Goal 3 If unconscious, client will remain free from complications (refer to General Nursing Goal 2, p. 225).

Goal 4 Client will become as independent as possible.

Implementation
1. Refer to General Nursing Goals 3 and 4, p. 225.
2. Explain prognosis: lengthy rehabilitation, potential lifetime implications.
3. Expect labile emotions (depression is common).
4. Prevent deformities.
5. Make referral to speech therapist as indicated.
6. Arrange for gait training; if fatigued from exercises, monitor for potential injury.

Evaluation
Client participates in rehabilitation activities; regains ability to walk.

✠ MENINGITIS
See Nursing Care of the Child, p. 443

✠ SPINAL CORD INJURIES (SCI)

1. Definition: fracture or displacement of one or more vertebrae, causing damage to spinal cord and nerve roots with resulting neurologic deficit (altered sensory percep-

tion, paralysis, or both). There will be total or partial absence of motor or sensory function below the level of the injury.
2. Incidence: estimated 10,000 to 20,000 people affected annually; usually younger age group.
3. Predisposing factors:
   a. Trauma: car or motorcycle accidents, falls, or diving accidents
   b. Tumors
   c. Congenital defects; spina bifida
   d. Infectious and degenerative diseases
   e. Ruptured intervertebral disks
4. Types of injuries:
   a. Fracture of vertebral body (excessive vertical compression)
   b. Compression of vertebral body (excessive flexion of vertebral column)
   c. Spinal malalignment or vertebral body displacement (rotational injury)
   d. Partial or complete dislocation of one vertebra onto another
   e. Disruption of intervertebral disk and compressed interspinous ligament (hyperextension injury)
5. Most common sites are cervical and lumbar vertebrae.
6. Immediately after an accident, care must be taken to prevent further neurologic damage while patent airway and circulation are maintained.

Nursing Process

ASSESSMENT
1. Respiratory function
2. Cardiovascular function
3. Loss of sensation and motor function in body parts below injury level (Table 3-56)
4. Loss of perspiration below injury level with resultant inability to cool body (autonomic responses become unpredictable)
5. Bowel and bladder control (assess for paralytic ileus and urinary retention)
6. Pain
7. Edema
8. Nutritional status
9. Fever
10. Psychologic needs
11. Remaining sensory and motor function
12. Diagnostic tests
    a. Neurologic exam
    b. X-ray of spine

ANALYSIS/NURSING DIAGNOSIS (see p. 224)
PLANNING, IMPLEMENTATION, AND EVALUATION

Goal 1 Client will be free from further injury to spinal cord.

Implementation
1. Immobilize the head and entire spine.
2. Keep client's body and head in alignment.
3. "Log-roll" client if moving is necessary.
4. Use specialized equipment for turning: Stryker frame, Foster frame, or CircOlectric bed.
5. Apply cervical traction for cervical lesion.
6. Know that a laminectomy may be done to prevent further compression of spinal cord.
7. Administer steroids (dexamethasone sodium [Decadron]) or osmotic diuretic (e.g., mannitol) IV as ordered, to reduce cerebral and spinal cord edema (see Tables 3-20 and 3-45).

Evaluation
Client shows no signs of progression of paralysis.

Goal 2 Client will maintain adequate respiratory function.

Implementation
1. Observe respirations frequently (client may have spontaneous respirations after an accident but lose them later).
2. Maintain respiratory function through use of a respirator if necessary.
3. If respirations are spontaneous, have client deep breathe and cough qh.
4. Care for and suction secretions from tracheostomy tube if in place. (Refer to Tracheostomy Care, Goal 3, p. 151)

Evaluation
Client's respiratory rate remains within normal limits.

Goal 3 Client will be free from undetected spinal shock.

Implementation
1. Expect spinal shock to develop 30 to 60 minutes after injury and to last from 2 to 3 days to 3 months.
2. Observe for signs and symptoms caused by suppression

Table 3-56 Spinal cord

Area of spinal cord	Gross movements controlled
Upper cervical	Neck and head movement; elevation of the shoulders.
Middle cervical	Movement of the upper arms and forearms, diaphragmatic breathing.
Lower cervical	Movements of fingers and hands.
Thoracic	Intercostal muscles involved in respiration; muscles involved in abdominal contractions.
Upper lumbar	Leg flexion at hip; adduction of thigh.
Lower lumbar	Remaining thigh movements; movements in lower legs.
Sacral	Foot and toe movements; sphincter and perineal muscle contraction.

of reflexes at all spinal segments below the level of injury.
   a. Hypotension
   b. Dyspnea
   c. Flaccid paralysis
   d. Urinary retention
   e. Absence of sweating
3. Administer colloid fluids and analgesics prn as ordered.

Evaluation

Client's spinal shock is detected promptly.

Goal 4 Client with a cervical or high-thoracic injury will remain free from life-threatening autonomic dysreflexia.

Implementation

1. Observe for signs and symptoms caused by marked sympathetic stimulation.
   a. Severe hypertension
   b. Bradycardia (30 to 40 beats per minute)
   c. Severe pounding headache
   d. Flushing
   e. Diaphoresis
   f. Piloerection
2. Take preventive measures.
   a. Prevent bladder distention and colorectal impaction (most common precipitating causes of autonomic dysreflexia).
   b. Maintain urinary drainage from patent catheter.
   c. Prevent pressure sores, pain in lower extremities, or pressure on penis or testes when client is in prone position.
3. Initiate treatment immediately (medical emergency).
   a. Check the bladder for distention and colorectal impaction.
   b. Look for stimuli other than bladder distention or colorectal impaction (e.g., cold air, drafts, sharp objects pressing on skin below level of injury).
   c. Remove the cause (e.g., empty bladder by catheterization or irrigation of Foley catheter).
   d. Elevate head of bed to lower blood pressure.
   e. Administer antihypertensive ganglionic blocking agent (e.g., trimethaphan [Arfonad]) as ordered.

Evaluation

Client remains free from autonomic dysreflexia; maintains bowel and bladder function.

Goal 5 Client will ingest adequate fluids and nutrition.

Implementation

1. Give liquid diet until possibility of paralytic ileus has passed, then diet as tolerated.
2. Administer vitamin supplements as ordered.
3. Encourage fluid intake.
4. Monitor I&O.

Evaluation

Client's weight remains within desired range; skin turgor is normal.

Goal 6 Client will be free from urinary tract infection.

Implementation

1. Insert Foley catheter or use intermittent catheterization as ordered, using sterile technique.
2. Give aseptic care to Foley catheter.
3. Observe client for signs of bladder infection (e.g., fever; abnormal urinalysis [UA].
4. Encourage fluid intake to 3 L per day.
5. Observe odor, appearance, and amount of urine.
6. Monitor I&O carefully.

Evaluation

Client's urinary catheter drains normal urine; client has no fever.

Goal 7 Client will be free from stress ulcer.

Implementation

1. Monitor for complaints of ulcerlike pain.
2. Observe for melena, hematemesis.
3. Administer antacids and peptic ulcer drugs as ordered to prevent gastric irritation (see Table 3-26).

Evaluation

Client has no abdominal pain; has stools negative for occult blood.

Goal 8 Client will be free from pain in paralyzed limbs.

Implementation

1. Handle the affected limbs gently to avoid muscle spasms.
2. Identify and eliminate stimuli that cause spasms.
3. Medicate as ordered to control spasms and pain.

Evaluation

Client experiences relief of pain in affected limb.

Goal 9 Client will become as independent as possible. Refer to General Nursing Goal 4, p. 225.

PARKINSON'S SYNDROME (PARKINSONISM)

1. Definition: a progressive debilitating syndrome in which there is degeneration of nerve cells in the basal ganglia that impairs (Table 3-57)
   a. Important centers of coordination, especially control of associated automatic movements
   b. Control of muscle tone to produce finely coordinated movements
   c. Control of initiation and inhibition of gross, intentional movements
2. Incidence: one of the major causes of neurologic disability; estimated to affect more than a half-million people in the United States; more common in men
3. Onset: usually 50 to 60 years of age
4. Etiology
   a. Unknown
   b. It is hypothesized that these clients have a deficiency

Table 3-57   Comparison of chronic degenerative neurologic diseases

	Parkinsonism	Multiple sclerosis	Amyotrophic lateral sclerosis	Myasthenia gravis
Onset age	50-60 years	20-40 years	40-70 years	20-50 years
Sex	Male > female	Female > male	Male > female	Female > male
Etiology	Unknown	Unknown; virus/ autoimmune origin suspected	Unknown; virus/ autoimmune origin suspected	Unknown; autoimmune origin suspected; occurs in cool climates
Area affected	Substantia nigra cells in basal ganglia	Disseminated demyelinated plaques in white matter of brain and spinal cord	Motor neurons in brain and spinal cord	Myoneural junction of voluntary muscle
Pathophysiology	Impaired coordinated muscle movement and autonomic dysfunction because of deficiency of dopamine	Impaired nerve impulse conduction because of destruction of myelin	Impaired nerve impulse conduction because of degeneration of motor neurons	Impaired transmission of nerve impulse to skeletal muscle possibly because of acetylcholine deficiency
Signs and symptoms	Rigidity Slow movements Nonintentional tremor Autonomic dysfunction	Depends on site of plaque: Visual problems Spastic weakness/ paralysis Poor coordination Paresthesias Speech defects Intentional tremor Bowel/bladder dysfunction Emotional disorders Exacerbations and remissions	Twitching Muscle weakness, progressing to atrophy and paralysis of upper and lower extremities Usually fatal 2-15 years after onset	Profound muscle weakness and fatigue Can progress to respiratory failure (myasthenic crisis)
Treatment	Supportive Medication	Symptomatic	Symptomatic	Supportive Medication Surgery sometimes: thymectomy
Medication	Levodopa Carbidopa/levodopa (Sinemet)	Muscle relaxants Antiinflammatory (steroid) during exacerbation	Antibiotics for respiratory and urinary tract infections	Anticholinesterase: Diagnosis—Edrophonium chloride (Tensilon) Maintenance— Pyridostigmine bromide (Mestinon) Antiinflammatory (steroids) during acute phase

of dopamine, which is required for normal functioning of the basal ganglia; drug therapy aims at returning dopamine levels to normal to control symptoms of the syndrome

5. Precipitating factors
   a. Drug induced: phenothiazines and rauwolfia alkaloids
   b. Atherosclerosis
   c. Trauma (e.g., midbrain compression)
   d. Encephalitis
   e. Toxic poisoning: carbon monoxide

Nursing Process
ASSESSMENT
1. Muscle rigidity
   a. Major disability
   b. Bradykinesia and akinesia
2. Resting tremor (nonintentional)
   a. Especially of hands (pill rolling), arms, and head
   b. Rhythmic: regular and rapid
3. Facial mask
4. Speech difficulty
5. Difficulty chewing and swallowing (drooling)
6. Loss of automatic movements (e.g., blinking of eyes)
7. Shuffling propulsive gait
8. Emotional changes (mood disturbances), depression, and confusion
9. Autonomic nervous system dysfunction
   a. Perspiration, heat intolerance
   b. Increased lacrimation (tearing)
   c. Constipation

d. Incontinence
e. Decreased sexual activity
ANALYSIS/NURSING DIAGNOSIS (see p. 224)
PLANNING, IMPLEMENTATION, AND EVALUATION

Goal 1 Client will have optimal function of muscles and joints.

Implementation
1. Administer prescribed medications (Table 3-58).
2. Observe for side effects of medications.
3. Help client remain as active as possible (see General Nursing Goal 4, p. 225).
   a. Frequent ambulation
   b. Attention to grooming
Evaluation
Client maintains movement in muscles and joints; continues to ambulate and participate in ADL.

Goal 2 Client will be free from injury.

Implementation
1. Use ambulatory aids such as hand rails in all rooms and near bathtub or shower.
2. Instruct client to walk slowly and carefully.
3. Balance activity and rest to avoid fatigue.
Evaluation
Client is free from cuts, abrasions, and falls.

Goal 3 Client will maintain gastrointestinal integrity.

Implementation
1. Provide adequate fluid intake.
2. Give high-fiber diet.
3. Restrict protein as indicated.
4. Observe for constipation.
5. Administer stool softeners or laxatives as ordered prn (see Table 3-49).
6. Give oral hygiene to relieve dryness of the mouth.
7. Keep urinal and bedpan available in case client is unable to reach bathroom in time.

Table 3-58 Drugs used to treat parkinsonism

Name	Action	Side effects	Nursing implications
Levodopa (Larodopa)	Converts to dopamine in basal ganglia	Gastrointestinal irritation (e.g., nausea, anorexia, vomiting); gastrointestinal hemorrhage; psychiatric symptoms; orthostatic hypotension	Begin with low dosage; gradually increase to therapeutic level. Give medication with meals. Use cautiously in clients with cardiovascular, respiratory, endocrine, or hepatic peptic ulcer disease. Avoid vitamin B_6 (reverses effects of levodopa).
Carbidopa and levodopa (Sinemet)	Combined drugs provide same action as above at lower levels	Same as levodopa	Same as levodopa.
Amantadine (Symmetrel)	Unknown	Restlessness; mental and emotional changes	Well tolerated (less effective than levodopa).
Trihexyphenidyl (Artane)	Anticholinergic: blocks muscarinic receptors at cholinergic synapses with CNS; relieves tremor, rigidity. Minimal effect on akinesia	Dry mouth; blurred vision; constipation; urinary retention; mental dullness, confusion. Sudden withdrawal precipitates sudden, incapacitating increase in symptoms	Begin using small doses; increase dosages gradually. Avoid sudden withdrawal of medications; withdrawal of drug reverses side effects. Monitor client with psychosis, wide-angle glaucoma, diabetes. Administer after meals to avoid GI irritation.
Procyclidine (Kemadrin)	Same as trihexyphenidyl	Same as trihexyphenidyl	Same as trihexyphenidyl.
Benztropine mesylate (Cogentin)	Same as trihexyphenidyl	Same as trihexyphenidyl	Same as trihexyphenidyl.
Selegiline hydrochloride (L-deprenyl or Eldepryl)	Irreversibly, selectively inhibits monoamine oxidase type B	May exacerbate parkinsonism manifestations. Toxicity: nausea, dizziness, fainting	Used to delay the onset of severe disability in clients in early stages of parkinsonism; can be given with Sinemet. Avoid concurrent use of meperidine; interacts with L-deprenyl; rapidly absorbed and metabolized.

Evaluation

Client is free from constipation and impactions; has adequate bowel function.

> **Goal 4** Client will maintain positive body image and self-concept.

Implementation

1. Provide devices to assist in ADL.
2. Teach about or provide clothes that are simple and easy to put on.
3. Allow sufficient time for meals.
4. In general, do not hurry client.
5. Supervise and assist in skin care and personal hygiene.
6. Allow expression of depression and hopelessness (Refer to Depression, Nursing Care of the Client with Psychosocial and Mental Health Problems, p. 51).
7. Reward client's attempts at activity.
8. Arrange for speech therapy for dysarthria.
9. Refer to community agency (e.g., American Parkinson's Disease Association).

Evaluation

Client's grooming projects positive self-concept; client accepts responsibility for ADL to the fullest extent possible.

> **Goal 5** Client and significant others will express fears and other feelings about the present and future.

Implementation

1. Assess level of anxiety.
2. Give emotional support and relieve anxiety (see Anxious Behavior, p. 34).
3. Explain disease and drug therapy.
4. Clarify misconceptions and lack of information.
5. Explain prognosis.

Evaluation

Client and significant others express feelings (e.g., fear, sadness, anger); state realistic expectations for the future.

✠ MULTIPLE SCLEROSIS

1. Definition: chronic progressive disease of the central nervous system characterized by unpredictable exacerbations and remissions; typically, demyelinization of the white matter of the spinal cord and brain occurs in multiple areas (see Table 3-57)
2. Incidence
   a. Disease of young adults
   b. More common in women
3. Risk factors
   a. Living in the temperate zone 40 to 60 degrees north or south of the equator
   b. Higher incidence among higher socioeconomic classes
4. Etiology
   a. Unknown
   b. May be a virus that is latent for months or years before some other factor initiates disease
   c. Possibly an autoimmune disorder
   d. Mineral deficiency or toxic substances

Nursing Process
ASSESSMENT

1. At onset: vague symptoms
   a. Diplopia
   b. Awkwardness in handling articles and frequent dropping of articles
   c. Stumbling or falling with no apparent cause
2. Symptoms vary depending on location of myelin or nerve fiber destruction
   a. Classic symptoms
      1. nystagmus (rapid, involuntary movements of eyes)
      2. intention tremors, absent at rest
      3. scanning speech (slow enunciation with tendency to hesitate at beginning of a word or syllable, speech with pauses between syllables)
   b. Sensory disorders
      1. paresthesias (numbness, tingling, "dead" feeling, "pins and needles")
      2. diminished vibration sense
      3. impaired proprioception
   c. Visual disorders
      1. optic neuritis
      2. diplopia
      3. scotomas (blind spots)
   d. Motor disorders: spastic weakness or paralysis of limbs
   e. Cerebellar dysfunction: cerebellar ataxia
   f. Bowel and bladder dysfunction
      1. hesitancy, urgency, frequency
      2. retention, incontinence
      3. constipation
   g. Emotional disorders: euphoria, mood swings
3. Long-term effects of progressive disease
   a. Spasticity
   b. Paraplegia
   c. Speech defects
   d. Eating difficulties
   e. Extreme fatigue
   f. Vision difficulties
   g. Complete paralysis

ANALYSIS/NURSING DIAGNOSIS (see p. 224)
PLANNING, IMPLEMENTATION, AND EVALUATION

> **Goal 1** Client will have optimal function of muscles and joints.

Implementation

1. Arrange for physical therapy (muscle stretching and strengthening).
2. Assist with gait retraining if ataxic.
3. Encourage client to remain active and to do as many ADL as possible.

Evaluation

Client's joints and muscles function well; participates in ADL.

> **Goal 2** Client will maintain health-promoting habits in daily living.

Implementation
1. Determine and encourage optimal activity level.
2. Promote adequate rest periods to prevent exhaustion.
3. Use safety devices such as hand rails and walkers to prevent falls.
4. Maintain good nutrition and fluid intake.
5. Supply self-help devices for eating, ambulation, and reading.
6. Provide pain medication and muscle relaxants (e.g., baclofen [Lioresal]) as ordered.
7. Attend to incontinence and pressure areas to maintain integrity of skin and mucous membranes.
8. Make referral to community agencies (e.g., VNA, local branch of National Multiple Sclerosis Society) to help client and significant others in long-term management.
9. Educate client and significant others about these aspects of care.

Evaluation
Client maintains good personal hygiene; eats a nutritious, well-balanced diet.

Goal 3 Client will maintain positive body image and self-concept.

Implementation
1. Provide devices to assist in ADL.
2. Promote as much independence in client as possible; teach significant others to do the same.
3. Encourage hobbies and other pleasurable distractions.
4. Do *not* hurry client.
5. Supervise and assist in skin care and personal hygiene.
6. Reward client's attempts at activity.
7. Encourage and reinforce perseverance and hope.
8. Help client identify realistic goals.

Evaluation
Client's grooming projects positive self-image; performs ADL within own limits.

Goal 4 Client and significant others will express fears about present and future.

Implementation
1. Set aside time to talk to client and significant others together and separately.
2. Encourage expression of feelings.
3. Clarify misconceptions and lack of information about present status and prognosis.
4. Allow expression of depression and hopelessness.
5. Emphasize what the client can still do.

Evaluation
Client and significant others express fear about the diesase; state what to expect realistically in the future.

Goal 5 Client and significant others will learn to cope with illness-related problems and prevent complications.

Implementation
1. Evaluate knowledge and skills that client and significant others have and go over areas where they have not retained information.
2. Teach knowledge and skills related to Goals 1 and 2.

Evaluation
Client and significant others describe care needed because of disabilities; explain how to avoid complications related to disabilities.

✖ EPILEPSY

See Seizure Disorders in Nursing Care of the Child, p. 441).

✖ AMYOTROPHIC LATERAL SCLEROSIS (ALS)

1. Definition: progressive, degenerative disorder of motor neurons in the brain, spinal cord, and motor cortex; remissions are uncommon; death occurs 2 to 15 years after onset. (see Table 3-57)
2. Incidence
   a. Disease of middle age
   b. More common in men
   c. 3000 new cases in United States annually
3. Major complication: aspiration pneumonia
4. Etiology: unknown
5. Diagnosis
   a. Electromyography (EMG)
   b. Muscle biopsy to confirm diagnosis
   c. Elevated serum creatinine phosphokinase (CPK)

Nursing Process
ASSESSMENT
1. At onset
   a. Awkward fine-hand movements
   b. Weakness, wasting of hand muscles
   c. Twitching, cramping
2. Atrophy of hand, forearms; hyperactive reflexes
3. Progresses to upper arms, neck, shoulders
4. Late stage: weakness involves lower extremities
5. Remains alert and oriented
6. Bulbar palsy may be accompanied by erratic affective behavior (e.g., uncontrollable crying outbursts)
7. Impaired swallowing, palate, tongue, and pharynx

ANALYSIS/NURSING DIAGNOSIS (see p. 224)
PLANNING, IMPLEMENTATION, AND EVALUATION
Refer to Multiple Sclerosis Goals 1 through 5, p. 233.

✖ MYASTHENIA GRAVIS

1. Definition: a chronic, progressive neuromuscular disorder that affects lower motor neurons and muscles; characterized by rapid exhaustion of voluntary muscles; caused by a defect at the myoneural junction (see Table 3-57)
2. Pathophysiology: transmission of impulse from nerve to muscle is impaired because of inadequate acetylcholine at the myoneural junction; contractions of voluntary muscles become progressively weaker and cease when the muscle is stimulated

Table 3-59 Drugs used to treat myasthenia gravis

Name	Action	Side effects	Nursing implications
Neostigmine bromide Neostigmine methylsulfate (Prostigmin)	Anticholinesterase; blocks breakdown of acetylcholine at myoneural junction	Nausea, vomiting, diarrhea, abdominal cramps, muscle twitching, weakness, hypotension *Toxic effect: cholinergic crisis*— increased myasthenia symptoms, vomiting, perspiration, salivation, bradycardia, muscle tightness, fasciculations May cause skin rash	Give smallest dose that provides greatest strength; may give anticholinergics (e.g., atropine sulfate) to prevent side and toxic effects. Monitor vital signs; note CNS signs, irritability. Increased potassium levels potentiate drug's effects.
Pyridostigmine bromide (Mestinon)	As above	As above	Give 20-30 minutes before meals.
Ambenonium chloride (Mytelase)	As above	As above	Less commonly used than above drugs; drug of choice if client is sensitive to bromides.
Edrophonium chloride (Tensilon)	As above Short duration of action	As above	Useful in emergency treatment and as diagnostic agent. Differentiates disease from cholinergic crisis—watch for immediate relief of symptoms vs. increased weakness because of medication overdose.

3. Etiology
   a. Unknown
   b. Possibly an autoimmune disorder
   c. Client may have a genetic predisposition

Nursing Process

ASSESSMENT
1. Onset of symptoms insidious and gradual
2. Progressive voluntary-muscle weakness
3. Incapacitating fatigue
4. Ocular symptoms: ptosis, inability to open eyes, diplopia
5. Expressionless appearance with facial muscle involvement; characteristic "snarl" when client attempts to smile
6. Respiratory distress
7. Muscle weakness, documented by neurologic testing
8. Diagnostic test: positive Tensilon test (anticholinesterase): edrophonium chloride (Tensilon) injected IV produces increase in strength (Table 3-59)

ANALYSIS/NURSING DIAGNOSIS (see p. 224)
PLANNING, IMPLEMENTATION, AND EVALUATION

Goal I Client will have control of voluntary muscles.

Implementation
1. Administer anticholinesterase medications to control symptoms (e.g., neostigmine methylsulfate [Prostigmin], pyridostigmine bromide [Mestinon]) (Table 3-59).

2. Administer corticosteroids (e.g., prednisone) as ordered; may be used as adjuvant drug therapy.
3. Administer medications on individually adjusted schedule.

Evaluation
Client has control of voluntary muscles.

Goal 2 Client will remain free from respiratory impairment.

Implementation
1. Observe respiratory status.
2. Use postural drainage; turn frequently.
3. Give prophylactic antibiotics to prevent respiratory infections.
4. Instruct client to avoid exposure to people with URIs.
5. Teach client diaphragmatic breathing exercises, to maintain strength with maximum ventilation and minimum energy expenditure.
6. Balance physical activities with rest.
7. Have client eat only in sitting position.
8. Put client in a rocking bed if client unable to turn self.
9. Have tracheostomy set at bedside.
10. Know that client may require endotracheal intubation and mechanical ventilation.

Evaluation
Client's lungs are clear; no respiratory distress.

Goal 3 Client will remain well nourished.

Implementation
1. Give anticholinesterase medications (e.g., pyridostigmine bromide [Mestinon]) 20 to 30 minutes before meals for full advantage (see Table 3-59).
2. Provide small, frequent, semisolid, or fluid meals that are nutritious and high in potassium (adequate serum levels of potassium potentiate anticholinesterase effect).
3. Provide IV or NG feedings if needed.
4. Observe for aspiration; have suction equipment available.
5. Allow client to eat meals without rushing.
6. Observe for anorexia, nausea, diarrhea, abdominal cramping (common side effects of anticholinesterase drugs).
7. Provide adequate fluid intake (at least 2000 ml per day).

Evaluation
Client's weight remains stable.

Goal 4 Client will receive psychologic and rehabilitative support.

Implementation
1. Evaluate client and significant others' attitudes toward and knowledge of disease.
2. Provide careful explanations of disorder.
3. Offer opportunities for expressions of feelings.
4. Promote a balance of rest and activities.
5. Encourage healthy lifestyle.
6. Refer to Myasthenia Gravis Foundation for information and support.

Evaluation
Client expresses positive outlook for future; has a plan for balancing activities with adequate rest periods.

Goal 5 Client remains free from an undetected "cholinergic crisis."

Implementation
1. Know that a cholinergic crisis (medical emergency) occurs when client cannot tolerate the dosage of anticholinesterase medications (see Table 3-59).
2. Carefully monitor vital signs, including pupil checks, of client receiving increasing doses of anticholinesterase agents.
3. Observe for signs and symptoms of excessive parasympathetic stimulation (see toxic effect: cholinergic crisis, under Side Effects, Table 3-59).
4. Discontinue medications and give IV anticholinergic drug as ordered (e.g., atropine sulfate).

Evaluation
Client is free from symptoms of cholinergic crisis (e.g., no diarrhea, pallor).

SELECTED HEALTH PROBLEMS RESULTING IN AN INTERFERENCE WITH PERCEPTUAL FUNCTION

✳ CATARACTS

1. Definition: total or partial opacity of the normally transparent crystalline lens; the opacity of the lens interferes with light passage through the lens to the retina
2. Incidence
   a. Common after age 55
   b. Third leading cause of blindness
3. Etiology: unknown
4. Risk factors
   a. Aging
   b. Diabetes mellitus
   c. Intraocular surgery
   d. Previous injury to the eye
5. Medical treatment: surgical removal of lens, one eye at a time
   a. Intracapsular extraction by cryosurgery or extracapsular extraction by ultrasound fragmentation (phacoemulsification)
   b. Partial iridectomy commonly done with lens extraction to prevent acute secondary glaucoma
   c. Lens implantation commonly done

Nursing Process
ASSESSMENT
1. Distorted, blurred vision
2. Gradual and painless loss of vision
3. Absence of red reflex (the red reflection seen when the retina is viewed through an ophthalmoscope)
4. Knowledge of treatment modalities
5. Knowledge of procedure and expected outcome

ANALYSIS/NURSING DIAGNOSIS (see p. 224)

PLANNING, IMPLEMENTATION, AND EVALUATION

Goal 1 Client and significant others will be able to explain preoperative and postoperative care and the OR-PACU environment.

Implementation
1. Refer to Perioperative Period, p. 115.
2. Instill preoperative eye medications (mydriatics and cycloplegics) as ordered (Table 3-60).
3. Teach about postoperative procedures.
   a. Bed position varies with type of surgery (usually head of bed up 30 degrees).
   b. No turning, or turn only to unaffected side, postoperatively.
   c. Prevent falls (e.g., bed rails up, assist with ambulation).
   d. Keeps hands away from eyes to prevent infection (eye patch often used on first 2 postoperative days).
   e. Perform ROM exercise routine.

Table 3-60   Eye medications

Name	Action	Side effects	Nursing implications
CYCLOPLEGICS/MYDRIATICS			
Atropine sulfate	Parasympatholytic (anticholinergic) Dilation of pupil and paralysis of accommodation	Dryness of mouth, tachycardia, light sensitivity, inability to focus on near objects	Used to measure refractive errors, inflammations of the eye. Monitor for side effects, increased intraocular pressure (e.g., nausea, vomiting, pain). Inform of inability to accommodate for close-by objects, long duration of action, and photophobia. Contraindicated in glaucoma. Store in safe place out of reach of children.
Homatropine hydrobromide	As above Slow onset, prolonged action	As above	As above, plus use cautiously with older adults.
Scopolamine hydrobromide	As above	As above	As above.
MIOTICS			
Pilocarpine hydrochloride	Cholinergic causes: contraction of sphincter muscle of the iris, resulting in pupil constriction (miosis); spasms of ciliary muscle and deepening of the anterior chamber; and vasodilation of vessels where intraocular fluids leave the eye	Headache	Drug of choice in treatment of glaucoma. Monitor for side effects, individual duration of action and tolerance or resistance. Inform of difficult adjustment to changes in illumination. Instruct regarding frequent instillation.
Carbachol (Carbacel, Isopto Carbachol, Miostat)	As above Produces intense and prolonged miosis	Headache, conjunctival hyperemia	Used for glaucoma if pilocarpine is ineffective. As above.
Physostigmine salicylate (Eserine)	Anticholinesterase Pupil constriction Spasm of accommodation Short duration of action	Conjunctivitis, allergic reactions	As above, plus give very 4-6 hr for wide-angle glaucoma.
Isoflurophate (Floropryl)	Anticholinesterase Pupil constriction Spasm of accommodation	Vomiting and diarrhea, tenesmus	Used for wide-angle glaucoma; plus as above.
Neostigmine bromide (Prostigmin)	As above Short duration of action	Conjunctivitis	As above.
BETA-BLOCKING AGENT			
Timolol maleate (Timoptic)	Beta-adrenergic blocker Reduces intaocular pressure by decreasing aqueous formation Acts in ½ hour	Headache, bronchospasm, cardiac failure, hypotension, muscle weakness, dizziness	Generally well tolerated. Contraindicated in clients with COPD; used cautiously in those with hyperthyroidism. Monitor for side effects. Preferred for clients with pulmonary problems.
Betaxolol hydrochloride (Betoptic)	Cardioselective beta-adrenergic blocker		
CARBONIC ANHYDRASE INHIBITORS			
Acetazolamide (Diamox) Ethoxzolamide (Carase) Methazolamide (Neptazane) Dichlorphenamide (Daranide)	Inhibit carbonic anhydrase, an enzyme necessary for formation of aqueous humor Result in reduced intraocular pressure	Lethargy, anorexia, numbness, tingling of face and extremities, acidosis, ureteral stones	Used for treatment of glaucoma. Monitor for side effects. Prohibit use in first trimester of pregnancy.

Table 3-60   Eye medications—cont'd

Name	Action	Side effects	Nursing implications
OSMOTIC AGENTS (See Table 3-45)			
ANTIINFECTIVES			
Bacitracin ophthalmic oint-ment* (Baciguent)	Bactericidal antibiotic; effective against gram-positive bacteria	No systemic effects	Preserve solutions with refrigeration; potency remains for 3 weeks. Ointment stable for 1 year at room temperature.
Neomycin sulfate (Myciguent)	Broad-spectrum bactericidal antibiotic	Minimal allergic effects	Use cautiously with other systemically used antibiotics because of cross-sensitivity reactions. Effective for conjunctival and corneal infections.
Polymyxin B sulfate* (Aero-sporin)	Bactericidal antibiotic, effective against gram-negative bacteria	Minimal	Often used in combination with above two to produce broader effects.
Tetracyclines (Achromycin) (Aureomycin) (Terramycin)	Bacteriostatic antibiotic for superficial infections	Rare	Monitor for effects.
Sulfacetamide sodium (Bleph-10) (Sulamyd)	Bacteriostatic sulfonamide for surface infections	Local irritation	Monitor for ocular purulent drainage or exudate (interferes with sulfonamide's action).
ANTIINFLAMMATORIES			
Cortisone acetate Fludrocortisone acetate	Decrease defense mechanisms and reduce resistance to pathogenic organisms Inhibit inflammatory response	Prolonged use increases susceptibility to glaucoma, cataracts, and fungus infection	Indicated for all allergenic reactions, nonpyogenic inflammation, and severe injury. Use for limited period. Monitor for increased intraocular pressure and secondary fungus function.

*See Table 3-21.

Evaluation
Client correctly describes plan of treatment and postoperative care; explains what will happen in OR-PACU.

Goal 2 Client will be able, preoperatively, to explain how to prevent increasing intraocular pressure (IOP).

Implementation
1. Teach client before surgery:
   a. No straining.
   b. No coughing or sneezing.
   c. No bending or heavy lifting.
   d. Prevent vomiting.
   e. No squeezing eyelids shut.
2. Evaluate client knowledge after teaching.
3. Continue to explain areas client does not remember or understand.
Evaluation
Client correctly explains how to prevent increased intraocular pressure.

Goal 3 Client will remain free from postoperative complications.

Implementation
1. Refer to Perioperative Period, p. 115.
2. Provide adequate fluids.
3. Deep breathe qh; no coughing.
4. Elevate head of bed 30 to 45 degrees.
5. Turn only to unaffected side if turning is permitted.
6. Check dressing frequently for bleeding (q15min for 2h, then qh for 8h).
7. Prevent increased IOP.
8. Give antiemetics (Table 3-61) and laxatives or stool softeners (see Table 3-49) prn.
9. Observe and report severe eye pain immediately.
Evaluation
Client's vital signs are stable; has no complaints of pain.

Goal 4 Client will know the characteristics of the type of lenses or glasses to be used after surgery for optimal vision.

Table 3-61   Antiemetic drugs

Generic name (trade name)	Action	Side effects	Nursing implications
PHENOTHIAZINES			
Prochlorperazine (Compazine)	Acts on chemoreceptor trigger zone to inhibit nausea and vomiting	Drowsiness, dizziness, extrapyramidal symptoms, orthostatic hypotension, blurred vision, dry mouth	Dilute oral solution with juice, etc. Give deep IM only. Obtain baseline BP before administration. Monitor BP carefully
Perphenazine (Trilafon)	Same as above	Same as above	Same as above.
Thiethylperazine (Torecan)	Same as above	Same as above	Same as above.
NONPHENOTHIAZINES			
Dimenhydrinate (Dramamine)	Inhibits nausea and vomiting by means of unknown mechanism	Drowsiness	Warn client of decreased alertness. Dilute (very irritating to veins).
Benzquinamide (Emete-con)	Acts on chemoreceptor trigger zone to inhibit nausea and vomiting	Drowsiness	Do not give IV in clients with cardiovascular disease or with preanesthetic drugs. Do not reconstitute with 0.9% saline. Use large muscle for IM injection.
Trimethobenzamide (Tigan)	Same as above	Drowsiness	Do not give to children with viral illness (may contribute to Reye's syndrome). Warn client of drowsiness. Give deep IM.
Diphenidol (Vontrol)	Inhibits vestibular cerebellar pathways and possibly chemoreceptor trigger zone to inhibit nausea and vomiting	Drowsiness, dry mouth, confusion	Monitor BP carefully. Use only on hospitalized client. Observe for visual and auditory hallucinations.
Metoclopramide (Reglan)	Stimulates motility of upper GI tract; blocks dopamine receptors at chemoreceptor trigger zone to inhibit nausea and vomiting	Restlessness, anxiety, drowsiness, extrapyramidal symptoms, headache, and dry mouth	Give IV slowly over 15 min. Warn client of decreased alertness. Avoid alcohol and other depressants. Give oral dose ½-1 hr before meals for better absorption.
Ondansetron HCL (Zofran)	Selective 5-HT3 receptor antagonism; acts on the chemoreceptor trigger zone and vagus nerve terminal	Diarrhea, headache	May increase AST, ALT levels; monitor daily bowel activity and stool consistency.

Implementation
1. Teach according to client's situation.
   a. Cataract glasses (wear old glasses until curvature changes are complete: 12 to 14 weeks postoperatively)
      1. magnify objects by one third
      2. clear vision only through center of lens
   b. Contact lenses (less vision distortion than glasses; more costly)
   c. Intraocular lens
      1. synthetic lens implanted in eye
      2. designed for distance vision
      3. for near vision, corrective glasses needed

2. Discuss a plan for obtaining new glasses or contact lenses.

Evaluation
Client correctly describes type of corrective eyewear prescribed.

Goal 5 Client will be discharged with a written rehabilitation plan and a physician's appointment for follow-up.

Implementation
1. Refer to Perioperative Period, p. 115.
2. Develop a written plan that explains

a. Strenuous activity restrictions for 6 to 8 weeks.
b. Progressively increased activity.
c. Return to sexual activity.
d. Driving restrictions.
e. Dressing changes as required.
f. Eye medications as ordered.
g. Dark glasses when exposed to bright sunlight.
3. Instruct significant others in dressing change and medication administration.
4. Secure physician or clinic appointment for client.

Evaluation

Client correctly states activity limitations after discharge; significant others administer eye medications correctly.

RETINAL DETACHMENT

1. Definition: accumulation of fluid between the rod and cone layer and the underlying pigment epithelial layer of the retina. Partial separation becomes complete (if untreated) with subsequent total loss of vision.
2. Pathophysiology: vitreous humor seeps through opening and separates retina from pigment epithelium and choroid. Blindness results.
3. Types:
   a. Rhegmatogenous: break, hole, or tear in retina (e.g., postcataract extraction, severe myopia, ocular trauma)
   b. Nonrhegmatogenous: no retinal break or hole; caused by inflammation (e.g., proliferative diabetic retinopathy)
4. Medical treatment: early surgical repair is imperative to avoid irreparable damage and irreversible blindness.
   a. Cryotherapy: freezing stimulates inflammatory response leading to adhesions
   b. Photocoagulation: laser beam stimulates inflammatory response
   c. Diathermy: heat creates inflammatory response
   d. Scleral buckling
   e. Gas or fluid instillation

Nursing Process

ASSESSMENT
1. Gradual or sudden onset
2. Sudden flashes of light
3. Blurred vision that becomes progressively worse
4. Loss of portion of visual field
5. Ophthalmologic examination: retina hangs like a gray cloud; one or more tears

ANALYSIS/NURSING DIAGNOSIS (see p. 224)
PLANNING, IMPLEMENTATION, AND EVALUATION

Goal I Client will be able to explain preoperative and postoperative care and the OR-PACU environment.

Implementation
1. Prepare client for surgery (see Perioperative Period, p. 115).
   a. Apply bilateral eye patches preoperatively, if ordered.
   b. Protect client from injury.
   c. Minimize stress on eye (e.g., avoid sneezing, coughing, sudden jarring).

d. Instill preoperative medications as ordered (cycloplegics, mydriatics) (see Table 3-60).
2. Teach client postoperative positions and care.

Evaluation

Client correctly explains surgical plan, preoperative and postoperative care, and the OR-PACU environment.

Goal 2 Client will be able, preoperatively, to explain how to prevent increasing IOP (see Cataracts Goal 2, p. 238).

Goal 3 Client will recover free from postoperative complications.

Implementation
1. Refer to Perioperative Period, p. 115.
2. Position and ambulate client as ordered. (A specific position may be prescribed to promote reattachment by allowing the retina to fall back against the pigment epithelium.)
3. Have client avoid jerky head movements.
4. Speak before approaching client.
5. Check eye patches frequently.
6. Give antiemetics (see Table 3-61), analgesics (see Table 3-6) prn.

Evaluation

Client is stable and free from postoperative complications.

Goal 4 Client will be discharged with a written plan for rehabilitation.

Implementation
1. Refer to Perioperative Period, p. 115.
2. Inform client of activities after discharge.
   a. May watch television.
   b. Avoid reading for 2 to 3 weeks.
   c. Continue to avoid straining, injury to head.
   d. May shave, comb hair, bathe, and ambulate.
3. If pinhole glasses are prescribed, provide client with instructions for use.

Evaluation

Client correctly describes activities and limitations after discharge.

GLAUCOMA

1. Definition: abnormal increase in IOP caused by any obstruction of the outflow channels of aqueous humor; uncontrolled glaucoma causes irreversible blindness as a result of atrophy of the optic nerve
2. Types
   a. Chronic (wide-angle) glaucoma: most common
      1. resistance to flow because of thickening of collecting channels, trabecular network, and canal of Schlemm
      2. insidious onset characterized by a decrease in peripheral vision
   b. Acute (narrow-angle) glaucoma
      1. occurs when iris is abnormally structured in an anterior position

2. exerts pressure on collecting channels and decreases size of anterior chamber
3. sudden onset characterized by severe eye pain and rapid loss of vision
3. Risk factors
   a. Heredity
   b. Trauma
   c. Tumor or inflammation of the eye
   d. Vascular disorders
   e. Diabetes
   f. Prior eye surgery
4. Other information
   a. One of the leading causes of blindness
   b. Early detection is crucial (vision destroyed by optic nerve atrophy cannot be restored)
   c. Regular eye exams that include tonometry (measurement of IOP) are recommended for persons over age 35

Nursing Process
ASSESSMENT
1. Difficulty adjusting to dark rooms (early symptom)
2. Difficulty focusing on close work
3. Halos around lights
4. Loss of peripheral vision; loss of central vision with progression
5. Increased IOP (normal = 12 to 20 mm Hg)
6. Client's support system
7. Client's and significant others' coping mechanisms

ANALYSIS/NURSING DIAGNOSIS (see p. 224)
PLANNING, IMPLEMENTATION, AND EVALUATION

Goal 1 Client's IOP will remain within normal limits.

Implementation
1. Teach client
   a. How to instill eyedrops correctly (e.g., timolol maleate).
   b. How miotic eyedrops decrease intraocular pressure (e.g., pilocarpine); see Table 3-60.
   c. That emotional or stressful events can increase IOP.
   d. To avoid lifting, shoveling, wearing constrictive clothing around the neck.
   e. To avoid excessive sodium intake.

Evaluation
Client's IOP remains between 12 to 20 mm Hg with medication.

Goal 2 Client will be free from further visual impairment.

Implementation
1. Teach client that ocular damage that has already occurred is not reversible, but further visual impairment can be prevented by lifelong compliance with prescribed regimen.
2. Emphasize importance of routine eye exams and follow-up care.

Evaluation
Client develops no further visual impairment.

✻ EAR PROBLEMS REQUIRING SURGERY

1. Definition: corrective surgery of the middle ear; usually performed under local anesthesia
2. Precipitating factors
   a. Chronic otitis media (see Nursing Care of the Child, p. 417)
   b. Perforated tympanic membrane
   c. Otosclerosis: pathologic condition in which the normal bone of the bony labyrinth (inner ear) is replaced with spongy bone causing immobilization of the footplate of the stapes (middle ear) in the oval window; causes conductive hearing loss
3. Types of surgery
   a. Tympanoplasty: repair of tympanic membrane with a graft
   b. Stapedectomy: excision of immobile stapes and insertion of prosthesis

Nursing Process
ASSESSMENT
1. Pain: character and intensity
2. Isolation: withdrawal
3. Hearing impairment: bone conduction better than air conduction (see Nursing Care of the Child, Renne and Weber tests, p. 409)
4. Vertigo
5. Purulent discharge
6. Tinnitus
7. Fever

ANALYSIS/NURSING DIAGNOSIS (see p. 224)
PLANNING, IMPLEMENTATION, AND EVALUATION

Goal 1 Client and significant others will understand preoperative and postoperative care and the OR-PACU environment.

Implementation
1. Refer to Perioperative Period, p. 115.
2. Teach about postoperative procedures.
   a. Avoid blowing nose.
   b. Avoid coughing, sneezing.

Evaluation
Client and significant other can correctly explain preoperative and postoperative care. Postoperatively client avoids coughing and sneezing.

Goal 2 Client will remain free of postoperative complications.

Implementation
1. Monitor bleeding and drainage from ear; report excessive bleeding or pain immediately.
2. Elevate head of bed 30 degrees.
3. Monitor temperature.
4. Assess ear pain.
   a. Administer analgesic as ordered (see Table 3-6).
   b. Report excessive pain immediately.
5. Assess facial (seventh cranial) nerve function (i.e., wrinkle eyebrows, close eyelids, smile).

6. Prevent injury caused by decreased hearing.
   a. Determine hearing level.
   b. Identify environmental risk factors.
7. Prevent injury caused by balance disturbance.
   a. Assess dizziness.
   b. Administer antiemetic as needed (see Table 3-61).
   c. Encourage client to avoid sudden movement.
   d. Use side rails as needed.
   e. Assist with ambulation.

Evaluation

Client remains free from postoperative complications.

> **Goal 3** Client will be able to receive verbal communication.

Implementation

1. Assess ability to receive verbal communication.
2. Use communication techniques (e.g., slowed speech, lip reading).

Evaluation

Client is able to receive messages by using communication techniques.

> **Goal 4** Client and significant others will be prepared for discharge.

Implementation

1. Provide written instructions.
2. Teach client
   a. To avoid blowing nose or coughing.
   b. To sneeze with mouth open to prevent fluctuation of air pressure in middle ear.
   c. To avoid smoking.
   d. Self-care (e.g., no water in ear while bathing).
   e. Symptoms of complications to report immediately (e.g., fever, excessive ear pain or drainage).

Evaluation

Client correctly describes self-care measures and symptoms to report immediately.

NASAL PROBLEMS REQUIRING SURGERY

1. Definition: bone and soft tissue deformities requiring corrective surgery (usually under local anesthesia)
2. Precipitating factors
   a. Fracture
   b. Tumor
   c. Foreign body
   d. Deviated septum
   e. Polyps
   f. Cosmetic problems
3. Types of surgery
   a. Submucous resection (rhinoplasty)
   b. Reduction of a nasal fracture
   c. Removal of polyps, tumors, foreign bodies

Nursing Process

ASSESSMENT

1. Nasal obstruction
2. Pain (fractures)
3. Nasal congestion
4. Bleeding
5. Allergies
6. Self-concept/body image

ANALYSIS/NURSING DIAGNOSIS (see p. 224)

PLANNING, IMPLEMENTATION, AND EVALUATION

> **Goal 1** Client and significant others will understand preoperative and postoperative care and the OR-PACU environment.

Implementation

1. Refer to Perioperative Period, p. 115
2. Teach about postoperative procedures.
   a. Mouth breathing (nasal packing)
   b. No nose blowing
   c. Fowler's position
   d. Ice packs
3. Prepare for postoperative appearance (black eyes, dressing).

Evaluation

Client and significant others describe the surgery and postoperative course.

> **Goal 2** Client will remain free from any postoperative complications.

Implementation

1. Refer to Perioperative Period, p. 115.
2. Observe for frequent swallowing (hemorrhage).
3. Check dressing frequently for bleeding.
4. Change gauze pad under nose when saturated and note amount of bleeding.
5. Apply ice continuously to the area for first 24 hours.
6. Give frequent oral hygiene.
7. Maintain Fowler's position to prevent aspiration.

Evaluation

Client has vital signs within normal limits; has minimal periorbital edema and discoloration.

EPISTAXIS

1. Definition: nosebleed
2. Risk factors
   a. Trauma
   b. Hypertension
   c. Acute sinusitis
   d. Deviated nasal septum
   e. Nasal surgery

Nursing Process

ASSESSMENT

1. Bleeding from nose
2. Frequent swallowing
3. Bright red vomitus

ANALYSIS/NURSING DIAGNOSIS (see p. 224)
PLANNING, IMPLEMENTATION, AND EVALUATION

Goal 1 Client will experience control of epistaxis.

Implementation
1. Use first-aid interventions: direct pressure, Fowler's position, and ice pack.
2. Know that cautery may be used.
3. Monitor anterior and posterior nasal packing (removed in 48 to 96 hours to prevent infection).
4. Give vasoconstrictors as ordered (e.g., topical phenylephrine hydrochloride [Neo-Synephrine]).
5. Observe frequently for bleeding.

Evaluation
Client has no further bleeding from nose.

Goal 2 Client will remain free from future attacks.

Implementation
1. Teach client and significant others first-aid measures to use in event of future attack.
2. Demonstrate proper nasal care.
3. Help client identify precipitating factors.
4. Monitor BP for hypertension.

Evaluation
Client correctly states methods to prevent future attacks.

SELECTED HEALTH PROBLEMS RESULTING IN AN INTERFERENCE WITH PROTECTION

✕ BURNS

See Nursing Care of the Child, p. 430.

✕ SEXUALLY TRANSMITTED DISEASES

See Nursing Care of the Child, p. 422.

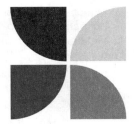

Mobility

OVERVIEW OF PHYSIOLOGY

1. Musculoskeletal system
   a. Muscles: contract and relax under the control of the nervous system to produce movement of the body as a whole or of its parts
      1. *fascia:* surrounds and divides muscles, main blood vessels, and nerves
      2. *tendons:* fibrous attachment between muscles and bones
      3. *ligaments:* fibrous connective tissue connecting bones and cartilage and serving as support for or attachment of muscles and fascia
   b. Bones: for support and protection
      1. *joints:* junction between two bones
         a. synovium: lining of joints that secretes fluid to lubricate
         b. bursa: a closed cavity containing a gliding joint
      2. *cartilage:* dense connective tissue covering the ends of bones and at other sites where flexibility is needed
2. Terminology (Fig. 3-28)
   a. *Adduction:* movement toward the main axis of the body
   b. *Abduction:* movement away from the main axis of the body
   c. *Flexion:* act of bending
   d. *Extension:* stretching out into a straightened position
   e. *Strain:* trauma to the muscle caused by violent contraction or excessive forcible stretch
   f. *Sprain:* trauma to a joint with some degree of injury to the ligaments
3. Range-of-motion (ROM) exercises (Fig. 3-28)
   a. Uses
      1. prevent atrophy
      2. prevent weakness
      3. prevent contracture
      4. prevent degeneration of muscles and joints
   b. Types
      1. active
      2. passive
   c. Procedure
      1. stress importance of performing full ROM exercises
      2. perform ROM exercises at least twice daily, especially for clients on bed rest
      3. breathing to be as normal as possible (e.g., client not to hold breath)
      4. perform movements slowly and gently, especially with active ROM
      5. provide rest between each exercise; do not force movement against a resistant or painful joint or muscle
      6. perform each exercise same number of times on both sides of body; initially do each exercise three times, then work up to five times
      7. teach significant others to do ROM exercises for client
         a. demonstrate exercises
         b. allow return demonstration
         c. provide written instruction
4. Massage (centripetal: toward the heart)
   a. Uses
      1. increases circulation
      2. reduces edema
      3. relieves spasm
   b. May be used with heat
5. Isometric exercises
   a. Definition: alternately tightening and relaxing muscles without moving the joints
   b. Uses
      1. maintain muscle tone
      2. increase muscle strength

APPLICATION OF THE NURSING PROCESS TO THE CLIENT WITH MOBILITY PROBLEMS

ASSESSMENT

1. Health history
   a. Current health status
   b. History of present complaint (e.g., weakness, stiffness, pain, or swelling)
   c. Usual activities (e.g., work, social and recreational pursuits)
   d. Diet and sleep patterns
2. Physical examination
   a. General inspection
      1. symmetry of the two sides of the body
      2. presence of spinal deformities, skin lesions, and masses
      3. posture
   b. Gait and balance: watch for specific gait patterns associated with specific disorders
   c. Joints: active and passive ROM
   d. Muscle strength and bulk
   e. Vascular system of extremities
      1. pulses

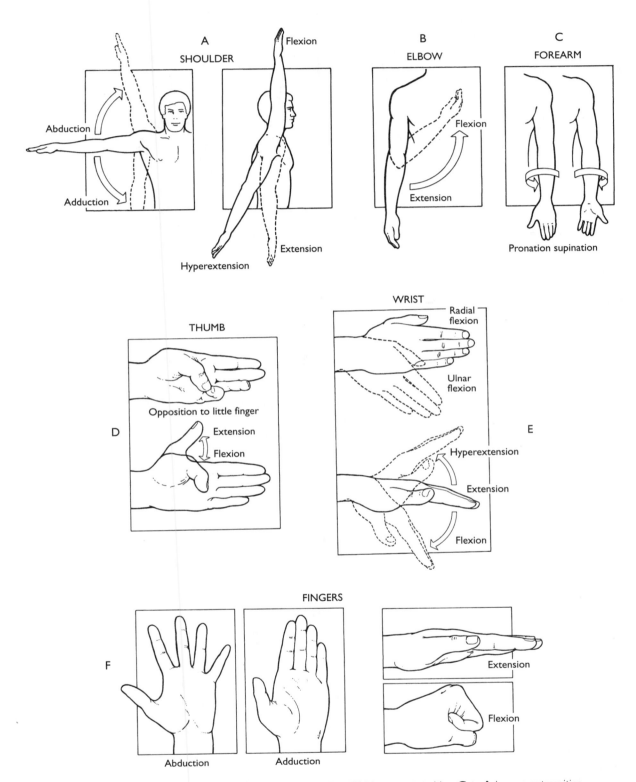

Fig. 3-28 Range-of-motion standards for mobility. **A** to **F,** Upper extremities. **G** to **J,** Lower extremities. (From Beare P, Myers J: *The principles and practice of adult health nursing,* ed 2, St Louis, 1994, Mosby.)

Continued.

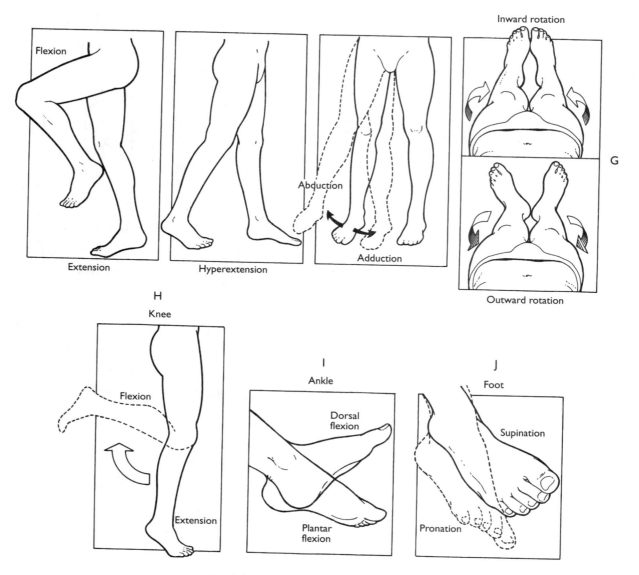

Fig. 3-28, cont'd   For legend see p. 245.

2. varicosities
3. edema
f. Deep-tendon reflex testing (do not test in painful or arthritic joints)
   1. upper extremities
      a. biceps
      b. triceps
      c. radial
   2. lower extremities
      a. patellar
      b. Achilles
3. Diagnostic tests
   a. Radiologic studies
      1. x-rays: detection of bone and soft-tissue injury
      2. bone scan: detection of bone tumors
      3. myelogram
         a. inspection of the spinal column

      b. radiopaque medium injected into subarachnoid space of the spine
      c. nursing care pretest
         ▪ check for iodine allergy
         ▪ teach client regarding spinal tap and x-ray procedure
      d. nursing care posttest
         ▪ keep flat in bed for 6 to 8 hours if client complains of a headache or if an oil-based medium was used
         ▪ keep head of bed elevated at least 30 degrees if a water-based medium was used
         ▪ force fluids
      4. CT scan
      5. MRI
   b. Hematologic studies
      1. increased sedimentation rate and serum globulin (nonspecific for inflammatory process)

2. C-reactive protein (CRP): arthritis
3. elevated serum uric acid: gouty arthritis
4. CBC (increased WBC with gouty arthritis)
5. antinuclear antibodies (ANA): positive with systemic lupus erythematosus (SLE)
   c. Electromyogram (EMG): a graphic record of the contraction of a muscle as a result of electric stimulation

ANALYSIS/NURSING DIAGNOSIS

1. Safe, effective care environment
   a. Risk for trauma
   b. Impaired physical mobility
   c. Knowledge deficit
2. Physiologic integrity
   a. Pain
   b. Impaired physical mobility
   c. Risk for disuse syndrome
3. Psychosocial integrity
   a. Anxiety
   b. Ineffective individual coping
   c. Body-image disturbance
4. Health promotion/maintenance
   a. Altered health maintenance
   b. Impaired adjustment
   c. Diversional activity deficit

GENERAL NURSING PLANNING, IMPLEMENTATION, AND EVALUATION

Goal 1 Client will achieve a maintenance of maximum physical mobility.

Implementation

1. Teach client the proper use of assistive devices.
2. Help client learn proper use of prosthetic devices.
3. Provide needed support and encouragement.

Evaluation

Client expresses and demonstrates proper use of assistive devices; maintains maximum physical mobility.

Goal 2 Client will adapt to changes in body image.

Implementation

1. Encourage client to verbalize concerns.
2. Provide client with correct information about extent of body-image alteration.

Evaluation

Client expresses self-acceptance; engages in usual social activities.

Goal 3 Client will be knowledgeable about disease process, medications, and the prevention of complications.

Implementation

1. Outline symptoms of disease.
2. Outline progression of disease if applicable.
3. Explain the rationale for ordered treatment regimen.
4. Provide information regarding the administration and side effects of all medications.

5. Discuss interventions that prevent the development of complications, including musculoskeletal damage and deficits.

Evaluation

Client is able to discuss disease process; takes medications as prescribed; returns for follow-up appointments; remains free from preventable complications.

Goal 4 Client will be free from complications of immobility.

Implementation

1. See Sensation and Perception, General Nursing Goal 2, p. 225
2. Prevent constipation.
   a. Increase fluid intake, unless contraindicated.
   b. Increase dietary roughage.
3. Assist with active ROM exercises as appropriate (see Fig. 3-28).
4. Prevent urinary calculi with increased fluids.
5. Prevent pressure sores.
   a. Turn q2h.
   b. Gently massage skin.
   c. Keep skin clean and dry.
6. Prevent thrombophlebitis.
   a. Apply antiembolic hose.
   b. Encourage isometric exercises.
   c. Avoid pillows behind the knees or use of Gatch bed.
7. Prevent atelectasis by having client cough and deep breathe.

Evaluation

Client remains free from complications of immobility.

SELECTED HEALTH PROBLEMS RESULTING IN AN INTERFERENCE WITH MOBILITY

✶ FRACTURES

1. Types (can be assigned both classifications)
   a. Classified according to severity
      1. *compound:* open
      2. *closed:* simple
      3. *complete*: bone broken into two pieces
      4. *comminuted:* fragmented
      5. *compression:* depressed
      6. *stress:* fatigue or sudden violent force
      7. *pathologic:* disease related, spontaneous
   b. Classified according to direction of fracture line
      1. *linear, longitudinal (vertical):* fracture runs parallel to long axis of the bone
      2. *transverse, horizontal:* fracture line runs straight across the bone
      3. *spiral:* twisted along shaft of the bone
      4. *oblique:* 45-degree angle
2. Risk factors
   a. Older adults
   b. Younger adults—active sports

   c. All ages—accidents
   d. Osteoporosis from disease or steroid therapy
3. Medical treatment
   a. Closed reduction (external fixation)
     1. manual manipulation of bone fragments into anatomic alignment
     2. immobilized in cast or traction
   b. Open reduction (internal fixation)
     1. surgical procedure with direct visualization
     2. realignment of fracture fragments and immobilization with metallic device (e.g., plate, intramedullary rod)
     3. advantages: allows early weight bearing
     4. complications include postoperative infections and delayed union
   c. Ambulation with assistive devices
     1. crutches (Fig. 3-29)
     2. cane carried in hand opposite affected leg for support
     3. walker
     4. sling for arm
   d. Traction (refer to Nursing Care of the Child, p. 480)
4. Emergency care of suspected fractures
   a. Control of evident hemorrhage (most important problem); sterile bandage to open wound
   b. Immobilize affected part (splint) before moving client
   c. Do not attempt to reduce fracture
   d. Apply ice pack to reduce swelling, hematoma, pain
   e. Transport to medical facility as soon as possible

Nursing Process

ASSESSMENT
1. Age, developmental consideration
2. Usual activity, recreational needs
3. Circumstances of fracture occurrence (most result from accidents)
4. Concurrent health problems (will affect healing)

ANALYSIS/NURSING DIAGNOSIS (see p. 247)

PLANNING, IMPLEMENTATION, AND EVALUATION

Goal 1 If closed reduction is used, client's cast will dry properly.

Implementation
1. Support cast on pillows along length of cast until dry (usually 24 hours).
2. Know that drying creates heat, which causes cast to harden; heat should be uniform in nature, not felt as isolated hot spots.
3. Use fan to stir air, but do not direct fan on the cast.
4. *Never use heat lamp or hair dryer on plaster cast.*
5. Do not completely cover the cast; when dry it is porous and will allow skin underneath to "breathe."
6. Avoid bearing weight on cast for 48 hours.
7. Do not handle cast when wet, if possible; handle with palms, not fingertips.
8. Do not place on hard surface while drying.
9. Know that x-ray will be taken after cast application to ensure proper alignment.

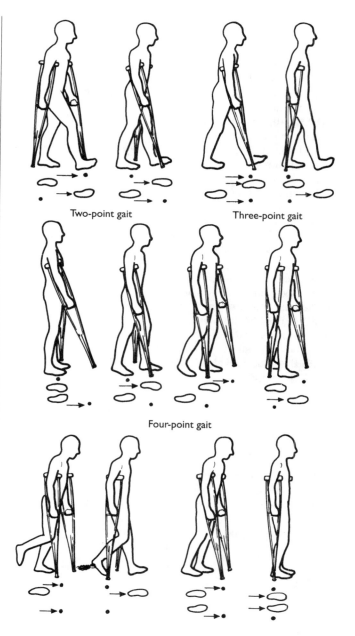

Two-point gait   Three-point gait

Four-point gait

Fig. 3-29 Crutch gaits. (From *Mosby's medical, nursing, and allied health dictionary,* ed 4, St Louis, 1994, Mosby.)

Evaluation
Client's cast dries completely with fracture in proper alignment.

Goal 2 Client will demonstrate appropriate circulation after cast is applied.

Implementation
1. Assess for the five *P*'s of neurovascular status for muscle ischemia.
   a. Pain: progressive pain on movement of the affected extremity
   b. Pallor: in the affected extremity

c. Paralysis: inability to move the affected part
d. Paresthesia: numbness and tingling
e. Pulselessness
2. Assess circulatory status in exposed fingers or toes when assessing vital signs, or at least every 2 hours.
    a. Color: equal to other extremity
    b. Temperature: warm and dry; equal to other extremity
    c. Swelling: minimal or none
    d. Circulation: appropriate blanching; capillary refill less than 3 seconds; palpable pulses
3. Assess for neurologic impairment.
    a. Presence of persistent, localized pain
    b. Ability to move digits
    c. Degree of sensation
4. Avoid pressure areas on extremity.
    a. Position client on opposite side of cast.
    b. Support cast, elevated the length of the cast on 1 or 2 pillows.
    c. "Petal" cast edges to eliminate rough, abrasive edges (see Fig. 5-5).

Evaluation
Client will have appropriate neurovascular status to exposed fingers or toes.

Goal 3 Client's activity level will be safely maintained to the extent allowed.

Implementation
1. Know the instruction client has been given for crutch walking and reinforce teaching.
2. Reinforce the principles of non–weight bearing or use of affected extremity.
3. Instruct client in principles of safe movement (e.g., no hopping around).
4. Instruct client in isometric, ROM exercises as appropriate.

Evaluation
Client's activity is safe and optimal.

Goal 4 Client will experience relief of pain.

Implementation
1. Administer pain medications as ordered.
2. Know that pain should decrease after fracture is set. Increasing pain may indicate that the cast is too tight or infection is beginning.
3. Instruct client to notify nurse of any new pain or pain unrelieved by analgesics.
    a. Unrelenting pain not relieved by analgesics is the first and most common finding associated with compartment syndrome.
    b. Pain increased by elevating the extremity is another common assessment finding associated with compartment syndrome.
4. Have client ambulate on crutches only with assistance after administration of pain medication.

Evaluation
Client is free from discomfort.

Goal 5 Client's rehabilitation course will remain free from complications.

Implementation
1. Teach client signs and symptoms of complications (e.g., poor circulation, infection, nerve damage).
    a. Check for "hot spots," which indicate an area of inflammation beneath them.
    b. Note odor under cast (necrotic tissue will produce malodor).
2. Teach client principles of cast care (Table 3-62).
    a. Keep clean and dry.
    b. Do not put objects (e.g., for scratching) down the cast.
3. Alert client to possible side effects of decreased mobility (e.g., weight gain, constipation).
    a. Increase fluids.
    b. Readjust diet to include more protein and roughage, fewer carbohydrates.

Evaluation
Client demonstrates methods of cast care; maintains weight; remains free from infection and constipation.

Goal 6 If open reduction with a cast or skeletal traction is used, client will be free from postoperative complications.

Implementation
1. Observe for postoperative bleeding.
    a. Draw circle around evidence of bleeding on cast; mark with date and time.
    b. Check when assessing vital signs.

Table 3-62 Client education guide to cast care

PLASTER OF PARIS CAST

Do not wash the cast because washing can weaken the cast and allow mildew to form. A slightly damp rag with cleanser may be used if moisture is wiped away afterward.

Protect the cast with a plastic wrap during bathing or if in rain or snow.

Remove loose plaster crumbs from under cast edges and brush them away from the area.

SYNTHETIC CAST

Cover any rough edges by petaling, or smooth them by lightly filing with a nail file or emery board.

Use only a small amount of mild soap in the area of the cast if getting the cast wet is allowed; rinse the cast well after bathing.

Try to keep all particles, such as dirt or sand, out of the cast; rinse out any particles that may get into the cast.

After swimming in a chlorinated pool or lake, flush the cast thoroughly with water.

Thoroughly dry padding and stockinette each time the cast gets wet, so that skin maceration will not result:
1. Remove excess water by blotting cast with a towel.
2. Use a hand-held hair dryer (on cool or warm setting) in sweeping motion over cast surface to reduce drying time.
3. Continue drying cast for about 1 hour; the cast will be dry when it no longer feels cold and clammy.

From Beare P, Myers J: *Principles and practice of adult health nursing*, ed 2, St Louis, 1994, Mosby.

2. Apply ice pack if ordered to reduce swelling and pain (protect cast from moisture).
3. Administer analgesics as ordered.
4. Maintain traction in proper alignment, with correct amount of weight.
5. Prevent complications of immobilization.
   a. Give meticulous skin care to prevent pressure ulcers; use sheepskin or egg-crate mattress.
   b. Perform isometric and ROM exercises on unaffected extremities to prevent contractures, thrombophlebitis, footdrop.
   c. Know that if the fracture occurred in the middle third of the femur, client may exercise ankle; if fracture is in the lower third, no ankle exercise.
   d. Increase fluids, roughage to prevent constipation, urinary calculi.
6. Observe carefully for postoperative wound infection.
   a. If skeletal traction or external fixation, pin sites cleansed q8h.
   b. If client has a cast, observe for increased pain, swelling, or a malodor coming from cast.
7. Provide bedridden client with age-appropriate diversions or activities, if possible.
   a. Arrange for schoolwork for child or adolescent.
   b. Arrange private time for adult clients and their visitors.
8. Be aware that prolonged bed rest may lead to sleep disturbances, sensory deprivation.

Evaluation

Client is free from complications during the recovery phase; maintains proper alignment, skin integrity; performs ROM exercises on unaffected extremities.

FRACTURED HIP (PROXIMAL END OF FEMUR)

1. Definition: "broken hips" include fractures that are within the head of the femur, associated with osteoporosis and minor trauma; extracapsular fractures that occur below the capsule and are caused by severe trauma or a fall; and those of the greater or lesser trochanter
2. Incidence
   a. Increases after age 60
   b. More common in women than men
3. Precipitating factors
   a. Falls associated with osteoporotic and degenerative changes of the bone
   b. Age-related physiologic changes in balance and perception
4. Medical treatment
   a. Medical intervention: closed reduction achieved with traction (rare in older clients)
   b. Surgical intervention: open reduction and internal fixation, or a prosthetic head-of-the-femur

Nursing Process

ASSESSMENT

1. Affected leg
   a. Shortened
   b. Externally rotated
   c. Abducted
   d. Severe pain and tenderness
2. Age of client and circumstances of injury
3. Current health and mental status, including degree of orientation
4. Availability of family support mechanisms

ANALYSIS/NURSING DIAGNOSIS (see p. 247)

PLANNING, IMPLEMENTATION, AND EVALUATION

Goal 1 Preoperatively, client will have prevention from further injury or pain.

Implementation

1. Administer analgesics as ordered.
2. Use skin traction (Buck's) to relieve muscle spasms and reduce edema.
3. Turn only 45 degrees to affected side; may turn only slightly to unaffected side, with or without traction.
4. Use fracture pan for elimination.
5. Prevent external rotation of affected hip.
6. Assess and monitor coexisting medical problems.

Evaluation

Client remains free from preoperative pain with affected leg in good alignment.

Goal 2 Postoperatively, client will maintain the proper position for functional healing of the hip.

Implementation

1. Prepare client's bed (e.g., firm mattress, bed board, overhead trapeze, adjustable footboard, bed rails, and other pressure ulcer–prevention aids).
2. Know that rapid onset of sharp hip pain may indicate dislocation.
3. For femoral head prosthesis: prevent internal rotation and maintain abduction of affected leg at all times (e.g., use an abductor splint or pillows between legs).
4. For internal fixation with nails or pins: prevent external rotation by placing a trochanter roll along affected side from hip to knee.
5. Turn every 2 hours alternating unaffected side and back.
6. Apply an antiembolic stocking from toes to groin on unaffected leg.
7. Monitor Hemovac, a continuous portable suction device, drainage; ensure that tubes remain patent.
8. Prevent acute flexion of hip by keeping head of bed low (e.g., not higher than 35 to 40 degrees); elevate only for meals.

Evaluation

Client's affected leg is maintained in proper position and alignment.

Goal 3 Client will remain free from complications of immobility.

Implementation

See General Nursing Goal 4, p. 247.

Evaluation

Client's postoperative course is free from complications (e.g., no fever, skin is intact).

Goal 4 Client's activity level will increase progressively (depending on type of surgery and degree of bone healing).

Implementation

1. Internal fixation with nails or pins:
   a. Have client stand first.
   b. Sit client up in chair 1 to 2 days postoperatively.
   c. Allow only partial weight bearing for 3 months.
   d. Allow full weight bearing in 6 months.
2. Femoral-head prosthesis:
   a. Use measures to prevent dislocation at all times.
   b. Have client stand at side of bed, starting 2 to 4 days postoperatively.
   c. Allow partial weight bearing 4 to 10 days postoperatively.
   d. Allow full weight bearing 2 to 6 months postoperatively.
   e. Do not use wheelchair for 2 weeks to prevent hyperflexion of the hip.
   f. Prevent flexion greater than 90 degrees.
3. Consult physician regarding muscle-setting exercises for gluteal and quadriceps muscles, movements of the affected leg, ambulation, and weight bearing on the unaffected leg.
4. Work with physical therapist to coordinate exercise and mobilization regimen.
5. Perform full ROM exercises at least twice daily on unaffected limbs.
6. Lead with unaffected leg when using transfer techniques.

Evaluation

Client ambulates with or without assistance and with or without partial weight bearing, depending on surgical intervention.

> **Goal 5** Client will remain free from psychosocial complications of hospitalization and immobility.

Implementation

Refer to Depression, p. 51, and Confused Behavior, p. 43.

Evaluation

Client maintains contact with reality; is minimally confused, disoriented, and dependent.

> **Goal 6** Client will regain use of joint to the maximum degree possible.

Implementation

1. Refer to General Nursing Goal 4, p. 247.
2. Teach client and family about precautions after discharge.
   a. Avoid sleeping on operative side.
   b. Use cane, walker, or crutches for support and partial weight bearing; wear sturdy shoes when walking.
   c. Do not cross or twist legs.
   d. Do not lift heavy objects.
   e. Observe carefully for signs of wound infection.
3. Reinforce need for continued exercise and maintenance of normal activities as possible.

Evaluation

Client uses rehabilitative measures to enhance recovery; pursues activities within range of ability, age, and level of interest.

> **Goal 7** Client will develop a workable plan for long-term convalescence.

Implementation

1. Help client and significant others decide about home care or where client will go after discharge (e.g., home, extended-care facility).
2. Teach client and significant others about
   a. Length of convalescence and progress of weight-bearing ambulation.
   b. General health measures to be followed (e.g., medications, exercise, diet).
   c. Correct safety precautions for use of cane, walker, or wheelchair.
   d. Persons and agencies who can be contacted for services.
3. Help client and significant others develop a plan to eliminate unsafe environmental conditions that may have contributed to fracture.

Evaluation

Client makes adequate arrangements for long-term convalescence.

�֎ LUMBAR HERNIATED NUCLEUS PULPOSUS (RUPTURED DISK)

1. Definition: a protrusion of the gelatinous cushion between the vertebrae (intervertebral disk) through the surrounding cartilage causing pressure on nerve roots with resultant pain; most common sites are L3-4, L4-5, L5-S1
2. Incidence: more frequent in men
3. Predisposing/risk factors
   a. Sedentary occupations
   b. Long-term driving (e.g., truck driver)
   c. Infrequent physical exercise, certain sports (e.g., bowling, baseball)
4. Medical treatment
   a. Medical intervention
      1. bed rest on a firm mattress with bed board
      2. pelvic traction
      3. proper body alignment (e.g., no prone position)
      4. medications
         a. muscle relaxants
         b. analgesics
         c. nonsteroidal antiinflammatory agents
         d. steroids
      5. physical therapy
         a. diathermy
         b. back exercises
         c. braces
      6. weight reduction as needed
   b. Surgical intervention
      1. indications
         a. prevention of further nerve damage and deficits
         b. severe back and leg pain that does not respond to conservative therapy
         c. a totally extruded disk that causes sensory and motor deficits in the lower extremities, bowel, and bladder (an emergency)

2. procedures
   a. *laminectomy:* removal of the posterior arch of the vertebra to relieve pressure on the nerve root
   b. *spinal fusion* (for additional stability): bone graft from iliac crest or synthetic bone graft used to fuse two or more vertebrae together
   c. *percutaneous lateral diskectomy:* local anesthesia allows for insertion of a metal cannula through which a cutting tool can be inserted; the pieces of the disk that are compressing nerves can be removed through the cannula
3. success rate ranges from 50% to 90%

Nursing Process

ASSESSMENT

1. Low-back pain radiating down posterior thigh (sciatic nerve involvement)
2. Paresthesia of affected nerve roots
3. Muscle weakness, muscle spasm in lumbar region
4. Numbness, weakness, paralysis, or decreased reflexes along affected nerve pathway of leg, ankle, and foot
5. Character of pain
   a. Intermittent; more frequent and severe depending on degree of herniation
   b. May be related to a single traumatic event
   c. Gets progressively worse
   d. Worsened by anterior and lateral flexion of the spine; rotational movements, laughing, sneezing, coughing, straining; straight leg raising to 80 or 90 degrees while supine
6. Client's occupation, exercise routine, physical status
7. Diagnostic tests
   a. CT scan
   b. MRI scan

ANALYSIS/NURSING DIAGNOSIS (See p. 247)
PLANNING, IMPLEMENTATION, AND EVALUATION

Goal 1 Client will be relieved of pain.

Implementation
1. Place on bed rest on a firm mattress with bed board; traction as ordered.
2. Administer analgesics, muscle relaxants as ordered; note client's response.
3. Prevent twisting and straining.
4. Use noninvasive methods to relieve pain (e.g., frequent back rubs, diversion).

Evaluation
Client experiences decreased pain; requires infrequent analgesia; maintains bed rest.

Goal 2 Client will learn how to care for back to prevent future episodes.

Implementation
1. Observe and reinforce physical therapy regimens.
2. Give warm bath and muscle relaxants prn before exercise sessions.

3. Help client apply back supports in a side-lying position and observe for any signs of skin irritation.
4. Teach client to use appropriate body mechanics.
   a. Use broad base of support.
   b. Use large body muscles.
   c. Maintain good posture.
   d. Bring object close to the body before moving.
   e. Pull rather than push an object.
   f. Do not lift items.
   g. Squat, do not bend over.
5. Walk rather than stand, but stand rather than sit.

Evaluation
Client demonstrates back exercises correctly and states a willingness to do them regularly; demonstrates use of appropriate body mechanics.

Goal 3 If surgery is required, client will be physically and psychologically prepared for surgery.

Implementation
1. Refer to Perioperative Period, p. 115.
2. Explain importance and demonstrate postoperative positioning, log roll turning, and body alignment.
3. Explain that if spinal fusion is to be done, a turning frame may be used.
4. Tell client about incision needed for bone graft and continuous portable suction device that may be in place.
5. Obtain preoperative neurologic assessment for postoperative comparison.

Evaluation
Client verbalizes a positive attitude toward the surgical outcome; demonstrates understanding of planned procedure and immediate postoperative care.

Goal 4 Client will remain free from postoperative complications.

Implementation
1. Refer to Perioperative Period, p. 115.
2. Keep client flat in bed for first 12 hours; then may raise head of bed to 30 degrees.
3. Know that client will usually get out of bed on first or second postoperative day (unless spinal fusion done).
4. Use turning sheet and turn client by log rolling.
5. Tell client to report numbness or tingling in feet or legs.
6. Give medications as ordered for pain and frequent muscle spasms.
7. Provide laxative to avoid straining.
8. When client is allowed to be up, have client stand and not sit.
9. Apply antiembolic stockings and have client do leg exercises to prevent thrombophlebitis.
10. For better support when client is ambulating, have client wear shoes and not slippers.
11. Prepare client for 3 to 6 months with body cast or brace postoperatively if fusion was done. A brace is applied in a side-lying position.

Evaluation
Client has uneventful postoperative course; maintains dry and intact dressing; has adequate sensation in toes; ambulates frequently with minimal discomfort.

Goal 5 Client and significant others will be adequately prepared for discharge.

Implementation
1. Refer to General Nursing Goal 3, p. 247.
2. Provide client and significant others with written instructions regarding care of operation site, back care regimen, and back exercises.
3. Ensure that client knows proper application of back brace, if ordered.
4. Provide client with a list of instructions or a timetable to resume activities such as driving, sexual intercourse, sports, housework, or job responsibilities.
5. Ensure that client knows to report signs of illness, fever, increasing back pain, or muscle spasms to physician.

Evaluation
Client states schedule for exercising; applies back brace correctly; knows when to resume additional activities.

AMPUTATION

1. Definition: removal of an appendage or limb
2. Indications
   a. Certain tumors
   b. Severe traumatic injuries (usually affects upper extremities)
   c. Arterial occlusive disease leading to gangrene; usually affects lower extremities

Nursing Process
ASSESSMENT
1. Physical and psychologic strengths of client
2. Support systems (e.g., family and friends)
3. Health status, risk factors (i.e., smoking habits, cardiovascular disease, diabetes, cancer)
4. Condition of affected appendage or limb
   a. Color of skin
      1. necrotic tissue may be blue or gray-blue
      2. turns dark brown or black
   b. Presence of infection
      1. red streaks along lymphatic channels
      2. systemic symptoms

ANALYSIS/NURSING DIAGNOSIS (see p. 247)
PLANNING, IMPLEMENTATION, AND EVALUATION

Goal I Client will be physically and emotionally prepared for surgical outcome.

Implementation
1. Refer to Perioperative Period, p. 115.
2. Explain that surgery is performed above level of healthy tissue.
3. Explain that grieving is normal.
4. Allow client and significant others opportunities to express anger and fears.

5. Initiate exercises to develop strength in muscles that will be used in rehabilitation.
6. Prepare client for postoperative stump care and prosthesis if appropriate.
7. Give prophylactic antibiotics as ordered.

Evaluation
Client is prepared physically and emotionally for the outcome of surgery.

Goal 2 Client's stump will remain free from contractures and will be reduced in size.

Implementation
1. Elevate stump for 24 hours (to hasten venous return and prevent edema).
2. Avoid elevation of stump after first 48 hours postoperatively to prevent hip contracture (most common postoperative complication).
3. Keep stump in an extended position; have client with a leg amputation lie prone for short periods 2 to 3 times daily to prevent flexion contractures.
4. Use "shrinker sock" or elastic bandage if prosthetic fitting is delayed; apply in a figure-eight fashion to reduce size of stump in preparation for prosthesis; teach client how to apply properly (elastic bandages applied to above-the-knee amputations are also wrapped around the waist).
5. Know that an immediate prosthetic fit reduces the incidence of postoperative complications, particularly incisional pain and phantom limb sensation.

Evaluation
Client applies shrinker sock properly; stump is clean, free from contractures; client experiences minimal pain.

Goal 3 Client will recover from surgery free from complications.

Implementation
1. Refer to Perioperative Period, p. 115.
2. Know that pain may be sharp and acute in the incisional area.
3. Assess for phantom limb sensation vs. phantom limb pain (limb sensation subsides with time).

Goal 4 Client will adapt to altered body image.

Implementation and Evaluation
1. Refer to General Nursing Goal 2, p. 247.

Goal 5 Client will use prescribed prosthetic device.

Implementation
1. See General Nursing Goal 1, p. 247.
2. Know that a good prosthetic fit takes time and adjustments.
3. Reinforce teaching done by the prosthetist.

4. Teach client to observe stump for signs of infection, irritation.
5. Teach client proper skin care: wash and dry daily, avoid use of skin creams.
6. Continue to offer encouragement and support to client and significant others throughout the rehabilitation process.
7. Reinforce client's efforts at maintaining balance and posture and increasing auxiliary muscle strength.
8. If prosthesis is not an option, instruct client in safe use of wheelchair, transfer techniques.

Evaluation
Client adapts to prosthesis with few problems; transfers from bed to wheelchair safely.

✠ ARTHRITIS

1. Rheumatoid arthritis
   a. Definition: a chronic, systemic, diffuse, collagen disease characterized by inflammatory changes in joints and related structures, resulting in crippling deformities
   b. Incidence
      1. occurs three times more frequently in women
      2. peak incidence between 30 and 40 years of age
      3. primarily affects proximal joints and synovial membranes before involving larger weight-bearing joints
   c. Predisposing factors
      1. possibly an autoimmune disorder
      2. possibly genetic and metabolic factors
   d. Pathophysiologic sequence: synovitis → pannus formation → fibrous ankylosis → bony ankylosis (frozen joint)
   e. Osteoporosis is common
2. Osteoarthritis
   a. Definition: a chronic disease involving the weight-bearing joints; nonsystemic
   b. Incidence
      1. occurs five times more frequently in women
      2. peak incidence between 50 and 70 years of age
   c. Predisposing factors
      1. aging
      2. trauma
      3. excessive use of joint (e.g., worker who types)
      4. obesity
   d. Pathophysiologic sequence: degeneration of articular cartilage → new bone formation: Heberden's nodes (bony nodules or spurs on the dorsolateral aspects of distal joints of fingers)
3. Gouty arthritis
   a. Definition: inflammation of a joint caused by gout (uric acid crystals deposited in joint)
   b. Incidence
      1. 19 times more frequent in men
      2. peak incidence between ages 20 and 40
      3. often affects a terminal joint (e.g., great toe)
   c. Predisposing factors
      1. hyperuricemia
      2. several metabolic disorders
   d. Pathophysiology
      1. metabolic disorders of purine metabolism
      2. urate deposits in and around joints

4. Surgical interventions: for rheumatoid arthritis, osteoarthritis
   a. *Tendon transplant:* from a normal muscle to another location to assume function of a damaged muscle
   b. *Osteotomy:* cutting bone to correct bone or joint deformity
   c. *Synovectomy:* removal of synovial membrane; helps prevent recurrent inflammation
   d. *Arthroplasty*
      1. hemiarthroplasty: one part of a joint is replaced (e.g., head of femur)
      2. total hip replacement: head of the femur and the acetabulum are replaced
      3. total knee replacement: both articular surfaces of the knee are replaced
      4. interphalangeal joint replacement

Nursing Process: Rheumatoid Arthritis and Osteoarthritis
ASSESSMENT
1. Rheumatoid arthritis
   a. Stiffness, especially in morning
   b. Proximal joint pain that decreases with use; fingers usually involved
   c. Swollen joint
   d. Limitation of muscle strength and atrophy; functional impairment caused by pain and muscle irritation
   e. Acute and chronic episodes with remissions and exacerbations
   f. Systemic symptoms (e.g., anemia, fatigue, elevated body temperature)
   g. Elevated sedimentation rate, serum rheumatoid factors
2. Osteoarthritis
   a. Stiffness, especially in morning
   b. Joint pain that increases with use
   c. Limitation of joint motion; no systemic symptoms
   d. Aggravation of symptoms with temperature, humidity change, and weight bearing

ANALYSIS/NURSING DIAGNOSIS (see p. 247)
PLANNING, IMPLEMENTATION, AND EVALUATION

Goal I Client will function as comfortably and normally as possible.

Implementation
1. Teach client to balance rest and activity.
   a. Encourage to optimum level of functioning.
   b. Exercise joint to point of pain—never beyond.
   c. Perform physical and occupational therapy activities as prescribed.
   d. During acute phase maintain complete bed rest and wear splints on affected joints as prescribed.
2. Apply heat to provide analgesia and relax muscles.
3. Teach client about medications and their side effects; see Table 3-63.
4. Help client modify environment to accomplish activities easily.

Evaluation
Client maintains activity without undue stress; can state side effects of ordered medications.

Table 3-63 Antiinflammatory drugs

Type	Side effects	Nursing implications
Acetylsalicylic acid (aspirin)	Tinnitus, GI distress, nausea, vomiting, prolonged bleeding time	Give with food, milk, or antacids. Avoid use with oral or parenteral anticoagulants.
Ibuprofen (Motrin)	Epigastric distress, nausea, vomiting, occult blood loss	Give with food, milk, or antacids, Monitor for GI distress, weight gain. Check renal and hepatic function in long-term therapy.
Indomethacin (Indocin)	Headaches, dizziness, blurred vision, nausea, vomiting, severe GI bleeding, hemolytic anemia, bone marrow depression	Give with food, milk, or antacids. Contraindicated for clients with aspirin allergy and GI disorders. In long-term drug therapy, monitor CBC and renal function, and encourage eye examinations.
Naproxen (Naprosyn)	Epigastric distress, nausea, occult blood loss	Monitor for GI distress.
Sulindac (Clinoril)	Epigastric distress, nausea, occult blood loss, aplastic anemia	Give with food, milk, or antacids. Monitor for bleeding. Watch for edema and periodically check blood pressure.
Piroxicam (Feldene)	Same as indomethacin (Indocin)	Same as indomethacin.
Gold salts (Myochrysine)	Renal and hepatic damage, corneal deposits, ulcerations in mouth, dermatitis	Monitor for skin eruptions, metallic taste in mouth, oral lesions.
Corticosteroids (see Table 3-20)		
Oxaprozin (Daypro)	Nephrotoxicity, blood dyscrasias, GI distress, cholestatic hepatitis, toxicity; blurred vision, tinnitus	Give with food. Teach: therapeutic effects may take up to 1 month; to report changes in voiding pattern, edema, fever, or signs of toxicity. Monitor labs: Creatinine, ALT/AST, Hgb, BUN

Goal 2 Client will adjust to the chronicity of the condition.

Implementation
1. Allow client to express fear and concerns.
2. Encourage as much activity as possible.
3. Teach client that continuous immobilization may cause increased pain.
4. Teach client to avoid sudden jarring movements of joints.
5. Warn client about "quacks" who promise miracle cures.
6. Encourage continued follow-up to reevaluate progression of disease and efficacy of drug therapy.
7. Counsel client and family regarding the need for a well-balanced diet and, if obesity is a problem, weight reduction.

Evaluation
Client states a willingness to continue with therapeutic regimen as prescribed; expresses concerns about chronicity of the disease; maintains maximum activity level.

Goal 3 Client will be prepared for surgery.

Implementation
1. Refer to Perioperative Period, p. 115.
2. Usually joint surgeries require multiple preps. After the final prep the area is covered with a sterile towel.

Evaluation
Client is physically and psychologically prepared for surgery.

Goal 4 If surgery is performed on the affected hip, client will remain free from postoperative complications.

Implementation and Evaluation
1. Refer to Perioperative Period, p. 115.
2. See Goal 2, Fractured Hip, p. 250.

Goal 5 Client will regain use of joint to the maximum degree possible.

Implementation and Evaluation
Refer to Goal 6, Fractured Hip, p. 251.

Nursing Process: Gouty Arthritis
ASSESSMENT
1. Pain, swelling, and inflammation of affected joint (usually great toe)
2. Increased serum uric acid, sedimentation rate, WBC count
ANALYSIS/NURSING DIAGNOSIS (see p. 247)
PLANNING, IMPLEMENTATION, AND EVALUATION

Goals 1 and 2 Refer to Rheumatoid Arthritis, p. 254.

Goal 3 Client will adjust diet and lifestyle to prevent future attacks.

Table 3-64   Antigout medications

Types	Uses	Action	Side effects	Nursing implications
Colchicine	Gout	Inhibits renal tubular reabsorption of urate	Nausea, vomiting, abdominal pain, diarrhea, aplastic anemia, and agranulocytosis with prolonged use	Monitor for GI distress. Monitor fluid I&O. Keep daily output at 2000 ml; force fluids (6-8 glasses/day).
Allopurinol (Zyloprim)	Gout	Reduces the production of uric acid	GI distress, drowsiness, headache, dizziness, agranulocytosis, aplastic anemia, and skin rash	Monitor for rash (may be first sign of severe hypersensitivity reaction). Give with or immediately after meals. Monitor I&O. Keep daily output at 2000 ml; force fluids (6-8 glasses/day). Periodically check CBC, hepatic and renal function.

Indomethacin (Indocin)—see Table 3-63

Implementation
1. Teach client about use of medications and their side effects (Table 3-64).
2. Obtain dietary counseling for client; instruct in a low-purine diet (i.e., restrict meats, especially organ meats, beer, wine, and legumes).
3. Encourage daily high intake of fluids to prevent precipitation of uric acid crystals in the kidney.
4. Advise regarding weight control as needed.

Evaluation
Client lists foods to be restricted; has a plan for weight reduction, if indicated.

✳ COLLAGEN DISEASE
1. Definition: a group of diseases characterized by widespread pathologic changes in connective tissue; these are difficult to diagnose, have no cure, and cannot be prevented
2. Systemic lupus erythematosus (SLE): generalized connective tissue disorder
   a. Incidence
      1. affects women four times more frequently than men
      2. more likely to occur in young adults and adolescents
   b. Etiology and risk factors are unknown; an autoimmune disease
3. Medical treatment: aim is temporary remission or slowing of collagen destruction
   a. High doses of steroids for exacerbation
   b. Nonsteroidal antiinflammatory drugs
   c. Plasmapheresis (plasma exchange)

Nursing Process
ASSESSMENT
1. Arthritis-like symptoms
2. Sensitivity to sun

3. Presence of erythematous "butterfly" rash across bridge of nose
4. Alopecia
5. Dysfunctions of organ systems
   a. Renal (leading cause of death from glomerulonephritis)
   b. Cardiovascular (pericarditis)
   c. Peripheral vascular insufficiency
   d. Nervous (neuritis)
   e. Respiratory (pleuritis)
6. Polymyositis (inflammation of skeletal muscle)
7. Raynaud's phenomenon
8. Diagnostic test results
   a. Positive lupus erythematosus prep
   b. Anemia
   c. Proteinuria

ANALYSIS/NURSING DIAGNOSIS (see p. 247)
PLANNING, IMPLEMENTATION, AND EVALUATION

Goal I Client will follow correct medication regimen.

Implementation
1. Outline plan for steroid therapy.
2. Minimize side effects through diet modification, time of administration.
3. Teach client safety precautions for steroid therapy (see Table 3-20).

Evaluation
Client describes medications, expected side effects, and ways to minimize them.

Goal 2 Client will exhibit an understanding the disease and its complications.

Implementation and evaluation
1. See General Nursing Goal 3, p. 247.

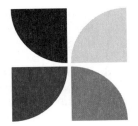

Cellular Aberration

OVERVIEW OF PHYSIOLOGY

1. Terms pertaining to neoplasia
   a. *Cancer:* a group of diseases in which cells multiply without restraint, destroy healthy tissue, and endanger life.
   b. *Metastasis:* spread of cancer from its original site to other parts of the body
   c. *Dysplasia:* bizarre cell growth resulting in cells that differ in size, shape, or arrangement from other cells of the same type of tissue
   d. *Hyperplasia:* increase in cell number
   e. *Neoplasia:* the new and abnormal development of cells that may be benign or malignant.
   f. *Differentiation:* degree to which neoplastic tissue resembles the parent tissue
   g. *Carcinoma:* a malignant tumor arising from epithelial tissue
   h. *Sarcoma:* a malignant tumor arising from connective tissue
   i. *Adjuvant therapy:* therapy designed to be adjunctive or supplemental to primary therapy
   j. *Palliation:* relief or alleviation of symptoms without cure
2. Tumors are characterized by tissue of origin
   a. Adeno: glandular tissue
   b. Angio: blood vessels
   c. Basal cell: epithelium, mainly sun-exposed areas
   d. Embryonal: gonads
   e. Fibro: fibrous tissue
   f. Lympho: lymphoid tissue
   g. Melano: pigmented cells of epithelium
   h. Myo: muscle tissue
   i. Osteo: bone
   j. Squamous cell: epithelium
3. Incidence
   a. Second leading cause of death in the United States (after cardiovascular disease)
   b. One of every four Americans can expect to develop cancer
   c. Occurs in all age groups; incidence increases with age
   d. Most cancer occurs in adults age 65 or older
4. Etiology: *no single cause*
5. Risk factors
   a. Tobacco: smoking or chewing
   b. Alcohol: excessive intake
   c. Hormones (e.g., estrogen, diethylstilbestrol [DES])
   d. Genetic predisposition

   e. Immune deficiency
   f. Age
   g. Occupational: exposure to carcinogens (e.g., asbestos, vinyl chloride, or benzene)
   h. Environmental factors: (ionizing radiation; sun exposure; radon; electromagnetic field effects; chemical pollutants; air polution.
   i. Diet: high fat or high total calories, lack of fiber
   j. Viruses
   k. Sexual practices
6. Characteristics of malignant cells
   a. Anaplastic (loss of differentiation)
   b. Disorderly division
   c. Uncontrolled growth pattern
   d. Loss of normal growth-limiting mechanisms (expands in all directions)
   e. Infiltrative growth
   f. Nonencapsulated
   g. Tend to metastasize
   h. May be necrotic from poor vascular supply
   i. Often recur after treatment
7. Metastasis
   a. Modes
      1. lymphatic
      2. vascular
      3. direct extension
      4. seeding
   b. Sites
      1. usually determined by the lymph and blood drainage patterns of the original cancer site (e.g., primary tumors entering systemic venous circulation are apt to lodge in the lung)
      2. most common (in order): liver, lungs, bone marrow, brain, adrenal glands
8. Classification
   a. Grading: the degree of malignancy; tumor cells are classified from grade 1 to grade 4 (the higher the grade, the poorer the prognosis)
   b. Staging: classification that describes the gross extent of the tumor and its spread
      1. TNM classification: a widely used classification system that stages the primary tumor (T), regional lymph nodes (N), and evidence of metastasis (M)
9. Prognosis depends on
   a. Tumor size
   b. Nodal involvement
   c. Metastasis

APPLICATION OF THE NURSING PROCESS TO THE CLIENT WITH CANCER
ASSESSMENT
1. Health history
   a. Seven warning signs (CAUTION)
      1. *C*hange in usual bowel and bladder habits
      2. *A* sore that does not heal
      3. *U*nusual bleeding or discharge (hematuria, tarry stools, ecchymosis, bleeding mole)
      4. *T*hickening or a lump in the breast or elsewhere
      5. *I*ndigestion or dysphagia (difficulty swallowing)
      6. *O*bvious change in a wart or mole
      7. *N*agging cough or hoarseness
   b. Family history
   c. Presenting symptoms
      1. decreased appetite
      2. weight loss
      3. decreased energy level
      4. pain: the incidence and severity of cancer pain depends on
         a. site of the cancer
         b. stage of the disease
         c. presence and location of metastasis
2. Physical exam
   a. General appearance
   b. Inspection
      1. total body skin inspection
      2. visible masses or thickening under skin
   c. Palpation
      1. masses (breast/testicular exam)
      2. lymph nodes
      3. fluid wave for ascites
   d. Percussion
      1. abdomen percussion (masses, ascites)
      2. chest percussion (masses)
3. Diagnostic tests
   a. Lab tests
      1. CBC, platelet count
      2. blood chemistries
      3. carcinoembryonic antigen (CEA): a tumor marker used to monitor response to antineoplastic therapy and to determine the client's prognosis in a variety of cancers (lung and gastrointestinal)
      4. alpha-fetoprotein (AFP) titer: presence suggests testicular, ovarian, gastric, pancreatic, or hepatocellular cancer
      5. CA-125 tumor marker: tumor marker for ovarian cancer (epithelial tumors of the ovary)
      6. CA 15-3 tumor marker: used in detecting advanced metastatic breast cancer
      7. CA 19-9 tumor marker: tumor marker for pancreatic cancer
      8. Prostate-specific antigen (PSA): a glycoprotein found in prostatic epithelial cells; increased levels found in prostatic cancer
      9. Bence Jones protein (urine study): increased levels seen in multiple myeloma and advanced metastatic cancer to the bone
      10. human chorionic gonadotropin (HCG): increased levels seen in gestational tumors and uterine choriocarcinomas
   b. Cytologic studies (microscopic exam of body secretions for cancer cells) (e.g., Pap smear, sputum cytology)
   c. Biopsy of mass (incisional or aspiration biopsy)
   d. Radiologic and scanning procedures
      1. x-rays (e.g., mammogram): avoid the use of antiperspirants before study because they may cast shadow on the x-ray
      2. CT scans
      3. radioisotope scanning
      4. ultrasound
      5. thermography
      6. tomography
      7. MRI
      8. positron emission tomography (PET)
   e. Endoscopic examinations (e.g., bronchoscopy, gastroscopy)
4. Medical treatment
   a. Surgery
      1. principles
         a. excision/radical excision: tumor plus margin of healthy tissue must be excised
         b. often results in some significant defect or loss of function
      2. uses
         a. diagnosis
         b. cure
         c. palliation
            - remove obstruction
            - debulk large unresectable tumors
            - control pain (e.g., cordotomies, nerve blocks)
         d. ablation: removal of hormone-producing organs to effect a response in hormone-dependent tumor
         e. reconstruction
         f. prophylaxis: removal of lesions that are likely to develop into cancer (e.g., polyps)
   b. Radiation
      1. definition: the use of ionizing radiation to cause damage and destruction to cancerous growths
      2. effect: radiation causes damage at the cellular level
         a. indirectly: water molecules within the cell are ionized
         b. directly: causes strand breakage in the double helix of DNA
         c. not every cell is damaged beyond repair
      3. uses
         a. cure
         b. palliation
         c. combined with surgery
            - preoperatively: to reduce size of the tumor
            - postoperatively: to retard or control metastasis of tumor cells
         d. combined with chemotherapy
      4. administration
         a. external
            - orthovoltage machines: delivers radiation dose to superficial lesions

- megavoltage (cobalt-60): delivers radiation to deeper body structures
- linear accelerators: delivers radiation dosage to deep lesions without harming skin and with less scattering of radiation within body tissues

b. brachytherapy (internal radiation therapy)
- sealed internal radiotherapy
  - implants
  - high dose rate remote after loader
- unsealed internal radiotherapy (radioactive iodine, I-131)

5. side effects
  a. radiation syndrome: systemic effects not related to site treated
  - fatigue, malaise
  - headache
  - anorexia, nausea, vomiting
  b. specific side effects: related to site treated
  - cranium: transitory or permanent hair loss (i.e., alopecia)
  - mouth, rectum: mucositis, stomatitis
  - mouth, head, and neck: taste alteration, reduced saliva production (xerostomia), dental caries
  - throat, esophagus: dysphagia
  - GI tract: nausea, vomiting, diarrhea
  - abdomen: malnutrition, anorexia
  - pelvis, long bones, sternum: bone marrow suppression
    - thrombocytopenia (decrease in platelets), which leads to bleeding
    - leukopenia (decrease in WBCs), which leads to infection
    - erythropenia (decrease in RBCs), which leads to anemia
  - bladder, pelvis: cystitis
  - testicles, ovaries: sterility
  - rectum: proctitis
  - lungs, chest wall: pneumonitis
  - skin: dry desquamation
  - vagina: shortening and narrowing, loss of lubrication

c. Chemotherapy
  1. definition: the use of drugs to retard the growth of or destroy cancerous cells
  2. classification/effect (see Table 5-25).
    a. antineoplastics
    - cell-cycle specific: attack cells at a specific point in the process of cell division
    - cell-cycle nonspecific: act at one time during cell division
    b. hormones
    - alter the hormone balance
    - modify the growth of some hormone-dependent tumors
  3. combination chemotherapy
    a. two or more drugs used simultaneously
    b. each drug has different effect
    c. increases the effectiveness of the destruction or retardation of cancerous cells

d. smaller doses of drugs can be given because of the cumulative effect

4. uses
  a. cure
  b. palliation
  c. combined with surgery
  d. combined with radiation

5. administration
  a. intravenous infusion
  - most common route
  - diffuses drug throughout the entire body
  b. arterial infusion
  - drug is introduced through a catheter directly into the tumor via the main artery that supplies it
  - advantage: high proportion of drug is absorbed by tumor before it reaches systemic circulation
  c. regional perfusion
  - one extremity is isolated from the general circulation
  - advantage: systemic circulation of drug is diminished, thus systemic toxic effects are reduced
  d. intraperitoneal chemotherapy
  - allows for high drug concentration in the peritoneal cavity for treatment of ovarian cancer and some colorectal cancers
  - advantage: keeps systemic toxicity at a lower level because of the peritoneal cavity's cellular barrier
  - procedure is time consuming: requires infusion of chemotherapy diluted in 2 L of warmed normal saline, a 4-hour dwell time, and 2 hours for drainage
  e. oral, IM (less common)

6. drug-specific side effects (see Table 5-25)
  a. nausea and vomiting
  b. bone marrow depression (leukopenia, thrombocytopenia, anemia)
  c. alopecia
  d. fatigue, anorexia
  e. stomatitis
  f. menstrual irregularities, aspermatogenesis
  g. renal damage

d. Biologic response modifiers
  1. definition: treatments that have the ability to alter the immunologic relationship between a tumor and the client with cancer to provide a therapeutic benefit; main purpose is to help modify the host's biologic responses to tumor cells
  2. types
    a. interferons
    - have antiviral and antitumor properties
    - help restore and strengthen immune mechanisms
    - effective on hairy-cell leukemia, renal cell cancer, and Kaposi's sarcoma
    b. monoclonal antibodies: the growth and production of specific antibodies to fight specific malignant cells

    c. lymphokines and cytokines (interleukin-2)
- stimulate the production and activation of T-lymphocytes
- help improve the cell-killing activity of the killer cells and cytotoxic T-cells

    d. colony-stimulating factors
- help regulate blood cell differentiation and proliferation
- used after bone marrow transplant

  3. side effects
    a. common side effects include, influenza-like symptoms, fatigue, leukopenia, nausea, and vomiting

e. Bone marrow transplant (BMT)
  1. used to treat
    a. acute lymphoblastic leukemia
    b. acute myelogenous leukemia
    c. aplastic anemia
    d. chronic myelogenous leukemia
  2. types
    a. allogeneic BMT: bone marrow comes from a healthy donor (usually an immediate family member)
    b. autologous BMT: client is given own bone marrow

f. Supportive (e.g., nutrition, comfort measures)

ANALYSIS/NURSING DIAGNOSIS
1. Safe, effective care environment
  a. Risk for infection
  b. Risk for injury
  c. Sensory-perceptual alterations: visual, auditory, kinesthetic, gustatory, tactile, olfactory
2. Physiologic integrity
  a. Pain
  b. Fatigue
  c. Altered nutrition: less than body requirements
  d. Altered oral mucous membranes
  e. Diarrhea
  f. Sexual dysfunction
3. Psychosocial integrity
  a. Anxiety
  b. Body-image disturbance
  c. Ineffective individual coping
  d. Anticipatory grieving
4. Health promotion/maintenance
  a. Knowledge deficit
  b. Altered family processes
  c. Diversional activity deficit

GENERAL NURSING PLANNING, IMPLEMENTATION, AND EVALUATION

Goal 1 Client will identify strategies for reducing the risk of developing cancer.

Implementation
Teach client strategies for the primary prevention of cancer (Table 3-65).
Evaluation
Client lists strategies for reducing the risk of developing cancer.

Table 3-65   Primary prevention of commonly occurring cancers

BREAST CANCER
Avoid high-fat foods.
Reduce weight; avoid obesity.

LUNG CANCER
Do not smoke.
Avoid secondhand smoke.
Avoid exposure to occupational/environmental carcinogens (asbestos, hydrocarbons, radon).
Wear protective clothing and masks when exposed to occupational/environmental carcinogens.

PROSTATE CANCER
Avoid high-fat foods.
Limit intake of alcohol.
Avoid exposure to occupational carcinogens (cadmium, fertilizers, rubber).

COLORECTAL CANCER
Avoid salt-cured and nitrite-cured foods.
Reduce weight; avoid obesity.
Increase fiber-containing foods.
Reduce dietary fat intake to no more than 30% of calories.

SKIN CANCER
Cover exposed skin.
Use protective sunscreen (SP 15 or more).
Limit sun exposure between 10 AM and 3 PM.
Avoid artificial sources of ultraviolet light (sunlight and tanning booths).
Avoid occupational/environmental exposure (arsenicals, pesticides, coal tar products).
Clean skin carefully if exposed to chemicals.
Avoid frequent exposure to ionizing radiation, x-rays, and radioisotopes.

Goal 2 Client will list/implement guidelines for early detection of cancer.

Implementation
1. Schedule client to use detection or screening services.
2. Explain importance of American Cancer Society guidelines for early detection in asymptomatic individuals (Table 3-66).
3. Refer client to American Cancer Society for information.
Evaluation
Client lists guidelines for early detection of cancer; implements guidelines.

Goal 3 Client undergoing cancer surgery will be physically and psychologically prepared.

Implementation
1. Refer to Perioperative Period, p. 115.
2. Help client deal with body-image changes.

Table 3-66   American Cancer Society guidelines for early detection of cancer

Exam	Age 20-40	Age 40-50	Age 51-plus
CANCER-RELATED CHECKUP			
	Every 3 years	Every year	Every year
BREAST EXAM			
Self-exam	Monthly	Monthly	Monthly
Physician exam	Every 3 years	Every year	Every year
Mammogram	Single baseline between 35-39	Every 1-2 years *(or as directed by physician)*	Every year
UTERUS			
Pelvic exam	Every 3 years	Every year	Every year
Pap smear	Every 3 years *after 3 initial negative tests that are 1 year apart* (from onset of sexual activity)	Every 3 years *(or as directed by physician)*	Every 3 years *(or as directed by physician)*
COLON AND RECTUM			
Digital rectal	none	Yearly	Yearly
Guaiac test	none	none	Yearly
Proctosigmoidoscopy	none	none	Every 3-5 years *after 2 initial negative exams that are 1 year apart*

3. Arrange referral to appropriate agency (e.g., Lost Chord, Reach-to-Recovery).

Evaluation

Client describes surgery in own terms; expresses fears and concerns.

> **Goal 4** Client will be knowledgeable about planned radiation treatment and how to minimize side effects.

Implementation

1. Discuss reasons for radiation therapy and type to be used (e.g., external or brachytherapy).
2. External radiation:
   a. Tell client that although he or she will be alone during the treatment, someone will be watching closely.
   b. Explain that skin (ink) markings must not be washed off for duration of therapy.
   c. Teach proper skin care.
      1. avoid soaps and bathing the area unless approved by physician
      2. avoid exposing area to sun, temperature extremes, and heat lamps
      3. expose area to air
      4. wear nonconstrictive clothing; cotton clothing is preferred
      5. do not apply cosmetics, lotions, deodorant, or powder to area unless directed to do so
      6. do not rub area
      7. do not apply tape over area
      8. do not shave area

   d. Maintain or improve client's nutritional status
      1. administer antiemetics as needed before vomiting occurs (see Table 3-61)
      2. Use nutritional counseling resources
      3. observe for signs of mucositis
      4. teach good oral hygiene; perform every 2 hours with a soft toothbrush and toothpaste for sensitive gums
      5. teach use of prescribed medications (e.g., viscous lidocaine [Xylocaine], oral antibiotics such as nystatin [Mycostatin] suspension)
      6. record daily weights
      7. avoid the use of commercial mouthwashes that contain alcohol
      8. advise small, low-residue meals if diarrhea develops
      9. encourage fluid intake
      10. advise sweet foods if taste is altered
   e. Protect client from bleeding and infection.
   f. Help client balance activity with rest.
3. Brachytherapy (internal radiation):
   a. *Intracavitary irradiation* for cancer of the endometrium, vagina, or cervix. A radioactive substance is put into a sealed metal capsule and placed into a body cavity to deliver radiation.
      1. place client in a private room
      2. restrict visitors: no pregnant women or children under age 18; others are allowed one 15-minute visit each day. Visitors should stay at least 6 feet from the source.
      3. wear radiation badges (dosimeter film badges) when giving direct care

4. explain radiation precautions of *time, distance,* and *shielding*
5. mark room with signs regarding radiation therapy
6. monitor for displacement of radiation source every 4 to 6 hours; use long forceps to handle a dislodged implant and place in a lead-lined container
7. place client on strict bed rest while implant is in place
8. keep head of bed in low position to prevent dislodging cervical implant
9. maintain Foley catheter
10. give low-residue diet
11. monitor for uterine cramping if the implant extends into the uretus
12. change perineal pads frequently (may have foul-smelling discharge)
13. instruct client in the use of a vaginal dilator twice a week (adhesions and shortening of the vagina may occur) after implant is removed
14. tell client that sexual intercourse may be resumed 3 weeks after the implant is removed; advise use of a water-soluble lubricant because of loss of natural vaginal lubrication
   b. *Interstitial radiotherapy:* implant of radioactive needles, wires, or seeds into the tissues. Holding tubes for the radioactive source are inserted while the client is under local or general anesthesia.
1. follow routine precautions for individuals receiving irradiation (implant remains in place for 2 to 3 days)
2. limit to quiet activity
3. know that lead aprons do not provide adequate protection against the high radiation emitted by implant sources
4. place lead shields strategically around the bed
5. assess for possible esophagitis and pneumonitis with breast implants
6. avoid use of deodorants with breast implants

Evaluation

Client states reason for and undergoes radiation therapy with minimal side effects.

Goal 4 Client will state the goals of chemotherapy, names of drugs, anticipated side effects, and treatment of side effects.

Implementation

1. Discuss treatment plans with client.
2. Tell client names of drugs prescribed and probable side effects.
3. Maintain integrity of veins.
   a. Use arm veins.
   b. Discontinue infusion at first sign of infiltration. Check patency by aspirating every 2 to 3 ml during IV-push drugs.
   c. Know drugs that are vesicants (e.g., nitrogen mustard, doxorubicin).
4. Avoid prolonged, severe nausea and vomiting.
   a. Use antiemetics preventatively.
   b. Advise light food intake before treatments.
   c. Avoid dairy products and red meats.
   d. Encourage dry, bulky foods, sweet foods, clear fluids, and noncarbonated cola.
   e. Remove unpleasant sensory stimuli from the room.
5. Prevent infection.
   a. Monitor client's bone marrow function.
   b. Monitor CBC.
   c. Hold chemotherapy if WBC falls below 3000 mm^3.
   d. Hold chemotherapy if granulocyte count falls below 2000 mm^3.
   e. Monitor for increased temperature.
   f. Institute catagory-specific isolation, the immunocompromised, prn.
   g. Employ strict hand washing.
   h. Screen visitors for colds or other infectious diseases.
6. Prevent bleeding.
   a. Monitor platelet count daily.
   b. Institute bleeding precautions for a platelet count below 100,000. Spontaneous bleeding may occur when the platelet count falls below 20,000.
   c. Assess frequently for hematuria, bruising, and bleeding into joints.
   d. Avoid IM injections whenever possible.
   e. Use soft toothbrush or foam cleaner for oral hygiene.
   f. Use electric razor for shaving.
   g. Test all excreta for occult blood.
   h. Administer platelet transfusion as ordered.
7. Prepare client for possible hair loss.
   a. Explain that all body hair is susceptible to effects of chemotherapy but that the fastest growing hair is most affected.
   b. To reduce alopecia use a scalp tourniquet or scalp hypothermia cap 15 minutes before infusion is initiated and leave on until 30 minutes after the infusion ends.
   c. Advise client to purchase a wig, hats, or scarves before losing hair.
   d. Tell client that hair will grow back after chemotherapy is discontinued, but color and texture may be different.
   e. Teach client to use a wide-toothed comb, mild shampoo, and a protein-based conditioner and to avoid the use of chemical processing on hair as well as hair dryers and hair sprays.
8. Maintain good oral hygiene.
   a. Teach client good oral hygiene (use diluted hydrogen peroxide mouth rinse or diluted baking soda mouth rinse; use a soft toothbrush; avoid commercial mouthwashes).
   b. Use artificial saliva as needed (Salivart, Ora-lub).
   c. Teach client signs and symptoms of stomatitis.
   d. Teach client what to do if stomatitis develops.

Evaluation

Client states the goals of chemotherapy; lists the drugs; and measures to minimize side effects.

SELECTED HEALTH PROBLEMS

�֍ **CANCER OF THE LUNG** (see p. 151)
 CANCER OF THE LARYNX (see p. 152)
 CANCER OF THE BLADDER (see p. 195)
 CANCER OF THE PROSTATE (see p. 207)
 CANCER OF THE COLON (see p. 217)
 LEUKEMIA (see p. 491)
 SOLID TUMOR CANCERS IN CHILDREN
 (see p. 493)
 HODGKIN'S DISEASE

1. Definition: malignancy of the lymphoid system characterized by a generalized painless lymphadenopathy; unknown etiology
2. Incidence
   a. Peak incidence between 15 and 30 years of age and after age 50
   b. More common in males
   c. 5-year survival rate is 90% with early detection and treatment
   d. Non-Hodgkin's lymphomas include other lymphoid malignant diseases with different disease courses and responses to treatment; occur in young and middle-aged adults; possible viral etiology
3. Medical treatment
   a. Diagnostic tests
      1. lymphangiography
      2. inferior venacavogram
      3. lab tests
         a. erythrocyte sedimentation rate (ESR): elevated
         b. serum copper: elevated
      4. biopsies
         a. bone marrow
         b. liver
         c. spleen
   b. Clinical staging: surgical laparotomy to determine stage of the disease and best course of treatment; staging determines prognosis
      1. lymph node biopsy for characteristic cell (Reed-Sternberg cell)
      2. surgical clips are used to outline area for irradiation
      3. splenectomy
   c. Chemotherapy: combination drug MOPP (mechlorethamine [nitrogen mustard], vincristine [Oncovin], prednisone, procarbazine) for 6 to 18 months
   d. Radiation therapy

Nursing Process
ASSESSMENT
1. Enlarged, painless lymph nodes (most common sites: cervical, inguinal, mediastinal, axillary, retroperitoneal regions)
2. Fatigue, weakness
3. Unexplained fever
4. Anorexia, weight loss
5. Malaise
6. Night sweats
7. Pruritus

ANALYSIS/NURSING DIAGNOSIS (see p. 260)
PLANNING, IMPLEMENTATION, AND EVALUATION

> **Goal 1** Client will be prepared for lymphangiography and be without complications.

Implementation
Pretest:
1. Explain lymphangiography in terms of what the client and client's family can expect.
   a. Explain to client that lymphangiography is an x-ray examination of the lymphatic system.
   b. Food and drink are usually *not* restricted.
   c. Procedure lasts approximately 3 hours, may last longer.
   d. Feet are anesthetized and immobilized for lymphatic vessel catheterization.
   e. Client must lie still during procedure. A local anesthetic is usually given.
   f. The dye may cause the following *normal* reactions:
      1. unusual taste sensations
      2. fever
      3. headache
      4. insomnia
      5. retrosternal burning sensation
      6. bluish-green discoloration of urine or stools for several days
      7. Evans blue dye will stain the skin for up to 48 hours, occasionally a few weeks or longer
2. Check for allergies to iodine or seafood.
3. Ensure that a signed consent is on chart.
4. Have client void before test.
Posttest:
5. Monitor for signs of complications.
   a. Bleeding or infection from cutdown site
   b. Oil embolism (from oil-based dye)
      1. fever, chills
      2. dyspnea
      3. cough
      4. chest pain, soreness
      5. hypotension
6. Maintain bed rest for 24 hours or as ordered.
7. Monitor vital signs frequently until stable, then every 4 hours for 48 hours.
8. Assess incision site for infection; dressing is usually not changed for 48 hours. Sutures should be removed in 7 to 10 days.
9. Keep original dressing dry.
10. Check for leg edema; elevate lower extremities as necessary.
11. Report numbness or discomfort distal to the incision to the physician.
12. Repeat x-ray in 24 hours.

Evaluation
Client is prepared for lymphangiography; develops no complications.

> **Goal 2** Client and family are prepared for staging and splenectomy.

Implementation
1. Refer to Perioperative Period, p. 115.
2. Inform client of effects of splenectomy: increased susceptibility to infection.

Evaluation
Client and family state effects of splenectomy and implications for lifestyle changes (minimizing exposure to infection).

✴ TESTICULAR CANCER

1. Incidence
   a. Second most common malignancy among men 20 to 35 years of age.
   b. Accounts for 1% to 2% of all tumors in men.
   c. Renal cell cancer and prostate cancer are most likely to metastasize to the testis.
   d. Germ cell tumors are most common type.
2. Clinical stages
   a. Stage A: tumor limited to testes.
   b. Stage B: tumor in testes and retroperitoneal lymph nodes.
   c. Stage C: tumor above the diaphragm or involving solid abdominal organs.
3. Predisposing factors
   a. Cause is unknown.
   b. Common associated factors are testicular atrophy, cryptorchidism (failure of testicles to descend), and scrotal trauma.
4. Medical treatment
   a. Inguinal orchiectomy
   b. Radical retroperitoneal lymphadenectomy
   c. Radiation therapy
   d. Chemotherapy

Nursing Process

ASSESSMENT
1. Hard, painless lump in a testis
2. Enlargement and tenderness of affected testis
3. Enlargement of inguinal and pelvic lymph nodes
4. Diagnostic tests: intravenous pyelogram, blood tests for alpha-fetoprotein and beta human chorionic gonadotropin, chest x-rays, and CT scans

ANALYSIS/NURSING DIAGNOSIS (see p. 260)

PLANNING, IMPLEMENTATION, AND EVALUATION

Box 3-2	TESTICULAR SELF-EXAM

1. Perform exam on a monthly basis.
2. Perform exam after a warm bath or shower.
3. Visually inspect the scrotum for changes in color (reddening, darkening).
4. Roll each testicle gently between thumb and fingers of both hands. Feel for changes in firmness, consistency (lumps), or size.
5. Notify physician if any lumps, nodules, swelling, or changes in consistency are found.

Goal 1 Client will state correct technique with normal and abnormal findings for the testicular exam.

Implementation
1. Testicular self-exam (Box 3-2)
2. Teach all males to perform testicular self-examination monthly beginning at age 15.
3. Apply a warm compress to testes before examination to decrease discomfort.

Evaluation
Client states correct technique with normal and abnormal findings for the testicular exam.

Goal 2 Client and partner state strategies for coping with altered fertility potential.

Implementation
1. Provide client with information regarding sperm banking.
2. Inform client that sperm production may remain suboptimal for 2 years after chemotherapy or radiation therapy.
3. Provide client with information regarding alternative strategies for having children.

EVALUATION
Client and partner state at least one strategy for coping with a change in fertility potential.

✴ CANCER OF THE CERVIX

1. Incidence
   a. Second most common cancer location in women
   b. Usually occurs in women between 30 and 50 years of age
   c. 100% cure if detected early (stage 0)
   d. Squamous cell most common cell type
2. Classification: clinical stages
   a. Stage 0: carcinoma in situ (the most advanced premalignant change)
   b. Stage I: confined to cervix
   c. Stage II: spread from cervix to vagina
   d. Stage III: involves lower one third of vagina and has invaded paracervical tissue to pelvic wall on one or both sides and is associated with palpable lymph nodes in pelvic wall
   e. Stage IV: involves bladder and rectum and extends outside true pelvis
3. Predisposing factors
   a. Early, frequent coital exposure to multiple partners
   b. Pregnancy at young age
   c. History of sexually transmitted disease/herpes
   d. Venereal warts caused by human papilloma virus
4. Medical treatment
   a. Stage 0: conization of the cervix
   b. Stage I: hysterectomy or possible conization
   c. Stage II or III: intracavitary and external beam irradiation; possible radical hysterectomy
   d. Stage IV: radiation therapy followed by pelvic exenteration when there is persistent disease

Nursing Process

ASSESSMENT

1. Menstrual history
2. Pain in back, flank, and legs
3. Vaginal discharge
4. Pain after coitus, bleeding
5. Diagnostic tests: positive cytologic results (Pap smear), cervical biopsy, colposcopy

ANALYSIS/NURSING DIAGNOSIS (see p. 260)

PLANNING, IMPLEMENTATION, AND EVALUATION

Goal Refer to Uterine Fibroids, p. 301.

✖ CANCER OF THE ENDOMETRIUM OF THE UTERUS

1. Incidence
   a. Most common in postmenopausal women between the ages of 50 and 60
   b. Ratio of cervical cancer to endometrial cancer is 3:1
   c. About 50% of clients with postmenopausal bleeding have endometrial carcinoma
   d. Diagnosis is made only after development of overt symptoms
2. Predisposing factors
   a. History of infertility
   b. Dysfunctional uterine bleeding
   c. Long-term estrogen therapy
   d. Obesity
3. Medical treatment
   a. Total abdominal hysterectomy (removal of uterine body and cervix), bilateral salpingo-oophorectomy, and saline wash of the peritoneal cavity
   b. More advanced endometrial cancer may require a radical hysterectomy (removal of uterus, supporting tissue, uppermost section of vagina, and pelvic lymph nodes), and irradiation
   c. Chemotherapy may be used in advanced cancer

Nursing Process

ASSESSMENT

1. Menstrual history
2. Irregular uterine bleeding
3. Diagnostic tests: aspiration curettage; dilation and curettage; endometrial, cervical, and endocervical biopsies

ANALYSIS/NURSING DIAGNOSIS (see p. 260)

PLANNING, IMPLEMENTATION, AND EVALUATION

Goals Refer to Vaginal Wall Changes, p. 301.

✖ OVARIAN CANCER

1. Incidence
   a. Accounts for 6% of cancer found in women (20,000 cases diagnosed each year)
   b. Considered the most lethal gynecologic cancer
   c. Overall death rate from ovarian cancer: 70%
   d. 5-year survival rate 60% to 70% for stage I, 25% to 45% for stage II, 12% to 13% for stage III, and 0% to 4% for stage IV
   e. 70% of clients with ovarian cancer are diagnosed at stage III or later
2. Clinical stages
   a. Stage I: malignancy limited to ovaries
   b. Stage II: disease involves one or both ovaries and extends to the pelvic cavity
   c. Stage III: disease involves one or both ovaries with peritoneal implants found outside of the pelvis; lymph node involvement
   d. Stage IV: disease involves one or both ovaries with distant metastasis
3. Predisposing factors
   a. Postmenopausal
   b. Caucasian
   c. Celibate
   d. Nulliparous
   e. Infertile
   f. Family history of ovarian, endometrial, breast, or colorectal cancer (increases risk to 1 in 6)
   g. Exposed to asbestos or talc
4. Medical treatment
   a. Total abdominal hysterectomy with bilateral salpingo-oophorectomy
   b. Omenectomy
   c. Chemotherapy (cisplatin, cyclophosphamide, doxorubicin, carboplatin)
   d. Paclitaxel (Taxol) used for advanced ovarian cancer that is unresponsive to other chemotherapy
   e. Radiotherapy
      1. Radioactive isotopes injected directly into the peritoneal cavity (used for stage I)
      2. Total abdominal radiation
   f. Biologic response modifiers
      1. Filgrastim (Neupogen)—used for the myelosuppressive effects of chemotherapy

Nursing Process

ASSESSMENT

1. Increased abdominal girth and bloating
2. Abdominal discomfort after meals
3. Food intolerance
4. Changes in bowel or bladder function
5. Weight change
6. Fatigue
7. Diagnostic tests: rectal or rectovaginal examination; ultrasound; staging laparotomy.

ANALYSIS/NURSING DIAGNOSIS (see p. 260)

PLANNING, IMPLEMENTATION, AND EVALUATION

Goals Refer to Uterine Fibroids and Vaginal Wall Changes, p. 301.

✖ CANCER OF THE BREAST

1. Incidence
   a. Most common cancer in women
   b. Can be bilateral
   c. Highest incidence in ages 40 to 49 and 65 and older
   d. Incidence increasing, especially in women under age 40

2. Predisposing factors
   a. Family history of breast cancer on maternal side (sister, mother)
   b. Menarche before age 12; menopause after age 55
   c. Nulliparity or first child after age 35
   d. Previous breast cancer
   e. Increasing age
   f. Obesity in postmenopausal women
   g. Suspected risk factors: oral contraceptives, estrogen replacement therapy, high-fat diet, alcohol consumption, and radiation exposure
3. Breast cancer in men
   a. Incidence: 900 men each year in the United States
   b. Risk factors: history of gynecomastia, increased age
   c. Treatment: mastectomy
4. Surgical and medical treatment
   a. Surgical intervention (primary treatment)
      1. modified radical mastectomy: removal of breast, axillary lymph nodes, and lining of pectoralis minor muscle
         a. commonly performed surgery
         b. suitable for palpable, nonfixed tumors
      2. Segmental mastectomy
         a. wide local excision with removal of tumor and a lobe of breast where the tumor is growing
         b. suitable for small (less than 1 cm) or nonpalpable tumors
         c. usually followed by radiation and chemotherapy, hormonal manipulation
         d. often done in combination with axillary lymph node dissection or sampling
         e. remains somewhat controversial
      3. lumpectomy: removal of only the tumor and some surrounding tissue
         a. indicated when tumors are well defined, less than 5 cm in size, no involvement of nipple, and no metastasis
         b. usually involves dissection of the axillary lymph node closest to the affected breast
         c. radiation therapy follows lymphectomy to eliminate any remaining cancer cells; usually begins 2 weeks after surgery; is administered over 6½ weeks
         d. iridium implants (^{192}Ir) may be used to seed the cancer site
      4. Halsted radical mastectomy; removal of breast, axillary contents, pectoralis muscle
         a. for advanced, fixed tumors
         b. infrequently used
   b. Adjuvant therapy
      1. chemotherapy: specifics of therapy vary from institution to institution
      2. hormonal manipulation done if tumor is known to be estrogen-receptor positive (ER positive)
         a. ER-positive tumors tend to grow more slowly and respond well to hormonal therapy (most postmenopausal women are ER negative)
         b. tamoxifen (antiestrogen therapy) is given 10 to 20 mg bid for 2 to 5 years
         c. tamoxifen delays recurrence of cancer in 77% of women who are ER positive

      d. side effects include hot flashes, nausea, headache, vaginal discharge
   5. Sequence of surgery
      a. One-step surgery: biopsy, frozen section, and mastectomy if positive; one anesthetic (rarely done today)
      b. Two-step surgery: biopsy under local or general anesthetic; when pathology results are available (2 to 3 days) treatment options are discussed; mastectomy or definitive surgery under a second anesthetic
      c. Breast reconstruction can be done immediately after a mastectomy or scheduled later.

Nursing Process

ASSESSMENT
1. Dimpling of skin
2. Retraction of nipple
3. Hard lump; not freely movable
4. Change in skin color
5. Change in skin texture (peau d'orange)
6. Alterations of contour of breast
7. Discharge from nipple
8. Pain (late sign)
9. Ulcerations (late sign)
10. Diagnostic tests: positive mammography, biopsy, and frozen section
11. Hormonal receptor assay: determines if tumor is estrogen or progesterone dependent
12. Symptoms of bone, lung, and brain involvement (common areas of metastasis)

ANALYSIS/NURSING DIAGNOSIS (see p. 260)
PLANNING, IMPLEMENTATION, AND EVALUATION

Goal 1 Client will be able to explain proposed surgery, effects of surgery, and preoperative and postoperative care.

Implementation
1. Refer to Perioperative Period, p. 115.
2. Explore client's expectations of what surgical site will look like.
3. Discuss possibility of reconstructive surgery (not indicated for advanced metastatic cancer).

Evaluation
Client describes treatment options; expresses satisfaction with treatment decision.

Goal 2 Client will remain free from postoperative complications.

Implementation
1. Refer to Perioperative Period, p. 115, for common complications.
2. Check under dressing, under the insertion site of the continuous portable suction device, and under client's back for bleeding.
3. Expect sanguineous drainage during first 24 hours (normal 100 cc per 24 hours), turning to serous drainage thereafter (30 to 90 cc per 24 hours).
4. Report drainage of more than 200 cc in 8 hours.

5. Drain is often left in place for 7 to 10 days to prevent seroma.

Evaluation

Client is free from postoperative complications or evidence of bleeding.

> **Goal 3** Client will regain use of arm and joint movement on side of surgery.

> **Goal 4** Client will demonstrate postoperative exercise to increase range of motion and decrease lymphedema.

Implementation

1. Position arm on operative side on a pillow to decrease incidence of lymphedema; if the arm is not incorporated into the dressing, elevate hand higher than the elbow and keep arm elevated above the level of the heart.
2. Teach exercises beginning 24 hours after surgery (unless contraindicated) to prevent contracture of the shoulder and to promote lymphatic flow. Exercise must be slow and gentle to prevent seroma.
3. Have client perform range-of-motion exercises of hand, elbow, and upper arm.
4. Squeezing a ball is contraindicated in the early postoperative period because it increases arm swelling.
5. Have client use arm and hand for daily activities (e.g., brush hair).
6. Consult with physician regarding additional exercises.
7. Instruct client not to lift, carry, or push heavy objects for 6 to 8 weeks after the operation.

Evaluation

Client has full use of arm and joint movement; demonstrates appropriate postoperative exercises; knows schedule for exercising.

> **Goal 5** Client will be able to explain incision care and choices of available prosthetic devices.

Implementation

1. Encourage client to look at incision.
2. Teach client to inspect incision for redness, swelling, drainage, and separation of wound edges.
3. Teach client to wash incision with soft cloth using soap and water.
4. On discharge, have client wear own bra with cotton padding or Reach-to-Recovery prosthesis.
5. Discuss with client plans for obtaining a permanent prosthesis.

Evaluation

Client explains wound care; lists options for prosthetic devices.

> **Goal 6** Client will identify ways to prevent lymphedema.

Implementation

1. Teach client reasons for lymphedema.

2. Have client sleep with arm elevated on pillows.
3. Suggest to client to elevate arm throughout day. Keep arm supported. Avoid dependent positions.
4. Have client avoid any constriction around arm or wrist.
5. Have client apply elastic bandage, arm stocking as needed.
6. Suggest that client decrease sodium and fluid intake.
7. Obtain an order for a Jobst pressure machine if these methods are ineffective.

Evaluation

Client describes measures to prevent lymphedema.

> **Goal 7** Client will describe precautions necessary to prevent infections in arm on side of surgery.

Implementation

1. Teach client to:
   a. Avoid BP measurements, injections, blood drawing in affected arm.
   b. Wear gloves during activities such as gardening.
   c. Attend to any small cut or scrape immediately.
   d. Avoid biting or chewing nails; avoid cutting cuticles.
   e. Prevent sunburn and any kind of regular burn.
   f. Do not shave axilla on affected side for at least 2 weeks after the operation.
   g. Avoid carrying heavy objects with affected arm.

Evaluation

Client lists measures to avoid arm infection.

> **Goal 8** Client will demonstrate positive self-concept.

Implementation

1. Encourage return to normal activities.
2. Help plan for prosthesis fitting if client desires.
3. Discuss types of clothes client can wear.
4. Discuss reconstruction possibilities.
5. Encourage client to discuss operation and diagnosis with significant others.
6. Spend time with significant others to allow discussion of concerns and fears so that they can provide support for client's needs.
7. Arrange Reach-to-Recovery visit (contacted through the American Cancer Society).

Evaluation

Client discusses self in positive terms.

> **Goal 9** Client will experience normal grieving.

Implementation

1. Allow for privacy if client cries or withdraws.
2. Explain that these feelings are usual and expected, that other women in a similar situation feel the same way.
3. Help client focus on future, but discuss loss.
4. Let client know that sometimes grief is delayed 2 or 3 months, and that it is a normal experience nonetheless.

Evaluation

Client expresses grief over loss of breast and diagnosis.

Goal 10 Client and significant other can describe additional treatment when appropriate.

Implementation
Refer to General Nursing Goals 3 and 4, pp. 260-261.
Evaluation
Client lists anticipated side effects of planned adjuvant therapy.

⬛ ACQUIRED IMMUNODEFICIENCY SYNDROME (AIDS)

1. Definition: A syndrome characterized by a defect in cell-mediated immunity; may have a long incubation period (from 6 months to 7 to 15 years). As the cell-mediated immunity becomes more impaired, the client becomes more likely to develop any of the opportunistic infections characteristically seen with the syndrome. There is no known cure and the syndrome is predominantly fatal.
2. Incidence: less than 50% of adult HIV-positive clients are homosexual or bisexual males. At highest risk are heterosexual women and their children and intravenous drug users.
3. Causative agent: human immunodeficiency virus (HIV), a retrovirus that destroys T4 helper cells, CD4 glycoproteins; HIV-I is the predominant cause of AIDS in the United States. HIV-2 is most prevalent in West Africa.
4. Mode of transmission
   a. Intimate sexual contact
   b. Parenteral exposure to HIV-infected blood, blood products, and blood-containing body fluids.
   c. Perinatally from mother to child
   d. HIV found in blood, semen, vaginal secretions, saliva, tears, breast milk, cerebrospinal fluid, amniotic fluid, and urine; studies to date have implicated only blood, semen, vaginal secretions, and rarely breast milk in transmission
5. Diagnostic tests
   a. Diagnosis of AIDS requires presence of cellular immunodeficiency, opportunistic infection, or cancer and positive test result for antibody to HIV
   b. HIV antibody tests
      1. enzyme-linked immunosorbent assay (ELISA)
      2. Western blot assay: confirms positive ELISA test
      3. positive results indicate that the client has been exposed to HIV and has produced antibodies; it does not mean that client has the disease of AIDS
      4. negative results do not necessarily indicate that a client is free of HIV (if the test was done immediately after exposure to HIV, detectable levels of antibodies may not be present; "window period" ranges from 6 weeks to 6 months)
   c. Antigen tests
      1. HIVAGEN test: detects antigens to HIV as early as 2 weeks after infection
      2. presence of the HIV antigen along with the HIV antibody indicates that the virus is replicating
   d. Polymerase chain reaction (PCR): identifies genetic subunits of HIV
   e. CBC and differential

   f. Immune profile (T-cell assay)
   1. measures the number of T-cells
   2. there is usually an increase in number and percentage of T-suppressor cells (T8, CD8, lymphocytes) and a decrease in T-helper cells (T4, CD4, lymphocytes)
6. CDC classification system for HIV infection in adults
   a. Stage I: acute infection—occurs at time of initial HIV infection and lasts for days to weeks; flulike symptoms
   b. Stage II: asymptomatic infection—occurs after stage I and lasts for several years; client asymptomatic
   c. Stage III: persistent generalized lymphadenopathy—this stage involves lymphadenopathy, at two or more sites, lasting longer than 3 months
   d. Stage IV: other diseases—development of a constitutional disease, neurologic disease, secondary infectious disease, or secondary cancer
7. Opportunistic infections seen in HIV-positive clients
   a. Protozoal infections
      1. *Pneumocystis carinii* pneumonia (PCP)
      2. *Toxoplasma gondii* encephalitis
      3. *Cryptosporidium muris* enteritis
   b. Mycobacterial infections
      1. *Mycobacterium tuberculosis*
      2. *Mycobacterium avium complex*
   c. Fungal infections
      1. *Candida albicans*
      2. *Cryptococcus neoformans*
      3. *Histoplasma capsulatum*
      4. *Aspergillus*
   d. Viral infections
      1. herpes simplex virus
      2. varicella zoster virus (VZV)
      3. cytomegalovirus (CMV)
8. Cancers in HIV infection
   a. Kaposi's sarcoma (most common)
   b. Burkitt's-like lymphomas
   c. Non-Hodgkin's lymphoma
   d. Cervical cancer (occurs more frequently in women who are HIV positive)
9. Medical treatment (Table 3-67)
   a. Zidovudine (Retrovir), also called azidothymidine (AZT), is recommended when CD4 counts fall below 500 cells per microliter (normal is 1000 cells per microliter)
      1. slows the rate of virus reproduction so that additional cells will not become infected
      2. delays the onset of opportunistic infections
      3. does not eliminate the virus from the body; the person infected still has the virus and can transmit it
      4. dosage: 500 to 600 mg per day
      5. side effects: low WBC, nausea, headache, muscle pain, low RBC, and low hematocrit
      6. as many as 30% of persons with AIDS are unable to take Zidovudine because of bone marrow suppression; other antiretroviral agents, didanosine (ddl) or dideoxycitidine (ddC), are given for intolerance to AZT

Table 3-67   Drugs used to treat AIDS and AIDS-related infections

Generic name (trade name)	Action	Uses	Side effects	Nursing implications
Zidovudine (AZT, Retrovir)	Inhibits viral RNA synthesis Prevents viral replication Virustatic action against selected retroviruses	Management of AIDS and selected patients with AIDS-related complex (ARC). Helps increase CD4 cell counts and helps halt the progression of the HIV infection	Headache, weakness, dizziness, nausea, abdominal pain, diarrhea, anemia, granulocytopenia	Monitor CBC results every 2 weeks. Watch for decreasing granulocytes. Must take as directed, around the clock. Wake patient if necessary to administer dosage. Teach patient to avoid activities that require alertness. Inform patient that zidovudine does not reduce the risk of transmission of HIV to others. Teach patient to avoid crowds and notify physician if fever or sore throat occurs.
Didanosine (ddl, Videx, dideoxyinosine)	Inhibits viral replication Virustatic action	Treatment of HIV infections in AIDS patients who are unable to tolerate zodovudine Helps increase CD4 cell counts Used as an alternative in patients who cannot tolerate zidovudine	Headache, rhinitis, cough, pancreatitis, diarrhea, nausea, vomiting, anorexia, liver failure, granulocytopenia, peripheral neuropathy, chills, fever	Assess patient for signs of peripheral neuropathy and pancreatitis (abdominal pain, nausea, vomiting, elevated serum amylase level). Should be avoided in patients with alcoholism. Monitor CBC and hepatic functions tests throughout therapy. Administer on an empty stomach (administering with food decreases absorption by 50%). Teach patient to avoid activities that require alertness. Teach patient to avoid crowds and persons with known infections. Each packet of buffered powder contains 1380 mg of sodium. Use cautiously with patients on a sodium-restricted diet. Buffered powder should only be mixed in water. Do not mix in fruit juice or other acid-containing beverages.

Continued.

Table 3-67   Drugs used to treat AIDS and AIDS-related infections—cont'd

Generic name (trade name)	Action	Use	Side effects	Nursing implications
Pentamidine Isothionate (Nebupent, Pentam)	Disrupts DNA or RNA synthesis in protozoa	Used in the treatment of *Pneumocystis carinii* pneumonia	Anxiety, headache, hypotension, dysrhythmias, pancreatitis, nephrotoxicity, leukopenia, thrombocytopenia, anemia, bronchospasms, chills, hypoglycemia, hypocalcemia, nausea, vomiting	Obtain culture and sensitivity of sputum before initiating therapy. Monitor blood pressure and pulse rate frequently during administration. Administer drug with patient lying down. Teach patient to change positions slowly. Assess patient for hypoglycemia. Monitor BUN and serum creatinine daily. Monitor CBC and platelet count. Monitor liver function studies every 3 days (AST, ALT). Monitor serum calcium every 3 days. Institute bleeding precautions. Teach client to avoid crowds or persons with known infections. Inform patient that a metallic taste may occur during administration of drug.
Ganciclovir (Cytovene, DHPG)	Inhibits viral DNA polymerase	Treatment of cytomegalovirus retinitis in immunocompromised patients	Neutropenia, thrombocytopenia, phlebitis at IV site	Obtain a culture for CMV before administration. Monitor neutrophil and platelet count throughout therapy. Monitor serum creatinine every 2 weeks during treatment. Wear gowns, gloves, and mask while handling medication. Do not administer SQ or IM. This causes severe tissue irritation. Rotate IV infusion site frequently to prevent phlebitis.-

Table 3-67   Drugs used to treat AIDS and AIDS-related infections—cont'd

Generic name (trade name)	Action	Uses	Side effects	Nursing implications
Foscarnet sodium (Foscavir, Astra)	Inhibits viral DNA polymerase	Treatment of cytomegalovirus retinitis in immunocompromised patients	Headache, impaired renal function, seizures, anemia, granulocytopenia, fever, nausea, vomiting, diarrhea, hypocalcemia, hypomagnesemia, hypokalemia, hyperphosphatemia	Closely monitor patient for renal impairment. Creatinine clearance baseline and 2-3 times a week during initial therapy. Encourage fluid intake of 2000-3000 cc per day. Avoid concurrent use of nephrotoxic drugs. Monitor for seizures, cardiac disturbances, and abnormal electrolyte levels. Infuse IV via a central line or a large peripheral vein.
Amphotericin B (Fungizone)	Fungistatic action against aspergillosis, blastomycosis, disseminated candidiasis, coccidioidomycosis, histoplasmosis	Treatment of active fungal infections	Headache, hypotension, hypokalemia, nausea, vomiting, diarrhea, nephrotoxicity, fever, chills, hypersensitivity, thrombophlebitis, burning at injection site, seizures, thrombocytopenia, agranulocytosis, leukopenia	Monitor patient closely during IV administration. Assess IV site frequently for thrombophlebitis. Monitor pulse and blood pressure every 15-30 minutes and assess respiratory status daily. Encourage 2000-3000 cc fluid intake each day to minimize nephrotoxicity. Monitor hemoglobin, hematocrit, BUN, serum creatinine, liver function tests, and potassium during therapy. Administer through central line if available. Administer slowly over a 6-hour period. Weigh weekly. A weight gain of over 2 lb per week may indicate renal damage.

b. Drug therapy to treat HIV infections
  1. antimicrobial therapy
  2. chemotherapy
c. Supportive care
d. Other drugs (including a vaccine for HIV) are being researched
10. Centers for Disease Control and Prevention isolation guidelines
  a. Standard precautions (tier 1)
    1. uses major features of universal precautions and body substance isolation
    2. standard precautions apply to blood, all body fluids, nonintact skin, and mucous membranes
    3. standard precautions include hand washing, gloves, masks, eye protection, and gowns as needed
    4. all sharp instruments and needles are discarded in a puncture-resistant container
    5. private room is necessary only if clients' hygiene is unacceptable
  b. Transmission categories (tier 2)
    1. transmission categories—used in addition to standard precautions
    2. airborne precautions—used for diseases that have droplet nuclei smaller than 5 microns (measles, varicella, disseminated varicella zoster, TB); requires private room, negative airflow with six exchanges per hour, special mask

3. droplet precautions—used for diseases that have droplets larger than 5 μm (diphtheria, rubella, pneumonia); requires private room or cohort clients mask
4. contact precautions—used for clients who are infected with multidrug resistant or highly infectious microorganisms; requires a private room or cohort clients, gloves, and gowns

Nursing Process

ASSESSMENT
1. Fever and chills
2. Weight loss
3. Fatigue and malaise
4. Lymphadenopathy
5. Diarrhea
6. Night sweats
7. Dry, productive cough
8. Dyspnea
9. Oral lesions
10. Skin rashes
11. Confusion
12. Signs and symptoms of opportunistic infections or cancer

ANALYSIS/NURSING DIAGNOSIS (see p. 260)
PLANNING, IMPLEMENTATION, AND EVALUATION

Goal I Significant others and staff will be protected from client's infection.

1. Ensure implementation of CDC isolation guidelines (standard precautions).
2. Use protective barriers to prevent skin and mucous membrane exposure to blood and body fluids (e.g., gloves, masks, protective eyewear, gowns, and face shields).
3. Wash hands after removing gloves and between client contacts.
4. Exercise care when handling sharp instruments.
   a. Do not recap needles.
   b. Do not clip or bend needles.
   c. Dispose of sharps in a puncture-resistant container.
5. Use disposable mouthpieces and airways instead of giving mouth-to-mouth resuscitation.
6. Do not rewash gloves to use with another client.
7. Use airborne, droplet, or contact precautions as client's condition necessitates.

Evaluation
Significant others and staff remain free from the client's infection.

Goal 2 Client will be free from respiratory infection and subsequent respiratory distress.

Implementation
1. Provide oxygen as needed.
2. Place in comfortable position for best respiratory effort.
3. Pace activities so as not to cause or increase fatigue.
4. Assess for signs and symptoms of respiratory infection, distress, and failure.

5. Administer pharmacologic therapy as ordered for PCP.
   a. Pentamidine isethionate (IV or aerosolized)
   b. Trimethoprim-sulfamethoxazole (TMP-SMX) (PO or IV)
6. Teach client and family signs and symptoms of respiratory complications.

Evaluation
Client breathes easily, has no reports of shortness of breath, and remains afebrile.

Goal 3 Client will have adequate nutrition and hydration.

Implementation
1. Monitor I&O, nutritional status, and electrolyte balance closely.
2. Provide appropriate calorie intake if oral nutrition is tolerated.
3. Provide antidiarrheal drugs prn.
4. Administer TPN as ordered.
5. Provide meticulous mouth care.
6. Provide pain relief from mouth lesions if present, before attempts at oral feedings.

Evaluation
Client eats prescribed diet; has adequate calorie intake; maintains good urine output and moist mucous membranes; maintains desired weight.

Goal 4 Client will exhibit an understanding of the goals of therapy, anticipated side effects of drugs, and methods to prevent HIV transmission to others.

Implementation
1. Assess client's knowledge of syndrome.
2. Encourage client to discuss feelings; concerns about plan of therapy; changes in work, home, and lifestyle environment.
3. Use a nonjudgmental approach during care.
4. Tell client names of drugs prescribed and possible side effects.
5. Teach signs and symptoms of infection and what steps to take if these symptoms occur.
6. Teach how to avoid transmission of the illness. Counsel client on safe sex practices and methods to decrease intravenous risk.
7. Warn not to share toilet articles or donate blood or organs.
8. Advise client to inform physicians, dentists, other appropriate health care workers, and sexual partners of diagnosis and required precautions.

Evaluation
Client discusses goals of therapy, lists side effects of prescribed drugs; employs methods to prevent spread of virus.

BIBLIOGRAPHY

The healthy adult

American Nurses Association: *Nursing: a social policy statement,* Publ. No. NP-63, Kansas City, 1980, ANA.

Andreoli T et al: *Cecil essentials of medicine,* ed 3, Philadelphia, 1993, Saunders.

Burke M, Walsh M: *Gerontological nursing: care of the frail elderly,* St Louis, 1992, Mosby.

Carnevali D, Patrick M, editors: *Nursing management for the elderly,* ed 3, Philadelphia, 1993, Lippincott.

Centers for Disease Control: Mortality patterns—United States, 1992, *MMWR* 43:915, 1994.

Couig M: The new food label, *Am J Nurs* 93(2):68, 1993.

Ebersole P, Hess P: *Toward healthy aging: human needs and nursing response,* ed 4, St Louis, 1994, Mosby.

Edelman C, Mandle C: *Health promotion throughout the lifespan,* ed 3, St Louis, 1994, Mosby.

Eliopoulos C: *Manual of gerontological nursing,* St Louis, 1994, Mosby.

Fuller J, Schaller-Ayers J: *Health assessment: a nursing approach,* ed 2, Philadelphia, 1994, Lippincott.

Haymaker SR, editor: Health promotion, *Nurs Clin North Am* 26(4):805, 1991.

Leavell HR, Clark EG: *Preventive medicine for the doctor in his community,* ed 3, New York, 1965, McGraw-Hill.

Malasanos L, Barkauskas V, Stoltenberg-Allen, K: *Health assessment,* ed 4, St Louis, 1990, Mosby.

McFarland G, Darland, TM: *Psychiatric mental health nursing: application of the nursing process,* Philadelphia, 1991, Lippincott.

Pender N et al: Health promotion and disease prevention: toward excellence in nursing practice and education, *Nurs Outlook* 40(3):106, 1992.

Phipps W et al: *Medical-surgical nursing: concepts and clinical practice,* ed 5, St Louis, 1995, Mosby.

Potter P: *Pocket Guide to Health Assessment,* ed 3, St Louis, 1994, Mosby.

Seidel H et al: *Mosby's guide to physical examination,* ed 3, St Louis, 1994, Mosby.

Thompson JM, Bowers AC: *Health assessment: an illustrated pocket guide,* ed 3, St Louis, 1992, Mosby.

Williams S: *Basic nutrition and diet therapy,* ed 10, St Louis, 1994, Mosby.

World Health Organization: *Constitution of the World Health Organization: chronicle of the World Health Organization 1,* Geneva, 1947, World Health Organization.

The adult client undergoing surgery

Agency for Health Care Policy and Research: *Acute pain management: operative or medical procedures and trauma. Clinical practice guidelines,* Washington, DC, 1992, Department of Health and Human Services

Agency for Health Care Policy and Research: *Acute pain management in adults: operative procedures. Quick reference guide for clinicians,* Washington, DC 1992 Department of Health and Human Services.

American Pain Society: CE: relieving pain: an analgesic guide, *Am J Nurs* 88:816, 1988.

Brooks-Brunn J: Postoperative atelectasis and pneumonia, *Heart Lung* 24(2):94, 1995.

Copp LA: The spectrum of suffering, *Am J Nurs* 90(9):35, 1990.

Coyle N: Analgesics and pain: current concepts, *Nurs Clin North Am* 22(3):727, 1987.

Drago SS: Banking on your own blood, *Am J Nurs* 92(3):61, 1992.

Fitzgerald JJ, Shamy P: Let your patient control his analgesic, *Nursing* 17(7):48, 1987.

Gray M: NSAIDs revisited, *Orthop Nurs* 14(1):52, 1995.

Hambleton N: Dealing with complications of epidural analgesia, *Nursing* 24(10):55, 1994.

Hardy E: Steroid management in orthopaedic patients, *Orthop Nurs* 11(6):27, 1992.

Jacox A et al: Managing acute pain: a guideline for the nation, *Am J Nurs* 92(5):49, 1992.

Jurf J, Nirschel A: Acute postoperative pain management: a comprehensive review and update, *Crit Care Nurs Q* 16(1):26, 1993.

Kleinman R et al: PCA versus regular IM injections for severe post-op pain, *Am J Nurs* 87:1491, 1987.

McCaffery M, Beebe A: *Pain: clinical manual for nursing practice,* St Louis, 1989, Mosby.

McCaffery M, Ferrell B: How to use the new AHCPR cancer pain guidelines, *Am J Nurs* 94(7):42, 1994.

McConnell E: Minimizing respiratory problems, *Nursing* 21(11):32, 1991.

McConnell E: Nurses and technology: partners in care, *Nursing* 24(8):32D, 1995.

Meeker J, Rothrock J: *Alexander's care of the patient in surgery,* ed 10, St Louis, 1994, Mosby.

Millam D: How to teach good venipuncture technique, *Am J Nurs* 93(7):38, 1993.

Nash C, Jensen P: When your surgical patient has hypertension, *Am J Nurs* 94(12):38, 1994.

Pasero C, McCaffrey M: Avoiding opioid-induced respiratory depression, *Am J Nurs* 94(4):24, 1994.

Phippen M, Wells M: *Perioperative nursing practice,* Philadelphia, 1994, Saunders.

Phipps W et al: *Medical-surgical nursing: concepts and clinical practice,* ed 5, St Louis, 1995, Mosby.

Posa P: Nutritional support of the critically ill patient: bedside strategies for successful patient outcomes, *Crit Care Nurs Q* 16(4):61, 1994.

Rowland MA: Myths and facts about postoperative discomfort, *Am J Nurs* 90(5):60, 1990.

Saleh K, editor: Post anesthesia care nursing, *Nurs Clin North Am* 28(3):483, 1993.

Tiernan P: Independent nursing intervention: relaxation and guided imagery in critical care, *Crit Care Nurse* 14(5):47, 1994.

Willens J: Giving fentanyl for pain outside the OR, *Am J Nurs* 94(2):24, 1994.

*Willey T: Use a decision tree to choose wound dressings, *Am J Nurs* 92(2):43, 1992.

Oxygenation

Anderson S: ABGs: six easy steps to interpreting blood gases, *Am J Nurs* 90(8):42, 1990.

Aragon D, Martin M: What you should know about thrombolytic therapy for acute MI, *Am J Nurs* 93(9):24, 1993.

Avey M: TB skin testing: how to do it right, *Am J Nurs* 93(9):42, 1993.

Bolgiano C et al: Administering oxygen therapy: what you need to know, *Nursing* 20(6):47, 1990.

Bright LD, Georgi S: CE: peripheral vascular disease: is it arterial or venous? *Am J Nurs* 92(9):34, 1992.

Bright L, Georgi S: How to protect your patient from DVT, *Am J Nurs* 94(12):28, 1994.

Brown K: Critical interventions in septic shock, *Am J Nurs* 94(10):20, 1994.

Buskirk M, Gradman A: Monitoring blood pressure in ambulatory patients, *Am J Nurs* 93(6):44, 1993.

Cannobbio MM: *Cardiovascular disorders,* St Louis, 1990, Mosby.

Caruthers D: Infectious pneumonia in the elderly, *Am J Nurs* 90(2):56, 1990.

*Highly recommended.

Centers for Disease Control: *Core curriculum on tuberculosis,* ed 3, Atlanta, 1994, Department of Health and Human Services.

Centers for Disease Control: Guidelines for preventing the transmission of *Mycobacterium tuberculosis* in health-care facilities, 1994, *MMWR* 43(RR-34), 1994.

Clark WG, Brater DC, Johnson AR: *Goth's medical pharmacology,* ed 13, St Louis, 1992, Mosby.

Emergency Cardiac Care Committee and Subcommittees, American Heart Association: Guidelines for cardiopulmonary resuscitation and emergency cardiac care, *JAMA* 268(16):2171, 1992.

Erickson R: Mastering the ins and outs of chest drainage. part 1, *Nursing* 19(5):37, 1989.

Fifth report of the Joint National Committee on Detection, Evaluation, and Treatment of High Blood Pressure, NIH Publication No. 93-1088, 1993.

Finney CP, editor: Coronary artery disease, *Nurs Clin North Am* 27(1):141, 1992.

Fowler J et al: How to manage diuretic therapy, *Am J Nurs* 95(2):38, 1995.

Gleeson B: Loosening the grip of anginal pain, *Nursing* 21(1):33, 1991.

Gustaferro CA, Steckelberg JM: Cephalosporin antimicrobial agents and related compounds, *Mayo Clin Proc* 66:1064, 1991.

Green E: Solving the puzzle of chest pain, *Am J Nurs* 92(1):32, 1992.

Hayden KL: What keeps oxygenation on track? *Am J Nurs* 92(12):32, 1992.

Hill MN, Grim CM: How to take a precise BP, *Am J Nurs* 91(2):38, 1991.

Hochrein M, Sohl L: Heart smart: a guide to cardiac tests, *Am J Nurs* 92(12):22, 1992.

Hockenberry B: Multiple drug therapy in the treatment of essential hypertension, *Nurs Clin North Am* 26(2):417, 1991.

How to work with chest tubes (programmed instruction), *Am J Nurs* 80:685, 1980.

Johannsen J: Update: guidelines for treating hypertension, *Am J Nurs* 93(3):42, 1993.

Kinney M et al: *Andreoli's comprehensive cardiac care,* ed 8, St Louis, 1995, Mosby.

Levin R: Caring for the cardiac spouse, *Am J Nurs* 93(11):50, 1993.

Lewis SM, Collier IC: *Medical-surgical nursing: assessment and managment of clinical problems,* ed 3, St Louis, 1992, Mosby.

Malasanos L et al: *Health assessment,* ed 4, St Louis, 1990, Mosby.

McCormac M: Managing hemorrhagic shock, *Am J Nurs* 90(8):22, 1990.

Murphy T: Digoxin toxicity: ventricular dysrhythmias to watch for, *Am J Nurs* 93(12):37, 1993.

*Murphy TG, Bennett EJ: CE: low tech, high-touch perfusion assessment, *Am J Nurs* 92(5):36, 1992.

1995 Physicians GenRx, ed 5, St Louis, 1995, Mosby.

O'Brien LM, Bartlett KA: TB plus HIV spells trouble, *Am J Nurs* 92(5):28, 1992.

O'Neal P: How to spot early signs of cardiogenic shock, *Am J Nurs* 94(5):36, 1994.

Pagana K et al: *Mosby's diagnostic and laboratory test reference,* ed 2, St Louis, 1994, Mosby.

Phipps W et al: *Medical-surgical nursing: concepts and clinical practice,* ed 5, St Louis, 1994, Mosby.

Powell A: Milking time is over, *Am J Nurs* 93(2):16, 1993.

Price SA, Wilson LM: *Pathophysiology: clinical concepts of disease processes,* ed 4, St Louis, 1992, Mosby.

Robinson K: Emergency! Pulmonary edema, *Am J Nurs* 93(12):45, 1993.

Roger V et al: Stress echocardiography, *Mayo Clin Proc* 70(1):5, 1995.

Saver C: Decoding the ACLS algorithms, *Am J Nurs* 94(1):26, 1994.

Sawyer D, Bruya M: Care of the patient having radical neck surgery or permanent laryngostomy: a nursing diagnostic approach, *Focus Crit Care* 17(2):167, 1990.

Springhouse: *Illustrated manual of nursing practice,* Springhouse, Pa, 1991, Springhouse Corporation.

Steismeyer J: A four-step approach to pulmonary assessment, *Am J Nurs* 93(8):22, 1993.

Stoy D: Controlling cholesterol with diet, *Am J Nurs* 89(12):162, 1989.

Stringfield Y: Back to basics: acidosis, alkalosis, and ABGs, *Am J Nurs* 93(11):43, 1993.

Thompson J et al: *Mosby's clinical nursing,* ed 3, St Louis, 1993, St Louis, Mosby.

Trottier D, Kochar M: Hypertension and high cholesterol: a dangerous synergy, *Am J Nurs* 92(11):40, 1992.

Trottier D, Kochar M: Managing isolated systolic hypertension, *Am J Nurs* 93(10):50, 1993.

Viall C: Your complete guide to central venous catheters, *Nursing* 20(2):34, 1990.

Walsh L, Johnson CC: Update on antimicrobial agents, *Nurs Clin North Am* 26(2):342, 1991.

Weilitz P, Dettenmeier P: Back to basics: test your knowledge of tracheostomy tubes, *Am J Nurs* 94(2):46, 1994.

Wilson S et al: *Respiratory disorders,* St Louis, 1990, Mosby.

Wright AJ, Wilkowske CJ: The penicillins, *Mayo Clin Proc* 66:1047, 1991.

Yeaw EM: Positioning and oxygenation: good lung down? *Am J Nurs* 92(3):26, 1992.

Nutrition and metabolism

Anderson FP: Portal systemic encephalopathy in the chronic alcoholic, *Crit Care Q* 8(4):40, 1990.

Anderson S: Seven tips for managing patients with diabetes, *Am J Nurs* 94(9):36, 1994.

Batcheller J: Disorders of antidiuretic hormone secretion, *Crit Care Nurse* 3(2):370, 1992.

Bockus S: Troubleshooting your tube feedings, *Am J Nurs* 91(5):24, 1991.

Bryce J: SIADH, *Nursing* 24(4):33, 1994.

Cagno J: Diabetes insipidus, *Crit Care Q* 9(6):86, 1991.

Chin R: Adrenal crisis, *Crit Care Clin* 7:23, 1991.

Christensen MH et al: How to care for the diabetic foot, *Am J Nurs* 91(3):50, 1991.

Deakins DA: Teaching elderly patients about diabetes, *Am J Nurs* 94(4):38, 1994.

Diehl AK: Laparoscopic cholecystectomy: too much of a good thing? *JAMA* 270(12):1469, 1993.

Doherty MM, Carver DK: Transjugular intrahepatic portosystemic shunt: new relief for esophageal varices, *Am J Nurs* 93(4):58, 1993.

Draszkiewicz C: Comprehensive care of the diabetic foot, *Orthop Nurs* 10(2):79, 1992.

Gardner SS, Messner RL: Gastrointestinal bleeding, *RN* 55(12):43, 1992.

Gurevich I: Enterically transmitted viral hepatitis: etiology, epidemiology and prevention, *Heart Lung* 22(4):370, 1993.

Holmgren C: Abdominal assessment, *RN* 55(3):28,1992.

Isley WL: Thyroid disorders, *Crit Care Nurs Q* 13(3):39, 1990.

Jackson DC et al: Endoscopic laser cholecystectomy, *AORN J* 51(6):1546, 1990.

Jess LW: Acute abdominal pain: revealing the source, *Nursing* 23(9):34, 1993.

Johns JL: When the patient has an ulcer, *RN* 54(11):44, 1991.

Juliano J: *When diabetes complicates your life,* Minneapolis, 1993, Chronimed.

Jurf JB et al: Cholecystectomy made easier, *Am J Nurs* 90(12):38, 1990.

Kestle F: Are you up to date on diabetes medications? *AM J Nurs* 94(7):48, 1994.

Kestle F: Using blood glucose meters, *Nursing* 23(3):34, 1993.

Krumberger JM: Acute pancreatitis, *Crit Care Nurse Clin North Am* 5(1):185, 1993.

Kurcharski SA: Fulminant hepatic failure, *Crit Care Nurse Clin North Am* 5(1):141, 1993.

Lee L, Grumowski J: Adrenocortical insufficiency: a medical emergency, *AACN Clin Issues Crit Care Nurs* 3(2):319, 1992.

Macheca MKK: Diabetic hypoglycemia: how to keep the threat at bay, *AM J Nurs* 93(4):26, 1993.

Massoni M: GI handbook, *Nursing* 20(11):65, 1990.

McConnell E: Auscultating bowel sounds, *Nursing* 20(6):76, 1990.

McMillan-Jackson M, Rymer TE: Viral hepatitis: anatomy of a diagnosis, *AM J Nurs* 94(1):43, 1994.

Miller D, Miller HW: Giving meds through the tube, *RN* 58(1):44, 1995.

Mudge C, Carlson L: Hepatorenal syndrome, *AACN Clin Issues Crit Care Nurs* 3(3):614, 1992.

Murray R: Home before dark, *Am J Nurs* 93(11):36, 1993.

O'Toole MT: Advanced assessment of the abdomen and gastrointestinal problems, *Nurs Clin North Am* 25(4):771, 1990.

Peterson A, Drass J: How to keep adrenal insufficiency in check, *Am J Nurs* 93(10):36, 19••.

Prevost SS, Oberle A: Stress ulceration in the critically ill patient, *Crit Care Nurs Clin North Am* 5(1):163, 1992.

Reasner CA II, Isley WL: Thyrotoxicosis in the critically ill, *Crit Care Clin* 7:57, 1991.

Reising DL: Acute hyperglycemia—putting a lid on the crisis, *Nursing* 25(2):33, 1995.

Reising DL: Acute hypoglycemia—keeping the bottom from falling out, *Nursing* 25(2):41, 1995.

Renkes J: GI endoscopy: managing the full scope of care, *Nursing* 23(6):50, 1993.

Robertson C, Cerrato PL: Managing diabetes, *RN* 56(10):26, 1993.

Saltiel-Berzin R: Managing a surgical patient who has diabetes, *Nursing* 22(4):34, 1992.

Sawin CT: Thyroid dysfunction in older persons, *Adv Intern Med* 37:223, 1991.

Shapiro B, Gross MD: Pheochromocytoma, *Crit Care Clin* 7(1):1, 1991.

Smith A: When the pancreas self-destructs, *AM J Nurs* 91(9):38, 1991.

Smith-Rooker JL, Garrett A, Hodges LC: Case management of the patient with a pituitary tumor, *Med Surg Nurs* 2:265, 1993.

Spittle L: Diagnoses in opposition: thyroid storm and myxedema coma, *AACN Clin Issues Crit Care Nurs* 3(2):300, 1992.

Steil CF, Deakins DA: Oral hypoglycemics, *Nursing* 22(11):34, 1992.

Tomky D: Diabetes 2000: advances in monitoring, *RN* 58(3):37, 1995.

Wardell TL: Assessing and managing a gastric ulcer, *Nursing* 21(3):34, 1991.

Webber-Jones J: How to declog a feeding tube, *Nursing* 22(4):62, 1992.

Welles DA et al: Gallstones: alternatives to surgery, *RN* 53(2):44, 1990.

Wilkinson M: Nursing implications after endoscopic cholangiopancreatography, *Gastroenterol Nurs* 13(2):105, 1990.

Wilkinson M: Your role in needle biopsy of the liver, *RN* 53(8):62, 1990.

Elimination

Bowel obstruction, *Am J Nurs* 93(5):51, 1993.

Brundage D: *Renal disorders,* St Louis, 1992, Mosby.

Campbell C: Diarrhea, not always linked to tube feedings, *Am J Nurs* 94(4):59, 1994.

Cooper C: What color is that urine specimen? *Am J Nurs* 93(8):37, 1993.

Doughty D: What you need to know about inflammatory bowel disease, *Am J Nurs* 94(6):24, 1994.

Doughty D, Jackson D: *Gastrointestinal disorders,* St Louis, 1993, Mosby.

Dunn S: How to care for the dialysis patient, *Am J Nurs* 93(6):26, 1993.

Faller N, Lawrence K: Obtaining a urine specimen from a conduit urostomy, *Am J Nurs* 94(1):37, 1994.

Fifield M: Relieving constipation and pain in the terminally ill, *Am J Nurs* 91(7):18, 1991.

Gray M: *Genitourinary disorders,* St Louis, 1992, Mosby.

Krasner D: What is wrong with this stoma? *Am J Nurs* 90(4):46, 1990.

Martin J: Transrectal ultrasound: a new screening tool for prostate cancer, *Am J Nurs* 91(2):69, 1991.

Meyer C: About-face on calcium and kidney stones, *Am J Nurs* 93(5):10, 1993.

Moore S, Newton M, Yancey R: How to irrigate a nephrostomy tube, *Am J Nurs* 93(7):63, 1993.

Moore S et al: Treating bladder cancer: new methods, new management, *Am J Nurs* 93(5):32, 1993.

Moore S et al: Nerve-sparing prostatectomy, *Am J Nurs* 92(4):59, 1992.

Murray S, Preuss M, Schultz F: How do you prep the bowel without enemas?, *Am J Nurs* 92(8):66, 1992.

New guidelines on prostate enlargement, *Am J Nurs* 94(4):10, 1994.

Ponteri-Lewis V et al: Post-operative management of patients undergoing radical cystectomy and urinary diversion, *Medsurg Nurs* 2(5):369, 1993.

Resnick B: Retraining the bladder after catheterization, *Am J Nurs* 93(11):46, 1993.

Schmelzer M, Wright K: Risky enemas: what's the ideal solution, *Am J Nurs* 93(7):16, 1993.

Stroud S, Dyer J: Sorbitol compares well with much costlier drugs, *Am J Nurs* 91(4):61, 1991.

Thayer D: How to assess and control urinary incontinence, *Am J Nurs* 94(10):42, 1994.

Warning: Smoking may be hazardous to kidneys, *Am J Nurs* 94(4):10, 1994.

Winslow E: Myth of the clean catch, *Am J Nurs* 93(8):20, 1993.

Winslow E: Continence cues, *Am J Nurs* 93(5):20, 1993.

Willis D: Taming the overgrown prostate, *Am J Nurs* 92(2):34, 1992.

Sensation and perception

Ceron GE, Rakowski-Reinhardt AC: Autonomic dysreflexia, *Nursing* 21(2):33, 1991.

Clark J et al: *Pharmocological basis of nursing practice,* ed 4, St Louis, 1993, Mosby.

Dyer J: Pros and cons of high-dose steroids in spinal trauma, *Am J Nurs* 93(12):51, 1993.

Finocchiaro DN, Herzfeld ST: Understanding autonomic dysreflexia, *Am J Nurs* 90:56, 1990.

Holt J: How to help confused patients, *Am J Nurs* 93(8):32, 1993.

Hydo B: Designing an effective pathway for stroke, *Am J Nurs* 95(3):44, 1995.

Kelly-Hayes M, Phipps MA, editors: Stroke, *Nurs Clin North Am* 26(4):1048, 1991.

Laskowski-Jones L: Acute spinal cord injury: how to minimize the damage, *Am J Nurs* 93(12):22, 1993.

Lower J: CE: rapid neuro assessment, *Am J Nurs* 92(6):38, 1992.

Morgan SP: Guillain-Barré: a passage through paralysis, *Am J Nurs* 92(10):70, 1992.

Olson EV et al: The hazards of immobility, *Am J Nurs* 90(3):43, 1990.

Parker C: Emergency! Fast action for subarachnoid hemorrhage, *Am J Nurs* 95(1):74, 1995.

Robinson K: Emergency! Early signs of epidural hematoma, *Am J Nurs* 94(4):37, 1994.

Sandler R: Clinical snapshot: glaucoma, *Am J Nurs* 95(3):34, 1995.

Subdural hematoma, *Am J Nurs* 93(10):54, 1993.

Vos H: Making headway with intracranial hypertension, *Am J Nurs* 93(2):28, 1993.

*Yen PK: Does a low-protein diet help with Parkinson's? *Geriatr Nurs* 11(1):48, 1990.

Mobility

Back belts don't enhance lifting power, *Am J Nurs* 94(6):10, 1994.

Carpal-tunnel syndrome, *Am J Nurs* 93(4):64, 1993.

Dykes P: Minding the five P's of neurovascular assessment, *Am J Nurs* 93(6):38, 1993.

Fecht-Gramley M: Recognizing compartment syndrome, *Am J Nurs* 94(10):41, 1994.

Hip dislocation, *Am J Nurs* 93(8):46, 1993.

Kuper B, Failla S: Shedding new light on lupus, *Am J Nurs* 94(11):26, 1994.

Mourad L: *Orthopedic disorders,* St Louis, 1991, Mosby.

Mudge-Grout C: *Immunologic disorders,* St Louis, 1992, Mosby.

Owen B, Garg A: Back stress isn't part of the job, *Am J Nurs* 93(2):48, 1993.

Pellino T: How to manage hip fractures, *Am J Nurs* 94(4):46, 1994.

Smith M: Two legs to stand on: left above-the-knee amputation, *Am J Nurs* 93(12):42, 1993.

Cellular aberration

Anastasi J, Lee V: HIV wasting: How to stop the cycle, *Am J Nurs* 94(6):18, 1994.

Anastasi J, Rivera J: Understanding prophylactic therapy for HIV infections, *Am J Nurs* 94(2):36, 1994.

Camp-Sorrell D: Controlling adverse effects of chemotherapy, *Nursing* 21(4):34, 1991.

Cancer update, *Nursing* 20(4):61, 1990.

Chapman K: When the prognosis isn't good, *RN* 58(7):55, 1994.

Dest V, Fisher S: Breast cancer: dreaded diagnosis, complicated care, *RN* 58(6):49, 1994.

Dillon P: Ovarian cancer: confronting the silent killer, *Nursing* 24(5):66, 1994.

Doane LS, Fischer LM, McDonald TW: How to give peritoneal chemotherapy, *Am J Nurs* 90(4):58, 1990.

Fox S, Haney L: Taxol: new hope for cancer patients, *RN,* 58(11):33, 1994.

Hussar DA: New drugs, *Nursing* 22(5):55, 1992.

Ivey C: When your patient has ovarian cancer, *RN* 58(11):26, 1994.

Ivey C, Gordon S: Breast reconstruction: new image, new hope, *RN* 58(7):48, 1994.

Johnson J: Caring for the woman who's had a mastectomy, *Am J Nurs* 94(5):25, 1994.

Lewis S, Collier I: *Medical-surgical nursing: assessment and management of clinical problems,* ed 3, St Louis, 1992, Mosby.

Pagana K, Pagana T: *Diagnostic testing and nursing implications: a case study approach,* ed 4, St Louis, 1994, Mosby.

Perdew S: *Facts about AIDS: a guide for health care providers,* Philadelphia, 1990, Lippincott.

Phipps W et al: *Medical-surgical nursing: concepts and clinical practice,* ed 5, St Louis, 1995, Mosby.

Rust DL, Dloppenborg EM: Don't underestimate the lumpectomy patient's needs, *RN* 53(3):58, 1990.

Scherer P: How AIDS attacks the brain, *Am J Nurs* 90(1):44, 1990.

Schuerman D: Clinical concerns: AIDS in the elderly, *J Geontol Nurs* 20(7):11, 1994.

Schweid L, Etheredge C, Werner-McCullough M: Will you recognize these oncological crises? *RN* 58(9):23, 1994.

Walbrecker J: Start talking about testicular cancer, *RN* 58(1):34, 1995.

Wikle T, Coyle K, Shapiro D: Bone marrow transplant: today and tomorrow, *Am J Nurs* 90(5):48, 1990.

BACK TO BASICS: ACIDOSIS, ALKALOSIS, AND ABGs

Do those arterial blood gas values mean the patient is acidotic or alkalotic? Do they indicate a respiratory or metabolic cause? Take this simple refresher course—then test yourself.

BY YVONNE N. STRINGFIELD

Over the last few hours, Albert Ruiz has taken a turn for the worse. He seems confused and disoriented. He's complaining of a severe headache and has been having seizures. He's been urinating copiously. His blood glucose level has soared, and his blood pressure has been dropping. You just got his arterial blood gas (ABG) results: pH is 7.23, $PaCO_2$ 32 mmHg, and HCO_3 15.5 mEq/L. What does it all add up to?

If you interpret ABG results every day, maybe you knew right away that Mr. Ruiz has compensated metabolic acidosis. But if you see them less often, chances are you had a harder time coming up with the answer. It's easy to get a bit "rusty" with lack of practice. In this quick review, we'll focus on using ABGs to determine acid-base balance and differentiate between respiratory and metabolic problems. Refresh your memory, then test your "ABG IQ" with the quick quiz that follows.

HOW TO INTERPRET THOSE NUMBERS

The body's acid-base balance (or, more precisely, the hydrogen ion concentration of extracellular fluid) is indicated by *pH*, which normally ranges from 7.35 to 7.45. A patient suffers from acidosis if his pH is below that range; if it's above, he has alkalosis (see *What's Normal, What's Not*).

ABGs tell you whether the regulatory mechanisms of the lungs and kidneys are successfully maintaining proper pH. Respiration's effect on pH is indicated by the partial pressure of carbon dioxide, or *$PaCO_2$*. Carbon dioxide, which reacts with water to become acidic, accumulates when respiration is impaired and is depleted in hyperventilation. $PaCO_2$ normally ranges between 35 and 45 mmHg; a lower value denotes *respiratory alkalosis,* a higher one *respiratory acidosis.*

Metabolic influences on pH are reflected in the level of the alkali bicarbonate (HCO_3), normally 22 to 26 mEq/L; less means *metabolic acidosis,* more *metabolic alkalosis.*

ALWAYS START WITH PH

To assess acid-base balance from ABG values, start with pH, to determine whether the patient is acidotic or alkalotic. Then move on to $PaCO_2$ and HCO_3, which will reveal whether the imbalance, if any, is respiratory or metabolic in origin. Let's consider some sample ABG values.

pH = 7.3, $PaCO_2$ = 35 mmHg, HCO_3 = 20 mEq/L. These values indicate metabolic acidosis. The pH and the HCO_3 are low, the $PaCO_2$ is normal. One common cause of metabolic acidosis is diabetic ketosis. Other situations where you might encounter it are renal failure, shock, and alcohol poisoning.

pH = 7.48, $PaCO_2$ = 38 mmHg, HCO_3 = 30 mEq/L. These values signal metabolic alkalosis. The pH and HCO_3 are high, and the $PaCO_2$ is normal. Vomiting, diarrhea, and excessive use of steroids and diuretics are possible causes.

pH = 7.3, $PaCO_2$ = 50 mmHg, HCO_3 = 24 mEq/L. Here, the numbers indicate respiratory acidosis. The pH is low, the $PaCO_2$ is high, and the HCO_3 is normal. Respiratory acidosis is caused by *hypoventilation* due to sedative overdose, chronic obstructive pulmonary disease, severe pulmonary edema, and various other conditions.

pH = 7.49, $PaCO_2$ = 30 mmHg, HCO_3 = 24 mEq/L. These values signal respiratory alkalosis. The pH is high, the $PaCO_2$ is low, and the HCO_3 is normal. Respiratory alkalosis results from *hyperventilation,* such as in adult respiratory distress syndrome, asthma, acute myocardial infarction, or congestive heart failure.

In the examples above, pH was abnormal, and so was either the $PaCO_2$ or HCO_3. One value was within normal range.

But in many cases, all three ABG values are abnormal. A patient may have both metabolic acidosis and respiratory alkalosis, for example. This happens when the body is trying to restore proper pH—a process called *compen-*

Yvonne N. Stringfield, RN, MS, EdD, is assistant professor of nursing at Christopher Newport University in Newport News, VA.

What's Normal, What's Not

ABG value	Normal	Acidosis	Alkalosis
pH	7.35-7.45	below 7.35	above 7.45
$PaCO_2$	35-45 mmHg	above 45 mmHg	below 35 mmHg
HCO_3	22-26 mEq/L	below 22 mEq/L	above 26 mEq/L

SELF-TEST

What conditions do the following ABGs reveal? Do the values indicate compensation or a fully compensated disorder? Check your answers against those at right.

1. pH = 7.31, $PaCO_2$ = 50 mmHg, HCO_3 = 22 mEq/L
2. pH = 7.31, $PaCO_2$ = 44 mmHg, HCO_3 = 20 mEq/L
3. pH = 7.47, $PaCO_2$ = 48 mmHg, HCO_3 = 30 mEq/L
4. pH = 7.3, $PaCO_2$ = 50 mmHg, HCO_3 = 30 mEq/L
5. pH = 7.33, $PaCO_2$ = 40 mmHg, HCO_3 = 21 mEq/L
6. pH = 7.48, $PaCO_2$ = 45 mmHg, HCO_3 = 30 mEq/L
7. pH = 7.33, $PaCO_2$ = 49 mmHg, HCO_3 = 26 mEq/L
8. pH = 7.48, $PaCO_2$ = 33 mmHg, HCO_3 = 24 mEq/L
9. pH = 7.31, $PaCO_2$ = 33 mmHg, HCO_3 = 20 mEq/L
10. pH = 7.48, $PaCO_2$ = 30 mmHg, HCO_3 = 20 mEq/L
11. pH = 7.45, $PaCO_2$ = 34 mmHg, HCO_3 = 20 mEq/L
12. pH = 7.35, $PaCO_2$ = 34 mmHg, HCO_3 = 20 mEq/L

ANSWERS

1. Respiratory acidosis (low pH, high $PaCO_2$, normal HCO_3)
2. Metabolic acidosis (low pH, normal $PaCO_2$, low HCO_3)
3. Metabolic alkalosis, compensation (high pH, high $PaCO_2$, high HCO_3)
4. Respiratory acidosis, compensation (low pH, high $PaCO_2$, high HCO_3)
5. Metabolic acidosis (low pH, normal $PaCO_2$, low HCO_3)
6. Metabolic alkalosis (high pH, normal $PaCO_2$, high HCO_3)
7. Respiratory acidosis (low pH, high $PaCO_2$, normal HCO_3)
8. Respiratory alkalosis (high pH, low $PaCO_2$, normal HCO_3)
9. Metabolic acidosis, compensation (low pH, low $PaCO_2$, low HCO_3)
10. Respiratory alkalosis, compensation (high pH, low $PaCO_2$, low HCO_3)
11. Respiratory alkalosis, fully compensated
12. Metabolic acidosis, fully compensated

sation. The abnormal pH indicates that compensation hasn't completely restored acid-base balance.

Sometimes, pH will be within the normal range while both $PaCO_2$ and HCO_3 are off. This means the primary disorder has been completely compensated for. For example, an initial metabolic acidosis may be completely balanced by compensating respiratory alkalosis.

As with uncompensated cases, pH is the key. See whether it falls to the alkalotic or acidotic side of 7.4. Now look at $PaCO_2$ and HCO_3: The one in the same state as the pH represents the patient's primary disorder. If you see low pH and high $PaCO_2$, for example, it means your patient's main problem is respiratory acidosis. The metabolic drive to compensate will be reflected in a high bicarbonate level.

Again, let's look at some sample numbers:

pH = 7.3, $PaCO_2$ = 49 mmHg, HCO_3 = 30 mEq/L. This indicates *respiratory acidosis with compensa-tion:* The pH is low, the $PaCO_2$ and HCO_3 are elevated. The pH and the $PaCO_2$ are both acidotic while the HCO_3 is alkalotic.

pH = 7.5, $PaCO_2$ = 30 mmHg, HCO_3 = 18 mEq/L. Here, the numbers show *respiratory alkalosis with compensation.* The pH is high, and the $PaCO_2$ and HCO_3 are low. The pH and the $PaCO_2$ are both alkalotic while the HCO_3 is acidotic.

pH = 7.48, $PaCO_2$ = 46 mmHg, HCO_3 = 30 mEq/L. These values indicate *metabolic alkalosis with compensation.* All three values are high: The pH and the HCO_3 are alkalotic while the $PaCO_2$ is acidotic.

pH = 7.3, $PaCO_2$ = 30 mmHg, HCO_3 = 18 mEq/L. This is an example of *metabolic acidosis with compensation.* All three values are low: The pH and the HCO_3 are acidotic while the $PaCO_2$ is alkalotic.

pH = 7.45, $PaCO_2$ = 46 mmHg, HCO_3 = 27 mEq/L. These values indicate *fully compensated metabolic alkalosis.* The pH is within the normal range, but on the high (alkalotic) side. The HCO_3 is high (alkalotic), and the $PaCO_2$ is also high (acidotic).

SELECTED REFERENCES

Anderson, S. ABGs: six easy steps to interpreting blood gases. *Am.J.Nurs.* 90: 42-43, 45, Aug. 1990.

Hartshorn, J., et al. *Introduction to Critical Care Nursing.* Philadelphia, W. B. Saunders, 1993.

AUTONOMIC DYSREFLEXIA

Spinal cord-injured patients can experience a life-threatening exaggeration of the sympathetic response to stimulation. Here's how to get them out of danger.

BY CAROL JORGENSEN HUSTON, RN, MSN, AND RENÉE BOELMAN, SN

Steve Crowley, age 24, has been a quadriplegic since a cervical spinal cord injury six months ago. He's been on your medical-surgical unit for two days for treatment of a sacral pressure ulcer.

When reviewing his recorded input and output measurements for the last 24 hours, you note that Mr. Crowley hasn't had a bowel movement in two days. You also find that his most recent urinary catheterization yielded only a small amount of urine.

You go to Mr. Crowley's room first during your initial rounds. When you arrive, he tells you through clenched teeth that he has a pounding headache, is nauseated, and feels "like his head is about to explode." His face and forehead are extremely diaphoretic and flushed. When you check his vital signs, you note that his heart rate, normally 70 to 80, is now only 48, and his blood pressure is elevated at 200/100.

DECIPHERING THE CLUES

Mr. Crowley is exhibiting some of the classic signs of autonomic dysreflexia—pounding headache, marked hypertension, diaphoresis (especially of the forehead), bradycardia, flushing, piloerection, nausea, and nasal congestion. A full bladder or bowel can put patients with spinal cord injury at risk for this condition.

WHAT CAUSES THE PROBLEM

When there's a spinal cord injury above the thoracic sympathetic outflow (T6 or T7), the feedback system between the sympathetic and parasympathetic branches of the autonomic nervous system is disrupted. If an irritant below the level of spinal cord injury

overstimulates the autonomic nervous system, the resulting sympathetic response—profound vasoconstriction, producing a rapid rise in blood pressure—is exaggerated because the parasympathetic response is partially disabled. Baroreceptors in the cerebral vessels, carotid sinus, and aorta detect the rising blood pressure and attempt to trigger visceral and peripheral vasodilation, but the impulses can't pass through the damaged spinal cord. The parasympathetic response is limited to vagal slowing of the heart rate and vasodilation, flushing, and diaphoresis above the level of spinal cord injury.

Anything that can cause discomfort to a neurologically intact person can trigger autonomic dysreflexia in a patient with spinal cord injury. The most common stimulus is a distended bladder or rectum. Stimulation of the skin from pressure, pain, heat or cold is another common cause.

HOW TO INTERVENE

Rapidly identifying and removing the cause of the dysreflexia and lowering Mr. Crowley's blood pressure are your first priorities. If left unchecked, systolic blood pressure can reach 300 mmHg in patients with this condition, risking stroke, myocardial infarction, and ocular hemorrhage that may lead to blindness. (In clinical situations where these risks are imminent, drug treatment may be used to reduce blood pressure before identifying and removing the cause of the dysreflexia.)

After calling the physician, you remove anything that may be stimulating Mr. Crowley's skin, such as constricting bed linens or sneakers worn to decrease foot drop. You help him sit up, while keeping his feet down, to promote orthostatic reduction of blood pressure. (For patients who can't sit up, elevate the head of the bed to 90°.)

You assess Mr. Crowley's abdomen

for evidence of a distended bladder (which causes autonomic dysreflexia more often than a full bowel does) and conclude that he needs catheterization. You insert the catheter after lubricating it liberally with Xylocaine to reduce stimulation. While monitoring and slowly draining the bladder, you check Mr. Crowley's blood pressure every few minutes.

Five minutes after his bladder was fully drained, there's no change in his blood pressure, so you suspect that his constipation is the primary factor. A repeat abdominal assessment indicates bowel distension. You gently insert 1 oz of Xylocaine, as ordered, into his rectum. When the anesthetic takes effect, you manually check for fecal impaction and remove all accessible stool.

The physician arrives as you're checking Mr. Crowley's blood pressure again. It's still elevated, so he orders hydralazine hydrochloride (Apresoline), 20 to 40 mg iv, an arteriolar vasodilator used to lower blood pressure and raise heart rate. (Sublingual nifedipine [Procardia], 10 to 20 mg, is a common alternative treatment.) You continue to check Mr. Crowley's blood pressure every two to three minutes until it returns to normal.

FOLLOWING UP

Within five minutes, Mr. Crowley's blood pressure has fallen to 100/60 and his symptoms have abated. A strict bowel and bladder regimen is planned to prevent overdistension.

Before he's discharged, Mr. Crowley and his primary caregiver are taught how to prevent another episode of autonomic dysreflexia by maintaining a bowel- and bladder-emptying program at home. He's also instructed about the other possible triggers of the condition and reminded to call for help immediately if he experiences any of its warning signs.

Carol Jorgensen Huston is a professor of nursing at California State University, Chico, and Renée Boelman is an interim permittee registered nurse.

TB SKIN TESTING: HOW TO DO IT RIGHT

The Mantoux test is the gold standard for tuberculosis screening. Here's a step-by-step guide to performing this test properly.

BY M. ANN AVEY

Nearly 15 million people in the United States are infected with the organism that causes tuberculosis (TB). Approximately 30,000 new diagnoses are reported annually, and by the year 2000 this figure is expected to jump to over 50,000 per year. So if it hasn't happened already, you may soon find yourself administering a test you learned long ago but haven't performed in years—the Mantoux tuberculin skin test, using purified protein derivative (PPD) of tuberculin.

The Mantoux test is known to be far more accurate than the multiple-puncture (tine) test, once widely used. That's because it uses known quantities of tuberculin and produces reactions that can be more precisely evaluated. Consequently, it's become the preferred method of screening for TB. Today, the Mantoux test usually provides the first evidence of clinical infection. And when meticulously administered, it can result in prompt treatment and help stop the resurgence of TB.

To help you refine your Mantoux skills, here's a brief review of the procedure—when to use the test, how to perform it, and how to interpret the results.

WHAT THE MANTOUX TELLS YOU

The Mantoux test is not diagnostic of active TB. Pulmonary tuberculosis is usually diagnosed by sputum cultures. To diagnose extrapulmonary TB, other specimens, such as urine, cere-

brospinal fluid, or pleural fluid, are usually required. In most cases, however, a positive Mantoux test does signify infection with the bacillus *Mycobacterium tuberculosis*. It may or may not mean the disease is active. But if an infection is new, a positive reaction allows you to treat the asymptomatic patient prophylactically.

The test works by revealing a person's hypersensitivity—and, therefore, exposure—to the bacillus. Hypersensitivity results from the interaction of antibodies or T lymphocytes and certain antigens; it's the price we sometimes pay for having a healthy immune system. And hypersensitivity is what makes TB so deadly. The bacillus isn't inherently toxic, but when a person is infected, both *M. tuberculosis* and its product, tuberculin, can induce very damaging, delayed, allergic—or hypersensitive—reactions. These reactions can destroy entire organs.

The Mantoux test is based on the fact that a person infected with *M. tuberculosis* will display a limited, local hypersensitivity when a small amount of tuberculin is injected between the layers of his skin. Unfortunately, it may take as long as 10 weeks after initial infection for the skin to react to the test. And even at that point, the test is neither 100% sensitive nor 100% specific.

WHY RESULTS ARE SOMETIMES FALSE

Although the Mantoux is the gold standard of TB tests—and is considered reliable when properly administered to the general population—as many as 60% of people infected with the human immunodeficiency virus

(HIV) have false negative Mantoux test results. False negatives occur more often among older people than younger people—generally because of suppressed immunity brought on by illness. In other words, a weakened immune system or advanced age can diminish hypersensitivity, producing anergy (lack of response to an injected antigen).

That's why people at high risk for TB exposure are usually retested in two weeks if they produce negative Mantoux test results and are over 35 years old (see chart). The second test heightens the subclinical hypersensitive response. Of course, any time pulmonary signs or symptoms (such as cough, chest pain, or blood-tinged sputum) are present, you'd refer the patient for further evaluation.

With the Mantoux test, false positives are rare. A false positive may indicate infection with mycobacteria other than *M. tuberculosis*. Or it could mean that the patient was vaccinated with the bacillus Calmette-Guérin (BCG), a TB immunization of questionable reliability. Many U.S. residents who were born outside of the country received this vaccine. It's not always possible to distinguish reactions caused by BCG from those caused by TB infection. But BCG vaccination is no guarantee that a positive skin test is false. Whether or not the patient has been vaccinated for TB, a positive result requires follow-up physical examination (often including chest X-rays and specimen samples) to rule out active disease.

Once a person reacts positively to the test, do not in repeating it. Positivity is almost always permanent.

M. Ann Avey, RN, BS, works as a public health nurse for the North East Tri-County Health District in Newport, WA.

Skin Reactions: How TB Risk Factors Affect the Reading

Tuberculosis is transmitted by droplets produced by coughing, sneezing, or speaking, usually during prolonged, close contact with an infected person. This chart tells you who's at highest risk for TB, when to do skin screening, how to interpret initial Mantoux test results, and when to retest. (Of course, any patient with suspicious signs and symptoms, such as an unexplained cough, chest pain, or blood-tinged sputum, should be tested, regardless of risk factors.)

TB risk factors	Skin screening	0-4 mm induration	5-9 mm induration	10-14 mm induration	15 mm or more induration
Compromised immune system	Once a year	Retest immediately if patient shows anergy		Positive	
Close contact with TB-infected person	Yes, immediately	Retest 10 weeks after last exposure and again in three months		Positive	
Abnormal chest X-ray consistent with TB	No (immediate sputum culture necessary)	Test unnecessary (sputum culture is diagnositic)			
Living or working in a hospital, long-term care facility, drug-treatment center, homeless shelter, or prison	Once a year	Retest two weeks after initial test if over 35 years old (in most states; 55 in some)			Positive
Substance abuse	On admission to any health care facility	Retest two weeks after initial test if over 35 years old (in most states; 55 in some)			Positive
Born in area where TB is prevalent (such as Asia, Africa, or Latin America)	On admission to any health care facility	Retest two weeks after initial test if over 35 years old (in most states; 55 in some)			Positive
Prolonged cortisone treatment, immuno-suppressive therapy, or gastrectomy	Not routinely needed	Retest two weeks after initial test if over 35 years old (in most states; 55 in some)			Positive
Diabetes, advanced renal disease, carcinoma, or being 10% or more below normal body weight	Not routinely needed	Retest two weeks after initial test if over 35 years old (in most states; 55 in some)			Positive
None (including immunization with BCG)	Not routinely needed	Negative			Positive

PREPARING FOR THE TEST

Before administering a Mantoux test, you might want to practice by giving intradermal injections of normal saline solution to a colleague. Follow the same procedure you'd use if you were giving PPD to a real patient.

Prepare for the test as you would for any injection—by washing your hands. Since you'll be using a needle, follow universal precautions and wear gloves—even though the risk of exposure to body fluids is minimal. Seat your patient comfortably, resting his exposed left arm on a firm, well-lighted surface. (Even with left-handed patients, using the left arm is standard procedure.) Clean the injection site with an alcohol swab and allow it to dry completely.

The Mantoux test requires you to give the patient an intradermal injection of 0.1 mL of 5 tuberculin units (TUs) of stabilized PPD. You'll use a single-dose tuberculin syringe and a ½-inch, 26- or 27-gauge needle with a short bevel.

Prepare the syringe out of the patient's sight. After filling it with just over 0.1mL, hold it upright and tap it lightly to remove air, then expel one drop. Check that a full 0.1mL remains in the syringe.

Although you may use any flat body surface as an injection site, skin reactions are usually easiest to assess when you avoid sites that are red or swollen. Also avoid visible veins—both to make it easier to assess reactions and to avoid accidental iv injection in patients with very shallow veins. The preferred injection site is on the volar or dorsal surface of the left forearm, about four inches below the elbow. If this site is unavailable, you might find it helpful to circle the injection site with a pen, so when it's time to evaluate the test it's easy to locate.

HOW TO PERFORM THE INJECTION

Start by stretching the skin taut with your nondominant hand. Then, while holding the syringe parallel to (almost resting on) the skin surface, insert the needle, bevel up, under the first one or two layers of skin. Positioned correctly, the tip of the needle will be visible just below the surface of the skin.

As you slowly inject the contents of the syringe, you'll feel a slight resistance. A firm, white wheal or bubble, about 6 to 10 mm in diameter, should appear at the injection site immediately. Test results will be reliable only if this distinct wheal appears. If injectate leaks out onto the skin and no wheal appears, it means you didn't place the needle deeply enough. If the wheal is shallow and diffuse, you've given the injection too deeply. In either case, you'll need to administer a second injection at least two inches from the first site.

You may see a drop of blood when you withdraw the needle. That's normal.

Afterward, as with any injection, place the syringe in a puncture-resistant container without recapping the needle. Tell the patient it will take 48 to 72 hours before his skin reaction can be assessed.

You can evaluate patients with suppressed immunity for delayed-type hypersensitivity (DTH) anergy when you perform the Mantoux screening. This involves testing the patient with two or more DTH antigens (*Candida,* mumps, or tetanus toxoid) using the Mantoux method. Like the PPD reaction, DTH anergy can be evaluated at 48 to 72 hours after injection.

MEASURING THE REACTION

If your patient's reaction is positive, you'll probably see both erythema and induration at the injection site. Carefully locate the perimeter of the indurated area by lightly palpating the site with a finger. Sometimes the precise edge of induration is difficult to palpate. Use a pen to help you mark the beginning and end points of induration. Use a flexible ruler to measure only the

area of induration—across the width of the forearm (never from elbow to wrist).

Document the time when you read the patient's reaction (the number of hours since you administered the injection), and note the lot number, if known. Then record the size of the induration in millimeters, disregarding any erythema. (No matter how much redness is present, it's clinically insignificant.) If a measurement falls between two millimeter demarcations on the ruler, record the smaller of the two, so the patient won't be unnecessarily treated with potent antituberculosis agents. And if the patient has no induration, record the results as "0 mm of reaction"—not simply as "negative"—so you have a baseline for future readings.

If you performed the test for DTH anergy, any induration from that injection after 48 to 72 hours is considered evidence of DTH responsiveness. No induration indicates anergy.

INTERPRETING THE RESULTS

Whether a person's Mantoux results are considered positive or negative depends a great deal on his risk of exposure to TB and general health. For those in good health with no risk factors, an induration of 15 mm is usually considered positive. But because those at risk for TB will probably have diminished hypersensitivity—through exposure or suppressed immunity—an induration as small as 5 mm may be

considered positive. When a patient's history or physical condition indicates a need to retest him, despite negative results, a second test should be done within three weeks.

If the results are positive, tell the patient that the test indicates TB infection, but the disease may or may not be active. Refer him for follow-up examination. And let him know that his physician may prescribe drugs to prevent the TB from becoming active.

No screening test is perfect. But when administered correctly, the Mantoux test can be an invaluable tool—leading to early detection, treatment, and containment of TB.

SELECTED REFERENCES

Pierce, N. R. "TB's insidious return: did we ask for it?" *Washington Post Writer's Group, County News,* Oct. 12, 1992.

Price, S. A., and Wilson, L. M. *Pathophysiology: Clinical Concepts of Disease Processes.* 4th ed. St. Louis, Mosby-Year Book, 1992, pp. 58-59, 600-603.

Tuberculosis morbidity in the United States: final data, 1990. *MMWR* 40[SS-3]:23-27, 1991.

U.S. Centers for Disease Control and Prevention. *Administering and Reading the Mantoux Test.* (videotape) Atlanta, The Centers, 1992.

U.S. Centers for Disease Control and Prevention. *Core Curriculum On Tuberculosis.* Atlanta, The Centers, 1991.

Washington State Health Division, Tuberculosis Division. *Tuberculosis Update '93;* a two-day workshop sponsored by Sacred Heart Hospital, Spokane, WA, June 1993.

7 CARE TIPS FOR MANAGING PATIENTS WITH DIABETES

Advice on how to avoid complications and keep patients satisfied with their diabetes care in the hospital.

BY SANDIE ANDERSON, RN, BSN, CDE

Marge Halloway, age 42, is admitted to a medical-surgical unit with right upper-quadrant abdominal pain. Her history reveals that she's had type I or insulin-dependent diabetes mellitus (IDDM) since age 23. Her last hospitalization was 13 years ago when she gave birth, and she's anxious about the care she'll receive during this hospital stay. When you're used to being in charge of your own diabetes care, it can be frightening to give up some of that control to others.

Ms. Halloway is scheduled for an intravenous (iv) cholangiogram, which requires her to be NPO after midnight. Her blood glucose level at 6:30 am is 135 mg/dL (normal is 70 to 115 mg/dL).

The nurse checks Ms. Halloway's medication administration record. She's scheduled for a morning dose of 33 units of NPH and seven units of Regular insulin, plus a sliding-scale dose before meals. Concerned that her patient's glucose level will fall below normal while she's NPO, the nurse consults Ms. Halloway's physician, who agrees that she should hold the morning insulin.

Ms. Halloway expresses concern that she hasn't received her insulin. The nurse explains: "I'm not giving you insulin this morning because I'm afraid your blood sugar will drop too low if I did, since you're not eating. I've already notified your doctor."

This nurse had frequently held insu-

lin for her patients who had diabetes and were NPO, with physician approval. None ever experienced any adverse effects. But most of those patients—like the 90% of the 14 million Americans with diabetes—had type II or non-insulin-dependent diabetes mellitus (NIDDM). Because they produce some endogenous insulin, these patients don't require exogenous insulin to sustain life.

Type I patients, however, produce no insulin at all. Their only source of insulin is exogenous. One delayed or missed dose can produce severe hyperglycemia.

That's what happened to Ms. Halloway. By 11:30 AM, after her cholangiogram, her blood glucose level had risen to 328 mg/dL.

How can you avoid problems like this when caring for patients with diabetes? The following seven tips will help.

1: KNOW WHAT TYPE OF DIABETES YOUR PATIENT HAS.

A quick review of the pathophysiology will clarify why knowing what type of diabetes your patient has is so important. In normal glycemic homeostasis, beta cells in the pancreas continuously secrete small amounts of insulin, maintaining an average fasting blood glucose level of 70 to 115 mg/dL. A continuous low-level secretion of insulin, called basal insulin, prevents hyperglycemia during periods of fasting. In the fasting state— when a patient is NPO, for example—the liver releases stored glucose to feed cells through gluconeogenesis and glycogenolysis. This process will rapidly increase blood glucose levels if basal

levels of insulin aren't present to check the liver's glucose production. That's why Ms. Halloway still needs her insulin even though she's NPO.

Because they have no effective insulin production, patients like Ms. Halloway need exogenous insulin to maintain metabolism and prevent rapid dehydration, catabolism, ketoacidosis, and death. For them, survival depends on the availability of exogenous insulin 24 hours a day to mimic normal patterns of insulin secretion.

If you don't know what type of diabetes your patient has, ask her. Patients with type I are usually well aware of their diabetes classification. If your patient doesn't know and her medical history doesn't help, ask her about her weight and age when she first learned she had diabetes. Most people who were thin or under age 30 at diagnosis are likely to have type I diabetes. Other indicators of type I include a history of ketonuria or ketonemia with hyperglycemia and a history of ketoacidosis. You can also learn your patient's diabetes type from laboratory test results, such as C-peptide levels, insulin autoantibodies, and islet cell antibodies.

2: BE SURE THAT YOUR PATIENT WITH TYPE I DIABETES HAS INSULIN "ON-BOARD" 24 HOURS A DAY.

Never hold insulin doses. You might get away with a reduced dose when your patient isn't eating much or is fasting, but her need for insulin around-the-clock continues. And if you know the duration of action of the insulins you're administering, you can anticipate when their effects will be abating, indicating a need for a

Sandie Anderson is a diabetes nurse clinician at the International Diabetes Center, Kansas City Regional Affiliate, located at Research Medical Center, Kansas City, MO.

new dose (see *Insulin Actions* on page 38).

For example, let's say you have an order to discontinue a Regular insulin drip. The insulin's effects will peak in 15 to 30 minutes, then diminish over the next one to two hours. So you'll want to give a second insulin dose subcutaneously before the iv insulin action stops. The onset of action of subcutaneous Regular insulin is about 30 minutes. If you give the subcutaneous dose about 30 minutes before the drip runs out, it will take effect just as the effects of the iv insulin are terminating.

3: COORDINATE REGULAR INSULIN ADMINISTRATION WITH MEALS.

Whether Regular insulin is given as a standard dose or on a sliding scale, schedule it for 30 minutes before the patient eats. Because hospital meal times are usually controlled by the dietary department, you'll need to accommodate their schedule of meal delivery. If the tray arrives before the 30 minutes have elapsed, explain to the patient why she needs to delay eating. (This will also serve to reinforce the interrelationship between good diabetes management and meal planning.) If trays are frequently late, hold off administering insulin until after the meal cart has arrived since tray delivery usually takes about 30 minutes.

The timing of insulin doses—for 30 minutes before meals—should be written in the patient's medication administration record. That way, each nurse can individualize her patient's insulin doses and meals. Avoid giving insulin after meals; the delayed onset will be too late to curb postprandial hyperglycemia.

One last point here: Try to arrange for any procedures to be scheduled early in the day. That way, insulin and nourishment can be resumed as soon as possible. Diabetes management requires consistency in the timing of meals and medications. The sooner your patient can resume her normal meals/medications schedule, the sooner her blood glucose levels can be balanced.

4: PERFORM CAPILLARY BLOOD GLUCOSE FINGERSTICKS 30 TO 60 MINUTES BEFORE ADMINISTERING INSULIN.

The results of fingerstick tests are used to determine sliding-scale insulin doses. Since glucose levels can vary after 60 minutes, repeat the test if an hour has elapsed without insulin being given.

A long delay between fingerstick tests and insulin doses may be of particular concern in the early morning. Often, night shift nurses perform morning fingerstick tests as early as 5 AM, when breakfast is still several hours away. If the insulin is given properly 30 minutes before breakfast, based on an hours-old glucose reading, the dose may not be the right one for the patient.

Following this fourth care tip might require that night shift nurses perform fingerstick tests no earlier than 6:30 AM, or that the day shift do all these tests.

5: PREPARE SLIDING-SCALE DOSES OF REGULAR INSULIN AND STANDARD DAILY DOSES IN THE SAME SYRINGE.

Let's say you have a type I patient who's scheduled for a standard dose of Regular insulin every morning. This patient also has an order for a sliding-scale dose of Regular insulin. The order calls for both doses to be given 30 minutes before meals.

To avoid an extra injection, prepare both doses in the same syringe. (One exception: Mixing Lente and Regular insulin will slow the action of the Regular insulin, so two injections would be necessary.)

6: DON'T OVERTREAT HYPOGLYCEMIA.

Hypoglycemia develops when there's too much insulin or not enough glucose available in the patient's bloodstream. Signs and symptoms of hypoglycemia include shakiness, headache, anxiety, and sweating, all of which indicate that cells aren't receiving enough glucose.

For initial treatment, the American Diabetes Association recommends 10 to 15 grams of a simple oral carbohydrate, such as four to six ounces of fruit juice or a nondiet carbonated drink, five or six Lifesavers, or two or three glucose tablets. (Adding sugar to fruit juice is unnecessary and may raise blood glucose levels too high.)

After this initial treatment, wait 15 to 30 minutes before doing another blood glucose check. This isn't easy— for you or your patient—especially if the patient continues experiencing signs and symptoms of hypoglycemia. But testing her glucose level too soon may prompt an unnecessary second administration of carbohydrate.

If the patient's signs and symptoms haven't improved by this time or her glucose level remains below the parameters set by the physician (usually 60 to 70 mg/dL), repeat the treatment.

7: MAKE SURE THAT YOUR PATIENT IS RECEIVING AN ADA DIET.

To illustrate this last point, let's return to Ms. Halloway. We left her with a blood glucose level of 328 mg/dL, which resulted from her nurse holding her standard morning dose of mixed insulin. It's now 11:30 AM. Ms. Halloway's cholangiogram has been done. A fingerstick reveals her high glucose level, which is treated with a sliding-scale dose. About a half hour later, Ms. Halloway starts eating her lunch.

"This gelatin tastes so much better than the sugar-free kind I use at home," Ms. Halloway says to her nurse. "I wonder what brand it is."

The nurse looks at the dish. It's not the kind the hospital uses to serve sugar-free gelatin. She calls the dietitian and confirms that Ms. Halloway

Insulin Actions

Insulin type	Onset of action	Peak effects	Effective duration
Regular	*sc:* 30-minutes-1 hour	2-3 hours	3-6 hours
	iv: immediate	15-30 minutes	1-2 hours
NPH	*sc* (only): 2-4 hours	4-10 hours	10-16 hours
Lente	*sc* (only): 3-4 hours	4-12 hours	12-18 hours
Ultralente	*sc* (only): 6-10 hours	minimal (effects tend to remain constant)	18-20 hours

NOTE: ABSORPTION RATES MAY VARY, DEPENDING ON SUCH FACTORS AS INJECTION SITE, TISSUE PERFUSION, AND ACTIVITY.

has received regular gelatin. In fact, her diet order is for an 1,800-calorie, low-fat diet—no mention of restrictions for diabetes.

Checking the original medical order, the nurse discovers that the physician had never ordered any diabetes restrictions. She calls the physician, who orders an 1,800-calorie ADA diet.

Remember that the cornerstone of diabetes control is the meal plan. If your patient isn't eating properly, glycemic control will be difficult, if not impossible. Diets for persons with diabetes are usually labeled "ADA," indicating that the meal plan follows the American Diabetes Association's current nutritional recommendations. Check the medical order for this hallmark. If an ADA diet isn't ordered, question the physician.

To go a step further, find out how your facility identifies sugar-free gelatins, puddings, juices, and the like. Sometimes they're marked "sugar-free" or "diet." Other times they're served in different containers. Check the tray when your patient's food arrives. If the foods appear to be highly concentrated sweets or unusually high in saturated fat, contact the dietitian for your unit and discuss your concerns.

These seven tips will help you manage your patients with diabetes effectively. Many of them involve interdependent functions that require a physician's order or the cooperation of other departments. But no one is more qualified to coordinate this team effort than you.

SELECTED REFERENCES

American Diabetes Association. Clinical Practice Recommendations, 1992-1993. *Diabetes Care* 16(Suppl. 2):3, 31-34, May 1993.

American Diabetes Association. *Physician's Guide to Insulin-Dependent (Type I) Diabetes: Diagnosis and Treatment.* Alexandria, VA, The Association, 1988.

American Diabetes Association. *Therapy for Diabetes Mellitus and Related Disorders. "Hypoglycemia in Patients with Type I Diabetes."* Alexandria, VA, The Association, 1991.

National Center for Chronic Disease Prevention and Health Promotion. *Diabetes Fact Sheets.* Atlanta, GA, Centers for Disease Control, 1990.

National Center for Chronic Disease Prevention and Health Promotion. *Diabetes Surveillance.* Atlanta, GA, Centers for Disease Control, 1991.

VIRAL HEPATITIS: ANATOMY OF A DIAGNOSIS

This interesting case study illustrates the clinical detective work required to diagnose viral hepatitis. It also underscores the importance of protecting yourself against the risk of contracting this disease as a health care professional.

BY MARGUERITE McMILLAN JACKSON, RN, MS, FAAN, AND
THÉRÈSE E. RYMER, RN, FNP-CS, COHN

Sue Nguyen, a 26-year-old registered nurse, had been feeling miserable for three days. She'd been vomiting and had abdominal pain and achy joints. Linda Johnson, her roommate who was also a nurse, brought her at 11 PM on the night of February 1 to the emergency department of the hospital where they both worked.

Dr. Marcella Juarez, the physician on duty, took Ms. Nguyen's history. While questioning her about other symptoms besides the nausea, she discovered that Ms. Nguyen was passing dark urine and light stools. She'd also recently given up smoking. In fact, she volunteered that now she had a strong distaste for cigarettes. Ms. Nguyen had lost five pounds in the last week, had no appetite, was exhausted, and reported difficulty in thinking clearly.

Dr. Juarez found that Ms. Nguyen had slight tenderness over her liver, but no evidence of enlargement. Her abdomen was soft and her spleen wasn't enlarged. Dr. Juarez also noted no lymph node enlargement.

Ms. Nguyen had been well before her present illness except for dry, cracked skin on her hands, thought to be related to a latex allergy. She was being treated by a dermatologist, but wasn't taking any systemic medica-

tions. She'd been using 1% hydrocortisone cream for about a week. Dr. Juarez didn't believe the topical treatment was related to her complaint. She hadn't injected drugs of any kind, didn't use alcohol, and wasn't pregnant.

Dr. Juarez suspected that Ms. Nguyen had some type of hepatitis because she had the classic signs and symptoms. Most notable were the changes in urine and stool, nausea, weight loss, exhaustion, and distaste for cigarettes. Her liver tenderness also supported this assessment.

IDENTIFYING POSSIBLE EXPOSURES

Because Ms. Nguyen was a nurse, Dr. Juarez first investigated potential exposures common to health care professionals. Ms. Nguyen couldn't recall any needlesticks or lacerations. Her roommate, Ms. Johnson, reminded her of the emergency care they'd given to a patient on the psychiatric unit where they both worked in early December. That patient, Walt Barlow, had collapsed in the unit hallway after experiencing bright red bloody vomiting. He was later diagnosed with esophageal varices thought to be related to his chronic alcohol abuse.

Mr. Barlow had a long-standing history of IV drug abuse in New York City, too, but was documented as HIV-negative on this and previous admissions. He was also known to be a chronic hepatitis B virus (HBV) and hepatitis C virus (HCV) carrier. Ms. Nguyen remembered not wearing

gloves and getting blood on her hands during this emergency, but she hadn't had needlestick, so she didn't consider the situation to require follow-up.

Dr. Juarez asked Ms. Nguyen whether she could have had a sexual exposure to hepatitis, particularly HBV. Ms. Nguyen said that she was engaged to a physician, Jim Li, who learned he had immunity to HBV when he was tested in medical school several years ago. Because he'd grown up in China, where HBV is common, it was likely he'd been infected perinatally. Although Ms. Nguyen was from Southeast Asia, another area where HBV is common, she didn't know her antibody status. She'd also had no sexual partners except her fiancé for the past three years.

Dr. Juarez questioned Ms. Nguyen and her roommate about international travel, any other sick household members, eating raw shellfish, or hepatitis A virus (HAV) exposures from patients known to be infected. Ms. Nguyen and Ms. Johnson remembered a young homeless patient, Wendy Anders, who was diagnosed with hepatitis A in early January. Ms. Anders had helped prepare and serve a salad during a unit Christmas party about two weeks before she was diagnosed. The staff and other patients had been given immune globulin as a precaution against HAV exposure. As with all cases of hepatitis, Ms. Anders' diagnosis was reported to the local health department.

Ms. Nguyen, however, had gone to San Francisco over the holidays to visit her fiancé and didn't return until about

Marguerite McMillan Jackson is administrative director of the University of California at San Diego Medical Center, epidemiology unit, and Thérèse E. Rymer is director of clinical service for the UCSD Center for Occupational and Environmental Medicine, San Diego.

A GLOSSARY OF SUE NGUYEN'S HEPATITIS MARKERS

Anti-HAV IgM	This antibody of the IgM class appears early in the disease but decreases within weeks. It indicates acute HAV infection.
Anti-HAV IgG	Presence of this antibody in the IgG class indicates previous infection with HAV and immunity to subsequent infection.
HBsAg	This antigen, associated with the viral coat or surface, is usually the first indicator of HBV infection. Characteristically, this appears during incubation and disappears during recovery. However, in chronic carriers it will persist.
Anti-HBc	Antibody to the core antigen. It can indicate previous infection or a chronic carrier state. This antibody doesn't develop in HBV vaccine recipients.
Anti-HBs	Antibody to HBV surface coat appears months after HBsAg. Usually appears after clinical recovery and persists for life. It doesn't develop in chronic carriers. It does develop in HBV vaccine recipients.
Anti-HCV	Antibodies to HCV typically take months to develop after acute infection.

three weeks after this potential exposure. When she did, the hospital's infection surveillance nurse explained that immune globulin wouldn't be effective so late after the exposure. She was advised to watch for signs and symptoms of viral hepatitis and to see her physician if she became ill.

To Dr. Juarez, this information confirmed her suspicion of viral hepatitis as the likely cause of Ms. Nguyen's illness. She ordered a complete blood count (CBC), urinalysis, a chemistry panel to include liver function studies, and hepatitis A, B, and C panels. Ms. Nguyen was sent home with an antiemetic and instructions for oral fluid replacement and rest. She was also advised to make a follow-up appointment with her primary physician. Dr. Juarez said that she would call Ms. Nguyen at home with the laboratory results in about three days.

FOCUSING ON HAV

Sue Nguyen's case isn't unusual. Health care professionals are frequently faced with multiple exposures and workplace injuries that put them at risk for contracting viral hepatitis.

Dr. Juarez thought that Ms. Nguyen might have contracted HAV because she'd eaten some of the salad prepared by Ms. Anders. No one could say for sure whether Ms. Anders had washed her hands before handling the salad. The fact that Ms. Nguyen hadn't received prophylactic immune globulin was also a concern.

Hepatitis A virus is primarily transmitted by fecal-to-oral route. Poor handwashing by food handlers after stool contact is a common way that food is contaminated. The incubation period for HAV is about two to six weeks, with an average of 28 days. The highest concentration of the virus is found in the stool of infected persons about two weeks prior to the onset of jaundice. This is when HAV is most likely to be transmitted. Ms. Anders handled the salad during that time.

The onset of HAV is usually acute, as was the case with Ms. Nguyen. It's marked by abdominal pain, vomiting, and changes in the color of urine and stool. The skin may feel itchy, especially if bilirubin levels are elevated, and jaundice may or may not be present. Smokers often lose interest in cigarettes and may even have a strong distaste for them.

Hepatitis A virus infection is rarely fatal and, unlike HBV, there's no possibility of becoming an asymptomatic carrier, but permanent liver damage may occur. The illness is usually brief, with symptoms lasting from one to three weeks. Some infections may last up to six months, but that's rare.

Hepatitis A is the most common form of viral hepatitis in the world. Antibodies to HAV have been found in 50% to 60% of adults over age 50 in developed countries. The disease is so common in some developing countries that virtually the whole population is exposed, primarily due to poor sanitation and contaminated water. Up to 95% of adults in developing countries have been infected and have HAV antibodies.

Immune globulin, when given within two weeks of exposure, provides passive antibody protection that's 80% to 90% effective. But it doesn't provide lifelong immunity, so future exposures will require additional doses. Immune globulin is recommended for people with known exposures, members of their households, and their sexual contacts.

ANTIBODY TESTING FOR HAV

Two laboratory tests are used to diagnose HAV infection. The test for anti-HAV IgG can tell you whether the person has ever been infected before. If so, the results of this test will be positive indefinitely. A positive finding also indicates lifetime immunity. Anti-HAV IgM antibody is detectable shortly after the person starts shedding virus in stool and is almost always positive by the time clinical illness becomes evident. It indicates recent infection and may be detectable for four to six months.

Ms. Anders, the patient who'd handled the salad, had a positive anti-HAV IgM that confirmed she had acute HAV infection. Ms. Nguyen had a negative anti-HAV IgM but a positive anti-HAV IgG. This indicated previous infection, probably dating back to her early life in Southeast Asia. So Dr. Juarez could rule out HAV as the cause of Ms. Nguyen's illness.

Because HAV is the most communicable form of viral hepatitis, Dr. Juarez was relieved by Ms. Nguyen's test results. If she'd tested positive, immune globulin would have been advised for her fiancé and her roommate. Additionally, an assessment of her work responsibilities and potential for exposing others would have been necessary.

WHAT ABOUT HBV?

You may wonder why HBV should even be considered as a possible diagnosis since Ms. Nguyen should have previously been vaccinated. The Occupational Safety and Health Administration (OSHA), in its 1991 Bloodborne Pathogens Standard, mandated that the HBV vaccine be offered to health care professionals at risk for exposure. Unfortunately, Ms. Nguyen hadn't gotten around to receiving the vaccine, even though it's provided free by her employer and she'd been encouraged to obtain it during in-service classes.

While Ms. Nguyen didn't receive a needlestick, she did get blood on her hands during Mr. Barlow's emergency and wasn't wearing gloves. Even worse, there were openings in her skin due to her dermatitis. Hepatitis B virus can be transmitted through needlesticks, broken skin, or at birth from an infected mother.

It's also commonly transmitted by sexual contact. Ms. Nguyen could have been infected in this way since she was sexually active and her fiancé also had occupational risks as a physician. But Dr. Li had been screened in medical school for HBV infection and had both anti-HBc and anti-HBs, indicating previous resolved disease. He was also negative for HBsAg, which would have indicated a chronic carrier state.

The incubation period for HBV is 45 to 180 days, with an average of 60 to 90 days. Ms. Nguyen became ill about 60 days after her exposure to Mr. Barlow's blood.

Generally, HBV has a more gradual onset than HAV, but its signs and symptoms are the same. One-third to one-half of persons with HBV develop jaundice. Many infected persons with HBV infection aren't diagnosed because they remain free of symptoms.

Up to 10% of infected persons may become chronic carriers and sources of infection for others. In addition, they're at risk for serious complications that can develop over time—for example, liver cancer and cirrhosis.

TEST RESULTS TO CONFIRM HBV

Besides the anti-HAV IgG and anti-HAV IgM tests, Dr. Juarez ordered several other laboratory tests for Ms. Nguyen, including HBsAg, anti-HBs, anti-HBc, and anti-HCV. Unfortunately, both the HBsAg and anti-HBc were positive, indicating acute illness from HBV. Dr. Juarez wasn't surprised to see that the anti-HBs was negative because this antibody develops only after the acute illness resolves. Anti-HBs also doesn't develop in persons who are chronic HBV carriers, though the reason for this isn't known.

The anti-HCV test was also negative for Ms. Nguyen and represented a baseline value for her. If it had been positive, it could be interpreted as resulting from a previous exposure. This test is rarely positive until at least five months after an acute exposure. Ms. Nguyen experienced her exposure to Mr. Barlow's blood in early December—two months before her illness. There hadn't been enough time for her to develop anti-HCV from this exposure, even if she was infected.

Additionally, Ms. Nguyen's aspartate aminotransferase (AST or SGOT) level was 430 IU/L (normal, 5 to 40); alanine aminotransferase (ALT or SGPT) was 640 IU/L (normal, 5 to 35); and total bilirubin was 9 mg/dL (normal, 0.1 to 1). However, her alkaline phosphatase, albumin, globulin, and prothrombin times were all normal. Dr. Juarez was pleased to see a normal prothrombin time because elevations could suggest liver necrosis and a poor prognosis.

FOLLOW-UP: LIVING WITH HBV

Three days after Ms. Nguyen's emergency department visit, the test results were available. Dr. Juarez called Ms. Nguyen at home to see how she was feeling and to discuss the results with her.

"I'm not nauseated any more," Ms. Nguyen said, "and I'm able to take liquids, but I feel so dragged out. My roommate says my eyes are beginning to look yellow. Did you get the results of my tests?"

"Your laboratory tests showed that you're already immune to hepatitis A," Dr. Juarez told her. "However, you do have evidence of current HBV infection and your liver function values are elevated. Your HCV antibody test results were negative. And I'm pleased there's no evidence of a bleeding disorder, based on your prothrombin time. You'll need to be followed carefully by your doctor, whom I understand you'll see tomorrow. You can expect your doctor to recheck your laboratory values periodically. Also, I've reported your case of HBV to the health department, as required by law, and they may contact you for additional information."

"How long do you think I'll feel like this? I'm getting married in March," Ms. Nguyen said.

"Full recovery can be expected over the next six weeks, although some people may be sick as long as six months. Your current illness may interfere with your wedding plans, so you and your fiancé should talk about that right away."

Ms. Nguyen knew that some people become chronic carriers and even need liver transplants. "Do I need to worry about that?" she asked.

"There's a risk that you may become a chronic carrier," Dr. Juarez said, "but I believe it's far too early to consider this in your case. The important treatment now is proper diet, rest, and close follow-up."

Ms. Nguyen then asked her about the possibility of HIV infection.

Dr. Juarez noted that Mr. Barlow had been HIV-negative on at least three occasions. "Unless Mr. Barlow is currently incubating HIV infection from a recent exposure, you aren't at risk. But you're eligible to have confidential follow-up for HIV through our hospital's employee health service. Even if Mr. Barlow was HIV-positive, the risk of infection from a needlestick with HIV-infected blood is about one in 300. It's much less with an exposure such as yours. Your primary physician will no doubt discuss this with you as well."

"I'm not too concerned about HIV right now," Ms. Nguyen said, "since Mr. Barrow is negative, but I don't want to give hepatitis to anyone else. Are there any precautions my roommate, fiancé, or co-workers need to take? Could I have given it to my patients?"

"Your fiancé isn't at risk, he's already immune to HBV. Your roommate already completed her HBV vaccine series and knows she has a positive antibody test—anti-HBs—so she's safe. Nonsexual transmission among adults within households is very rare anyway. We're not concerned about your co-workers or patients because your work doesn't expose them to your blood."

Guide to the Five Types of Viral Hepatitis

	Hepatitis A virus (HAV)	Hepatitis B virus (HBV)	Hepatitis C virus (HCV)	Hepatitis D virus (HDV)	Hepatitis E virus (HEV)
Mode of transmission	Fecal-to-oral route primarily; poor sanitation and contaminated water contribute to the risk; many outbreaks are traced to infected food handlers; intimate contact within households; sexual contact	Sexual contact; blood-to-blood contact; perinatal (at birth); contaminated blood products; occupational risks from needlesticks and other blood exposures	Blood-to-blood contact; contaminated blood products; risks not well defined for sexual or perinatal transmission; occupational risks to health care professionals are similar to HBV	Can cause infection only together with HBV; routes of transmission the same as for HBV	Fecal-to-oral route; contaminated water and poor sanitation contribute to risk as with HAV; seen in Asia, Africa, and Mexico, but not common in the U.S.
Incubation period	15 to 50 days (average: 28 days)	45 to 180 days (average: 60 to 90 days)	14 to 180 days (average: 40 to 60 days)	Not firmly established in humans; HBV infection must precede HDV; chronic carriers of HBV are at risk throughout their carrier state	15 to 64 days (average: 26 to 42 days in different epidemics)
Infectiousness	Most infectious during two weeks before onset of illness; in most cases, unlikely to be infectious after first week of jaundice	Begins before symptoms appear and persists for four to six months after acute illness; persists for the lifetime of chronic carriers	Begins one to two weeks before symptoms appear; continues throughout clinical course and indefinitely in chronic carriers	Blood is potentially infectious during all phases of active HDV infection; although HDV may fall rapidly to undetectable levels, it may be present in the blood of chronic HBV carriers for an extended period	Not known; may be similar to HAV
Laboratory tests (Note: All tests are done on blood serum.)	Anti-HAV IgM (indicates current infection) Anti-HAV IgG (indicates past, resolved infection)	HBsAg (indicates current or chronic infection) HBeAg (a marker for increased infectivity) Anti-HBc (a marker for infection at some time) Anti-HBe (a marker for decreased infectivity) Anti-HBs (a marker for immunity and the antibody produced in response to the HBV vaccine)	Anti-HCV (a marker for infection with HCV virus)	Anti-HDV IgM (indicates current infection) Anti-HDV IgG (indicates past infection)	Serologic tests are currently under development

Continued

Guide to the Five Types of Viral Hepatitis—cont'd

	Hepatitis A virus (HAV)	Hepatitis B virus (HBV)	Hepatitis C virus (HCV)	Hepatitis D virus (HDV)	Hepatitis E virus (HEV)
Postexposure management	Immune globulin within two weeks of exposure; if given early in incubation period, it has 80% to 90% effectiveness	In the unimmunized person exposed, give HBV vaccine and high-titer immune globulin (HBIG) to reduce the risk of HBV infection	The value of immune globulin is unclear; no other treatment is presently available	Focus of management is to prevent HBV; HBIG, immune globulin, and HBV vaccine don't protect HBV carriers from HDV infection	Exposures unlikely in the U.S. and immune globulin available in U.S. isn't likely to contain protective antibodies
Complications	Rare, but can be fatal if fulminant hepatitis develops; protracted cholestasis can occur	With acute HBV infection, death from fulminant hepatitis is possible; up to 10% become chronic carriers and may be at risk for cirrhosis, liver cancer, and death; anyone with HBV is at risk for HDV infection	Chronic carrier state in as many as 50% of those infected via blood transfusions or IV drug abuse; chronic liver disease; cirrhosis; liver cancer; death	Those with HBV and HDV have greater risk of serious morbidity or mortality	Similar to HAV
Prognosis	Good; generally full recovery; no chronic carrier state	Good; generally, a full recovery, except for chronic carriers	Chronic carrier rate high; generally, a full recovery in others	Infection may be acute and short-lived or become chronic; HDV should always be suspected in patients with fulminant HBV or when chronic HBV carriers have sudden exacerbations	Good; full recovery likely; no chronic carrier state
Prevention	Handwashing prior to food preparation; proper personal hygiene; environmental sanitation measures; food and water sanitation; immune globulin for travelers into areas where HAV is common; HAV vaccine (not yet licensed in the U.S.)	HBV vaccine for all infants, health care professionals, and others at risk; condom use, screening donated blood; devices to minimize risk to health care professionals (such as needleless IV access devices); personal protective devices for health care professionals (such as aprons, eye and mucous membrane protection, gloves, gowns)	Screening donated blood; avoidance of blood-to-blood exposure for at-risk individuals and health care professionals with the same measures as for HBV. Note: There is no HCV vaccine.	HBV vaccine for all at risk will also prevent HDV infection; other prevention measures same as for HBV Note: HDV infection isn't possible without HBV infection	Handwashing; food and water sanitation measures; improved personal hygiene; other measures as for HAV Note: It's unlikely that immune globulin from U.S. donors would provide protection.

HEPATITIS C, D, AND E

During Ms. Nguyen's recovery, she and Ms. Johnson learned more about HCV, which is a parenterally transmitted form of non-A, non-B hepatitis. The incubation period for HCV is from two weeks to six months, with an average of six to nine weeks. But antibodies take several months to develop and serologic tests don't detect them until five months to a year after exposure.

Fortunately, the amount of circulating HCV in the blood is far less than the amount of virus found in the blood during HBV infections. This means that HCV is more difficult to transmit through needlesticks and other occupational blood exposures than is HBV. In the United States, most cases of HCV are reported in recipients of blood products and IV drug abusers.

Dr. Juarez told Ms. Nguyen she needed to have her anti-HCV checked again in six and 12 months because Mr. Barlow was known to be anti-HCV positive. There was a small chance that her exposure could also result in transmission of HCV.

Over the next few weeks, Ms. Nguyen was followed closely by her primary physician. Her physician told her that as long as her blood was positive for HBsAg, she was at some risk for hepatitis D virus (HDV) infection—particularly if over the next few months she received a needlestick injury from a patient with HBV and HDV coinfection. If her own HBV infection resolved as expected, her HBsAg should clear within four to six months and anti-HBs should appear shortly thereafter. The appearance of anti-HBs would indicate recovery from HBV infection and that she wasn't a chronic carrier.

Her physician explained that you must have HBV to be infected with HDV, a defective RNA virus that requires HBV for its survival and replication. Hepatitis D virus infection occurs only with HBV infection and can't outlast the HBV infection. It's most common among IV drug abusers, hemophiliacs, and persons who have received multiple blood transfusions. Vaccination against HBV also prevents infection with HDV because you can't have HDV independently from HBV.

Hepatitis E virus (HEV) is another type of non-A, non-B virus that's transmitted through the fecal-to-oral route, like HAV. It occurs in epidemics and sporadically in parts of Asia, Africa, and Mexico. It hasn't been identified as a problem disease in the United States or Western Europe. Ms. Nguyen's physician also reminded her that since she and Dr. Li are from Asia, they need to be aware of HEV should they plan future visits there.

INSTRUCTIVE LESSON

Sue Nguyen eventually recovered fully from her HBV and never developed HCV. She and Jim Li postponed their wedding until June and decided not to honeymoon in a developing country. Both Sue Nguyen and Linda Johnson learned a lot about viral hepatitis and became expert resources for their hospital's psychiatric unit.

As a nurse, you're at risk for exposure to infectious diseases. Fortunately, all five types of viral hepatitis are largely preventable if the right steps are taken. Sue Nguyen's story is an instructive lesson on that important point.

SELECTED REFERENCES

Benenson, A.S. (ed.) *Control of Communicable Diseases in Man*. 15th ed. Washington, DC, American Public Health Association, 1990.

Centers for Disease Control. Hepatitis B virus: A comprehensive strategy for eliminating transmission in the United States through universal childhood vaccination: Recommendations of the Immunization Practices Advisory Committee (ACIP). *MMWR* 40(No. RR-13):1-25, 1991.

Gerberding, J.L., and Henderson, D.K. Management of occupational exposures to bloodborne pathogens: hepatitis B virus, hepatitis C virus, and human immunodeficiency virus. *Clin.Infect.Dis.* 14: 1179-1185, June 1992.

Gilchrist, E. Hepatitis B—it will never happen to me. *Today's OR Nurse* 13:15-18, Oct. 1991.

Jackson, M.M., and McPherson, D.C. Hepatitis A through E: current and future trends. *Today's OR Nurse* 13:7-11, Oct. 1991.

Jackson, M.M., and Pugliese, G. The OSHA bloodborne pathogens standard. *Today's OR Nurse* 14:11-16, July 1992.

Kiyosawa, K, et al. Hepatitis C in hospital employees with needlestick injuries. *Ann.Intern.Med.* 115:367-369, Sept. 1, 1991.

Lettau, L.A. The A, B, C, D, and E of hepatitis: spelling out the risks for health care workers. *Infect.Control Hosp.Epidemiol.* 13:77-81, Feb. 1992.

Poss, J.E. Hepatitis D virus infection. *Nurse Pract.* 14:12, 14-15, 18, Aug. 1989.

Stein, J.H. (ed). *Internal Medicine*. 3rd ed. Boston, Little, Brown, and Co., 1990.

U.S. Department of Labor, Occupational Safety and Health Administration. 29 CFR Part 1910: Occupational exposure to bloodborne pathogens: final rule. *Fed.Reg.* 56(235):64004-64182, 1991.

Wormser, G.P., et al. Hepatitis C infection in the health care setting; Part 1. Low risk from parenteral exposure to blood of human immunodeficiency virus-infected patients. *Am.J.Infect.Control* 19:237-242, Oct. 1991.

Contents

Chapter *4*

Nursing Care of the Childbearing Family

COORDINATOR

Marybeth Young, RNC, PhD

Contributors

Gita Dhillon, RN, MA, MS, MEd, CNM

B. Patricia Grace, RN, MSN

Roberta A. Kordish, RN, MSN

Marianne Scharbo-DeHaan, RN, BSN, MN, CNM, PhD

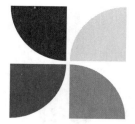

Women's Health Care

NOTE: The concept development in the sections on the adult, child, and the client with psychosocial problems also applies to the mother and her newborn. However, this section has been organized according to the normal childbearing cycle, from conception to postpartum.

OVERVIEW OF PHYSIOLOGY

1. Structure of the female pelvis (Fig. 4-1)
   a. Pelvic structure (four united bones): two hip bones (right and left innominate), the sacrum, and the coccyx
   b. Pelvic divisions: two parts divided by the inlet or brim
      1. false pelvis: upper portion above brim; supports uterus during late pregnancy
      2. true pelvis: located below brim; composed of three parts: the pelvic inlet, the midcavity, and the pelvic outlet; forms birth canal through which fetus passes during parturition
   c. Pelvic variations: pelvic structures differ in shape and size (may be combination of shapes)
      1. gynecoid: true female type; slightly ovoid or rounded inlet; influence on labor and delivery *most favorable*
      2. android: normal male type; heart-shaped inlet, narrow pubic arch; influence on labor and delivery is not favorable
      3. platypelloid: flattened anteroposteriorly, oval-shaped inlet; influence on labor and delivery not favorable
      4. anthropoid: apelike type; oval-shaped inlet; influence on labor and delivery favorable
   d. Pelvic measurements
      1. diagonal conjugate (DC): distance between sacral promontory and lower margin (inferior border) of symphysis pubis; adequate size for childbirth is 12.5 cm or more, depending on fetal size, position *estimated on pelvic exam*
      2. true conjugate or conjugate vera (CV): distance between upper margin, superior border of symphysis pubis to sacral promontory; adequate size for childbirth 11 cm or more (1.5 to 2 cm less than diagonal conjugate); *measured accurately by x-ray*
      3. obstetric conjugate: the shortest distance between the inner surface of the symphysis and the sacral promontory; *measured by x-ray or estimated if diagonal conjugate is known*

4. tuberischial diameter: transverse diameter of the outlet, the distance between the ischial tuberosities; adequate size for childbirth 9 to 11 cm or more; *estimated on pelvic exam*
5. assessment of size
   a. estimate of pelvic dimensions: diagonal conjugate and tuberischial diameter on pelvic exam
   b. x-ray or internal pelvimetry: use is limited to suspected pelvic bony contractions and suspected cephalopelvic disproportion (in late pregnancy or labor)
   c. ultrasonography: employs high-frequency sound waves for determination of gestational age; used most frequently of all assessments

2. Female external organs
   a. Mons veneris or pubis: rounded, soft, fatty pad over symphysis pubis, covered by coarse hair in adult
   b. Labia majora: two folds of skin containing fat and covered with hair; located on either side of the vaginal opening
   c. Labia minora: two thin folds of delicate tissue without hair; located within labia majora
   d. Glans clitoris: a small body of erectile tissue partially hidden between the anterior ends of the labia minora; highly sensitive to touch, temperature, and pressure
   e. Hymen: thin mucous membrane; located at the opening of the vagina, can be stretched or torn during intercourse, physical activity, tampon insertion, or vaginal examination
   f. Urinary meatus: external opening of the urethra
   g. Openings of vulvovaginal or Bartholin's glands: two small glands situated between the vestibula on either side of the vaginal orifice; secrete alkaline mucus during coitus
   h. Openings of Skene's ducts: two paraurethral glands open onto posterior urethral wall
   i. Perineum: area between vagina and rectum consisting of fibromuscular tissue

3. Female internal organs (Fig. 4-2)
   a. Ovaries: two oval-shaped organs located on either side of the uterus in the upper pelvic cavity; responsible for producing the ovum and the female hormones estrogen and progesterone
   b. Fallopian or uterine tubes: two thin, muscular canals extending from the cornua of the uterus to the ovaries; responsible for transport of the ovum from the

ovaries to the uterus; fertilization occurs in middle third (ampulla) of either fallopian tube

c. Uterus: a hollow muscular organ that is the site of implantation, retainment, and nourishment of the products of conception; organ of menstruation in the nonpregnant female. The larger, upper portion of the uterus is known as the *body* and the smaller, lower segment is called the *cervix;* the convex, upper part between the insertion of fallopian tubes is the *fundus;* in the nonpregnant female the uterus is located in the pelvic cavity between the bladder and rectum and weighs approximately 60 g; the uterus is composed of smooth muscle (myometrium) and an inner mucoid lining (the endometrium) that responds to estrogen and progesterone during the menstrual cycle

d. Vagina: a thin-walled, dilatable canal located between the bladder and rectum that serves as the passageway for menstrual discharge, copulation, and the fetus

e. Accessory structures (breasts): two mammary glands composed of glandular tissue and fat, which are capable of producing and secreting milk for nourishment of the infant

4. Menstrual cycle

a. Reproductive hormones (all are affected by thyroid function)

1. follicle-stimulating hormone (FSH): secreted by anterior pituitary gland during the first half of the menstrual cycle; stimulates development of graafian follicles

2. interstitial cell-stimulating hormone (ICSH) or luteinizing hormone (LH): secreted by the anterior pituitary gland; stimulates ovulation and development of the corpus luteum

3. estrogen: secreted primarily by the ovaries, corpus luteum, adrenal cortex (in small amounts), and the placenta in pregnancy; assists in maturation of ovarian follicles, stimulates thickening of the endometrium, causes suppression of FSH secretion, and is responsible for development of secondary sex characteristics; in pregnancy it maintains the endometrium, causes fatigue, and stimulates contraction of smooth muscle

4. progesterone: secreted by corpus luteum and by the placenta during pregnancy; supplements estrogen effect on endometrium by facilitating secretory changes; relaxes smooth muscle; decreases uterine motility; has thermogenic effect (i.e., increases temperature); causes cervical secretion of thick viscous mucus; allows pregnancy to be maintained

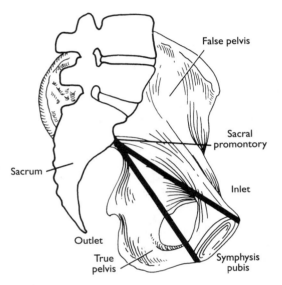

Fig. 4-1   Female pelvis.

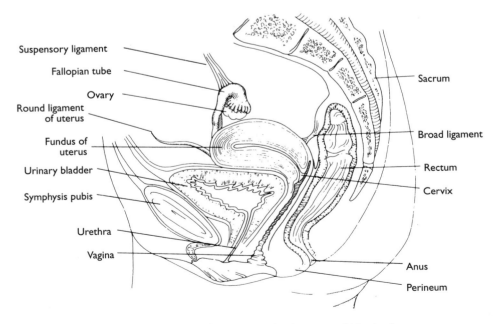

Fig. 4-2   Female internal reproductive organs (side view).

5. prostaglandins: fatty acids categorized as hormones, produced by many organs of the body, including the endometrium; affect the menstrual cycle and may influence the onset and maintenance of labor

b. Ovulation: growth and release of a nonfertilized ovum from the ovary after puberty; generally occurs 13 to 15 days before next menses in regular cycle; presence of stretchable cervical mucus (spinnbarkeit) observed at ovulation (enhances sperm motility and permits fertilization)

c. Menstruation: cyclic vaginal discharge of blood and superficial fragments of endometrium and other secretions in response to falling levels of estrogen and progesterone after puberty
   1. amenorrhea: absence or abnormal cessation of the menses
      a. primary (menses have never occurred)
      b. secondary (menses occurred at puberty but have since stopped)
   2. hypomenorrhea: abnormally short menstruation
   3. hypermenorrhea: abnormally long menstruation
   4. oligomenorrhea: infrequent menstruation
   5. polymenorrhea: too frequent menstruation
   6. dysmenorrhea: painful menstruation

5. Fertilization: impregnation of an ovum by a spermatozoon, occurring in the ampulla of the fallopian tube; egg life span is 24 to 36 hours after ovulation; sperm life span is 48 to 72 hours or more after ejaculation; usual sperm count is 250 to 400 million per ejaculation

6. Implantation: the imbedding of the fertilized ovum into the uterine mucosa (usually in the upper segment); occurs approximately 7 to 10 days after ovulation (also known as nidation)

7. Menopause: cessation of menses at end of fertility cycle
   a. Occurrence: normal developmental process that occurs naturally between the ages of 35 and 60 (average age is 53)
   b. Alterations: early menopause may be stimulated by
      1. multiple, frequent pregnancies or abortions
      2. hypothyroidism with obesity
      3. surgical removal of ovaries
      4. hard physical work or extremely active exercise
      5. overexposure to radiation
   c. Assessment
      1. vaginal epithelium thins; vaginal pH increases, resulting in dryness, burning, irritation, and dyspareunia
      2. urinary frequency and incontinence
      3. osteoporosis risk factors: low calcium intake during adolescence, smoking, excessive protein or caffeine, sedentary lifestyle, nulliparity, early menopause
      4. decline in serum levels of high-density lipoprotein (HDL) cholesterol and an increase in low-density lipoprotein (LDL), placing women at risk for coronary heart disease
      5. vasomotor instability, night sweats, and emotional disturbances
   d. Hormone replacement therapy (HRT)
      1. estrogen replacement therapy (ERT) relieves symptoms and is recommended for women with no contraindication to estrogen
      2. ERT decreases the risk of cardiovascular disease but increases risk of endometrial cancer; adding progestin greatly decreases this risk
      3. HRT should be continued indefinitely for women at high risk for osteoporosis
      4. benefits of HRT outweigh risk for most women if combined with general health promotion strategies
   e. Alternative methods of management
      1. Bellergal-S tablets relieve symptoms related to autonomic system activity
      2. vitamin E relieves hot flashes, leg cramps, and energy loss
      3. Chinese herbal medicines (Ginseng)
      4. Kegel exercises to increase muscle tone
      5. K-Y lubricating jelly and coconut oil (water soluble)
      6. calcium supplementation
      7. weight-bearing exercises

Application of the Nursing Process to Reproductive Health Maintenance/Health Promotion of Adult Women

ASSESSMENT

1. Health history: onset of menarche, duration of menstrual periods, menstrual problems, premenstrual tension, osteoporosis (decrease in skeletal bone mass), use of family planning, past and current pregnancies, infertility problems (Table 4-1), symptoms such as hot flashes, dizzy spells, palpitations; identification of risk factors (e.g., history of sexually transmitted disease [STD])
2. External reproductive organs (by physician or nurse); breast palpation for masses; mammography; bimanual internal examination; observation of cervical-vaginal discharge; Pap smear
3. Knowledge of progesterone-to-estrogen ratio, hormonal effects (mild or severe episodes of irritability, depression, anxiety, fatigue, exhaustion, or food cravings)

ANALYSIS/NURSING DIAGNOSIS

1. Safe, effective care environment; altered health maintenance related to
   a. Knowledge deficit
   b. Risk for infection
2. Physiologic integrity
   a. Altered nutrition: less than body requirements
   b. Sleep pattern disturbance
3. Psychosocial integrity
   a. Fear
   b. Anxiety
   c. Self-esteem disturbance
   d. Altered sexuality patterns
4. Health promotion/maintenance
   a. Health-seeking behaviors
   b. Impaired adjustment

GENERAL NURSING PLANNING, IMPLEMENTATION, AND EVALUATION

Goal I Client will understand her reproductive system; will report gynecologic problems to her health care provider.

Table 4-1   Assessment of fertility/infertility

Test	Purpose	Nursing implications
MALE		
Semen analysis	To determine sperm count, motility	Take careful lifestyle and sexual history of both partners, chronic health problems, medications, smoking, drug use, exposure to chemicals, radiation
FEMALE (SIMPLEST TO MORE COMPLEX)		
Basal body temperature	To determine time of ovulation	
Cervical-mucus examination (self-performed, basis for natural family planning)	To determine elasticity for sperm motility	Provide detailed explanation of all tests to couple
Pelvic examination (bimanual)	To identify obvious reproductive problems	Know that process of assessment of fertility and subsequent interventions may be lengthy and, for the couple, frustrating
Ultrasonography		
Blood hormone levels and thyroid function tests	To measure levels of estrogen and progesterone, and influence of the thyroid	
Sims-Huhner test (postcoital cervical mucus test)	To determine pH of cervical mucus, effects of hormones	
Tubal patency tests hysterosalpingogram (x-ray) laparoscopic exam (direct visualization)	To determine condition, patency of fallopian tubes	
Endometrial biopsy	To determine condition of endometrium	
Culdoscopy (examination through cul-de-sac with dye injection)	To determine function of fallopian tubes	

Implementation

1. Discuss anatomy and physiology of female reproductive system.
2. Review menstrual cycle, ovulation, and fertilization.
3. Teach client reportable problems.

Evaluation

Client gives a basic explanation of reproductive anatomy and physiology; explains relationship of menstrual cycle, ovulation, and fertilization; reports problems to health care provider.

Goal 2 Client will plan appropriate healthy lifestyle changes before conception.

Implementation

1. Assess client's learning needs.
2. Provide instruction on lifestyle changes that improve client's health and promote good fetal outcome.
3. Explain the importance of a balanced diet related to client and fetal health.
4. Advise client of the benefits of physical fitness.
5. Teach client the importance of discontinuing oral contraceptives 3 months before conception.
6. Assist client to select another method of conception control, such as barrier method.
7. Assess family coping and potential for growth related to pregnancy and body-image changes.
8. Discuss impact of chronic illness (e.g., diabetes) and measures to ensure optimal health before conception.

Evaluation

Client describes health promotion activities; discusses with partner the decision to have a baby; knows the importance of avoiding oral contraceptives for 3 months before conception.

Goal 3 Client and partner will be knowledgeable about various methods of family planning.

Implementation

1. Assess client's/couple's learning needs.
2. Assess client's/couple's contraceptive history, lifestyle, age.
3. Provide information as needed (Table 4-2).
4. Emphasize need for effective protection from STDs.

Evaluation

Client describes family planning options; asks questions about them; uses chosen method consistently and according to directions; lists potential problems with specific method; reports problems associated with use.

Goal 4 Client will discuss risk factors relating to genetic disorders.

Implementation

1. Assess for genetic risk factors.
2. Teach the couple about genetic disorders before conception.
3. Demonstrate sensitivity to the couple concerned about or at risk of having a child with a genetic disorder (see the section on anxious behavior).
4. Collaborate with other health care team members in evaluating risk factors.
5. Prepare couple for assessment procedures.

Evaluation

Client makes an informed decision to become pregnant and understands risk factors and assessments.

Table 4-2 Family planning

Method and mode of action	Characteristics	Nursing implications
TEMPORARY METHODS		
Oral contraceptives (birth control pills): may be single hormone or combination of estrogen and progesterone Prevent ovulation by inhibiting FSH Change cervical mucus	*Effectiveness:* 99% if used as directed *Advantages:* convenient, effective *Disadvantages:* increased risk over age 35; smokers; women with risk/history of vascular disease hypertension, respiratory problems, breast cancer in family	Teach proper and regular use; action to take if one or more pills are missed; side effects; reportable signs (e.g., headaches, chest or calf pain, heavy bleeding). Recommend regular Pap smears. Caution against use of antibiotics unless physician is aware that client uses oral contraceptives. Increase folic acid, vitamins B and C. Advise client to notify physician and discontinue oral contraceptives if pregnancy is suspected.
Progestin implant (Norplant) Prevents some ovulatory cycles Alters cervical mucus	*Effectiveness:* greater than 99% over 5 years	Teach benefits for specific women. Help to make informed choice. Teach reportable problems, e.g., heavy bleeding.
Intrauterine device (IUD) Causes local inflammatory response, inhibiting implantation Several IUD products have been withdrawn by manufacturers Copper IUD most effective	*Effectiveness:* 90%-99% *Advantages:* convenient, long-term, effective *Disadvantages:* increased risk for pelvic infection, ectopic pregnancy; subsequent infertility	Teach compliance with regular health care visits; reportable signs (e.g., abdominal pain, foul discharge); to check for presence of string before coitus. Recommended for multiparas in monogamous relationships. Must be removed by health care provider.
Diaphragm Barrier to seminal fluid, sperm when used with spermicidal cream	*Effectiveness:* 83%-95% if correctly fit and properly used *Advantages:* side effects, UTI rare *Disadvantages:* requires motivation and planning; may interfere with spontaneity; must remain in place several hours after coitus	Teach proper cleansing and use with spermicide (not K-Y jelly). Suggest that client be refitted after pregnancy, weight changes. Report problems with fit, removal, vaginal discharge/infection. Promote good hygiene. Leave in place 6-8 hr after intercourse.
Vaginal contraceptive sponge	*Effectiveness:* 84%-97% *Advantages:* convenient; no additional creams needed; may leave in place up to 24 hours; barrier to seminal fluid, sperm; economical *Disadvantages:* increased risk of allergies, toxic shock; removal may be difficult	Teach proper use and insertion. Avoid use for over 30 hr. Avoid use during menses. Urge immediate reporting of problems/symptoms. Leave in place 6 hr after intercourse.
Cervical cap Barrier to seminal fluid and sperm Extended wear Used with spermicidal cream	*Advantages:* side effects are rare; unlikely to dislodge during coitus *Disadvantages:* increased risk of cervical erosion, inflammation; may be difficult to remove	Teach proper use. Check position of cap before and after intercourse. Seek regular health care; refit after pregnancy, weight change, gynecologic surgery. Report signs of vaginal infection or other problems. Seek regular health care. Teach proper use. Discuss role in prevention of transmission of STDs, AIDS.
Condom Barrier to passage of sperm when slipped over erect penis	*Effectiveness:* 64%-98% when used with spermicides; addition of nonoxyl 9 increases contraceptive effectiveness and protection against STDs *Advantages:* involves male in family planning; protects against some STDs; easily available *Disadvantages:* requires motivation and planning; may tear during use; rare allergic reactions	Teach proper use. Discuss role in prevention of transmission of STDs, AIDS.

Table 4-2 Family planning—cont'd

Method and mode of action	Characteristics	Nursing implications
Vaginal sheath Combination of diaphragm and condom	*Advantages:* protection against STDs if applied well before intercourse	Use with spermicidal jelly.

Spermicides
  Immobilize or destroy sperm
	Effectiveness: 70%-98% depending on use; more effective with other methods (e.g., condom, diaphragm)
	  Advantages: easily available; few side effects
	  Disadvantages: inconvenient; may cause allergic reaction; there is concern (unproven) about potential risk of birth defects in some users
		Teach proper use after reading specific product directions.
		Avoid douching after coitus.
		Report problems (e.g., itching, burning).

Natural family planning
  Abstinence from coitus during the fertile (ovulation) phase of the menstrual cycle (the couple trying to conceive may also plan optimal time for coitus to achieve pregnancy)
  Assessment of ovulation if based on
    Daily basal body temperature (BBT) (Fig. 4-3) to monitor changes before and at ovulation (slight drop, then rise after ovulation)
    Cervical mucus characteristics: clear, slippery, elastic at ovulation (Billings method)
    Calendar recording based on usual menstrual pattern
    Symptothermal method: a combination of calendar tracking of monthly fertility cycle, BBT, and cervical mucus self-exam
    On speculum exam os dilates, cervix softens, rises
  Predictor test for ovulation for home use detects surge of LH
	Effectiveness: 75%-98% depending on accuracy of observations, motivation of both partners
	Advantages: inexpensive: involves both partners; no chemical or mechanical barrier to sperm movement; no health risk
	Disadvantages: requires motivation of both partners; may be less effective in presence of infection or during menopause
		Teach and reinforce information to both partners.

PERMANENT METHODS		
Tubal ligation/vasectomy Ligation/severance of fallopian tube or vas deferens for permanent sterilization (some procedures are reversible)	*Effectiveness:* greater than 99.5% (reversing the procedure is difficult, outcome is not guaranteed) *Advantages:* prevents pregnancy permanently *Disadvantages:* requires informed consent; rare complications; use of bands or clips allows possible return of patency	Teach couple alternative methods if permanent sterility is not desired. Caution that pregnancy is still possible for a short period of time after vasectomy. Use contraception until sperm count is zero on two occasions.

> **Goal 5** Client will understand the importance of periodic examinations in reproductive health maintenance.

Implementation

1. Explain the need for periodic Papanicolaou (Pap) smears (cells taken from squamocolumnar junction) to detect cancer of the uterus and abnormalities of cervical, vaginal cells (frequency varies according to sexual activity, age, and risk).

2. Explain importance of regular breast self-examination after cessation of menstrual period (days 5 to 7 of menstrual cycle) or after menopause on regular monthly basis.

3. Demonstrate breast self-examination (palpation and inspection of breasts and nipples while standing and reclining); ask client for return demonstration; emphasize reporting any changes or suspicious findings immediately.

4. Tell client to see physician for regular breast examination.

5. Explain value of mammography.
6. Discuss meaning, purposes, and interpretation of various tests (Table 4-3).
7. Provide supplemental reading materials to increase client's knowledge.

Evaluation
Client performs breast self-examination regularly at end of each menstrual cycle; schedules appointments for periodic checkups and Pap smears.

Goal 6 Client will be knowledgeable about premenstrual tension syndrome; will discuss any concerns with health care provider.

Implementation
1. Assess client's learning needs.
2. Provide information as needed.
3. Review hormones and their effects.

Evaluation
Client gives basic description of hormones and their effects; asks questions; uses a method to relieve symptoms.

Goal 7 Client will be physically and psychologically prepared for menopause; will participate in treatment decisions as an informed consumer.

Implementation
1. Allow client to voice feelings about menopause.
2. Teach client how to maintain and promote health and prevent osteoporosis (Table 4-4).
3. Discuss normal developmental changes that occur with menopause.
4. Dispel "myths" concerning menopause.
5. Discuss sexuality needs and family planning until ovulation ceases.
6. Provide emotional support, anticipatory guidance.

Table 4-3   Interpretation of Pap test results

Old terminology	Current terminology	Characteristics
Class I	Within normal limits	Minimal or no inflammation; no malignant cells
Class II	Inflammatory atypia	Inflammation; mild atypia
Class III	Cervical intraepithelial neoplasia	
Mild dysplasia	CIN grade I	Abnormal nucleus; normal cytoplasm
Moderate dysplasia	CIN grade II	Abnormal nucleus; minimal cytoplasm abnormalities
Severe dysplasia	CIN grade III	Abnormal chromosome and cytoplasm; abnormal cells predominate; many
Carcinoma in situ		undifferentiated cells

From Beal MW: Cervical cytology, *NAACOG's Clin Issu Perinat Womens Health Nurs* 1(4):475, 1990.

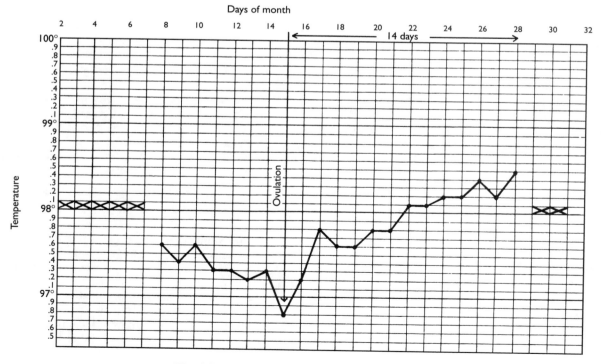

Fig. 4-3   Basal body temperature (30-day cycle).

Evaluation

Client lists the signs and symptoms of menopause; participates in decisions about treatment as an informed consumer.

SELECTED HEALTH PROBLEMS

✖ UTERINE FIBROIDS

1. Definition: benign uterine tumors of connective tissue and muscle
2. Incidence
   a. 20% to 25% of women over age 30 have myomas
   b. Higher incidence in black women
3. Predisposing factors
   a. Infertility
   b. Hormone usage
   c. Age (myomas often disappear with menopause)
4. Medical treatment: depends on symptoms such as bleeding, pressure, and client's age and reproductive status
   a. Medical intervention
      1. close supervision
      2. no hormone administration
      3. reassess after menopause
   b. Surgical intervention
      1. simple myomectomy (subsequent pregnancies may require delivery by cesarean section)
      2. hysterectomy
         a. vaginal approach
         b. abdominal approach

Nursing Process

ASSESSMENT

1. Menorrhagia
2. Dysmenorrhea
3. Low-back and pelvic pain

Table 4-4 Health teaching to reduce risk of osteoporosis

ALL ADULT WOMEN SHOULD

Eat a balanced diet to ensure adequate vitamin and mineral intake (especially sufficient fruits and vegetables).

Increase daily food sources of calcium (dairy products, seafood, yogurt, greens) to prevent or compensate for bone loss.

Decrease fats and excess phosphorus intake (animal proteins, dairy products, diet soda) to prevent calcium excretion. (Aluminum antacids may be suggested as phosphorus binders.)

Maintain adequate vitamin D intake (sunlight, fortified milk products) to balance calcium and phosphorus.

Exercise regularly to strengthen bones.

MENOPAUSAL AND POSTMENOPAUSAL WOMEN SHOULD

Take calcium carbonate or calcium gluconate supplements as prescribed by a physician.

Avoid calcium preparations purchased in health food stores that contain lead, bone meal, and dolomite.

Follow physician recommendations on estrogen replacement therapy to prevent further bone loss.

4. Constipation
5. Uterine enlargement
6. Presence of predisposing factors

ANALYSIS/NURSING DIAGNOSIS (see p. 296)

PLANNING, IMPLEMENTATION, AND EVALUATION

> **Goal** Client will be free from problems during conservative management until pregnancy and birth are achieved.

Implementation

1. Explain effects of hormones on fibroids.
2. Support client's decision about pregnancy.
3. Monitor for increased severity of symptoms.

Evaluation

Client experiences no increase in symptoms; is able to conceive and sustain a pregnancy with minimal difficulty.

✖ VAGINAL WALL CHANGES ASSOCIATED WITH CHILDBEARING OR AGING

1. Definitions
   a. *Cystocele:* relaxation of the anterior vaginal wall with prolapse of the bladder
   b. *Rectocele:* relaxation of the posterior vaginal wall with prolapse of the rectum
   c. *Uterine prolapse:* downward displacement of uterus
2. Predisposing factors
   a. Multiparity
   b. Pelvic tearing during childbirth
   c. Inappropriate bearing down during labor
   d. Congenital weakness
   e. Vaginal-muscle weakness associated with aging
   f. Race: less common in ethnic women of color
3. Management
   a. Preventive
      1. correctly performed episiotomy
      2. postpartum perineal exercises (Kegel)
      3. spaced pregnancies
   b. Surgical intervention
      1. vaginal hysterectomy
      2. anterior or posterior vaginal repair (colporrhaphy)
   c. Postoperative care
      1. no hormones needed
      2. evaluate success of repair

Nursing Process

ASSESSMENT

1. Cystocele
   a. Incontinence or dribbling with cough, sneeze, or any activity that increases intraabdominal pressure
   b. Retention
   c. Cystitis
2. Rectocele
   a. Constipation
   b. Hemorrhoids
   c. Sensation of pressure
3. Uterine prolapse
   a. Dysmenorrhea
   b. Cervical ulceration

c. Pelvic pain

d. Dragging sensation in pelvis and back

ANALYSIS/NURSING DIAGNOSIS (see p. 296)

PLANNING, IMPLEMENTATION, AND EVALUATION

> **Goal** Client will remain free from undetected complications after anterior and posterior colporrhaphy or vaginal hysterectomy; will regain normal patterns of urinary and bowel elimination.

Implementation

1. Refer to general preoperative and postoperative care, p. 115.
2. Administer cleansing douche and enema preoperatively as ordered.
3. Instruct client to refrain from coughing, sneezing, or straining postoperatively.
4. Promote perineal healing as in postpartal care (see p. 350).
5. Note amount and character of vaginal drainage.
6. Apply vaginal creams as ordered.
7. Monitor urinary output.
8. Provide Foley catheter care.
9. Teach perineal (Kegel) exercises qh and gradual bladder training.
10. Observe for abdominal distention.
11. When Foley catheter is removed, monitor output.
12. Avoid rectal tubes and taking rectal temperatures.
13. Check Homans' sign.
14. Ambulate as soon as possible.
15. Instruct on gradual increase of residue in diet.
16. Administer stool softeners or mineral oil before first bowel movement.
17. Provide emotional support.

Evaluation

Client heals postoperatively free from complications; demonstrates normal control and elimination patterns.

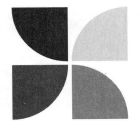

Antepartal Care

NORMAL CHILDBEARING

1. Definition: care provided to a woman and her family during pregnancy
2. Normal adaptations: changes that occur in body systems of childbearing women because of the influence of hormones and growth of the embryo/fetus (Table 4-5)
   a. Integumentary system
      1. changes in skin pigmentation stimulated by elevated levels of melanocyte-stimulating hormone (may include acne)
         a. chloasma (mask of pregnancy): brown blotches that appear on face and neck, often visible in second trimester; usually fade after delivery
         b. linea nigra: a dark line that extends from umbilicus to mons veneris; will lighten after delivery
      2. striae gravidarum: pink or slightly reddish streaks on abdomen, thighs, or breasts, resulting from stretching of underlying connective tissue because of adrenal cortex hypertrophy; grow lighter after delivery but never disappear completely
      3. vascular spider angiomas and palmar erythema
   b. Reproductive system
      1. changes in the uterus
         a. size: increases in length (6 to 32 cm), width (4 to 24 cm), and depth (2.5 to 22 cm)
         b. weight increase: 60 to 1000 g
         c. shape: from globular to oval; wall thickens and then becomes thin at term
         d. location: rises out of pelvis at twelfth week; near xiphoid process at term
         e. structure
            ▪ body of uterus
               • three distinct uterine segments in pregnancy
               • vascularity increases
               • muscle fiber changes, mainly enlargement of preexisting fibers; longitudinal fibers will shorten with contraction of labor to cause effacement; middle-layer fibers constrict blood vessels in labor; add to force of labor; inner fibers exert pressure on blood vessels in lower uterus; prevent hemorrhage
               • new fibroelastic tissue develops and strengthens uterine wall
            ▪ softening of the lower uterine segment (Hegar's sign)
            ▪ cervix: softens (Goodell's sign) and increases in vascularity (Chadwick's sign)
            ▪ formation of mucus plug (prevents bacterial contamination)
         f. contractility: Braxton Hicks contractions occur intermittently throughout pregnancy
      2. changes in the vagina
         a. increased vascularization, which results in purplish discoloration (Chadwick's sign) beginning in sixth week of pregnancy
         b. thickening of mucosa
         c. loosening of connective tissue
         d. increased vaginal discharge (thick, whitish leukorrhea) without signs of itching or burning
      3. changes in the breasts
         a. enlargement and prominence of superficial veins
         b. increase in size and firmness
         c. Montgomery's glands in areolas enlarge
         d. nipples become more prominent, areolas darken and increase in diameter
         e. colostrum may be secreted in fourth or fifth month (16 to 20 weeks) and subsequently in small amounts until delivery
         f. alveoli and duct system enlarge
      4. changes in joints and ligaments
         a. relaxation of pelvic joints and ligaments
         b. hypertrophy and elongation of
            ▪ broad, round ligaments (stabilize uterus)
            ▪ uterosacral ligaments (support cervix)
      5. changes in abdomen: occur to accommodate progressive growth in uterine size
         a. at end of twelfth week the uterus is at level of symphysis pubis
         b. by 22 to 24 weeks uterus is at level of umbilicus
         c. by 38 weeks the uterus is at level of xiphoid process until lightening occurs
         d. decrease in fundal height after lightening in primigravidas
   c. Endocrine system (placenta)
      1. function of placenta
         a. secretes hormones from early weeks of pregnancy: estrogen, progesterone, human chori-

Table 4-5 Signs and symptoms of pregnancy

Subjective	Objective
PRESUMPTIVE	
Amenorrhea	Chadwick's sign (8-12 wk)
Breast sensitivity	Breast enlargement
Nausea, vomiting (5-12 wk)	Skin pigmentation, striae
Urinary frequency (6-12 wk)	
Fatigue	
Quickening (16-20 wk)	
PROBABLE	
Enlarged abdomen	Ballottement
Hegar's sign	
Goodell's sign	Positive pregnancy tests
Braxton Hicks contractions	
POSITIVE	By examiner:
	Fetal movements
	Fetal outline—sonography
	Fetal heart tones (10-16 wk)

onic gonadotropin (HCG), and human placental lactogen (HPL), also called human chorionic somatomammotropin

b. acts as a barrier to some substances and organisms (e.g., heparin in large doses does not cross; bacteria are less likely to cross placenta than a virus is); barrier is not effective for nicotine, alcohol, depressants, stimulants, antibiotics, cocaine, caffeine, heroin

c. nutrition: transports nutrients and water-soluble vitamins to fetus and eliminates wastes from fetus

d. exchanges: fluid and gas transport
   ▪ diffusion, such as O_2 and CO_2, water, electrolytes (low molecular weight)
   ▪ facilitated transport (e.g., glucose)
   ▪ active transport: amino acids, calcium, iron (high molecular weight)
   ▪ pinocytosis (e.g., gamma globulin, albumin, fat particles)
   ▪ usually there is no mixing of maternal and fetal red blood cells
   ▪ leakage because of slight placental defects allows fetal and maternal blood cells to mix slightly

2. dimensions
   a. 15 by 3 cm
   b. discoid
   c. 400 to 600 g at term
   d. covers quarter of uterine wall
   e. fetal-placental weight ratio at term is 6:1

3. structure and development
   a. fully developed by twelfth week from the decidua basalis and chorion of the embryo; functions most effectively through 40 to 41 weeks; may be dysfunctional after maturity or in women with health problems

b. normally develops in the posterior surface of the upper uterine segment

c. two surfaces
   ▪ fetal (amniotic) surface: chorionic villi and their circulation; membranes: amnion (inner) and chorion (outer) fused
   ▪ maternal surface: decidua basalis (hypertrophied endometrium of pregnancy) and its circulation; cotyledons present

d. umbilical cord: 55 cm at term; most commonly is inserted centrally into fetal surface of placenta; contains one vein to oxygenate fetus and two arteries to carry deoxygenated blood from fetus to placenta to mother

4. hormones
   a. estrogen and progesterone: after first 2 months of gestation, placenta is major source of production; responsible for growth of uterus and development of breasts

   b. HCG: secreted by third week after fertilization, detected in urine 10 days after missed period (basis for simple pregnancy tests); HCG prolongs life of corpus luteum; radioimmunoassay (RIA) for HCG will be positive the second day after implantation

   c. human chorionic somatomammotropin (human placental lactogen): secreted by third week after ovulation; prepares breasts for lactation, influences somatic cell growth of fetus; antagonist to insulin, considered principal maternal diabetogenic factor

d. Musculoskeletal system
   1. relaxation and increased mobility of pelvic joints result in a waddling gait and instability
   2. increase in normal lumbosacral curve because of enlarging uterus; poor posture may increase problem
   3. stress on ligaments and muscles of middle and lower spine
   4. backache and leg cramps may occur

e. Cardiovascular system
   1. heart and vessels
      a. heart rate increases 10 to 15 beats per minute in second trimester; persists to term
      b. blood pressure should remain constant during pregnancy with a decrease in the second trimester (possible postural hypotension)
      c. increase in vasculature: dilation of pelvic veins, varicose veins, varicosities of the vulva, hemorrhoids
   2. cardiac output increases 20% to 30% during first and second trimesters to meet increased tissue demands
   3. blood volume altered in pregnancy; total increase approximately 20% to 30%, peaking in third trimester; increases immediately after delivery because of fluid shift; placental shift no longer present
      a. plasma volume increases out of proportion to the red-cell increase, resulting in hemodilution; this causes normal physiologic anemia

b. hemoglobin range 10 to 16 g/dl; may decrease; problematic if it falls below 10 g/dl

c. hematocrit range 35% to 42%; may decrease approximately 10% in second and third trimesters; anemia if it falls below 35%

d. average white blood cell (WBC) count 5000 to 11,000 per mm^3 (may be as high as 25,000)

4. palpitations: common in early and late pregnancy because of sympathetic nervous system disturbance and increased intraabdominal pressure

f. Renal system

1. elimination/fluid transport greatly increased because of circulatory changes and need to excrete fetal waste products

2. glomerular filtration rate increases 50%

3. renal functioning is compromised in standing or sitting position; lateral recumbent position enhances kidney function

4. reduced renal threshold for glucose glycosuria may occur; reflection of kidneys' inability to absorb glucose; appears to have little relationship to serum glucose

5. increased amount of urine; decreased specific gravity; increased pH

6. dilation of ureters, especially on the right, may lead to urinary stasis and urinary tract infection (UTI)

7. decreased bladder tone, caused by progesterone effect

8. increased pressure on bladder by enlarging uterus (first and third trimesters), therefore decreased capacity and increased frequency

g. Respiratory system

1. diaphragm rises as much as 1 inch; slight dyspnea may occur until lightening (60% of pregnant women)

2. thoracic cage is pushed upward and widened

3. increased vital capacity, tidal volume, respiratory minute volume to supply maternal and fetal needs

4. increased vascularization because of elevated estrogen can cause nasal stuffiness; nosebleed, voice changes, eustachian tube blockage

h. Digestive system

1. gastrointestinal motility and digestion slowed because of progesterone effects

2. delayed emptying time of stomach; reflux of food

3. upward displacement and compression of stomach

4. displacement of intestines as fetus develops

5. decreased secretion of HCl

6. slower emptying of gallbladder and high cholesterol levels may lead to gallstone formation

7. common problems

a. nausea and vomiting (morning sickness, 50% to 75% of pregnant women)

b. pica: food or substance cravings (e.g., laundry starch, clay)

c. acid indigestion or heartburn

d. constipation

e. hemorrhoids

f. bleeding, swollen gums because of estrogen

i. Psychosocial adaptations in pregnancy

1. factors influencing a woman's response to pregnancy (varies with developmental stage)

a. memories of her own childhood

b. cultural background

c. existing support systems

d. socioeconomic conditions

e. perceptions of maternal role

f. impact of mass media

g. coping mechanisms

h. knowledge of pregnancy changes

2. maternal adaptations to pregnancy

a. first trimester: initial ambivalence about pregnancy; pregnant woman places main focus on self (i.e., physical changes associated with pregnancy and emotional reactions to pregnancy)

b. second trimester: relatively tranquil period; acceptance of reality of pregnancy; increased awareness and interest in fetus; introversion and feeling of well-being

c. third trimester: anticipation of labor and delivery and assuming mothering role, viewing infant as reality vs. fantasy; fears, fantasies, and dreams about labor are common; "nesting" behaviors (e.g., preparing layette)

3. psychologic tasks of pregnancy (Rubin, 1961)

a. acceptance of pregnancy as a reality and incorporation of fetus into body image

b. preparation for physical separation from fetus (birth)

c. attainment of maternal role

4. developmental tasks of pregnancy

a. accept the biologic fact of pregnancy (i.e., "I am pregnant")

b. accept the growing fetus as distinct from self and as a person to care for (i.e., "I am going to have a baby")

c. prepare realistically for the birth and parenting of the child (i.e., "I am going to be a mother")

5. paternal reactions to pregnancy

a. vary with developmental stage, sociocultural factors (as with woman), and involvement

b. first trimester: ambivalence and anxiety about role change; concern or identification with mother's discomforts (couvade)

c. second trimester: increased confidence and interest in mother's care; difficulty relating to fetus; "jealousy"

d. third trimester: changing self-concept; concern about body changes; active involvement common; fears about delivery, mutilation, or death of partner or fetus

6. sibling reactions to pregnancy

a. normal rivalry dependent on developmental stage

b. may need increased affection and attention

c. regression in behavior (may appear in bed-wetting and thumb-sucking); rejection

3. Fetal development
   a. During first lunar month (1 lunar month = 4 weeks)
      1. after fertilization, the ovum (zygote) begins a process of rapid cell division (mitosis or cleavage) leading to formation of *blastomeres,* which eventually become a ball-like structure called the morula
      2. the *morula* changes into a *blastocyst* after entering the uterus
      3. implantation occurs within 5 to 9 days, when the exposed cells of the trophoblast (cellular walls of the blastocyst) implant in the anterior or posterior fundal portion of the uterus
      4. the cells of the embryo will differentiate into three main groups: an outer covering (ectoderm), a middle layer (mesoderm), and an internal layer (entoderm)
         a. ectoderm: later differentiates into epithelium of skin, hair, nails, nasal and oral passages, sebaceous and sweat glands, mucous membranes of mouth and nose, salivary glands, the nervous system
         b. mesoderm: later differentiates into muscles; bones; circulatory, renal, and reproductive organs; connective tissue
         c. entoderm: differentiates into epithelium of gastrointestinal and respiratory tracts, the bladder, thyroid
   b. Subsequent lunar months
      1. end of first lunar month (4 weeks): heart functions; beginning formation of eyes, nose, digestive tract; arm and leg buds
      2. end of second lunar month (8 weeks): recognizable human face, rapid brain development, appearance of external genitalia
      3. end of third lunar month (12 weeks): placenta fully formed and functioning; sex determination apparent; bones begin to ossify; less danger of teratogenic effects after this time; length: 3½ inches (9 cm), weight: ½ oz (2 g)
      4. end of fourth lunar month (16 weeks): external genitalia obvious; meconium present in intestinal tract; eyes, ears, and nose formed; fetal heartbeat heard with fetoscope; length: 6½ inches, weight: 4 oz
      5. end of fifth lunar month (20 weeks): lanugo present; fetus sucks and swallows amniotic fluid; quickening (mother can feel movement); length: 10 inches, weight: 8 oz
      6. end of sixth lunar month (24 weeks): vernix present; skin reddish and wrinkled; considered viable, but usually does not survive if born now; length: 12 inches, weight: 1 lb 5 oz
      7. end of seventh lunar month (28 weeks): iron stored; surfactant production begins; nails appear; better chance of survival if delivered than in earlier gestation; length: 15 inches, weight: 2 lb 8 oz (1000 g)
      8. end of eighth lunar month (32 weeks): iron, cal-cium stored; more reflexes present; good chance of survival if delivered preterm
      9. end of ninth lunar month (36 weeks): well padded with subcutaneous fat; survival same as term
      10. end of tenth lunar month (39 to 40 weeks or full term): lanugo shed, nails firm, testes fully descended; length: 18 to 22 inches (45 to 55 cm), weight: average 7 lb 8 oz (3400 g)
   c. Fetal circulation
      1. fetus receives oxygen through placenta
      2. oxygenated blood enters fetal circulation through umbilical vein of cord to the ductus venosus and liver; ductus venosus attaches to inferior vena cava and allows blood to bypass liver
      3. from inferior vena cava, blood flows into right atrium and goes directly to the left atrium through the foramen ovale
      4. blood enters right atrium through superior vena cava, flows to right ventricle, to pulmonary artery (small amount enters lungs for nourishment); the ductus arteriosus shunts blood from pulmonary artery into the aorta, allows bypass of fetal lungs
      5. two umbilical arteries return deoxygenated blood from fetus to placenta
   d. Amniotic fluid
      1. multiple origins; composition changes in pregnancy; from maternal serum to fetal urine toward term
      2. appearance: clear, pale, straw colored, with faint characteristic odor; neutral to slightly alkaline (pH 7.0 to 7.25) while vaginal secretions are normally acidic
      3. volume: about 30 ml at 10 weeks, 350 ml at 20 weeks, approximately 1000 ml at term; specific gravity 1.007 to 1.025
         a. *oligohydramnios* is less than 500 ml of fluid
         b. *polyhydramnios* is greater than 1500 ml of fluid
      4. contains albumin, urea, uric acid, creatinine, lecithin, sphingomyelin, bilirubin, epithelial cells, fat, fructose, leukocytes, enzymes, lanugo
      5. functions
         a. protects fetus from injury
         b. separates fetus from fetal membrane
         c. allows fetus freedom of movement
         d. provides source of oral fluids
         e. serves as excretion-collection system
         f. exchanges at rate of 500 ml/hr (at term)
         g. regulates fetal body temperature

Overview of Management

1. Interdisciplinary health team: nurses, nurse practitioners, midwives, physicians, social workers, dietitians, and other health care providers
2. Schedule of visits
   a. Routine if no complications
      1. every 4 weeks, up to 32 weeks
      2. every 2 weeks from 32 to 36 weeks (more frequently if problems exist)
      3. every week from 36 to 40 weeks

b. Initial visit
1. obtain family and obstetric history
   a. personal and social profiles of childbearing family, including cultural patterns, education, support systems, coping methods, economic level (low income level may mean little or no antenatal care, inadequate nutrition, or high risk for preeclampsia)
   b. maternal factors affecting course of pregnancy: viral infections, smoking, use of alcohol or drugs, activities of daily living, sleep patterns, bowel habits, nutrition (inadequate diet increases risk of anemia, preeclampsia), weight, age, and living at high altitude (increased hemoglobin), medical treatments such as x-rays or anesthetics, exposure to environmental hazards, infections
   c. preexisting medical disorders: diabetes mellitus, cardiac disease, anemia, hypertension, thyroid disorders; immune deficiency
   d. family planning measures; health history during pregnancies; history of infertility
   e. attitudes toward present pregnancy
   f. history of preceding pregnancies and perinatal outcomes (TPAL)
      - T: number of term births (i.e., born at 37 weeks gestation or beyond)
      - P: number of premature births
      - A: number of abortions (spontaneous or induced)
      - L: number of living children
      - *gravida:* all pregnancies regardless of duration or outcome, including present pregnancy
      - *parity:* past pregnancies resulting in viable fetus (20 to 24 weeks), whether born dead or alive (twins considered as one)
      - cesarean births
      - Rh or ABO sensitization; RhoGAM given
      - serious emotional or psychologic distress
      - stillborns
   g. past personal and family medical history
2. calculate expected date of birth (EDB) using Nagele's rule: count back 3 calendar months from the first day of the last regular menstrual period (LMP) and add 7 days (Table 4-6)
c. Initial and subsequent visits
1. assess vital signs and blood pressure for normal range or baseline
2. check urine for albumin and glucose: ideally not more than 1+ glucose with protein negative
3. monitor weight gain: a total gain of 24 to 32 lb is recommended, depending on prepregnant nutritional state and maternal age
   a. 2 to 4 lb in the first trimester
   b. 11 to 14 lb in the second trimester
   c. 8 to 11 lb in the third trimester (i.e., 0.5 lb weekly)
4. assess fetal growth and development over duration of pregnancy
   a. fetal heart rate (FHR)
   b. abdominal palpation
   c. fundal height (McDonald's rule)
5. allow time for client to express concerns, problems or discomfort, and learning needs
6. document accurately

Application of the Nursing Process to Normal Childbearing, Antepartal Care

ASSESSMENT
1. Refer to Initial and Subsequent Visits, left

ANALYSIS/NURSING DIAGNOSIS
1. Safe, effective care environment
   a. Risk for injury
   b. Knowledge deficit
2. Physiologic integrity
   a. Fatigue
   b. Altered nutrition: less than body requirements
3. Psychosocial integrity
   a. Self-esteem disturbance
   b. Altered role performance
4. Health promotion/maintenance
   a. Health-seeking behaviors
   b. Altered family processes

PLANNING, IMPLEMENTATION, AND EVALUATION

Goal I Client will participate in regular prenatal care; fetus will be well oxygenated and nourished throughout gestation.

Implementation
1. Measure vital signs, including temperature, blood pressure, pulse, and respiration.
2. Assess client: general physical assessment including height and weight (initial visit).
3. Help with/perform physical examination and bimanual pelvic examination.
   a. Prepare and arrange necessary equipment (gloves, lubricant [for digital exam], vaginal speculum, materials for Pap smear [no lubricant used], light, and pelvimeter).
   b. Prepare client for procedure by providing explanation, instructing her to empty bladder, and placing her in lithotomy position, position hands across chest.
   c. Provide emotional support and maintain comfort of client before and during examination (using relaxation, breathing, and focusing techniques).
4. Measure fundal height using McDonald's rule (in second and third trimester): symphysis pubis to fundus (Table 4-7).
5. Estimated fetal weight (EFW): rump-to-crown length in utero in centimeters × 100 = EFW (g)

Table 4-6 Nägele's rule

If first day of last menstrual period was
January 17
subtract 3 months
+
add 7 days
Estimated date of delivery is October 24

Table 4-7 McDonald's rule

Height of fundus (cm)
   × 2/7 = duration of pregnancy in *lunar months*
   × 8/7 = duration of pregnancy in *weeks*

6. Check for fetal heartbeat, detectable as early as 16 weeks with fetoscope and by 10 to 12 weeks with Doppler device.
7. Assist in obtaining samples for laboratory studies.
   a. Clean-catch urine for urinalysis, albumin, glucose, and asymptomatic bacteriuria.
   b. Blood for hemoglobin, hematocrit, type, Rh, rubella titer (greater than 1:8 shows immunity).
   c. Sickle cell disease or trait in black women.
   d. Standard tests for sexually transmitted diseases (serology for syphilis; smears for gonorrhea, herpes).
   e. Schedule glucose 50 g test during 24 to 28 weeks
8. Encourage regular antepartal care.
   a. Explain need for continuity.
   b. Describe *danger signals* (e.g., vaginal bleeding, dizziness or visual spots, swelling of face or fingers, epigastric pain, physical trauma) or reportable signs that require immediate medical care.
9. Promote health through anticipatory guidance: rest and exercise, personal hygiene, sexual activity, dental care, clothing, travel, immunizations, smoking, alcohol use, substance abuse.
   a. Tell couple to expect an increased need for sleep during entire pregnancy, with fatigue common in first trimester; needs vary among individuals; plan rest times during day.
   b. Teach relaxation methods in preparing for sleep.
   c. Advise to continue usual exercise regimen; avoid introduction of strenuous sports; avoid exercise leading to fatigue, exhaustion, overheating, dehydration.
   d. Explain exercise limitations related to the changing center of gravity (e.g., high-impact aerobics, jogging) and temperature elevations.
   e. Avoid sauna/whirlpool, hot tub.
   f. Suggest that client may continue to work except if exposed to toxic chemicals, radiation, or biologic or safety hazards (if job requires sitting for a long period of time, encourage frequent position changes).
   g. Teach hygiene and skin care; daily baths if desired (caution on safely getting into and out of bathtub); avoid soap on nipples; towel-dry breasts; for vaginal discharge: daily bathing, wear cotton underwear (douching not recommended).
   h. Suggest that changes in sexual desire/response may occur, related to discomforts or anxieties of pregnancy; encourage couple to share their concerns and feelings; alternative coital positions may be helpful, as may be other methods of satisfying sexual needs; coitus may be continued throughout pregnancy unless premature labor, rupture of membranes, or bleeding occur.
   i. Encourage dental checkup early in pregnancy and delay extensive dental work and x-ray examinations when possible; hypertrophy and tenderness of gums is a common problem.
   j. Recommend comfortable, nonrestricting maternity clothing, well-fitting bra, and low-heeled, supportive shoes.
   k. Advise client to stop or reduce cigarette consumption; *maternal smoking is associated with low birth weight* (related to vasoconstriction).
   l. Advise client to *avoid alcohol consumption* during pregnancy because alcohol, even in minimal to moderate amounts, is harmful to fetus; linked to fetal alcohol syndrome.
   m. Warn client to avoid medication, particularly in the first trimester (over-the-counter, prescription drugs, and street drugs may cross placental barrier and cause congenital anomalies).
   n. Suggest that while traveling long distances by automobile, stop, get out, and walk frequently; use seat belts for safety.
   o. Teach couple that attenuated, live vaccines (e.g., mumps, rubella) are contraindicated for immunizations during pregnancy.

Evaluation

Client receives initial and regular antepartal care to prevent or detect any early complications; avoids substances that may potentially harm the fetus; fetus maintains a growth and development pattern appropriate for gestational age as evidenced by maternal weight gain, fundal height, activity level, and other antenatal screening techniques; is protected from environmental hazards and stresses (e.g., alcohol, nicotine).

Goal 2 Client will be able to differentiate between normal discomforts and danger signals that require immediate attention.

Implementation

1. Teach health maintenance and relief of common discomforts.
   a. *Morning sickness:* eat dry crackers or toast before slowly arising; eat small, frequent meals; avoid greasy, highly seasoned food; take adequate fluids between meals; eat a protein snack at bedtime.
   b. *Nasal stuffiness:* use cool-air vaporizer.
   c. *Excessive saliva:* rinse mouth with astringent mouth wash.
   d. *Breast tenderness:* wear a well-fitted, supportive bra with wide, adjustable straps.
   e. *Heartburn and indigestion:* avoid overeating, ingesting fatty or fried food; take small, frequent meals; avoid taking sodium bicarbonate; remain upright 3 to 4 hours after eating.
   f. *Backache:* maintain proper body alignment (pelvic tilt) and use good body mechanics; use maternity girdle in selected situations; wear comfortable shoes; use proper mattress; rest frequently; do pelvic-rock exercise and tailor sitting.
   g. *Leg cramps:* stretch involved muscles (i.e., extension of leg with dorsiflexion of the foot); may be related to alterations in calcium, phosphorus.

h. *Varicose veins:* elevate legs frequently when sitting or lying down in bed; avoid sitting or standing for prolonged periods or crossing legs at the knees; avoid tight or constricting hosiery or garters (physician may suggest wearing supportive hose).

i. *Vaginal discharge:* clean perineum daily; wear cotton-crotch underwear; report any burning or redness or change in vaginal discharge.

j. *Hemorrhoids:* apply warm compresses; if recommended by physician, reinsert hemorrhoids (place client in a side-lying or knee-chest position; use gentle pressure and a lubricant), avoid constipation; take sitz baths.

k. *Constipation:* increase fluid intake (ideal is 6 to 8 glasses per day), roughage; develop good daily bowel movement habits; exercise.

l. *Urinary frequency:* empty bladder regularly; report any burning, dysuria, cloudiness, or blood in urine; restrict fluids in the late afternoon (not below 8 glasses daily); do Kegel exercises in sets of 10 to tighten sphincter muscles.

m. *Ankle edema:* change position, lie on left side; rest with legs and hips elevated (report any edema in face and in hands).

n. *Uterine contractions* (Braxton Hicks): normal during late pregnancy; report if they progressively increase and are accompanied by signs of labor.

o. *Faintness:* avoid staying in one position over a long period; arise from bed from a lateral position to prevent supine hypotension.

p. *Shortness of breath:* use proper posture when erect; sleep with head elevated by several pillows (left lateral position preferred).

Evaluation
Client identifies own basic discomforts of pregnancy and appropriately relieves them.

> **Goal 3** Client will follow a balanced diet to meet her own developmental needs, the physical requirements of pregnancy, and fetal growth and development.

Implementation
1. Obtain complete nutritional profile (suggest client use 24-hour recall).
   a. Prepregnant and current nutritional status (e.g., overweight, underweight, anemic)
   b. Physical symptoms possibly indicative of poor nutrition (e.g., dry scaly skin, lack of skin turgor, fatigue)
   c. Socioeconomic status: available finances for a balanced diet; food storage and preparation; customs and cultural/religious restrictions
   d. Dietary habits: regularity of meals, junk-food intake, pica, peer pressure
   e. Knowledge of nutritional needs, food pyramid, recommended allowances during pregnancy.
2. Assess for nutritional risk factors at the onset of pregnancy.
   a. Adolescence
   b. Frequent pregnancies

c. Poor reproductive history
d. Economic deprivation
e. Bizarre food patterns
f. Vegetarian diet
g. Smoking, drug addiction, or alcoholism
h. Chronic systemic disease
i. Prepregnant weight problems, including anorexia and bulimia

3. Assess for nutritional risk factors during pregnancy.
   a. Anemia of pregnancy
   b. Pregnancy-induced hypertension
   c. Inadequate or excessive weight gain
   d. Demands of lactation
4. Teach based on consideration of mother's age, routine activity, developmental needs, cultural dietary patterns, and risk factors.
5. Encourage good nutritional practices; see Tables 4-4 and 4-8.
   a. Discuss well-balanced diet, adapted during pregnancy.
   b. Recommend that pregnant adolescents take in additional calories, protein, and calcium for own developmental needs.
   c. Suggest a minimum fluid intake of 6 to 8 glasses of fluids or water each day.
   d. Discuss possible vitamin and mineral supplements (e.g., iron or folic acid).
   e. Caution against overdose of vitamins A and D (may cause fetal deformities).
   f. Monitor weight gain each antepartal visit; a total weight gain of 24 to 32 lb is usually recommended.
   g. Recognize when restrictions in salt may be indicated (e.g., high-sodium foods such as carrots, spinach, celery, carbonated beverages, canned soup, bacon, ham, monosodium glutamate, pickles, and olives).
   h. Refer to nutritionist or assistance programs for additional teaching/counseling and services.

Evaluation
Client knows the nutrients and calories needed each day; follows a balanced diet; gradually and steadily gains 24 to 32 lb during the pregnancy; fetus maintains a growth and development pattern appropriate for gestational age.

> **Goal 4** Client and family will participate in preparation for childbirth classes.

Implementation
1. Explain the purpose and scope of childbirth education (decrease fear and anxiety through knowledge, effective use of relaxation techniques to reduce pain perception during labor and lead to a *satisfying birth experience*).
2. Discuss various methods (Table 4-9).
3. Offer direct instructions (Leboyer) or referral to appropriate resources (e.g., ASPO Lamaze or International Childbirth Education Association).

Evaluation
Couple expresses a positive attitude toward pregnancy and is adequately prepared for birth experience; openly expresses concerns and provides emotional support to each other; begins the role transition to parenthood.

Table 4-8 Nutritional recommendations during pregnancy and lactation

Nutrient	RDA for nonpregnant female (25-50 yr)	RDA during pregnancy	RDA for lactation* (first 6 mo/second 6 mo)	Reasons for increased need	Food sources
Calories	2200	2200 (first trimester); 2500 (second and third trimesters)	2700/2700	Increased energy needs for fetal growth and milk production	Carbohydrate, fat, protein
Protein (g)	50	60	65/62	Synthesis of the products of conception: fetus, amniotic fluid, placenta; growth of maternal tissue: uterus, breasts, red blood cells, plasma proteins, secretion of milk protein during lactation	Meats, eggs, milk, cheese, legumes (dry beans and peas, peanuts), nuts, grains
Minerals					
Calcium (mg)	800	1200	1200/1200	Fetal skeleton and tooth bud formation; maintenance of maternal bone and tooth mineralization	Milk, cheese, yogurt, sardines or other fish eaten with bones left in, deep green leafy vegetables except spinach or Swiss chard,† tofu, baked beans
Phosphorus (mg)	800	1200	1200/1200	Fetal skeleton and tooth bud formation	Milk, cheese, yogurt, meats, whole grains, nuts, legumes
Iron (mg)	15	30	15/15	Increased maternal hemoglobin formation, fetal liver iron storage	Liver, meats, whole or enriched breads and cereals, deep green leafy vegetables, legumes, dried fruits
Zinc (mg)	12	15	19/16	Component of numerous enzyme systems; possibly important in preventing congenital malformations	Liver, shellfish, meats, whole grains, milk
Iodine (μg)	150	175	200/200	Increased maternal metabolic rate	Iodized salt, seafood, milk and milk products, commercial yeast breads, rolls, and donuts
Magnesium (μg)	280	320	355/340	Involved in energy and protein metabolism, tissue growth, muscle action	Nuts, legumes, cocoa, meats, whole grains
Selenium (mg)	55	65	75/75	Antioxidant (protects cell membranes), tooth component	Organ meats, seafood, whole grains, legumes, molasses

RDA, Recommended daily allowance.

*Milk production generally declines during the second 6 months of lactation as the infant's diet increasingly begins to include other foods. Thus maternal needs for many nutrients decrease.

†Spinach and chard contain calcium but also contain oxalin acid, which inhibits calcium absorption.

Table 4-8 Nutritional recommendations during pregnancy and lactation—cont'd

Nutrient	RDA for nonpregnant female (25-50 yr)	RDA during pregnancy	RDA for lactation* (first 6 mo/second 6 mo)	Reasons for increased need	Food sources
Fat-soluble vitamins A (RE)†	800	800	1300/1200	Essential for cell development, thus growth; tooth bud formation (development of enamel-forming cells in gum tissue); bone growth	Deep green leafy vegetables, dark yellow vegetables and fruits, chili peppers, liver, fortified margarine and butter
D (mg)‡	5	10	10/10	Involved in absorption of calcium and phosphorus, improves mineralization	Fortified milk, fortified margarine, egg yolk, butter, liver, seafood
E (µg)	8	10	12/11	Antioxidant (protects cell membranes from damage), especially important for preventing hemolysis of red blood cells	Vegetable oils, green leafy vegetables, whole grains, liver, nuts and seeds, cheese, fish
Water-soluble vitamins C (mg)	60	70	95/90	Tissue formation and integrity, formation of connective tissue, enhancement of iron absorption	Citrus fruits, strawberries, melons, broccoli, tomatoes, peppers, raw deep green leafy vegetables
Folic acid (µg)	180	400	280/260	Increased red blood cell formation, prevention of macrocytic or megaloblastic anemia	Green leafy vegetables, oranges, broccoli, asparagus, artichokes, liver
Thiamin (mg)	1.1	1.5	1.6/1.6	Involves in energy metabolism	Pork, beef, liver, whole or enriched grains, legumes
Riboflavin (mg)	1.3	1.6	1.8/1.7	Involved in energy and protein metabolism	Milk, liver, enriched grains, deep green and yellow vegetables
Pyridoxine (B₆) (mg)	1.6	2.2	2.1/2.1	Involved in protein metabolism	Meat, liver, deep green vegetables, whole grains
B₁₂ (µg)	2.0	2.2	2.6/2.6	Production of nucleic acids and proteins, especially important in formation of red blood cells and prevention of megaloblastic or macrocytic anemia	Milk, egg, meat, liver, cheese
Niacin (mg)	15	17	20/20	Involved in energy metabolism	Meat, fish, poultry, liver, whole or enriched grains, peanuts

*Milk production generally declines during the second 6 months of lactation as the infant's diet increasingly begins to include other foods. Thus maternal needs for many nutrients decreases.
†RE, Retinol equivalents. Replaces international units (IU). 1 RE = 5 IU.
‡As cholecalciferol. 10 µg cholecalciferol = 400 IU of vitamin D.

Table 4-9 Childbirth preparation

Method	Chief focus	Breathing/relaxation techniques
G.D. Read	Earliest modern physician to identify fear-tension-pain cycle	
	Avoidance of medication; removed childbirth from illness orientation	
Gamper	Based on Read; use of uterus as focal point	Abdominal/natural breathing
Bradley	Based on Read/Gamper	Diaphragmatic breathing
	Focus on individual relaxation methods	
	Mother-centered; coached by partner	
	Emphasis of client decision making	
Lamaze	Conscious application of conditioned responses to stimuli	Chest breathing in early labor
(psychoprophylactic)	Use of focal point outside mother's body	Increasing rate as labor progresses
		Cleansing breaths

HIGH-RISK CHILDBEARING

1. Definition: any existing or developing condition or factor that prevents or impedes the normal progress of pregnancy to the delivery of a viable, healthy, term infant.
2. Assessment of risk factors
   a. Age: under 17 or over 35 (greater risk over 40)
      1. pregnant adolescents have a higher incidence of prematurity, pregnancy-induced hypertension, cephalopelvic disproportion, poor nutrition, social/economic instability, and inadequate antepartal care
      2. women over 35 are at increased risk for chromosomal disorders in infants (e.g., Down syndrome), pregnancy-induced hypertension, and cesarean delivery; those over 35 for first pregnancy may be at increased risk
   b. Parity
      1. multiparity: two or more pregnancies (may not be significant)
      2. grand multiparity: women with six or more pregnancies at greater risk for postpartal hemorrhage
      3. short intervals between pregnancies: greater risk for iron-deficiency anemias
   c. Past health history
      1. diabetes
      2. heart disease
      3. renal conditions
      4. essential hypertension
      5. anemias
      6. thyroid disorders
      7. physical abuse
   d. Past obstetric history
      1. lack of antepartal care; poor compliance with visit schedule (may be a factor in late detection of health problems); contributes to high infant mortality rate in this country
      2. abortions: spontaneous
      3. ectopic pregnancy
      4. preterm labor and delivery
      5. intrauterine growth retardation
      6. congenital malformations: result of genetic disorders
      7. cesarean births
      8. previous fetal loss
      9. pregnancy-induced hypertension
      10. gestational diabetes
      11. vaginal bleeding in pregnancy
      12. isoimmunization
      13. multiple gestation
      14. large infants
   e. Current obstetric history
      1. pregnancy-induced hypertension (21% of maternal deaths)
      2. infections (18% of maternal deaths)
         a. sexually transmitted diseases
         b. TORCH syndrome (*T*oxoplasmosis, *O*ther, *R*ubella, *C*ytomegalovirus infection, *H*erpes)
         c. other viral diseases (e.g., hepatitis or HIV)
         d. bacterial infections (e.g., tuberculosis; Beta-strep)
      3. hemorrhage (14% of maternal deaths)
      4. exposure to toxic environmental agents
      5. use of drugs
      6. multiple gestation
      7. placental abnormalities
      8. abnormal presentations
      9. premature rupture of membranes
      10. chronic health problems (e.g., diabetes, cardiac disease, anemia)
      11. coexisting medical problems
      12. abnormal antenatal test results (e.g., on amniotic-fluid analysis, ultrasound)
   f. Socioeconomic-cultural status
      1. low socioeconomic status: often associated with
         a. inadequate nutrition
         b. lack of general knowledge about health care needs
      2. incidence of small-for-gestational-age (SGA) babies is common in some Asian and black women and adolescents
   g. Malnutrition or deprivation: less than 4 kg weight gain by 30 weeks of gestation; may be related to eating disorders
   h. Drug or alcohol addiction: associated with congenital anomalies, intrauterine growth retardation, and numerous other problems
   i. Smoking: associated with low-birth-weight and SGA infants
3. Diagnostic tests, biophysical and biochemical, to evalu-

ate fetal-placental function or fetal maturity; critical in high-risk pregnancy

a. Fetal movement or fetal kick count
   1. definition: daily recording of fetal movements to assess active and passive fetal states
   2. indications: in all pregnancies; started earlier with high-risk clients
   3. procedure: a noninvasive test that may be done by pregnant woman while resting on side
   4. interpretation (optimal number of fetal movements varies with source)
      a. normally three or more movements felt in an hour; fetal states normally vary (cyclic periods of rest and activity)
      b. sharp decrease in fetal activity (unrelated to sleep) of two or fewer movements per hour should be reported, and a nonstress test (NST) may be scheduled
   5. reassure client that there are fetal rest and sleep states with minimal or no fetal movement
b. Nonstress testing
   1. definition: observation of FHR related to fetal movement (accelerations suggest fetal well-being with good prognosis)
   2. indications: for fetal evaluation, especially in postterm pregnancies, uteroplacental insufficiency, poor fetal history
   3. procedure
      a. performed in an ambulatory setting or in the hospital obstetric unit by nurse trained in test administration
      b. requires external electronic monitoring (indirect) using ultrasound transducer to measure FHR and tocodynamometer to trace fetal activity or spontaneous uterine activity
      c. pregnant woman placed in semi-Fowler's or left lateral position after light snack.
      d. maternal blood pressure (BP) recorded initially
      e. requires 30 to 50 minutes to administer test
      f. client must activate "mark button" with each fetal movement
   4. interpretation
      a. reactive (normal): two FHR accelerations (greater than 15 beats per minute) above baseline—lasting 15 seconds or more—occur with fetal movement in a 10- or 20-minute period
      b. nonreactive (abnormal): failure to meet the reactive criteria indicates the need for additional evaluation, perhaps using contraction stress test (CST) or biophysical profile
      c. unsatisfactory result: uninterpretable FHR or fetal activity recording; additional testing performed in 24 hours or CST done
c. Contraction stress test: oxytocin challenge test (OCT) or nipple stimulation test
   1. definition: the response of the fetus (FHR pattern) to induced uterine contractions is observed as an indicator of uteroplacental and fetal physiologic integrity
   2. indications: in all pregnancies after 28 weeks

with high-risk clients; avoid if history of preterm labor
   3. procedure
      a. performed on an outpatient basis in or near the labor and delivery unit
      b. requires external electronic monitoring (indirect) using ultrasound transducer to measure FHR and tocodynamometer to trace uterine activity
      c. pregnant woman placed in semi-Fowler's or left lateral position
      d. maternal blood pressure recorded initially and at intervals during test
      e. requires 60 minutes to 3 hours to complete test
      f. increasing doses of oxytocin are administered as a dilute intravenous (IV) infusion according to hospital protocol or physician's orders or nipple stimulation until uterine contractions occur
      g. provide emotional support during and after procedure
   4. interpretation
      a. negative (normal): the absence of late decelerations of FHR with each of three contractions during a 10-minute interval; known as "negative window"
      b. positive (abnormal): the presence of late decelerations of FHR with three contractions during a 10-minute interval; known as "positive window"
      c. equivocal or suspicious: the absence of a positive or negative window (i.e., criterion of three contractions in a 10-minute interval is not achieved)
      d. unsatisfactory tests occur when interpretable tracings are not obtained or adequate uterine contractions are not achieved
      e. high-risk pregnancies are usually allowed to continue if a negative OCT is obtained; test is repeated weekly for these clients
d. Nipple stimulation-contraction stress test
   1. baseline data obtained through monitoring as in CST procedure
   2. nipple stimulated by warm towel application or nipple rolling, causing release of oxytocin and producing uterine contractions
   3. interpretation: as with CST, uterine contraction with absence of late decelerations is the desired result
e. Ultrasonography
   1. definition: a noninvasive procedure involving the passage of high-frequency sound waves through the uterus to obtain an outline of the fetus, placenta, uterine cavity, or any other area under examination
   2. purposes
      a. confirm pregnancy (first trimester)
      b. determine fetal viability
      c. estimate fetal age through measuring the biparietal diameter of the fetal head; most accurate at 12 to 24 weeks

    d. monitor fetal growth

    e. determine fetal position

    f. locate placenta

    g. detect fetal abnormalities

    h. identify multiple gestation

    i. confirm fetal death

    j. fetal biophysical profile

  3. procedure

    a. advise pregnant woman to consume 1 quart of water 2 hours before procedure and avoid emptying bladder (important in first trimester); scanning is done when the bladder is full (exception: before amniocentesis)

    b. transmission gel spread over maternal abdomen

    c. sonographer scans vertically and horizontally in sections across abdomen

  4. possible risk

    a. none known with brief, infrequent exposure to high-intensity sound

    b. couple and physician together should discuss indications, benefits, and potential risks

 f. Chorionic villi sampling (research ongoing)

  1. definition: removal of a small sample of chorionic villi for examination

  2. purposes

    a. detect chromosomal defects

    b. detect biochemical abnormalities

  3. procedure

    a. done at 8 to 10 weeks of gestation

    b. catheter passed through cervix into the uterus (guided by sonography)

    c. sample aspirated under negative pressure

  4. advantages

    a. early detection of abnormalities allowing for first-trimester termination of the pregnancy if desired

    b. results available within 2 to 10 days

  5. disadvantages

    a. risk of abortion

    b. infection

    c. embryo-fetal/placental damage

 g. Biophysical profile

  1. surveillance of fetal well-being is based on five categories

    a. NST

    b. amniotic fluid index

    c. fetal breathing movements

    d. fetal movement

    e. fetal tone

  2. each category carries a score of 2; a score of 8 to 10 is reassuring, provided amniotic fluid level is within normal limits

 h. Amniocentesis

  1. definition: an invasive procedure for amniotic fluid analysis to assess fetal health and maturity; done from 14 weeks of gestation

  2. procedure

    a. ultrasonography is first performed to locate the placenta

    b. pregnant woman must empty bladder before procedure if greater than 20 weeks of gestation

    c. baseline vital signs and FHR are assessed; monitor every 15 minutes

    d. pregnant woman is placed in supine position and given an abdominal prep

    e. a needle is passed through the abdominal and uterine walls into the amniotic sac, and a small amount of amniotic fluid is withdrawn

  3. possible risks: overall, less than 1%

    a. maternal: hemorrhage, infection, Rh isoimmunization, abruptio placentae, labor

    b. fetal: death, infection, hemorrhage, abortion, premature labor, injury from needle

  4. observe client closely for 30 to 40 minutes after procedure; instruct client to report any side effects (e.g., unusual fetal activity, vaginal bleeding, leakage of amniotic fluid, uterine contractions, fever, or chills); give Rh-negative woman RhoGAM

  5. provide emotional support/counseling as needed

 i. Laboratory studies

  1. serum estriol determination: to assess placental functioning

    a. steroid precursor produced by the adrenals of the fetus is synthesized into estriols in the placenta and is excreted by the maternal kidneys; mother's levels normally rise during pregnancy

    b. serial estriol determinations are obtained with repeat blood samples

    c. a sudden drop in estriol level is associated with fetal hypoxia; continuous low levels associated with compromise of fetus

  2. Serum placental lactogen

    a. hormone produced by placenta; levels rise through 36 weeks of gestation, then stabilize

    b. low values indicate possible fetal distress; values low in threatened abortion, toxemia, intrauterine growth retardation, and postmaturity

  3. maternal serum alpha-fetoprotein (AFP)

    a. maternal blood sampling between 16 and 20 weeks of gestation is used

    b. low values may indicate chromosomal defects (e.g., Down syndrome); high values may indicate defects such as neural tube defects, anencephaly, absence of the ventral abdominal wall

  4. Triple screen

    a. Maternal blood sampling between 16 and 18 weeks of gestation

    b. Increases sensitivity of maternal AFP screening by including estriol and serum chorionic gonadotropin levels to screen for Down syndrome

  5. Analysis of amniotic fluid (Table 4-10)

    a. chromosomal studies to assess genetic disorders (e.g., Down syndrome, cell culture for karyotype)

Table 4-10   Laboratory studies of fetal well-being

Study	Purpose/indication	Interpretation
Urinary serum estriol	Assess placental functioning	Sudden drop = fetal hypoxia
		Continuous low levels = fetal compromise
Amniotic fluid analysis	Chromosomal studies	Detection of genetic disorders
	Determination of sex chromatin	Detection of sex-linked disorders
	Biochemical analysis of fetal-cell enzymes	Detection of inborn errors of metabolism
	Fetal lung maturity (lecithin/sphingomyelin ratios)	L/S ratio of 2:1 or greater = fetal lung maturity in nondiabetics
	Alpha-fetoprotein (AFP) levels	High levels = neural-tube defects, anencephaly
	Creatinine levels	More than 2.0 mg = fetal age greater than 36 wk
	Identification and evaluation of Rh incompatibility	Increased bilirubin = evaluate for intrauterine transfusion or delivery
	Lipid cells (Nile blue stain)	20% of cells stained orange = fetal weight at least 2500 g
	Meconium presence	Fetal hypoxia (except with breech)

b. determination of sex chromatin in fetal cells to assess sex-linked disorders

c. biochemical analysis of fetal-cell enzymes to assess inborn errors of metabolism

d. determination of lecithin-to-sphingomyelin ratios (L/S ratios) to assess fetal lung maturity (most reliable)
- lecithin and sphingomyelin are important components of surfactant, a phosphoprotein that lowers surface tension in the fetal lungs and facilitates extrauterine expiration
- an L/S ratio of 2:1 or greater is generally associated with fetal lung maturity except for selected high-risk neonates (e.g., infants of diabetic mothers)

e. evaluation of phosphatidyl glycerol (PG): provides greater confidence, especially for diabetics, that respiratory distress will not occur; values equal to or greater than 3% needed

f. determination of creatinine level: 2.0 mg or greater suggests fetal age greater than 36 weeks

g. identification and evaluation of isoimmune disease; usually done after 24 weeks to assess bilirubin levels and optical density

h. determination of AFP levels in weeks 16 to 20 to assess neural-tube defects such as anencephaly and spina bifida; high levels also associated with congenital nephrosis, esophageal atresia, fetal demise

i. identification of meconium (often indicative of fetal hypoxia)

Application of the Nursing Process to the High-Risk Pregnant Client

ASSESSMENT
1. Risk factors (see p. 312)
2. Results of diagnostic tests

ANALYSIS/NURSING DIAGNOSIS
1. Safe, effective care environment
   a. Risk for fetal injury
   b. Risk for infection
2. Physiologic integrity
   a. Ineffective airway clearance/risk for aspiration
   b. Actual/risk for fluid volume deficit
3. Psychosocial integrity
   a. Anxiety
   b. Anticipatory grieving
4. Health promotion/maintenance
   a. Altered family processes
   b. Actual/risk for altered parenting
   c. Health-seeking behaviors

PLANNING, IMPLEMENTATION, AND EVALUATION

> **Goal** The pregnant woman and partner will verbalize an understanding of symptoms (danger signals) of high-risk conditions to be reported immediately.

Implementation
1. Teach woman and partner to immediately report any of the following danger signals.
   a. Infection
   b. Vaginal bleeding
   c. Generalized edema
   d. Trauma
   e. Leaking amniotic fluid
   f. Elevated temperature
   g. Headache (continuous)
   h. Visual changes (e.g., blurred vision, spotting before eyes)
   i. Abdominal, epigastric pain
   j. Projectile vomiting
   k. Decreased fetal activity
2. Reinforce the importance of keeping appointments as scheduled and complying with therapeutic regimen.
3. Provide emotional support, especially during and after diagnostic tests and fetal screening.
4. Assess client and fetal heart rate at each subsequent visit for potential or actual problems.
5. Document accurately.

Evaluation
The pregnant woman or partner reports danger signals immediately on detection.

SELECTED HEALTH PROBLEMS IN THE ANTEPARTAL PERIOD

✼ ABORTION

1. Definition: one of the bleeding disorders of pregnancy, it is termination of pregnancy before viability (fetus less than 20 weeks of gestation or less than 500 g) as a result of elective procedures or reproductive failure. Approximately 75% of all spontaneous abortions occur during the first 12 weeks of gestation. See Fig. 4-4.
2. Types:
   a. *Spontaneous:* natural termination of pregnancy
   b. *Threatened:* possible loss of the products of conception; slight bleeding, mild uterine cramping, cervical os closed, no passage of tissue
   c. *Inevitable:* threatened loss of the products of conception that cannot be prevented or stopped; moderate bleeding, cramping; open cervical os; no passage of tissue
   d. *Incomplete:* the expulsion of part of the products of conception and the retention of other parts in utero; heavy bleeding, severe cramping, open cervical os, passage of tissue
   e. *Complete:* the expulsion of all the products of conception; slight bleeding, mild cramping, closed cervical os, passage of tissue
   f. *Missed:* retention of the products of conception in utero after the fetus dies; slight bleeding, no cramping, closed cervical os, no passage of tissue
   g. *Habitual:* spontaneous abortion in three or more successive pregnancies
   h. *Therapeutic* (or induced): pregnancy that has been purposely terminated
3. Predisposing factors (spontaneous abortion): often unknown (20% to 25%), may be associated with
   a. Embryonic/fetal problems (50% to 60%): disorganization of germ plasma, ovular defects, chromosomal aberration, faulty placental development
   b. Maternal problems (15% to 20%): systemic infections, severe nutritional deprivation, abnormal pathologic conditions of the reproductive tract, endocrine dysfunction, trauma, medical diseases

Nursing Process
ASSESSMENT
1. Identify symptoms (spontaneous vaginal bleeding, uterine cramping, contractions)
2. Evaluate blood loss: save pads; assess saturation, frequency of change; save tissue passed
3. Recognize signs and symptoms of shock and sepsis (see p. 129)

ANALYSIS/NURSING DIAGNOSIS (see p. 315)
PLANNING, IMPLEMENTATION, AND EVALUATION

Goal Client will be free from complications.

Implementation
1. Note and record blood and tissue loss.
2. Institute nursing measures to treat shock if necessary (see Shock, p. 129).
3. Monitor I&O.
4. Replace fluids as ordered.
5. Prepare for dilation and curettage (D&C) as necessary (incomplete abortion).
6. Give RhoGAM to Rh-negative woman.
7. Provide emotional support of grieving process (refer to Loss and Death and Dying, p. 29).

Evaluation
Client is free from excessive blood loss; maintains fluid balance.

✼ INCOMPETENT CERVICAL OS/PREMATURE DILATION OF THE CERVIX

1. Definition: mechanical defect in the cervix, often a cause of habitual second trimester abortions or preterm labor (premature cervical dilation)
2. Predisposing factors: anatomic deviation of the cervix, cervical trauma from D&C, conization, cauterization, or cervical lacerations with previous pregnancies
3. Medical treatment: physician determines preferred surgical intervention, suturing of cervix during 14 to 18 weeks of gestation, or before next pregnancy
   a. Permanent suture (Shirodkar procedure); subsequent delivery by cesarean section
   b. Cerclage (temporary purse string McDonald procedure); suture removed at term, with vaginal delivery

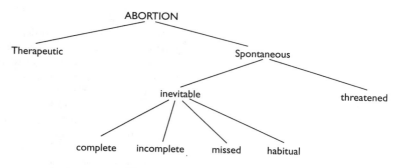

Fig. 4-4   Types of abortion.

Nursing Process

ASSESSMENT

1. History of spontaneous abortions
2. Relaxed cervical os on pelvic examination

ANALYSIS/NURSING DIAGNOSIS (see p. 315)

PLANNING, IMPLEMENTATION, AND EVALUATION

> **Goal** Client with an incompetent cervical os will report problems, seek treatment, and comply with restricted activity; will maintain gestation to term.

Implementation (postoperative)

1. Suggest limited activity for 2 or more weeks after surgical procedure.
2. Tell client to report signs of labor.
3. Monitor fetal growth to term and continue prenatal assessment and care as needed.
4. Observe for signs of labor, infection, and premature rupture of the membranes.

Evaluation

Client complies with activity restrictions after treatment; carries fetus to term.

ECTOPIC PREGNANCY

1. Definition: an *extrauterine* pregnancy, implantation occurring most often in ampulla of the fallopian tubes (Fig. 4-5)
2. Incidence: 1 in 80 to 1 in 100 live births; seventh highest cause of maternal mortality (from rupture of tube leading to hemorrhage, infection, and shock)
3. Predisposing factors: any condition that causes constriction of the fallopian tube (e.g., pelvic inflammatory disease, puerperal and postabortion sepsis, developmental defects, prolonged use of an IUD)
4. Medical treatment: diagnosis, ultrasound, surgical intervention (laparoscopy, laparotomy, salpingotomy, salpingectomy); management may include methotrexate

Nursing Process

ASSESSMENT

1. Signs and symptoms
   a. Lower unilateral abdominal tenderness, cramps related to stretching of the tube
   b. Knifelike pain in lower quadrant (only when tube has ruptured)
   c. Profound shock, if ruptured
   d. Vaginal spotting (may be inconsistent with degrees of shock observed)

2. History: last menstrual period
3. Prior history of infection, IUD use

ANALYSIS/ NURSING DIAGNOSIS (see p. 315)

PLANNING, IMPLEMENTATION, AND EVALUATION

> **Goal** Client will report early signs of ectopic pregnancy; will be free from complications after surgery; will return to a homeostatic state.

Implementation

1. Monitor vital signs; carry out an ongoing assessment for shock.
2. Maintain IV infusion for administration of plasma/blood, antibiotics, or other required medication.
3. Prepare client for surgery, physically and emotionally.
4. Postoperatively, continue to monitor vital signs, fluid intake and output (I&O); have client cough and deep breathe q2h; monitor for infection.
5. Support grieving process.

Evaluation

Client seeks treatment before rupture of tube, is free from other complications; regains postoperative homeostasis.

HYDATIDIFORM MOLE

1. Definition: a developmental anomaly of the chorion causing degeneration of the villi and formation of grapelike vesicles; fertilized ovum is initially present but usually no embryo develops (Fig. 4-6)
2. Incidence: 1 in 1500 pregnancies
3. Predisposing factors: unknown; however, it is associated with induction of ovulation by clomiphene therapy, adolescence, or maternal age greater than 40 years
4. Medical treatment
   a. Surgical intervention (D&C or, in women over 45 or with profuse bleeding, hysterectomy)
   b. Medical intervention: monitor HCG levels; chemotherapy, if indicated
   c. Close supervision for 1 year to detect signs of choriocarcinoma

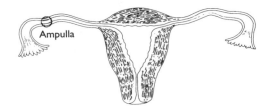

Fig. 4-5   Common site of ectopic pregnancy.

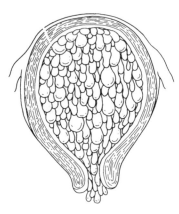

Fig. 4-6   Hydatidform mole.

Nursing Process

ASSESSMENT

1. Signs and symptoms
   a. Initially appears as a normal pregnancy
   b. Uterus larger than expected for reported gestational age
   c. Lower uterine segment soft and full on palpation
   d. Excessive nausea and vomiting (hyperemesis gravidarum)
   e. Brownish discharge or vaginal spotting; passing of vesicles; onset around 12 weeks of gestation
   f. Hypertension and other symptoms of preeclampsia (e.g., proteinuria) before twentieth week
2. Pregnancy test: HCG often high

ANALYSIS/NURSING DIAGNOSIS (see p. 315)

PLANNING, IMPLEMENTATION, AND EVALUATION

> **Goal** Client will report abnormal signs, seek treatment; will comply with physician's plan for supervision for 1 year to detect signs of choriocarcinoma; will delay subsequent pregnancy.

Implementation

1. Administer plasma or blood replacement as ordered.
2. Maintain fluid and electrolyte balance through replacement.
3. Emphasize need for follow-up supervision for 1 year with HCG measurement, examination to detect choriocarcinoma, chemotherapy if indicated.
4. Emphasize that pregnancy should be avoided for at least 1 year.
5. Provide emotional support.

Evaluation

Client has hydatidiform mole removed; complies with regular schedule of visits after therapy; avoids pregnancy until cleared by physician.

✖ PLACENTA PREVIA

1. Definition: abnormal implantation of placenta in lower uterine segment
2. Incidence: 1 in 170 pregnancies; most common cause of bleeding in late pregnancy
3. Predisposing factors: decreased vascularity of upper uterine segment, multiparity, scarring from prior surgery, use of cocaine
4. Degrees of placenta previa (Fig. 4-7)
   a. *Partial:* placenta partially covers the internal cervical os
   b. *Complete:* placenta totally covers the cervical os (cesarean birth necessary)
   c. *Low-lying or marginal:* placenta encroaches on margin of internal cervical os
5. Placental abnormalities in formation or implantation: associated with maternal bleeding during the third trimester or intrapartum period; hemorrhage is the leading cause of maternal mortality
6. Medical intervention: diagnosis; blood and fluid replacement and cesarean birth if placental placement prevents vaginal birth of fetus

Nursing Process

ASSESSMENT

1. Signs and symptoms
   a. Painless, bright red, vaginal bleeding in the third trimester (often begins in seventh month); early episodes may have small amount of bleeding; several episodes of profuse bleeding may occur
   b. Soft uterus
   c. Manifestations of hemorrhage, shock
2. Diagnosis is confirmed by ultrasound

ANALYSIS/NURSING DIAGNOSIS (see p. 315)

PLANNING, IMPLEMENTATION, AND EVALUATION

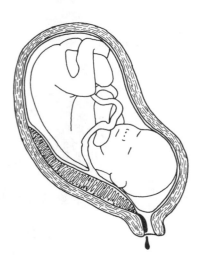

Marginal implantation

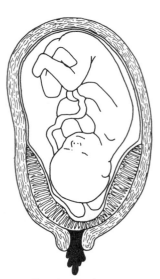

Complete implantation

Fig. 4-7 Placenta previa.

> **Goal** Client will report signs of bleeding from abnormal placental implantation; will maintain fluid balance, experience minimal blood loss; will understand need for cesarean birth for total placenta previa; will deliver healthy newborn.

Implementation
1. Maintain bed rest, avoid vaginal examinations, and observe carefully (conservative management).
2. Monitor blood loss closely.
3. Assess maternal vital signs and FHR frequently.
4. Institute appropriate nursing measures if shock develops (i.e., administer fluids, transfusions).
5. Give physical and emotional preparation for possible cesarean birth; physician may perform "double setup."
6. Observe for associated problems (e.g., prematurity of newborn, disseminated intravascular coagulation [DIC]).

Evaluation
Couple is adequately prepared for possible cesarean birth; client is free from frank hemorrhage and shock; delivers a healthy newborn at or near term.

✖ ABRUPTIO PLACENTAE
1. Definition: premature partial or complete separation of normally implanted placenta; also known as accidental hemorrhage or ablatio placentae
2. Incidence: 1 in 80 to 1 in 200 pregnancies
3. Predisposing factors: pregnancy-induced hypertension, fibrin defects, accidents (motor vehicle accident [MVA], abuse); associated with older multigravidas, cocaine use
4. Types (Fig. 4-8)
   a. *Marginal* (overt): evident external bleeding; placenta separates at margin
   b. *Central* (concealed): bleeding not evident or inconsistent with extent of shock observed; placenta separates at the center

5. Medical intervention: diagnosis; blood and fluids replacement; cesarean birth as necessary to save fetal or maternal lives

Nursing Process
ASSESSMENT
1. Bleeding: third trimester; amount of bleeding is not an accurate indicator of degree of separation
   a. Mild to moderate bleeding: uterine irritability and hypertonicity
   b. Severe bleeding
      1. severe abdominal pain
      2. rigid, distended uterus
      3. enlarged uterus
      4. shock
      5. associated problems (e.g., renal failure)
      6. hypofibrinogenemia, DIC
   c. Fetal assessment: late decelerations caused by uteroplacental insufficiency
2. Diagnosis: ultrasound

ANALYSIS/NURSING DIAGNOSIS (see p. 315)
PLANNING, IMPLEMENTATION, AND EVALUATION

> **Goal** Client will maintain homeostasis despite signs of placental separation; will maintain fluid balance, have blood loss replaced; couple will understand the need for emergency surgery or vaginal delivery as indicated; will deliver a viable, well-oxygenated newborn.

Implementation
1. Maintain bed rest.
2. Monitor FHR and maternal vital signs.
3. Assess blood loss and uterine pain.
4. Administer blood replacement as ordered by physician.
5. Monitor I&O.

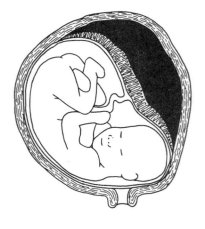

Concealed bleeding

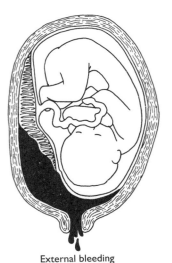

External bleeding

Fig. 4-8 Abruptio placentae.

6. Institute nursing measures for shock (e.g., flat in bed, monitor vital signs frequently, keep warm, increase IV fluids); see also Shock, p. 129.
7. Provide emotional support; explain what is happening and all procedures; encourage expression of feelings.
8. Prepare physically and emotionally for emergency cesarean birth or prompt delivery.
9. Observe for associated problems after delivery (e.g., DIC, poorly contracted uterus, neonatal hypoxia).

Evaluation

Couple is prepared for emergency birth; client delivers a viable newborn; has blood loss controlled; maintains fluid balance.

✖ PREGNANCY-INDUCED HYPERTENSION (HYPERTENSIVE DISORDERS)

1. Definition: a group of disorders characterized by presence of hypertension, with onset during last 10 weeks of pregnancy or in preceding pregnancy
2. Incidence: 6% to 7% of all gravidas; one of three major causes of maternal mortality and a significant cause of fetal and neonatal deaths
3. Common types
   a. Pregnancy-induced hypertension (toxemia)
      1. preeclampsia
      2. eclampsia
   b. chronic essential hypertension
      1. antecedent to pregnancy
      2. with superimposed preeclampsia (coincidental with pregnancy)
4. Predisposing factors: age (less than 17 or more than 35 years), primiparity, low socioeconomic class, inadequate protein intake, diabetes, previous history of hypertension; absence of early or regular antepartal care is a factor in late detection and treatment
5. Etiology: unknown
   a. Vasospasm and ischemia believed to be underlying mechanism
   b. Impaired placental function may result from vasospasm
   c. Development of uteroplacental changes leading to decreased oxygen and nutrition to fetus
   d. May lead to degenerative changes in renal, endocrine, and hematologic systems and the brain
6. HELLP syndrome (*h*emolysis, *e*levated *l*iver enzymes, *l*ow *p*latelet count)
   a. 2% to 12% of women with untreated or uncontrolled preeclampsia develop this syndrome
   b. Maternal mortality: 0% to 24%
   c. Perinatal mortality: 8% to 60%
7. Medical interventions: bed rest, increased protein in diet, possible salt reduction, medications to prevent convulsions and reduce blood pressure
8. The only cure for preeclampsia is delivery of all of the products of conception

Nursing Process

ASSESSMENT

1. Third trimester onset of hypertension, edema, rapid weight gain, and proteinuria
2. Classification (Table 4-11)

ANALYSIS/NURSING DIAGNOSIS (see p. 315)
PLANNING, IMPLEMENTATION, AND EVALUATION

Goal I Client will report excessive weight gain, edema, headaches, visual changes.

Implementation

1. Detect preeclampsia through early and regular antepartal care.

Table 4-11 Classification of pregnancy-induced hypertension

MILD PREECLAMPSIA

Elevated BP	A systolic increase of 30 mm Hg and diastolic increase of 15 mm Hg or more above baseline × 2 at least 6 hours apart or a BP above 140/90
Weight gain	More than 1 lb/wk in the third trimester
Edema	Hands and in front of tibia (1+ or 2+)
Proteinuria	≥1 g/24 hr (1+ or 2+ on qualitative testing)
Hyperreflexia	3+

SEVERE PREECLAMPSIA

All changes associated with mild preeclampsia, plus:

Elevated BP	Systolic ≥ 160 mm Hg or diastolic ≥ 110 mm Hg × 2 at least 6 hours apart with client restricted to bed rest
Weight gain	More than 5 lb/wk
Edema	Generalized edema, puffiness of face (3+ or 4+)
Proteinuria	≥5 g/24 hr (3+ or 4+ on qualitative testing)
Hyperreflexia	4+, clonus
Oliguria	≤400-500 ml
Other	Severe headaches, dizziness, blurred vision, retinal arteriolar spasm, spots before eyes, nausea and vomiting, epigastric pain, irritability, pulmonary edema, elevated liver enzymes, hemolysis

ECLAMPSIA

All changes associated with preeclampsia, plus tonic and clonic convulsions, coma, and hypertensive shock or crisis

2. Prevent severe preeclampsia/eclampsia by promoting regular antepartal care and good nutrition (with adequate protein).
3. Monitor BP, weight, I&O, edema, urine, and reflexes (each antepartal visit).
4. Instruct to take daily weight at home.
5. Provide bed rest lying on left side if signs of pregnancy-induced or preexisting hypertension occur (at home for milder forms of preeclampsia; hospitalization for severe preeclampsia).
6. Provide specific dietary information; may include reduced sodium.
7. Monitor I&O and FHR for hospitalized client.
8. Monitor administration of magnesium sulfate (anticonvulsant and sedative) if ordered (Table 4-12); assess for signs of toxicity.
   a. Symptoms of central nervous system (CNS) depression (anxiety followed by drowsiness or lethargy)
   b. Respirations less than 12 per minute
   c. Reduced BP
   d. Deep-tendon reflexes absent or less than 1+
   e. Signs of paralysis
   f. Stop administration if there are signs of toxicity or if urinary output less than 30 ml/hr; antidote is calcium gluconate (10%) solution
9. Administer sedatives, antihypertensives, and anticonvulsants (e.g., phenobarbital, diazepam [Valium], hydralazine [Apresoline]) as ordered by physician to control symptoms and to prevent eclampsia and cerebrovascular accident (CVA).
10. Monitor progress of labor.
11. Have airway/suction available.
12. Provide emotional support to couple.

Evaluation

Client complies with prenatal teaching; maintains pregnancy as long as possible without compromising herself or fetus; is safely delivered of a healthy newborn; has blood pressure controlled both before and after delivery.

> **Goal 2** Client will be free from physical injury in the event of seizure; will regain homeostasis; will maintain fetal oxygenation.

Implementation

If convulsion occurs:
1. Maintain patent airway.
2. Use suction to prevent aspiration.
3. Protect mother from injury.
4. Note nature, onset, and progression of seizure.
5. Monitor for signs of abruptio placentae.
6. Administer O_2.
7. Monitor FHR.
8. Administer medications as ordered.

Evaluation

Client recovers from convulsions without physical injury; remains stable; FHR is within normal limits.

✖ DIABETES

1. Definition: an inherited metabolic disorder characterized by a deficiency in insulin production from the beta cells of the islets of Langerhans in the pancreas (see also p. 179)
2. Incidence: 1 in 100 pregnancies; the condition may be a concurrent disease in pregnancy or have its first onset during gestation
3. Predisposing factors
   a. Family history of diabetes
   b. Glucosuria
   c. Obesity
   d. History of repeated spontaneous abortions or fetal loss (stillbirth)
   e. History of delivery of infants over 10 lb
4. Classifications
   a. Class A1: onset at any age in pregnancy; diet controlled
   b. Class A2: onset at any age in pregnancy; insulin controlled
   c. Class F: presence of nephropathy
   d. Class R: presence of proliferative retinopathy
   e. Class H: presence of heart disease
5. Effects of diabetes: maternal risk and fetal loss increase as classes change from A1 to H
   a. Effects of maternal diabetes on the fetus/infant
      1. overall perinatal mortality increases when mother has diabetes
      2. as classes change from A to E, increased incidence of ketoacidosis for mother resulting in high risk for fetus

Table 4-12 Magnesium sulfate

Action	Side effects	Nursing implications
Anticonvulsant that decreases amount of acetylcholine (IV or IM) liberated with nerve impulse, relaxes smooth muscle, depresses CNS Especially valuable in lowering seizure threshold in women with pregnancy-induced hypertension; may be used in preterm labor to decrease uterine activity (no FDA approval for this use at this time)	*Maternal:* severe CNS depression, hypereflexia, flushing, confusion *Fetal:* tachycardia, hypoglycemia, hypocalcemia	Monitor for seizures. Observe for signs of CNS depression. Monitor fetal heart rate. Monitor magnesium levels regularly. Have calcium gluconate available to counteract toxicity of magnesium sulfate. Discontinue infusion if respirations are below 12/min, reflexes are severely hypotonic, output is below 20-30 ml/hr, or in event of mental confusion or lethargy or fetal distress.

3. greater risk of congenital abnormalities (3 to 4 times), especially when hyperglycemia exists in early pregnancy (during embryogenesis)
4. hypoxia and fetal death more common
5. infants large for gestational age (classes A, B, C) or growth retarded in severe diabetes
6. neonatal hypoglycemia common as a result of fetal response to hyperglycemia of mother
7. newborn injury at birth
8. neonatal respiratory distress
   b. Effects of diabetes on the mother
   1. uteroplacental insufficiency often complicates pregnancy
   2. higher incidence of dystocia
   3. susceptibility to infections
6. Effects of pregnancy on diabetes
   a. Insulin resistance progressively increases in most pregnant diabetics
   b. Blood glucose less easily controlled
   c. Insulin shock common
7. Medical treatment: preconception testing in the diabetic woman is critical
   a. Diagnostic tests (with *criteria* for *high risk* as seen in gestational diabetes or insulin-dependent diabetes)
      1. screening of all pregnant women at 24 to 28 weeks of gestation for gestational diabetes
         a. 50 g oral glucose: normal value: <140 mg/dl at 1 hour
      2. 100 g glucose tolerance test (GTT): highly sensitive, used if screening is abnormal; normal values as follows
         a. fasting blood glucose: <105 mg/dl
         b. 1 hour: <190 mg/dl
         c. 2 hours: <165 mg/dl
         d. 3 hours: <145 mg/dl
      3. 2-hour postprandial blood glucose
         a. <120 mg/dl
         b. used to randomly evaluate diet and compliance
      4. mean blood glucose test (HbA$_{1c}$ [glycosylated hemoglobin]): at risk over 8.8%; indicates recent hyperglycemia
      5. chem strip blood-glucose testing may be advised
      6. urine glucose monitoring inaccurate during pregnancy; test for ketones
      7. repeat GTT on gestational diabetics at 6 weeks postpartum to evaluate status
   b. Nutritional counseling with calories and sucrose ingestion altered
   c. Insulin therapy as indicated based on blood glucose; the use of oral hypoglycemics is contraindicated
   d. Hospitalization to stabilize condition if necessary
   e. Monitor fetal/placental oxygenation with nonstress testing, CST, ultrasound, biophysical profile, L/S ratio, phospholipids PG and PI, estriol levels
   f. Anticipate emotional impact
   g. Cesarean birth or induction at 36 to 37 weeks if evidence of fetal compromise; attempt made to maintain pregnancy until fetal lungs are mature

Nursing Process

ASSESSMENT

1. Signs and symptoms of hypoglycemia and hyperglycemia (refer to Table 3-37)
2. Indications of hydramnios, preeclampsia, infection
3. History of large-for-gestational-age (LGA) newborns
4. Insulin requirements

ANALYSIS/NURSING DIAGNOSIS (see p. 315)

PLANNING, IMPLEMENTATION, AND EVALUATION

> **Goal** Client will follow prescribed diet/insulin plan and monitor glucose levels, reporting problems immediately.

Implementation

1. Stress importance of ongoing, regular, and more frequent antepartal care.
2. Assist in performing diagnostic tests.
3. Demonstrate accurate glucose-testing technique; have client return demonstration, learn to record results.
4. Educate client regarding nutritional needs: strict adherence to prescribed dietary regimen.
5. Teach to give own insulin (regular insulin preferred); observe for accuracy and correct as necessary.
6. Regulate insulin dose as prescribed by blood glucose levels, not by urine tests, because of lowered renal threshold; expect altered requirements in intrapartal and postpartal periods.
7. Recognize and share changes in diabetic state with client.
   a. As pregnancy develops, insulin need increases.
   b. Insulin need will decrease postpartum.
8. Promote good personal hygiene to prevent infection.
9. Monitor for early signs of infection; pregnancy-induced hypertension (PIH).
10. Assure mother that she will be able to breast-feed her infant, if she wishes.
11. Initiate ophthalmologic referral.
12. Discuss birth control options.

Evaluation

Client complies with diet and insulin regimen during pregnancy; prevents complications of diabetes during pregnancy and the puerperium; carries pregnancy as close to term as possible; delivers a newborn with minimal problems.

✖ CARDIAC DISORDERS

1. Definition: includes a number of heart diseases/defects, which include both congenital and acquired conditions. Pregnant women with heart disease are seen more frequently today because of better care, screening, and surgical correction of defects. Refer also to Congestive Heart Failure, p. 135.
2. Effects of pregnancy on heart disease: alters heart rate, blood pressure, and volume of cardiac output.
3. Incidence: 0.5% to 2% of all pregnant women.
4. Predisposing factors: arteriosclerosis, renal and pulmonary disease, rheumatic fever, congenital defects of the heart, surgical repair of defects; syphilis.
5. Types: New York Heart Association's functional classification system for clients with heart disease (based on

client history of past and present disability and uninfluenced by presence or absence of physical signs); used in current obstetric management:

    a. Class 1: no limitation of activity; no symptoms of cardiac insufficiency.

    b. Class 2: slight limitation of activity; asymptomatic at rest; ordinary activities cause fatigue, palpitations, dyspnea, or angina.

    c. Class 3: marked limitation of activities; comfortable at rest; less than ordinary activities cause discomfort.

    d. Class 4: unable to perform any physical activity without discomfort; may have symptoms even at rest.

6. Prognosis depends on

    a. Functional capacity of heart.

    b. Complications that further increase cardiac load.

    c. Quality of health care provided.

    d. Maternal and fetal risk (increases from classes 1 to 4; women in classes 3 and 4 will have serious problems in pregnancy).

      1. maternal heart failure

      2. spontaneous abortion or premature labor, caused by maternal hypoxia

      3. maternal dysrhythmias

      4. intrauterine growth retardation

7. Medical treatment:

    a. Confirm diagnosis.

      1. difficult to differentiate heart disease because of normal cardiac changes that occur with pregnancy

        a. functional systolic murmurs common

        b. edema and some dyspnea frequently present in last trimester

        c. changes in position of heart suggest cardiac enlargement

      2. criteria for establishment of diagnosis of heart disease

        a. continuous diastolic or presystolic heart murmur

        b. a loud, harsh systolic murmur, especially if associated with a thrill

        c. unequivocal cardiac enlargement

        d. severe dysrhythmia

    b. Hospitalization may be necessary 1 to 4 weeks before delivery.

    c. Prophylactic antibiotic treatment required to prevent subacute bacterial endocarditis.

    d. Vaginal delivery is the method of choice, using regional anesthesia and forceps.

Nursing Process

ASSESSMENT

1. History; fetal heart rate; maternal vital signs
2. Compliance with prescribed therapeutic regimen
3. Cardiac and respiratory status both at rest and with activity

ANALYSIS/NURSING DIAGNOSIS (see p. 315)

PLANNING, IMPLEMENTATION, AND EVALUATION

Goal Client will maintain regimen of rest, exercise, and nutrition to prevent anemia and cardiac decompensation.

Implementation

1. Encourage early and more frequent antepartal care; monitor vital signs, FHR, and weight.
2. Promote compliance with therapeutic regimen.
3. Teach proper nutrition with adequate iron intake to prevent anemia.
4. Emphasize need for additional rest and stress reduction.

    a. Classes 1 and 2: some limits on strenuous activity

    b. Classes 3 and 4: bed rest with expert medical supervision

    c. Semi-Fowler's position in bed if helpful for breathing; left lateral preferred

5. Prevent exposure to persons with upper respiratory infections (URIs); provide early treatment of URIs.
6. Observe the subtle changes in condition indicative of congestive heart failure (e.g., rales with cough, decreased ability to carry out household tasks, increased dyspnea on exertion, hemoptysis, tachycardia, progressive edema).
7. Administer medications as ordered by physician (e.g., diuretics, digitalis); explain actions, side effects and possible fetal effects.
8. Maintain continuous maternal and fetal monitoring during the intrapartum period; advise client to avoid pushing; position in semi-Fowler's.
9. Postpartum, assess for signs of hemorrhage, puerperal infection, thromboembolism, and congestive heart failure; avoid giving ergonovine and other oxytocics.

Evaluation

Client complies with regimen of rest, exercise, and care; is free from the complications of cardiac disease during pregnancy/puerperium; delivers a healthy newborn.

✠ ANEMIA

1. Definition: decrease in the oxygen-carrying capacity of the blood
2. Cause: often because of low iron stores and reduced dietary intake
3. Incidence: 20% of all pregnant women; 90% of anemias caused by iron deficiency; most frequently encountered complication of pregnancy
4. Predisposing factors: heredity and malnutrition
5. Prognosis: maternal and fetal mortality and morbidity rates are increased; specifically

    a. Anemia aggravates existing problems such as cardiac disease during pregnancy

    b. Anemic women have increased incidence of abortion, premature labor, infection, pregnancy-induced hypertension, and postpartum hemorrhage

    c. Maternal anemia is associated with intrauterine growth retardation

    d. Severe anemia may cause heart failure

6. Types of disorders

    a. Iron deficiency: most common

    b. Folic acid deficiency (megaloblastic anemia): less than 3% of all gravidas; caused by poor diet and malabsorption

    c. Hemoglobinopathies (e.g., sickle cell anemia [higher mortality in pregnancy]; crises common; refer to Nursing Care of the Child, p. 458), thalassemia

Nursing Process

ASSESSMENT

1. Signs and symptoms are usually absent in mild to moderate iron-deficiency anemia
2. Diagnosis based on
   a. Hgb < 11 g/dl or Hct < 37%
   b. Hgb < 10.5 g/dl or Hct < 35% in second trimester
   c. Hgb < 10 g/dl or Hct < 33% in third trimester
3. Nutritional intake

ANALYSIS/NURSING DIAGNOSIS (see p. 315)
PLANNING, IMPLEMENTATION, AND EVALUATION

> **Goal** Client will maintain an optimal Hgb and Hct; will be free from severe anemia; will comply with diet, treatments, and medication; will maintain adequate fetal oxygenation.

Implementation

1. Monitor Hgb or Hct levels at initial antepartal visit and in later pregnancy.
2. Provide dietary counseling regarding importance of iron-rich diet (minimum of 18 mg per day).
3. Instruct to take oral iron compounds (ferrous sulfate or gluconate) as daily supplement as ordered; teach regarding side effects.
   a. Change in color of stools (become black).
   b. Take with a source of vitamin C to facilitate absorption.
   c. Take with food only if gastric distress occurs (better absorbed between meals).
4. Provide folic acid supplement of 5 mg per 24 hr orally for folate deficiency, as ordered.
5. Observe for symptoms of hemolytic crisis (e.g., chills, fever, pain in back and abdomen, prostration, shock) with hemoglobinopathies.
6. Refer for genetic counseling (women with inherited disorders).

Evaluation

Client eats a balanced, adequate, iron-rich diet during pregnancy; takes prescribed iron medications; maintains health; delivers newborn of appropriate size for gestational age.

✳ HYPEREMESIS GRAVIDARUM (PERNICIOUS VOMITING OF PREGNANCY)

1. Definition: excessive vomiting during pregnancy, leading to dehydration, starvation, and electrolyte imbalance
2. Cause: not always clear; may be psychologic, or result from multiple pregnancy, hormonal abnormalities, or hydatidiform mole
3. Prognosis: severe cases may lead to dehydration and fluid-electrolyte complications

Nursing Process

ASSESSMENT (SIGNS AND SYMPTOMS ARE RELATED TO SEVERITY)

1. Mild: slight dehydration and weight loss
2. Severe: metabolic acidosis, hypoproteinemia, hypovitaminosis, jaundice, hemorrhage

ANALYSIS/NURSING DIAGNOSIS (see p. 315)
PLANNING, IMPLEMENTATION, AND EVALUATION

> **Goal** Client will retain food and fluids; will maintain hydration.

Implementation

NOTE: Hospitalization may be necessary.

1. Administer parenteral fluids or total parenteral nutrition (TPN).
2. Promote a quiet environment.
3. Provide frequent, small meals when oral feedings are tolerated.
4. Refer to psychologic consultant if necessary.

Evaluation

Client is free from vomiting; maintains fluid and electrolyte balance; eats adequate diet; begins to gain weight.

✳ INFECTIONS

1. Definition: a variety of infectious agents can affect maternal and fetal health, leading to increased morbidity and mortality. Maternal disease that is mild or even asymptomatic can cause severe anomalies or death in the embryo/fetus/neonate.
2. Types of infectious diseases:
   a. The TORCH syndrome (*t*oxoplasmosis, *o*ther, *r*ubella, *c*ytomegalovirus infection, *h*erpes)
      1. *toxoplasmosis* (protozoa)
         a. transmitted through ingestion of raw or undercooked meat; through improper hand washing after handling cat litter that has been contaminated with infected cat's feces
         b. maternal symptoms may be absent or nonspecific
         c. possible to detect by serologic screening
         d. organism readily crosses placenta
         e. fetal effects include hydrocephaly, chorioretinitis, mental retardation, neurologic damage
      2. *other*
         a. *beta-hemolytic streptococcal* infection: streptococci estimated to be present in genital tract of approximately 15% of women of childbearing age; associated with urinary tract infection; premature rupture of the membranes, premature labor, chorioamnionitis; may cross placenta and cause septic abortion, puerperal sepsis, stillbirth, neonatal sepsis, meningitis, sensory impairment, retardation
         b. *syphilis:* prenatal serologic screening test is important for prevention of congenital syphilis; associated with late abortion, stillbirth, prematurity, severe anemia, and congenital syphilis
         c. *gonorrhea:* may cause postpartum infection, pelvic inflammatory disease, sterility; danger to newborn is ophthalmia neonatorum, sepsis, pneumonia; refer to Sexually Transmitted Diseases, p. 422.
         d. *human immunodeficiency virus (HIV)/acquired immunodeficiency syndrome (AIDS):* viral infection with severe depression of immune sys-

tem; perinatal transmission from infected mother to fetus; high mortality rate; precautions as for hepatitis B (see also Newborn Care, p. 372)
   e. *nongonococcal urethritis* (NGU)
      - mild; may be asymptomatic
      - increasingly common STD
      - organism: chlamydia
      - partner should be treated; erythromycin often used for pregnant client
      - may cause stillbirth, pneumonia, conjunctivitis in newborn
   3. *rubella:* extremely teratogenic in first trimester
      a. transmitted transplacentally
      b. congenital rubella syndrome in the neonate includes cataracts, hemolytic anemia, heart defects, mental retardation, deafness (first-trimester exposure)
      c. exposure after the first trimester can lead to intrauterine growth retardation, sepsis
      d. infected infant can shed live viruses for many months after birth
      e. women with low titers should receive attenuated vaccine in early postpartum period and avoid pregnancy for at least 3 months
   4. *cytomegalovirus* (CMV); also called cytomegalic inclusion disease (CMID): member of herpesvirus group
      a. adult usually asymptomatic or has mononucleosis-like symptoms; common
      b. transmission in adults is respiratory, possibly venereal
      c. transmission to fetus is transplacental; occasionally may be transmitted during passage through birth canal
      d. no effective treatment
      e. effects on neonate include mental retardation, intrauterine growth retardation, congenital heart defects, deafness, microcephaly
   5. *herpes simplex virus* (HSV II)
      a. sexually transmitted, painful vesicles present on cervix, vaginal wall, vulva, and thighs; last 10 days to 2 weeks; remissions, exacerbations; primary outbreak most virulent.
      b. usual mode of transmission to neonate is passage through birth canal; may occur transplacentally in rare cases
      c. infection results in high infant mortality, preterm births
      d. cesarean birth, if pregnant woman has primary outbreak or has symptoms or visualized lesions
   b. Tuberculosis (TB)
      1. rarely transmitted to fetus
      2. may be asymptomatic
      3. disease must be arrested by usual methods of care for client with TB
      4. infant usually kept from close contact with mother, if the disease is active, to protect from infection
   c. Urinary tract infections
      1. affect approximately 10% of gravidas, generally as a result of *Escherichia coli;* may be asymptomatic

   2. predisposing factors: urinary stasis, related to anatomic changes during pregnancy; poor hygiene
   3. increased incidence of pyelonephritis if bacteria present
   4. associated with increased incidence of premature labor
   5. treated with appropriate antibiotic after culture
   d. Condylomas (genital warts)
      1. viral transmission
      2. may be transmitted to fetus at birth
      3. should be treated with laser beam, antibiotics, cautery, cryosurgery
      4. biopsy indicated for large warts (potential malignancy)
   e. Candidal infections
      1. caused by fungus *Candida albicans*
      2. present in about 20% of pregnant women
      3. fetus may contract thrush if infection not cured before delivery
   f. *Trichomonas vaginalis*
      1. protozoan
      2. treated with metronidazole (Flagyl), which may possibly be teratogenic and should not be used during first half of pregnancy
   g. Hepatitis
      1. may cause abortion, preterm birth, fetal or newborn hepatitis
      2. precautions depending on type A or B; refer to Hepatitis, p. 167 and universal precautions

Nursing Process

ASSESSMENT
1. Routine smears, cultures, serologic studies for sexually transmitted disease; selected laboratory tests as indicated
2. Signs and symptoms of infectious diseases

ANALYSIS/NURSING DIAGNOSIS (see p. 315)

PLANNING, IMPLEMENTATION, AND EVALUATION

> **Goal** Client will be free from infection in pregnancy; will seek medical care and will comply with treatment if exposed to infection; when indicated, partner will comply with treatment; fetal effects will be minimized.

Implementation
1. Review precautions in order to minimize exposure to infection.
2. Teach client to report any symptoms (e.g., vesicles, discharge, rash, elevated temperature).
3. Administer drugs as ordered for sexually transmitted diseases (e.g., penicillin for syphilis).
4. Promote compliance of partner.
5. Instruct to take drugs as ordered (e.g., isoniazid [INH], PAS); explain expected actions, side effects; avoid self-medication.
6. Implement standard precautions or isolation as indicated by organism and mode of transmission.

Evaluation
Client is free from infectious disease; maternal or fetal risks are minimized; client and partner comply with therapeutic regimen.

✕ MULTIPLE GESTATION

1. Definition: gestation of two or more fetuses. Twins may be produced from a single ovum (monozygotic or identical twins) or from separate ova (dizygotic or fraternal). Fraternal twinning is an inherited autosomal recessive trait and is more common (70%) than identical twins (30%). Triplets result from one, two, or three separate ova.
2. Incidence: 2% to 3% of all viable births.
3. Predisposing factors:
   a. Black women: higher incidence of multiple pregnancies than white women
   b. Family history of dizygotic twins
   c. Fertility drugs
4. Prognosis
   a. Increased risk of premature labor, pregnancy-induced hypertension (25%), hemorrhage, placenta previa
   b. Increased risk of delivery of low-birth-weight infants, often premature (50%)
   c. Increased risk of maternal anemia (40% to 50%)
   d. Increased risk of uterine inertia (10%), hydramnios (5% to 10%), intrauterine asphyxia (5%)
   e. Increased risk of secondary cessation or weakening of effective uterine contractions
   f. Monozygotic twins have higher mortality and morbidity rates than dizygotic twins because of increased congenital anomalies, twin-to-twin transfusion syndrome, and intrauterine growth retardation

Nursing Process
ASSESSMENT
1. 1. Early identification of multiple pregnancy based on
   a. History
   b. Weight gain
   c. Abdominal palpation
   d. Fundal height greater than expected for dates
   e. Asynchronous fetal heartbeats
   f. Ultrasonography
2. Maternal and fetal status: prenatal visits every 2 weeks
3. Nutritional status
ANALYSIS/NURSING DIAGNOSIS (see p. 315)
PLANNING, IMPLEMENTATION, AND EVALUATION

Goal Client with a multiple pregnancy will report early signs of health problems; will comply with health regimen and keep regular antepartal appointments; will deliver as close to term as possible.

Implementation
1. Advise frequent rest periods; left lateral position provides oxygenation for fetal/placental unit.
2. Teach balanced diet, with adequate protein; iron and vitamin supplements as ordered.
3. Monitor FHR carefully for indication of fetal distress.
4. Prepare for vaginal delivery unless complications arise (e.g., fetal distress, cephalopelvic disproportion).
5. Administer oxytocic agent as ordered immediately after birth to prevent postpartum hemorrhage (secondary to overdistention of the uterus).

Evaluation
Client is free from complications (e.g., anemia); carries multiple pregnancy to term (or close to term), with delivery of healthy newborns.

✕ ADOLESCENT PREGNANCY

1. Definition: pregnancy in a female under 17 years of age (see also The Healthy Child, p. 408)
2. Incidence: worldwide, one third of all births are to girls under 17 years of age; one million teenage pregnancies occur each year (10% of all teenagers) (World Health Organization, 1987)
3. Predisposing factors: teenage pregnancies are associated with
   a. Changing age of menarche
   b. Early sexual experimentation
   c. Poor family relationships
   d. Poverty
4. Prognosis
   a. For pregnant girls under 15 years, a high risk of stillbirths, low-birth-weight infants, neonatal mortality, and cephalopelvic disproportion
   b. Increased maternal risk of pregnancy-induced hypertension, prolonged labor, iron-deficiency anemia, and urinary tract infections

Nursing Process
ASSESSMENT
1. Nutrition status
2. Knowledge of physiology of pregnancy
3. Emotional status
4. Support systems
ANALYSIS/NURSING DIAGNOSIS (see p. 315)
PLANNING, IMPLEMENTATION, AND EVALUATION

Goal The pregnant teen will maintain good health; will eat a balanced diet with adequate protein; will prepare for birth and care of newborn; will achieve developmental tasks of adolescence and pregnancy; fetus will develop appropriately for gestation.

Implementation
1. Help pregnant teen achieve developmental tasks of adolescence (in addition to those of pregnancy).
   a. Develop sense of identity.
   b. Accept changing body image.
   c. Develop close, mature relations with peers (male and female).
   d. Socialize into appropriate gender role.
   e. Establish an independent and satisfying lifestyle.
2. Provide dietary counseling regarding
   a. Importance of well-balanced meals.
   b. Selection of nutritionally valuable yet acceptable food.
   c. Increased protein, calcium, and iron intake.
3. Prepare for childbirth; arrange for support person during labor.
4. Refer to social service for
   a. Career and educational counseling.

b. Options regarding child care/adoption.
c. Support services in community (e.g., parenting classes, supplemental food programs).
5. Instruct in child care.
6. Teach family planning.

Evaluation
Client is free from preventable complications; has a positive birth experience; delivers a healthy newborn; cares safely for newborn or arranges for alternative placement; achieves appropriate developmental tasks.

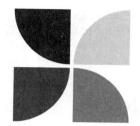

Intrapartal Care

THE LABOR PROCESS

1. Definitions
   a. Labor: a series of processes by which the products of conception are expelled from the maternal body
   b. Delivery: the actual event of birth
2. Essential factors in labor: the four *P*'s
   a. *Powers:* uterine contractions, voluntary bearing down, abdominal muscle contractions, and contractions of levator ani muscle
   b. *Passageway:* bones, tissues, ligaments
      1. type of pelvis: gynecoid, android, anthropoid, and platypelloid; refer to structure of the female pelvis, p. 295
      2. adequacy of planes of true pelvis
         a. true pelvis forms the birth canal through which fetus must pass
         b. three distinct levels
            ▪ plane of inlet
            ▪ midplane (plane of least dimensions)
            ▪ plane of outlet
      3. condition of soft tissues (lower uterine segment, cervix, and vaginal canal)
   c. *Passenger:* the fetus
      1. attitude (habitus or posture): the relation of the fetal parts to its own trunk; normal attitude of the fetus in utero is complete flexion
      2. engagement: the entrance of the greatest diameter of the presenting part through the plane of inlet and the beginning of the descent through the pelvis (biparietal diameter of head is at the inlet)
      3. lie: the relation of the long axis of the fetus to the long axis of the mother; it is either longitudinal, transverse, or oblique
         a. transverse lie: long axis of fetus is at right angle to mother's long axis; it is a pathologic lie if present at term
         b. longitudinal lie: long axis of the fetus is parallel to mother's long axis; it has two alternatives
            ▪ cephalic presentation (head first)
            ▪ breech presentation (buttocks first)
      4. presentation and presenting part: that part of the fetal body that enters the true pelvis and presents itself at the internal cervical os for delivery; the presentation depends on the attitude of the fetal extremities to its body and the fetal lie
         a. in cephalic presentations (95% of term deliver-

ies), the fetal head is the presenting part: the head may be
   ▪ completely flexed on the fetal chest (vertex presentation)
   ▪ moderately flexed (sinciput presentation)
   ▪ partially extended (brow presentation)
   ▪ hyperextended with chin presenting (face presentation)
      b. in breech presentations (3% of term births)
   ▪ the fetus' knees and hips both may be flexed, positioning the thighs on the abdomen and calves on the posterior thighs (complete breech)
   ▪ the hips may be flexed and the knees extended (frank breech)
   ▪ extension of the knees and hips (footling breech)
   ▪ shoulder presentation is commonly known as transverse lie
      5. position: the relationship of a specific established point (i.e., occiput, sacrum, brow, or mentum) of the fetus to the right or left of the mother's pelvis and to the anterior or posterior aspect (Fig. 4-9)
         a. cephalic (vertex) presentation: occiput (O); mentum (M)
         b. breech presentation: sacrum (S)
         c. shoulder presentation: scapula (Sc)
      6. station: the relationship of the presenting part of the fetus to the ischial spines of the mother (i.e., the degree of engagement); measured in centimeters above or below the pelvic midplane from the presenting part to the ischial spines (Fig. 4-10)
   d. *Person:* pregnant woman's general behavior and influences on her (psyche)
      1. maternal response to uterine contractions
      2. cultural influences and perceptions about labor and delivery
      3. antepartal or childbirth education
      4. ability to communicate feelings to significant others and staff
      5. support system
3. Signs of labor
   a. Premonitory signs of labor: changes indicating that labor will be approaching shortly
      1. increased Braxton Hicks contractions: intermittent contractions of the uterus occurring throughout pregnancy; generally painless but may cause discomfort in late pregnancy

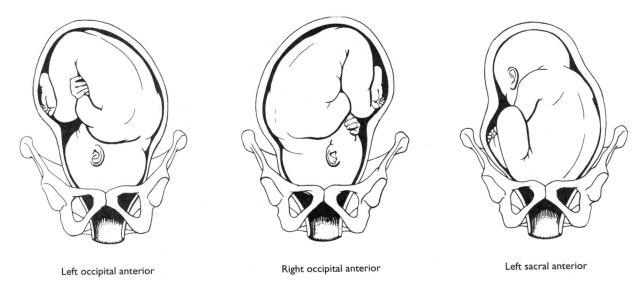

Left occipital anterior   Right occipital anterior   Left sacral anterior

Fig. 4-9 Selected categories of presentation. (From *Clinical education aids,* Columbus, Ohio, Ross Laboratories.)

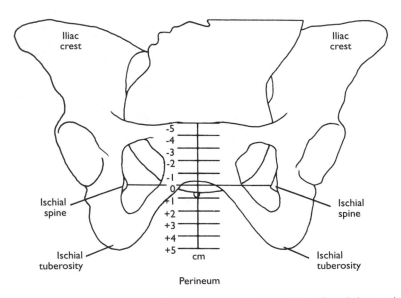

Fig. 4-10 Station. (From *Clinical education aids,* Columbus, Ohio, Ross Laboratories.)

2. lightening or engagement: the descent of the fetus into the pelvic cavity; generally occurs 2 to 3 weeks before the onset of labor in primigravidas; causes increased bladder pressure and reduced diaphragm pressure
3. show: blood-tinged mucus discharged from cervix shortly before or during labor
4. sudden burst of energy
5. weight loss resulting from fluid loss and electrolyte shifts
6. increased backache and sacroiliac pressure caused by fetal pressure
7. spontaneous rupture of membranes may occur; woman will be advised to enter hospital immediately

b. True vs. false labor
  1. true labor
    a. contractions increase progressively in strength, duration, and frequency
    b. regular pattern, not relieved by walking (walking may increase the strength of the contractions)
    c. felt in back or radiating toward front
    d. *effacement and dilation of the cervix*
    e. fetal membranes
      ▪ intact: generally in early labor, indicated by negative nitrazine paper test (yellow to yellow-olive paper) or negative ferning
      ▪ ruptured: generally in active labor, indicated by positive nitrazine paper test (blue-green to

blue paper or positive ferning); false readings may be obtained if contaminated by blood; meconium staining may indicate fetal distress, except in breech presentation

2. false labor
   a. an exaggeration of the periodic uterine contractions normally occurring during pregnancy
   b. does not produce progressive dilation, effacement, or descent
   c. contractions are irregular and do not increase in frequency, duration, or intensity
   d. walking gives relief
   e. discomfort felt in lower abdomen and groin
   f. absence of bloody show

4. Labor onset theories
   a. Oxytocin stimulation: alone or in combination with other factors
   b. Progesterone withdrawal: allowing uterine contractions to progress
   c. Estrogen stimulation: causing hypertrophy of myo-metrium and increased production of contractile proteins
   d. Prostaglandin secretion: effect on uterine muscle (increased uterine irritability)
   e. Fetal endocrine secretion of cortical steroids
   f. Distention of uterus: with subsequent pressure on nerve endings stimulating contractions and increased irritability of uterine musculature

5. Physiologic alterations occurring during labor (Fig. 4-11)
   a. Dilation to 10 cm: the process by which the cervix opens
   b. Effacement to 100%: thinning, shortening, and obliteration of cervix
   c. Physiologic retraction ring: the separation of the upper (active, thicker) and lower (passive, thinner) uterine segments in labor

6. Fetal positional response to labor (mechanisms of labor)
   a. Engagement: passage of fetus into true pelvis
   b. Descent: the progress of the presenting part through the pelvis

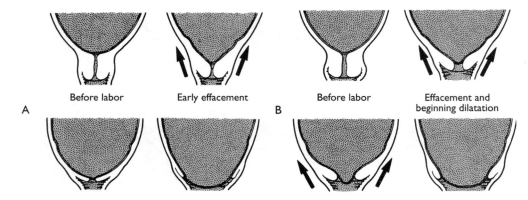

Fig. 4-11 Cervical dilation and effacement. **A,** Primigravida. **B,** Multigravida. (From *Clinical education aids,* Columbus, Ohio, Ross Laboratories.)

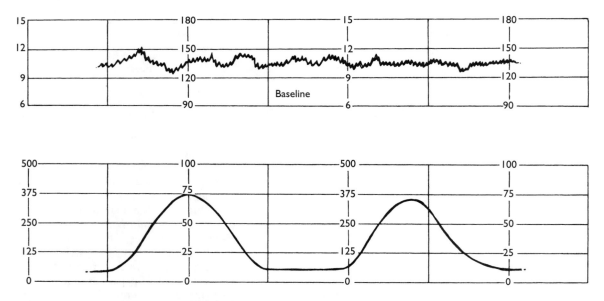

Fig. 4-12 Tracing of normal fetal heart rate.

c. Flexion: further contact of fetal chin to chest when head meets resistance from the pelvic floor

d. Internal rotation: the process by which the long axis of the fetal skull changes from the transverse diameter to an anteroposterior diameter at the outlet

e. Extension: birth of the head as it leaves the outlet

f. External rotation (restitution): realignment of head with back and shoulders

g. Expulsion: delivery of shoulders, trunk, extremities

7. FHR during labor

a. Baseline FHR: FHR when there are no contractions or in between contractions; normally between 120 and 160 beats per minute; see Fig. 4-12 and Table 4-13

b. Baseline variability: normal irregularities of FHR caused by autonomic nervous system stimuli; may be altered in normal fetal sleep, prematurity, medications; see Fig. 4-12

  ▪ short-term variability (STV): unevenness from one heartbeat to another (NOTE: true beat-to-beat variability can be determined only by direct fetal or internal monitor)

  ▪ long-term variability (LTV): rhythmic cycles from baseline (usually 3 to 5 per minute)

  ▪ minimal or absent variability: less than 5 beats per minute (ominous sign)

c. Periodic changes: FHR changes during contractions

  1. accelerations: transient rise in FHR greater than 15 beats per minute for more than 15 seconds related to uterine contractions; see Fig. 4-13

  2. decelerations: transient decrease in FHR; see classifications in Table 4-14 and Fig. 4-14

Table 4-13 Baseline fetal heart rate (normal range: 120-160 beats/min) over 10 minutes of FHM strip

	Tachycardia	Bradycardia
Mild	161-180 beats/min	100-119 beats/min
Marked	Greater than 180 beats/min	Less than 100 beats/min
Causes	Maternal fever	Maternal hypotension
	Early fetal hypoxia	Late fetal hypoxia
	Drugs	Drugs
	Amnionitis	

NOTE: Any rise or fall in baseline heart rate of more than 30 beats per minute persisting longer than 10 minutes is classified as tachycardia/bradycardia.

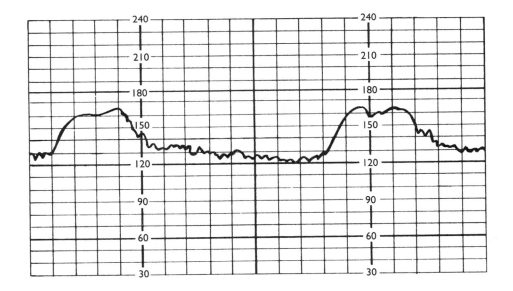
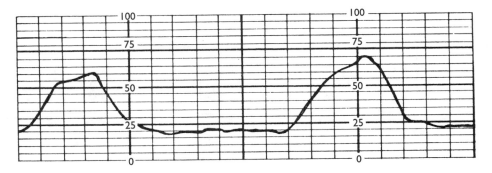

Fig. 4-13 Acceleration of fetal heart rate in response to uterine activity.

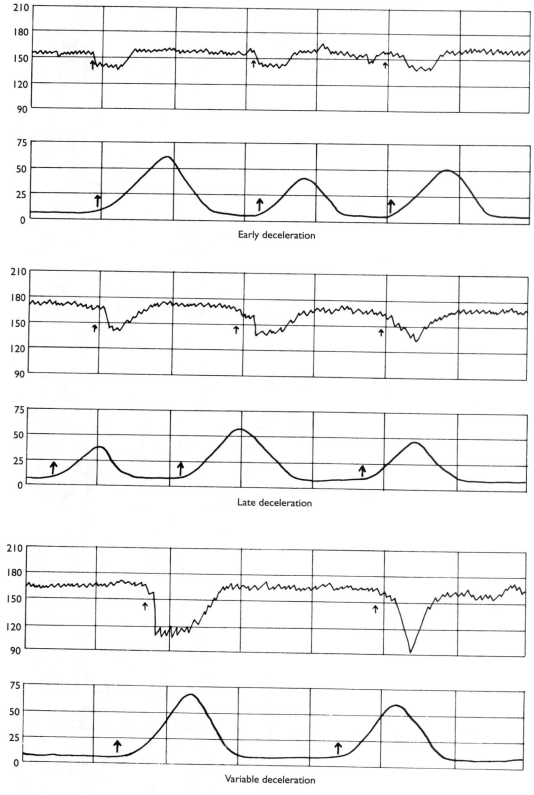

Early deceleration

Late deceleration

Variable deceleration

Fig. 4-14   Types of deceleration in fetal heart rate.

Table 4-14 Decelerations in fetal heart rate (see Fig. 4-14)

TYPE 1 (EARLY DECELERATIONS)

Cause: fetal head compression

FHR decreases with onset of contraction and mirrors the pattern of contractions

FHR returns to baseline as the contraction ends

Range of drop in FHR within normal parameters

Has a uniform shape

Innocuous

Nursing implications: continue observation

TYPE 2 (LATE DECELERATIONS)

Cause: uteroplacental insufficiency causing fetal hypoxia

FHR decreases *after* the onset of contraction

FHR deceleration persists beyond completion of contraction

Range of drop in FHR within normal

Has a uniform shape

Ominous

Nursing implications: turn client to left side, give O_2, and summon physician

TYPE 3 (VARIABLE DECELERATIONS)

Cause: umbilical cord compression

FHR decreases at any point *during* or *between* contractions

Decelerations may be jagged V or U shape

Range of drop in FHR is large and extends below normal

Not uniform in shape

Ominous

Nursing implications: turn client to left side, give O_2, and summon physician

Ongoing Management and Nursing Care

1. Fetal monitoring: monitor FHR by either
   a. Periodic auscultation: count for 1 full minute during and immediately after uterine contractions
   b. Electronic fetal monitor
      1. external or indirect electronic monitoring: applied when membranes intact
         a. *tocodynamometer:* disk attached over fundus and secured with belt; provides continuous record of external pressure created by contractions, allows measurement of frequency and duration of contractions
         b. *ultrasonic transducer:* applied at site of loudest fetal heartbeat, secured with belt (conducting gel is spread over transducer); provides continuous FHR recording, which is interpreted in relation to uterine activity; phonocardiography also may be used for indirect fetal electrocardiography
      2. internal or direct monitoring: applied when membranes have ruptured and cervix has dilated 2 to 3 cm
         a. *pressure transducer:* an intrauterine catheter filled with water is inserted beyond presenting part; allows measurement of frequency, duration, and intensity of contractions
         b. *internal spiral electrode:* applied to fetal scalp; provides continuous measurement of FHR, baseline variability, and periodic changes
   c. Fetal blood sampling: a small volume of fetal blood is taken (from a small puncture into the fetal scalp) to assess fetal hypoxia during labor
      1. procedure
         a. an invasive technique requiring rupture of the fetal membranes and cervical dilation (3 to 4 cm); performed when fetus is in jeopardy
         b. pregnant woman generally placed in a lithotomy position
         c. an amnioscope (truncated plastic or metal cone) is employed for visualization of presenting part of fetus during the procedure
         d. electronic fetal monitoring is desirable during the procedure
         e. after procedure, observe for vaginal bleeding (of fetal origin) and fetal tachycardia
      2. laboratory analysis of fetal pH, Po_2, and Pco_2 is done from blood sample (normal pH: 7.25 to 7.35; pH of 7.20 is associated with hypoxia)
2. Uterine contractions: refer to Table 4-15 and Fig. 4-15; monitor
   a. Frequency: timed from beginning of one to beginning of next contraction
   b. Duration: timed from beginning to end of one contraction
   c. Intensity: degree of muscle contraction; may be mild, moderate, or strong (50 to 100 mm Hg)
   d. Tonus: pressure within the uterus in between contractions; only measurable with an intrauterine catheter (5 to 15 mm Hg)
3. Analgesics: drugs that relieve pain or alter its perception may alter level of consciousness and reflex activity; administer as ordered and monitor effects; common obstetric analgesics include
   a. Central nervous system (CNS) depressants
      1. produce sedation; may depress fetus
      2. examples: secobarbital sodium (Seconal) and pentobarbital sodium (Nembutal) may be given in early labor
   b. Narcotics (e.g., meperidine [Demerol])
      1. may initially slow labor, have depressive effect on neonatal respirations
      2. administered when client is in active labor (4 to 5 cm); avoid use in transition
   c. Narcotic agonist-antagonists (e.g., Stadol, Nubain)
      1. produce analgesia with only limited respiratory depression
      2. can produce withdrawal symptoms in drug-dependent client
   d. Tranquilizers
      1. produce sedation and relaxation; often given with narcotics because of potentiating effects; when given alone, there may be little or no analgesia; may cause excitement and disorientation in presence of pain
      2. examples: promethazine hydrochloride (Phenergan), hydroxyzine pamoate (Vistaril), proma-

Table 4-15 Stages and phases of labor

First stage (onset of regular contractions to complete dilation)

	LATENT: PHASE I	ACTIVE: PHASE II	TRANSITION: PHASE III
Time			
Primipara	8½ hours	4 hours	1 hour
Multipara	5½ hours	2 hours	10-15 minutes
Cervix			
Effacement	0%-50%	Completed	
Dilation	0-3 cm	4-7 cm	8-10 cm
Contractions			
Frequency	More than 10 minutes apart	3-5 minutes	2-3 minutes
Duration	30 seconds	45 seconds	60-90 seconds
Intensity	Mild: less than 50 mm Hg	Moderate: 50-75 mm Hg	Strong: 75-100 mm Hg
Manifestations	Abdominal cramps; backache; client generally excited, alert, talkative, and in control; may rupture membranes	Show; moderate increase in pain; client more apprehensive; fear of losing control; focusing on self; skin warm and flushed	Client may be irritable and panicky; may lose control; amnesic between contractions; perspiring, nausea, and vomiting common; trembling of legs; pressure on bladder and rectum; backache; increased show; circumoral pallor

Second stage (complete dilation to birth of newborn)

Time	
Primipara	30-50 minutes
Multipara	20 minutes
Contractions	
Frequency	2-3 minutes
Duration	60-90 seconds
Intensity	Very strong; 100 mm Hg
Manifestation	Decrease in pain from transitional level; increased bloody show; pressure on rectum; urge to bear down; bulging perineum; client excited, eager, and in control

Third stage (delivery of newborn to delivery of placenta)

Time	5-30 minutes
Contractions	Strong uterus changing to globular shape
Manifestation	Gush of blood; apparent lengthening of cord; client focuses on newborn; excited about birth; feeling of relief

Fourth stage (delivery of placenta to homeostasis)

Time	Usually defined as first hour postpartum
Uterus	Firm, at midline, 2 finger breadths above umbilicus
Manifestations	Lochia rubra; exploration of newborn; parent-infant bonding begins; newborn alert and responsive, first period of reactivity

zinehydrochloride (Sparine) and diazepam (Valium)
   3. effects
     a. peak action within 60 minutes
     b. may last 6 to 8 hours depending on stage of labor and activity of client
  e. Amnesics (rarely used today)
   1. produce sedation and alter memory
   2. example: scopolamine (belladonna alkaloid)
   3. may cause dysrhythmias and fetal tachycardia
4. Anesthetics: produce a local, regionalized, or generalized loss of sensation
  a. Local infiltration
   1. examples: lidocaine hydrochloride (Xylocaine), chloroprocaine (Nesacaine)

   2. used for pain relief during second stage of labor: episiotomy and perineal repair
   3. temporarily interrupts nerve impulses and pain in the perineum
   4. any agent may cause an allergic response
  b. Regional blocks
   1. paracervical block (seldom used)
     a. agent: a dilute, local anesthetic solution
     b. used during first stage, active phase of labor to produce rapid relief of contraction pain; no perineal effect
     c. blocks nerves to lower uterine segment, cervix, and upper vagina for about 1 hour
     d. may cause fetal intoxication: bradycardia or CNS depression and apnea at delivery

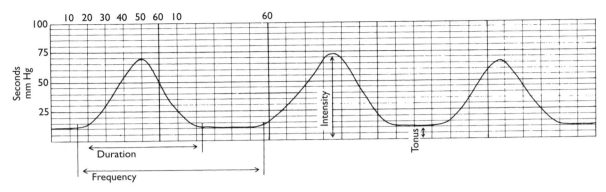

Fig. 4-15   Assessment of uterine contractions.

2. pudendal block
   a. agent: a dilute, local anesthetic solution
   b. used during second stage of labor to relieve vaginal and perineal pain
   c. blocks nerves at the cervix and perineum for about 30 minutes
   d. safe for newborn; does not affect contractions, but diminishes bearing-down reflex
3. peridural block
   a. agent: a suitable local anesthetic or morphine
   b. used during first stage, active phase, and during second stage of labor to relieve uterine and perineal pain; used to prevent pain during and after cesarean birth
   c. may be single injection or repeated doses (continuous) through an indwelling catheter
   d. types
      ▪ epidural: lumbar epidural anesthesia (LEA)
         • site: between lumbar vertebrae into epidural space; does not pierce dura mater of spinal cord
         • possible untoward effects: maternal hypotension, depression of contractions, fetal distress, diminished bearing-down reflex
      ▪ caudal
         • site: through the sacral hiatus and the sacral canal into the lowest part of the peridural space
         • possible untoward effects: same as for epidural
4. intradural block (spinal block)
   a. agent: local anesthetic mixed with dextrose solution
   b. used during second stage of labor or for abdominal surgery to produce instant loss of sensation and muscle relaxation; loss of bearing-down reflex
   c. injected between lumbar vertebrae, *through* dura mater of spinal cord, *between contractions,* and mixes with cerebrospinal fluid; duration of 1 to 3 hours
   d. possible untoward effects: maternal hypotension, respiratory inadequacy from high level, spinal headache from leakage of cerebrospinal fluid at puncture site; mother remains flat for

8 to 12 hours after dose to prevent leakage (limited value)
   e. types
      ▪ spinal block: into third, fourth, or fifth lumbar interspace
      ▪ saddle block or low spinal block: dermal anesthetic level at or below umbilicus; anesthetizes low back, pudendum, symphysis pubis, and pelvic viscera
   c. General—inhalation
      1. examples: thiopental sodium (Pentothal), halothane (Fluothane) inhalation, combination (thiopental, nitrous oxide and oxygen, succinylcholine)
      2. rarely used for uncomplicated vaginal births; can be used to relax the uterus for intrauterine manipulation or version or can be used for cesarean birth
      3. produces sleep and general loss of sensitivity to touch, pain, and stimulation
      4. possible untoward effects: aspiration, respiratory depression, newborn depression

Application of the Nursing Process to Normal Childbearing, Intrapartal Care
ASSESSMENT
1. History; confirm due date
2. Membranes intact or ruptured
3. Premonitory signs of labor
4. Labor status: true labor; stage and phase (Table 4-16)
5. Uterine contractions
6. Fetal response to labor
7. Psychologic factors: preparation for childbirth; support systems; culture and religious beliefs
8. Newborn adaptation at birth
9. Maternal homeostasis after delivery
ANALYSIS/NURSING DIAGNOSIS
1. Safe, effective care environment
   a. Anxiety related to knowledge deficit
   b. Risk for infection
2. Physiologic integrity
   a. Pain
   b. Fatigue
   c. Impaired skin integrity
3. Psychosocial integrity
   a. Anxiety

b. Ineffective individual coping
c. Powerlessness
4. Health promotion/maintenance
   a. Impaired adjustment
   b. Self-care deficit: bathing/hygiene

PLANNING, IMPLEMENTATION, AND EVALUATION

> **Goal I** The client will verbalize understanding of status and ask questions as need arises.

Implementation
1. Orient client and partner to physical setting and review basic procedures to be performed.
2. Obtain baseline vital signs and BP.
3. Determine onset, duration, and frequency of contractions.

4. Perform Leopold's maneuver (Fig. 4-16). Have client empty bladder and flex knees for abdominal relaxation; warm hands; then
   a. Proceed with fundus palpation: note breech or cephalic presentation.
   b. Proceed with lateral palpation: note back and small parts of fetus.

Table 4-16   Uterine dysfunction in labor

	Hypertonic	Hypotonic
Contractions	Intense, high tonus	Weak, ineffective
Symptoms	Painful	Painless
Fetal distress	Fetal hypoxia	Tendency for sepsis
Treatment	Sedation	Stimulation of labor

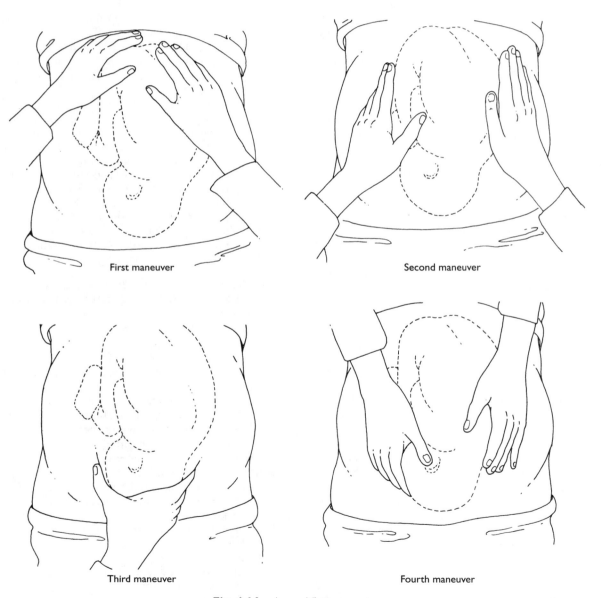

First maneuver

Second maneuver

Third maneuver

Fourth maneuver

Fig. 4-16   Leopold's maneuvers.

c. Just above symphysis pubis, note position and mobility of fetal head.

d. Midline about 2 inches above Poupart's ligaments, note position and descent of head, location of back.

5. Observe FHR and pattern changes in relation to contractions. (NOTE: The use of electronic fetal monitoring is determined by hospital policy or physician. Obtain consent to use an internal electrode.)

6. Determine client's knowledge of the labor and delivery process; childbirth preparation.

7. Prepare and position client appropriately for initial vaginal exam and reinforce the rationale for exam; explain the results of exam.

8. Note color, consistency, amount, and gross appearance of amniotic fluid.

9. Obtain laboratory specimens: urine for protein (normally negative), glucose (normally negative), and ketones (normally negative); blood for Hgb (normal range 12 to 16 g/dl), Hct (normal range 38% to 45%), WBC (normal range 4500 to 11,000 ml), Venereal Disease Research Laboratory (VDRL) test.

10. Determine time of last food ingestion.

11. Document all assessments.

12. Review process of labor.

13. Provide emotional support to client and coach.

14. Perform vulvar or perineal preparation as ordered.

15. Administer cleansing enema if ordered by physician; check FHR after procedure.

Evaluation

Client is admitted to labor and delivery unit; verbalizes an understanding of status; displays minimal anxiety.

> **Goal 2** Client will be comfortable and safe during the first stage of labor; will be supported by support person; will maintain optimal fetal oxygenation.

Implementation

1. Take maternal vital signs qh, if stable and within normal limits.

2. Monitor temperature qh if membranes ruptured more than 24 hours previously or if temperature is greater than 37.5°C (may indicate infection or dehydration).

3. Observe blood pressure between contractions.

4. Watch for supine-hypotensive syndrome caused by pressure of enlarged uterus on vena cava (decreased BP, pulse, pallor, clammy skin); condition may be prevented or corrected by placing client in left lateral position.

5. Monitor fetal status.

   a. Auscultate FHR using a fetoscope q30min (early labor) to q5min (transition) (Fig. 4-17); count rate for 1 full minute (normal is 120 to 160 per minute) or observe FHR tracing from electronic monitor for baseline changes, variability, and periodic changes related to contractions.

   b. Check FHR immediately after rupture of membranes.

   c. Check for prolapse of cord; client may feel cord slither down vagina, nurse may see cord outside vagina or palpate cord on vaginal examination; if cord

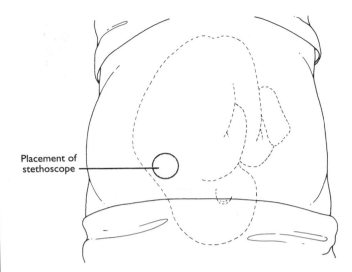

Fig. 4-17 Site of auscultation of FHR.

Placement of stethoscope

is prolapsed, place in Trendelenburg's or knee-chest position or lift head off cord through vagina (to minimize pressure of presenting part on cord), give O₂, and notify physician immediately; grave danger of fetal hypoxia because of cord compression; prepare for immediate delivery.

6. Monitor uterine contractions through abdominal palpations q30min (in early labor) to q5min (in transition); note regularity, frequency, intensity, and duration, or observe uterine tracings from electronic monitor for tonus, frequency, duration, and intensity of contractions.

7. Document all assessments.

8. Assist with or perform periodic vaginal examination to assess dilation and effacement of cervix, fetal descent, presentation, and lie.

9. Monitor fluid and electrolyte balance.

   a. Record I&O.

   b. Encourage voiding q2h; catheterize for bladder distention.

   c. Observe for signs of dehydration.

   d. Note diaphoresis.

   e. Monitor parenteral therapy; specific use determined by medical regimen and duration of labor.

10. Provide sufficient nourishment according to medical policy and client need.

    a. NPO routine in many hospitals, especially if client is receiving medication; observe for signs of hypoglycemia and dehydration.

    b. Ice chips or liquid diet may be given in some settings. (NOTE: Gastrointestinal [GI] absorption and motility are decreased during labor.)

    c. Observe for nausea and vomiting during transition (common).

11. Maintain a safe environment.

    a. Client may ambulate in early labor if desired, unless there are contraindications (e.g., membranes ruptured and fetal head not engaged, medications).

    b. Keep side rails up as necessary to prevent injury during active labor.

12. Administer basic comfort measures: oral hygiene; pillows to support body; frequent position change; bathe face and body as necessary; back rubs; effleurage for abdominal discomfort; change linen and pads frequently.
13. Assist client with breathing techniques or provide direct coaching as necessary.
    a. Use appropriate techniques taught in antepartal or childbirth classes or instruct as necessary (e.g., abdominal breathing, shallow chest breathing, panting).
    b. Advise client to relax and rest between contractions but assist with breathing techniques at onset of next contraction.
    c. Observe for symptoms of hyperventilation (lightheadedness, dizziness, and tingling and numbness of lips); if it occurs, slow breathing; have client breathe into paper bag or into cupped hands.
    d. Support coach by giving periodic relief for a break and nourishment.
    e. Praise efforts and keep client and significant other informed about progress in labor.
14. Assess ability to manage pain, desire for medications.
15. Administer analgesics (or assist with anesthetic administration) as ordered by physician, in accordance with client's preference or decision.
    a. Provide relaxing environment by maintaining calm manner and reducing external stimuli.
    b. Administer and record administration of medications ordered.
    c. Note client and fetal response to medication; report any undesired side effects.
    d. Monitor client's vital signs and FHR q5-15min, depending on drug given.
    e. Place client in appropriate position for administration of anesthetic.
    f. Place client in lateral position; increase IV fluids if hypotension develops.
    g. Administer 6 to 10 L of O_2 per minute for maternal hypotension or late decelerations in FHR.

Evaluation
During the first stage of labor, the client maintains homeostasis, is as comfortable as possible; is supported effectively by coach or nurse; fetal heart rate is normal in response to contractions.

Goal 3 Client will be maintained during the second stage of labor; will assist with birth by effective pushing, supported by coach; a healthy newborn will be delivered with minimal trauma.

Implementation
1. Maintain a safe environment.
   a. If transfer to delivery room is required, plan move between uterine contractions (multiparas may be transported at 8 to 9 cm dilation, primiparas at full dilation with perineal bulging).
   b. Wear appropriate apparel and goggles; assist significant other in proper hand washing and obtaining ap-

propriate scrub attire for delivery room; birthing room regulations may be flexible.
   c. Place client in optimal position for birth of newborn.
      1. for lithotomy position: pad stirrups; maintain equal height of legs; ensure no pressure on popliteal space
      2. alternate positions may include semi-Fowler's on birthing table, side lying, squatting, birthing chair.
2. Prep vulvar and perineal area as indicated, wearing sterile gloves; use standard precautions.
3. Palpate fundus for uterine contractions, or assess electronically.
4. Monitor FHR by either auscultation with a fetoscope or electronically.
5. Monitor BP at frequent intervals.
6. Encourage strong pushing with contractions.
   a. Instruct client to begin by taking two cleansing breaths, then hold and bear down or push as desired with contractions; legs should be spread with knees slightly flexed.
   b. Show the client which muscles are to be used by showing or touching those muscles in the pelvic floor.
   c. Use blow-blow breathing pattern to prevent pushing between contractions and during delivery of head.
7. Assist physician or nurse midwife as necessary.
8. Promote emotional well-being of client and support person.
   a. Inform them about progress and all procedures.
   b. Position mirror so delivery may be viewed if desired.
   c. Encourage rest and relaxation between contractions.
   d. Praise frequently for efforts.

Evaluation
Client is positioned appropriately and safely for delivery; pushes and bears down effectively; is supported by coach; delivers fetus with minimal trauma.

Goal 4 Client will remain stable during the third stage; will expel placenta intact; will be free from excessive bleeding; newborn will remain stable and have early contact with mother.

Implementation
1. Note time of delivery of infant.
2. Provide immediate newborn care; refer to p. 365.
3. Place newborn close to client or to breast, on uncovered abdomen if possible.
4. Allow client to touch and explore infant after cord is cut.
5. Assess for signs that placenta has separated.
   a. Uterus rises up in abdomen.
   b. Uterus changes to globular shape.
   c. Sudden trickle of blood appears.
   d. Umbilical cord lengthens.
6. Observe time and mechanism of placental delivery; chart on delivery record.
   a. Duncan mechanism: maternal surface of the placenta presents on delivery; appears dark and rough; increased risk of retained placental fragments.
   b. Schultze mechanism: fetal surface of the placenta presents on delivery; appears shiny, smooth.

7. Inspect placenta for intactness and three blood vessels.
8. Palpate uterus to check for muscle tone and location at frequent intervals (firm and contracted).
9. Administer and document oxytocic agents as ordered (Tables 4-17 and 4-18).
   a. Drug and dose determined by individual need and physician's order; may be given intramuscularly (IM) or added to existing IV
   b. Used to prevent or control postpartum hemorrhage by stimulating uterine contractility
   c. Important with overdistention or poor muscle tone
10. Measure BP at 5- to 15-minute intervals (decreases in BP are often associated with blood loss and administration of oxytocic drugs).
11. Send cord blood to lab; especially important if client is Rh-negative or O-positive (for direct Coombs' test).
12. Allow client (and significant other if present) opportunity to see and directly touch newborn (promotes bonding) after initial stabilization.
13. Initiate breast-feeding (hospital policies may vary).

Evaluation

Client remains stable during the third stage of labor; delivers placenta intact; maintains firmly contracted uterus; has minimal bleeding; parent-infant bonding begins.

Goal 5 Client will remain stable during recovery period; will be free from complications; will maintain homeostasis; will bond with newborn.

Implementation

1. Take vital signs q15min until stable (take temperature on admission and subsequently as indicated).
2. Check height of fundus.
   a. Palpate q15min during first hour.
   b. Note position in relation to umbilicus (at or just above umbilicus, 1 to 2 finger breadths).
   c. Note consistency: should be firmly contracted; if boggy, massage until firm (avoid overmassaging).
3. Palpate bladder for distention; measure initial voiding; catheterize if necessary (full bladder displaces the uterus).
4. Observe lochia q15min during first hour; note amount (small, moderate, or heavy), color (rubra), consistency; presence of large clots may indicate retained placental fragments; flow is considered excessive if bleeding saturates pad within 15 minutes (flow may increase as oxytocics wear off).
5. Check perineum: note general appearance, any swelling, redness, bruising, drainage, or condition of episiotomy; assess for pain.
6. Assess for afterpains.
7. Promote general comfort.
8. Provide contact with newborn, if not possible in delivery room.
9. Assist with breast-feeding if client desires.
10. Perform and teach perineal care (see p. 350); reinforce that pad should be applied from front to back.

Table 4-17   Uterine smooth muscle stimulants

Drug name	Action	Side effects	Nursing implications
Ergonovine maleate (Ergotrate)	Reduces risk of or treats postpartum hemorrhage by stimulating uterine contraction	Nausea, vomiting, dizziness, hypotension, hypertension	Monitor BP before and during administration. Palpate fundus and note lochia. Monitor contractions, lochia, BP.
Methylergonovine maleate (Methergine)	Stimulates uterine contraction, increases uterine muscle tone, prevents/controls postpartum hemorrhage	Nausea, vomiting, dizziness, slight changes in BP (less likely than with ergonovine maleate), headaches	

Table 4-18   Oxytocin (Pitocin)

Action	Side effects	Nursing implications
Stimulates uterine smooth muscle to contract; increases intracellular calcium. Used in dilute concentrations IV (10 units in 500 or 1000 ml normal saline or D_5W or balanced electrolytes); infusion rate gradually increased to induce or augment labor contractions and stimulate cervical effacement and dilation before delivery.	**IN LABOR** Maternal: overstimulation of uterus resulting in rapid labor, delivery; tetany and uterine rupture; abruptio placentae, water intoxication Fetal: hypoxia, distress, trauma with precipitous delivery	Monitor and record vital signs and contractions (frequency, duration, and strength). Discontinue infusion if contractions exceed 70-90 seconds; signs of tetany or abruptio placentae. Record I&O. Monitor FHR; discontinue infusion if evidence of distress; turn client to left side and give O_2 Report problems immediately to responsible physician.
After delivery acts to stimulate uterine contraction and prevent hemorrhage as a result of atony.	**FOLLOWING DELIVERY** Water intoxication, uterine atony (if overused)	Monitor BP, uterine contraction, lochia, output.

11. Maintain adequate fluid intake; state specific amounts of fluids to be taken in 8-hour period.
12. Transfer to postpartum care when condition stable (usually within 1 to 2 hours); may remain in birthing room.

Evaluation

Client is physiologically and psychologically stable; couple gazes at, holds, touches, and cuddles newborn.

Application of the Nursing Process to the High-Risk Intrapartal Client

ASSESSMENT
1. Risk factors in pregnancy
2. Problems identified in the intrapartal period
3. Alterations of labor progress

ANALYSIS/NURSING DIAGNOSIS
1. Safe, effective care environment
   a. Risk for infection
   b. Risk for injury
2. Physiologic integrity
   a. Pain
   b. Impaired gas exchange
3. Psychosocial integrity
   a. Anxiety
   b. Ineffective individual coping
4. Health promotion/maintenance
   a. Knowledge deficit

PLANNING, IMPLEMENTATION, AND EVALUATION

> **Goal** Client and fetus will experience no undetected complications; will receive immediate treatment for problems; will have a safe birth experience. Newborn and mother will maintain physiologic and psychosocial integrity.

Implementation
1. Observe for potential and actual problems in labor and delivery.
2. Act immediately to maintain fetal and maternal well-being.
3. Report problems to physician or nurse-midwife.
4. Administer therapy and medications as ordered.
5. Document assessments and care.
6. Support couple in difficult birth situation.

Evaluation

Client and fetus at risk have problems detected and treated immediately; return to a homeostatic state after a safe delivery.

SELECTED HEALTH PROBLEMS IN THE INTRAPARTAL PERIOD

✷ DYSTOCIA

1. Definition: difficult, painful labor or delivery characterized by abnormally slow progress (more than 24 hours)
2. Incidence: approximately 5% of intrapartum women (largely primigravidas) experience some type of dystocia

3. Types: fall into four categories, which may exist alone or in combination
   a. The *powers* (or forces): the main ones are
      1. hypertonic uterine dysfunction (primary inertia); see Table 4-17
         a. the uterine muscle is in a state of greater than normal muscle tension; contractions are of poor quality, and the force of the contraction is distorted
         b. increased tonus
         c. no cervical changes
         d. treatment: sedation
      2. hypotonic uterine dysfunction
         a. the tone or tension of the muscle is defective or inadequate, resulting in failure of cervical dilation and effacement
            ▪ primary inertia: inefficient contractions from onset of labor
            ▪ secondary inertia: well-established contractions become weak, inefficient, or stop
         b. treatment: oxytocics if no cephalopelvic disproportion (CPD)
      3. inadequate voluntary expulsive forces or anesthesia
         a. may be a result of exhaustion, position
         b. treatment: coach woman in bearing down; cesarean delivery if necessary
   b. The *passageway*: abnormalities in the size or character of the birth canal that form an obstacle to the descent of the fetus
      1. CPD: disproportion between the size of the fetal head and that of the birth canal
         a. most frequently caused by a contracted pelvis: slight irregularities in the structure of the pelvis may delay the progress of labor; severe deformities often make delivery through the natural passages impossible
            ▪ contraction of the inlet
            ▪ contraction of the midpelvis
            ▪ contraction of the outlet
            ▪ a combination
      2. soft-tissue dystocia: obstruction of birth passage by an anatomic abnormality (e.g., myoma or tumor, placenta previa)
   c. The *passenger*: variations in position, presentation, or development of the fetus; includes a variety of conditions that are associated with prolonged labor, failure to progress, lack of engagement
      1. abnormal position: persistent occiput posterior position (25% of pregnancies)
      2. faulty presentation
         a. shoulder or face presentation
         b. breech presentation
      3. excessive size of fetus
         a. weight: a fetus over 4000 g (8 lb 13½ oz) may be too large to pass through the birth canal of some pregnant women; the fetal head also becomes less malleable when fetal weight increases
         b. enlargement of head (hydrocephalus): excessive accumulation of cerebrospinal fluid in the

ventricles of the brain with consequent enlargement of the cranium; incidence: 1 in 2000 births; enlargement of fetal body (e.g., tumors, abdominal distention)

d. The *person*
   1. position of mother: restrictions of position or upright position, walking
   2. psychologic response: lack of emotional readiness, educational preparation, support, environment, confinement to bed

Nursing Process

ASSESSMENT
1. Vaginal exam, pelvimetry, or ultrasound to establish diagnosis
2. False labor vs. true labor
3. Fetal status
4. Cause of dystocia
5. Complications of uterine dysfunction
   a. Maternal exhaustion
   b. Intrapartum infection
   c. Traumatic operative delivery
   d. Uterine rupture
   e. Fetal death and injury
6. Presentation of fetus by palpation (Leopold's maneuver)
7. Meconium staining of amniotic fluid (normal when associated with breech presentation)
8. Anxiety

ANALYSIS/NURSING DIAGNOSIS (see p. 340)
PLANNING, IMPLEMENTATION, AND EVALUATION

Goal 1 Client will have dystocia detected; the client with dystocia will remain stable during the intrapartal period; will not experience undetected complications; fetal distress will be identified.

Implementation
1. Assess uterine contractions/pattern and maternal vital signs.
2. Plot individual labor pattern, compare with Friedman curve (average labor curve of cervical dilation and hours in labor; see Fig. 4-18).
3. Assist with ultrasonographic or radiographic studies for laboring woman who has previously suspected CPD.
4. Immediately assess FHR when fetal membranes rupture (spontaneously or artificially); observe for cord prolapse (see p. 337).
5. Monitor fluid/electrolyte replacement.
6. Administer broad-spectrum antibiotics as ordered for treatment of intrauterine infection.
7. Promote rest and pain relief.
8. Support family.
9. Document assessments.

Evaluation
Abnormalities in the powers, passageway, or passenger are identified during the antepartal or early intrapartal period; client with dystocia is promptly treated; client and fetus remain stable during difficult labor; healthy newborn is delivered.

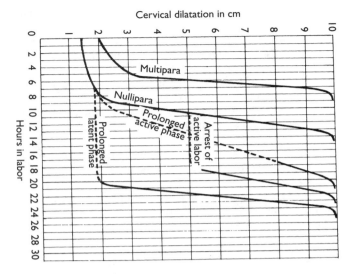

Fig. 4-18 Friedman curve.

Goal 2 Client will be stable during oxytocin augmentation or prostaglandin gel (PGE) administration.

Implementation
1. Administer oxytocin (Pitocin) according to physician's order or hospital's protocol and client's condition (see Table 4-18); the physician must consider the following criteria before administration:
   a. There must be true hypotonic dysfunction; oxytocin ABSOLUTELY CONTRAINDICATED for *hypertonic* uterine dysfunction.
   b. The client must be in true labor (progressed to at least 3 cm dilation and cervix thinning).
   c. No mechanical obstructions to safe delivery exist (e.g., cephalopelvic disproportion, placenta previa).
   d. The condition of the fetus must be good: regular fetal heart rate, no meconium staining.
   e. Pitocin is used judiciously in the following circumstances:
      1. grand multiparity
      2. overdistention of uterus
      3. history of uterine surgery
      4. previous cesarean birth
2. Monitor administration of oxytocin.
   a. Use infusion pump.
   b. Increase infusion rate as ordered or by established protocol.
   c. Monitor vital signs, infusion rate q30 minutes.
   d. Continue electronic fetal monitoring; observe and document fetal heart rate pattern with contractions (duration, intensity, tonus, and frequency).
   e. Place client in a left lateral position to maximize uterine blood flow by reducing pressure on vena cava and aorta.
   f. Never leave client unattended (physician must be available).

g. Assess for problems (e.g., rigid abdomen, intense pain).
h. If uterine tetany occurs, contractions exceed 90 seconds in duration, or there is fetal distress or bradycardia, discontinue oxytocin.
i. Give O_2 8 to 10 L for signs of fetal distress.
j. Monitor for abruptio placentae.

3. Monitor client receiving PGE (gel or suppository).
   a. Perform maternal and fetal assessments as with oxytocin.
   b. Maintain bed rest for 1 hour after PGE administration.
   c. Observe for diarrhea (common side effect).

Evaluation

Client is free from complications related to oxytocin or PGE administration; has effective uterine contractions; maintains optimal fetal status.

> **Goal 3** Client will verbalize understanding of the induction process and will cope effectively with the assistance of support person/nurse.

Implementation

1. Inform client about her status and measures taken to help her.
2. Provide basic comfort measures as in normal labor.
3. Assess level of fatigue and ability to cope with pain.
4. Provide emotional support to client and significant other.
5. Assist with administration of anesthetic to relax uterus (hyperactive uterine contractions).
6. Discuss rationale and expected outcomes with client and partner if cesarean birth indicated.

Evaluation

Client experiences minimal anxiety; knows the status of labor and the fetus; rests comfortably between contractions, treatments; is supported by coach and nurse.

> **Goal 4** If malpresentation requires cesarean birth, client will verbalize understanding of risks/benefits and cooperate with surgical preparation. Newborn will be delivered in a timely fashion with minimal risk.

Implementation

1. Assist with vaginal or rectal exam to determine presenting fetal part.
2. Explain and prepare client for ultrasonic or radiographic studies to confirm previously unsuspected malpositions (anomalies often undetected before intrapartum period).
3. Assess effectiveness of labor and fetal well-being by continuous electronic monitoring.
4. Encourage lateral recumbent position.
5. Provide emotional support and coaching as indicated (labors are often prolonged).
6. Support significant other.
7. Apply sacral pressure and frequent back rubs to keep pressure of fetal occiput off client's sacrum (occiput posterior presentation).
8. Observe for cord prolapse (occurs in 1 in every 400 births) when membranes rupture (see p. 337).
9. Assist with cesarean birth.

Evaluation

Client safely is delivered of a healthy newborn; has problems such as abnormal fetal position identified early.

PRETERM LABOR

1. Definition: onset of labor between 20 and 37 weeks of gestation
2. Predisposing factors that may cause premature labor; pregnancy complications that may necessitate delivery of preterm infant
   a. Maternal
      1. diabetes
      2. cardiovascular or renal disease
      3. pregnancy-induced or chronic hypertension
      4. infection: chorioamnionitis
      5. uncontrolled hemorrhage associated with placenta previa or abruptio placentae
      6. prematurely ruptured membranes
      7. incompetent cervix
      8. smoking
      9. severe isoimmunization
      10. diethylstilbestrol (DES) exposure
      11. abdominal surgery during pregnancy
      12. iatrogenic causes
      13. previous preterm deliveries
      14. history of previous pregnancy losses
      15. unknown
   b. Fetal
      1. multiple gestation
      2. hydramnios
      3. infection
      4. intrauterine growth retardation (IUGR)
3. Prognosis: fetal/neonatal mortality is less than 5% in pregnancies when gestation has lasted 35 or more weeks and fetus is larger than 2500 g

Nursing Process

ASSESSMENT

1. Identify women at risk.
2. Assess for true labor (contractions of increased frequency and duration, effacement and dilation of cervix).
3. Estimate gestation.

ANALYSIS/NURSING DIAGNOSIS (see p. 340)

PLANNING, IMPLEMENTATION, AND EVALUATION

> **Goal** Client in preterm labor will experience a cessation of labor; will carry fetus as close to term as possible.

Implementation

1. Maintain bed rest, lateral recumbent position in a quiet environment, hydrate, empty bladder.
2. Administer selected tocolytic agents to suppress labor as prescribed by physician (e.g., beta-adrenergic drugs: ritodrine, terbutaline; magnesium sulfate).
   a. Assess the effects of drugs on the pattern of labor (uterine contractions) and fetal well-being with electronic monitoring system.
   b. Avoid these drugs for control of preterm labor if contraindicated (e.g., client has a cardiac condition, gestation less than 20 weeks).

c. If administering ritodrine or terbutaline: assess for specific cardiovascular side effects (Table 4-19).

d. If administering magnesium sulfate: assess BP, reflexes, respirations, and urinary output before and during administration (see Table 4-12).

3. Document response to therapy; alter dose as ordered.
4. Maintain adequate hydration through oral or parenteral intake.
5. Monitor I&O.
6. Monitor client's vital signs.
7. Provide emotional support to client and significant other.
8. Plan for home maintenance if indicated.
9. Administer glucocorticoid therapy (betamethasone) if indicated to prevent respiratory distress syndrome in newborn.
   a. Drug is effective if delivery can be delayed 48 hours or more.
   b. Avoid use if delivery is imminent or if maternal hypertensive or cardiovascular disorders exist.
   c. Observe for signs of pulmonary edema (reported in rare cases when ritodrine and corticosteroids are used together).
10. Administer minimal analgesics for pain during labor and delivery.
11. Prepare for preterm delivery if maternal complications are present (e.g., diabetes, hemorrhage, eclampsia) or dilation progresses.

Evaluation

Client carries the pregnancy as close to term as possible and is safely delivered of the newborn.

EMERGENCY BIRTH (UNASSISTED BY PHYSICIAN, NURSE, OR NURSE WIDWIFE)

1. May occur in a hospital or community setting
2. Predisposing factors: precipitate labor, environmental problems, absence of physician and midwife
3. Prognosis: increased maternal and fetal risk associated with possible
   a. Intrauterine hypoxia (precipitate labor or delivery)
   b. Laceration of the perineum
   c. Infection

Nursing Process

ASSESSMENT
1. Fetal status
2. Stage and phase of labor

ANALYSIS/NURSING DIAGNOSIS (see p. 340)

PLANNING, IMPLEMENTATION, AND EVALUATION

Goal Client is safely delivered of newborn, free from complications, despite an emergency situation.

Implementation
1. Remain with client; have another adult (if present) call for assistance; remain calm and give simple instructions to mother.
2. Provide as clean an environment as possible.
3. Assist client into side-lying position.
4. Instruct client to pant when head crowns.
5. Rupture amniotic sac (if intact) when fetal head crowns.
6. Apply gentle downward pressure on fetal head to pre-

Table 4-19 Ritodrine hydrochloride

Drug name	Action	Side effects	Nursing implications
Ritodrine hydrochloride IV (Yutopar—oral) (only drug with current FDA approval for preterm labor)	Relaxes arterioles in uterine muscle; vasodilator As a beta-sympathetic agent, stops uterine contractions in preterm labor of at least 20 weeks (membranes should be intact) IV solution (150 mg to 500 ml fluid) is given at increasing rates until desired effect is achieved	Maternal: tachycardia, tremors, palpitations, PVCs; pulmonary edema, widening pulse pressure, headache, hyperglycemia, hypokalemia, anxiety, diarrhea (contraindicated if history of CV, thyroid disease; asthma) Fetal: tachycardia, hypoxia, acidosis	Maintain infusion rate; increase as ordered. Monitor apical pulse; report and document pulse above 120 (should not exceed 140). Check BP frequently. Record I&O; observe for side effects. Monitor glucose and potassium levels. Teach client to expect responses such as nervousness. Explain that the value of therapy is to allow time for fetal lung development (glucocorticoids may be ordered to stimulate surfactant). Monitor for signs of pulmonary edema. Have antidote (propranolol) available. Monitor and document FHR (should not exceed 180).

vent head from "popping out," damaging fetal head, and causing maternal lacerations.

7. Deliver fetal head between contractions.
8. Check for cord around neck; if wrapped around neck, slip cord over newborn's head; then deliver shoulders
9. Clear airway and facilitate mucus drainage; do not hold upside down by feet or ankles.
10. Dry newborn rapidly (maintain at level of uterus).
11. Cover newborn with blanket or towel to prevent heat loss.
12. Clamp cord in two places and cut between the two clamps; use sterile or clean scissors or knife; leave intact if medical assistance will be available shortly or if clamps/scissors are not available.
    a. Do not pull on cord.
    b. Instruct client to gently push out placenta.
13. Place newborn on client's abdomen or breast to stimulate uterine contractions.
14. Assess client after birth: prevent hemorrhage.
15. Congratulate parents.

Evaluation
Client is safely delivered of a healthy newborn; is free from complications.

NOTE: The next four selected health problems are classified as "Operative Obstetrics."

EPISIOTOMY

1. Definition: an incision made into the perineum to facilitate delivery
2. Indications: any condition that places the woman at risk for perineal tearing, such as
   a. Rapid labor
   b. Large baby
   c. Malposition of the fetus
3. Prognosis: generally heals within 2 to 4 weeks after delivery; may cause mild to moderate discomfort in the postpartum period
4. Types (Fig. 4-19)
   a. Median (midline)
      1. advantages: easily repaired; generally less painful; minimal blood loss
      2. disadvantages: may extend into rectal sphincter (third degree) or rectum (fourth degree)
   b. Mediolateral (right or left)
      1. advantage: less likely extension into rectum
      2. disadvantages: greater blood loss; repair more difficult; area more painful during healing; possible damage to pubococcygeal muscle

Nursing Process

See Postpartal Care, Nursing Goal 1, p. 350.

FORCEPS

1. Definition: obstetric instruments used to extract the fetal head during delivery; each consists of a blade, shank, handle, and lock
2. Predisposing factors
   a. Maternal
      1. to shorten second stage of labor in dystocia
      2. expulsive efforts that are ineffective or deficient because of anesthesia or maternal exhaustion

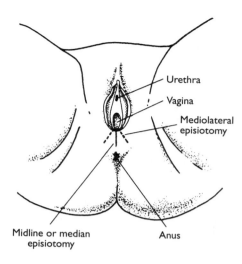

Fig. 4-19 Types of episiotomies.

      3. if pushing is contraindicated because of a chronic disease or cardiac problem
   b. Fetal
      1. premature labor (to protect fetal head)
      2. fetal distress
      3. arrested descent
      4. abnormal presentation
3. Prognosis
   a. Perineal lacerations may occur with a difficult forceps delivery or may occur after a precipitate delivery
      1. first-degree laceration involves fourchette, perineal skin, and vaginal mucosa
      2. second-degree laceration involves skin, mucous membrane, muscles of perineal body
      3. third-degree laceration involves skin, mucous membranes, muscles of perineal body, and rectal sphincter
      4. fourth-degree laceration involves all features of third-degree lacerations plus tearing into the lumen of the rectum
   b. Pressure by forceps on fetus' facial nerve may cause temporary paralysis of one side of the face
   c. Perinatal morbidity and mortality increased, particularly with midforceps delivery
   d. Increased risk of postpartum hemorrhage with midforceps delivery
   e. Maternal complications after forceps or other traumatic delivery may include cystocele, rectocele, or uterine prolapse later in life
4. Types of forceps deliveries
   a. Outlet or low forceps: fetal head on perineal floor
   b. Midforceps: fetal head at the level of ischial spines

Nursing Process
ASSESSMENT

1. Cervix fully dilated before use of forceps
2. Head engaged
3. Fetus in vertex presentation (or face with mentum anterior)
4. Membranes ruptured
5. No cephalopelvic disproportion

6. Bowel and bladder empty
7. Fetal heart rate stable
ANALYSIS/NURSING DIAGNOSIS (see p. 340)
PLANNING, IMPLEMENTATION, AND EVALUATION

> **Goal** Client and fetus will experience minimal trauma despite forceps delivery.

Implementation
1. Explain procedure to client and significant other.
2. Provide physician with selected forceps.
3. Monitor fetal heart rate continuously during procedure.
4. Assess newborn for forceps bruises and facial paralysis.

Evaluation
Client is free from the complications of forceps delivery; is delivered of a healthy newborn with minimal trauma.

VACUUM EXTRACTION

NOTE: This technique is used infrequently in current practice.
1. Definition: use of an obstetric instrument consisting of a suction cup attached to a suction pump for extraction of the fetal head; employs negative pressure and traction
2. Predisposing factors
   a. Prolonged labor
   b. Fetal distress
   c. Fetal malposition
   d. Chronic maternal disease or complications that contraindicate pushing
   e. Maternal fatigue
3. Prognosis
   a. Increased risk of tissue necrosis of the fetal head, cephalhematoma, and cerebral trauma
   b. Increased risk of trauma to vagina and cervix
   c. Increased risk of postpartum hemorrhage

Nursing Process

ASSESSMENT
1. Fetal status
2. Fetal position
ANALYSIS/ANALYSIS (see p. 340)
PLANNING, IMPLEMENTATION, AND EVALUATION

> **Goal** Client will verbalize understanding of the procedure; experiences no undetected complications.

Implementation
1. Clarify procedure after physician's explanation.
2. Assemble and set up necessary equipment.
3. Monitor fetal heart rate continuously.
4. Assist the physician with the suction apparatus.
5. Assess newborn for caput and cerebral swelling.

Evaluation
Newborn is delivered safely; mother is free from undetected problems.

CESAREAN BIRTH

1. Definition: delivery of a newborn through abdominal wall and uterine incisions. The procedure may be prear-ranged and performed before the onset of labor (elective) or unplanned and initiated after the onset of labor (emergency).
2. Indications
   a. Cephalopelvic disproportion
   b. Abnormal presentation (e.g., breech)
   c. Dystocia
   d. Fetal distress
   e. Weakened or defective uterine scar caused by previous cesarean birth or uterine surgery (VBAC may be an option: refer to p. 346)
   f. Placenta previa or abruptio placenta
   g. Severe preeclampsia, eclampsia, or diabetes out of control
   h. Pelvic tumors
   i. Prolapsed cord
   j. Fetal abnormalities
   k. Vaginal infection (e.g., active herpes lesions)
   l. Multiple gestation
3. Prognosis
   a. Related to the reasons the cesarean delivery was performed, the type of procedure used, length of time membranes were ruptured, and the nature of complications occurring
   b. Perinatal mortality increases with fetal immaturity and complications compromising uteroplacental blood exchange
4. Types (Fig. 4-20)
   a. Classical: vertical incision is made through the visceral peritoneum and into the full body of the uterus above the bladder; performed infrequently
      1. advantages: simple and rapid to perform, useful when there is an anterior placenta previa
      2. disadvantages
         a. potential for rupture of the scar with subsequent pregnancy
         b. increased risk of small bowel adhesion to the suture line
   b. Lower segment: incision made into the lower segment of the uterus
   c. Extraperitoneal: incision is made into the lower uterine segment without entering the peritoneal cavity

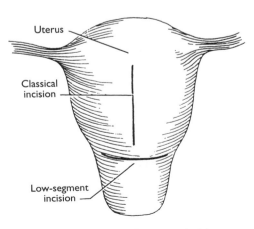

Fig. 4-20   Types of cesarean incisions.

Nursing Process

ASSESSMENT

1. History and indications for surgery
2. Maternal and fetal well-being
3. Pain and anxiety

ANALYSIS/NURSING DIAGNOSIS (see p. 340)

PLANNING, IMPLEMENTATION, AND EVALUATION

Goal 1 Preoperatively, client and fetus will be free from problems; client will be physically and emotionally prepared for the cesarean birth.

Implementation

1. Provide care as for any surgical procedure; refer to Perioperative Period, p. 115 (preoperative care will vary with an elective vs. an emergency cesarean birth).
2. Request/evaluate laboratory studies: type and cross-match, complete blood cell count (CBC), Hgb, and Hct, Rh, chemistry.
3. Insert Foley catheter.
4. Monitor fetal heart rate.
5. Administer antacid or other medications as ordered.
6. Prepare emergency equipment for resuscitation of mother and newborn.

Evaluation

Client and fetus are in no distress; couple is prepared for cesarean birth.

Goal 2 Client will tolerate surgery; will achieve postoperative homeostasis; will initiate maternal-infant bonding; newborn will be free from preventable complications.

Implementation

1. Refer to Perioperative Period, p. 115; Goal 5, p. 339; and Postpartal Care, p. 350.
2. Assist physician with surgical procedure as necessary.
3. Monitor maternal-fetal status.
4. Assess for signs and symptoms of hemorrhage.
5. Administer oxytocic agents as ordered by physician.
6. Provide assistance as necessary during mother-infant interactions.
7. Monitor recovery from anesthesia.
8. Anticipate client's possible feelings of failure and grief response.
9. Provide emotional support to help mother and significant other integrate the experience.
10. Assess newborn's status.

Evaluation

Client is free from complications; remains stable and comfortable during the postoperative period; initiates bonding; newborn is in good condition.

VAGINAL BIRTH AFTER CESAREAN BIRTH (VBAC)

1. Incidence: VBAC is increasing: 60% to 75% of women who attempt vaginal deliveries after cesarean births are successful; should be hospital birth

2. Contraindications
   a. Upper segment uterine incision (classical)
   b. Any contraindication for vaginal delivery (e.g., CPD, complete placenta previa, active herpes)

Nursing Process

ASSESSMENT

1. Maternal status; history
2. Fetal responses to contractions

ANALYSIS/NURSING DIAGNOSIS (see p. 340)

PLANNING, IMPLEMENTATION, AND EVALUATION

Goal Client will be free of complications with labor and vaginal delivery after previous cesarean birth; is delivered of a newborn in good condition.

Implementation

1. Monitor uterine contractions frequently.
2. Monitor fetal status continuously.
3. Assess for threatened rupture or rupture of uterus (see Rupture of the Uterus, following).

Evaluation

Client experiences normal labor free from complications; client and newborn both are in satisfactory condition.

✖ RUPTURE OF THE UTERUS

1. Definition: the uterus ruptures from the stress of labor; rupture may be complete or partial
2. Occurrence: rare, 1 in every 2000 births
3. Predisposing factors
   a. Previous surgery of myometrium or cesarean birth
   b. Oxytocin (Pitocin) induction (second most common cause)
   c. Nonprogressive labor
   d. Intense contractions
   e. Faulty position or fetal abnormalities
   f. Injudicious use of forceps
   g. Trauma
4. Prognosis
   a. Maternal mortality 5% to 10%
   b. Fetal mortality is high: 50% to 75%

Nursing Process

ASSESSMENT

1. Sharp abdominal pain (during contractions); onset sudden
2. Tachypnea, tachycardia, anxiety, cool and clammy skin, confusion (shock), rapid change in condition
3. Sudden absence of uterine contractions (with complete rupture)
4. Uterus palpated as a hard mass adjacent to fetus
5. Hemorrhage into the abdominal cavity or vagina
6. Abdominal tenderness

ANALYSIS/NURSING DIAGNOSIS (see p. 340)

PLANNING, IMPLEMENTATION, AND EVALUATION

Goal Client will be free from hemorrhage caused by uterine rupture; will maintain fluid and electrolyte balance; will verbalize an understanding of the need for emergency surgery; will maintain oxygenation of fetus.

Implementation
1. Assess carefully during labor; report any signs of an impending rupture.
2. Monitor fetal status.
3. Provide immediate treatment for shock.
4. Prepare client and significant other for possible emergency cesarean birth or hysterectomy.
5. Provide emotional support to couple.

Evaluation
Client is delivered of a newborn in stable condition; has hemorrhage controlled; is in good condition after emergency surgery.

AMNIOTIC FLUID EMBOLISM

1. Definition: the entrance of amniotic fluid into the maternal circulation through the placental site and venous sinuses

2. Occurrence: extremely rare complication that occurs in the intrapartum or early postpartum period
3. Predisposing factors: rapid, intense contractions from oxytocin infusion; multiparity with large fetus
4. Prognosis
   a. Fetal death will result if delivery is not implemented immediately
   b. Maternal death may occur within 1 to 2 hours if emergency interventions are ineffective
   c. Presence of meconium or mucus in amniotic fluid is indicative of increased lethality, grave outlook

Nursing Process
Refer to Pulmonary Embolus, p. 147.

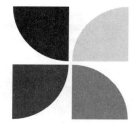

Postpartal Care

NORMAL CHILDBEARING

1. Definition: the postpartum period (puerperium) starts immediately after delivery and is completed when the reproductive tract has returned to the nearly prepregnant state and family readjustment has occurred (usually defined as 6 weeks)
2. Length of stay (LOS) in hospital or birth center has declined
   a. Current LOS
      1. for vaginal births 6 to 48 hours
      2. for cesarean births 48 to 96 hours
   b. Postpartum follow-up/home care varies to meet needs of childbearing families to
      1. monitor recovery
      2. reduce risks
      3. meet learning needs
3. Maternal physiologic status
   a. Uterine involution
      1. process of involution takes 4 to 6 weeks to complete
         a. weight of uterus decreases from 2 pounds to 2 ounces
         b. hormones decrease
         c. autolysis occurs (enzyme action)
         d. contractions increase muscle tone
         e. vasoconstriction occurs at placental site
         f. endometrium regenerates
         g. fundus steadily descends into true pelvis; fundal height decreases about 1 finger breadth (1 cm) per day; by 10 days postpartum, cannot be palpated abdominally
      2. factors delaying involution
         a. multiparity
         b. conditions causing overdistention of uterus
         c. infection
         d. retained placenta or membranes
         e. hormonal deficiencies
      3. cervical involution
         a. after 1 week, muscle begins to regenerate
         b. small lacerations may heal or need cauterization
         c. external cervical os remains wider than in a nonparous woman
         d. internal cervical os closed after 1 week
      4. lochia (Table 4-20)
         a. constituents: blood, mucus, particles of decidua, cellular debris, leukocytes, red blood cells (RBCs)
         b. changes from rubra (delivery day to day 3: bright red) to serosa (days 4 to 10: brownish pink) to alba (days 10 to 14: white, as a result of increased leukocytes); normally has fleshy odor; decreases daily in amount; increases with ambulation; lochia disappearance coincides with healed internal reproductive tract
         c. signs of abnormal lochia
            ▪ foul smell
            ▪ excessive amount (any stage)
            ▪ scant (during rubra stage)
            ▪ return to rubra after serosa or alba
            ▪ large clots
      5. afterbirth pains resulting from contraction of uterus occur primarily in multiparas and in mothers who
         a. have a history of blood clots
         b. were treated with oxytocic drugs
         c. breast-feed their infant
         d. had an overdistended uterus during pregnancy (large baby, multiple gestation, polyhydramnios)
   b. Perineal healing
      1. vaginal distention decreases, although muscle tone is never restored completely to its pregravid state
      2. vaginal rugae begin to reappear around third week
      3. lacerations or episiotomy suture line gradually heals
      4. hemorrhoids common; generally subside
   c. Bladder and bowel function: physiologic adaptations include
      1. increased urinary output resulting from normal diuresis
      2. increased bladder capacity and relative insensitivity to pressure; trauma to the bladder during delivery may diminish urge to void; asymptomatic urinary retention common in early postpartum period
      3. urine may show increased acetone, nitrogen, albumin, and lactose
      4. edema of the urethra and vulva
      5. GI tract motility sluggish because of
         a. relaxed abdominal and intestinal muscles
         b. decreased intraabdominal pressure because of distention of the abdominal wall
   d. Restoration of abdominal wall
      1. abdomen may be soft and flabby; usually returns to normal state by 6 to 8 weeks

2. striae fade to silvery-white; linea nigra fades
3. diastasis recti may be marked
e. Breast changes: condition of breasts during pregnancy maintained for first 2 days postpartum; physiologic adaptations include
   1. establishment of lactation
      a. colostrum secreted during first 2 to 3 days postpartum
      b. prolactin released from anterior pituitary gland
      c. oxytocin (released from posterior pituitary) causes let-down reflex
   2. engorgement
      a. onset usually day 3
      b. lasts 24 to 48 hours
      c. caused by venous and lymphatic stasis of the breasts
   3. mechanism of lactation: sucking activates nerve impulses from nipple to spinal cord to pituitary gland
      a. anterior pituitary gland produces prolactin only if breasts are emptied; seems to inhibit FSH and LH
      b. posterior pituitary gland secretes oxytocin, causing let-down reflex or milk ejection from ducts
   4. effect on mother
      a. increased metabolic-system stress
      b. loss of large amounts of stored protein and fats
      c. increased need for calcium, phosphorus, and all nutrients and fluids; see Table 4-8 (note the increased need of the lactating woman)
      d. hastens involution of uterus, may decrease incidence of breast cancer
      e. enhances physical closeness with infant (usually pleasurable)
   5. infant's sucking stimulates milk production of 200

to 300 ml (6 to 10 oz) by day 4; by end of 6 weeks, about 600 ml per day (20 oz)
f. General physiologic status
   1. restoration of energy reserves
      a. immediate need for sleep
      b. subsequent need for sleep and rest increased
   2. blood
      a. decrease in volume
      b. moderate anemia if excessive blood loss at delivery
      c. leukocytosis immediately after delivery
      d. elevated fibrinogen levels during first week postpartum; may contribute to thrombophlebitis
   3. weight loss
      a. usually 11 to 15 pounds immediately because of baby, placenta, amniotic fluid, and diuresis
      b. 5 pounds in following week
   4. vital signs
      a. temperature first day may be 38°C (100.4°F)
      b. pulse: initially decreases postpartum, range 50 to 70
      c. blood pressure: normal limits
4. Maternal psychologic adaptation (Table 4-21)
   a. Adaptive responses to parental role (Rubin, 1961)
      1. taking-in phase: first 2 to 3 days postpartum
         a. passive and dependent behavior
         b. mother focuses on own needs rather than baby's (e.g., sleeping and eating)
         c. verbalizations center on reactions to delivery (help integrate experience)
         d. beginning to recognize child as an individual
      2. taking-hold phase: third to tenth day postpartum
         a. mother strives for independence; wants to care for self and child
         b. strong element of anxiety
            ▪ unsure of mothering role (primipara)
            ▪ unsure of own ability to physically care for child
         c. stage of maximum readiness for learning
         d. interested in learning baby care
         e. may show mood swings
      3. letting-go phase: 10 days to 6 weeks
         a. achieves independent, realistic role transition
         b. learns to accept baby as separate person and establishes new norms for self

Table 4-20 Lochia changes

Time postpartum	Characteristics
Delivery-day 3	Lochia rubra (red)
4-10 days	Lochia serosa (brownish to pink)
10-14 days	Lochia alba (white)

Table 4-21 Maternal psychologic adaptation (Rubin)

Phase	Characteristics	Nursing implications
Taking in (1-2 days postpartum)	Mother passive, dependent, concerned with own needs; verbalizes delivery experience	Assist mother in meeting physical needs. Begin teaching. Allow verbalization.
Taking hold (3-10 days postpartum)	Mother strives for independence, strong anxiety element; maximal stage of learning readiness; mood swings may occur.	Provide positive reinforcement of parenting abilities. Continue teaching.
Letting go (10 days to 6 weeks postpartum)	Mother achieves interdependence; realistic regarding role transition; accepts baby as separate person; new norms established for self	Assist mother in providing for her increased energy requirements, provide positive reinforcement as she identifies her roles with her support system. Allow her to verbalize her new role.

b. Postpartum blues (see Table 4-21 and Postpartum Depression, p. 356).

Application of the Nursing Process to Normal Childbearing, Postpartal Care

ASSESSMENT

1. Degree of homeostasis achieved
2. Vital signs
3. Fundus: height, consistency, and position
4. Lochia: amount, color, consistency, and odor
5. Perineum: REEDA, comfort, hemorrhoids
6. Bladder: distention and displacement
7. Bowel: constipation
8. Breasts/nipples: secretions, engorgement; nipple variations/condition; color, support
9. Psychologic status
10. Homans' sign: thrombophlebitis
11. Costovertebral angle (CVA) tenderness: kidney infection
12. Nutrition
13. Rest/activity
14. Bonding/attachment; role attainment

ANALYSIS/NURSING DIAGNOSIS

1. Safe, effective care environment
    a. Ineffective individual management of therapeutic regimen
    b. Impaired home maintenance management
2. Physiologic integrity
    a. Altered nutrition
    b. Pain
3. Psychosocial integrity
    a. Altered sexuality patterns
    b. Anxiety
4. Health promotion maintenance
    a. Altered family processes
    b. Altered parenting

PLANNING, IMPLEMENTATION, AND EVALUATION

Goal I Client will achieve homeostasis; will be comfortable; will be knowledgeable about self-care.

Implementation

1. Review antepartum and intrapartum records for history.
    a. Antepartal care, labor and delivery, and chronic conditions
    b. Lab values: Hgb, Hct, VDRL, blood type, Rh factor, rubella titer
2. Monitor vital signs on admission to postpartum unit, then every 4 to 8 hours.
    a. BP may drop initially after birth, then returns to normal.
    b. Bradycardia (50 to 70 beats per minute) is common the first 10 days postpartum.
    c. Temperature may be elevated within first 24 hours because of dehydration.
    d. Temperature of 38°C (100.4°F) or above on any 2 consecutive days is considered febrile (excluding first 24 hours); possible causes: endometritis, urinary tract infection.

3. Monitor ongoing postpartal progress by daily assessment.
4. Observe abdomen for muscle tone, diastasis recti abdominis; measure degree of any diastasis; teach corrective exercise to client.
5. Promote perineal healing and relief of perineal and hemorrhoidal discomfort.
    a. Inspect episiotomy daily for normal healing; observe for redness, edema, ecchymosis, discharge, approximation (REEDA), and hematoma.
    b. Apply ice pack during first 12 to 24 hours to reduce edema (as ordered).
    c. Encourage use of sitz baths, cool astringent compresses, and topical anesthetic creams as ordered to promote comfort and healing.
    d. Teach proper technique for frequent perineal care (e.g., dry perineal area from front to back, blot rather than wipe; apply perineal pad carefully; cleanse area front to back in shower daily).
    e. Reinforce teaching of perineal care and comfort measures.
6. Promote bowel and bladder function.
    a. Encourage frequent voiding.
    b. Ambulate to bathroom.
    c. Measure initial voidings.
    d. Recognize signs of bladder distention and catheterize if necessary.
    e. Check for signs of urinary infection (e.g., frequency, burning).
    f. Encourage adequate fluid intake and a balanced diet, high in fiber to avoid constipation.
    g. Use stool softeners, cathartics, and enemas as ordered by physician (enemas/suppositories contraindicated for clients with third or fourth degree tears).
7. Promote breast comfort in nonlactating mother.
    a. Encourage binding bra until milk is gone.
    b. Apply ice bags for 24 to 48 hours to minimize engorgement.
    c. Demonstrate methods to release foremilk for extreme tension.
    d. Give analgesics as ordered.
8. Treat afterbirth pains.
    a. Encourage frequent voiding.
    b. Advise mother to lie on her abdomen.
    c. Give analgesics as ordered.
9. Administer Rho(D) immune globulin if ordered; indicated for unsensitized (negative indirect Coombs' test) Rh-negative women bearing an Rh-positive child; given within 72 hours of delivery (antepartal Rho(D) immune globulin is used for selected clients) (Table 4-22).
10. Teach self-assessment and self-care.

Evaluation

Client has stable vital signs, expected involution and healing, adequate output; minimal pain; expected psychologic progression; performs self-care.

Goal 2 Client will verbalize and demonstrate knowledge of lactation, breast changes, and breast care.

Table 4-22 Rho(D) human immune globulin

Drug name	Action	Side effects	Nursing implications
RhoGAM	Provides temporary passive immunity by destroying fetal cells in the maternal circulation before sensitization occurs, therefore blocking antibody production. Effective if administered to an Rh-negative woman after each abortion, ectopic pregnancy, amniocentesis and within 72 hr of delivery of an Rh-positive, Coombs'-negative infant. Also given prophylactically at 28 weeks of gestation.	Transfusion reaction; lethargy myalgia; contraindication if antibodies are present.	Teach to carry identification card and to inform health care providers of RhoGAM history. Instruct that Rh-negative women will need addition dose during subsequent pregnancies, miscarriage/abortion, amniocentesis, or delivery of Rh-positive, Coombs'-negative infant.

Implementation

1. Observe nipple type/condition and breast fullness/secretion.
   a. Use pump or shells to draw out flat or inverted nipples.
   b. Expect colostrum for 24 to 48 hours, then transitional milk; then mature milk.
2. Explain and demonstrate mechanisms of lactation.
   a. Supply and demand: supply established by feeding on demand 8 to 12 times in 24 hours; supplemental bottles in first 2 to 3 weeks may cause nipple confusion and interfere with adequate supply.
   b. Positions: cradle, football, side lying.
   c. Correct latch: mouth wide open, tongue under nipple; as much of areola as possible in mouth.
   d. Coordinated suck-swallow.
   e. Break suction before detaching by gentle compression of infant's cheeks and finger in mouth.
   f. Adequate intake: observe elimination (six to eight wet diapers and one stool in 24 hours), satisfaction between feedings.
3. Encourage air-drying of nipples after breast-feeding.
4. Teach daily cleansing of nipples with clear water (natural antiseptic lysosome cleanses as well).
5. Teach prevention/resolution of sore nipples: correct latch, position changes.
6. Teach prevention/resolution of engorgement: frequent emptying of breasts through nursing every 2 to 3 hours; softening through manual expression or pumping of foremilk; application of warm packs before nursing and ice packs between feedings; analgesics as ordered.
7. Teach resolution of cracked nipples: application of expressed breast milk or pure lanolin after feedings.

Evaluation

Lactating woman verbalizes understanding of lactation, feeds newborn effectively, demonstrates correct care of breasts, demonstrates correct technique in using breast pump.

Goal 3 Client will verbalize knowledge of nutrition to meet own needs for recovery and lactation.

Implementation

1. Obtain diet history.
2. Compare intake to national recommendations from food pyramid and suggest options for deficiencies.
3. Encourage nutritious snacks and increased fluids.
4. Advise lactating mothers to take in adequate protein, calcium, iron, phosphorus, and vitamins (see Table 4-8).
5. Advise increased intake of iron-rich foods for mothers with low hemoglobin or history of hemorrhage.

Evaluation

Client verbalizes understanding of dietary recommendations; selects foods from the food pyramid to meet recovery and lactation needs.

Goal 4 Client will be knowledgeable about rest and exercise in the immediate postpartal period.

Implementation

1. Encourage early ambulation to prevent thrombophlebitis and constipation. NOTE: If client had regional or spinal anesthesia, maintain recumbent position as ordered; accompany mother when ambulating the first time in case of syncope.
2. Restrict dangling of feet for long periods while sitting on side of bed (constricts popliteal arteries and veins).
3. Encourage frequent rest periods during day with minimal interruptions.
4. Teach postpartum exercises to strengthen muscles of back, pelvic floor, and abdomen; Kegel or pelvic-floor exercises increase vaginal tone.
5. Advise client to wait 6 weeks before resuming strenuous activities.

Evaluation

Client ambulates safely, takes several rest periods during the day; performs postpartum exercises correctly.

Goal 5 Parents will continue to bond and attach to the newborn.

Implementation

1. Encourage physical closeness between newborn and parents; facilitate eye-to-eye contact and an en face position.
2. Encourage physical examination: exploration with fingertips/palms, touching, and stroking.
3. Compare newborn's likeness to and differences from other family members.
4. Encourage addressing newborn by name.
5. Explain normal newborn appearance, cues, and responses.
6. Allow parents to verbalize their feelings, concerns, and questions about newborn.
7. Stay with parents during initial feeding and care activities as needed.
8. Provide positive reinforcement of parenting abilities.

Evaluation

Parents exhibit bonding/attachment behaviors (e.g., gaze at, cuddle, fondle, talk to newborn); make positive statements about newborn, demonstrate increasing confidence in caring for newborn.

Goal 6 Client will discuss conflicts about role changes.

Implementation

1. Explain that conflicts are common.
   a. Independence vs. dependence
   b. Idealized vs. realistic role
   c. Love vs. resentment of newborn
   d. Self-fulfillment vs. motherhood
   e. Love for significant other vs. love for newborn
2. Promote maternal psychologic adaptation.
   a. Listen to mother and help her to interpret events of labor and delivery.
   b. Clarify any misconceptions about the birth experience.
   c. Encourage rooming-in with newborn.
   d. Obtain information for evaluating the future parent-child relationship (i.e., plans to integrate newborn into family).
   e. Act as a role model in assisting the mother with maternal tasks.

Evaluation

Client discusses conflicts about maternal role; asks questions; shares feelings and concerns about caring for baby and incorporating newborn into family.

Goal 7 Parents will verbalize understanding about home care of mother and newborn.

Implementation

1. Provide discharge planning and teaching information about
   a. Normal uterine involution
   b. Lochia: may last up to 3 to 6 weeks
   c. Perineal healing: episiotomy sutures absorb in about 3 weeks
   d. Maintaining lactation
   e. Expected weight loss
   f. Changes in abdominal wall
   g. Diaphoresis common in first 2 to 3 weeks ("night sweats")
   h. Return of menses and ovulation (if mother not nursing, menses return within 6 to 12 weeks; if nursing, menses returns within 4 to 18 months; no menses while mother is exclusively breast-feeding)
2. Teach maternal self-care, needs (e.g., rest, sleep, nutrition, and adequate fluids); proceed slowly with activities.
3. Instruct to report any of the following:
   a. Temperature above 100.4° C
   b. Reverse in trend in lochia characteristics or passage of large clots
   c. Signs of infection: bladder, uterus, episiotomy, breasts
   d. Pain in calf
   e. Signs of pregnancy-induced hypertension
4. Discuss and demonstrate newborn care (see p. 367).
5. Provide opportunity for client to care for newborn in hospital.
6. Review approaches to manage sibling rivalry: extra attention and special times needed for other children.
7. Discuss sexual adjustment; encourage open communication between partners.
   a. Sexual intercourse may be resumed after cessation of lochia and when comfort permits (except if hematoma or infection); physician may suggest delay until after postpartal examination.
   b. Breast-feeding mothers may experience decreased vaginal lubrication or breasts leaking/spurting milk during orgasm.
   c. Fatigue and hormonal changes may influence desires.
   d. Altered body image may affect satisfaction.
8. Discuss family planning.
   a. Evaluate goals (time desired until next conception).
   b. Review methods (Table 4-2).
      1. breast-feeding is not a form of contraception unless used exclusively without supplementary bottles and solid foods
      2. barrier methods provide protection against early postpartum infection
      3. diaphragms must be refitted after delivery as weight changes
      4. oral contraceptives may affect lactation or harm newborn
   c. Facilitate decision making.
9. Review need for follow-up care.
   a. Home visit by RN if possible
   b. Visit to office or clinic
   c. Referral (e.g. social service; support group)

Evaluation

Parents describe and demonstrate skills for maternal self-care, newborn care; identify reportable danger signs; describe plans to manage sibling rivalry and altered sexuality; identify choices for family planning and keep appointment for follow-up care.

Application of the Nursing Process to the High-Risk Postpartal Client

ASSESSMENT

1. Risk factors in pregnancy, labor, and delivery
2. Potential/actual problems following delivery

ANALYSIS/NURSING DIAGNOSIS

1. Safe, effective care environment
   a. Risk for injury
   b. Risk for infection
   c. Knowledge deficit
2. Physiologic integrity
   a. Interrupted breast-feeding
   b. Fluid volume deficit
   c. Impaired gas exchange
3. Psychosocial integrity
   a. Fear
   b. Body-image disturbance
   c. Ineffective individual coping
4. Health promotion/maintenance
   a. Self-care deficit
   b. Altered family process
   c. Risk for altered parent-infant attachment

PLANNING, IMPLEMENTATION, AND EVALUATION

Goal Client will be free from undetected problems; will maintain physiologic and psychosocial integrity.

Implementation

1. Teach client normal postpartal adaptation.
2. Observe for actual/potential problems in immediate post-partal period (e.g., signs of developing hemorrhage/hematoma, infection).
3. Administer treatment or medication as ordered.
4. Instruct on reportable signs at discharge.
5. Reinforce importance of postpartal check-up.

Evaluation

Abnormal findings are identified early; treatment is effective; client is empowered to monitor self and access to necessary care.

SELECTED HEALTH PROBLEMS IN THE POSTPARTAL PERIOD

POSTPARTUM HEMORRHAGE

1. Definition: postpartum bleeding of more than 500 ml after delivery
2. Incidence: third highest cause of maternal mortality
3. Predisposing factors
   a. *Uterine atony:* lack of uterine muscle tone often associated with
      1. conditions that overdistend the uterus
         a. delivery of a large infant
         b. multiple gestation
         c. hydramnios
      2. multiparity
      3. use of deep general anesthesia
      4. premature separation of the placenta
      5. obstetric trauma

      6. abnormal labor pattern (e.g., prolonged labor)
      7. oxytocin stimulation or augmentation during labor
      8. overmassage of an already contracted uterus
      9. low platelet levels secondary to PIH
   b. *Lacerations:* more common after operative obstetrics
      1. perineum
      2. vagina
      3. cervix
   c. *Retained placenta fragments:* predicted by Duncan mechanism or manual removal by physician; associated with
      1. entrapment by uterine constriction ring
      2. premature uterine contraction by massage or ergot administration
      3. abnormal adherence of all or part of placenta to uterine wall (e.g., placenta accreta)
4. Prognosis: 14% of all maternal deaths are from hemorrhagic complications
5. Types
   a. *Early* postpartum hemorrhage occurs within the first 24 hours after birth; incidence is 1 in 200 births
   b. *Late* postpartum hemorrhage occurs between the second day and sixth week postpartum; incidence is 1 in 1000 births; more common in women with history of abortions or uterine bleeding during pregnancy

Nursing Process

ASSESSMENT

1. Inspect placenta to determine intactness.
2. Evaluate vaginal bleeding after delivery.
   a. Bleeding may be slow and continuous (most common) or rapid and profuse.
   b. Blood may escape from the vagina or accumulate in the uterus or maternal tissues.
   c. Bleeding from a laceration often appears bright red in presence of a well-contracted uterus.
   d. Blood may contain large clots.
3. Palpate fundus for firmness, height, and position.
4. Recognize signs of shock; see Shock, p. 129.
5. Assess bladder distention.
6. Assess any unusual pelvic discomfort or backache.

ANALYSIS/NURSING DIAGNOSIS (see right)

PLANNING, IMPLEMENTATION, AND EVALUATION

Goal Client will be free from undetected hemorrhage and shock; will have blood volume restored; will regain homeostasis; will understand discharge teaching.

Implementation

1. Remain with the client.
2. Massage boggy fundus gently but firmly, cupping uterus between two hands; avoid overmassage.
3. Administer oxytocic agents in fourth stage of labor as prescribed by physician (Tables 4-17 and 4-18).
4. Monitor closely during acute phase of hemorrhage (e.g., vital signs, intake, output, level of consciousness, fundal firmness, bleeding, and central venous pressure [CVP]).
5. Encourage frequent voiding.

6. Replace fluid and blood as ordered.
7. Administer O₂ through face mask at 4 to 7 L.
8. Maintain asepsis because hemorrhage predisposes to infection.
9. Give prophylactic antibiotics as ordered.
10. Support significant other.
11. Assist with preoperative preparation (for surgical removal of retained placental fragments), suturing as indicated.
12. Before discharge, teach client signs of possible late hemorrhage (critical because of increasingly early discharge).
13. Counsel client to increase iron in diet; iron supplements; administer iron dextran (Imferon) if ordered.
14. Arrange for follow-up care.

Evaluation
Client is free from hemorrhage or complications of excessive blood loss; regains homeostasis; lists signs and symptoms of late hemorrhage; identifies foods high in iron or need for iron supplement; agrees to planned follow-up care.

✖ HEMATOMA

1. Definition: a collection of blood, often on the external genitalia, as a result of injury to a blood vessel during spontaneous or forceps delivery; most common site of a genital tract hematoma is the lateral wall in the area of the ischial spines
2. Incidence: occurs once in every 300 to 1500 births
3. Predisposing factors: prolonged pressure of fetal head on vaginal mucosa; forceps delivery

Nursing Process

ASSESSMENT
1. Complaints of severe perineal pain or intense rectal pressure
2. Visible large mass at the introitus or labia majora
3. Bruising, ecchymosis
4. Pain on palpation
5. Inability to void because of pressure of hematoma on the urethra
6. Signs and symptoms of shock in presence of well-contracted uterus and no visible vaginal bleeding

ANALYSIS/NURSING DIAGNOSIS (see p. 353)

PLANNING, IMPLEMENTATION, AND EVALUATION

Goal Client will experience minimal discomfort while the hematoma is treated/absorbed.

Implementation
1. Monitor changes/enlargement of hematoma.
2. Notify physician of condition.
3. Promote general comfort.
   a. Apply cold to site.
   b. Administer analgesics as ordered.
4. Prepare woman for surgery, if indicated, to evacuate the hematoma.
5. Assess for further vaginal bleeding, signs of DIC.

Evaluation
Client's hematoma does not enlarge or is evacuated; client experiences only minimal discomfort; is free from excessive bleeding, DIC.

✖ PULMONARY EMBOLUS

1. Definition: the passage of a thrombus, often originating in one of the uterine or other pelvic veins, into a lung, where it obstructs the circulation of blood; usually occurs at end of first week postpartum
2. Predisposing factors
   a. Infection
   b. Hemorrhage
   c. Thrombosis
3. Prognosis: maternal mortality high with large and undetected clots (refer to Pulmonary Embolus, p. 147)

✖ PUERPERAL INFECTION

1. Definition: any inflammatory process in the genital tract within 28 days after abortion or delivery of a newborn
2. Incidence: associated with 4% to 8% of maternal deaths
3. Criterion: an elevation in temperature to 38°C (100.4°F) for two consecutive days, with the onset after the first 24 hours postpartum
4. Origin
   a. *Endogenous:* infection from within or other preexisting infection/sexually transmitted disease
   b. *Exogenous:* infection introduced by others, poor technique, or both
5. Predisposing factors
   a. Debilitating antepartal conditions
      1. anemia
      2. malnutrition
   b. Debilitating conditions related to labor and delivery
      1. prolonged labor after membranes rupture
      2. soft-tissue trauma or hemorrhage
      3. operative obstetric procedures (e.g., cesarean delivery, forceps delivery)
      4. invasive procedures (e.g., multiple vaginal examinations, internal fetal monitoring
      5. prolonged labor resulting in weakness and exhaustion of client
   c. Retention of placental fragments
6. Prognosis
   a. One of three leading causes of maternal mortality
   b. Outcome improved with early detection and appropriate medical and nursing management
7. Types of infection
   a. Localized lesions of perineum, vulva, and vagina
   b. Endometritis: localized infection of lining of uterus, usually beginning at placental site
   c. Local infection may extend through venous circulation, resulting in
      1. infectious thrombophlebitis
      2. septicemia
   d. Local infection may extend through lymphatic vessels to cause
      1. peritonitis
      2. parametritis
      3. salpingitis

8. Bacterial causative agents
   a. *Streptococcus hemolyticus:* virulent, early onset, and rapid progression; less common today
   b. *E. coli*
   c. *Staphylococcus aureus*
   d. *Chlamydia trachomatis*
   e. Mixed aerobic-anaerobic infection: low virulence, two or more species of bacteria present

Nursing Process

ASSESSMENT

1. Temperature greater than 38°C (100.4°F) after the first 24 hours
2. Abnormal lochia
   a. Remains rubra longer or becomes brown
   b. May have foul odor
   c. Scant or profuse in amount
3. Tachycardia (may be 100 to 120 beats per minute)
4. Delayed involution
   a. Fundal height does not descend as rapidly
   b. Uterus may feel larger and softer
   c. Client may have pain or tenderness over the uterus
5. Pain, tenderness, or inflammation of perineum
6. Malaise
7. Fatigue
8. Chills
9. Abnormal lab results: leukocytosis, increased sedimentation rate
10. Calf tenderness, positive Homans' sign

ANALYSIS/NURSING DIAGNOSIS (see p. 353)
PLANNING, IMPLEMENTATION, AND EVALUATION

Goal Client will be free from local or systemic infection; will have infection treated early; will participate in prescribed treatment; will have homeostasis restored.

Implementation

1. Determine source of infection and take measures to prevent further problems.
2. Use standard precautions and body substance isolation for blood, body fluids, nonintact skin, and mucous membranes.
3. Obtain specimens for culture and sensitivity as ordered.
4. Take vital signs frequently.
5. Isolate client if indicated by causative organism (may be separated from newborn).
6. Encourage semi-Fowler's position to facilitate lochia drainage.
7. Change perineal pads frequently.
8. Reinforce perineal hygiene techniques; encourage hand washing.
9. Provide comfort measures (e.g., sitz baths to promote perineal healing).
10. Administer analgesics as ordered.
11. Maintain adequate hydration with oral or intravenous fluids (2000 to 4000 ml per day).
12. Administer antibiotic therapy as prescribed by physician.
13. Administer oxytocic medications as prescribed by physician.
14. Encourage high-caloric fluid intake; high-protein diet.
15. Inform client about condition of newborn if separated.
16. Maintain bed rest with leg elevated for suspected thrombophlebitis; give anticoagulants if prescribed.

Evaluation

Client responds to treatment for infection (e.g., falling temperature, negative cultures, relief of symptoms, increasing energy).

✖ MASTITIS

1. Definition: an inflammation of the breast as a result of an infection, usually caused by *Staphylococcus aureus* or *Streptococcus hemolyticus;* mainly seen in breast-feeding mothers; 10% of women with mastitis develop an abscess.
2. Predisposing factors include nipple fissure, erosion of the areola, overdistention, milk stasis.
3. Prognosis: condition is generally preventable; prompt and appropriate treatment with antibiotic therapy significantly decreases maternal morbidity.

Nursing Process

ASSESSMENT

1. Blocked milk duct: hard, warm, reddened, and tender site; often in the outer, upper quadrant of the breast
2. Mastitis
   a. Fever
   b. Breast may have red area, be warm to touch, and be tender; lump may be visible
   c. Pain, chills
   d. Engorgement
   e. Axillary adenopathy
   f. Tachycardia often present (usual time of occurrence is 2 to 4 weeks after delivery)
   g. Headache

ANALYSIS/NURSING DIAGNOSIS (see p. 353)
PLANNING, IMPLEMENTATION, AND EVALUATION

Goal Client will be free from undetected mastitis; will participate in treatment to prevent further complications; will maintain lactation, if desired.

Implementation

1. Administer antibiotics as ordered by physician.
2. Promote comfort.
   a. Suggest supportive bra.
   b. Apply local heat or cold.
   c. Administer analgesics as prescribed by physician.
3. Maintain lactation in breast-feeding mothers.
   a. Regular nursing of infant (controversial, will vary with physician)
   b. Manual expression of breast milk
   c. Use of a breast pump
4. Encourage good hand washing and breast hygiene.
5. Offer emotional support.
6. Prepare client for incision and drainage of abscess if necessary.

Evaluation

Client is free from symptoms of mastitis; maintains milk supply; resumes lactation as able.

Table 4-23 Postpartum depression

Types	Characteristics	Incidence
Blues	Mild, brief; originates 2-10 days after birth	80%
Atypical	Moderate, longer lasting; physical as well as psychologic symptoms	10%
Psychosis	Severe; may be long-term risks of suicide, infanticide	0.5%-3.0%

✣ POSTPARTUM CYSTITIS

1. Definition: an infection of the bladder occurring in about 5% of postpartum women; usually caused by coliform bacteria
2. Predisposing factors: trauma to the bladder during vaginal delivery or cesarean birth; catheterization during or after labor

✣ PSYCHOLOGIC MALADAPTATIONS

Postpartum depression occurs in some new mothers; physical as well as psychologic symptoms may be evident. It is usually benign and self-limiting but can last for years in its most severe form.
1. Definitions on continuum (Table 4-23)
   a. *Postpartum blues:* mild and brief; originates 2 to 10 days after birth; affects up to 80% of new mothers
   b. *Atypical depression:* moderate and longer lasting; more disabling; affects 10% or more of new mothers
   c. *Psychosis:* severe and long-term risks of suicide and infanticide; affects 0.5% to 3.0% of new mothers
2. Manifestations (see also Elated-Depressive Behavior, p. 46)
   a. Feelings of sadness, guilt, or irritation
   b. Tearfulness, crying
   c. Decreased energy, decision-making ability
   d. Insomnia
   e. Decreased appetite, anorexia
3. Theories of etiology
   a. Hormonal changes
   b. Fatigue, discomfort
   c. Immaturity
   d. Sensory deprivation or overload

   e. Nonsupportive environment
   f. Unrealistic expectations of maternal role

Nursing Process
ASSESSMENT
1. Behavioral and psychologic responses (e.g., depression, anger, blues that persist)
2. Maladaptations in attachment
3. Delusions, hallucinations
ANALYSIS/NURSING DIAGNOSIS (see p. 353)
PLANNING, IMPLEMENTATION, AND EVALUATION

> **Goal** Client and family will recognize common postpartum psychologic changes; client will be free from psychologic maladaptation or psychosis postpartum; will seek medical care and will participate in treatment; will function adequately as a parent.

Implementation
1. Recognize early signs of problems.
2. Refer client to obstetrician to evaluate physiologic status.
3. Support positive parenting behaviors.
4. Refer client to resource: psychiatrist, nurse psychotherapist, pediatrician, support group, public health nurse.
Evaluation
Client and family list expected emotional changes; report deviations in normal responses; client receives prompt treatment and support for maladaptive responses or psychosis; shows signs of attachment to newborn and increased feelings of self-worth.

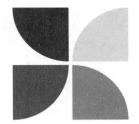

Newborn Care

THE NORMAL NEWBORN

1. Definition: full-term newborn
2. Gestational age: 38 to 42 weeks; between 10th and 90th percentiles on growth curves
3. A newborn may have a higher-than-normal risk of morbidity and mortality related to a maternal condition during the antepartal or intrapartal period (e.g., bleeding; poor nutritional status; maternal drug, smoking, and alcohol history; hypertension; infection; diabetes; complications of labor and birth; and use of anesthetic/analgesic)
4. Risk of morbidity and mortality may also be increased; related to problems at birth or to the transition from intrauterine to extrauterine life

General Characteristics

1. Transition period
   a. Phase one: first period of reactivity
      1. birth through first 30 minutes (initial alert stage)
         a. awake, active
         b. strong sucking reflex
         c. rapid and irregular respirations and heart rate
         d. falling body temperature
      2. sleep period follows
   b. Phase two: second period of reactivity
      1. onset from end of first sleep period for 2 to 5 hours
      2. awakens; alert; mild cyanosis may occur
      3. frequent gagging with mucus regurgitation
      4. frequently passes first meconium stool
2. Stabilization with wakeful periods about every 3 to 4 hours
3. Behavior
   a. Sleeping and waking (Brazelton, 1973)
      1. individuality from birth: each normal newborn has unique, *usually predictable* behavioral responses in the first days of life
      2. state patterns
         a. pattern is a predictor of newborn's receptivity and cognitive response to stimuli
         b. sleep-wake states (alternate periods of physiologic state and behavior)
            - deep sleep
            - light sleep
            - drowsiness
            - quiet alert (best for learning)
            - active alert (high activity level)
            - crying

3. unique ability to "comfort" self by finger or thumb sucking (self-quieting) and to shut out stimuli (habituation)
   b. Sensory responses to environmental stimuli
      1. *sight*: response to visual stimulation
         a. pupillary and blink reflexes present
         b. vision present but limited; optimal range for visual acuity is 7 to 8 inches
         c. some degree of color and pattern discrimination: prefers dim colors, contrasting patterns, medium complexity, reflecting objects
         d. can fixate and track for short distance to midline; greatest ability is in first hour after birth
         e. focuses on human face
      2. *hearing*: response to auditory stimulation
         a. *in utero*: responds to music and to sound of mother's voice
         b. *newborn*: within hours of birth, responds to sound by generalized activity depending on reactive state
            - loud sounds elicit Moro's reflex
            - low-frequency sounds elicit decreased motor activity; high-frequency sounds elicit alerting reaction
      3. *taste*: response to feeding
         a. differentiates between sweet and sour and bitter
         b. vigor of sucking may vary with arousal
      4. *smell*: response to olfactory stimulation
         a. present as soon as nose is cleared of mucus and amniotic fluid
         b. sensitive, discriminates (e.g., odor of mother's breast milk)
      5. *touch*: response to tactile stimulation
         a. well developed; face, hands and soles most sensitive
         b. reacts to painful and soothing stimuli
4. Posture
   a. May assume prenatal position
   b. Assumes partially flexed position
   c. Resists having extremities extended
5. Size (compared for length, weight, and weeks of gestation on growth curves)
   a. Length
      1. normal ranges 48 to 53 cm (19 to 21 inches)
      2. average: 50 cm (20 inches)
      3. rapid growth in first 6 months

b. Weight
1. normal range 2500 to 4000 g (5 lb 8 oz to 8 lb 13 oz)
2. average weight 3400 g (7 lb 8 oz)
3. 10% of birth weight may be lost in first few days of life because of
a. minimal intake of nutrients
b. loss of excess fluid
c. passage of meconium
4. regains birth weight within first 2 weeks
c. Head circumference
1. normal range 33 to 35 cm (13 to 14 inches)
2. approximately 1 to 2 cm more than chest circumference after resolution of molding
3. essential assessment for suspected hydrocephalus
d. Chest circumference
1. normal range 30 to 33 cm (12 to 13 inches)
2. shape and measurements change as newborn grows
e. Symmetry
1. face symmetric
2. ears symmetric; placed at level of outer canthus of eyes
3. bilateral, asynchronous movements of extremities
6. Vital signs
a. Blood pressure: normal range 60 to 80/40 to 50 mm Hg
b. Pulse: normal range 120 to 160 per minute (apical) if newborn is quiet
c. Respirations
1. normal range 30 to 60 per minute
2. irregular and shallow
3. diaphragmatic and abdominal breathing normal
4. periodic apnea (<15 seconds) may be present
d. Temperature
1. normal axillary range 36.4°C to 37.2°C (97.5°F to 99°F)
2. temperature should stabilize within several hours of birth

Specific Body Parts: Usual Findings and Common Variations

1. Skin
a. Texture: smooth, elastic
b. Color
1. bright red at birth, turning to pink; ethnic variations
2. normal changes
a. localized cyanosis of extremities (acrocyanosis): peripheral circulation not well established
b. mottling (transient discoloration of skin when exposed to decreased temperature) resulting from vasoconstriction, lack of fat and hypoxia
3. physiologic jaundice (icterus neonatorum)
a. yellow discoloration of newborn skin and sclera often appearing 48 to 72 hours after birth (Refer to Neonatal Jaundice, p. 368)
b. common, appearing in 50% to 70% of newborns
c. disappears in 7 to 10 days

c. Characteristics
1. Vernix caseosa
a. white, odorless, cheeselike substance on skin, usually found in folds of axillae, groin
b. produced in utero; diminishes close to term
c. is gradually absorbed or washed off after birth
2. Lanugo
a. fine, downy hair on shoulders, back, upper arms, forehead, and cheeks
b. gradually disappears close to term
3. Desquamation
a. dry peeling of skin, particularly on palms and soles
b. requires no treatment
c. more pronounced in postmature newborn
d. Variations
1. Milia
a. pinpoint white papules on cheeks, across bridge of nose, or on chin; caused by blocked sebaceous glands
b. require no treatment
c. disappear in a few weeks
2. Erythema toxicum (newborn rash)
a. pink papular rash anywhere on the body, appearing within 24 to 48 hours of birth
b. harmless and disappears within a few days
c. must be differentiated from rashes found in infections
3. Mongolian spots
a. areas of grayish-blue pigmentation most often found on buttocks and sacrum; increased frequency in specific racial groups
b. may disappear by school age
4. Nevi (stork bite)
a. red spots found on back of neck and eyelids
b. usually disappear spontaneously between first and second years of life
5. Birthmarks
a. vary in type and location (e.g., port-wine stain, strawberry mark)
b. may or may not disappear with age, depending on type and location
2. Head
a. Appears round and symmetric by 2 to 3 days of life; full movement to right and left, up and down; may be covered by silky hair in varying amounts
b. Molding: the shaping of the fetal head to accommodate passage through the birth canal as a result of overriding of the cranial bones; the head will return to its normal shape in about 2 to 3 days
c. Cephalhematoma: a collection of blood between the periosteum and the bone of the skull
1. caused by rupture of blood vessels from pressure during the birth process
2. swelling usually severe but does not cross suture lines
3. spontaneously resolves in 3 to 6 weeks
d. Caput succedaneum
1. localized, edematous area of the scalp, usually caused by birth process

2. extends across suture lines
3. is absorbed and disappears in 3-4 days
e. Fontanels (soft spots) (Fig. 4-21)
  1. anterior
    a. diamond shaped, palpable
    b. 3 to 4 cm long, 2 to 3 cm wide
    c. found between frontal and parietal bones
    d. closes within 18 months
  2. posterior
    a. triangular, usually palpable
    b. 1 to 2 cm
    c. found between occipital and parietal bones
    d. closes within 3 months
3. Eyes
  a. Appearance
    1. blue or grey-blue/black
    2. bright and clear
    3. pupils equal in size
    4. eyes evenly placed on face
    5. lacrimation in 50% of neonates not evident until 2 to 4 weeks old
  b. Movement
    1. to all directions
    2. poor neuromuscular control
  c. Common variations
    1. subconjunctival hemorrhage: red spot on sclera, rupture of small capillaries during delivery; will be absorbed in about 2 weeks
    2. chemical conjunctivitis: inflammation with discharge, resulting from reaction of eye prophylaxis (must be differentiated from infectious process)
  d. Vision (refer to Sensory responses, p. 357)
4. Nose
  a. Shape: varies; may appear flattened because of delivery process
  b. Placement: evenly placed in relation to eyes and mouth
  c. Nares: bilateral patency; newborns are nose-breathers (without flaring)
  d. Sneezing common
5. Mouth
  a. Lips: appear equal on both sides of facial midline; symmetry of movement
  b. Tongue
    1. in midline; moves freely in all directions
    2. size proportional to mouth
    3. color pink (varies with ethnic group); white, cheesy coating may indicate thrush (related to maternal candida vaginal infection)
  c. Palate: intact and highly arched
  d. Epstein's pearls: small epithelial cysts on hard palate or gums; will disappear in 1 to 2 weeks
  e. Saliva: small quantity present
6. Ears
  a. Well-formed cartilage by term; recoil rapidly; may be flattened against skull because of pressure during birth
  b. Placement: same level and position on both sides of head; top of pinnae in line with outer canthus of eyes (low-set ears are associated with trisomy 13 or 18 and renal agenesis)
  c. Hearing: refer to Sensory responses, p. 357
7. Neck
  a. Appears short and thick; head moves freely
  b. Skin folds present; no webbing
  c. Clavicles should be intact; crepitus indicates fracture
8. Chest
  a. Shoulders: sloping; width greater than length
  b. Chest movements: bilateral expansion equal with respiration; no retractions

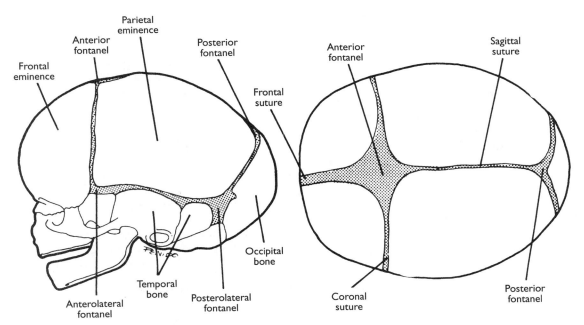

Fig. 4-21 Bones, fontanels, and sutures of newborn's skull.

c. Breath sounds: loud and equal bilaterally; clear on crying

d. Cough reflex: absent; appears by second or third day of life

e. Heart: rhythm regular, normal rate; usually heard to left of midclavicular space at third or fourth interspace; may have functional murmurs (refer to p. 358 for normal vital sign values)

f. Breasts
    1. flat; nipples symmetric; breast-tissue diameter greater than 5 mm
    2. breast engorgement common in both sexes; occurs by third day of life and may last up to 2 weeks; may have some nipple discharge resulting from maternal hormonal influence in utero and subsequent withdrawal after birth

9. Abdomen
    a. Prominent: cylindrical; movements synchronous with respirations
    b. Umbilical cord stump
        1. two arteries and one vein apparent at birth, surrounded by Wharton's jelly; clamped at birth
        2. cord begins drying within 1 to 2 hours after birth, shed by 7 to 10 days after birth
        3. protrusion of umbilicus possible; assess for umbilical hernia
    c. Diastasis recti (separation of rectus muscles): common in some races and preterm neonates
    d. Bowel sounds: audible
    e. Liver palpable 1 to 3 cm below right costal margin
    f. Femoral pulses: palpable and equal bilaterally

10. Genitalia
    a. Female
        1. labia majora cover labia minora; symmetric, slightly edematous
        2. clitoris enlarged
        3. vaginal tag (hymen) may be evident
        4. a mucoid, vaginal discharge is common
        5. pseudomenstruation: blood-tinged discharge is normal
        6. some vernix caseosa may be between labia
    b. Male
        1. urethral meatus evident at tip of penis
        2. foreskin covers glans; prepuce not totally retractable; forcible retraction is unnecessary for hygiene and may cause adhesions
        3. extensive rugae on scrotum
        4. testes descended and palpable bilaterally in scrotal sac; if not, check inguinal, femoral, or abdominal areas for undescended testes

11. Buttocks and anus
    a. Buttocks: symmetric; anus patent
    b. Gluteal folds: symmetric; asymmetry associated with hip dislocation

12. Extremities and trunk
    a. Muscle tone: good; equal bilaterally
    b. Position: extremities slightly flexed; full range of motion
    c. Arms and legs: arms equal in length; legs equal in length; legs shorter than arms

d. Five digits on each hand and foot; freely movable, nails present

e. Normal palmar crease (simian line indicative of Down syndrome)

f. Fat pads and creases covering anterior two thirds of soles of infant's feet

g. Spine: straight and flat (prone position) and intact

Systems Adaptations

1. Neuromuscular: normal neonatal reflexes
    a. Sucking: newborns tend to suck any object that comes in contact with lips; essential for nutritional intake, oral satisfaction, begins to disappear at 12 months
    b. Rooting: newborns tend to turn head in direction of stimulus (object touching cheek or mouth); usually disappears at 3 to 4 months but may persist up to 12 months
    c. Spontaneous reflexes
        1. swallowing: usually follows sucking
        2. gagging: lifelong reflex
        3. yawning: lifelong reflex
        4. sneezing: lifelong reflex
        5. hiccoughing: lifelong reflex
        6. stretching
    d. Moro: newborns tend to symmetrically extend both arms and legs and then draw them up in normal flexed position in response to sudden movement or loud noise; most significant reflex indicative of CNS status; disappears by 6 months; strongest during first 2 months
    e. Grasp
        1. palmar grasp; newborn's tendency to grasp an examiner's finger when palm is stimulated; lessens at 3 to 4 months
        2. plantar grasp: newborn's tendency to curl toes downward when sole of foot is stimulated; lessens at 8 months
    f. Tonic neck: newborns tend to assume a fencer's position when head is turned to one side; the extremities on the same side extend, while flexion occurs on the opposite side; response sometimes more dominant in leg than arm; disappears at 3 to 4 months
    g. Stepping or walking: newborns tend when held upright to take steps in response to feet touching a hard surface; disappears at 4 weeks
    h. Babinski's: newborns tend to hyperextend toes with dorsiflexion of big toe when one side of sole is stimulated from heel upward across ball of foot; disappears at 1 year
    i. Motor function: head may be maintained erect for short periods of time; head lag less than 45 degrees; movement of extremities may be jerky

2. Cardiorespiratory
    a. Circulatory adaptations occurring after birth and ligation of umbilical cord (Fig. 4-22)
        1. closure of ductus arteriosus, foramen ovale, and ductus venosus
            a. caused by changes in pressure in the first days of life
            b. allows oxygenation of all body systems
        2. closure of umbilical vessels after clamping of cord

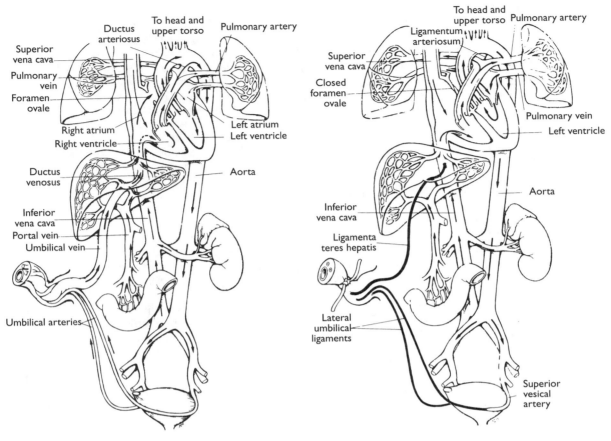

Fig. 4-22   Fetal circulation.

b. Pulses (reflect systemic circulation)
   1. femoral, brachial; easily palpable
   2. radial, temporal; more difficult to palpate
c. Respirations
   1. initiation of respirations
      a. first breath; inflation of lungs in response to increased Pco_2 and lower pH (chemical factors); tactile and sudden chilling (thermal factor); questionable impact of tactile stimulation
      b. reduction of pulmonary-vascular resistance
      c. increased pulmonary blood flow
      d. recoil of chest causing replacement of fluids
      e. surfactant reduces alveolar surface tension
   2. respiratory secretions may be abundant
   3. may be irregular with short periods of apnea (<15 seconds)
d. Blood pressure
   1. highest immediately after birth; at lowest level at 3 hours
   2. crying and moving cause changes in BP (up to 20 mm Hg)

3. Hematologic
a. Blood values (venous samples): average ranges for a normal, full-term newborn
   1. hemoglobin: 14 to 20 g/dl (reflects oxygenation of tissues); broken down to bilirubin
   2. hematocrit: 42% to 61%
   3. RBC: 5 to 7.5 million/mm^3
   4. WBC: approximately 20,000/mm^3 (10,000 to 30,000/mm^3)
   5. platelets: 100,000 to 280,000
   6. blood volume: 78 to 98 ml/kg depending on cord clamping
b. Leukocytosis: normal; related to birth trauma
c. Fetal RBCs: have short life (80 to 100 days); hemolyzed RBCs increase bilirubin levels
d. Coagulation
   1. inability to synthesize vitamin K because of absence of intestinal flora normal in older people
   2. supplementary injection of vitamin K (e.g., Aqua-MEPHYTON, given prophylactically to promote normal clotting) IM-thigh, vastus lateralis

4. Thermoregulation (temperature regulation)
a. Adaptive factors
   1. newborn responds to cold with increased motor activity, restlessness, increased respirations
   2. increased metabolism compensates for cold stress (newborn does not shiver)
   3. brown fat (or brown adipose tissue) is the newborn's major source of thermogenesis (2% to 6% of body weight) (located between scapulae, around kidneys, sternum, adrenals, and in the axillae); reserves are rapidly depleted with cold stress

b. Heat loss: disproportionate to adult because of large skin surface to body mass; mechanisms of heat loss include
   1. *convection:* loss of heat from body surface to cooler surrounding air (e.g., newborn placed in cool incubator)
   2. *evaporation:* loss of heat from body occurring when fluid converts to vapor (e.g., wet newborn loses heat immediately after birth in delivery room)
   3. *conduction:* transfer of heat from warm object to a cooler surface (e.g., newborn placed on a cold object)
   4. *radiation:* indirect transfer of heat from a warmer object to a cooler one (e.g., newborn loses heat to cool wall of incubator)
5. Elimination (gastrointestinal and renal)
   a. Stools: change according to feeding
      1. meconium stool: viscous, dark green or black; formed of mucus, vernix, lanugo, hormones, carbohydrates; first one usually passed within 24 to 48 hours (if no stool passed, assess for imperforate anus, intestinal obstruction)
      2. transition stools: loose, green-brown, seedy: second to sixth day
      3. breast-fed newborns: golden-yellow, mushy stools, often after each feeding
      4. bottle-fed newborns: soft, yellow-brown stools; more formed; 4 to 6 per day
   b. Stomach capacity: 50 to 60 ml; empties in about 3 hours
   c. Urination: newborn usually urinates in first 24 hours; if newborn unable to void, assess for fluid intake and distention
      1. frequency: initially 6 to 10 per day, then up to 20 per day
      2. color: pale yellow (immature kidneys cannot concentrate); may appear cloudy if decreased fluid intake
      3. uric acid excretion is high; appears as red spots on diaper ("brick spots")
6. Immunologic
   a. In utero: full-term fetus has had IgG (immunoglobulins) transferred; maternal antibodies may be present (depending on mother's immunity) for tetanus, diphtheria, pertussis, measles, mumps, rubella
   b. At birth: immunologic system immature
      1. capable of some antibody response to immunizing agents
      2. phagocytosis ineffective
      3. cannot localize infection or respond with a well-defined, recognizable inflammatory response, as can older child
      4. breast milk: contains IgA; gives immunologic protection from some infections
      5. infection may not be reflected by elevated temperature
7. Nutrition
   a. Sucks, swallows, and digests feedings; these reflexes may be weak in premature infants
   b. Digestion
      1. unable to digest complete carbohydrates because of insufficient quantities of amylase
      2. can absorb simple carbohydrates and protein
      3. fat absorption poor because of insufficient lipase
   c. Regurgitation is common
      1. cardiac sphincter is immature, nervous control of stomach incomplete
      2. newborns often spit up mucus in first 24 hours after birth
   d. Blood sugar normally 30 to 50 mg/dl (full term)
   e. Benefits from immunoglobulins, enzymes, and lactobacilli in breast milk
   f. Psychologic factors
      1. both bottle-feeding and breast-feeding can be satisfying
      2. attachment facilitated by breast-feeding
      3. stress can inhibit successful breast-feeding
   g. Initial feedings: breast milk or sterile water given after birth to assess sucking reflex and absence of structural anomalies
   h. Subsequent feedings
      1. bottle-fed newborns: q3-4h or on demand
      2. breast-fed newborns: on demand or about q2-3h; may cluster feed, then sleep for longer period
   i. Fluid needs vary with age and size of newborn; average intake of 17½ oz per day for 7-lb baby
   j. Calories: 80 to 120 cal/kg/day (birth to 5 months); most commercial formulas contain 20 calories per oz (Table 4-24)

Gestational Age Variations Based on Neuromuscular Responses and External Physical Characteristics (Fig. 4-23)

1. Preterm newborn
   a. Definition: born before 38 weeks of gestation, regardless of birth weight
   b. Etiology: associated with chronic hypertensive disease, toxemia, placenta previa, abruptio placentae, incompetent cervix, infections, smoking, multiple gestation, inadequate maternal nutrition, maternal age under 20; premature rupture of membranes
   c. General appearance: will vary with gestational age
      1. head large in proportion to body

Table 4-24 Nutritional comparison of human and cow's milk

| Nutrients | Amounts per liter | | |
	Human milk (breast)	Cow's milk* (whole)	Common formulas†
Protein (g)	10.12	32‡	15
Carbohydrate (g)	67.82§	45.4	72
Lipid	43.12	35.7	36
Calories	684.00	626.0	640

*Not given to newborns.
†Examples are Similac, Enfamil.
‡Because of the higher percentage of protein, cow's milk must be diluted to avoid kidney overload.
§Breast milk is higher in lactose, which limits pathogenic growth.

Estimation of gestational age by maturity rating
Symbols: X - 1st exam   O - 2nd exam

Neuromuscular maturity

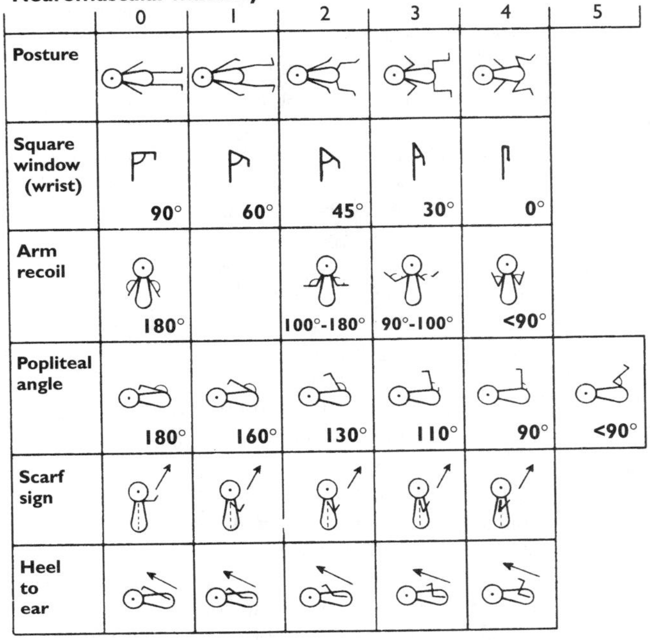

	0	1	2	3	4	5
Posture						
Square window (wrist)	90°	60°	45°	30°	0°	
Arm recoil	180°		100°-180°	90°-100°	<90°	
Popliteal angle	180°	160°	130°	110°	90°	<90°
Scarf sign						
Heel to ear						

Gestation by dates _____ wks

Birth date _____ Hour _____ am / pm
APGAR _____ 1 min _____ 5 min
Weight _____ Length _____
Head _____ Chest _____

Maturity Rating

Score	Wks
5	26
10	28
15	30
20	32
25	34
30	36
35	38
40	40
45	42
50	44

Physical maturity

	0	1	2	3	4	5
Skin	gelatinous red, transparent	smooth pink, visible veins	superficial peeling &/or rash, few veins	cracking pale area, rare veins	parchment, deep cracking, no vessels	leathery, cracked, wrinkled
Lanugo	none	abundant	thinning	bald areas	mostly bald	
Planter creases	no crease	faint red marks	anterior transverse crease only	creases ant. 2/3	creases cover entire sole	
Breast	barely percept.	flat areola, no bud	stippled areola, 1-2 mm bud	raised areola, 3-4 mm bud	full areola 5-10 mm bud	
Ear	pinna flat, stays folded	sl. curved pinna, soft with slow recoil	well-curv. pinna, soft but ready recoil	formed & firm with instant recoil	thick cartilage, ear stiff	
Genitals male	scrotum empty, no rugae		testes descending, few rugae	testes down, good rugae	testes pendulous, deep rugae	
Genitals female	prominent clitoris & labia minora		majora & minora equally prominent	majora large, minora small	clitoris & minora completely covered	

Scoring section

	1st exam=X	2nd exam=O
Estimating gest. age by maturity rating	_____ Weeks	_____ Weeks
Time of exam	Date_____ Hour_____ am/pm	Date_____ Hour_____ am/pm
Age at exam	_____ Hours	_____ Hours
Signature of examiner	_____ M.D.	_____ M.D.

Fig. 4-23 Newborn maturity rating and classification. (From Mead Johnson & Co., Evansville, Ind. Scoring section adapted from Ballard JL: *Pediatr Res* 11:374, 1977. Figures modified from Sweet AY: Classification of the low-birth-weight infant. In Klaus MH, Fanaroff AA: *Care of the high-risk infant,* Philadelphia, 1977, Saunders.

2. transparent appearance to skin
3. lack of subcutaneous fat
4. excessive lanugo
5. immature neurologic system
6. minimal flexion of extremities
7. fontanels large; sutures prominent
d. Associated problems (Table 4-25)
   1. *high mortality rate*
   2. *respiratory distress syndrome* (RDS), related to immaturity of lungs and deficiency of surfactant (NOTE: L/S ratio and presence of PG determined by amniocentesis is helpful before delivery to determine lung maturity)
   3. *infection:* low WBC count, increased polymorphonuclear cells

Table 4-25 High-risk conditions for newborns by gestational age and growth classifications

Growth class	Gestational age		
	SGA	Average	LGA
PRETERM			
Apnea of prematurity	X	X	X
Brain damage	X		
Congenital abnormalities	X	X	X
Hyperbilirubinemia	X	X	X
Hypoglycemia	X	X	X
Infection	X	X	X
Intracranial hemorrhage	X	X	X
Meconium aspiration	X		
Neonatal asphyxia	X		
Polycythemia	X		X
Pulmonary hemorrhage	X		
Respiratory distress syndrome	X	X	X
Temperature instability	X	X	X
TERM			
Brain damage	X		
Birth injuries			X
Congenital abnormalities	X		X
Hypoglycemia	X		X
Polycythemia	X		X
Infection	X		
Meconium aspiration	X		
Neonatal asphyxia	X		
Pulmonary hemorrhage	X		
Temperature instability	X		
POSTTERM			
Brain damage	X	X	X
Congenital abnormalities	X		X
Hypoglycemia	X		
Infection	X		
Meconium aspiration	X	X	X
Neonatal asphyxia	X	X	X
Polycythemia	X	X	X
Pulmonary hemorrhage	X		
Temperature instability	X		

4. *feeding problems*
   a. regurgitates food easily
   b. may aspirate because of weak or absent suck-swallow reflexes
   c. may require gavage feedings
   d. breast milk or 24-calorie/ml formula advised
5. *hypoglycemia* (glucose less than 20 mg/dl), caused by decreased glycogen and fat stores, decreased glyconeogenesis
6. *hypothermia* and cold stress, owing to poor temperature control, increased surface area for cooling, extension of extremities, lack of brown fat, lack of subcutaneous fat
7. *jaundice* because of impaired bilirubin conjugation in liver
8. *intracranial hemorrhage,* related to birth trauma or hypoxia after birth; fragility of blood vessels
9. *apnea,* related to fatigue or immaturity of respiratory mechanism
10. *oxygen therapy complications:* retrolental fibroplasia (ROP—retinopathy of prematurity); BPD—bronchopulmonary dysplasia (alveolar-bronchial necrosis)

2. Postmature newborn
   a. Definition: born after 42 weeks of gestation regardless of birth weight
   b. General appearance: related to advanced gestational age and placental insufficiency
      1. thin, long newborn
      2. dry, parchmentlike skin
      3. decreased or absent vernix
      4. little subcutaneous tissue; loose skin
      5. meconium staining of amniotic fluid (nails and skin stained yellow) related to hypoxia
      6. lanugo absent
      7. alert, wide-eyed (sign of hypoxia)
      8. nails lengthened
   c. Associated problems: higher morbidity and mortality (Table 4-25)
      1. *hypoxia:* may be related to placental insufficiency
      2. *hypoglycemia:* caused by decreased glycogen stores
      3. *postmaturity syndrome* with intrauterine asphyxia and fetal distress
      4. *polycythemia:* response to hypoxia
      5. *seizure disorders:* related to hypoxia (chronic)
      6. *cold stress* related to minimal subcutaneous fat
      7. *meconium aspiration*
3. Small-for-gestational-age (SGA) newborn
   a. Definition: significantly underweight for gestational age (i.e., birth weight at or below the 10th percentile on intrauterine growth Denver curve); also known as intrauterine growth retardation or small-for-dates newborn
   b. Etiology: associated with maternal malnutrition, pregnancy-induced hypertension, diabetes, drug addiction, alcoholism, smoking, maternal viral infections, prescribed or over-the-counter drugs, placental abnormalities or acute hypoxia, and other conditions affecting uteroplacental sufficiency

c. General appearance (varies based on symmetric or asymmetric growth retardation)
1. little subcutaneous tissue
2. loose, dry skin
3. loss of muscle mass in trunk and extremities
4. desquamation
5. length often normal, yet weight decreased
6. polycythemia: may be related to intrauterine hypoxia
7. meconium staining of nails, skin
8. appears alert because of hypoxia
d. Associated problems (see Table 4-25)
1. *intrauterine infection* if exposed to organisms while in utero
2. *asphyxia at birth:* associated with intrauterine hypoxia
3. *hypoglycemia:* caused by decreased glycogen stores and decreased glyconeogenesis (increased metabolic rate resulting from heat loss)
4. *hypothermia:* related to decreased subcutaneous tissue and fat and poor thermal regulation
5. *congenital anomalies* (10 to 20 times more frequent)
6. *respiratory distress:* often follows perinatal asphyxia
7. *hypocalcemia:* may be related to asphyxia and respiratory diseases
8. *meconium aspiration:* subsequent possible minimal brain dysfunction
4. Large-for-gestational age (LGA) newborn
a. Definition: significantly overweight for gestational age (birth weight at or above 90th percentile on intrauterine growth curve; usually over 9 lb 15 oz)
b. Etiology: unclear; may be genetic predisposition associated with multiparity and maternal diabetes; large parents; certain ethnic groups
c. General appearance
1. fat and puffy
2. may be edematous
3. poor muscle tone
d. Associated problems
1. *birth trauma* because of CPD
2. *hypoglycemia* related to lack of maternal glucose (after birth)
3. *hypocalcemia*
4. *polycythemia*
5. *congenital birth defects (especially heart)*

Application of the Nursing Process to the Normal Newborn

ASSESSMENT
1. Immediate (in delivery room, birthing room, or other setting)
a. Airway
1. patency
2. secretions: may contain mucus, blood, and amniotic fluid
b. Apgar score: provides index of infant's initial condition at 1 minute and baseline for subsequent assessment at 5 minutes; the 5-minute score is the better indicator of adaptation (Table 4-26)
1. 0 to 2: severe asphyxia, extremely poor condition
2. 3 to 6: mild to moderate asphyxia, fair condition
3. 7 to 10: mild or no distress, good condition
c. Gross appearance: appears to be free from obvious birth defects
d. Umbilical cord
1. early clamping: less possibility of placental transfusion
2. late clamping: expansion of newborn's blood volume, high systolic BP, higher Hgb, possibly greater jaundice
3. blood vessels: two arteries, one vein
2. Ongoing
a. Vital signs
b. Passage of meconium, urine, or both
c. Umbilical cord
d. Tracheoesophageal fistula or esophageal atresia, manifested by
1. cyanosis during feeding
2. immediate regurgitation
3. inability to swallow feeding
e. Parent-infant bonding

ANALYSIS/NURSING DIAGNOSIS
1. Safe, effective care environment
a. Risk for caregiver role strain
b. Diversional activity deficit
2. Physiologic integrity
a. Ineffective airway clearance
b. Ineffective thermoregulation
c. Ineffective infant feeding pattern
3. Psychosocial integrity
a. Organized infant behavior
b. Risk for altered parent-infant attachment

Table 4-26   Agar scoring chart

Sign	Score		
	0	**1**	**2**
Heart rate	Absent	Slow (below 100 beats/min)	Over 100 beats/min
Respiratory effort	Absent	Slow, irregular, weak cry	Good, strong cry
Muscle tone	Flaccid	Some flexion of extremities	Well flexed
Reflex irritability			
Catheter in nostril	No response	Grimace	Cough or sneeze
Slap to sole of foot	No response	Grimace	Cry and withdrawal of foot
Color	Blue, pale	Body pink, extremities blue	Completely pink

4. Health promotion/maintenance
   a. Effective breast-feeding
   b. Health-seeking behaviors

PLANNING, IMPLEMENTATION, AND EVALUATION

Goal 1 Newborn will adapt successfully to extra-uterine life during the immediate period after birth; will have early contact with mother/father.

Implementation

1. Facilitate the immediate establishment of respiration.
   a. Clear air passages before onset of respirations (suction with DeLee or bulb syringe).
   b. Have oxygen ready if distress develops.
   c. Assist physician with resuscitation as necessary (ratio of heartbeat to respiratory ventilation rate is 5:1).
2. Prevent hypothermia: maintain newborn's body temperature and minimize heat loss; metabolic rate and O_2 consumption are minimized.
   a. Dry rapidly.
   b. Place on mother's skin, in warmed Isolette, under radiant heater, or in warm blanket; cover head
   c. Leboyer or admission bath may be given when temperature becomes stable.
3. Promote bonding/attachment in first hour after birth.
4. Provide prophylactic treatment of eyes with a 1% silver nitrate or other antibacterial agent such as erythromycin (0.5%) for protection against ophthalmia neonatorum, which may be caused by gonococcal infection; may also be effective for chlamydial ophthalmia neonatorum.
5. Place appropriate identification bands on newborn and mother; footprint may be taken.
6. Weigh and measure newborn.
7. Administer a single dose of vitamin K IM, as ordered, to prevent hypoprothrombinemia.
8. Send cord blood to lab as ordered.

Evaluation

Newborn maintains adequate oxygenation and body temperature; bonds with parents; receives prophylactic medications; is identified, weighed, and measured.

Goal 2 Newborn will continue to maintain homeostasis free from respiratory, cardiovascular, nutritional, and elimination difficulties.

Implementation

1. Check identification on admission to nursery.
2. Monitor newborn's condition (frequency of assessment determined by condition).
   a. Assess apical pulse and respiration for 1 full minute; assess axillary temperature.
   b. Note periods of apnea (should not exceed 15 seconds); note cyanosis or distress.
   c. Use suction if mucus is excessive.
   d. Position on side to promote drainage, especially after feedings.
   e. Observe skin, sclera, mucosa color (jaundice or cyanosis).
   f. Observe for respiratory changes or fatigue during feedings.
3. Maintain adequate nutrition
   a. Assist mother with breast-feeding or bottle-feeding
   b. Weigh daily; after initial loss infant may take up to 10 days to regain birth weight
   c. Avoid routine water or supplemental feedings for breast-fed infants
4. Note time of first urination and passage of meconium; then monitor elimination.
5. Obtain blood sample for phenylketonuria (PKU) (Guthrie test).
   a. A recessive hereditary disorder characterized by deficiency in the liver enzyme phenylalanine hydroxylase that is needed for conversion of phenylalanine into tyrosine
   b. Leads to mental retardation if undetected
   c. Newborn must have protein feedings 48 hours before test is accurate; with early discharge, newborn must be retested between 48 hours and 2 weeks of age

NOTE: in some states, screening for hypothyroidism and other metabolic tests may be required.

Evaluation

Newborn has vital signs within normal range; achieves initial respiratory and cardiovascular stability; has metabolic disorders detected accurately; ingests nutritional fluids appropriate for size; voids and passes meconium.

Goal 3 Newborn will remain infection free.

Implementation

1. Prevent infections from developing in newborn and spreading within nursery and mother-baby unit.
   a. Use proper hand-washing and scrub techniques.
   b. Use standard precautions and body substance isolation for blood, body fluids, nonintact skin, and mucous membranes.
   c. Exclude personnel with known infections from caring for newborns.
   d. Instruct parents about importance of hand washing and proper technique.
   e. Isolate newborns with any signs of infection, elevated temperature, or known risk.
2. Bathe newborn and maintain newborn's personal hygiene.
   a. Use plain water on face and mild soap on body for daily care.
   b. Proceed from clean to dirty areas (i.e., eyes to face to genitals).
   c. Assess/clean newborn's cord daily with alcohol and a designated antibacterial agent.
3. Assess condition of circumcised penis: keep clean and observe for bleeding; a sterile petroleum jelly or antibiotic ointment may be applied during first 24 hours; check for voiding.

NOTE: There is much controversy about risks and benefits of circumcision. Since 1989 the American Academy of Pediatrics Task Force on Circumcision has neither condemned nor recommended routine circumcision for health/medical reasons. The task force concluded that circumcision should be an elective procedure performed only on stable neonates. Cultural/religious practices may influence decision making.

Evaluation

Newborn has stable temperature; no signs of infection; is protected from exposure to infectious agents.

> **Goal 4** Parents will verbalize an understanding of principles and techniques of newborn care; will demonstrate proper, safe care and feeding.

Implementation

1. Assess parents' knowledge and past experience with child care.
2. Offer modified or complete rooming-in.
3. Encourage new parents' involvement in newborn care (to foster bonding/attachment).
4. Demonstrate cue-response patterns in interacting with infant
5. Discuss the importance of touch and stimulation in developing trust.
6. Demonstrate techniques of bathing and daily care.
   a. Emphasize safety and asepsis.
   b. Teach bathing, diapering, clothing.
   c. Teach cord and circumcision care.
7. Reinforce knowledge of feeding
   a. Benefits of breast-feeding vs. bottle-feeding (should be discussed in antepartal classes)
   b. Frequency of feeding
   c. Amount and length of feeding
   d. Position of newborn for nursing
   e. Common feeding problems (e.g., burping, regurgitation, hiccoughs)
   f. Position on side after feeding; position on side or back for sleep to minimize risk for sudden infant death syndrome (SIDS)

Evaluation

Parents verbalize infant communication and stimulation capabilities and needs; demonstrate correct care and feeding techniques.

> **Goal 5** Parents will know what to expect at home regarding newborn's behavior, sleep patterns, stools, weight gain, feeding; will verbalize an understanding of reportable problems; will discuss adjustments of siblings.

Implementation

NOTE: Criteria for discharge teaching vary with gestational age, weight, age at discharge, general health status of newborn and mother, home environment, ages of siblings, and available resources.

1. Share common characteristics/variations of newborns.
2. Identify unique characteristics of newborn with parents and siblings.
3. Counsel on breast-feeding or formula preparation and nutrition at home.
   a. Discuss common concerns (sore nipples, supplementary feedings, expression of milk).
   b. Review methods of formula preparation, care of bottles and nipples
   c. Discuss newborn's daily needs: intake of approximately 50 calories per pound per day

d. Delay solids until 6 months.
e. Avoid cow's milk until 12 months.
f. Discuss expected weight gain (birth weight doubles by 5 to 6 months, triples by 1 year).

4. Discuss newborn behavior and development in discharge teaching.
   a. Sleep needs: average 20 hours per day with wide variations; intermittent alertness
   b. Crying: newborn's method of communicating basic needs
   c. Teach *reportable signs* of problems (e.g., constipation, diarrhea, fever, vomiting, hypothermia, hyperthermia, and behavioral changes)
   d. Refer to home health nurse for necessary care
   e. Discuss plans for health care follow-up of newborn (with clinic, physician, or nurse practitioner)
5. Counsel on sibling adjustments to newborn.

Evaluation

Parents verbalize realistic expectations of infant capabilities and behavior; express confidence in ability to care for newborn; list reportable signs; discuss plans for dealing with sibling adjustments.

Application of the Nursing Process to the Newborn at Risk

ASSESSMENT

1. Maternal risk factors
2. Actual/potential problems identified during fetal life
3. Immediate adaptation to extrauterine life
4. Actual/potential problems noted after birth

ANALYSIS/NURSING DIAGNOSIS

1. Safe, effective care environment
   a. Risk for injury
   b. Risk for infection
2. Physiologic integrity
   a. Impaired gas exchange
   b. Altered cerebral tissue perfusion
   c. Altered nutrition; less than body requirements
   d. Altered growth and development
3. Psychologic integrity
   a. Disorganized infant behavior
   b. Altered parenting
4. Health promotion/maintenance
   a. Altered health maintenance
   b. Knowledge deficit

PLANNING, IMPLEMENTATION, AND EVALUATION

> **Goal** Newborn will be free from undetected problems; will have problems treated immediately and will maintain physiologic integrity. Family will comply with teaching for health maintenance and promotion.

Implementation

1. Perform ongoing assessment.
2. Notify physician of problems/changes in status.
3. Document altered condition.
4. Implement specific therapy as ordered.
5. Inform family of infant status.
6. Maintain a safe environment.

7. Promote asepsis.
8. Teach parents specific care for problem.

Evaluation

Newborn has problems detected and treated immediately; maintains homeostasis. Family understands recommended follow-up care.

SELECTED HEALTH PROBLEMS IN THE NEWBORN

✖ HYPOTHERMIA

1. Definition: a drop in the newborn's body temperature below 36.4°C (97.5°F), produced by rapid heat loss to the environment. All newborns are at risk for heat loss because of their limited subcutaneous fat and large surface area in relation to body weight
2. Predisposing factors
   a. Newborns with reduced stores of subcutaneous fat (e.g., premature, postmature, SGA newborns)
   b. Newborns with reduced glycogen reserves (e.g., premature, nutritionally deprived, SGA newborns)

Nursing Process

ASSESSMENT
1. Newborn's body temperature
2. Signs of cold stress
   a. Increased activity level
   b. Crying
   c. Increased respiratory rate
   d. Cyanosis
   e. Mottling of skin

ANALYSIS/NURSING DIAGNOSIS (see p. 367)
PLANNING, IMPLEMENTATION, AND EVALUATION

> **Goal** Newborn will expend a minimum amount of extra energy in the production of heat; will be free from periods of hypothermia.

Implementation
1. Prevent heat loss in delivery room (refer to Goal 1, p. 366).
2. Administer warmed air or O_2 to newborn prn.
3. Monitor newborn's temperature frequently; maintain axillary temperature at 36.5°C (97.8°F), abdominal skin temperature at 36.1°C to 36.7°C (97°F to 98°F).
4. Place crib or incubator away from draft and windows.
5. Keep portholes of incubator/Isolette closed.
6. Wrap in blankets if in crib.

Evaluation

Newborn maintains a skin temperature in normal range.

✖ NEONATAL JAUNDICE (HYPERBILIRUBINEMIA)

1. Definition: yellow color resulting from accumulation of bilirubin in the blood and tissues of the newborn (bilirubin is a product derived from the breakdown of erythrocytes and hemoglobin) and inability of the newborn's liver to bind it for excretion.

2. Extent:
   a. Fills sites from cephalad to caudal progression
   b. Resolves from caudal to cephalad direction
3. Predisposing factors
   a. Ethnic background (Asian, Native American, Eskimo)
   b. Prematurity
   c. Isoimmunization: maternal red blood cell–destroying antibodies are transferred to the fetus, resulting in fetal erythrocyte destruction; after initial maternal sensitization occurs, the effects on subsequent pregnancies with blood incompatibilities increase in severity
      1. Rh-negative mother and Rh-positive father may produce an Rh-positive fetus; this leads to antigen-antibody response affecting subsequent fetus
      2. mother with type O blood and father with type A, B, or AB (Fig. 4-24) produce a fetus with type A, B, or AB (generally results in less severe disease than Rh incompatibility)
   d. Polycythemia
   e. Exposure to drugs in utero
   f. Sepsis
4. Common forms
   a. Physiologic jaundice (affects 50% to 70% of all infants)
      1. onset
         a. full-term newborn: jaundice appears after 24 hours and disappears by end of seventh day
         b. preterm newborn: jaundice appears after 48 hours and disappears by ninth or tenth day
      2. lab values
         a. bilirubin is unconjugated (indirect); below 6 mg/dl on first day and not increasing by more than 5 mg/dl per day; newborn is without evidence of hemolytic disease or infection
         b. RBCs and WBCs are normal
   b. Pathologic jaundice (hyperbilirubinemia)
      1. onset: occurs within first 24 hours after birth
      2. lab values: characterized by rising bilirubin level in excess of normal
         a. in full-term newborn: rises 6 mg/dl in 24 hours

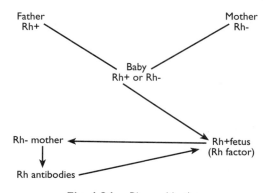

Fig. 4-24 Rh sensitization.

b. in premature newborn: higher levels; longer lasting

c. direct bilirubin greater than 1.0 mg/dl

3. severe sequela is kernicterus (deposit of unconjugated bilirubin in basal ganglia of brain) when bilirubin levels rise over 20 mg/dl in full-term newborns; signs and symptoms include

a. lack of interest in feeding

b. sluggish Moro's reflex with incomplete flexion of extremities

c. opisthotonic posturing

d. vomiting

e. bulging fontanels

f. twitching convulsions (late symptom)

c. Breast-milk jaundice: yellowing of newborn's skin caused by high concentration of enzyme lipoprotein lipase, which breaks down lipids to form free fatty acids and glycerol; increasing the amount of free fatty acids is thought to inhibit conjugation and excretion of bilirubin; may affect 1% to 4% of breast-fed newborns

1. onset: after mature milk is secreted; 4 to 5 days after delivery

2. lab values: bilirubin level begins to rise on about fourth day, peaks at 10 to 15 days of age, returns to normal between 3 and 12 weeks of age

5. Associated problems

a. Hydrops fetalis (erythroblastosis fetalis) related to Rh or ABO incompatibility: generalized edema, pleural and pericardial effusions, ascites

b. Hepatosplenomegaly

c. Progressive hemolytic anemia

Nursing Process

ASSESSMENT

1. Prenatal history

a. Positive hemantigen test (maternal blood serum)

b. Positive indirect Coombs' test (maternal blood serum)

c. No prior history of RhoGAM use

2. Early identification of newborns at risk; includes those with

a. Predisposing factors (e.g., prematurity, birth trauma)

b. Delayed passage of meconium

c. Placental enlargement (may weigh one half to three fourths of newborn's weight)

d. Visible jaundice of skin (bilirubin greater than 5 mg/dl): blanch bridge of nose or chest

e. Abnormal bleeding (e.g., extensive bruising or cephalhematoma)

f. Positive direct Coombs' test (neonatal cord blood)

g. Yellow-stained vernix on cord

3. Signs and symptoms of polycythemia, especially in large-for-gestational-age newborns

a. Decrease in peripheral pulses

b. Plethoric ruddy appearance

c. Tachycardia

d. Respiratory distress

4. Newborn pallor with jaundice, appearing within 24 to 36 hours after birth

5. Increased optical density of amniotic fluid

ANALYSIS/NURSING DIAGNOSIS (see p. 367)
PLANNING, IMPLEMENTATION, AND EVALUATION

> **Goal** Newborn at risk for jaundice will be identified; will be free from kernicterus.

Implementation

1. Interpret laboratory values and recognize deviations from normal (i.e, rise in serum bilirubin, Hgb decrease, rapid decrease in hematocrit, positive Coombs' test).

2. Offer early feedings (prevent reabsorption of bilirubin).

3. Give appropriate dose of vitamin K as ordered (decreases prothrombin time).

4. Give appropriate care to newborn undergoing phototherapy (method of treatment in which bilirubin is transported from skin to blood to bile and excreted). For traditional light unit:

a. Remove clothing.

b. Protect eyes with eye patches over closed lids (to prevent retinal damage).

c. Turn every 2 hours for maximum skin exposure.

d. Provide adequate fluids (needs increase 25% to 200%.

e. Feed q2-3h to prevent metabolic disorders (may be removed from light for feedings).

f. Assess for signs of dehydration (e.g., sunken fontanels); specific gravity of urine.

g. Maintain lights 16 inches away.

h. Monitor temperature every 2 hours.

i. Monitor weight gain and loss.

j. Observe for side effects (e.g., bronze skin, peripheral vasodilation, temperature and metabolic disturbances, diminished activity, loose stools). Fiberoptic phototherapy blanket may be used for home therapy.

5. Assist with exchange transfusion as indicated. (Newborn receives O-negative blood if problem is related to Rh incompatibility because no A, B, or Rh antigens are present in O-negative blood. Antibodies remaining are gradually removed; no further hemolysis occurs.

a. Observe for signs of transfusion reaction.

b. Educate parents about procedure.

Evaluation

Newborn shows signs of decreasing jaundice (e.g., falling serum bilirubin level, decreasing yellow color of skin); is free from kernicterus.

✖ RESPIRATORY DISTRESS

1. Definition: difficulty in maintaining respiratory function adequate to meet oxygen needs; caused by a variety of problems

2. Predisposing factors

a. Dysmaturity (SGA newborns)

b. Prematurity

c. Postmaturity

d. Maternal diabetes

e. Maternal bleeding

f. Fetal asphyxia

g. Birth asphyxia

h. Pregnancy-induced hypertension

i. Prolonged labor after rupture of the amniotic membranes

j. Meconium-stained amniotic fluid
k. Low Apgar score
l. Cesarean birth
3. Common respiratory disorders
   a. Respiratory distress syndrome, also known as hyaline membrane disease (HMD)
      1. definition: deficiency of surfactant activity leading to atelectasis, which prevents adequate gas exchange
      2. characterized by collapse of the alveoli
      3. most frequently affects preterm newborns, especially those weighing between 1000 and 1500 g; also observed in newborns of diabetic mothers and newborns of mothers whose pregnancies were complicated by antepartum vaginal bleeding
   b. Meconium-aspiration syndrome
      1. aspiration of meconium-stained amniotic fluid into the lungs may occur with asphyxic or placental disturbances in utero
      2. associated with intrauterine growth retardation (SGA newborns) and postmaturity (postterm newborns)
4. Associated problems
   a. Hypoxia
   b. Atelectasis
   c. Bronchopulmonary dysplasia, retrolental fibroplasia (complications of O_2 administration)

Nursing Process

ASSESSMENT

1. Use *Silverman-Andersen scale:* index of respiratory distress (scores of 0 are indication of good respiratory function) (Fig. 4-25)
   a. Grunting: sound of air pushing past partially closed glottis, heard during expiration

   b. Retractions: sternal and intercostal; result from use of accessory muscles to aid in breathing
   c. Flaring nares: result from newborn's effort to lessen resistance in narrow nasal passages
   d. Seesaw respirations: flattening of chest with inspiration and bulging of abdomen; caused by use of abdominal muscles during prolonged, forced respirations
2. Cyanosis
3. Alterations in respiratory rate, rhythm, and depth
   a. Tachypnea: respiratory rate greater than 60 per minute or greater than 15 per minute over baseline
   b. Bradypnea: respiratory rate less than 30 per minute
   c. Apneic spells: absence of respiration for 15 seconds or more
4. Falling body temperature

ANALYSIS/NURSING DIAGNOSIS (see p. 367)
PLANNING, IMPLEMENTATION, AND EVALUATION

Goal Newborn will maintain adequate oxygen levels to meet physiologic demands; will be free from undetected respiratory distress or further complications.

Implementation

1. Collect blood-gas samples and pH from umbilical line; interpret results of studies.
2. Administer prescribed oxygen (dependent on results of blood-gas study).
   a. Give warmed and humidified oxygen.
   b. Monitor concentration and pressure of oxygen.
3. Monitor oxygen concentration through oximeter, blood gas and pH studies, and transcutaneous oxygen tension.
4. Maintain newborn in supine position, with head slightly

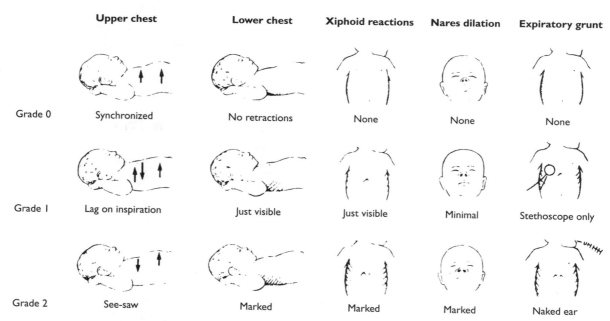

	Upper chest	Lower chest	Xiphoid reactions	Nares dilation	Expiratory grunt
Grade 0	Synchronized	No retractions	None	None	None
Grade 1	Lag on inspiration	Just visible	Just visible	Minimal	Stethoscope only
Grade 2	See-saw	Marked	Marked	Marked	Naked ear

Fig. 4-25 Silverman-Andersen scale. (From *Nursing inservice aid #2,* Columbus, Ohio, Ross Laboratories; Silverman W, Andersen D: *Pediatrics* 17:1, 1956, American Academy of Pediatrics.)

extended to improve respiratory function, or leave newborn flat.

5. Evaluate skin color.
   a. Pallor
   b. Plethora
   c. Cyanosis: circumoral, generalized, at rest or with activity
6. Maintain thermoneutral environment.
7. Minimize energy expenditure by keeping newborn warm.
8. Facilitate newborn's respiratory efforts.
   a. Continuous positive airway pressure (CPAP): controlled pressure exerted on expiration to prevent collapse of alveoli
   b. Oxygen hood (to provide controlled oxygen and humidity)
9. Suction endotracheal tube q1-2h as needed; protect from extubation.
10. Protect skin on nasal septum from breakdown and undue pressure from endotracheal tube.
11. Provide for nutritional needs (IV, gavage, hyperalimentation) with minimal energy expenditure.
12. Prevent and detect complications.
13. Give supportive care to parents.

Evaluation

Newborn adequately meets oxygen needs of body; maintains respiratory rate between 30 and 60 without dyspnea; is free from complications from therapy.

✖ NEONATAL NECROTIZING ENTEROCOLITIS (NEC)

1. Definition: a disorder of vascular ischemia, affecting the gastrointestinal mucosa, often associated with perforation
2. Incidence: approximately 5% of all newborns in intensive care nurseries; morbidity and mortality can be reduced by early detection and treatment of asphyxia (within 30 minutes of birth)
3. Predisposing factors
   a. Neonatal asphyxia and hypoxia
   b. Pregnancy-induced hypertension
   c. Maternal vaginal bleeding
   d. Excessive amounts of feeding
   e. Immature immunologic system
   f. Prematurity
4. Associated problem: sepsis

Nursing Process

ASSESSMENT
1. Abdominal distention
2. Pallor
3. Poor feeding
4. Gastric residuals (2 ml or more) before feedings
5. Occult blood in stool (positive guaiac test)
6. Increased apneic periods

ANALYSIS/NURSING DIAGNOSIS (see p. 367)
PLANNING, IMPLEMENTATION, AND EVALUATION

> **Goal** Newborn will be free from necrotizing enterocolitis, or complications from NEC.

Implementation
1. Check bowel sounds.
2. Monitor stools and gastric secretions for blood.
3. Monitor abdominal distention by measuring abdominal girth.
4. Record I&O, nature and type of gastric secretion.
5. Administer parenteral therapy or hyperalimentation as ordered.
6. Monitor for signs of dehydration.
7. Maintain nasogastric suction on low, intermittent suction.
8. Test urine for glucose to monitor tolerance for hyperalimentation solution.
9. Administer antibiotic therapy as indicated.
10. Provide appropriate preoperative and postoperative care when surgery is required (resection or colostomy).

Evaluation
Newborn receives prompt and appropriate treatment of any abnormalities (e.g., asphyxia, feeding problems); is free from sepsis and other complications of NEC.

✖ HYPOGLYCEMIA

1. Definition: decreased blood glucose level: less than 30 mg/dl (full-term) in first 72 hours of life or 45 mg/dl thereafter; less than 20 mg/dl in premature infants (NOTE: Dextrostix below 45 mg in term newborn, at 1 hour, warrants further testing)
2. Etiology: beta cells in the fetal pancreas become overstimulated in utero because of high levels of circulating maternal glucose; after birth, insulin production remains higher than needed for circulating glucose
3. Predisposing factors
   a. Malnourished newborns
      1. prematurity
      2. intrauterine growth retardation
      3. postmaturity
      4. twin pregnancy (smaller newborn affected)
   b. Newborns of diabetic mothers (usually LGA)
   c. Large-for-gestational age newborns (i.e., greater than 8.8 lb)
   d. Newborns of mothers with pregnancy-induced hypertension
   e. Severe Rh incompatibility
   f. Severely stressed newborns (e.g., newborns with cold stress, infections, fetal or respiratory distress)
4. Associated problems
   a. Jaundice
   b. Hypocalcemia (serum calcium less than 7 to 7.5 mg/dl); those at risk include preterm infants, newborns of diabetic mothers, newborns with birth trauma and perinatal asphyxia

Nursing Process

ASSESSMENT
1. Note any predisposing factors
2. Signs and symptoms of hypoglycemia
   a. Apnea
   b. Lethargy
   c. Irregular respiration
   d. Feeding difficulties
   e. Jitteriness

f. Twitching
g. Weak, high-pitched cry
3. Signs and symptoms of hypocalcemia
   a. Neonatal tetany
   b. Twitching from central nervous system irritability
   c. Jerking tremors
   d. Seizures
   e. Cyanosis
   f. High-pitched cry
   g. Respiratory distress
   h. Poor feeding
4. Laboratory values for deviations from normal
5. Behavior and reflexes
   a. Daily weight
   b. Note frequency and amount of urination and stools

ANALYSIS/NURSING DIAGNOSIS (see p. 367)

PLANNING, IMPLEMENTATION, AND EVALUATION

> **Goal** Newborn will maintain normal blood glucose level for gestational age; will have hypoglycemic reactions detected before complications develop; will maintain adequate nutrition and fluid and electrolyte balance.

Implementation

1. Perform Dextrostix or laboratory blood glucose test on admission to nursery, and for newborns at risk for hypoglycemia [q30min 3 times, then q2h 2 times until stable]; notify physician if Dextrostix result is less than 30 mg (full term) and less than 20 mg (preterm).
2. Provide adequate calories for all newborns.
3. Feed newborns at risk for hypoglycemia sterile water within first hour after birth, followed with glucose water, formula (oral or tube feeding as indicated), or breast milk.
4. Administer 10% to 25% glucose, IV or orally, as ordered.
5. Minimize handling of newborn; maintain warmth.
6. Observe carefully for signs of seizure related to low blood glucose.
7. Recommend regular pediatric care throughout childhood.

Evaluation

Newborn maintains normal blood-glucose level; has hypoglycemic reactions detected early; ingests calories appropriate for size; maintains fluid and electrolyte balance (e.g., moist mucous membranes, good skin turgor).

NEWBORN INFECTION

1. Definition: an invasion of the fetus or newborn by bacterial or viral microorganisms during pregnancy or during or after birth
2. Predisposing factors
   a. Poor maternal nutrition
   b. TORCH syndrome
   c. Intrauterine growth retardation (SGA)
   d. Prematurity, especially gestational age less than 34 weeks
   e. Prolonged labor after rupture of membranes
3. Modes of transmission
   a. Chronic transplacental infection, acquired in utero through the placenta
      1. usually resulting from viruses; others include bacteria, protozoa
      2. onset early in gestation
      3. may lead to growth retardation
   b. Ascending intrauterine infection, acquired through the cervix after rupture of membranes
      1. onset late in gestation
      2. usually resulting from bacteria, often *E. coli;* beta-hemolytic streptococcus
      3. may lead to premature labor and subsequent premature birth
   c. Newborn infection, acquired after birth from organisms in the environment by way of transmission from another person or newborn (sepsis is most common infection seen in newborn)
      1. often resulting from staphylococcus, streptococcus, or *E. coli*
      2. preterm newborns at greatest risk for infection because of lower immunologic defenses
      3. more common in boys than in girls
4. Associated problems
   a. Generalized sepsis
   b. Septic shock (evidenced by fall in BP and tachypnea)
   c. Hyperbilirubinemia
   d. Meningitis (evidenced by bulging anterior fontanel)
   e. Increased mortality rate, especially in premature newborns

Nursing Process

ASSESSMENT

1. Antenatal and intrapartal history to identify newborns at risk
2. Septic workup if infection suspected (blood culture, lumbar puncture, gastric aspiration, umbilical-stump culture, stool culture, amniotic-membrane culture)
3. Signs and symptoms
   a. Lethargy
   b. Newborn does not "look right"
   c. Poor feeding and sucking
   d. Increased respiratory rate
   e. Jaundice
   f. WBC increase
   g. Loss of weight
   h. Restlessness, tremors, convulsions
   i. Diarrhea and vomiting
   j. Abdominal distention
   k. Skin rashes or skin lesions
   l. Hypothermia or hyperthermia

ANALYSIS/NURSING DIAGNOSIS (see p. 367)

PLANNING, IMPLEMENTATION, AND EVALUATION

> **Goal** Newborn will be free from undetected infection, will not experience complications or generalized sepsis.

Implementation
1. Treat immediately by administering antibiotics as ordered (e.g., ampicillin, kanamycin, polymyxin); observe for side effects.
2. Prevent spread of infection by isolating septic newborns; use standard precautions and body substance isolation for blood, body fluids, nonintact skin, and mucous membranes.
3. Monitor thermal environment.
4. Monitor body temperature (temperature rise is *not an early sign of sepsis); in later stages, observe for severe hyperthermia or hypothermia.*
5. Take daily weight.
6. Monitor I&O; observe for dehydration.
7. Provide adequate nutrition
8. Promote respiratory function.
9. Observe for central nervous system involvement (lethargy, apnea, seizures, tremors).

Evaluation
Newborn shows signs of decreasing infection (e.g., decreasing respirations, skin temperature between 36.1°C and 36.7°C); does not develop generalized sepsis.

❖ NEONATAL DRUG AND ALCOHOL ADDICTION

1. Fetal alcohol syndrome
   a. Definition: a group of disorders characterized by teratogenesis as a result of chronic maternal alcoholism during pregnancy or moderate drinking; high incidence in female newborns
   b. Associated problems
      1. intrauterine growth retardation; microcephaly
      2. ocular structural defects
      3. limb anomalies
      4. cardiovascular disturbances and anomalies (e.g., atrial and ventricular septal defects)
      5. mental retardation
      6. fine-motor dysfunction
      7. prematurity
      8. convulsions
      9. developmental delays
2. Cocaine
   a. Exposure of the fetus during pregnancy may adversely affect the health and the growth and development of the neonate
   b. Associated problems
      1. congenital malformations
      2. intrauterine growth retardation
      3. prematurity
      4. poorly organized infant state
      5. decreased interactive behavior
      6. irregular sleep behavior
      7. increased risk of acute hypertension, cerebral artery injury/infarction, SIDS (not confirmed)

Nursing Process
ASSESSMENT (ALCOHOL)
1. Signs and symptoms: onset according to time of last maternal use, type of combinations of drug taken, amount of drug taken, and length of addiction (onset of withdrawal generally occurs within 24 hours in

alcohol addiction; can be up to 72 hours with some drugs)
   a. CNS signs
      1. restlessness
      2. jittery and hyperactive reflexes (e.g., constant sucking)
      3. high-pitched, shrill cry
      4. convulsions
      5. difficult to console
   b. GI system signs
      1. feeds poorly
      2. vomiting
      3. diarrhea
      4. dehydration
   c. Respiratory system signs
      1. nasal stuffiness
      2. yawning and sneezing
      3. apnea
      4. tachypnea
      5. excessive secretions
2. Fluid-balance status

ASSESSMENT (COCAINE)
1. Newborn urine testing can detect cocaine exposure within the preceding 6 to 9 days
2. Signs and symptoms vary with the degree of maternal substance abuse and time and dose of most recent exposure; may occur 4 to 5 days after birth
   a. CNS: tremulousness, irritability, muscular rigidity, increased startle response, disturbed sleep pattern, poor response to stimuli, avoids eye contact
   b. GI: feeds poorly, vomiting, diarrhea, dehydration
   c. Cardiorespiratory: elevated respiratory and heart rate
   d. Fluid balance: alterations
   e. Genitourinary: congenital defects
   f. Muscular: prune-belly syndrome

ANALYSIS/NURSING DIAGNOSIS (see p. 367)
PLANNING, IMPLEMENTATION, AND EVALUATION

> **Goal** Newborn will remain free from injury; will have minimal symptoms associated with withdrawal; limited seizures; parents will understand the need for follow-up care.

Implementation
1. Reduce stimuli in environment and minimize handling.
2. Protect from injury (swaddle newborn in snug-fitting blanket).
3. Promote bonding/attachment.
4. Ensure that newborn receives required fluid and caloric intake; use pacifier between feeding.
5. Feed on demand; give small amounts at frequent intervals.
6. Administer IV therapy as ordered.
7. Position on side to avoid aspiration.
8. Measure I&O; watch for signs of dehydration resulting from vomiting, loose stools, poor feeding.
9. Weigh frequently.
10. Give skin care with special attention to body folds; expose to air.

11. Protect skin from injury (mittens on hands, sheepskin on crib, pads on sides of crib).
12. Give medications as ordered.
    a. Phenobarbital (6 mg/kg/day IM or 2 mg PO qid)
    b. Paregoric (2 to 4 gtt/kg orally q4-6h; dose may increase to 20 to 30 gtt/kg q4-6h)
13. Maintain patent airway if seizure occurs.
14. Maintain adequate warmth.
15. Teach parents the importance of long-term follow-up health care.
16. See also Substance Use Disorders, p. 77, and journal articles, p. 101.

Evaluation

Newborn is comfortable and free from seizures, complications of withdrawal; has homeostasis restored; parents have an appointment with physician or clinic for follow-up care.

✜ ACQUIRED IMMUNODEFICIENCY SYNDROME (AIDS)

1. Definition: a disease that affects the immune system (T-cells) and renders infant unable to fight disease or infection. High mortality rate in the first 3 years of life; no known cure. Currently 50% of infants born to HIV-positive women will show HIV-positive after 1 year.
2. Modes of transmission to newborn:
   a. Transplacental
   b. Through breast milk
   c. Contact with body fluids

Nursing Process

ASSESSMENT

1. Often SGA
2. Hepatosplenomegaly
3. Neurologic abnormalities (e.g., microcephaly)
4. Prominent, boxlike forehead
5. Increased distance between inner canthi; flattened nasal bridge
6. Recurrent infections (e.g., interstitial pneumonia)
7. Evidence of Epstein-Barr viral infection; thrush

ANALYSIS/NURSING DIAGNOSIS (see p. 367)

PLANNING, IMPLEMENTATION, AND EVALUATION

Goal Risk of HIV/AIDS will be identified early; standard precautions will protect family and caregivers; newborn will be free from complications of AIDS; parents will understand need for referral and follow-up care.

Implementation

1. Assess infants of mothers at risk (e.g., IV drug users and their partners, prostitutes, those with positive HIV test) for signs and symptoms of AIDS.
2. Promote bonding/attachment.
3. Use standard precautions and body substance isolation for blood, body fluids, nonintact skin, and mucous membranes.
4. Educate parents about disease process, transmission, current treatment, follow-up care.
5. Provide emotional support to family.

Evaluation

Newborn is free from complications; parents keep all follow-up care appointments.

✜ BIRTH INJURIES/CONGENITAL ANOMALIES

1. Birth injuries
   a. Definition: physical trauma to the newborn resulting from the birth process
   b. Predisposing factors: large-for-gestational-age newborn, dystocia
   c. Common types of injuries
      1. brachial plexus injuries
      2. cephalhematomas
      3. fractures (commonly of clavicle)
      4. intracranial hemorrhage
2. Congenital anomalies
   a. Definition: a variety of defects or disorders, which may be evident or concealed at birth; the physical and developmental consequences will vary with selected problems
   b. Incidence: 6 in 1000 total births
   c. Predisposing factors
      1. past personal or family history of congenital anomalies, genetic factors (e.g., chromosomal aberrations)
      2. exposure to toxic agents, viruses, or drugs during pregnancy
      3. genetic-environmental interaction

Nursing Process

ASSESSMENT

1. Birth injuries
   a. Decreased mobility of arm, abnormal positioning (brachial-plexus injuries)
   b. Swelling of head caused by rupture of the blood vessels between a cranial bone and the periosteum; does not cross suture lines (cephalhematoma)
   c. Swelling, irritability associated with pain, decreased mobility of affected extremity, abnormal positioning at rest (fractures)
   d. Respiratory irregularities with cyanosis, reduced responsiveness, high-pitched cry, tense fontanel, or convulsions (intracranial hemorrhage resulting from hypoxia and hypovolemia seen mainly in premature infants)
2. Congenital anomalies
   a. Antepartum/intrapartum high-risk factors, including maternal history of
      1. chronic alcoholism or drug addiction
      2. family members born with congenital defects
      3. exposure to toxic agents in environment
      4. infections (e.g., TORCH)
      5. high-altitude resident
   b. Hydramnios: associated with
      1. neurologic defects such as hydrocephalus, anencephalus, and spina bifida
      2. gastrointestinal malformation such as esophageal atresia, cleft palate, pyloric stenosis
      3. Down syndrome
      4. congenital heart disease

5. maternal diabetes
6. prematurity
c. Oligohydramnios, associated with anomalies of the renal system

ANALYSIS/NURSING DIAGNOSIS (see p. 367)

PLANNING, IMPLEMENTATION, AND EVALUATION

> **Goal 1** Newborn will not develop undetected complications of birth injury.

Implementation
1. Assess for asymmetric movements by placing newborn on back and observing movements of arms and legs.
2. Screen all LGA newborns for birth injuries; listen for high-pitched, weak cry; observe muscle tone (poor), hypertonicity, hyperactivity, flaccidity.
3. Palpate fontanels for bulging, tenseness.
4. Observe pupillary response.
5. Position head higher than hips (for intracranial hemorrhage); minimize handling; provide warmth; maintain adequate nutrition.
6. Implement specific treatment, which varies with nature and extent of insult.
7. Document observations.

Evaluation

Newborn receives early treatment of birth injury; is free from long-term sequelae (e.g., mental retardation) when possible.

> **Goal 2** Newborn will have anomalies recognized and treated early; will be free from complications; will maintain homeostasis; parents will understand need for referral.

Implementation
1. Screen for apparent and hidden congenital anomalies (often done on admission to nursery).
2. Implement appropriate therapeutic measures (interdisciplinary health care team approach essential).
3. Refer family for care and genetic counseling.

Evaluation

Newborn adapts successfully to extrauterine life; receives appropriate treatment for defect; parents have an appointment for appropriate referral.

PARENTAL REACTION TO A SICK, DISABLED, OR MALFORMED NEWBORN

1. The grief and mourning process is initiated by abnormality (parents grieve over the loss of normalcy in their newborn)
2. Stages of grief and mourning (refer to Loss and Death and Dying, p. 29)
   a. First stage
      1. initial sadness
      2. guilt feelings ("What did I do to cause this? What happened?")
      3. shock over reality of situation
      4. denial
      5. general anger at situation; overprotectiveness of the newborn
      6. neglect of other family members
      7. isolation/loneliness (increases after mother's discharge from hospital)
   b. Second stage: developing awareness of reality of situation
   c. Restitution: coming to terms with situation

Nursing Process

ASSESSMENT
1. Stage of grief and mourning
2. Parental behavior: adaptive or maladaptive

ANALYSIS/NURSING DIAGNOSIS (see p. 367)

PLANNING, IMPLEMENTATION, AND EVALUATION

> **Goal** Parents will grieve their loss; accept support in their grief over the ill, disabled, or malformed newborn.

Implementation
1. Allow parents to express grief (may be shown as anger, denial, depression, or crying); be supportive.
2. Modify hospital policies when possible to allow early contact with newborn and frequent visitation; encourage parents to see newborn, to touch and hold newborn in neonatal intensive care unit.
3. Point out normal characteristics of their newborn to parents.
4. Encourage parental participation in care (e.g., providing breast milk, bathing, and feeding).
5. Recognize signs of maladaptive responses.
   a. Possibility of abuse or neglect
   b. Overwhelming guilt
6. Expect repeated periods of sadness.
7. Provide simple explanations for procedures.
8. Refer parents to social worker for follow-up while newborn is in hospital, according to family need.
9. Encourage parents who are unable to visit to call nursery for progress reports.
10. Refer to visiting nurse for health supervision after discharge of newborn.
11. Plan for follow-up or institutionalization as necessary.

Evaluation

Parents grieve for their newborn's condition; express feelings of sadness and anger; allow nursing staff, family, and friends to support them.

BIBLIOGRAPHY

Women's health care

Barrett-Connor E, Bush T: Estrogen and coronary disease in women, *JAMA,* 265(14):186, 1991.

Bobak I et al: *Maternity nursing,* ed 4, St Louis, 1995, Mosby.

Bobak I, Jensen M: *Maternity and gynecologic care,* ed 5, St Louis, 1993, Mosby.

Breast cancer screening guidelines remain unchanged, *Cancer News* 19:2, Summer 1993.

Contraception choices for women over 35: Focus on benefits and risks, *Contracept Rep* 3(2):4, 1992.

Davis D, Dearman C: Coping strategies of infertile women, *J Obstet Gynecol Neonatal Nurs* 20(3):221, 1991.

Davis M: Natural family planning, *Perinat Women Health Nurse* 3(2):280, 1992.

Elwood J, Cox B, Richardson A: The effectiveness of breast cancer screening by mammography in younger women, *Online J Curr Clin Trials* 2:25, 1993.

Harlan L, Berstein A, Kessler L: Cervical cancer screening: who is not screened and why? *Am J Public Health* 81(7):885, 1991.

Hatcher R et al: *Contraception technology: 1994-1996*, ed 16, New York, 1994, Irvington.

Libbus M: Condoms as primary prevention in sexually active women, *MCN Am J Matern Child Nurs* 17(5):256, 1992.

Urrows S, Freston M, Pryor D: Profiles in osteoporosis, *Am J Nurs* 91:33, 1991.

Antepartal care

Acosta Y et al: HIV disease and pregnancy. Part 1: epidemiology, pathogenesis and history, *J Obstet Gynecol Neonatal Nurs* 21(2):86, 1992.

Bernstein J: Parenting after infertility, *J Perinat Neonat Nurs* 4:11, 1990.

Bobak I et al: *Maternity nursing* ed 4, St Louis, 1995, Mosby.

Bobak I, Jensen M, Zalar M: *Maternity and gynecologic care*, ed 5, St Louis, 1993, Mosby.

Cook P, Peterson R, Moore D: Alcohol, tobacco and other drugs may harm the unborn, *U.S. Department of Health and Human Services DHHS Pub No (ADM) 90-1711*, Rockville, Md, 1990, Office for Substance Abuse Prevention.

Conner G, Denson F: Expectant fathers' response to pregnancy. *J Perinat Neonat Nurs* 4:33, 1990.

Cunningham F et al: *Williams' obstetrics*, ed 19, Norwalk, Conn, 1993, Appleton & Lange.

Eganhouse D, Burnside S: Nursing assessment and responsibilities in monitoring the preterm pregnancy, *J Obstet Gynecol Neonatal Nurs* 21(5):355, 1992.

Harris B, Sandelowski M, Holditch D: Infertility and new interpretation of pregnancy loss, *MCN Am J Matern Child Nurs* 16(4):217, 1991.

Haire D: Patient education in childbirth; a long way in forty years, *Int J Childbirth Educ* 6:7, 1991.

Leff E, Gagne M, Jefferis S: Type I diabetes and pregnancy, *MCN Am J Matern Child Nurs* 16(2):83, 1991.

Mackey M: Womens' preparation for the childbirth experience, *Matern Child Nurs J* 19(2):143, 1990.

McDonald A, Armstrong B, Sloan M: Cigarette, alcohol and coffee consumption and congenital effects, *Am J Public Health* 82(1):91, 1992.

Merlin R: Understanding bulimia and its implications in pregnancy, *J Obstet Gynecol Neonatal Nurs* 21(3):199, 1992.

Nichols F, editor: *Perinatal education, AWHONN's Clinical Issues in Perinatal and Women's Health Nursing*, Philadelphia, 1993, Lippincott.

Patterson E, Freese M, Goldberg R: Seeking safe passage: utilizing health care during pregnancy, *Image J Nurs Sch* 22(1):27, 1990.

Peters H, Theorell C: Fetal and maternal effects of maternal cocaine use, *J Obstet Gynecol Neonatal Nurs* 20(2):121, 1991.

Tinkle M, Amaya M, Tamayo O: HIV disease and pregnancy. Part 2: antepartum and intrapartum care, *J Obstet Gynecol Neonatal Nurs* 21(2):97, 1992.

Intrapartal care

Bobak I et al: *Maternity nursing*, ed 4, St Louis, 1995, Mosby.

Bobak I, Jensen M, Zalar M: *Maternity and gynecologic care*, ed 5, St Louis, 1993, Mosby.

Clark J, Queener S, Karb V: *Pharmacologic basis of nursing practice*, St Louis, 1990, Mosby.

Cunningham F et al: *Williams' obstetrics*, ed 19, Norwalk, Conn, 1993, Appleton & Lange.

Johnson S: Ethical dilemma: a patient refuses a life saving cesarean, *MCN Am J Matern Child Nurs* 17(3):121, 1992.

Wild L, Coyne C: Epidural analgesia: the basics and beyond, *Am J Nurs* 92(4):26, 1992.

Postpartal care

Association of Women's Health, Obstetric and Neonatal Nurses (AWHONN): Position statement, issues: shortened maternity and newborn hospital stays, *Voice* 2(5):20, 1994.

Bobak I et al: *Maternity nursing*, ed 4, St Louis, 1995, Mosby.

Bobak I, Jensen M, Zalar M: *Maternity and gynecologic care*, ed 5, St Louis, 1993, Mosby.

Bostin N et al: HIV disease in pregnancy. Part 3: postpartum care of the HIV positive woman and her newborn, *J Obstet Gynecol Neonatal Nurs* 21(2):105, 1992.

Cohen S et al: *Maternal, neonatal and women's health nursing*, Springhouse, Pa, 1991, Springhouse.

Cunningham F et al: *William's obstetrics*, ed 19, Norwalk, Conn, 1993, Appleton & Lange.

Eidelman A et al: Cognitive deficits in women after childbirth, *Obstet Gynecol* 81(5, part 1):764, 1993.

Olds S et al: *Maternal-newborn nursing: a family centered approach*, ed 4, Redwood City, Calif, 1994, Addison-Wesley.

Riordan J, Auerbach K: *Breastfeeding and human lactation*, Boston, 1993, Jones & Bartlett.

Rubin R: Puerperal change, *Nurs outlook* 9:753, 1961.

Williams L, Cooper M: Nurse-managed postpartum home care, *J Obstet Gynecol Neonatal Nurs* 22(1):25, 1993.

Newborn care

Bobak I et al: *Maternity nursing*, ed 4, St Louis, 1995, Mosby.

Bobak I, Jensen M, Zalar M: *Maternity and gynecologic care*, ed 5, St Louis, 1993, Mosby.

Brazelton T: *Neonatal behavioral assessment scale*, Philadelphia, 1973, Lippincott.

Cohen S et al: *Maternal, neonatal and women's health nursing*, Springhouse, Pa, 1991, Springhouse.

Cunningham F et al: *Williams' obstetrics*, ed 19, Norwalk, Conn, 1993, Appleton & Lange.

Driscoll J: Maternal parenthood and the grief process, *J Perinat Neonat Nurs* 4:1, 1990.

Lund M: Perspectives on newborn male circumcision, *Neonat Net* 9:7, 1990.

Newman T, Maisels M: Evaluation and treatment of jaundice in the newborn: a kinder gentler approach, *Pediatrics* 89:809, 1992.

Olds S et al: *Maternal-newborn nursing: a family centered approach*, ed 4, Redwood City, Calif, 1994, Addison-Wesley.

Seidel H et al: *Primary care of the newborn*, St Louis, 1993, Mosby.

Williams L, Cooper M: Nurse-managed postpartum home care, *J Obstet Gynecol Neonatal Nurs* 22(1):25, 1993.

Wong D: *Whaley and Wong's nursing care of infants and children*, ed 5, St Louis, 1994, Mosby.

CAN WE ENCOURAGE PREGNANT SUBSTANCE ABUSERS TO SEEK PRENATAL CARE?

Hawaii's nurses created a positive response.

BY JANE STARN, KATHRYN PATTERSON, GARDNER BEMIS, OLIVIA CASTRO,
AND PATRICIA BEMIS

Perinatal substance abuse, with its potential for compromised child development, is an increasing problem in the United States (1,2). State laws addressing drug use in pregnancy respond to this illegal activity with punitive or public health approaches or both (3). When a punitive approach is taken, the woman who uses drugs during pregnancy may be prosecuted and jailed for illicit activities associated with the drug use or for delivering drugs to the fetus in utero. Fear of punitive action often drives women away from seeking health care. The result is late or no prenatal care, with all the attendant perinatal risks.

States using the public health approach emphasize legislation for a controlled and safe environment within

Jane Starn, RN, DrPH, and Kathryn Patterson, CNM, PhD, are associate professors at the School of Nursing at the University of Hawaii at Manoa. Dr. Starn is also an associate researcher at the Center for Youth Research of the University of Hawaii and serves as principal investigator on the DISC project. Gardner Bemis, MD, is a pediatrician; Olivia Castro, RN, MPH, is a women's health nurse practitioner and clinical nurse specialist; and Patricia Bemis, RN, is the nursery supervisor, all at Kaiser Permanente Medical Care System, Honolulu. For copies of consent forms, contracts, and protocols used by the DISC program, write to Dr. Jane Starn, 1532 Kamole Street, Honolulu, HI 96821, and enclose a stamped, self-addressed envelope and $2.50 to cover handling.

which women cease drug use. Physical, psychological, and social needs of the woman and baby are met by providing comprehensive health and social services, such as drug cessation therapy, parenting support, and skill building. These programs require consent for random toxicology screening and may include written contract agreements between the woman and the agency (4).

The state of Hawaii considers drug-exposed or addicted newborns to be abused or neglected children and requires referral to Children's Protective Services (CPS) when a positive maternal or neonatal drug toxicology screen is obtained (3). Because this focus limits legal and social action, the state has instituted several programs to intervene at an earlier phase to prevent punitive outcomes. It creates a comprehensive public health approach to substance abuse that serves both publicly and privately insured clients, using existing programs and new ones where needed.

A blind screening of all women admitted to Hawaiian hospitals while in labor demonstrated that substance abuse is found in all populations and in all zip codes (5). Moreover, a state health task force found gaps at various levels of service to substance-abusing families. First noted was a lack of consistent and organized effort to identify substance-abusing women during the prenatal period. Once identified, there

was frequently a lack of follow-through from obstetrical care to pediatric care, from ambulatory care to inpatient care, and from hospital-based care to community follow-up services (6).

To address these gaps, the Hawaii Department of Health used federal and state matching funds to start Baby S.A.F.E. (Substance Abuse Free Environment), a community outreach program for perinatal drug users limited to four geographic areas of documented high drug use. The Salivation Army also developed an inpatient treatment program with ten residential treatment beds for substance-abusing women and children that women may join during pregnancy. All other substance abuse programs in the state do not admit women into services unless they leave their children with another caregiver while they receive rehabilitation.

In addition, to address the unmet needs of both public and private health care recipients, the Hawaii Department of Health funded the Drug Identification, Screening and Counseling (DISC) project for the island of Oahu. DISC represents the first effort to coordinate both public and private health and social services for perinatal substance users.

A SYSTEMATIC APPROACH TO INTERVENTION

The DISC project is a systematic program to detect, assess, and inter-

A HEROIN-ADDICTED MOTHER

Sarah, a 34-year-old white woman, was referred to the DISC project in her fourth month of pregnancy. She was married, had a four-year-old son, and worked with her husband in a small business as the office manager. Learning that she was pregnant, Sarah was concerned about the baby and reported her heroin addiction. She willingly began methadone maintenance with an outpatient treatment program after referral by DISC and her physician.

Sarah was worried because she had been arrested twice for drug use and dealing. She had two hearings pending and talked about the need to get her life back in order for the sake of her family.

Six months into the pregnancy, Sarah developed severe right-sided facial pain and headaches. Her obstetrician hesitated to prescribe pain medication because of her history of drug use, despite the neurologist's diagnosis of Bell's palsy. After intervention by the Kaiser maternal-child clinical nurse specialist and the DISC project nurse, the obstetrician prescribed propoxyphene (Darvocet-N). The medication brought Sarah some relief from the facial pain, but it also brought hassles from the drug rehabilitation program when the presence of the medication appeared in the urine toxicology screen. A phone call by the DISC project nurse to the rehabilitation program clarified the need for the pain medication.

Sarah gave birth one month early to a 4 pound, 8 ounce daughter named Barbara. Sarah was contacted while on the postpartum unit by the pediatric nurse practitioner (PNP) of the DISC staff, who explained the contract for continued home visits and weekly phone calls. Child Protective Services was notified of the baby's birth and the DISC follow-up of the family.

Barbara tested positive for methadone metabolites but not for "street drugs." At birth, she appeared thin, with jittery movements and an intense cry. She responsed well to swaddling and decreased stimulation. She went home with her mother three days after birth.

The PNP visited at Sarah's workplace when the baby was six days old. On this first visit, Sarah looked very tired. She explained that she had returned to work immediately after her son was born and expected to handle it with this birth, too. She had set up an area for Barbara at the office and spent a lot of time holding the baby when she was fussy. Sarah explained that her husband was unable to read when she first met him. Although she had taught him to read, he still relied on her for assistance in the business.

Completion of the NCAST Feeding Scale while Sarah fed Barbara revealed that Sarah was sensitive and responsive as a mother (11). She learned quickly to sense when Barbara needed decreased stimulation and swaddled her and laid her in the crib so that she could fall asleep.

During the subsequent months, the baby's jitteriness and fussy cry decreased, and she began to sleep longer at night. Sarah and her husband Jim continued to be sensitive to the baby's needs. The Bell's palsy gradually began to subside, and Sarah experienced decreased pain and a slight return of right-sided facial mobility and expression. At the three-month visit, she looked less tired.

Sarah utilized the Baby's First year calendar in playing with her daughter (12). Completion of the Difficult Life Circumstances and Parenting Stress Index stimulated Sarah to talk about her earlier life, her father's death in prison and the two years she was subjected to incest by her uncle (8,13). She also talked about her inability to make friends as a teenager, except with peers who used drugs.

Her present extended family circumstances were still full of abusive and substance-abusing situations, which increased her stress but seemed to reinforce her determination to stay off street drugs. Sarah said that she thought of herself as a person who had taken a bad path, not as a bad person. She was able to think of drugs as repulsive and could recognize that friends who offered her drugs were not truly friends.

As her trial dates approached, six months after Barbara was born, Sarah became anxious. The PNP wrote a letter to her defense attorney, describing her parenting abilities, her contributions to the family business, and her diligence in rehabilitation. By this time, Sarah was on minimal methadone and was expressing the need to wean herself from this dependence. Fortunately, the trials went well. Sarah was sentenced to probation, follow-up drug testing, and 500 hours of community service.

Because of the support of the PNP during this period, Jim became more trusting. Both parents began to share their lives and concerns during the monthly visits. Barbara and Sarah came to the University PNP office for completion of the Fagan Test for Early Intelligence and the Mullen Scale of Early Learning (14, 15). Sarah and Jim were delighted to learn that Barbara tested normally on both scales. When the four-year-old son, Brent, began to experience problems in kindergarten, the PNP was able to talk with the family about school readiness. She encouraged the parents to consider having Brent repeat kindergarten the following year because he was one of the youngest members of his class.

When Barbara was eight months old, Sarah's grandmother, who had been the most nurturing figure in her life, had a stroke. Sarah and Barbara flew to her mother's home and stayed for the grandmother's death and funeral. Sarah decided to stay an additional three weeks while she stopped using methadone. Her mother and new stepfather were supportive and helpful during this time.

Sarah returned home free of drugs and really pleased to be "clean." Believing that it was no longer safe to have Barbara at work, she arranged to have her sister-in-law watch the baby during work hours. Brent was ready to restart kindergarten and seemed adjusted to the decision.

By the 11-month visit, Barbara was saying several words, crawling, and cruising around furniture. Her only abnormality involved her walking. She walked on tiptoes rather than with her feet touching down. The PNP recommended minimal walker use and putting her in shoes. At this visit, Sarah and Jim gave the PNP an invitation to the baby's 12-month birthday luau, a Hawaiian tradition. The parents seemed to have weathered the storms of drug use, criminal prosecution, an unexpected pregnancy, their son's difficulty in school, their infant's initial fussiness, a grandmother's death, and drug rehabilitation well.

At one year (13 months because of her premature birth) Barbara's walking was normal and she was able to squat and recover to standing. She tested in the 14- to 18-month range for the gross motor, visual receptive and expressive, and language receptive and expressive scales of the Mullen Scales of Early Learning (15). In addition, she tested low risk on the Fagan Test of Infant Intelligence, which assesses infant perception (14). She was not referred for further services based on her excellent test scores. However, early intervention therapy services are available in Hawaii for children until the age of three if they are needed.

vene with mothers and their infants who are exposed to drugs. The University of Hawaii's nursing faculty, as grantees, sought Hawaii's Kaiser Permanente Medical Care System as the sight of implementation because the agency was proactive in its response to the increasing numbers of drug-exposed newborns. Kaiser Permanente is a health maintenance organization that serves patients from both privately funded and publicly (Medicare, Medicaid) funded sectors. It also serves a wide geographic area and consists of seven community health centers and its own hospital. Initial funding was for a two and one-half year period.

The nursing faculty at the university of Kaiser's interdisciplinary staff worked together to develop a blueprint for addressing perinatal substance abuse from early pregnancy through the first year of the infant's life. The DISC project was structured around program implementation, provision of clinical services, and research evaluation.

The project required one year of planning and development prior to serving the first client in May 1991. The review boards of both the University of Hawaii and Kaiser approved the research evaluation. Counsel from Kaiser's legal staff worked with the state Department of Human Services and CPS to develop an *information only* report upon the birth of an infant with, or whose mother has, a positive toxicology screen. The DISC project's working agreement with CPS forestalls action by CPS for women who participate in the DISC contract agreement.

The consent form that the mother signs to participate in the project spells out requirements for participation. It advises that the consequence for failure to follow the agreement is referral to CPS. The Hawaii Department of Health, Maternal Child Health Branch, manages the contract and holds the project nursing faculty accountable for implementation. Such formalized cooperative agreements between private and state institutions are necessary to address the complex social, psychological, and health risks that substance abuse presents. These formal relationships also acknowledge that no one agency, program, or individual can meet all the needs of the perinatal substance-abusing family.

The Perinatal Task Force, a joint committee of Kaiser personnel and university nursing faculty, meets monthly to coordinate services between the clinic and the inpatient obstetric, pediatric, and family practice providers. The task force developed protocols and consent forms, which were approved by the Kaiser Forms Committee. The DISC screening tool to identify pregnant women using drugs was developed by the nursing faculty, refined by the task force, and approved as a pilot form by Kaiser Permanente.

Kaiser's obstetric, pediatric, and family practice physicians, nurse practitioners, and nursing staff were introduced to the goals of the program and received education in the new procedures and in the use of the new forms. The video, *Challenge to Care,* was used to demonstrate successful interviewing techniques to nurses assigned to interview new prenatal patients (7).* This video helps resensitize viewers about society's attitudes toward mothers on drugs.

IDENTIFYING THE PREGNANT DRUG USER

The prenatal phase of the DISC program involves screening all pregnant women within the Kaiser System on Oahu who use the outpatient services at seven community sites and the inpatient services at the Moanalua Hospital. The women complete the drug screening tool at the initial prenatal visit, when they also provide demographic information, insurance forms, and past obstetric and medical history. The interview nurses or nurse practitioners then review the screening forms for indicators of drug use.

Approximately 3 percent of the new obstetric patients are identified as using drugs. This rate corresponds favorably to the 1990 double-blind screen that revealed a rate of 4.2 percent of Hawaiian women testing positive for drug use while in labor (5).

Women identified as drug users are referred to the DISC program faculty or graduate student research assistants. Subsequent interviews by the research

To obtain Challenge to Care, *contact Vida Health Communications, Inc., 6 Bigelow St., Cambridge, MA 02139.*

assistants determine if the women meet the criteria for inclusion in the program. Criteria include significant and current use of cocaine, crystal methamphetamine, marijuana, or alcohol. Significant use means weekly or more frequently. Alcohol, although not illegal, was included because of potential harm to the fetus and because many women are polydrug users.

Smoking marijuana or trying cocaine once or twice prior to pregnancy is not considered serious and ongoing substance abuse. However, if there is an indication of recent use, follow-up contact is made by telephone and through home visits for further assessment. If included in the program, women are asked to sign consent forms, one from the university and one from Kaiser, stipulating program conditions.

CONTACT BEFORE AND AFTER THE BABY IS BORN

As with most prenatal patients at Kaiser, every effort is made to alternate visits between the physician and an ob/gyn nurse practitioner (NP). The NP provides weekly phone contact as a source of encouragement and support to remain drug free during the pregnancy. During follow-up visits, women are asked to complete demographic information, a depression scale, and the Difficult Life Circumstances Scale to determine levels of stress and disorganization in their daily lives (8). They are also assessed for preterm labor risk and other common obstetrical complications.

Many substance-abusing families face social problems and environmental stressors that contribute to their perinatal drug use. Beyond the immediate problem of substance abuse is the significant need to address poverty, malnutrition, and immature social development (9). The program encourages good nutrition, referring women to the Women and Infant Children (WIC) nutrition program.

During the prenatal visits, the nurse practitioners pay particular attention to the women's psychosocial needs, helping them work through the problems and pain in their lives and begin setting goals for the future. They listen, offer referrals and support, and help the women to improve their self-esteem and to believe in their ability to stop using drugs.

When the program first began, the women with positive toxicology screens were asked to participate in weekly group sessions led by recovered substance users. This format was not effective because the women chose not to attend. An alternate plan was devised whereby the women were given the responsibility for calling a support person from Alcoholics Anonymous (AA) or Narcotics Anonymous (NA). Two former users volunteered to help women locate a program near their residence and identify a "buddy" to follow them in recovery.

To date, only two out of 35 women have required residential treatment programs. These women were severely addicted and were without housing and social support. Currently in the program is a 20-year-old woman who uses crystal methamphetamines daily. Attempts are being made to encourage her to also enroll in a residential program.

Upon arrival of the baby, the pediatric nurse practitioner, a faculty member, or a graduate student visits the mother and infant in the hospital to make an initial pediatric assessment. This visit is meant to foster the transition for the woman to a different coordinator/provider during the follow-through period.

The faculty members and graduate students assume responsibility for the weekly phone calls and monthly home visits during the infant's first year of life. They assess the baby's development, parent–infant interaction, family coping and stress reduction, and drug abstinence. The program builds on the work of Kathryn Barnard and associates in the application of Newborn Nursing Models for optimizing parent–infant development (10). Follow-up is designed to ensure that the women participate in their own and their infant's health care appointments, enter and complete drug treatment programs or participate in support groups, and provide a nurturing environment for themselves and their babies.

A protocol outlines the responsibilities of each staff area—prenatal, labor and delivery, postpartum, and nursery. Contact among these areas is maintained through the patient's chart, with program personnel available to respond to questions.

ISSUES OF CONFIDENTIALITY

In order to facilitate the continuity of care from outpatient to inpatient care, it is necessary to identify the charts of the women participating in the program. There continue to be debates about the consequences of labeling patients' record with information that may have potentially negative consequences. The patient's right to confidentiality conflicts with the concept of the chart as a legal document containing obligations of disclosure. These issues are juxtaposed with concerns for the physical well-being of the mother and the baby, the need to communicate to maintain continuity of care, and the need to convey an expectation to the mother that she must continue to obtain care for herself and her child.

The decision was made to stamp the prenatal records of women consenting to DISC participation with the words "prenatal drug use" to identify them when they are admitted for hospital or clinic services. Urine toxicology is performed on both the mother and infant at the time of delivery.

As stated earlier, the DISC project's working agreement with CPS forestalls action by CPS for women who participate in the DISC contract agreement. Word-of-mouth knowledge of this arrangement has brought women out of hiding and back for prenatal care. Therefore, the short-term assessment is that labelling the chart is having a positive, rather than a negative effect, on these women's lives.

EARLY RESULTS

The DISC project is completing the first year of data collection. (Kaiser is presently determining how to continue the program internally.) Of the 1,350 women screened for perinatal drug use, 94 women (6.9 percent) were referred for further assessment and 35 (2.6 percent) entered the DISC program.

Many of the 94 women did not have significant drug use. Those eliminated reported drinking beer occasionally or using marijuana briefly during their teen years. Fourteen women who should have enrolled in the project did not consent to participate. Their charts were flagged for observation during labor and during the postpartum period.

Two chose to join the program after giving birth. Others, who had negative toxicology screens, did not join. Four women who did not indicate drug use were subsequently identified by positive toxicology after giving birth and they joined the program at that time.

Thirty-four percent of the 94 women admitted to the use of multiple drugs, ranging from marijuana and alcohol to crystal methaphetamine and crack cocaine. One woman is on methadone maintenance for heroin addiction (see A Heroin-Addicted Mother).

The women in the DISC program ranged in age from 15 to 39, with 35 percent between the ages of 15 and 19; 38 percent between the ages of 20 and 29; and 27 percent between the ages of 30 and 39. Only 8 percent of the women planned their pregnancy, with 47 percent having a first pregnancy, 26 percent a second pregnancy, and 19 percent a third or later pregnancy. Slightly over half (52 percent) of the women were married, another 22 percent were unmarried but living with a partner, 8 percent lived alone, and 17 percent were unmarried but living with family.

Fifty-four percent of the women had adequate to moderate family incomes, over $20,000 per year. Their circumstances varied, with 31 percent of the women living on less than $9,000 per year and 15 percent living on between $10,000 and $19,000. Twenty-four percent had incomes between $20,000 and $29,000, 15 percent between $30,000 and $39,000, and 15 percent more than $40,000. As expected for Hawaii, the mothers represented various ethnic groups. The largest number, 38 percent, were Hawaiian or part-Hawaiian, and 24 percent were white. The remaining were as follows: Japanese, 14 percent; Chinese, 10 percent; Korean, 5 percent; African American, 5 percent; and Filipino, 4 percent.

Future analysis of the data will examine whether these women have significant depression and/or stress in their lives. Postdelivery data will assess parent–infant interactions and infant developmental outcomes. The group with positive postpartum urine toxicology screens will be compared with the women who have negative drug toxicology screens at their infant's birth to determine if there are also differences in stressors, coping, and environmental factors between the two groups.

Early findings indicate that women will talk about their substance abuse during pregnancy when approached in a systematic, nonjudgmental manner and when they know that the program is helpful and safe, that is, they will not be referred to CPS. The data also reinforce the understanding that substance abuse crosses all ethnic and economic strata.

In offering systematic follow-up, including a home visitation program, DISC project staff members serve as resources who link pregnant drug users and their families to inpatient, ambulatory, and community services. Recognizing the need for coordinated care to meet the many needs of this population, DISC staff members build an atmosphere of respect, support, and trust that facilitates lifestyle change. This comprehensive approach to perinatal substance abuse is possible because of the cooperative efforts of public and private health care resources.

REFERENCES

1. Adams, C., and others. Nursing intervention with mothers who are substance abusers. *J. Perinat. Neonat. Nurs.* 3:43-52, Apr. 1990.
2. Alpert, J.J., and Zuckerman, B. Alcohol use during pregnancy: what is the risk? *Pediatr. Rev.* 12:375-381; [Discussion] 380-381, June 1991.
3. Moore, K.G., Substance abuse and pregnancy: state lawmakers respond with punitive and public health measures. *Am. College Obstet. Gynecol Legislet.* 9:1-7, Fall, 1990.
4. Free, T., and others. A descriptive study of infants and toddlers exposed prenatally to substance abuse. *MCN: Am J. Maternal/Child Nurs.* 15:245-249, July-Aug. 1990.
5. Yasuhara, J.S. Drug exposed infants. *Kapiolani Counseling Center Newsletter* (Honolulu, HI) 4(1):2, 1991.
6. American Hospital Association. *The Role of Hospitals in Caring for Pregnant Substance-Abusing Women.* Chicago, The Association, 1991.
7. Vida Health Communications. *Challenge to Care: Strategies to Help Chemically Dependent Women and Infants.* [videotape] Cambridge, MA: The Author, 1991.
8. Barnard, K.E. *Difficult Life Circumstances Scale, Nursing Child Assessment.* Seattle, WA: Satellite Training, University of Washington, COMRC.
9. Woodhouse, L.D. Women with jagged edges: Voices from a culture of substance abuse. *Qualitative Health Res.* 2:262-281, 1992.
10. Barnard, K.E., and others. Newborn nursing models: a test of early intervention of high-risk infants and families. In *Children and Families: Studies in Prevention and Intervention,* ed. by E. Higgs. Madison, WI.: International Universities Press, 1988, pp 63-82.
11. Barnard, K. *NCAST Feeding Scale, Nursing Child Assessment* Seattle, WA: Satellite Training, University of Washington, WS-10.
12. Stodden, N. *Baby's First Year: Calendar of Learning Games and Memories.* Honolulu: International Education Corp., 1986.
13. Abidin, R.R. *Parenting Stress Index.* 3rd ed. Charlottesville, VA: Pediatric Psychology Press, 1990.
14. Fagan, J.F., and Shepard P.A. *The Fagan Test of Infant Intelligence.* Cleveland: Infantest Corp, 1985.
15. Mullen, E.M. *Infant Mullen Scales of Early Learning.* Cranston, RI: T.O.T.A.L. Child, Inc., 1985.

CAN WE HELP THE SUBSTANCE-ABUSING MOTHER AND INFANT?

Yes, answered New Orleans' nurses in one perinatal acute care setting.

BY JOAN SULLIVAN, MARTHA BOUDREAUX, AND PATRICIA KELLER

More than half of the women who deliver infants in Charity Hospital in New Orleans, a hospital serving an urban and rural indigent population, receive limited or no prenatal care. Not surprisingly, many of these women use "crack" cocaine with varying frequency. The population served is comparable to many large public hospitals in metropolitan areas, where cocaine use is reported to occur in 3 to 18 percent of pregnant women (1).

In 1988, when substance abuse was reaching epidemic rates and cocaine was particularly dangerous because of its ready availability and low price, the hospital conducted a survey of pregnant women admitted for delivery during a three-month period. Eight percent of the women, between 28 and 32 per month, had positive urine toxicology screens for cocaine. Of these women, 85 percent were multiparas who were the primary caregivers for their other children; 58 percent were 25 years or older; and more than half presented for delivery with no history of prenatal care. The survey also disclosed that 11 percent of the newborns had low birth weight (<2000 gm), compared to 7.3 percent of the newborns born at the hospital and 3.5 percent of infants born in Louisiana (2).

CLINICIAN'S CONCERNS

The hospital staff experienced a sense of urgency to do something for the safety of the newborns. Reports of infants being rehospitalized and periodic newspaper accounts of neglected and dying infants and children contributed to their concerns. They questioned what they could do about this complicated and perplexing situation, particularly since most, if not all, of these women had not been identified as users of cocaine prior to the birth of their baby. Identification of drug use was made only through positive urine toxicology after delivery, and the mothers presented no special problems in labor.

Community treatment resources were limited and already strained by more referrals than could be adequately served. Substance abuse treatment facilities specifically for pregnant women and women with newborns were nonexistent. A creative intervention to provide nursing care in an acute care hospital for substance-abusing women who do not seek perinatal care was required.

In response to these concerns, clinical nurse specialists on the hospital staff developed the Perinatal Substance Abuse Intervention and Prevention Program, a well-defined, comprehensive, tertiary prevention and intervention program to address the nursing care of perinatal patients within the hospital setting and in future pregnancies. The program, which began in March 1990, had the support of hospital and community health care professionals. A grant from the local chapter of the March of Dimes provided substantial funds for the first year, helping to finance the clinical nurse specialist position and to pay for educational materials and research needs.

The initial goals of the Program were as follows:

1) To identify cocaine-abusing women and their newborns and to assess their needs,

2) To plan and implement interventions on behalf of these women and their newborns,

3) To conduct follow-up activities by collaborating with other community programs and resources, and

4) To educate the hospital staff and the wider community about the problem.

With no immediate prospect of additional financial resources, an assessment was made of Medicaid benefits, for which most of the women and newborns were eligible. It was determined that home visits by nurses are covered by Medicaid for "at risk" newborns and children when ordered by a physician. Therefore, home health referral was chosen as a plausible intervention and a cornerstone of the program. The rest of the program was developed around the available resources on the perinatal units and the creativity and the determination of the staff.

Joan Sullivan, RN, DNS, is now Director of Nursing Research and Evaluation at Charity Hospital and Medical Center of Louisiana, New Orleans, Louisiana. She developed the Perinatal Substance Abuse Intervention and Prevention Program when she was a clinical nurse specialist. Martha Boudreaux, RN, MN, is a clinical nurse specialist at Louisiana State University School of Medicine, Department of Obstetrics and Gynecology, New Orleans. Patricia Keller, RN, MN, is clinical nurse specialist of perinatal substance abuse, Charity Hospital and Medical Center of Louisiana.

<table>
<tr><td>

INTERVIEW PROTOCOL

Information About Other Children
Who helps with them
Age, grade, problems
Do they live with the mother

Information About the Mother
Medicines used during pregnancy
Numbers of cigarettes/day smoked
Alcohol: amount, frequency, last time for beer, wine, liquor
Street drugs: amount, frequency, route, and last time; alone or with others
How use of street drugs began, age that use started
Sensations achieved from drug use
This baby's father's drug use
Length of time drug free, if ever
Medical treatments: types, length of times drug free
Interest in treatment during this pregnancy and any follow-through
History of any abuse
Interest in home health for baby
Plans for contraceptive use
Information about her mother's pregnancy

</td></tr>
</table>

FIRST POSTPARTUM CONTACT

The resulting intervention program consisted of multiple components. All pregnant women admitted to the hospital were tested using a urine toxicology screen that tested for seven illicit drugs. (It did not test for the presence of alcohol.) During the first 24 to 48 hours postpartum, a clinical nurse specialist interviewed every woman who gave a history of or tested positive for cocaine, initiating the interactive phase of the intervention process.

During the interview, which took approximately one hour, the nurse expressed concern for the woman and her infant and, at the same time, confronted her with the results of the urine screen. After nurses interviewed more than 200 women, they created an interview protocol from topics that emerged frequently. (See Interview Protocol.)

Cocaine and other drug use was determined by asking women to "tell their stories," assuring them that anything they shared about their lives or experiences would be helpful. Most of the women, even those whom the staff felt were extremely hostile, seemed relieved to participate. Only a few were unwilling to talk with anyone, including their families.

The nurses also used the interview to explain the effects of cocaine on the newborn as well as on the mother. They described behaviors noted in infants exposed to cocaine and recommended ways for the mothers to comfort and nurture their babies. They then explained the availability and the benefits of the home health referral program from the point of view of the babies, encouraging the women to sign an agreement outlining the benefits and indicating their willingness to participate.

The home health referrals were restricted to newborns for reasons other than the organizational complexity of the hospital and of Medicaid. Mothers are concerned about possible effects of their prenatal drug use on their infants, and this concern provided a potent means to enlist their cooperation. Moreover, home health nurses could assess the babies and observe their environments on a regular basis. The assessments and observations would provide follow-up information that could be used for subsequent referrals as necessary.

On the agreement was space for the woman's address and telephone number and the addresses and phone numbers of friends or relatives. Both the clinical nurse specialist and the mother signed the agreement and each received a copy. The nursing staff used the written agreement as recognition of an adult-to-adult relationship between the two parties. It also provided valuable information for follow-up. (For a detailed description of the nurse-patient relationship with addicted women, see Communicating with Addicted Women in Labor, *MCN,* Jan./Feb. 1992.)

In addition, the staff developed an illustrated, simply worded, four-page booklet as a teaching tool and birth memento and as a list of community resources.* The booklet is personalized with the names of the mother and infant on the front cover. The back cover contains telephone numbers of hospital and community resources. The booklet serves as a valuable link with the hospital nurses for women who usually do not have private health care and demonstrates, in writing, that somebody cares—an important intervention for women using "crack" cocaine.

When the mothers were receptive, the interviews led to an exploration of giving up drug use. For many women, giving birth leads to motivation to change for the benefit of the child (3). Many of the women expressed how important it was for them to stop their substance abuse and to seek supportive treatment. The nurses encouraged the women to make changes in their lives for the benefit of their newborns and for themselves and helped them to investigate possible lifestyle alternatives.

Social workers also interviewed the women to assess their home situations and to provide additional services as appropriate. The information given to the social worker often differed from, but did not conflict with, the information collected by the nurse. Communication was maintained through an interdepartmental form attached to the mother's chart, and the nurses and social workers met for troubleshooting conferences.

Another part of the program involved the use of the Nursery Abstinence Score Sheet (NASS) to assess the newborns (4). The NASS was scored once per day. Newborns who exhibited higher than recommended scores were evaluated with the NASS on each shift and physicians were notified according to a standard protocol. Most term newborns were discharged to the care of their mothers within 3 to 10 days, but some remained hospitalized for a longer period of time to receive antibiotic therapy.

VISITING IN THE HOME

At the start of the program, only a limited number of mothers and newborns were referred for home visits. These referrals were voluntary and were made with the cooperation of the nursing, social services, and medical staffs of the hospital and six home health agencies. Their purpose was to monitor the infants for symptoms of

---

For one copy of the booklet, write to Dr. Joan Sullivan, Director of Nursing Research and Quality Improvement, Charity Hospital and Medical Center, 1532 Tulane Ave., New Orleans, LA 70140-1015. There is no charge.

Adapted from: Finnegan, L.P.
Neonatal Abstinence, In *Current
Therapy in Neonatal-Perinatal
Medicine,* ed. by N.M. Nelson,
Toronto, B.C. Decker, Inc., 1985,
p. 262.

NURSING ABSTINENCE SCORE SHEET—AREAS ASSESSED

Signs and Symptoms Numerically Scored

Central Nervous
Quality of cry
Hours of sleep after feedings
Moro reflex
Tremors disturbed/undisturbed
Muscle tone
Excoriation
Myoclonic jerks
Generalized convulsions

Metabolic/Respiratory
Sweating
Fever
Frequent yawning
Mottling
Nasal stuffiness
Sneezing
Respiratory rate (with retractions?)

Gastrointestinal
Excessive sucking
Poor feeding
Regurgitation
Stool quality

Weight

withdrawal, to ensure safe care, to support the caregiver mother, and to provide follow-up information to the hospital nursing staff. Immediately after discharge, there were three visits per week. Later visits were arranged with the mothers or caregivers according to need. The home health nurses used the NASS to assess the babies so that there could be a comparison of behaviors in the hospital and at home.

Prior to the inception of the referral program, nursery personnel and social workers met with home health nurses to offer guidance and to answer questions. They agreed to be available by telephone to answer questions from the home health nurses. The home health nurses agreed to visit referred newborns and their mothers.

After approximately two months of the pilot, the nursing staff extended the referrals to include all term and low-birth-weight infants born to mothers who had a history of or tested positive for cocaine. This natural extension of the pilot doubled the number of newborns referred.

Home visits with the first 40 term newborns from the initial months of the pilot program showed the following health and social conditions, some of which overlap.

• Several of the infants had minor health problems: Two had diaper rashes, two were constipated, and two had ear infections that were treated medically. One baby was "high strung" and another had trouble with sucking.

• One newborn was in the care of child protective services. One was admitted to another hospital for possible neglect.

• Five mothers left the home, leaving the new baby and older children in the care of family members; one left her children alone in the house; three were incarcerated; one was hospitalized with emotional problems; and several continued the previous pattern of cocaine use.

• Several mothers were reported lacking the basics of food, water, electricity, or adequate formula and diapers.

• Eight newborns and their mothers were no longer in the pilot home health program: Three had been discharged because the mothers were off drugs and home health services were no longer needed; one mother withdrew from the program after three home health visits; and four were lost to follow-up.

The follow-up information confirmed the initial assessment that these newborns were "at risk" because of their mothers' lifestyles. However, the mothers seemed to suffer more immediate deleterious effects because of their substance abuse than did their newborns. The home health nurses who discovered neglect in the course of their visits made the appropriate referrals, to Child Protective Services as needed, and to the relatives listed on the agreement signed by the mother.

A profile of a typical cocaine-abusing pregnant woman evolved from the implementation of the intervention. She is usually single, multiparous, and unemployed, with a history of having been pregnant as a teenager (ages 14-18), and has not completed high school. She often has unresolved grief issues, such as the death of close family members or significant others, and a history of child or sexual abuse.

Depression and low self-esteem are common, and the women report experiencing feelings of isolation and helplessness. Without exception, the present pregnancy was unplanned and relationships with male partners are inconsistent and without commitment. There is usually a history of illicit substance abuse by other family members, including parents and siblings, as well as family histories of addictive disorders, including alcohol, nicotine, and gambling. Poly-substance abuse (marijuana, nicotine, alcohol, cocaine) is the norm.

The neighborhoods of these women and children are unsafe. Crime and violence occur frequently. The housing is often crowded, with the women and their children sharing two bedrooms or less with other families.

EFFECTS ON STAFF MORALE

A sense of ownership and pride developed among the perinatal staff during the Program implementation. The Program was presented at medical staff rounds, in nursing meetings, and at educational offerings. There was extensive media coverage on television and in the newspaper. The clinical nurse specialist was a guest speaker or poster presenter at local and national meetings.

Feelings of anger, helplessness, and frustration among the staff began to dissipate as they participated in the development of the intervention and in educational programs, and as it became apparent that the babies were not more seriously affected by the drugs. The clinical nurse specialist helped nurses to develop relationships with the mothers. Hospital nurses felt satisfied that they were extending the intervention by working with home health nurses, who, in turn, appreciated being able to call the hospital nursery staff at any time during the day for information.

The referral process proceeded more smoothly as the intervention gained acceptance and was integrated into the workloads of the people and departments involved. The social service department in the central office and the social workers on the unit experienced a dramatic increase in the number of home health referrals, which put an initial strain on the staff. Regularly scheduled troubleshooting meetings were held with the social service personnel, the supervisors of maternal-child services and home health agencies, the nursery head nurse, other interested staff, and the clinical nurse specialist. During a five-month period when the clinical nurse specialist position was vacant, nurses who worked on the staff of the nursery for full-term babies took over the management of the newborn referrals.

The intervention developed within the hospital continues and a second phase, to help *prevent* cocaine exposure to fetuses in future pregnancies, is in the planning stages. This phase involves education and services related to realistic family planning options, including levonorgestrel implants, which may prove effective in the future. State funding is available for immediate postpartum insertion and outpatient funding is available through Medicaid.

Other positive results include system changes. The Coalition for Maternal and Infant Health, a state group of health care professionals and agencies, used information gained through the program to lobby for the establishment of formal state legislative action to address perinatal substance abuse problems. In response, the legislature formed and commissioned the Council to Prevent Chemically Exposed Infants, whose directed purpose is to recommend alternative and innovative strategies for solving the problems of these families. Both the present and former clinical nurse specialists have testified and were appointed members of this council.

Interventions for cocaine-abusing pregnant women initiated in acute care settings, while helpful, have their limitations. In order to achieve optimum outcomes, for the newborns and their mothers as well as for society, comprehensive treatment programs must be readily available and accessible, preferably prior to pregnancy but certainly during pregnancy. A national commitment to provide resources for the long-term treatment of substance-abusing women and their families is required. Nevertheless, Charity Hospital has demonstrated that a creative intervention program can foster beneficial changes when resources are limited and when nurses and other health professionals combine efforts for patients in an acute care setting.

REFERENCES

1. Lindenberg, C.S., and others, A review of the literature on cocaine abuse in pregnancy. *Nursing Research.* 40:69-75, Mar-Apr. 1991; Comment 40:235, July-Aug. 1991.
2. Office of Public Health Statistics, Louisiana Health Department, New Orleans, 1990.
3. Sullivan, J.M., *Adjusting expectations: A theory of maternal thinking.* Unpublished dissertation. New Orleans, Louisiana State University, School of Nursing, 1989.
4. Finnegan, L.P. Neonatal abstinence. In *Current Therapy in Neonatal-Perinatal Medicine,* ed. by N.M. Nelson. Philadelphia, B.C. Decker, 1985, p. 262.

TEACHING PREGNANT ADOLESCENTS TO COPE WITH ENVIRONMENTAL SMOKE

Culturally relevant materials and role playing are effective in a program for African American students. Initial results are promising.

BY MARILYN L. WINKELSTEIN

Several school-based educational programs have been developed to acquaint pregnant adolescents with the harmful effects of active smoking (1,2). Few such programs, however, have focused on the harmful effects of passive smoking, and none have included strategies to help pregnant adolescents cope with environmental exposure to tobacco smoke.

Strong support for such a program resulted from recent studies that demonstrated significant health risks for the pregnant woman, the developing fetus, and the young child from passive exposure to cigarette smoke. A program developed for African American students in an inner-city junior/senior high school for pregnant adolescents in Baltimore suggests several areas for further research.

THE PROBLEM

Nonsmoking pregnant women exposed to cigarette smoke accumulate and concentrate significant amounts of nicotine and its by-product, cotinine, in their own hair and the hair of the developing fetus (3). Cotinine has also been found in the meconium of infants born to mothers exposed to passive

smoke (4). These women are twice as likely to deliver low-birth-weight infants as unexposed women (5). Moreover, the infants are at risk for impaired neurodevelopment (6).

Infants exposed to passive smoking are at risk for slow neurological development, sudden infant death, respiratory tract illnesses, and chronic middle-ear infections (7-10). Passive smoking also aggravates childhood asthma, increasing symptoms, hospitalizations, and trips to the emergency room (11-13).

The decision to focus on the effects of passive smoking was based on a preliminary needs assessment of 115 pregnant students attending the junior/senior high school. While only four students, less than 3 percent, actively smoked, 74 percent reported that they lived in homes containing smokers and were exposed to cigarette smoke daily. This figure is consistent with other surveys of inner-city populations (14).

The purpose of the program was to help the students develop strategies to cope with situations involving smoking and environments containing smoke. The educational component was designed by a pediatric nurse in collaboration with American Lung Association staff and classroom teachers.

Four learning objectives and several learning activities were developed. (See Learning Objectives and Activities.) The content and learning activities were based on literature concerning the harmful effects of passive smoking, current recommendations for school-based smoking prevention pro-

grams, social learning theory, and the developmental needs of adolescents.

IMPLEMENTATION OF THE PROGRAM

The program consisted of two 45-minute classes delivered on two consecutive days during the Family Life and Parenting Class. Approximately 120 students (six groups of 20) ranging in age from 13 to 17 years participated. The majority of the students were unmarried and pregnant for the first time.

Part One. In the first class, delivered by the classroom teacher, the students completed a study guide containing questions relating to material presented in a 10-minute videotape. They then viewed the tape, "Beginning the Journey . . . to Control," which was developed by KCET public television of California and the California State Department of Health in cooperation with a community outreach group of African American women. Videotapes have been used previously in school-based smoking prevention programs (15,16). Those that are sensitive to the ethnic and cultural needs of their audience have been found to be particularly effective (17,18).

"Beginning the Journey . . . to Control" is geared toward young women. It uses colorful graphics and lively music and dance by the entertainer Janet Jackson to profile a young African American single mother as she struggles to overcome her dependence on cigarette smoking. The content of the video includes facts about health

Marilyn L. Winkelstein, RN, PhD, is an associate professor, Department of Maternal Child Health, University of Maryland School of Nursing, Baltimore, Maryland. The author thanks KarenAnn Bochau and Cathleen Kinnear of the American Lung Association of Maryland and the staff and students of the Laurence G. Paquin School for making this project possible.

LEARNING OBJECTIVES AND ACTIVITIES

Objectives

1. The students will identify the effects of passive smoking on the fetus, the young infant, child, and adolescent.

2. The student will participate in a role playing situation that requires decision making and the selection of coping skills to use when confronted with passive smoking in the environment.

3. The student will identify specific types of advertising used by tobacco companies to promote smoking dependence in African American communities.

4. The student will identify selected interventions and community resources that can be used to help family members who are trying to stop smoking.

Activities

Classroom discussion in second class
Pamphlet: "Please Don't Smoke. There's a baby in the house"
Role Playing Scenarios
Classroom discussion in first and second classes
"Beginning the Journey . . . to Control" Videotape Study Guide
Classroom discussion in first and second classes
"Beginning the Journey . . . to Control" Videotape Study Guide
Pamphlet: "Breathing for Two—Quit Smoking for You and Your Baby"
Listing of Community Smoking Cessation Programs

---

risks for women who smoke and for young children exposed to smoke; a discussion of the social and economic influences that promote tobacco dependence in the African American community; and several possible coping mechanisms for trying to stop smoking.

After the presentation, the teacher gave the students the answers to the questions on the study guide and conducted an informal discussion. (See "Beginning the Journey . . . to Control" Videotape Study Guide.) Each student then received two educational pamphlets: "Breathing for Two—Quit Smoking for You and Your Baby," published by the American Lung Association of Wisconsin, which contains information to help pregnant women quit smoking, and "Please Don't Smoke . . . There's a Baby in the House," published by the Missouri Department of Health, Office of Health Promotion. This pamphlet contains information concerning the effects of secondhand smoke on newborn infants and young children.*

Part Two. The pediatric nurse led the second class the following day. The students itemized the harmful effects of

* For a single copy of this pamphlet, write to the Missouri Department of Health, Office of Health Promotion and Special Supplemental Food Program for Women, Infants and Children (WIC), P.O. Box 570, Jefferson City, MO 65102. (Do not telephone.) For a copy of "Breathing for Two—Quit Smoking for You and Your Baby," contact your local chapter of the American Lung Association. To obtain a copy of the video "Beginning the Journey . . . to Control," contact the Tobacco Education Clearing House, P.O. Box 1830, Santa Cruz, CA 95061-1830.

passive smoking on the pregnant woman, the fetus, the newborn, and the young infant, and the nurse listed them on the blackboard.

The students also discussed how they might support family members who were trying to stop smoking. They identified smoking cessation programs located in churches and community centers as the most valuable type of support and were given a list of all such programs in their community. They were encouraged to refer family members to these programs.

The class also discussed advertising campaigns used by the tobacco industry. Students were encouraged to become active observers of advertising aimed at or located within the African American community.

During this class, the students participated in role playing scenarios involving exposure to environmental smoke. (See Role Playing Scenarios.) Content was based on the developmental and cognitive needs of adolescents and social learning theory.

Cognitive development during adolescence involves the development of formal operational thinking (19). As abstract thinking evolves, teenagers begin to focus on potentiality and possibilities. This is a slow and gradual process that may not be completed until the middle or end of adolescence. Young adolescents in the initial stages of formal operations need help problem solving, imagining the consequences of their actions, and moving from egocentric, concrete level thinking to more abstract reasoning.

Role playing in peer groups is an ef-

fective instructional strategy to help them translate abstract information into concrete and specific actions (20). In addition, role playing uses social learning principles by encouraging the expression of feelings, problem solving, and rehearsing decision making and coping skills (21,22). Female students, in particular, have benefited from school-based smoking prevention programs that include role playing led by a teacher or some other adult (23).

TEACHER AND STUDENT REACTIONS

The educational program was favorably received by teachers and students. By the end of the first class, each participant could correctly identify several harmful effects of secondhand smoking (Question 5, Videotape Study Guide). Most retained this knowledge and were able to discuss harmful effects of passive smoking with the pediatric nurse during the second class and in a question-and-answer session led by a pediatrician two days later. Teachers, school administrators, and the pediatrician were all impressed with the students' interest in this topic and their desire to protect themselves and their infants from cigarette smoke.

In addition, most of the students, 85 percent, identified at least three ways to help family members cope with urges to smoke (Question 3, Videotape Study Guide). In the second class, students described smoking cessation programs as the best way to help family members quit smoking. They found the list of community programs valuable and offered the following comments:

"This program is just down the street from my house"; "My Mom could easily attend this program"; and "This program is held at my church."

The discussion of tobacco advertising was especially relevant for this group. Although only a few students could remember the specific amount of money that the tobacco industry spends annually on advertising in the African American community (Question 6, Videotape Study Guide), all students could list several types of cigarette advertising seen in their community (Question 7, Videotape Study Guide). Every student knew the locations of the "Joe Camel" billboards and voiced anger and concern when they learned that tobacco companies target adolescent women and minority groups for advertising campaigns. Several students also commented on the tobacco industry's practice of distributing free packs of cigarettes at sporting events and rock concerts.

At the end of the two classes, students were able to meet all of the learning objectives. The most rewarding part of the program, however, was the reaction to the role playing scenarios. Each girl participated in at least one scenario, and all participated freely during the discussions that followed the role playing.

After the first scenario, the students identified the conflicting needs of the infant's parent and the maternal grandmother. This provided an opportunity for the students to explore the difficulties they would soon encounter as a result of their dual roles, that of parent and adolescent daughter. Several of the girls stated, "I don't think I could ever tell my Mom not to smoke around my baby. After all, I'm living in her house and she's supporting me." Others suggested statements or approaches that the daughter might use in response, such as stating that it was time for the baby's bath when the grandmother started to smoke.

As alternative approaches were modeled, students who were originally uncomfortable with this scenario became more relaxed and rehearsed new ways to express their feelings about smoking to their mothers. One student commented, "I will simply say, 'Gee Mom, please don't smoke around the baby'."

The second scenario provided an opportunity to rehearse decision making when confronted with peer pressure. By assuming different parts, the students could experiment with their role as a new mother while learning how to cope with the feelings of friends. As they participated, they became more comfortable expressing their own feelings and learned how to be assertive with their peers.

The third scenario provided practice in relating to the father of the baby while also acting as an advocate for the baby. Several students, rehearsing their future role as mothers, took pride in stating: "I'm the mother and I know what the doctor told me and what's best for my baby. I want to keep my baby well. You'll have to go outside the house if you want to smoke."

EXTENDING THE PROGRAM

Although the program was successfully implemented and enthusiastically received by this particular inner-city population, results cannot be generalized to all groups of pregnant adolescents without several modifications and plans for long-term evaluation. The program was not part of a longitudinal study, and the adolescents were not followed over time. Therefore, how successful they were in using the coping strategies to reduce their actual exposure to environmental smoke is not known.

To evaluate lasting impact, it will be necessary to include a survey of efforts made by pregnant adolescents to limit their exposure to passive smoke before and immediately following the program and at several points in time after giving birth. Program outcomes might also be evaluated by administering the survey to all pregnant students in the school, comparing the responses of students who received the educational program to those who did not.

To quantify long-term outcomes of the program, urinary cotinine analysis can be done at several points in time during the pregnancy. This method has been used effectively to document maternal exposure to tobacco smoke (24). Because pregnant adolescents who attend schools such as the one used for this project often receive their prenatal care at school-based clinics, the analysis can easily be done on routine prenatal urine specimens.

A further modification would be to

"BEGINNING THE JOURNEY . . . TO CONTROL" VIDEOTAPE STUDY GUIDE

DISCUSSION QUESTIONS:

1. Name two methods of quitting smoking.
   Answer: The cold turkey method and tapering off
2. List one way to relieve stress after you quit smoking.
   Answer: Begin walking or some other form of exercise
   Participate in a hobby
   Read a book
   Do activities that help you relax or take your mind off smoking
3. List five ways to cope with the urge to smoke once you have quit smoking (hint: all these ways begin with the letter D).
   Answer: *Delay* smoking the cigarette
   Deep-breathing exercises
   Drink water or other nutritional fluids
   Do something to occupy your mind
   Dialogue or talk with a supportive friend or family member
4. What is the primary reason why women continue to smoke?
   Answer: Fear of gaining weight
5. List all the harmful effects of breathing in secondhand smoke. (Effects can be on the pregnant woman, the unborn baby, the newborn infant, young children, and adolescents.)
   Answer: Low birth weight
   Sudden infant death
   Increased respiratory tract illnesses
   Increased middle ear infections in toddlers
   Earlier onset of asthma, and increased symptoms and number of emergency room visits for children with asthma
6. What percentage of the tobacco industry's U.S. advertising dollars are spent in the African American community?
   Answer: 40 percent, or approximately $3.2 million dollars a year
7. What types of cigarette advertising do you see in your community?
   Answer: Billboards in the community with "Joe Camel"
   Newspaper and magazine advertising

ROLE PLAYING SCENARIOS

Scenario 1:
You have just finished eating supper. Everyone is sitting around the table talking while drinking coffee. You are holding your baby in your lap. Your mother is sitting beside you. Your mother takes out a cigarette and starts to smoke. She does this every evening after supper. Your mother says her cigarette after supper is the best one of the day. You can smell the smoke. You can see the smoke drift above your baby's face.

Scenario 2:
You are at the mall with friends. You have your baby with you. Everyone is talking about how cute the baby is. You haven't been out of the house for days and this is the first time you have seen your friends since the baby was born. You need a baby-sitter for Saturday night. Your friend, Kim, offers to watch your baby. Kim is a smoker. She lives with her Mom and brother who also smoke.

Scenario 3:
Your baby is six months old. You and the baby's father are spending the evening together watching television. You took the baby to the clinic earlier in the day because the baby had a cold and was wheezing. The doctor told you that the baby has asthma. As you are watching television, the baby's father lights up a cigarette.

broaden the scope of the program by including family members, using "take home" educational materials or establishing a dialogue with the nurse. Smokers are often unaware of the potentially harmful effects of their habit on the pregnant woman, the developing fetus, and the young child as well as other adults (25).

Another approach would be to hold informal classes for family members, in the evening or as part of a parent-teacher meeting. During the class, the nurse can provide information about the harmful effects of environmental smoke, encourage smoking cessation, provide referrals to and lists of community smoking cessation programs, and establish support groups for family members who have recently stopped smoking.

With a minimal expenditure of money and energy, this program can be used in other settings, such as health maintenance organizations and ambulatory care clinics. For example, the video can be shown to women waiting for their prenatal, postpartum, or ambulatory pediatric appointments. Nurses can ask about family smoking habits and involuntary exposure to tobacco smoke as part of their routine assessment, answer questions about the videotape, and provide relevant educational materials and referrals to community smoking cessation programs.

The role playing scenarios can be used by nurse practitioners who work with pregnant adolescents and adolescent mothers in all prenatal health education and parenting classes. They can also be modified for use with both male and female adolescents in ambulatory care clinics, schools, and other community settings.

It is essential that all maternal-child health nurses recognize and acknowledge the harmful effects of passive smoke exposure on the pregnant woman, the fetus, and the young child. Educational activities that enable pregnant adolescents to learn more about these harmful effects and how to cope with environments that contain tobacco smoke will help to prevent tobacco-related illnesses in the future.

The early results of the school-based program in Baltimore demonstrate that students are motivated to learn and eager to provide a safe environment for their babies. Providing the facts they need in a format that is clear, enjoyable, and culturally relevant is important. Helping them explore new ways of communication may yield pleasantly surprising results.

REFERENCES

1. Sarvela, P.D., and Ford, T.D. Indicators of substance use among pregnant adolescents in the Mississippi Delta. *J. Sch. Health* 62:175-179, May 1992.
2. ———An evaluation of a substance abuse education program for Mississippi delta pregnant adolescents. *J. Sch. Health* 63:147-152, Mar. 1993.
3. Eliopoulos, C., and others. Hair concentrations of nicotine and cotinine in women and their newborn infants. *JAMA* 271:621-623, Feb. 23, 1994.
4. Ostrea, E.M., Jr., and others. Meconium analysis to assess fetal exposure to nicotine by active and passive maternal smoking. *J. Pediatr.* 124:471-476, Mar. 1994.
5. Rubin, D.H., and others. Effect of passive smoking on birth-weight. *Lancet* 2:415-417, Aug. 23, 1986.
6. Makin, J., and others. A comparison of active and passive smoking during pregnancy: long-term effects. *Neurotoxicol. Teratol.* 13:5-12, Jan.-Feb. 1991.
7. Haglund, B. and Cnattingius, S. Cigarette smoking as a risk factor for sudden infant death syndrome: a population-based study. *Am. J. Public Health* 80:29-32, Jan. 1990; Erratum 82:1489, Nov. 1992.
8. Fielding, J.E., and Phenow, K.J. Health effects of involuntary smoking. *N. Engl. J. Med.* 319:1452-1460, Dec. 1, 1988.
9. National Research Council Staff, Committee on Passive Smoking. *Environmental Tobacco Smoke: Measuring Exposure and Assessing Health Effects.* Washington, D.C., National Academy Press, 1986.
10. U.S. Office on Smoking and Health. *The Health Consequences of Involuntary Smoking, A Report of the Surgeon General.* [DHHS Publication No. (CDC) 87-8398] Washington, D.C., U.S. Government Printing Office, 1986.
11. Weitzman, M., and others. Maternal smoking and childhood asthma. *Pediatrics* 85:505-511, Apr. 1990.
12. Murray, A.B., and Morrison, B.J. Passive smoking and the seasonal difference of severity of asthma in children. *Chest* 94:701-708, October 1988.
13. Evans, D., and others. The impact of passive smoking on emergency room visits of urban children with asthma. *Am. Rev. Respir. Dis.* 135:567-572, Mar. 1987.
14. Weiss, S.T. Passive smoking and lung cancer. What is the risk? [editorial] *Am. Rev. Respir. Dis.* 133:1-3, Jan. 1986.
15. Biglan, A., and others. Videotaped materials in a school-based smoking prevention program. *Prev. Med.* 17:559-584, Sept. 1988.
16. Greer, R.O., Jr. Effectiveness of video instruction in educating teenagers about the health risks of smokeless tobacco use. *J. Cancer Educ.* 4:33-37, Jan. 1989.
17. Airhihenbuwa, C.O., and Pineiro, O. Cross-cultural health education: a pedagogical challenge. *J. Sch. Health* 58:240-242, Aug. 1988.

18. Ireland, D.F. New attitude/new look: an African-American adolescent health education program. *Pediatr. Nurs.* 16:175-178, 205, Mar.-Apr. 1990.

19. Inhelder, B., and Piaget, J. *The Growth of Logical Thinking from Childhood to Adolescence.* New York, Basic Books, l958.

20. Redman, B.K. *The Process of Patient Education.* 7th ed. St. Louis, Mosby–Year Book, 1993.

21. Glynn, T.J. Essential elements of school-based smoking prevention programs. *J. Sch. Health* 59:181-188, May 1989.

22. Best, J.A., and others. Preventing cigarette smoking among school children. *Annu. Rev. Public Health* 9:161-201, 1988.

23. Botvin, G.J., and others. A cognitive-behavioral approach to substance abuse prevention: one-year follow-up. *Addict. Behav.* 15:47-63, Jan.-Feb. l990.

24. Jordanov, J.S. Cotinine concentrations in amniotic fluid and urine of smoking, passive smoking and non-smoking pregnant women at term and in the urine of their neonates on 1st day of life. *Eur. J. Pediatr.* 149:734-737, July 1990.

25. Lavengood, T.D. Involuntary smoking—children in crisis. *Pediatr. Nurs.* 14:93-95, Mar.-Apr. l988.

KANGAROO CARE: SKIN-TO-SKIN CONTACT IN THE NICU

Having parents hold their infants in a carefully monitored environment is safe and well worth the extra nursing effort.

BY FRITZI DROSTEN-BROOKS

We designed our hospital nurseries without considering the parents. When I started working in the neonatal intensive care unit (NICU) 12 years ago, only two parents were allowed in at any one time, and they were permitted to stay for only 15 minutes. It was as if the infants were theirs only upon discharge, and professionals—because we had scrubbed and wore our hospital garments—were the only ones sanitary enough to handle the infants for more than a brief touch.

The rules have changed. We accept the parents, and now acknowledge that they must be able to hold their infants as soon as possible. If parents do not begin learning about the needs of their babies and establishing a relationship at this vulnerable time, they may have problems learning those needs and providing for them later.

We have always known that the best incubator is the mother's womb, so we hold off the birth as long as we can when the mother is in premature labor. Perhaps the mother, and even the father, are still the best incubators. Though the infant is ill, very small, and connected to invasive equipment, the parents must be encouraged to enter the nursery and hold their child as long as they want and when they want.

Fritzi Drosten-Brooks, RN, CLC, is a lactation consultant and staff nurse at the Kaiser Permanente Medical Center, Oakland, California. The medical editing department of the Kaiser Foundation Research Institute provided editorial assistance.

My experience with kangaroo care, skin-to-skin contact between infants and their parents, began during my years as a mother-infant recovery room nurse, with full-term infants. As I learned more, I began to include kangaroo care in my NICU nursing practice for much smaller infants. Observations of the babies during and after contacts with the parents led to the conclusion that this contact was good. At first the infants would open their eyes and look around; then they would settle down and sleep. As I put them back in their isolettes, I saw a relaxed look on their faces, and they would continue to sleep and rest well for a long time. The parents left the nursery smiling.

The advantages of kangaroo care have been documented in the literature (1-13). They include decreased oxygen requirements, longer quiet sleep periods, and shortened hospitalization. (For a brief review of some of the results that have been documented to date, see Safety and Effectiveness of Kangaroo Care: Summary of the Literature.)

TWO EARLY EXAMPLES

One of the first infants in our unit who received successful long-term skin-to-skin care was the daughter of an occupational therapist who had worked with developmentally disabled children. Shortly after birth, the baby girl (1480 g) had suffered a grade IV intraventricular hemorrhage. The mother, who had a keen understanding of high-risk infants, was enthusiastic when approached about kangaroo care for her daughter and read the literature I provided. With the knowledge and support of the physicians on the unit, I initiated skin-to-skin contact.

During lengthy daily visits, the mother and her husband buttoned the baby into her or his shirt. Being allowed to come in the nursery, visit at length, and provide a warm bed with a heartbeat gave a positive tone to the parents' visits. The infant had no problems when she was held.

The second baby was a 27-week infant girl, 1030 g, who squirmed and appeared uncomfortable while on the ventilator. The infant appeared to love kangaroo care; her oxygenation saturation remained in the high 90s when she was held. The nurses were moved as they watched the family's positive reactions, and both parents became active participants in the program.

The mother was the first to hold the infant, who was first held while intubated, then while receiving nasal continuous positive airway pressure, and finally while receiving oxygen by nasal cannula. When the mother held her daughter to her chest, she covered the other side of the baby with a special bulky blanket, the baby's own, to shield her from the lights and sounds of the nursery. The blanket was kept in the cabinet of the isolette and was used just for holding times.

After the parents and daughter experienced kangaroo care, the infant became part of a newer program, which started breast-feeding at around the age of 32 weeks if no other problems existed and delayed bottle-feeding as

SAFETY AND EFFECTIVENESS OF KANGAROO CARE: SUMMARY OF THE LITERATURE

Author	Safety	Effectiveness
Acolet (3)	Skin temperature maintained. No apnea or bradycardia during holding.	Some infants with chronic lung disease showed rise in $TcpO_2$.
Ludington (4,9)	Heart rate increased slightly. Temperatures were stable.	Quiet sleep and length of sleep increased. Activity level decreased. Prone position recommended.
Whitelaw (10,12)		Mothers lactated longer. At six months, infants cried less.
de Leeuw (13)	No change in transcutaneous oxygen level ($TcpO_2$), heart and respiration rates, apneic attacks, or temperature.	Apneic attacks diminished.
Affonso (6)		Kangaroo care infants were discharged sooner than other infants; infants were breast-fed longer; and mothers were confident of their ability to care for infant.
Anderson (1)		Infants (in Colombia, SA) were discharged while still quite small to avoid stay in overcrowded hospital with little equipment to maintain infants.

long as possible. The parents had long visits holding their daughter in the chair. The infant thrived on kangaroo care, and the presence of her parents in the nursery helped assure staff that the program was working.

CLINICAL CONCERNS

Close monitoring of the parent and child is necessary to alleviate clinical concerns. In addition, parents are taught to focus on the infant's responses to being held. Primary concerns relate to overstimulation, airway management, and temperature control.

Overstimulation: The nervous systems of the tiniest infants are constantly bombarded by the lights, sounds, handling by staff, and procedures of an NICU. The infants have had to experience all sorts of unexpected events and are just becoming used to this new environment. A sudden transfer to outside the incubator may be a rude shock, no matter how comfortable it may become in five or ten minutes.

Gently trying to awaken the infants to prepare them for handling helps to smooth the transition. When placed on their parents' skin, infants respond best when those in the area are as quiet and still as possible. This is sometimes difficult because the experience is so intensely emotional for the parents. They usually must stop themselves from crying, and from talking and rocking. Other nurses or family members may

want to come and make comments, but this must be avoided.

Being very quiet and whispering, dimming the lights, and providing a screen for privacy all help to remind parents to be quiet. It is easy to stop the rocking by placing a hand on the back of the chair, reminding the parents about the reasons not to rock the baby at this time. The observing nurse can sit behind the family so that monitors are in view and the family has a semblance of privacy.

As an infant grows and the parents become more confident, some parents become louder and more active with their baby, who may still be too young to tolerate the stimulation. Close observation of the infants' tolerance of activities must remain a nursing and a teaching priority. Infants not tolerating stimulation will display signs of stress, such as frowning, looking very tired, or becoming agitated.

Airway Management: Preventing problems is better than contending with the parental guilt that results when an infant has a problem the first time she is held by the parent. Endotracheal tubes can be managed by listening to breath sounds, assuring that the infant does not need suctioning, and by having a second or third nurse assist with the transfer. After the infant is in the parent's arms, the tubing can be secured with tape to the parent's clothing.

Handling recently extubated infants,

or those receiving intermittent nasal continuous positive airway pressure, is helped by awakening them and allowing them to first stretch and yawn. If needed, suctioning is done before the transfer, with some recovery time allowed. Infants are best placed in a vertical position, prone on the chest, between the breasts (1,2). Close observation of infants by NICU nurses is necessary and can be augmented by cardiorespiratory and oxygen saturation monitors.

Temperature Control: A main reason that parents have not been allowed to hold such small infants was the belief that the infants would be cold. Although this fear is still common among many physicians and nurses and often is a topic of discussion, no deleterious effects have been reported (3,4). It is important to remember that people have warm skin, so skin-to-skin contact is preferable to blankets alone for small infants.

We ask parents to wear button-front shirts. We button the shirt around the babies and perhaps place a blanket around the shirt. Skin probes on the infants can monitor the temperature. Infants not only stay warm but often perspire next to the parent's skin. They may even become uncomfortable because they are too hot and need a layer of blanket removed. If they become cold, a warming lamp or warm blanket may be used, but watching for drafts and keeping the

ELEMENTS OF KANGAROO CARE PROTOCOL

Candidates

Infants whose parents wish to hold them, who are stable enough to tolerate handling, and whose nurses feel comfortable encouraging the parents to hold them. In general, infants larger than 800 g may be kangaroo held.

Monitoring

All infants must be monitored while being held. Consider using heat lamps to help maintain temperature if infant is less than five days old and has never been out of a radiant warmer or isolette. Infants who are intubated, have an umbilical catheter, or chest tube must have a nurse at the bedside continuously. Observe infant for signs of stress, vital sign stability, and patency of all lines, and return to isolette as necessary. Monitor temperature every hour. Observe frequently during the session, especially while parents are gaining competence at observing their infant for signs of distress.

Positioning

Position infant carefully. Most infants tolerate this handling best in an upright position, prone, on the parent's breast, or between the breasts. Provide kangaroo care for infant as long as the baby is stable, and the parent desires, usually one to two times daily, for one hour or more. Do not disturb infant if at all possible while he is sleeping. Provide for privacy as much as possible. Place blanket over infant, or button shirt over infant as needed. Since a parent's temperature is usually 98.6° F, hats on infants are generally not necessary.

Infant Stimuli: Parent Teaching

Explain the kangaroo concept to parents when applicable, so they may choose to participate if they desire. Instruct skin-to-skin participants to wear a blouse or shirt that opens in front, so that the infant may be partially "buttoned on" and protected from heat loss. Parent teaching focuses on observing the infant's responses to being held. Reassure parents and provide support as needed, as many parents become very emotional during the initial holding, especially with an extremely small infant. Explain that transition to skin-to-skin contact is a big environmental change and the infant may not be able to tolerate added stroking, rocking, talking to, or eye contact with observers. The infant will become better equipped to handle more stimuli as he matures.

infant on the chest usually prevents this problem.

STAFF ADJUSTMENT

Another identified problem is staff resistance. Nurses tend to fear that problems will occur and that they will be blamed. The idea that the infant's condition may improve in a parent's arms is difficult to introduce (4,5). In addition, some nurses have difficulty incorporating parent teaching into the care of the infant in a critical care unit. However, such teaching early in the hospital stay reaps long-term benefits for infants, parents, and staff. In our hospital, we have had few line or tube problems during infant holding and have noted that parents' anxiety decreases as the level of attachment increases.

Nurses' attitudes tend to change as they observe the reactions of infants to skin-to-skin contact with parents. In our hospital, support for kangaroo care came from the unit supervisor, who had previous experience at a hospital where limited infant holding was encouraged. The nursery educator invited a nurse researcher to give a presentation on the practice, and a neonatologist brought in relevant literature. In general, the physicians and supervisors were supportive and recommended the preparation of guidelines for skin-to-skin holding in the nursery. A written protocol was developed. (See Elements of Kangaroo Care Protocol.)

Problems have centered around the presence of parents in the NICU for extended periods of time. While parents are typically asked to leave during nurses' reports and physicians' rounds, creative planning is possible so that the parent-baby couple may remain undisturbed. The reports may be given in another area or the parents, infant, and monitor may be taken to an empty breast-feeding room or isolation room when possible to avoid interrupting the visit. Some infants are irritable and difficult to care for and do better if they are held uninterrupted.

Our NICU, as a tertiary referral center, provides hands-on experience with kangaroo care for staff nurses doing preceptorships in our nursery. In addition, we actively share information with nurses and physicians from referring hospitals by providing outreach educational programs.

A SPACE FOR FAMILIES

When a father dozed off while holding his son, my first impulse was to tell him that he might drop the baby. Then I remembered that his son was buttoned into his shirt and still monitored. The father looked so comfortable with his feet up and the baby's head sticking out of the shirt, that we let him and his infant sleep.

The technology in the NICU has come a long way. By helping families cope with this technology and making it work for them, we are on our way to the ultimate desired outcome—a healthy infant going home to capable parents.

But we must redesign our nurseries. Parents need space to visit their babies and space for family privacy. They need easy chairs and rockers, screens, quiet corners, footstools, and pillows. Improved nursery environments will not come quickly, yet such improvements are not costly. Additional space or rockers will better fit the economic crisis that hospitals face today than will purchasing more expensive machinery. We have made tremendous progress in the last few years in neonatal intensive care. Widespread acceptance of kangaroo care will improve our practice even more.

REFERENCES

1. Anderson, G.C., and others. Kangaroo care for premature infants. *Am. J. Nurs.* 86:807-809; Erratum 86:1000, Sept. 1986.
2. Heimler, R., and others. Effect of positioning on the breathing pattern of preterm infants. *Arch. Dis. Child.* 67:312-314, Mar. 1992.
3. Acolet, D., and others. Oxygenation, heart rate and temperature in very low birthweight infants during skin-to-skin

contact with their mothers. *Acta. Paediatr. Scand.* 78:189-193, Mar. 1989.

4. Ludington, S. M. Energy conservation during skin-to-skin contact between premature infants and their mothers. *Heart Lung* 19(5 Pt 1):445-451, Sept. 1990.

5. Anderson, G.C. Current knowledge about skin-to-skin (kangaroo) care for preterm infants. *J. Perinatol.* 11:216-226, Sept. 1991.

6. Affonso, D.D., and others. Exploration of mothers' reactions to the kangaroo method of prematurity care. *Neonatal Netw.* 7:43-51, June 1989.

7. Anderson, G.C. Skin-to-skin: kangaroo care in western Europe. *Am. J. Nurs.* 89:662-666, May 1989.

8. Colonna, F., and others. The "kangaroo-mother" method: evaluation of an alternative model for the care of low birth weight newborns in developing countries. *Int. J. Gynaecol. Obstet.* 31:335-339, Apr. 1990.

9. Ludington, S.M., and others. Efficacy of kangaroo care with preterm infants in open-air cribs. [abstract] *Neonatal Netw.* 11:101, Sept. 1992.

10. Whitelaw, A. Kangaroo baby care: just a nice experience or an important advance for preterm infants? *Pediatrics* 85:604-605, Apr. 1990.

11. Whitelaw, A., and Sleath, K. Myth of the marsupial mother: home care of very low birth weight babies in Bogota, Colombia. *Lancet* 1:1206-1208, May 25, 1985.

12. Whitelaw, A., and others. Skin to skin contact for very low birthweight infants and their mothers. *Arch. Dis. Child.* 63:1377-1381, Nov. 1988.

13. de Leeuw, R., and others. Physiological effects of kangaroo care in very small preterm infants. *Biol. Neonate* 59(3):149-155, 1991.

GUIDELINES FOR ASSESSING HIV IN WOMEN

Many women are diagnosed late or not at all. A system-by-system physical assessment and specific questions about risk behaviors can lead to identification of HIV.

BY CAROLYN SIPES

As many as 110,000 women in the United States may be unaware that they are infected with human immunodeficiency virus (HIV), the virus that causes AIDS (1). The primary reason is that HIV is a silent disease, which can take 10 years to manifest symptoms (1). A careful examination—asking the right questions and examining the patient carefully, head to toe—will help identify signs and symptoms that are common indicators of HIV disease.

The Centers for Disease Control and Prevention (CDC) reports that HIV infection continues to increase at an alarming rate (2). Approximately 1 million persons in the United States are believed to be infected, a figure that remains constant because the rate of infection corresponds with the rate of deaths (3).

Many women are at risk because they are unaware of the modes of transmission of HIV and fail to recognize or acknowledge their own risk behaviors. Some consider HIV to be a "gay disease" or something that happens to others, such as prostitutes and intravenous drug users (4). Some fail to recognize how their sexual partners put them at risk. They may not ask the right questions or even question their partners at all. Or, perhaps, the partners are untruthful or uninformed.

Of those who are infected, many have been misdiagnosed, not diagnosed at all, or diagnosed in a late stage of HIV disease when they already have

developed AIDS. Moreover, infected women often do not trust nurses and other health care workers. They fear stigmatization, rejection, or abandonment and thus withhold information critical for rapid assessment and treatment (5-7).

Health care providers contribute to the problem by attributing symptoms to other causes (8). Some do not know the signs and symptoms of HIV disease as they specifically relate to women. Women have only recently been included in research studies, and much of the current information is extrapolated from studies of men (8,9). Kaposi's sarcoma, for example, is seen mostly in men, while affected women frequently suffer from gynecological infections.

There is also reluctance to ask personal questions regarding sexual practices and risk behaviors (5). These factors make it difficult to obtain a complete health and risk assessment and therefore impede important diagnoses.

The life expectancy of women after diagnosis of HIV is less than that of men. This results from the fact that women are frequently diagnosed at a late stage, when they are already very sick (10). Women with HIV are predominantly in the age group 15 to 44 and economically disadvantaged. They are less likely to seek health care than men, who usually have greater economic security and access to services (11).

HIV HEALTH HISTORY AND PHYSICAL ASSESSMENT

When woman are infected with HIV, their quality of life and life ex-

pectancy depend on early diagnosis and treatment. A complete head-to-toe physical assessment is needed, along with a health history and risk assessment.

HIV exhibits a variety of signs and symptoms caused by numerous organisms. The most common symptoms are outlined in the Summary of Common or Early Indicators of HIV in Women. The 1993 HIV Classification System for Adults and Adolescents lists conditions indicative of HIV infection with and without laboratory testing and helps clarify how the AIDS diagnosis is determined. Use of this system provides specific guidelines for early indicator diseases that alert the clinician to examine the patient further.

The health history and physical assessment start with a general review of the systems. First, obtain general information regarding weight loss, weakness, fatigue, and history of fevers and flulike symptoms during the past 6 to 12 months. Then start the physical assessment, using a system-by-system approach that incorporates health history questions.

General survey. In a succinct overview, record pulse, respiratory rate, blood pressure, temperature, and current weight. Ask questions about unexpected weight loss over the last few months, unexplained fevers, episodes of diarrhea, night sweats, and general nutrition. Ask for a dietary history related to any changes, particularly decreased intake, that might explain weight loss. Anorexia, poor appetite and the inability to eat, is frequently noted in HIV disease (12).

Skin. It is important to remember

Carolyn Sipes, MSN, CNS, is a doctoral candidate at Rush University, Chicago, Illinois.

that skin diseases most frequently seen in uninfected individuals will be more severe in HIV disease. Examine the facial skin for lesions and rashes. Eyelids and areas behind the ears are frequent sites for seborrheic dermatitis. Folliculitis, a rash caused by *Staphylococcus aureus,* is frequently seen in those who are HIV positive (13).

Small, pearly, blisterlike lesions on the face are *Molluscum contagiosum.* These frequently occurring lesions, caused by poxvirus, may be open and draining, requiring the use of gloves during the assessment (14,15).

Although rarely seen in women, cutaneus lesions that are painless, not itchy or ulcerated, and purple to red in color may be signs of Kaposi's sarcoma. Herpes zoster, known as shingles, is exhibited by a rash that follows nerve pathways. This condition is very painful (16).

Eyes. Examine the eyes for external lesions or rashes. Examine the retina for hemorrhagic areas and "cotton-wool" spots, caused by cytomegalovirus (CMV). A common early sign of CMV retinitis is decreased visual acuity or the presence of "floaters" (17,18).

Oropharyngeal. Among the earliest signs of HIV infection are white plaques on the oral mucosa and esophagus, known as candidiasis or thrush. This fungal infection gives the mouth a "cottage cheese" appearance and may cause dysphagia, painful swallowing, and sternal pain. It may contribute to inability to eat and consequent weight loss (19).

Other white lesions seen on the tongue, primarily on the dorsal surfaces, may be hairy leukoplakia. These lesions are painless and cannot be scraped off the tongue. Hairy leukoplakia is an AIDS indicator disease if the patient is HIV positive. It has been identified with rapid progression of HIV disease (20).

Lesions frequently seen in more advanced disease include recurrent aphthous ulcers (RAU). These are red with white borders and are found on the palate. They are extremely painful, making it difficult to eat and swallow (21).

The last oral lesion indicative of HIV and AIDS is recurrent oral herpes simplex that does not respond to treatment. These lesions manifest as painful ulcerating vesicles usually seen on the gingiva or palate (22).

Neck and lymph nodes. The next areas to assess are the lymph nodes of the upper torso, including the parotid, supraclavicular, axillary, and other nodes in this area. Examination of the nodes is of particular importance, because persistent generalized lymphadenopathy (PGL) is one of the earliest signs of HIV disease (23,24). The nodes most frequently involved, in decreasing order, are cervical, axillary, inguinal, supraclavicular, infraclavicular, and popliteal. These nodal chains need to be assessed in each system as those areas are examined.

Thorax and lungs. The thorax is evaluated for skin diseases, such as the rashes and lesions described above. Women with HIV disease may have two or more concurrent skin diseases.

Recurrent herpes zoster, involving more than one dermatome, is indicative of HIV infection and may present as a painful rash that follows the nerve pathways (3).

Lymph node involvement in this area, that is, PGL, may cause cellulitis and edema of the upper extremities. Evaluate for a history of recurrent bacterial, viral, and fungal pneumonias. An AIDS-defining diagnosis is *Pneumocystis carinii pneumoniae* (PCP), caused by a fungus. Early signs of PCP are fever and fatigue. Later signs include fever, nonproductive cough, and shortness of breath, first on exertion, then at rest (16,22).

Abdomen. Evaluation is needed for episodes of diarrhea, a common complaint in HIV that can be caused by numerous organisms. Cytomegalovirus (CMV) and *Mycobacterium avium*

SUMMARY OF COMMON OR EARLY INDICATORS OF HIV IN WOMEN

The Physical Exam by System	Symptoms	Causes
General	Weight loss, fever	*Mycobacterium avium,* AIDS-wasting syndrome, anorexia
Skin	Lesions, rashes	*Staphylococcus,* shingles, Kaposi's sarcoma (KS)
Eyes	Cotton-wool spots, floaters	Cytomegalovirus (CMV) retinitis
Oropharyngeal	White plaques, oral ulcers, dysphagia	Candidiasis, hairy leukoplakia, recurrent aphthous ulcers, herpes
Lymph nodes	Generalized lymphadenopathy	Persistent generalized lymphadenopathy (PGL), lymphoma
Thorax and lungs	Lesions, rashes, pneumonias, fever, shortness of breath, cough, cellulitis	*Staphylococcus,* shingles, PGL, *Pneumocystis carinii* pneumonia (PCP), tuberculosis (TB), bacterial and fungual infections
Abdomen	Diarrhea, abdominal pain, weight loss	*Mycobacterium avium* (MAC), CMV
Neurologic and mental status	Confusion, fever, headache	Central nervous system (CNS) toxoplasmosis, cryptococcosis
Genitourinary	Vaginal discharge, itching, fever, headache, dysuria, pain, lesions, warts, severe lower abdominal pain, tenderness, bleeding	Vaginal candidiasis, cervical intraepithelial neoplasia (CIN), human papilloma virus (HPV), genital herpes, pelvic inflammatory disease (PID), sexually transmitted disease (STD)

complex (MAC) are identified as co-factors of disease progression in men that may increase the rate of disease progression in infected women. They cause severe abdominal pain, diarrhea, and malabsorption with weight loss (25). These infections need to be assessed and treated properly.

Neurologic and mental status. Central nervous system (CNS) involvement associated with HIV results from a number of causes. The primary signs are usually due to *Toxoplasmosis gondii* infections, which cause encephalitis, and *Cryptococcus neoformans,* which causes meningitis.

The signs of toxoplasmic encephalitis are fever, headache, altered mental status, confusion, and cognitive impairment. There may also be focal neurological changes, as well as changes that resemble a cerebral vascular accident, such as hemiparesis (19). If toxoplasmosis is suspected, it is important to evaluate the patient's dietary habits with regard to eating raw or undercooked meats and contact with cat feces, for example, cleaning litter boxes.

The lung is frequently the primary site for cryptococcosis, while meningitis is the most prevalent life-threatening manifestation. Cryptococcal meningitis exhibits typical meningitis symptoms such as headache, nausea, vomiting, and confusion (26).

Genitourinary. In several studies of women, chronic, refractory vaginal candidiasis has been found to be the first clinical indicator of HIV infection (27). Common symptoms are complaints of vaginal discharge and itching. Treatments will control symptoms, but will not cure the infections.

In addition, women who are HIV positive are at increased risk for cervical intraepithelial neoplasia (CIN). Added to the CDC list in 1993, CIN manifests many of the same signs as sexually transmitted diseases (STDs) in women. A precursor of cervical neoplasia, human papilloma virus (HPV) has also been found to exacerbate cervical abnormalities in women who are HIV positive (11).

Other common complaints are related to herpes simplex type-2 infections, also known as genital herpes. They include fever, headache, dysuria, pain, and lesions or warts in the genital area. Pelvic inflammatory disease (PID) is frequently seen in women with

---

1993 HIV CLASSIFICATION SYSTEM FOR ADULTS AND ADOLESCENTS

Without laboratory evidence of HIV infection:
- Candidasis of esophagus, trachea, bronchi, or lungs
- Cryptococcosis, extrapulmonary
- Cryptosporidiosis with diarrhea persistent longer than one month
- Cytomegalovirus disease other than lymph nodes
- Herpes simplex virus infection longer than a month, bronchitis, pneumonitis, or esophagitis
- Kaposi's sarcoma (KS), less than 60 years of age
- Lymphoma of brain (primary), less than 60 years of age
- *Mycobacterium avium* complex (MAC), disseminated
- *Pneumocystis carinii pneumoniae* (PCP)
- Progressive multifocal leukoencephalopathy
- Toxoplasmosis of the brain

With laboratory evidence of HIV infection: symptomatic conditions occurring in an HIV-infected adolescent or adult that meet at least one of the following criteria: 1) the conditions are attributed to HIV infection and/or are indicative of a defect in cell-mediated immunity; or 2) the conditions are considered by physicians to have a clinical course or management that is complicated by HIV infection. Examples of conditions include, but are not limited to:
- Bacterial endocarditis, meningitis, pneumonia, or sepsis
- Candidiasis, vulvovaginal; persistent (longer than one month duration) or poorly responsive to therapy
- Candidiasis, oropharyngeal (thrush)
- Cervical dysplasia, severe; or carcinoma
- Coccidioidomycosis, disseminated
- Constitutional symptoms, such as fever (≥38.5°C) or diarrhea lasting longer than one month
- HIV encephalopathy (HIV dementia)
- HIV wasting syndrome
- Hairy leukoplakia, oral
- Herpes zoster (shingles), involving at least two distinct episodes or more than one dermatome
- Histoplasmosis, disseminated
- Idiopathic thrombocytopenic purpura
- Isosporiasis with diarrhea persisting longer than one month
- Invasive cervical cancers
- KS at any age
- Listeriosis
- *Mycobacterium tuberculosis,* pulmonary
- Nocardiosis
- Pelvic inflammatory disease
- Peripheral neuropathy

Adapted from Centers for Disease Control and Prevention. 1993 revised classification system for HIV infection and expanded AIDS surveillance case definition for adolescents and adults. *Morbidity and Mortality Weekly Report,* RR-7, 1992; 41:1-5.

HIV disease and is usually associated with STDs. Signs and symptoms include fever, severe lower abdominal pain, tenderness, vaginal discharge, and/or bleeding. Some women may have mild or no symptoms (28).

CONDUCTING A RISK ASSESSMENT

Because women tend to be uneducated regarding signs of HIV disease or deny the possibility of becoming infected, they need to be assessed at every opportunity. As patient advocates, nurses must be able recognize the signs of HIV and take appropriate actions, such as referrals for laboratory testing and providing follow-up for treatment. Those nurses working with pregnant women must complete the HIV assessment as quickly as possible, as treatment with zidovudine (Retrovir, also

RECOMMENDED RESOURCES FOR WOMEN

WARN (Women and AIDS Resource Network), 30 Third Avenue, Room 213, Brooklyn, NY 11217; call 718-596-6007. Provides HIV education, support, advocacy, and referrals.

National Women's Health Network, 1325 G Street NW, Washington, DC 20005; call 202-347-1140. An advocacy group that also provides information on HIV infection.

Sister Love Women's AIDS Project, 1237 R. Ralph Abernathy Blvd., SW, Atlanta, GA 30310; call 404-753-7733. An AIDS outreach group that provides training kits or training workshops for facilitation of "health love parties." The parties teach small groups of women about HIV infection and prevention.

known as AZT) will greatly reduce the risk of HIV transmission to the fetus. (For more information about vertical HIV transmission, see Keeping Up with Neonatal Infection: Designer Bugs, Part II, by J. W. Lott and C. Kenner, *MCN*, September/October 1994.)

Nurses must also take an active role in educating women about HIV disease and the factors leading to transmission. Those who have problems coming to terms with aspects of HIV will need to consider their feelings about the disease. They may benefit from spending time as observers in clinics, homes, or hospices for women. By watching women interact with others, they will acquire a clearer understanding of the psychosocial effects of the disease.

They also need to examine their own level of comfort when asking questions about sexual and potentially risky behaviors that put women at risk. Often, nurses believe the client will be untruthful or refuse to respond when answering questions. The following suggestions may be helpful:

• Role play with peers before conducting an assessment. Comfort levels improve as the number of interviews increases.

• View the process from the client's perspective. Correct misconceptions and point out risk behaviors, but don't be overly judgmental or critical.

• Tell the client that you are concerned for her safety. This will help establish trust.

• Conduct the risk assessment on all clients, treating everyone the same way. Asking all women the same questions—not only those suspected to be at high risk for HIV infection—will help eliminate bias. Women in their 50s, married for the second time, have

frequently been overlooked and found to be infected late.

• The woman may not have been tested for HIV but wants to be. If she asks about HIV testing, refer her for pre- and posttest counseling. In some states, counseling prior to being tested for HIV is required.

• Remember, HIV is considered a silent disease, and patients frequently do not show symptoms until the disease is advanced, 10 years on the average. When women do show symptoms of HIV, they may have fully developed AIDS.

RISK ASSESSMENT QUESTIONNAIRE

Knowledge of institutional policies and state laws regarding issues of confidentiality is essential before proceeding with risk assessment. Also essential is knowledge about which counseling services are available. Some questions may trigger strong emotions, especially if the client is revealing information for the first time. (For further information about counseling, see Recommended Resources for Women.)

The interview begins with the assurance that responses will be kept confidential. Written consent is requested, if that is the institution's policy, and the reasons for the assessment are outlined. The client is told that the assessment is needed to provide adequate services and treatment for women, identify the need for further health assessment and monitoring, and provide education about risk behaviors.

To get the most useful information, it is important to ask specific questions. Questions are categorized as general, HIV specific, sexual practices, drugs, and alcohol.

• *General.* Do you think you are at risk for becoming infected with HIV? Did you have a blood transfusion prior to 1985?

• *HIV/AIDS.* Have you ever been tested for HIV? Do you know how you can get HIV/AIDS? Have you participated in any behaviors that might be risky, such as having multiple partners, having sex with a bisexual male, or having sex with someone who has? Have you had sex for money? Have you had a new partner in the last year? Have you had any sexually transmitted diseases, such as herpes simplex virus (HSV) or chlamydia? Has your partner been tested for HIV?

• *Sexual practices.* Are you aware of your partner's past history and sexual orientation? How many partners has he had? Have any of his partners been gay or bisexual? How many sexual partners have you had in the past three to six months? Were any of these partners HIV positive? What types of sex have you had—vaginal intercourse, anal intercourse, or oral sex? How do you protect yourself when you have sex? Do you use condoms? If so, what kind and how often? How does your partner feel about using condoms? Do you use them with a spermicide?

• *Drugs.* Have you or your partner used any street or illegal drugs in the last week, month, year, or ever used drugs? If so, what kind? Do you "shoot up"? How do you clean your "works"? Do you share needles, "cookers," or other drug equipment?

• *Alcohol.* Do you use alcohol? How many glasses of wine or beer per day? per week? What kind of alcohol do you use?

After the assessment for the risk for HIV, be sure to refer the client to the appropriate service agencies for treatment or counseling.

As patient advocates, nurses have an important impact on women's health. Armed with the knowledge that women frequently do not know that they are infected with HIV, nurses must learn the signs and symptoms of the disease, from its earliest stages. And, sadly, as many women engage in behaviors that place them at risk, nurses must ask the right questions and provide accurate and timely information. These steps are critical to improving the length and quality of life of all women and their children.

REFERENCES

1. Novello. A. The HIV/AIDS epidemic: a current picture. *J. Acquir. Immune Defic. Syndr.* 6:645-654, 1993.
2. Hankins, C.A., and Handley, M.A. HIV disease and AIDS in Women: current knowledge and a research agenda. *J. Acquir. Immune Defic. Syndr.* 5:957-971, Oct. 1992.
3. U.S. Centers for Disease Control. Addendum to the proposed expansion of the AIDS surveillance case definition. *MMWR Morb. Mortal. Wkly. Rep.* 42:1-4, Oct. 1993.
4. Bennett, G., and others. A potential source for the transmission of the human immunodeficiency virus into the heterosexual population: bisexual men who frequent beats. *Med. J. Aust.* 151:309-314, Sept. 8, 1989.
5. Day, N. Training providers to serve culturally different AIDS patients. *Fam. Community Health* 13(2):46-53, 1990.
6. Schilling, R.F., and others. Developing strategies for AIDS prevention research with black and Hispanic drug users, *Public Health Rep.* 104:2-11, Jan.-Feb. 1989.
7. Thomas, S.B. Public health then and now: The Tuskegee Syphilis Study, 1932 to 1972: implications for HIV education and AIDS risk education programs in the black community. *Am. J. Public Health* 81:1498-1505, Nov. 1991.
8. Cohen, F. Clinical manifestations and treatment of HIV infection and AIDS in women. In *Women Children and HIV/AIDS,* edited by F.L. Cohen and J.D. Durham. New York, Springer Publishing Co., 1993, pp. 169-190.
9. Gwinn, M., and others. Prevalence of HIV infection in childrearing women in the United States. *JAMA* 265:1704-1708, Apr. 3, 1991.
10. Grant, I., and others. Gender differences in AIDS-defining illnesses. In *Abstracts of the VII International Conference on AIDS* held in Florence, Italy, 1991, Vol. 1, P346; abstract MC 3192.
11. Anastos, K., and Palleja, S.M. Caring for women at risk of HIV infection. *J. Gen. Intern. Med.* 6(1 Suppl.):S40-S46, Jan. 1991.
12. U. S. Centers for Disease Control. 1993 revised classification system for HIV infection and expanded surveillance case definition for AIDS among adolescents and adults. *MMWR Morb. Mortal. Wkly. Rep.* 41(RR-17):1-19, Dec. 1992.
13. Jacobson, M.A., and others. *Staphylococcus aureus* bacteremia and recurrent staphylococcal infection in patients with acquired immunodeficiency syndrome and AIDS-related complex. *Am. J. Med.* 85:172-176, Aug. 1988.
14. Farthing, C. Non-malignant cutaneous disease in AIDS and related conditions. *Clin. Immunol. Allergy* 6(3):559-567, 1986.
15. Franco, E.L. Viral etiology of cervical cancer: a critique of the evidence. *Rev. Infect. Dis.* 13:1195-1206, Nov.-Dec. 1991.
16. Long, I. *Womens AIDS Treatment Issues: 1991 Update.* New York, The author, 1991. (Available from Iris Long, PhD, c/o ACT-UP New York, 496 Hudson Street, Suite 4G, New York, NY 10014)
17. Schuman, J.S., and others. Acquired immunodeficiency syndrome (AIDS). *Surv. Ophthalmol.* 31:384-410, May-June 1987.
18. Drew, W. Cytomegalovirus infection in patients with AIDS. *J. Infect. Dis.* 158:449-456, Aug. 1988.
19. Glatt, A.E., and others. Current concepts. Treatment of infections associated with human immunodeficiency virus. *N. Engl. J. Med.* 318:1439-1448, June 2, 1988; Erratum 319:1166, Oct. 27, 1988.
20. U.S. Centers for Disease Control. Projection of the number of persons diagnosed with AIDS and the number of immunosuppressed HIV-infected persons—United States, 1992-1994. *MMWR Morb. Mortal. Wkly.Rep.* 41(RR18), 1993.
21. Greenspan, J., and others. Diagnosis and management of the oral manifestations of HIV infection and AIDS. In *The Medical Management of AIDS,* 2nd ed., edited by M.A. Sande and P.A. Volberding. Philadelphia, W.B. Saunders, 1990, pp. 131-144. (4th ed. 1994)
22. St. Louis, M.E., and others. Seroprevalence rates of human immunodeficiency virus infections at sentinel hospitals in the United States. *N. Engl. J. Med.* 323:213-218, July 26, 1990.
23. Levine, A. (1988). Reactive and neoplastic lymphoproliferative disorders and other miscellaneous cancers associated with HIV infection. In *AIDS Etiology. Diagnosis Treatment and Prevention,* 2nd ed., edited by V.T. DeVita, Jr. and others. Philadelphia: J.B. Lippincott, 1988, pp. 110-275. (3rd ed. 1992)
24. Yarchoan, R., and others. AIDS therapies. *Sci. Am.* 259:110-119, Oct. 1988.
25. Handsfield, H.H. Heterosexual transmission of human immunodeficiency virus. [editorial] *JAMA* 260:1943-1944, Oct. 7, 1988.
26. Price, R., and Brew, B. (1988). Management of the neurologic complications of HIV infection and AIDS. In *The Medical Management of AIDS,* 2nd ed., edited by M.A. Sande and P.A. Volberding. Philadelphia, W.B. Saunders, 1988, pp. 111-126. (4th ed. 1994)
27. Imam, N., and others. Hierarchical pattern of mucosal candida infections in HIV-seropositive women. *Am. J. Med.* 89:142-146, Aug. 1990.
28. Carpenter, C.C., and others. Human immunodeficiency virus infection in North American women: experience with 200 cases and a review of the literature. *Medicine* (Baltimore) 70:307-325, Sept. 1991.

BIBLIOGRAHY

Feinkind, L., and Minkoff H. HIV in pregnancy. *Clin. Perinatol.* 15(2):189-202, 1988.

Flaskerund. J.H., and Nyamathi, A.M. Black and Latina women's AIDS related knowledge, attitudes, and practice. *Res. Nurs. Health* 12:339-346, Dec. 1989.

Kurth, A., ed. *Until the Cure: Caring for Women with HIV.* New Haven, Yale University Press, 1993.

Raisler, J. Safer sex for women. *Clin. Issu. Perinat. Womens Health Nurs.* 1(1):28-32, 1990.

Contents

Chapter **5**

Nursing Care
of the Child

COORDINATOR
Susan Colvert Droske, RN, MN, CPN

Contributors

Karen S. Bernardy, RN, MSN

Susan Colvert Droske, RN, MN, CPN

Judith W. Gross, RN, PhD

Maribeth L. Moran, RN, BSN, MSN, CPN

The Healthy Child

INFANT (1 MONTH TO 1 YEAR)

1. Normal growth and development
   a. Psychosocial development—Erikson: trust vs. mistrust (see Table 2-1, p. 15)
      1. trust: infant's needs are met consistently, resulting in feelings of physical comfort and emotional security; learns to love and be loved
      2. depends on the quality of the relationship between the primary caregiver and infant
   b. Physical growth and development
      1. physical growth should follow standard growth curves
      2. length: 50% increase by 1 year (grows from average 20 inches at birth to 30 inches at 1 year)
      3. weight
         a. gains about 1½ pounds per month during the first 6 months; ¾ pounds per month the second 6 months
         b. doubles at 5 to 6 months
         c. triples by 1 year (18 to 25 pounds at 1 year)
      4. head circumference greater than chest circumference until age 2
      5. vital signs (Table 5-1)
         a. pulse 80 to 150 per minute; average 100 per minute
         b. respirations 20 to 50 per minute
      6. developmental characteristics
         a. cephalocaudal (head to tail): gross motor skills
            ▪ 3 months: lifts head and shoulders off table
            ▪ 5 months: turns over, no head lag when in sitting position
            ▪ 6 months: assumes tripod position; supports weight when held in standing position
            ▪ 7 months: sits alone with hands held forward for support
            ▪ 8 months: sits securely without support
            ▪ 9 months: able to "creep" and crawl, able to regain balance when sitting
            ▪ 10 months: pulls to standing position
            ▪ 1 year: stands upright, able to "cruise" about a room by holding onto objects; may take first "solo" steps
         b. proximal to distal (central axis of body outward) and general to specific (differentiate): fine motor skills
            ▪ 3 to 4 months: arm control; supports upper body weight; "rakes" objects with hands
            ▪ 6 to 7 months: transfers objects from one hand to the other
            ▪ 10 months: pincer (thumb and index finger) grasp intact
      c. fontanels
            ▪ anterior: closes at 12 to 18 months
            ▪ posterior: closes at 2 months (may be closed at birth)
      d. teeth: development begins in utero
            ▪ 4 to 8 months: central mandibular incisors
            ▪ 1 year: 8 teeth (average)
   c. Cognitive development—Piaget: sensorimotor stage (birth to 2 years)
      1. 1 month: reflexive
      2. 1 to 4 months
         a. visually follows objects 180 degrees
         b. recognizes familiar faces and objects
         c. turns head to locate sounds
         d. discovers parts of own body (hands, feet)
      3. 4 to 8 months: beginning object permanence
         a. searches for objects that have fallen
         b. imitates expressions and gestures of others
         c. smiles at self in mirror (mirror-image play)
         d. begins development of depth and space perception
      4. 9 to 12 months: searches for hidden objects
   d. Socialization
      1. 1 month: differentiates between face and object
      2. 2 months: social smile
      3. 4 months: recognizes primary caregiver
      4. 7 to 8 months: shy with strangers
      5. 9 to 10 months: separation anxiety
   e. Vocalization (language development)
      1. 2 months: differentiated cry
      2. 3 months: squeals with pleasure
      3. 5 months: simple vocal sounds (ooh, aah, goo-goo), turns to voice
      4. 6 months: begins to imitate sounds
      5. 9 months: first word (dada, baba); says "dada," "mama" specifically
      6. 12 months: two words besides mama and dada; uses gesture language (e.g., "up" [points] or "bye" [waves])
   f. Play (solitary)
      1. purposes: to stimulate sensorimotor development
      2. toys
         a. simple, easily handled

Table 5-1   Vital sign ranges in children (averages)

Pulse*	1 month-1 year	80-150 beats/min
	1-5 years	80-120 beats/min
	5-10 years	70-110 beats/min
	10-16 years	60-100 beats/min
Respiration*	1 month-1 year	20-50/min
	1-5 years	20-40/min
	5-10 years	18-30/min
	10-16 years	14-26/min
Blood pressure	1 month-1 year	80/50 mm Hg
	1-5 years	90/60 mm Hg
	5-10 years	100-110/60-70 mm Hg
	10-16 years	110-120/70-80 mm Hg

*Lower numbers in range represent values with child asleep.

Table 5-2   Average daily caloric needs of infants and children*

Age	Calories
Birth-6 months	53 × weight in pounds = kcal/day (400-800 kcal/day)
6 months-1 year	48 × weight in pounds = kcal/day (800-1200 kcal/day)
1-3 years	1300 kcal/day
4-6 years	1700 kcal/day
7-10 years	2400 kcal/day
11-16 years	
Boys	2700 kcal/day
Girls	2200 kcal/day

From the Food and Nutrition Board of the National Research Council, National Academy of Sciences.
*These daily averages may vary considerably for an individual child, depending on the child's activity level, length (height), and body build.

b. safe; no sharp points or small removable parts
c. stimulating
d. washable
e. nonlead paint
3. types of toys
  a. mobiles (black-and-white or bright colors)
  b. rattles, musical toys
  c. squeeze toys, sponge toys
  d. activity box for crib or playpen
  e. balls, blocks
  f. pots and pans (9 to 10 months)
4. games: peek-a-boo and patty-cake
2. Nutrition
  a. Caloric needs: approximately 400 (newborn) to 1200 (1-year-old) kcal per day (Table 5-2); actual caloric requirements depend on baby's activity and rate of growth.
  b. Introduction of solid foods
    1. when to start solids: variety of opinions; some evidence that early feeding of solids is linked to food allergies and overweight
    2. does not need solids first 4 to 6 months because
      a. salivary and intestinal enzymes that aid digestion not present until 4 to 6 months
      b. extrusion reflex lasts until 3 to 4 months
      c. tooth eruption begins at 4 to 8 months
      d. chewing movements begin at 7 to 9 months
    3. introduce foods one at a time; continue about 1 week before introducing another
    4. give small quantities (start with 1 tsp)
  c. Types of foods
    1. cooked cereals are introduced first at 4 to 6 months; rice cereal is preferable (high iron content, easily digested, less likely to cause allergic reaction)
    2. strained/cooked vegetables are introduced next at 6 to 7 months (before fruits, which have lower iron content)
    3. strained/mashed fruits are introduced at 7 to 8 months (bananas are preferable first fruit)
    4. ground/pureed meats are introduced at 8 to 9 months, egg yolks at 10 months (delay egg whites until 12 months because of possible allergies)

    5. chewable and finger foods are introduced when teething begins (6 to 9 months): zwieback, toast, crackers
    6. avoid nuts, raisins, popcorn, gum, candy, hot dogs (can be aspirated)
  d. Self-feeding: at 6 months infant begins handling spoon, finger foods; by 1 year, most infants are able to use a spoon; weaning—ready for introduction of a cup at 6 to 8 months, should be weaned gradually from breast or bottle; offer juice in a cup; drink independently from a cup at 1 year (may still want bottle or breast for security)
  e. Food allergies (a common health problem in infancy)
    1. common foods causing allergic responses include
      a. cow's milk
      b. foods containing wheat, corn, or soy (protein gluten)
      c. egg white (albumin)
      d. chocolate
      e. citrus foods
    2. indications of hypersensitivity to food
      a. urticaria
      b. abdominal pain, vomiting, and diarrhea
      c. respiratory symptoms
    3. diagnosis
      a. singular addition of food
      b. food diary or history
      c. skin testing not useful (because of immature immune system)
    4. treatment
      a. removal of causative food
      b. change to soy formula (if milk allergy)
      c. elimination diet
3. Sleep
  a. Most infants have nocturnal sleep pattern by 3 months
  b. 6 months: sleep through night
  c. 8 to 9 months: two naps during day, sleep 10 to 12 hours at night
  d. Anticipatory guidance for parents
    1. each infant's sleep patterns are unique

2. best indicators of adequate sleep are normal activity during waking hours and normal physical growth
3. sleeping arrangements are influenced by family's cultural beliefs and customs

4. Health care
    a. Immunizations
        1. see Table 5-3 for recommended schedule of the American Academy of Pediatrics
        2. contraindications
            a. febrile illness
            b. previous severe reaction to toxoid

Table 5-3   Recommended immunization schedule (1994)

Age	Immunization
Birth	Hepatitis B (HBV) #1 (can be given 0-2 months of age)
2 months	Diphtheria/tetanus/pertussis (DTP) #1 Oral poliovirus vaccine (OPV) #1 *Haemophilus influenzae* type B conjugate vaccine (Hib) #1 HBV #2 (can be given at 4 months)
4 months	DTP #2, OPV #2, Hib #2
6 months	DTP #3, Hib #3, HBV #3 (can be given 6-18 months of age), OPV #3
12-15 months	Hib #4, Measles-mumps-rubella (MMR), tuberculin testing may be done at same visit
15-18 months	DTP #4
4-6 years	DTP #5, OPV #4
11-12 years	MMR #2
14-16 years	Tetanus-diptheria toxoids (Td); should be repeated every 10 years

PRIMARY IMMUNIZATION FOR CHILDREN NOT IMMUNIZED IN THE FIRST YEAR OF LIFE

Under 7 years

First visit	DTP #1, Hib #1 (if less than 5 years of age) HBV #1, MMR #1 (if older than 15 months), OPV #1 (tuberculin testing can be done at same visit)

Interval after first visit

1 month	DTP #2, HBV #2
2 months	DTP #3, Hib #2 (if child received #1 when younger than 15 months), OPV #2
8 months or more	DTP #3, HBV #3, OPV #3
4-6 years	DTP #4, OPV #4 (not necessary if #3 was given after fourth birthday)
11-12 years	MMR
10 years later	Td (repeat every 10 years)

7 years and older

First visit	HBV #1, OPV #1, MMR, Td

Interval after first visit

2 months	HBV #2, OPV #2, Td
8-14 months	HBV #3, OPV #3, Td
11-12 years	MMR
10 years later	Td (repeat every 10 years)

c. presence of skin rash
            d. malignancy
            e. pregnancy
            f. poor immunologic response
            g. administration of gamma globulin, plasma, or blood in previous 6 to 8 weeks
        3. common side effects
            a. mild fever
            b. malaise
            c. soreness and swelling at injection site (DPT)
            d. mild rash (measles, rubella)
        4. advise parents of possible side effects; use of acetaminophen for fever (aspirin is contraindicated because of possible link between viral illness, aspirin, and Reye's syndrome)
    b. Accident prevention: accidents are the second leading cause of death in this age group
        1. aspiration/suffocation
            a. avoid propping bottles
            b. keep small objects out of reach
            c. check toys for small removable parts or sharp edges
            d. close pins when changing cloth diaper
            e. keep plastic bags away from all infants and children
        2. falls
            a. never leave unattended on elevated surface
            b. keep crib rails up
        3. auto accident: use infant car seats (crash tested, facing backward)
        4. burns: check water temperature before immersing infant; reduce temperature of water heater; keep hot substances away from infant (cigarette ashes, coffee, etc.); check temperature of foods/formulas; expose to sun gradually; use sunscreen of more than 15 SPF

TODDLER (1 TO 3 YEARS)

1. Normal growth and development
    a. Psychosocial development—Erikson: autonomy vs. shame and doubt
        1. all activities contribute to independence; expands independence by exploring environment and extending the child's limits
        2. verbally negative ("No!") even when agreeable to request; part of establishing identity as a separate entity
    b. Physical growth and development
        1. vital signs: pulse and respirations decrease, blood pressure increases with increasing size and age (see Table 5-1)
        2. teeth: all 20 deciduous present by 2½ to 3 years
        3. general appearance: potbellied, exaggerated lumbar curve, wide-based gait
        4. practices and increases muscle coordination and physical abilities
            a. jumps in place
            b. pushes and pulls toys
            c. scribbles spontaneously
            d. 15 months: climbs; goes up steps, cannot get down but will not accept help; builds a tower of cubes

e. 18 to 24 months: learns to undress self

f. 24 to 36 months: able to dress self with minimal help

c. Cognitive development—Piaget: sensorimotor and preconceptual stages

  1. 13 to 18 months

    a. extremely curious

    b. identifies geometric shapes

    c. opens doors and drawers

    d. points to body parts

    e. puts objects into holes, smaller objects into larger ones

  2. 19 to 24 months

    a. egocentric thinking and behavior

    b. beginning sense of time; waits in response to "just a minute"

  3. 24 to 36 months

    a. beginning magical thinking

    b. understands prepositions (e.g., over, under, behind, up)

    c. animism (attributes lifelike characteristics to inanimate objects)

    d. understanding of cause-and-effect relationships is determined by proximity of two events; therefore should be disciplined immediately

    e. increasing attention span

d. Socialization

  1. 15 months

    a. resistant to sitting still on laps

    b. wants to move independently

  2. 18 months to 2½ years: imitates parent behaviors (e.g., housework)

  3. dawdling and ritualistic behavior

  4. temper tantrums may be used to cope with frustration, assert independence, and gain control, especially when desires are thwarted

  5. may be attached to transitional objects, such as a favorite blanket or stuffed animal

  6. territorial: possessive of own toys and body

e. Vocalization

  1. understands simple commands

  2. 18 months: 20 words, names 1 body part

  3. 2 years: makes simple two- or three-word sentences; uses pronouns, plurals; knows full name

f. Play (parallel)

  1. purposes: to help child make transition from solitary to cooperative play, to stimulate motor development

  2. child will play beside, not with, another child

  3. types of toys should allow for self-play and be action oriented

    a. cars and trucks

    b. push-pull toys

    c. blocks, building toys, balls

    d. telephone

    e. stuffed toys and dolls

    f. books

    g. clay, finger paints

    h. wood puzzles

  4. games: likes to throw and retrieve objects, prefers "rough and tumble" play

2. Nutrition and dental care

a. Growth slows, appetite smaller; "physiologic anorexia" (may eat a great deal one day and little the next); needs an average of 1300 calories per day (see Table 5-2)

  1. ritualistic food preferences

  2. likes finger foods (crackers, green beans) and not foods that are "mixed up," such as casseroles

  3. drinks from cup

  4. self-feeds by 18 months

  5. prone to iron-deficiency anemia, especially if milk intake is high

  6. should consume foods from all food groups; lifelong eating habits are being formed

b. Anticipatory guidance for parents

  1. serve small portions

  2. recommended daily milk intake 24 to 32 oz

  3. do not give bottle as a substitute for solid foods; give solids before or with milk

  4. *do not use food as a reward*

  5. recognize ritualistic needs (e.g., same dishes, utensils, chair)

  6. do not force child to eat

c. Dental care guidelines

  1. brush and floss twice daily with help from parents

  2. first visit to dentist as soon as all primary teeth have erupted (2½ to 3 years)

  3. use fluoridated water or oral fluoride supplement (0.25 to 0.5 mg per day)

  4. limit concentrated sweets

  5. do not allow child to take a bottle containing juice or milk to bed because "bottle mouth caries" may result

3. Elimination: toileting practices

a. Learning bowel and bladder control is one of the major tasks of toddlerhood and is dependent on physiologic and cognitive factors as well as parent's positive attitudes and patience

b. Myelinization of nerve tracts occurs around 15 to 18 months of age (physiologic readiness)

c. Toddler uses toileting activities to control self and others

d. Independent toileting depends on

  1. physiologic readiness

    a. Ages

      ▪ 18 months: bowel control

      ▪ 2 to 3 years: daytime bladder control

      ▪ 3 to 4 years: nighttime bladder control (bladder must have at least an 8 oz capacity before child will be dry all night)

  2. ability to verbally communicate need to defecate or urinate, as well as indicate discomfort in soiled diapers

  3. ability to get to toilet and manage clothing

  4. psychologic readiness (desire to please)

4. Limit setting and discipline help child learn self-control and socially appropriate behavior; promote security

a. Enforcement of limits should be consistent and firm

b. Discipline should occur immediately after wrongdoing

c. Positive approach is best

d. Disapprove of the behavior, *not* the child

e. Types of discipline
   1. redirecting child's attention
   2. ignoring the behavior (often difficult)
   3. time-out
   4. reasoning and reprimanding, loss of privileges (for older children; not effective with toddlers)
   5. corporal punishment (controversial)
5. Accident prevention: accidents are leading cause of death from 1 to 15 years of age
   a. Falls
      1. Motor development is far ahead of judgment and perceptions
      2. climbs over side rails: change to regular bed
      3. climbs stairs: use safety gates
      4. supervise at playgrounds
   b. Poisonous ingestion (leading cause of injury and death): keep poisons and sharp objects locked up and out of reach
   c. Supervise when near cars; use car safety seats; never leave unattended in car
   d. Burns: cover electrical outlets; do not leave unattended in bathtub, near hot stove, fireplace, etc.; teach child what "hot" means
   e. Drowning: supervise near water (e.g., bathtub, toilet, pools, lakes)
   f. Aspiration: avoid foods such as popcorn, hard candy, nuts, uncooked vegetable chunks, hot dogs

PRESCHOOLER (3 TO 6 YEARS)

1. Normal growth and development
   a. Psychosocial development—Erikson: initiative vs. guilt
      1. learns how to do things, derives satisfaction from activities
      2. needs exposure to variety of experiences and play materials
      3. imitates role models
      4. active imagination
         a. reality vs. fantasy often blurred
         b. may have imaginary friends
         c. needs little guidance in play
      5. exaggerated fears (e.g., fear of mutilation, monsters)
   b. Physical growth and development
      1. body contours change: thinner and taller
      2. blood pressure 100/60 mm Hg; pulse 70 to 110 beats per minute
      3. motor skills: better control of fine and gross motor skills; posture more erect
         a. uses scissors and simple tools
         b. draws a person
            ▪ 4 years: three parts
            ▪ 5 years: six or seven parts
         c. rides a tricycle or Big Wheel
         d. skips and hops, throws and catches a ball well (5 years)
         e. walks downstairs as well as upstairs alternating feet on steps
         f. dresses self completely
         g. Right- or left-handedness usually established by end of preschool age

   c. Cognitive development—Piaget: preconceptual and intuitive thought stages
      1. increased sense of time and space (tomorrow, afternoon, next week)
      2. less egocentric
      3. perception dominates reasoning
      4. centration
         a. thinks of one idea at a time
         b. unable to think of all parts in terms of a whole
         c. conclusions based on immediate visual perceptions
      5. increased ability to think without acting out; anticipates events
      6. Regression: usually occurs in response to stress
   d. Socialization
      1. beginning social awareness
      2. capable of sharing; begins to have "best friends"
      3. may be physically aggressive
      4. boasts and tattles
      5. learns appropriate social manners
      6. separates easily from mother
   e. Vocalization
      1. 3-year-old: constantly asks "how" and "why" questions; vocabulary of 300 to 900 words
      2. 5-year-old: uses sentences of adult length
      3. knows colors, numbers, and alphabet
      4. understands analogies ("If fire is hot, ice is [cold]")
      5. stuttering (dysfluency) is fairly common among toddlers and preschoolers; normal variation of language development; parents should ignore stuttering so child does not become anxious; persistent stuttering beyond age 5 may require speech therapy
   f. Play (cooperative)
      1. purpose: to help child learn to share and to play in small groups, to learn simple games and rules, language concepts, and social roles
      2. play may be dramatic, imitative, or creative; expresses self through play
      3. types of toys
         a. housekeeping toys
         b. playground equipment
         c. wagons
         d. tricycles, Big Wheels
         e. dress-up clothes
         f. materials for cutting, pasting, and painting
         g. simple jigsaw puzzles
         h. books
         i. dolls, cars
         j. television (controversial but a contemporary reality)
2. Nutrition: a slow-growth period; needs an average of 1700 calories per day (see Table 5-2)
   a. Appetite remains decreased; has definite food preferences; less picky—foods from all food groups should be offered
   b. Self-feeding: 4-year-old uses fork, can use knife to spread; able to get snacks for self
   c. Sets the table; learns table manners; food habits are forming
   d. Able to pour from a pitcher

3. Sleep
   a. Sleep problems are most common in this age group
   b. Requires 9 to 12 hours each night
   c. May or may not take one nap during day
   d. May have fears of the dark, or may awaken with nightmares
   e. Guidelines for caregivers
      1. provide quiet time before bedtime
      2. use a nightlight
      3. adhere to a consistent bedtime pattern
4. Sexuality
   a. Knows sex differences by 3 years
   b. Imitates masculine or feminine behaviors; gender identity well established by 6 years
   c. Sexual curiosity and exploration
      1. masturbation is normal; especially common in pre-schoolers, may increase in frequency when child is under stress
      2. curious about anatomic differences and seeks to "investigate" them
   d. Guidelines for caregivers
      1. assess what child already knows when child asks a question
      2. answer questions simply, honestly, and matter-of-factly (avoid detailed explanations), using correct terminology
      3. masturbation: redirect child's attention without punishing or verbally reprimanding; teach child that touching genitals is not appropriate in public
5. Accident prevention
   a. Motor vehicle accidents (leading cause of injury and death)
      1. street safety: teach to wait at curb until told to cross; avoid riding cycles near street or driveways; wear bicycle helmet
      2. wear seat belt
   b. Drownings: teach to swim; supervise near pools, lakes
   c. Burns: teach not to play with matches or lights; supervise near fireplace; teach how to escape from burning home
   d. General safety: teach not to talk to strangers; child should know own name, address, telephone number, and how to seek help if lost; do not put child's name on clothing

SCHOOL AGE (6 TO 12 YEARS)

1. Normal growth and development
   a. Psychosocial development—Erikson: industry vs. inferiority
      1. develops a sense of competency and esteem academically, physically, and socially
      2. school phobias may occur as a result of increased competition, desire to succeed, fear of failure
      3. desire for accomplishment so strong that young school-age child may try to change rules of game to win
      4. gains competence in mastering new skills and tasks; assumes more responsibilities
      5. desires to get along socially; more responsive to peers; has "best friends"; may be involved in organized groups (e.g., Boy Scouts)
      6. still needs reassurance and support from family and trusted adults
   b. Physical growth and development
      1. growth is slow and regular (1 to 2 inches gain in height per year, 3 to 6 lb weight gain per year); prepubertal females are usually taller than males
      2. importance of daily exercise
      3. motor skills: increases strength and physical ability, refines coordination
         a. 6 years: jumps, skips, hops well; ties shoelaces easily, prints; "constant motion"
         b. 7 years: vision fully developed, can read regular-size print; can swim and ride a bicycle
         c. 8 years: writes rather than prints; increased smoothness and speed
         d. 9 years: fully developed hand-eye coordination; individual capabilities/talents emerge
         e. 10 years: increased strength, stamina, coordination
         f. 11 years: awkward; nervous energy (drumming fingers, etc.)
   c. Cognitive development—Piaget: concrete operations stage (7 to 11 years)
      1. decentering: can consider more than one characteristic at a time; leads to ability to empathize and sympathize
      2. reversibility: able to imagine a process in reverse
      3. conservation: able to conserve (mentally retain) physical properties of matter even when form is changed
      4. accommodation: limited ability to imagine self in another person's situation; to see the world from their viewpoint
      5. able to classify objects and verbalize concepts involved in doing so
      6. reasons logically; reasoning dominates perception
      7. able to think through a situation and anticipate the consequences; may then alter course of action; increased use of problem solving
   d. Socialization
      1. prefers friends to family; life is centered around school and friends
      2. relationships with peers and adults other than parents of increasing importance
      3. increasing social sensitivity
      4. more cooperative; improved manners
      5. school phobia: difficulty coping with the academic or social demands of school may result in psychosomatic complaints (stomachache, headache) and refusal to attend school; best managed by rewarding school attendance, withdrawing privileges and attention for school avoidance
      6. by 10 years enjoys privacy (e.g., own room, box that locks)
   e. Vocalization/language
      1. curious about meaning of different words; rapidly expanding vocabulary
      2. likes name-calling, word games (e.g., rhymes)
      3. develops a sense of humor; giggles and laughs a great deal; silly
      4. knows clock and calendar time

f. Play (cooperative, team, rule-governed, same sex together)
　　1. purposes: to learn to bargain, cooperate, and compromise; to develop logical reasoning abilities; to increase social skills
　　2. types of toys; entertainment
　　　　a. play figures, trains, model kits
　　　　b. games, jigsaw puzzles, magic tricks
　　　　c. books: joke and comic books, storybooks, adventure, mystery
　　　　d. television, video games, tapes, radio
　　　　e. riding a bicycle
　　　　f. structured activities (sports, scouting, music and dancing lessons, camping, slumber parties)
g. "Collecting" age (stamps, cards, rocks, etc.)
2. Nutrition and dental health
　a. Appetite increases; needs an average of 2400 calories per day (Table 5-2); breakfast is important for school performance
　b. More influenced by mass media; more likely to eat junk food because of increased time away from home; problems of obesity
　c. Nutrition education
　　1. teach food pyramid
　　2. teach basic cooking skills, meal planning
　　3. nutritious snacks
　d. Dental health
　　1. loss of deciduous teeth (begins at 5 to 7 years of age); eruption of permanent ones, including first and second molars
　　　　a. reassure permanent teeth will appear
　　2. many school-age children wear braces
　　　　a. good oral hygiene is important
　　　　b. self-image may be affected
　　3. dental caries are a major health problem
　　　　a. caused by poor nutrition, influence of television advertising contributing to increased intake of carbohydrates and concentrated sweets, inadequate dental hygiene
　　　　b. prevention: good brushing and flossing techniques, regular dental checkups, fluoridated water, good nutrition
3. Accident prevention
　a. Accepts increasing responsibility for own safety; safety education is essential
　b. Motor vehicle accidents
　　1. teach how to cross street
　　2. bike safety—helmet
　　3. use car safety belts
　c. Drowning
　　1. learn to swim; adopt a buddy system
　　2. teach water safety; wear a life vest
　d. Burns
　　1. teach safety around fires (e.g., fireplaces, campfires) and safe use of candles and matches
　　2. teach not to play with explosives, firearms
　e. Sports injuries: teach about appropriate protective equipment

ADOLESCENT (12 TO 20 YEARS)
1. Normal growth and development
　a. Psychosocial development—Erikson: identity vs. identity diffusion
　　1. "Who am I?"
　　2. "What do I want to do with my life?"
　　3. has many changes in body image
　　4. experiences mood swings; vacillates between maturity and childlike behavior
　　5. continually reassesses values and beliefs
　　6. begins to consider career possibilities
　　7. gains independence from parents
　b. Physical growth and development: time of rapid physiologic growth; two major milestones are puberty (average onset in males occurs 2 years later than in females) and cessation of body growth (females 16 to 17 years old and males 18 to 20 years old)
　　1. males: development of secondary sex characteristics
　　　　a. increase in size of genitalia
　　　　b. growth of pubic, axillary, facial, and chest hair
　　　　c. voice changes
　　　　d. increase in shoulder breadth
　　　　e. production of spermatozoa; nocturnal emissions
　　2. females: development of secondary sex characteristics
　　　　a. increase in transverse diameter of pelvis
　　　　b. development of breasts
　　　　c. change in vaginal secretions
　　　　d. growth of pubic and axillary hair
　　　　e. onset of menstruation: 12 years of age (average)
　　3. both sexes
　　　　a. acne
　　　　b. perspiration
　　　　c. blushing
　　　　d. rapid increase in height and weight
　　　　e. fatigue (because heart and lungs grow at slower rate)
　c. Cognitive development—Piaget: formal operations (11 years and older); attained at different ages and depends on formal education, experience, cultural background
　　1. abstract thinking
　　2. forms hypotheses, analytical thinking
　　3. can consider more than two categories at same time
　　4. generalizes findings
　　5. thinks about thinking; philosophical; concerned with social and moral issues
　d. Socialization
　　1. with adults
　　　　a. may resent authority
　　　　b. wishes to be different from parents: may ridicule them
　　　　c. has need for parent figures
　　　　d. develops crushes on adults outside the family, "hero worship"

2. with peers
   a. overidentifies with group: same dress, same ethical codes
   b. has close friendships with members of same sex
   c. develops sexual preferences
   e. Recreation, leisure activity: expanding variety
   1. parties, dances
   2. Video games, television, movies, and music (radio, tapes)
   3. telephone conversations, daydreaming
   4. sports, games, hobbies
   5. reading and writing
   6. part-time jobs (especially babysitting) to earn extra money
   f. Sexual activity
   1. estimated 50% of adolescents engage in sexual experimentation and activity
   2. educate about birth control methods, pregnancy, sexually transmitted disease, and safe sex
2. Nutrition
   a. Appetite increases with rapid growth; puberty changes nutritional requirements; needs complete nutrition (food pyramid)
   b. Caloric needs vary with activity level, sex, and body build (see Table 5-2)
   1. girls need approximately 2200 calories per day
   2. boys need an average of 2700 calories per day
   c. Increased need for protein, calcium, iron, and zinc
   d. Sports activity may increase nutritional requirements
   e. Eating habits are easily influenced by peer group
   1. intake of junk food
   2. fad diets and dieting: can lead to health problems, including anorexia nervosa and bulimia (especially in girls)
   3. overeating or inactivity: may result in obesity
   4. iron-deficiency anemia common
   f. nutritional education: approach must be nonjudgmental with emphasis on involving adolescent in making good choices
3. Accident prevention
   a. Motor vehicle accidents: enroll in driver-training programs, wear seat belts
   b. Drownings: teach water safety, first aid, cardiopulmonary resuscitation (CPR)
   c. Sports injuries: educate for prevention
   d. Alcohol and drug abuse: education, teach peer pressure resistance techniques
   e. Suicide: be alert for signs of depression

Application of the Nursing Process to the Healthy Child

ASSESSMENT
1. Health history
   a. General health status: incidence of illnesses in past year, visits to health care provider, immunization history, current medications
   b. Developmental history: parents' health status, mother's obstetric history with this child, child's neonatal history, achievement of developmental milestones, self-care abilities, behavior, and temperament
   c. Parents' perceptions and concerns
   d. Parents' knowledge of development, child care, safety, nutrition, and so on
   e. Child's home and school environments: safety, appropriate stimulation, barriers to development
   f. Nutrition: daily food and fluid intake, child's preferences and dislikes, self-feeding abilities, special needs (cultural/religious practices, allergies), eating patterns
   g. Dental care: number of teeth, tooth eruption (discomfort, management), daily oral hygiene, self-brushing and flossing, fluoride (water or daily supplement), dental visits
   h. Elimination: daily routine, toilet trained or diapers, problems (e.g., diarrhea, constipation, enuresis; how managed)
   i. Activity/sleep: exercise and activity patterns; sleep habits: sleep environment, daily total, special needs, problems
   j. Sexuality: gender knowledge and identity, sexual curiosity and exploration, sexual knowledge, primary and secondary sex characteristics; adolescent: knowledge, sexual activity, contraception, pregnancy, sexually transmitted disease
2. Clinical appraisal
   a. Development
   1. observation of age-appropriate developmental behavior and abilities
   2. administration of developmental screening tools when indicated to screen for delays (e.g., Denver II [a screening tool to detect developmental problems in four areas: personal-social, fine motor–adaptive, language, and gross motor; *not* an intelligence test; does not predict future developmental potential])
   3. home environment: visit to appraise for support of or barriers to development
   b. General physical appraisal
   1. growth: length, weight, head circumference; percentiles on standard growth curves
   2. vital signs: annual blood pressure screening (especially in high-risk children) (see Table 5-1)
   3. general health: skin, activity, attention span, ability to communicate, and so forth
   4. vision/hearing screening
      a. vision testing
      ▪ binocularity tests for strabismus; if strabismus is not detected and corrected by age 6 years, amblyopia (decreased visual activity, even blindness) may result
      • corneal light reflex test
      • cover test
      ▪ visual acuity tests; *Snellen E* (preschoolers or illiterate children) or Snellen alphabet chart
      ▪ head tilting or squinting may indicate visual impairment
      ▪ ophthalmoscopic exam

- referral criteria
  - 3 years: vision in one or both eyes 20/50 or worse
  - 4 to 6 years: vision in one or both eyes 20/40 or worse
  - 7 years and older: vision in one or both eyes 20/30 or worse
  - children with one-line or more difference between both eyes (example: 20/30 in left eye, 20/40 in right)
  - abnormal findings from cover test or corneal light reflex test
  b. hearing testing
  - otoscopic exam
  - conduction tests
    - Rinne test (comparison of bone and air conduction)
    - Weber's test (bone conduction)
  - pure tone audiometry (audiogram) to test for conductive or sensorineural hearing impairments

ANALYSIS/NURSING DIAGNOSIS

1. Safe, effective care environment
   a. Risk for injury
   b. Sensory-perceptual alteration: visual, auditory, kinesthetic, tactile, olfactory
   c. Knowledge deficit
2. Physiologic integrity
   a. Risk for activity intolerance
   b. Altered nutrition: risk for less/more than body requirements
   c. Fatigue
3. Psychosocial integrity
   a. Decisional conflict
   b. Altered role performance
   c. Body-image disturbance, self-esteem disturbance
4. Health promotion/maintenance
   a. Ineffective family coping
   b. Altered growth and development
   c. Health-seeking behaviors

GENERAL NURSING PLANNING, IMPLEMENTATION, AND EVALUATION

Goal 1 Child will achieve optimal development.

Implementation

1. Provide information to parents on normal growth and development.
   a. What to expect (skills, behavior)
   b. Age-appropriate play activities and materials
   c. Ways to stimulate development
2. Discuss child-rearing methods and styles, limit setting, and ways to cope with child-rearing problems.
3. Administer screening tools during well-child visits to detect developmental delays (e.g., language, speech, gross and fine motor skills, social, self-help).
4. Refer for further evaluation or to early intervention services if developmental delay detected.

Evaluation

Child grows and develops within expected range; is free from delays in development; parents cope effectively with child-rearing concerns and problems.

Goal 2 Child will experience a safe environment and will be free from accidental injury.

Implementation

Provide anticipatory guidance to parents concerning age-related safety hazards and ways to prevent accidental injury (safety proofing the home, auto safety restraints, swimming and bicycling safety, safe toys, driver education, firearm safety).

Evaluation

Child is free from accidental injury.

Goal 3 Child will receive optimal nutrition and dental care.

Implementation

Provide teaching and counseling to parents concerning child's nutritional requirements, feeding techniques, dental hygiene, tooth eruption, and food allergies.

Evaluation

Child's physical growth follows growth curve; child receives daily nutritional requirements (calories, protein, carbohydrates, fats, vitamins and minerals); feeds self in accordance with developmental abilities; receives appropriate dental hygiene and care and is free from dental caries; child's food allergies are detected and diet is adjusted as needed.

Goal 4 Child will get adequate rest and sleep.

Implementation

Provide anticipatory guidance to parents concerning child's sleep needs, patterns of sleep in childhood, and ways to cope with sleep problems.

Evaluation

Child gets amount of sleep required for optimal growth and development; parents cope with child's sleep problems.

Goal 5 Child will develop healthy sexuality.

Implementation

1. Provide anticipatory guidance to parents concerning child's developing sexuality.
   a. What to expect (questions, behaviors)
   b. How to answer child's questions matter-of-factly, honestly, accurately
   c. How to encourage open and honest communication with adolescent
2. Teach child about sex and sexuality appropriate to child's age and expressed interest.

Evaluation

Child develops gender-appropriate sexual identity and sexual behaviors.

> **Goal 6** Child will be free from preventable communicable diseases.

Implementation

1. Reinforce to parents the importance of childhood immunizations.

2. Administer immunizations according to recommended schedule.

Evaluation

Child receives immunizations according to recommended schedule; is free from preventable communicable diseases.

The Ill and Hospitalized Child

OVERVIEW

1. Hospitalization and illness are stressful for children
   a. Difficulty changing routines
   b. Limited coping mechanisms
   c. Reason for hospitalization is often less significant than consequences (e.g., separation from familiar persons and surroundings, painful procedures, restricted mobility)
2. Major stressors for the child
   a. Separation
   b. Loss of control
   c. Body injury
   d. Pain
   e. Immobility
3. Factors that affect responses to illness and hospitalization
   a. Developmental level (see following, Developmental Responses to Hospitalization)
   b. Past experiences, especially with hospitalization and surgery
   c. Level of anxiety: child and parents
   d. Relationship between parents and child
   e. Nature and seriousness of illness or injury; circumstances of hospitalization
   f. Family background: education, culture, support systems
4. Developmental responses to hospitalization
   a. Infant
      1. separation: before attachment (under 4 to 6 months) not as significant; older infant's response is significant with crying, rage, protest; stranger anxiety
      2. loss of control
         a. expects that crying will bring immediate response from caregiver (changed, fed, held); may interfere with development of trust
         b. in hospital
            ▪ immediate response may not occur
            ▪ need may be met by unfamiliar person
            ▪ unable to express needs or understand explanations
      3. immobility: restrictions and restraints interfere with activity and sucking (Table 5-4)
      4. pain: procedures cause discomfort; responds by crying and withdrawal
   b. Toddler
      1. separation
         a. fear of unknown and abandonment
         b. separation anxiety is similar to grief; so encourage protest behaviors as healthy response
            ▪ protest: cries loudly, rejects attentions of nurses, wants parent
            ▪ despair: monotonous cries, state of mourning, "settling in"
            ▪ denial: renewed interest in surroundings; seems adjusted to loss, but actually repressing feelings for parent
         c. disruption in routines (eating, sleep, toileting) decreases security and control
         d. regression: may attempt to seek comfort by returning to earlier, dependent behaviors
            ▪ clinging, whining
            ▪ bed-wetting after being toilet trained
            ▪ wanting bottle, pacifier
      2. loss of control: special concern because major task is to gain autonomy
      3. body injury: fears intrusive procedures (e.g., rectal temperature, injections) and reacts intensely
      4. immobility: cannot freely explore environment; may interfere with motor, language development if prolonged
      5. pain: becomes emotionally distraught and physically resistant to painful procedures
   c. Preschooler
      1. body injury/body integrity
         a. confusion between reality and fantasy
         b. casts and bandages are particular problems because child is not assured that all body parts that were there before are there now; much worry over body integrity
      2. loss of control: the child's active imagination may lead to exaggeration or misinterpretations of hospital experiences; fears and fantasies may get the best of the child
      3. separation
         a. may view as punishment for something thought or done
         b. more subtle responses than toddler (quiet crying, sleep problems, loss of appetite)
      4. pain
         a. recognizes cues that signal an impending painful experience
         b. able to anticipate pain: may try to escape, may become physically combative
      5. immobility: prevents mastery of fears; preschooler often feels helpless

Table 5-4 Commonly used pediatric protective devices

Type	Indications	Precautions
Jacket	In crib (alternative to crib net) In high chair To maintain horizontal position in crib	Tie in back. Secure ties underneath crib or high chair.
Crib net	To prevent infant or toddler from climbing over side rails	Avoid nets with tears or large gaps. Tie to bedsprings, not to crib sides.
Crib cover	To prevent toddler from climbing out of crib	Ensure that all latches are locked.
Mummy	For infant or small toddler needing short-term protection Venipuncture Gavage feedings Eye, ear, nose, and throat exams	Keep top of mummy sheet level with shoulder. Maintain arms and legs in anatomic position. Expose needed extremity only.
Clove hitch or commercial ties	For arm or leg protective devices to limit motion for venipunctures	Observe for adequacy of circulation. Place pad under protective device. Tie ends to crib springs. Remove q2h for range-of-motion exercise.
Elbow	To prevent touching of head or face, scalp vein infusions, after repair of cleft lip, palate	Use pad with stiff material. Use pins or ties to prevent slippage. Remove one at a time q2h for range-of-motion exercise.

d. School-age child
  1. separation
    a. from family and friends
    b. easier than other age groups because of cognitive level and better time concept
  2. fear of loss of control
    a. through immobility
    b. enforced dependence
    c. fear of injury and death; death anxiety peaks
    d. does not want others to see loss of control (e.g., crying), tries to appear brave
  3. pain: responses are influenced by cultural variables; usually uses passive coping strategies (lies rigidly still, shuts eyes, clenches teeth and fists)
  4. immobility: affects sense of physical achievement and need for competition
e. Adolescent: loss of control/enforced dependence when the need is to move toward own identity and independence

Application of the Nursing Process to the Ill and Hospitalized Child

ASSESSMENT
1. Child's development level and major fear associated with age group
   a. Infant: separation
   b. Toddler: separation, intrusive procedures
   c. Preschooler: body mutilation, pain
   d. School age: loss of control, separation from peers
   e. Adolescent: change in body image and self-identity, loss of esteem
2. Child's perceptions/understanding of illness and hospitalization
3. Family responses to child's hospitalization
   a. Parents may react with denial, disbelief, guilt, fear, anxiety, frustration, and depression
   b. Alterations in family routines and lifestyle

c. Parents' coping mechanisms
   1. support systems for parents (e.g., friends, extended family members)
   2. financial resources
   3. family's ability to cope with the child's illness
   4. ability to express reaction to child's illness
4. Child's response to pain: unable to express verbally; often results in underuse of pain-relief methods
   a. Through observation
      1. verbally: younger child often uses incorrect words (e.g., "bad," "funny," "hot"); older child often reluctant to complain because of fear of "shots"
      2. behaviorally: pulling at area (ear), irritable, loss of appetite, lying or moving in unusual position
      3. physiologically: vomiting, change in vital signs, flushed skin, increased sleep time, sleep disruptions
   b. Asking child to rate the pain (e.g., using happy/unhappy faces, or scale of 0 to 10)

ANALYSIS/NURSING DIAGNOSIS
1. Safe, effective care environment
   a. Risk for infection
   b. Risk for injury
   c. Sensory-perceptual alteration
2. Physiologic integrity
   a. Ineffective airway clearance/risk for aspiration
   b. Pain
   c. Fluid volume deficit
3. Psychologic integrity
   a. Ineffective individual coping
   b. Anxiety/fear
   c. Body-image disturbance
4. Health promotion/maintenance
   a. Altered growth and development
   b. Knowledge deficit
   c. Altered family processes

PLANNING, IMPLEMENTATION, AND EVALUATION

> **Goal 1** Child will be prepared psychologically for hospitalization.

Implementation

1. Encourage preadmission preparation.
   a. *Before 2 years:* explanation is ineffective; allow to take favorite toy and objects (e.g., blanket)
   b. *2 to 7 years:* usually tell child ahead in days equal to years of age (e.g., 2 years = 2 days ahead, 6 years = 6 days ahead)
   c. *Over 7 years:* tell child when parent knows (use judgment)
2. Orient child and family to surroundings (hospital tour, etc.).
3. Anticipate and alleviate age-related needs and fears.
   To develop trust in infant:
   a. Arrange for rooming-in.
   b. Ensure consistency of caregiver.
   c. Provide security objects (e.g., toy, blanket).
   d. Make routine patterns as similar as possible to home.
   e. Hold, cuddle, stroke; allow infant pacifier if possible.
   To help toddler maintain control:
   f. Use familiar words (e.g., child's word for toileting).
   g. Ask parents to leave familiar objects with child (e.g., toy, blanket).
   h. Encourage rooming-in and parental participation in care.
   i. Accept regressive needs but avoid promoting them (e.g., do not put toilet-trained child back in diapers).
   j. Provide explanations immediately before any procedure with use of simple, concrete words.
   k. Use time orientation in relation to familiar activities (e.g., "after naptime").
   l. Prepare parents to recognize and accept regressive behavior after discharge.
   m. Maintain limit setting to provide consistency for child.
   n. Do not offer choices when there are none.
   To help preschooler relieve body-mutilation anxiety:
   o. Allow child to wear underwear if possible.
   p. Provide reassurance regarding invasive procedures.
   q. Encourage play that incorporates equipment (such as BP cuff, stethoscope) and treatments.
   r. Concept of time is related to routine activities (e.g., when you wake up, after lunch).
   s. Allow some choices to promote feelings of control and mastery (choice of fluids, play activities).
   To help school-age child maintain a degree of control:
   t. Provide explanations of illness and treatment with pictures, simple anatomic diagrams, dolls (call them models or teaching models with older child), books, or step-by-step illustrations.
   u. Maintain educational level during long-term hospitalization to help meet need for accomplishment.
      1. homework; contact with own schoolteacher
      2. in-hospital teacher
   v. Allow to participate in planning care by choosing food, times for bath or treatments.

To help adolescent maintain esteem and identity:
   w. Maintain peer contacts.
      1. visiting should be open to adolescents
      2. place in adolescent unit or room
      3. make sure telephone is available
      4. respect privacy—knock before entering room
   x. Encourage participation in decision making regarding own body.
4. Provide honest explanations, information, and support.
   a. Determine level of understanding based on cognitive development and preexisting knowledge.
   b. Use age-appropriate language, terminology, and timing before instruction.
5. Foster a sense of safety and security.
   a. Encourage rooming-in, security objects for younger children.
   b. Determine child's routine, rituals, and nickname.
   c. Implement age-appropriate safety measures (e.g., bubble-top [covered] cribs, raised crib rails [see Table 5-4]).

Evaluation

Child maintains developmental level; expresses feelings/desires about hospital (e.g., wants to go home); maintains attachments (family, favorite objects, friends).

> **Goal 2** Parents will feel in control.

Implementation

1. Allow and encourage parents to participate in child's care; provide 24-hour open visiting and rooming-in facilities.
2. Foster family relationships between ill child for family members; include siblings.
3. Provide support; help family identify persons or community resources who can help.
4. Provide information about child's illness, treatment, and care at rate that parents are able to cope with and accept.
5. Provide information regarding home care.

Evaluation

Parents express satisfaction with caregivers and information provided; child and parents maintain/regain supportive relationships.

> **Goal 3** Child undergoing hospital procedures and surgery will be prepared.

Implementation

1. Refer to Perioperative Period, p. 115.
2. Measure child's height and weight (used for calculating medications and intravenous (IV) fluids).
3. Explain procedure, recovery room, and postoperative care to child (appropriate for age) and to parents.
   a. Use concrete words and visual aids.
   b. Use neutral words (e.g., "fixed" instead of "cut").
   c. Emphasize body part involved and any change in function.
   d. Use drawings and storytelling to evaluate child's understanding.

e. Take child and parent to see equipment and rooms if possible.

Day of surgery

4. Keep NPO (nothing by mouth—from Latin, *nil per os*) (shorter duration for a child compared with an adult).

5. Check for loose teeth and inform anesthesiologist of findings.
6. Allow favorite toy to accompany child to operating room (OR).
7. Encourage parents to remain with child as long as possible.

Table 5-5   Medication and temperature guide

Age group	Usual form of oral medication	Available injection sites	Usual route for temperature
Infant	L	VL	A R, tympanic
Toddler	L P (crush)	VL	A R, tympanic
Preschooler	L P (crush or chew)	VL VG GM	A R O (older child), tympanic
		D for all immunizations except DPT (give deep IM)	
School-age child	L P	VL VG GM D	O A, tympanic
Adolescent	L P C	VL VG GM D	O A, tympanic

P, pills; *L,* liquid; *C,* capsules; *VL,* vastus lateralis; *GM,* gluteus medius; *CG,* ventrogluteal; *D,* deltoid; *O,* oral; *A,* axillary; *R,* rectal.

Table 5-6   Medication administration for young children

Age	Developmental considerations	Nursing implications
1-3 months	Strong sucking reflex Extrusion reflex	Allow sucking for oral medications (e.g., nipples, syringes). Give medications in small amounts to allow for swallowing. Keep head upright. Place liquid on side of mouth, toward back.
	Reaches randomly Whole body reacts to painful stimuli	Control child's hands when giving oral medications. Use own body to control infant's arms and legs for parenteral medications.
3-12 months	Extrusion reflex disappears Drinks from cup Can finger-feed Can spit out medication	Use medicine cup and syringe rather than spoon. Offer physical comforting more than verbal.
12-30 months	Development of large motor skills Can spit out medications or clamp jaw shut Can use medicine cup Auditory canal is not straight Autonomy vs. shame/doubt Ritualistic Takes pride in tasks	Never leave medications where child can reach or throw. May need two adults to give injections (one to restrain). Be honest about taste/pain; use distractions. Give ear drops by pulling pinna down and back. Be firm, ignore resistive behavior. Give choices when possible.
2½-3½ years	Has eating likes and dislikes Little sense of time Tries to coerce, manipulate Has fantasies Body boundaries are unclear	Disguise medicinal taste. Use chewable medications. Use concrete and immediate rewards (e.g., stickers, badges). Give choices when possible, but do not offer if there are none. Be consistent. Give simple explanations; assure medicine is not for a punishment. Use Band-Aids for covering injection sites.
3½-6 years	Develops proficiency at tasks Refining senses Has loose teeth Can make decisions Has a sense of time Takes pride in accomplishment Developing a conscience Fears mutilation, punishment May master pill swallowing	Allow child to handle equipment (e.g., syringes). Will be unable to disguise tastes and smells. Consider teeth when deciding route. Allow choice about route, if possible. Allow participation in choice of administration time when possible (e.g., before or after meals). Explain in simple terms reason for medications. Avoid prolonged reasoning. Use simple command by trusted adult that medication is to be given. Allow control when possible. Praise after medication is given.

8. Clothe child for OR: diaper for non–toilet-trained child; permit older child to wear underwear under hospital gown, if possible.
9. Administer preoperative medications as ordered; oral or parenteral form is influenced by type, amount, age, and accessibility; see Tables 5-5 and 5-6.

Evaluation

Child and family understand rationale for NPO and comply; child is prepared correctly for surgery; child and family correctly verbalize understanding of postoperative care.

Goal 4 Postoperatively, child will maintain adequate pulmonary ventilation and circulation, fluid and electrolyte balance.

Implementation
1. Turn, position, and get child to cough at least q2h.
2. Allow some crying in infants to achieve deep breathing.
3. Use inspirometer, straw games with older child to ensure deep breathing.
4. Monitor IV closely.
   a. If microdrip (60 gtt/ml used), gtt/min = ml/hr
   b. Check for fluid overload (pulmonary rales)
5. Exercise limbs immobilized with protective devices q2h; fasten restraint ties to crib or bed (not to side rails); monitor circulatory status qh.
6. Monitor hydration status.
   a. Keep accurate intake and output (I&O).
   b. Check urine specific gravity.
   c. Weigh daily as ordered
   d. Check skin turgor.

Evaluation

Child has adequate ventilation and circulation, normal color, and no evidence of cyanosis or fluid volume deficit or overload.

Goal 5 Child will be free from pain.

Implementation
1. Be alert to nonverbal messages in a young child or child who may fear injections and not wish to communicate discomfort.
2. Anticipate pain; use routine dosing if available; if as required (prn) schedule, give on regular basis to prevent pain. Medicate for nausea and pain as ordered (analgesics such as acetaminophen are often used).
3. Determine correct medication dosage (Table 5-7).
4. Assess for response to medications every 1 to 2 hours.

Evaluation

Child experiences minimal pain.

Table 5-7   Estimating pediatric drug dosages

Pediatric medication dosages may be estimated using *body surface area (BSA)*: most reliable method; must plot child's height and weight on a nomogram (available in reference texts)

$$\frac{\text{Body surface area of child } (m^2)}{1.7 \ (m^2)} \times \text{Adult dose} = \text{Estimated pediatric dose}$$

Example: Child's BSA is 0.34; usual adult dose is 500 mg. What is the child's estimated dosage?

$$\frac{0.34}{1.7} \times 500 \text{ mg} = 100 \text{ mg}$$

Goal 6 Child will use diversionary activity and play to cope with the stress of hospitalization.

Implementation
1. Refer to The Healthy Child, p. 402.
2. Help child participate in nursing activities (e.g., tea party for fluid intake, inspirometer for deep breathing, bean bags for range of motion).
3. Use drawings, storytelling, or puppets to help child express feelings about illness.
4. Allow child to use syringes, needles with supervision.

Evaluation

Child expresses fears and feelings during play; adapts to hospital routine with minimal distress.

Goal 7 Child and family will receive appropriate discharge teaching.

Implementation
1. Provide oral and written instructions regarding
   a. Activities and restrictions
   b. Diet
   c. Procedures
   d. Medications: schedule, administration, storage, side effects
2. Teach parents procedures that must be performed at home.
3. Contact appropriate outside resources as needed (e.g., homebound teacher, Visiting Nurse Association).

Evaluation

Child (as appropriate) and parent describe medical regimen that must be carried on at home (e.g., medications, diet, restrictions); demonstrate how to do procedures or give medications; know how to obtain refills and arrange for follow-up appointments.

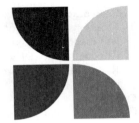

Sensation, Perception, and Protection

OVERVIEW OF PHYSIOLOGY

1. Immunologic differences in children
   a. Newborn receives passive immunity from mother for most major childhood communicable diseases (assuming mother is immune and infant is term).
   b. The young infant's immune system is not fully developed; therefore the infant is more prone to infectious disease.
   c. The eustachian tube in infants and young toddlers is shorter and straighter than in older children and adults, leading to increased risk of middle-ear infections.
   d. Increasing exposure of toddlers and preschoolers to infectious diseases in group settings and the immaturity of their immune system leads to increased incidence of infections.
2. Integumentary (skin) differences in children
   a. The skin is less thick during infancy.
   b. The epidermis is fragile and more prone to irritation.
   c. The infant's skin is more sensitive to changes in temperature (especially extremes of heat and cold) and is more susceptible to invasion by bacteria and other infectious organisms.
3. Neurologic differences in children
   a. The greatest neurologic changes occur during the first year of life.
   b. The brain reaches 75% of adult size by age 2, 90% by age 4.
   c. Cortical development is usually complete by age 4.
   d. Primitive neonatal reflexes disappear as higher centers of the brain take over; most neonatal reflexes disappear or diminish by 3 to 4 months of age; their persistence may indicate a neurologic problem.

Application of the Nursing Process to the Child with a Sensory Problem

ASSESSMENT

1. Nursing history
   a. Frequent earaches or sore throats, persistent nosebleeds, sinus problems, or allergies
   b. Eye crosses, deviates outward or inward, tears excessively; history of other vision problems
   c. Parental concerns about child's vision or hearing
2. Clinical appraisal
   a. Otoscopic exam, ear pain or "fullness," and hearing loss
   b. Ophthalmoscopic exam, head tilting or squinting
   c. Hypertrophy of tonsils, sore throat

3. Diagnostic tests
   a. Vision and hearing testing (refer to The Healthy Child, p. 409)

ANALYSIS/NURSING DIAGNOSIS

1. Safe, effective care environment
   a. Sensory-perceptual alteration: visual, auditory, tactile
   b. Risk for injury
   c. Risk for infection
2. Physiologic integrity
   a. Pain
   b. Actual/risk for impaired skin integrity
3. Psychosocial integrity
   a. Body-image disturbance
   b. Anxiety
4. Health promotion/maintenance
   a. Knowledge deficit
   b. Self-care deficit
   c. Altered growth and development

NURSING PLANNING, IMPLEMENTATION, AND EVALUATION

Refer to Selected Health Problems, following.

SELECTED HEALTH PROBLEMS: INTERFERENCE WITH SENSATION

OTITIS MEDIA

1. Definition: middle-ear infection; two types
   a. *Otitis media with effusion:* nonpurulent effusion of middle ear
   b. *Suppurative otitis media (acute or chronic):* accumulation of viral or bacterial purulent exudate in middle ear
2. Cause
   a. With effusion: unknown, but there appears to be a relationship with allergies
   b. Suppurative: pneumococci, *H. influenzae,* streptococci
3. Incidence: one of the most common illnesses of infancy and early childhood
4. Medical treatment
   a. Diagnosis
      1. otoscopic exam
         a. inflamed, bulging tympanic membrane (acute) or dull gray membrane (serous)
         b. no visible landmarks or light reflex
      2. tympanometry (measures air pressure in auditory canal): decreased membrane mobility

b. Antibiotic therapy: ampicillin (may cause diarrhea; given q6h) or amoxicillin (more expensive but fewer side effects; given tid) 10 to 14 days, Ceclor, Septra or Bactrim
c. Low-dose, long-term Septra or Bactrim for chronic, recurrent infections
d. Surgical intervention: incision of membrane (myringotomy) and insertion of myringotomy tubes in cases of recurrent chronic otitis media; adenoidectomy

Nursing Process

ASSESSMENT
1. *Suppurative otitis*
   a. Pain (infants may pull or hold ears)
   b. Irritability (nonspecific response to pain)
   c. High fever
   d. Lymphadenopathy
   e. Purulent discharge (indicates rupture of membrane)
   f. Nasal congestion, cough
   g. Anorexia, vomiting
   h. Diarrhea
   i. Perceived hearing loss in older child
2. *Serous otitis*
   a. Ear "fullness"
   b. Popping sensation when swallowing
   c. Conductive hearing loss

ANALYSIS/NURSING DIAGNOSIS (See p. 417)
PLANNING, IMPLEMENTATION, AND EVALUATION

Goal 1 Child will be free from infecting organism and recurrence of infection.

Implementation
1. Teach parents to administer antibiotics as prescribed.
2. Educate parents concerning importance of adhering to medication regimen for full course of therapy.
3. Clean drainage from ear with cotton balls and water.

Evaluation
Child shows no signs or symptoms of continuing infection (e.g., pulling at ears, fever); no discharge from ears; disease does not recur.

Goal 2 Child will receive comfort measures and be free from pain and fever.

Implementation
1. Monitor body temperature.
2. Teach parents to administer antipyretic analgesics (acetaminophen or ibuprofen).
3. Control fever with tepid baths or sponging.
4. Avoid foods that require chewing.
5. Apply external heat (warm water bottle or heating pad).

Evaluation
Child is free from pain, able to play and sleep comfortably; child's temperature returns to normal.

Goal 3 Child will have no permanent hearing impairment.

Implementation
1. Monitor for signs of hearing loss (decreased attention and responsiveness).
2. Conduct audiometry screening at routine intervals.
3. Refer child to appropriate resources if results are abnormal.

Evaluation
Child has normal hearing.

Goal 4 Family will receive appropriate information and support in dealing with chronic disease.

Implementation
1. Teach parents that chronic or recurrent otitis media is a problem that may take several months to resolve.
2. Reassure parents that there is no "quick fix" for the problem.
3. Encourage open communication between caregivers and health care personnel about frustration in dealing with problem.
4. Provide written materials about infections and treatment goals.

Evaluation
Caregiver is cooperative with length of treatment, implements treatment plan, and demonstrates understanding about variety of approaches.

Goal 5 Child and family will receive appropriate information concerning home care after a myringotomy and insertion of tubes.

Implementation
1. Tell parents to expect some drainage from the ear for several days postoperatively; obvious bleeding is not normal, so the physician should be notified.
2. Keep ear dry; use physician-recommended earplugs during all activities that might cause ear to become submerged in water (e.g., bathing, swimming).
3. Advise parents to notify physician if the child develops fever, headache, irritability, lethargy, or nausea/vomiting (meningitis).
4. Check the ears periodically in case the tubes become dislodged (they normally remain in approximately 6 months and then fall out spontaneously).

Evaluation
Child has uneventful recovery; family implements home care without problems or complications.

✠ TONSILLECTOMY, ADENOIDECTOMY, OR BOTH

1. Definition: surgical excision of the tonsils and adenoids; usually done after 3 years of age because of the danger of excessive bleeding and tonsillar regrowth if done earlier
2. Indications for surgery: controversy exists regarding the value of surgery; most widely accepted reasons are chronic tonsillitis (most common cause is beta-streptococci, group A), airway obstruction, and chronic otitis media

Nursing Process
ASSESSMENT
1. Airway obstruction: noisy or increased respiration; restless/change in behavior; diaphoretic; pale/cyanotic
2. Active infection: fever, sore throat, enlarged lymph nodes; elevated white blood cell (WBC) count
3. Bleeding disorders: bleeding and coagulation time: prothrombin time (PT), partial thromboplastin time (PTT)
4. Preoperative anxiety: child and family's knowledge concerning surgery

ANALYSIS/NURSING DIAGNOSIS (see p. 417)
PLANNING, IMPLEMENTATION, AND EVALUATION

Goal 1 Preoperatively, the child and family will be prepared psychologically for hospitalization and surgery (refer to The Ill and Hospitalized Child, Goal 1, p. 414)

Goal 2 Postoperatively, the child will remain free from excessive bleeding or hemorrhage; maintain a patent airway.

Implementation
1. Position child on side with knee on upper side flexed until alert and recovered from surgery.
2. Monitor vital signs frequently.
3. Observe for excessive swallowing, vomiting of fresh blood, restlessness, frequent clearing of throat.
4. Inspect surgical site for signs of oozing.
5. Discourage child from coughing, sneezing, crying, and sucking on straw (puts tension on suture line).
6. Employ comfort measures.
   a. Ice collar to promote vasoconstriction and reduce pain
   b. Analgesics prn (avoid aspirin)
   c. Nonirritating, cool liquids (ice chips, Popsicles, Jell-O); avoid milk products, citrus, red liquids
   d. Mouth care (no gargling or toothbrush)

Evaluation
Child maintains patent airway free from hemorrhage; experiences minimal pain and discomfort.

Goal 3 Child or family will receive appropriate information concerning home care.

Implementation
1. Observe for delayed hemorrhage (5 to 10 days postoperatively) caused by infection or tissue sloughing during healing process.
2. Limit child's activities for 1 to 2 weeks.
3. Provide daily rest periods.
4. Keep child away from anyone with an active infection (e.g., upper respiratory infection [URI]).
5. Provide nonirritating foods to child for 1 to 2 weeks; not hot, citrus, spicy, or rough foods; encourage clear liquids.
6. Have child refrain from coughing, clearing throat, or gargling (sore throat usually lasts 7 to 10 days).

Evaluation
Child's surgical site heals without complications; child resumes normal diet and activities 1 to 2 weeks postoperatively.

✖ STRABISMUS
1. Definition: neuromuscular defect of the eye that can cause visual impairment, either diplopia (double vision) or amblyopia (suppression of vision in one eye)
2. Incidence: normal in young infants; considered abnormal after 6 months of age, requiring evaluation and treatment
3. Medical treatment (done before age 6 to preserve or restore vision in affected eye)
   a. Eye muscle exercises (orthoptics)
   b. Corrective lenses
   c. Patching unaffected eye to strengthen muscles of affected eye
   d. Surgical correction

Nursing Process
ASSESSMENT
1. Eye crosses or deviates outward; may be unilateral or bilateral
2. Squinting; head tilting
3. Cover test: unaffected eye is covered while child focuses on an object, cover is removed, affected eye deviates
4. Corneal light reflex test: shine penlight on bridge of child's nose while child fixates on a distant object, light reflects from a different point on each pupil, indicating an imbalance

ANALYSIS/NURSING DIAGNOSIS (see p. 417)
PLANNING, IMPLEMENTATION, AND EVALUATION

Goal 1 Child and parents will implement treatment plan (exercises, patching, or corrective lenses).

Implementation
1. Teach child and parents how to carry out prescribed treatment measures.
2. Emphasize importance of adhering to treatment plan for specified length of time.

Evaluation
Child cooperates with and adheres to corrective measures; has vision restored; experiences no worsening of visual impairment.

Goal 2 Child will be prepared for eye surgery; complications will be prevented.

Implementation
1. Assist child in becoming familiar with postoperative environment (e.g., call light, bedside table).
2. Minimize changes in child's postoperative environment.
3. Speak to child in normal voice tones; identify self and purpose *before proceeding with care.*
4. Maintain eye patches or shields as prescribed.
5. Keep bed's side rails up; pad as necessary.

6. Teach child to avoid straining, coughing, sudden movement, rubbing eyes (use elbow restraints if necessary).
7. Assess for nausea—administer antiemetics (if ordered) prn.
8. Observe and report ocular redness, discharge, itching, or pain.
9. Instill eye ointments or drops as prescribed (inner to outer canthus).
10. Provide auditory and tactile play activities (music, reading to child, story tapes, favorite attachment objects).

Evaluation

Child's eye heals without injury or infection; child cooperates with care and maintains age-appropriate play activities.

Application of the Nursing Process to the Child with an Interference with Protection: Communicable Disease

ASSESSMENT

1. Nursing history
   a. Immunization history
   b. History of exposure to disease
   c. Previous communicable disease, how treated
   d. Signs and symptoms of current illness
      1. alterations in skin sensation
      2. skin lesions
      3. pain or tenderness
      4. itching
      5. fever
      6. infestations
2. Clinical appraisal
   a. Skin lesions: size, color, distribution (general, localized), configuration (single, clustered, diffuse, linear), type of lesion (macule, papule, vesicle, pustule, crust)
   b. Description of infestation (lice, scabies, ringworm, pinworms)
3. Diagnostic tests
   a. Microscopic exam of lesions
   b. Culture of organism

ANALYSIS/NURSING DIAGNOSIS

1. Safe, effective care environment
   a. Risk for poisoning
   b. Risk for infection
2. Physiologic integrity
   a. Pain
   b. Fluid volume deficit
   c. Impaired skin integrity
3. Psychosocial integrity
   a. Body-image disturbance
   b. Social isolation
   c. Anxiety
4. Health promotion/maintenance
   a. Knowledge deficit
   b. Self-care deficit
   c. Altered health maintenance

GENERAL NURSING PLANNING, IMPLEMENTATION, AND EVALUATION

Goal Child will be free from communicable disease (infection, infestation) and will not spread communicable diseases to others.

Implementation

1. Ensure that child's immunizations remain up-to-date.
2. Explain prescribed treatment to parents and child, and encourage them to comply with therapy.
3. Prevent child's exposure to others during communicable period.
4. Identify contacts who also may require treatment.

Evaluation

Child is free from communicable disease; does not transmit disease to others.

SELECTED HEALTH PROBLEMS: COMMUNICABLE DISEASES, SKIN PROBLEMS, INFESTATIONS

✖ COMMUNICABLE DISEASES

1. Definition: a disease caused by a specific agent or its toxic products, transmitted by direct contact or indirectly through contaminated articles; the incidence of communicable disease has significantly decreased with availability and widespread use of immunizations
2. Types of immunity
   a. Active: antibodies formed by body as a result of having had the disease or through immunization
   b. Passive: introduction of antibodies formed outside the body, such as by placental transfer, breast milk, or gamma globulin injection
3. Medical treatment
   a. Prevent through immunization (see Table 5-3)
   b. Antibiotic therapy for scarlet fever (penicillin/erythromycin), Rocky Mountain spotted fever (tetracycline/chloramphenicol), and Lyme disease (doxycycline/tetracycline)
   c. Rubella titer before pregnancy or during first trimester

Nursing Process

ASSESSMENT

1. Prodromal period
   a. Malaise
   b. Anorexia
   c. Coryza
   d. Sore throat
   e. Fever
   f. Lymphadenopathy
   g. Headache
2. Specific characteristics
   a. *Chickenpox (varicella zoster):* rash begins as macule, progresses to papule and vesicle that breaks open and crusts over; all stages present in varying degrees at same time; rash begins on trunk and spreads to extremities and face; intense pruritus; child communicable until all lesions crusted
   b. *Mumps (parotitis):* enlarged parotid glands, earache; after puberty, sterility in males is major complication; encephalitis is frequent complication of mumps for any age group
   c. *German measles (rubella):* discrete pink maculopapular rash, first on face, then downward to neck, arms, trunk, and legs; greatest concern is teratogenic

effect on fetus during first trimester of pregnancy; rubella titer on women of childbearing age highly recommended

d. *Rocky Mountain spotted fever (RMSF):* transmitted by ticks; found primarily along Atlantic coast and Rocky Mountain region; high fever and rash beginning on ankles, wrists, soles of feet; may see edema and central nervous system (CNS) problems; methods for tick removal include withdrawing tick by turning counterclockwise with tweezers or pulling gently at 45-degree angle

e. *Lyme disease:* transmitted by deer ticks throughout the continental United States; most common in late spring and early summer; spreading red-pink ring-like rash develops around tick bite 3 to 4 weeks after exposure accompanied by flulike symptoms—fever, fatigue, myalgias, nausea; if untreated, child may develop arthralgias, synovitis, neuropathy, and dysrhythmias 6 weeks to 3 years after exposure

f. *Roseola (exanthema subitum):* seen in children ages 6 months to 2 years; high fever for 3 to 4 days; temperature returns to normal with onset of rosy-pink, macular rash; rash fades with pressure and lasts 1 to 2 days; febrile convulsions

g. Rubeola: caused by virus from respiratory secretions, urine, and blood; anorexia, lymphadenopathy, rash from face downward, photophobia

h. *Diphtheria (corynebacterium diphtherae):* from mucous membrane and skin; strict isolation required

i. *Fifth disease (erythema infectiosum):* caused by human parvovirus B19; affects preschool and school age; characterized by "slapped-cheek" erythematous rash lasting 10 to 20 days; greatest concern is risk of severe fetal anemia, hydrops, and fetal death secondary to maternal infection

j. *Scarlet fever:* caused by beta-hemolytic streptococcus group A; high fever, strawberry tongue, and red pinpoint rash, especially in skin folds; rheumatic fever or acute glomerulonephritis may follow

k. *Hepatitis:* caused by several viruses; spread by fecal/oral or sexual contact; increasing incidence in children (see Hepatitis, p. 167)

l. *Mononucleosis:* highly communicable, acute syndrome caused by Epstein-Barr virus; usually mild in children but can cause fever, lymphadenopathy, elevated SGOT, and jaundice; duration 6 to 14 days.

m. *Reye's syndrome:* not communicable, but a serious complication that may occur after a viral infection (e.g., chickenpox, flu); child appears to have recovered from viral infection and then usually begins to vomit; may see changes in level of consciousness (LOC): combativeness, increased intracranial pressure (ICP), and seizures; increased risk in children who received aspirin during viral illness; acetaminophen is drug of choice for this reason

ANALYSIS/NURSING DIAGNOSIS (see p. 420)
PLANNING, IMPLEMENTATION, AND EVALUATION

Goal I Child will be prepared for isolation, will not spread disease.

Implementation
1. Explain reason for isolation to child, parents, and significant family members.
2. Provide age-appropriate play.
   a. Diversion
   b. Plan time to play with child
   c. Television in room (except if photophobic)
3. Accept expressions of fear, anger, restlessness, boredom.
4. If child is hospitalized, use appropriate isolation procedures (Table 5-8).
5. Discontinue isolation as soon as period of communicability is over.

Evaluation
Child accepts restrictions of isolation (stays in room); engages in age-appropriate activities; other cases of disease do not occur.

Goal 2 Child will be free from complications and long-term sequelae.

Implementation
1. Observe and report signs of encephalitis: headache, bizarre behavior changes, seizures, fever, muscle weakness.
2. Observe and report signs of vision or hearing loss.
3. Observe and report signs of respiratory or cardiac complications: pneumonia, laryngotracheitis, otitis media, rheumatic fever.
4. Observe and report signs of orchitis in mumps.

Evaluation
Child is free from complications and long-term sequelae (e.g., neurologic disability, sensory impairment, sterility, or cardiac damage).

Goal 3 Child will ingest adequate food and fluids to meet nutritional needs.

Implementation
1. Avoid rough or acidic foods; offer bland foods.
2. Use colorful glasses, straws, or liquids to enhance appetite.
3. Offer favorite foods and fluids (ice cream, pudding, gelatin).
4. Advance from liquids to regular diet as tolerated.

Evaluation
Child ingests adequate daily intake; is free from dehydration; eats a soft diet of sufficient caloric content.

Goal 4 Child will experience minimal discomfort.

Implementation
1. Give antipyretics for fever or discomfort (acetaminophen dose: 1 grain for every year of age up to 10 years q4h prn). *Do not give aspirin. Acetaminophen dose is 5 to 10 mg/kg.*
2. Place on bed rest until fever subsides.
3. Change bed linen and clothing daily.
4. Provide cool humidifer as needed.
5. Use tepid baths to relieve fever and itching; keep skin clean; observe for signs of secondary skin infection.

Table 5-8 Types of isolation

Mode of transmission	Isolation	Nursing responsibilities
Direct contact; airborne (droplets)	Strict	Private room Hand washing Gown, gloves, and mask Double-bag linen and trash Sterilize all reusable equipment Lab specimen precautions
Airborne (droplets)	Respiratory	Private room Hand washing Mask Double-bag respiratory trash Lab specimen precautions
Direct/indirect contact with feces	Enteric	Private room Hand washing Gowns and gloves when in contact with feces or materials contaminated with feces Double-bag contaminated articles Lab specimen precautions
Direct/indirect contact with purulent material or drainage from infected body sites	Drainage/secretions precautions	Hand washing Gown and gloves when in contact with contaminated linen, dressings, etc. Double-bag linen/trash
Direct/indirect contact with infected blood or body fluids	Standard (universal) precautions	Hand washing Gowns and gloves when in contact with body fluids, soiled linens, clothes, dressings, etc. Protective eyewear when splashing of body fluids can be expected Double-bag contaminated articles Avoid needle-stick injuries Dispose of used needles correctly Keep emergency ventilation devices at bedside if indicated Health care personnel with open skin lesions should avoid all direct client care
	Severely compromised client (reverse)	Private room with positive pressure airflow Hand washing Gowns, gloves, and mask Sterilize linen, clothing, etc.

6. Apply calamine lotion for itching (wash off completely once a day to prevent maceration of skin); administer antihistamines or antipruritic medications.
7. Keep fingernails short and clean; apply mittens if needed.
8. Dim lights if photophobia is present.
9. Use warm compresses or irrigations of saline to eyes (measles).
10. Local applications of heat or cold to relieve parotid discomfort (mumps).

Evaluation

Child rests and sleeps comfortably; has only minimal fever and itching.

SEXUALLY TRANSMITTED DISEASES

1. Definition: a communicable disease transmitted by direct genital contact or sexual activity; sexually transmitted diseases (STDs) are the most prevalent communicable diseases in the United States; majority of cases occur in adolescents and young adults; some STDs are contracted by newborns *(Candida [thrush], herpes, chlamydial conjunctivitis and pneumonia); STDs in infants and children may indicate sexual abuse and should be investigated*
2. Cause (Table 5-9)
3. Medical treatment (Table 5-9)

Nursing Process

ASSESSMENT (see Table 5-9)

ANALYSIS/NURSING DIAGNOSIS (see p. 420)

PLANNING, IMPLEMENTATION, AND EVALUATION

Goal 1 Client will participate in treatment of STD; will not transmit the disease to others.

Implementation

1. Use a straightforward, nonjudgmental approach when taking nursing history.
2. Reassure client of confidentiality of information and exam.
3. Teach signs, symptoms, and transmission mode of STD.

Table 5-9   Sexually transmitted diseases

Disease/cause	Incidence	Symptoms	Treatment
Gonorrhea *Neisseria gonorrheae*	Most commonly reported communicable disease	Males: dysuria, frequency, purulent urethral discharge Females: purulent vaginal discharge; 60% asymptomatic Diagnosis: by Gram stain or culture (Thayer-Martin medium) Complications if untreated: prostatitis and epididymitis in males; pelvic inflammatory disease, infertility, and arthritis in females	Penicillin or other antibiotics Probenecid may be given to delay excretion of penicillin
Herpes *Herpesvirus hominus* type 2	300,000-500,000 new cases each year	Active lesions: painful vesicular lesions that ulcerate Signs and symptoms of systemic illness: fever, headache, general adenopathy Diagnosis: isolation of virus in tissue culture; demonstration of multinucleated giant cells on microscopic exam	Viscous lidocaine to ease pain Keep lesions clean and dry apply cornstarch use warm air blower wear loose clothing Females: dysuria may be eased by voiding in warm water Acyclovir (Zovirax) may decrease duration of the initial or subsequent episodes but does not prevent recurrences
Syphilis *Treponema palidum*	Third most commonly reported communicable disease	Primary (3 weeks after exposure): classic chancre (painless, red, eroded lesions with indurated border at point of entry) Secondary (1-3 months after exposure): cutaneous, nonpruritic, diffuse lesions on face, trunk, or extremities Tertiary (10-30 years after exposure): cardiac and neurologic destruction Diagnosis: positive darkfield slide of organism; VDRL, RPR, or FTA	Penicillin
Trichomoniasis *Trichomonas vaginalis*	May be the most frequently acquired sexually transmitted disease in the United States	Symptoms range from none to frothy, greenish-gray vaginal discharge Diagnosis: microscopic identification of motile protozoan	Metronidazole (Flagyl)
Candidiasis *Candida albicans*	Overall incidence in United States is unknown	Yeastlike fungus causing monilial infection in the vagina; not associated with sexual transmission; seen in birth control pill use, pregnancy, and other nonsexual sources; often an early indication of diabetes in girls and women Erythematous, edematous, pruritic vulva Thick, white, "cottage cheese"–like discharge	Nystatin (Mycostatin) vaginal suppositories or cream; if this fails, clotrimazole 1% (Lotrimin)

Continued

4. Teach client to avoid sexual contact with partner while infected.
5. Provide clear, specific, written and oral explanations of medical treatment.
6. Counsel women of childbearing age concerning transmission of STD to newborn.
   a. Gonorrheal conjunctivitis (may cause blindness)
   b. Neonatal herpes infection (may cause blindness, deafness, mental retardation, or may be fatal)
   c. Congenital syphilis (passively transmitted through placenta)
   d. Oral candidiasis (thrush)
   e. Chlamydia (conjunctivitis and pneumonia)
7. Assist with identification and treatment of sexual contacts.
8. Report cases of gonorrhea, syphilis to health department.
9. Teach how to reduce risk of reinfection.

Evaluation

Client participates in treatment plan; is free from disease recurrence; does not transmit disease to others.

Goal 2 Client will resolve feelings of embarrassment, shame, guilt, and negative self-worth resulting from diagnosis

Implementation

1. Treat with respect, dignity.
2. Ensure confidentiality.
3. Provide sexuality education to dispel myths and misinformation.
4. Encourage to express any feelings of shame, embarrassment, guilt, loss of esteem.

5. Refer to self-help groups (herpes) in community as appropriate.

Evaluation

Client resolves negative feelings about diagnosis; uses support group (when appropriate); client's confidentiality is protected.

Goal 3 Client will be aware of sexual practices that will reduce the chances of acquiring an STD.

Implementation

1. Avoid sex with individuals who have multiple partners.
2. Follow strict personal hygiene habits (e.g., bathing, diet).
3. Use only water-soluble lubricants.
4. Use latex condoms lubricated with nonoxynol-9.
5. Avoid douching before and after sex (increases the risk of infections because the body's normal defenses are reduced or destroyed).
6. Be aware of symptoms of STD (fever, weight loss, persistent diarrhea, enlarged lymph nodes, unusual discharge, dysuria, bruising).

Evaluation

Client remains free from STD.

✖ COMMON SKIN PROBLEMS AND INFESTATIONS

1. Definition: inflammatory responses, bacterial infections, or insect infestations of the skin, hair, or scalp; common in preschoolers and school-age children, whose close contact increases their susceptibility
2. Cause (Table 5-10)
3. Medical treatment (Table 5-10)

Table 5-9 Sexually transmitted diseases—cont'd

Disease/cause	Incidence	Symptoms	Treatment
Scabies *Sarcoptes scabiei*	Epidemic in United States	Intense, nocturnal genital itching Diagnosis: microscopic examination of shave excision lesion	1% gamma benzene hexachloride lotion (Kwell) A-200 Pyrinate, RID in children under 5
Chlamydia *Chlamydia trachomatis*	More prevalent than gonorrhea Affects approximately 3 million Americans a year	Major cause of nongonococcal urethritis in men (frequency, dysuria) Accounts for 20%-30% of all pelvic inflammatory diseases May be transmitted to the newborn during delivery and result in conjunctivitis and pneumonia Many women are asymptomatic; others may complain of frequency, dysuria, urgency, abnormal vaginal discharge, even bleeding Diagnosis: identification of organism through culture	Tetracycline/erythromycin; should take medication at least 7-10 days; sexual partners should also be treated
Acquired immunodeficiency syndrome (AIDS) *Human immunodeficiency virus (HIV)*	See p. 268	See p. 268	See p. 268

Nursing Process

See Table 5-10.

PINWORMS (HELMINTHS)

1. Definition: parasitic infestation primarily of the intestinal tract; worms deposit eggs in anal area, causing severe itching; eggs attach to child's fingers, causing reinfection when fingers are put in mouth
2. Incidence: approximately half of all school-age children will have pinworms at some time
3. Medical treatment
   a. Examine stool for ova and parasites (not a reliable test for pinworms)
   b. Cellophane-tape test; child should be rechecked 2 or 3 times because of false-negative findings; tape test should be done in early morning (i.e., 5 AM to 6 AM)

Table 5-10 Common skin problems and infestations

Cause	Assessment	Medical treatment	Plan/implementation
ACNE VULGARIS: SKIN LESIONS (COMEDOS) CAUSED BY INCREASED SEBACEOUS SECRETIONS DURING PUBERTY AND ADOLESCENCE; MORE THAN THREE FOURTHS OF ALL ADOLESCENTS ARE AFFECTED			
Corynebacterium acnes Dietary factors (chocolate, iodine) have not been substantiated Exacerbated by menstruation, stress, oil-based cosmetics, and oral contraceptives	Sebum blocks skin pores, resulting in local inflammation Blackheads, papules, cysts, or nodules appear on face, back, chest, arms, and neck	Topical antibiotics Tetracycline or prednisone for severe cases Ultraviolet light Isotretinoin (Accutane)	Teach adolescent to avoid picking or squeezing lesions (may cause infection and scarring). Encourage regular cleansing of skin, especially when sweaty (hot weather, after exercise). Avoid using caps, headbands. Recommend over-the-counter antiacne cleansers and cover creams (contain alcohol and benzoyl peroxide, a peeling and drying agent) to help keep skin dry. Encourage a healthy lifestyle: balanced diet, exercise, rest; minimize stress.
ATOPIC DERMATITIS (ECZEMA): ALLERGIC REACTION TO FOODS, ENVIRONMENTAL INHALANTS, AND POLLEN			
Unknown	Disease of remissions and exacerbations Lesions appear as papules, vesicles, and crusts; begin on cheeks and spread to face and flexor surfaces of body Intense itching that may lead to secondary skin infection Some consider eczema a precursor to asthma	Elimination diet Topical steroids Nonsoap preparations (Cetaphil) Wet soaks with Burow's solution Antihistamines for itching	Teach parents the importance of adhering to the diet. Teach administration of medications Steroids may mask infections; may see rebound effect when ointment discontinued Antihistamines may cause drowsiness Control itching by Administering medications as ordered Avoiding soap preparations Keeping nails cut; covering hands with mittens; may need to use elbow restraints Cotton clothing Avoiding overheating Exposure to ultraviolet light (irritates and dries the lesions) Wet soaks with Burow's prn (e.g., nap time)
IMPETIGO CONTAGIOSA: SUPERFICIAL BACTERIAL SKIN INFECTION			
Staphylococcus, Streptococcus	Vesicles that rupture to form honey-colored crusts; erupt most often on face, axillae, and extremities; itches, highly contagious	Removal of crusts with Burow's solution Topical bactericidal ointment (Neosporin, Bactroban) Penicillin in severe cases	Teach child and parent how to soften and remove crusts, apply antibiotic ointment. Teach administration of oral antibiotics (penicillin/erythromycin). Prevent scratching by keeping nails clipped, using mitts or elbow restraints as necessary. Teach child to use own towels and washcloths until lesions heal.

Continued

Table 5-10 Common skin problems and infestations—cont'd

Cause	Assessment	Medical treatment	Plan/implementation
LICE (PEDICULOSIS): PARASITIC INFESTATION OF HEAD (PEDICULOSIS CAPITIS), BODY (PEDICULOSIS CORPORIS), OR PUBIC AREA (PEDICULOSIS PUBIS)			
Pediculus humanus	Ova (nits) on hair shafts Itching, skin excoriation Enlarged lymph nodes	Kwell (Lindane 1%) shampoo or lotion (not recommended for children younger than 5) A-200 Pyrinate, RID (Pyrethrin) and NIX (permethrin)	Teach parents how to apply prescribed shampoo or lotion; caution against Kwell overuse (neurotoxicity); should repeat treatment in 7-10 days. May need to cut long hair. Use fine-tooth comb dipped in vinegar to remove nits. Discard contaminated combs and brushes. Teach children not to exchange such personal items as towels, combs, brushes, and hats. Launder bed linens and towels. Use gamma benzene spray on upholstered furniture.
RINGWORM (TINEA): SUPERFICIAL FUNGAL INFECTION OF HEAD (TINEA CAPITIS), BODY (TINEA CORPORIS), "JOCK ITCH" (TINEA CRURIS), OR "ATHLETE'S FOOT" (TINEA PEDIS)			
Various fungi	Scaly, _Capitis_ circumscribed patches Areas of patchy hair loss Itching Green concentric ring under Wood's light (ultraviolet) illumination Positive culture	Oral griseofulvin: 20 mg/kg/day for 7-14 days Local antifungal preparations Whitfield's ointment Tolnaftate (Tinactin)	Teach parents how to administer oral and local antifungal agents. Shampoo frequently using clean towels, combs, and brushes. Keep child's hair short. _Corporis and cruris_ Avoid wearing nylon underwear and tight-fitting clothes. Keep affected areas clean and dry. Identify and treat source (often from household pets). _Pedis_ Wear clean, light, cotton socks. Wear well-ventilated shoes. Apply topical antifungal powder containing tonaftate. Avoid bare feet in public places (such as school gym) until infection has cleared.

c. Anthelmintics
   1. pyrvinium pamoate (Povan), single dose 5 mg/kg; stools turn red; tablets should not be chewed because they stain teeth
   2. piperazine citrate 65 mg/kg daily for 3 days; contraindicated in children with impaired renal/hepatic function or seizure disorders

Nursing Process
ASSESSMENT
1. Intense anal itching (worsens at night)/vaginitis
2. Enuresis
3. Irritability/restlessness
4. Night waking/insomnia

ANALYSIS/NURSING DIAGNOSIS (see p. 420)
PLANNING, IMPLEMENTATION, AND EVALUATION

> **Goal** Child will be free from infestation, will not reinfest self or infest others.

Implementation
1. Identify other family members and close contacts who may also need treatment.
2. Teach good hand washing and personal hygiene (after toileting, before eating, and on arising from sleep).
3. Wear tight-fitting diapers or panties.
4. Change and launder underwear, pajamas, and bed linens daily.
5. Have child sleep alone.
6. Wear mitts or socks to prevent scratching.
7. Carry out proper disposal of feces.
8. Ensure that parents understand importance of carrying out these measures.

Evaluation
Child is free from infestation; does not reinfest self or transmit infestation to others; parent establishes adequate sanitation.

Application of the Nursing Process to the Child with an Interference with Protection: Safety

See Selected Health Problems, following.

SELECTED HEALTH PROBLEMS RESULTING IN AN INTERFERENCE WITH PROTECTION: SAFETY

✖ POISONOUS INGESTIONS

1. Definition: the swallowing of common nonnutritive materials that can cause health problems or poisoning; common ingested substances include lead, corrosives, hydrocarbons, aspirin, acetaminophen, and sedatives/hypnotics
2. Incidence: poisonous ingestions are fifth leading cause of death between 1 and 4 years of age; peak incidence is during toddler years
3. Cause: developmental curiosity; incorrect storage of potentially toxic substances
4. Aim of treatment is to
   a. Remove ingested toxic substance from body *or*
   b. Neutralize its effects as quickly as possible
5. Vomiting or use of an emetic is contraindicated when
   a. Child is comatose, convulsing, or in severe shock (increases risk of apsiration)
   b. Substance is a hydrocarbon (aspiration may cause a chemical pneumonia)
   c. Substance is a corrosive (acid or alkali) (emesis may further damage or perforate esophageal mucosa); see Table 5-11 for general information, treatment, and assessment of specific ingestions

Nursing Process

ASSESSMENT (see Table 5-11)
ANALYSIS/NURSING DIAGNOSIS (see p. 420)
PLANNING, IMPLEMENTATION, AND EVALUATION (FOR ALL INGESTIONS)

Goal 1 Child will receive emergency treatment for acute poisonous ingestion.

Implementation

1. Instruct parent to contact poison control center (provide telephone number) or take child to nearest emergency facility.
2. Instruct to induce vomiting (if appropriate) by stimulating gag reflex and giving syrup of ipecac; do not use salt water as an emetic.
3. Position child to avoid aspiration when vomiting; give physical support while child is vomiting.
4. Tell parent to keep original container label for determining antidote.
5. Analyze ingested substance and child's output.
   a. Bring in container and any remaining substance.
   b. Bring in any vomitus or urine output since ingestion.
6. Make appropriate referrals (e.g., social service).

Evaluation

Parent institutes correct emergency care of child; child receives appropriate follow-up care.

Goal 2 Child will maintain adequate oxygenation.

Implementation

1. Monitor vital and neurologic signs at least q15min until stable and as indicated.
2. Administer O_2 therapy as ordered.
3. Assess color of skin, nail beds, and mucous membranes.
4. Report difficulty breathing or swallowing immediately; may require a tracheotomy; keep laryngoscope, endotracheal tube, and tracheotomy tray at bedside.
5. Observe for seizure activity.
6. If breathing is labored, stay with child to reduce fear and anxiety.

Evaluation

Child remains free from respiratory distress; maintains normal respiratory rate, color.

Goal 3 Child's ingestion will be recognized and treated early to prevent complications; child will be kept safe during treatment regimen.

Implementation

1. Institute seizure precautions.
2. Check vital signs frequently until stable; if temperature elevated, sponge with tepid water; may need to use cooling blanket; observe for febrile seizures.
3. If child is confused, provide safety measures as appropriate.
4. Record I&O accurately qh.
5. Monitor urine output hourly (EDTA is potentially toxic to kidneys).
6. Prepare child for painful injections (EDTA and BAL); mix with local anesthetic (procaine hydrochloride); rotate injection sites.
7. Increase fluid intake to 1 to 2 times maintenance (aspirin).

Evaluation

Child returns to normal activities with no residual effects; is free from acquired injuries, and damage to body systems kept to minimum.

Goal 4 Child will regain fluid and electrolyte balance.

Implementation

1. Observe and report signs of respiratory alkalosis (deep and rapid breathing, light-headedness, tetany, convulsions, and coma).
2. Observe and report signs of metabolic acidosis (deep breathing, shortness of breath, disorientation, coma).
3. Observe and report signs of metabolic alkalosis (depressed respirations, hypertonicity, and tetany).

Table 5-11   Commonly ingested poisonous substances

General information	Nursing assessment	Medical treatment
ASPIRIN (SALICYLATE POISONING)		

Toxic dose: 2 grains/kg of body weight
Lethal dose: 4 grains/kg
Effects: stimulates respiratory center, which leads to respiratory alkalosis; increases metabolism, leading to fever, metabolic acidosis (from high level of ketones)
	GI effects
	  Vomiting
	  Thirst
	CNS effects
	  Hyperventilation
	  Confusion, dizziness
	  Staggered gait
	  Coma
	Hematopoietic effects
	  Bleeding tendencies
	Metabolic effects
	  Sweating
	  Hyponatremia
	  Hypokalemia
	  Dehydration
	  Hypoglycemia
		Induce vomiting with syrup of ipecac:
		  6-12 months of age: 10 ml (2 tsp) and as much water as possible.
		  over 1 year: 15 ml (1 tbst) and 2-3 glasses of water.
		Gastric lavage.
		IV fluids, sodium bicarbonate (enhances excretion), electrolytes.
		Vitamin K for hypoprothrombinemia.
		Glucose for hypoglycemia.
		Diuretics: acetazolamide (Diamox).
		Dialysis when potentially lethal doses have been ingested.

ACETAMINOPHEN (TYLENOL)		

Most common cause of childhood poisoning
Toxic dose: uncertain, do not exceed recommended levels
Effects: cellular necrosis of the liver resulting in liver dysfunction and, in some cases, hepatic failure
	First stage (first 24 hours)
	  Nausea
	  Vomiting
	  Sweating
	  Pallor or cyanosis
	  Weakness
	Second stage (24-48 hours)
	  SGOT, SGPT elevated
	  Liver tenderness (RUQ)
	  Prolonged prothrombin time
	Third stage (1 week)
	  Liver necrosis
	  Hepatic failure
	  Possible death
		Induce vomiting or gastric lavage (see aspirin).
		Acetylcysteine (Mucomyst) as an antidote, given PO with fruit juice or cola, or via NG tube (offensive odor).
		IV fluids.
		Sodium-restricted, high-calorie, high-protein diet.

CORROSIVES (LYE, BLEACH, AMMONIA)		
Extent of damage depends on the causticity of the substance and the amount ingested	Grossly visible whitish burns of mouth and pharynx; color darkens as ulcerations form Edema Respiratory distress Difficulty swallowing Excess drooling Severe pain Shock	DO NOT INDUCE VOMITING; DO NOT LAVAGE Activated charcoal may be given. Dilute with small amounts of water. Tracheostomy if respiratory distress is severe. IV fluids while child is NPO. Analgesics, steroids, antibiotics, antacids. Possible gastrostomy. Possible esophageal dilations to prevent strictures (or maintain patency of esophagus). Colon transplant if esophageal damage is severe (done when child is older).
HYDROCARBONS (GASOLINE, KEROSENE, TURPENTINE, MINERAL SEAL OIL)		
Immediate concern is aspiration, which can cause severe (or fatal) chemical pneumonitis Systemic effects from GI absorption of hydrocarbons are relatively mild	Burning sensation in mouth and throat Characteristic breath odor Nausea, anorexia, vomiting Lethargy Fever	DO NOT INDUCE VOMITING Supportive measures for respiratory effects, pneumonitis (O_2, antibiotics, IV fluids).

Table 5-11   Commonly ingested poisonous substances—cont'd

General information	Nursing assessment	Medical treatment
LEAD (CHRONIC POISONING)		

Approximately 4%-10% of children under age 6 years have excessive blood lead levels (BLLs); BLLs greater than 40 μg/dl cause symptoms; African American children are at 6 times greater risk	Acute poisoning
	  Anemia
	  GI symptoms: anorexia, nausea, vomiting, constipation
	Chronic poisoning
	  CNS effects: irritability, lethargy, hyperactivity, developmental delays, clumsiness, seizures, disorientation, coma, possible death
	  Sketetal effects: increased density of long bones, lead lines in long bones
	  Renal effects: glycosuria, proteinuria, possible acute or chronic renal failure
		All children in at-risk settings should be screened in toddler years.
		Remove child from lead source; hospitalize if BLL is greater than 10 μg/dl.
		Chelating agents: EDTA usually used in combination with BAL; given IM q4h for 5 days (causes lead to be deposited in bone and excreted via kidneys); monitor kidney function because EDTA is nephrotoxic; monitor calcium levels because EDTA enhances excretion of calcium.
		Oral chelating agents: succimer if BLL > 45 μ/dl; monitor for transient increases in liver function tests, rashes, GI disturbances.
		Calcium phosphorus, and vitamin D aid lead excretion.
		Anticonvulsants for seizure control.
		Oral or IM iron for anemia.
		Follow-up lead levels to monitor progress (lead is excreted more slowly than it accumulates in the body).

4. Observe and report signs of hypokalemia: malaise, thirst, polyuria, cardiac dysrhythmias, decreased BP, thready pulse, depressed reflexes.
5. Observe and report signs of hypoglycemia or hyperglycemia.
6. Monitor vital signs frequently until stable.
7. Offer clear liquids in small amounts (if child is able to swallow); observe for nausea, ability to swallow.
8. Evaluate hydration status frequently.

Evaluation
Child is well hydrated without electrolyte imbalance.

Goal 5 Child will rest comfortably and be free from pain.

Implementation
1. Administer analgesics as ordered.
2. Soothe child with gentle touching and soft voice.
3. Encourage parental contact and involvement to reduce anxiety and to induce relaxation.
4. Provide opportunities for age-appropriate play.

Evaluation
Child rests and sleeps normally; is free from pain.

Goal 6 Parents will receive appropriate information to prevent or reduce recurrences.

Implementation
1. Provide anticipatory guidance concerning developmental issues and accidents.
2. Teach the essentials of prevention (childproofing environment).
   a. Do not place substances in unmarked containers.
   b. Keep harmful substances out of child's reach, in locked cabinets.
   c. Teach child that medication is not candy.
   d. Emphasize poisonous quality of abused over-the-counter drugs.
3. Provide appropriate supervision of the child.
4. Provide love and attention to the child.
5. Observe child for pica.
6. Obtain continued medical care as appropriate.
7. Support parents and child in dealing with feelings about ingestion (guilt and anger).
8. Assist parents to identify and remove sources of lead in environment (paint, dust from dump site, ceramics, drinking water)

Evaluation
Parent modifies home environment to prevent recurrence of ingestion.

✖ COCAINE AND DRUG-ADDICTED INFANTS

1. Definition: physical dependence and addiction appearing at birth in neonates whose mothers use and abuse illicit drugs; common drugs include cocaine, crack, heroin, PCP, opiates, alcohol, and CNS depressants
2. Incidence: estimates indicate 7% to 16% of women of childbearing years are addicted to drugs: 2% to 3% are cocaine dependent
3. Cause: many drugs freely cross the placental barrier and are incorporated into the fetal circulation; the fetus metabolizes these drugs differently, often resulting in delayed excretion
4. Pathophysiology: crack and cocaine cause hypertension, tachycardia, and vasoconstriction in mothers that may result in abruptio placentae and fetal hypoxia; chronic maternal blood flow restrictions can cause fetal anoxia,

prematurity, intrauterine growth retardation, precipitous delivery, and fetal demise
5. Medical treatment
   a. Diagnosis: antepartal history of drug abuse; blood and urine testing of mother and neonate
   b. Treatment: life-sustaining measures include cardiac and respiratory support, social services and law enforcement assistance as needed

Nursing Process

ASSESSMENT
1. Antepartal history: maternal crack and cocaine or other drug use
2. Intrapartal history: abruptio placentae, meconium staining, prematurity, intrauterine growth retardation, microcephaly, positive blood and urine drug screens in mother or infant
3. Neonatal period: increased startle reflex, tremulousness, seizure activity, irritability, muscular rigidity, poor feeding patterns, ineffective suck-swallow coordination, and transient electroencephalograph (EEG) abnormalities
4. Infancy and childhood: developmental delays, delayed language acquisition, increased incidence of sudden infant death syndrome (SIDS), asymmetric muscle development, and poor interactive capabilities

ANALYSIS/NURSING DIAGNOSIS (see p. 420)
PLANNING, IMPLEMENTATION, AND EVALUATION

Goal I Child will experience love and physical contact without overstimulation.

Implementation
1. Decrease stimulation to child: lower lights, minimize sudden noises and movements, and remove from stimuli as much as possible.
2. Swaddle infant; hold closely and securely when providing care; use rhythmic movements (e.g., rocking, swaying).
3. Be observant and responsive to cues of overstimulation, including gazing away, tremors, increased irritability.
4. Provide totally darkened, quiet environment if necessary.
5. Support parent in learning caretaking role.

Evaluation
Child responds appropriately to external stimuli; is able to form attachments to primary caretakers.

Goal 2 Child will maintain adequate nutrition.

Implementation
1. Wake for feedings q4-6h if needed (infant may sleep 20 to 22 hours if allowed).
2. Provide small feedings in upright position.
3. Establish quiet environment, calm routine surrounding feedings.
4. Monitor height and weight.

Evaluation
Child follows growth curve for height and weight, participates in self-feeding as appropriate.

Goal 3 Child will achieve optimum level of growth and development.

Implementation
1. As negative reactions to environment decrease (by 3 to 4 months of age), provide appropriate developmental stimulation with specific attention to language skills.
2. Provide massage therapy.
3. Hold child with child's arms in midline position to aid in development of hand coordination.

Evaluation
Child achieves normal developmental milestones within first year of life.

Goal 4 Child, family, and caretaker will receive appropriate teaching and follow-up.

Implementation
1. Assess family's ability to safely care for infant at home.
2. Contact social service immediately after birth to arrange involvement of foster parents as needed.
3. Provide information to caretaker about infant's difficulty responding to environment.
4. Explain to families possible short- and long-term effects of prenatal drug exposure.

Evaluation
Family states effects of drug exposure; demonstrates ability to safely provide physical and emotional care for infant.

✴ BURNS

1. Definition: tissue damage that results from thermal, chemical, electrical, or radioactive agents (Table 5-12)
2. Incidence
   a. Third-leading cause of accidental injury and death in children
   b. Over 50% of burns occur in children 5 years of age or younger
   c. Thermal burns are most common
3. Classification: severity of burn based on both surface area and depth of burn
   a. Percentage of body surface burned
      1. rule of nines (adults) (Fig. 5-1)
      2. modified rule of nines (children) (Fig. 5-1)
   b. Degree of damage (depth of burn injury)
      1. first degree: superficial partial thickness; pain, redness, no tissue or nerve damage, superficial epidermis affected
      2. second degree: deep-dermal partial thickness; pain, pale to red edematous skin, vesicles, entire affected area of epidermis and varying amounts of dermis affected
      3. third degree: full thickness; painless; skin white, red, or black; edematous; bullae; nerves, epidermis, dermis destroyed; subcutaneous adipose tissue, fascia, muscle and bone may also be destroyed or damaged

Table 5-12 Systemic responses to burn injury

Alterations in fluid volume	Altered capillary permeability results in shifts of water, protein, and electrolytes from the intravascular to interstitial spaces, which reduces the circulating blood volume. The body adapts through vasoconstriction, tachycardia, and conservation of fluid volume by renal reabsorption. However, this is temporary, and unless the deficit is corrected, burn shock will result. Fluid losses continue for 3-4 days with major losses in the first 12 hours. Severe edema of burned tissue occurs with mild to moderate edema to the rest of the body; once fluid begins to shift back to intravascular spaces, diuresis occurs (within 48 hours), and the edema subsides. Sodium and potassium are exchanged with sodium entering the cell and potassium entering intravascular spaces; once diuresis occurs, potassium is excreted, child becomes hypokalemic, and replacement therapy is essential. Fluid volume deficit results in decreased renal blood flow, which impairs glomerular filtration; acute renal failure may develop if fluid replacement is not adequate. Hemolysis of RBCs may lead to anemia and renal tubular obstruction.

Alterations in metabolism	Increased metabolic rate and oxygen consumption are the body's usual responses to major burns.
	1. The stress of a burn injury causes
	  Glycogen breakdown leading to depletion of energy stores within 24 hours after burn, followed by gluconeogensis (breakdown of protein stores)
	  Negative nitrogen balance (elevated BUN and urine area nitrogen)
	  Increased blood glucose levels
	2. Elevated aldosterone and antidiuretic hormone (ADH) levels
	3. Metabolic acidosis (often compensated for by respiratory alkalosis)

Potential complications related to multisystem effects of burn injury	The body's response to a burn is systemic in nature and carries the potential of affecting every system of the body. Respiratory problems: inhalation injury, aspiration, bacterial pneumonia, pulmonary edema Wound infection (usually occurs within 3-5 days after burn; most often caused by gram-negative organisms, especially *Pseudomonas*) Curling's ulcer (gastric or duodenal stress ulcer) Paralytic ileus (most common when burned surface is greater than 20%) Arterial hypertension CNS disturbances: disorientation, personality changes, seizures (especially in burned children), coma

4. Medical treatment (moderate to severe burns)
   a. Medical intervention
      1. immediate emergency care
         a. extinguish fire (teach children to "Stop, drop, and roll")
         b. slowly immerse burn injury in cool water if possible (relieves pain, inhibits edema formation, slows tissue damage)
         c. do *not* use ice water, ice packs, or topical ointments
         d. cover burn with clean cloth (e.g., clean bed sheet)
         e. cover with blankets (uninvolved areas) if child is hypothermic
         f. remove constrictive clothing and jewelry before swelling occurs
         g. if child is alert and oriented, provide warm liquids
         h. transport to nearest medical facility if burn is extensive
      2. admission care
         a. establish airway (O_2, intubation if laryngeal edema is a risk)
         b. *frequently* assess blood gases
         c. initiate fluid and electrolyte therapy based on body weight and percent of surface area burned
            ▪ one half of total estimated fluid requirements for the first 24 hours is usually replaced in the first 8 hours after the burn injury
            ▪ types of solutions used may vary
               • first 24 hours: crystalloid solutions, such as normal saline or Ringer's lactate
               • after diuresis, colloid solutions such as albumin or plasma
         d. assess other injuries
         e. insert urinary indwelling catheter for accurate assessment of urinary output
         f. insert nasogastric (NG) tube to prevent vomiting, abdominal distention, and gastric aspiration
         g. administer IV pain medication as ordered
         h. administer antibiotics (penicillin or erythromycin) to prevent infection (broad-spectrum antibiotics are not used because of possibility of superimposed infections)
         i. immunize with tetanus toxoid (according to recommended schedule)
      3. care of burn wounds
         a. initial therapy
            ▪ cleaning with hypochlorite solution by immersion in Hubbard tank or "hosing" (flow of sterile solution from hose over wounds)
            ▪ minor debridement; do not break vesicles
            ▪ hair removal next to burn area

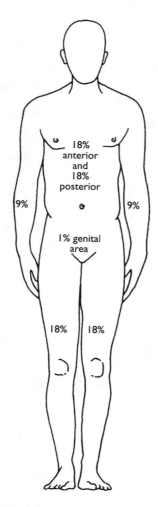

18%
anterior
and
18%
posterior

9%

9%

1% genital
area

18%   18%

a) Over 12 years: rule of nines (see figure
   at left)

b) Under 12 years: modified rule of nines

Head and neck   9% plus 1% for each year under
                age 12 years

Each arm   9%

Trunk   36%

Each leg   18% minus $\frac{1}{2}$% for each year
                under age 12 years

Genital area   1%

Fig. 5-1   Estimation of burn surface area. Percentages include anterior and posterior aspects, except for genital area.

b. open method: reverse isolation
  ▪ burn exposed to air; crust or eschar forms a protective barrier
  ▪ topical medication
    • silver sulfadiazine (Silvadene): penetrates wound slowly; is soothing, causes no acid-base complications, keeps eschar soft; debridement easier; may also be used with closed method
    • mafenide acetate (Sulfamylon): penetrates wound rapidly, is painful, causes mild acidosis; used when silver sulfadiazine is ineffective
c. closed method
  ▪ burn covered with nonadherent fine-mesh gauze and fluffed-gauze outer layer covered by stretch gauze bandages
  ▪ topical medication
    • nitrofurazone (Furacin): acts by interfering with bacterial enzymes; most frequent problem is allergic contact dermatitis; may see superinfections

    • silver nitrate: painless, bactericidal; liquid, must be kept moist; stains healthy skin and fabrics black
d. primary surgical excision: immediate surgical excision of burned tissue with grafting; reduces risk of infection; blood loss may be significant
e. debridement and hydrotherapy (hosing or Hubbard whirlpool tank): done regardless of method of treatment used
f. grafting and reconstructive surgery: long-term treatment; to improve function and cosmetic appearance

Nursing Process
ASSESSMENT
1. Respiratory status: patency of airway (burns of head, neck, and chest areas predispose child to respiratory distress)
2. Extent and depth of burn; location of burn injury
3. Observe for early signs of shock (behavioral changes, tachycardia, alterations in BP, diminished output)

4. Presence of pain (frequently manifested as irritability, depression, hostility, or aggression)
5. Observe for signs of hemorrhage (decreased BP; rapid, thready pulse; diaphoresis; pallor; decreased body temperature)
6. Monitor laboratory findings
   a. Hematocrit, arterial blood gases
   b. Sodium, chloride, potassium, CO_2
   c. Blood urea nitrogen (BUN), creatinine
   d. Serum protein
   e. Urine pH, specific gravity
7. Child's and parents' emotional responses to burn injury

ANALYSIS/NURSING DIAGNOSIS (see p. 420)
PLANNING, IMPLEMENTATION, AND EVALUATION

Goal I Child will maintain adequate oxygenation.

Implementation
1. Observe for respiratory distress (wheezing, rales, dyspnea, increased respiratory rate, nasal flaring, stridor, air hunger).
2. Monitor arterial blood gases.
3. Elevate burned extremities.
4. Assess arterial circulation in burned extremities qh.
5. Carefully monitor intubated child who is assisted by a ventilator; humidified O_2 as ordered.
6. Use suction qh or prn.
7. Prevent aspiration: maintain patency of nasogastric tube.
8. Have child turn, cough, and deep breathe; use inspirometer (to prevent hypostatic pneumonia); provide humidified air.
9. Check eschar on neck and chest for constriction; assist with escharotomy as needed.

Evaluation
Child is free from respiratory distress; has normal respiratory rate, normal color, adequate circulation (for age) in extremities.

Goal 2 Child will maintain adequate hydration and electrolyte balance.

Implementation
1. Monitor vital signs qh and as necessary; central venous pressure (CVP) line if appropriate.
2. Monitor I&O hourly (urine output 1 to 2 ml/kg/hr for children, 30 to 50 ml/hr for adult); check urine specific gravity and pH (may need to catheterize).
3. Observe for signs of hemorrhage (bleeding; decreased BP; decreased body temperature; rapid, thready pulse).
4. Observe for signs of dehydration (thirst, dry tongue, decreased urinary output, decreased BP, tachycardia, poor skin turgor).
5. Monitor IV therapy (NOTE: check for adequate urine output and serum K^+ level before adding potassium to IV).
6. Observe for signs of fluid overload (venous distention, increased BP, shortness of breath, rales, behavioral changes).

7. Observe for signs of electrolyte imbalance (e.g., abnormal lab results, cardiac dysrhythmias, tingling of fingers, abdominal cramps, convulsions, and spasms).

Evaluation
Child is free from shock, maintains adequate circulatory volume and electrolyte balance.

Goal 3 Child will be free from infection and have optimal wound healing.

Implementation
1. Use standard precautions or isolation as ordered.
2. Administer antibiotics and tetanus prophylaxis as ordered.
3. Use sterile technique with wound care; handle wound carefully to prevent damage to healing tissues.
4. Keep wounds and surrounding areas shaved.
5. Encourage self-care to increase child's sense of control and autonomy; encourage child (when possible) to participate in dressing changes.
6. Observe for and report any signs of wound infection (temperature elevation, redness at wound edge, purulent or green-gray drainage, offensive odor).
7. Observe for and report signs of systemic infection (increased body temperature, chills, tachycardia, hyperemia).
8. Observe for and report signs of respiratory infection (increased body temperature, signs of respiratory distress).

Evaluation
Child's wounds heal without complications; child assumes an active role in the wound care process.

Goal 4 Child will have minimal pain and discomfort.

Implementation
1. Administer analgesics as ordered around the clock if necessary (often given IV to ensure absorption; IM contraindicated); observe for response.
2. Medicate before painful procedures (debridement, PT, etc.).
3. Use comfort measures (e.g., pillows).
4. Teach child to change focus to music, television, friends; use imagery when appropriate.
5. Provide heat lamps, warmed blankets to assist with thermoregulation.

Evaluation
Child experiences no more than minimal pain or discomfort; develops coping strategies that reduce/modify painful experiences (e.g., dressing changes); maintains body temperature of 98°F to 100°F.

Goal 5 Child will maintain adequate nutritional intake to prevent nitrogen loss and gastrointestinal (GI) complications.

Implementation

1. Provide a high-protein, high-calorie diet; determine special likes and dislikes.
2. Weigh daily.
3. Offer small, frequent meals; encourage family to bring food from home.
4. Assess bowel sounds for possible paralytic ileus.
5. Observe for signs of Curling's ulcer (coffee-ground emesis, abdominal distention, occult blood in stool, anemia); usually occurs during the third and fourth weeks after the burn in children (first week after burn in adults).
6. Give supplemental vitamins and minerals (vitamins A, B, and C; iron and zinc), H_2 antagonists, and antacids as ordered.

Evaluation

Child ingests therapeutic diet as ordered; is free from gastrointestinal complications; maintains weight.

Goal 6 Child will achieve functional use of burned area and successful cosmetic results.

Implementation

1. Protect graft site from injury; if grafted area is exposed, child may need to be immobilized; help child not to scratch.
2. When pockets of fluid accumulate under graft site, gently "roll" the fluid out at the graft edges with a sterile cotton-tipped swab. Control bleeding from graft site with minimal pressure.
3. Do not change dressing on donor site (prevents tearing of underlying delicate epithelium).
4. Observe for signs of infection at graft sites.
5. Minimize scar formation by maintaining affected areas in a functional position; use splints when appropriate.
6. Assist with range-of-motion (ROM) exercises as ordered.
7. Encourage ambulation when appropriate.
8. Encourage child's participation in self-care and activities of daily living (ADL).
9. Provide explanations to child and family for positioning requirements.

Evaluation

Child has full (or increasing) ROM of affected and unaffected joints; has no footdrop, contractures; graft sites heal without complications.

Goal 7 Child will verbalize concerns and feelings about altered body image.

Implementation

1. Assess child's and parents' adjustment to altered body image (child's verbalizations and nonverbal behavior).
2. Spend time listening to concerns and feelings.
3. Use play therapy.
4. Offer preprocedure preparation according to age.
5. Use visual, auditory, and tactile simulation.
6. Use elastic bandages, camouflage clothes, and makeup to enhance appearance.
7. Refer to support groups.

Evaluation

Child talks about effect of burns on body; asks questions about what others will think of body; participates in activities appropriate for age and personal interest.

Goal 8 Child and family will receive appropriate information concerning home care of burns.

Implementation

1. Teach family how to change the burn dressing using clean technique; have family return demonstration; remember to adapt dressing change to family needs.
2. Instruct family to observe for signs of wound infection.
3. Review importance of vitamin C, protein, and increased calories in the healing process, and discuss ways to increase these nutrients in the child's diet.
4. Teach family appropriate care of a healed burn.
   a. Wash with mild soap and apply lubricating cream or jelly (nonperfumed).
   b. Avoid direct sunlight.
   c. Use medications prn for pruritus.
   d. Observe for signs of infection.
   e. Integrate ROM into daily routine.
   f. Teach parent pain relief strategies.
5. Discuss developmental aspects of disfiguring injuries; include extended family, peers, school teachers in rehabilitation; return child to school as soon as possible.
6. Stress importance of self-care activities to strengthen sense of self.

Evaluation

Child's burns heal with minimal contractures; child participates in routine ADL; returns to school.

Application of the Nursing Process to the Child with Developmental or Neurologic Disabilities

ASSESSMENT

Developmental and neurologic disabilities include any serious, chronic disability caused by an impairment of physical or mental functioning, or both, that occurs in childhood, is likely to persist throughout life, and results in limitations in daily functioning. It may cause significant and permanent interruptions in the child's physical, emotional, and social growth and development; early detection and appropriate intervention are essential to promote optimum development. Approximately 10% of all children and adolescents have some type of developmental disability.

1. Nursing history
   a. Achievement of developmental milestones; child's self-care abilities
   b. Developmental delays: motor, language, social, cognitive (such as persistent head lag, failure to roll over, delayed speech, impaired social functioning)
   c. Perceptual problems: vision and hearing
   d. Perinatal history (refer to Newborn Care, p. 357)
   e. Family history: congenital anomalies, hereditary factors, infections
   f. Child's health history: illnesses, allergies, medications, immunizations

g. Communication, memory, and attention problems; school performance

h. Current health problems: signs and symptoms, medical treatment, home management, concerns or problems

i. Parents' and family's perception of health problem
   1. child's adaptation to disability
   2. family's ability to cope with loss of "perfect child" (refer to Loss and Death and Dying, p. 29)
   3. stressors: economic, marital, lack of time and energy
   4. threats to self-esteem and control
   5. overprotectiveness or rejection of child

2. Clinical appraisal
   a. General: level of consciousness, affect, attention span; head circumference, cranial sutures and fontanels; vital signs, including BP
   b. Persistent or absent neonatal reflexes
   c. Posture: persistent extension and flexion of extremities, scissoring, frog-leg position, opisthotonos
   d. Motor function: muscle size and tone; symmetric, spontaneous movements of all extremities; involuntary movements such as tremors, spasticity, athetosis
   e. Developmental skills: assess for developmental progress (e.g., Denver Developmental Screening Test), gross and fine motor development, language, self-help skills (dressing, feeding, and toileting)
   f. Vision: infant's ability to focus on small objects; vision screening tests for older children (refer to The Healthy Child, vision/hearing screening, p.409)
   g. Hearing: startle reflex is a rough estimate of sound perception in infants; audiometry is unreliable with infants, toddlers, and mentally retarded children

3. Diagnostic tests (refer to Nursing Care of the Adult, diagnostic tests, p. 222)

ANALYSIS/NURSING DIAGNOSIS

1. Safe, effective care environment
   a. Risk for injury
   b. Sensory-perceptual alteration: tactile and visual
   c. Impaired home maintenance management
2. Physiologic integrity
   a. Impaired physical mobility
   b. Activity intolerance
   c. Altered nutrition: more/less than body requirements
3. Psychosocial integrity
   a. Anticipatory grieving
   b. Body-image disturbance
   c. Altered thought processes
4. Health promotion/maintenance
   a. Altered growth and development
   b. Self-care deficit
   c. Altered family processes
   d. Knowledge deficit

GENERAL NURSING PLANNING, IMPLEMENTATION, AND EVALUATION

Goal 1 Child will achieve optimum level of growth and development.

Implementation

1. Screen children at risk for developmental disabilities so that problems are detected and treated early to minimize developmental delays.
2. Keep child's activities in the mainstream as much as possible to promote self-sufficiency, adjustment, and mental development.
   a. Refer family to infant stimulation, developmental, and special education programs.
   b. Maintain open communication between family and all members of interdisciplinary team.
3. Treat child according to developmental (not chronologic) age.
4. Provide guidance for learning acceptable social behaviors.
5. Identify parenting concerns and ways to handle them (e.g., consistent discipline; needs for nurturing are identical to any other child).
6. Include activities that enhance child's self-esteem and self-worth.
7. Provide a variety of stimuli; help child pay attention to distinct stimuli.
8. Break tasks into small components; use positive reinforcement (verbal praise, hugs, stickers). Do not use food as a reward.
9. Provide visual and auditory cues and opportunities for practice (repetition enhances learning).
10. Teach self-care skills for activities of daily living (e.g., hygiene, feeding, and dressing).
    a. Allow child as much independence as possible, even if activities take longer (remember to stress that child is a family member, too).
    b. Acknowledge and positively reinforce parents' care of child and child's progress.
    c. Help parents provide a stimulating, healthful environment for the child (mainstreaming).

Evaluation

Child achieves and maintains optimum developmental potential; performs ADL as independently as possible; is maintained in a community setting.

Goal 2 Adolescent or young adult will receive appropriate education regarding sexuality.

Implementation

1. Emphasize that adolescent may understand more than he or she can communicate.
2. Provide appropriate information concerning developmental changes, menstruation, or birth control.
3. Provide explanations at level adolescent can understand.

Evaluation

Adolescent or young adult verbalizes age-appropriate knowledge regarding sexuality.

Goal 3 Parents and family members will express feelings about having a child with a developmental disability and their ability to cope.

Implementation

1. Allow parents and family members opportunities to express their grief; be supportive and anticipate repeated periods of sadness, anger; acknowledge that this is usually a lifetime process.
2. Help parents identify and reinforce child's capabilities and normal characteristics *(this is first a child, and then a child with a disability)*.
3. Encourage family discussion and coping with changes that may occur in the family system as a result of caring for the child.
4. Refer the family to appropriate community resources.

Evaluation

Parents and family express feelings and concerns regarding child's limitations; develop realistic plans to care for the child at home; include child as a member of the family constellation; involve all family members in child's care; use appropriate community resources (e.g., parent-support groups, available programs).

> **Goal 4** The family will remain cohesive and function at its optimal level.

Implementation

1. Identify families at risk for adapting poorly to disability and chronic illness.
   a. Recognize that certain family types (e.g., single-parent families, teen parents) may require more support and guidance in care of child.
   b. Consider the availability of extended-family members and their ability and willingness to participate in care of child.
   c. Consider access to care—financial and physical.
2. Determine the family's perception of the child's disability and encourage realistic discussion about the child's capabilities and limitations.
3. Identify support systems within the family and community (e.g., home health care).

4. Encourage activities that enhance individual and family development for *all family members*.
5. Provide respite care to family when necessary.

Evaluation

Family discusses realistic perceptions about the child; uses available support systems; participates in activities outside the home.

SELECTED HEALTH PROBLEMS: DEVELOPMENTAL OR NEUROLOGIC DISABILITIES

✦ MENTAL RETARDATION

1. Definition: below-average intellectual functioning that becomes apparent during childhood development and is associated with impairment in adaptive behavior; manifestations include impaired learning, inadequate social adjustment, and delayed or lowered potential capacity for achievement; see Table 5-13 for classification levels
2. Causes
   a. *Prenatal:* chromosomal and genetic variations (Down syndrome, PKU, Tay-Sachs), German measles or infection in mother during pregnancy, incompatible blood between mother and child (Rh or ABO), glandular disorders, toxic chemicals, nutritional deficiencies, excessive maternal drug or alcohol use
   b. *Perinatal:* birth injury such as anoxia or intracranial hemorrhage
   c. *Postnatal:* encephalitis, head trauma, glandular disturbances, inadequate developmental stimulation in early childhood, cardiac arrest, poisoning
3. Incidence: 3% of the U.S. population; 1 in 10 American families has a member with mental retardation (MR); 70% to 80% are in the borderline or mild (educable mentally retarded [EMR]) category (Table 5-13); 20% to 30% are moderately, severely, or profoundly retarded (the latter are most often cared for in residential institutions)

Table 5-13 Levels of retardation (classification system of American Association of Mental Deficiency)

Level	IQ range	Potential mental age	Rehabilitation potential
Level 0: Borderline	68-83	Close to normal	Usually capable of marriage, being *self-supporting* (probable low socioeconomic living standard).
Level 1: Mild or educable	52-67	8-12 years	Can usually be maintained in community. *Can work but needs supervision in financial affairs;* fourth- or fifth-grade academic possibilities (special classes for educable mentally retarded [EMR]) and vocational skills, but often has difficulty holding a job in a competitive market.
Level 2: Moderate	36-51	3-7 years	First- to third-grade academic potential (special classes for trainable mentally retarded [TMR]) or *vocational training in sheltered workshop in neighborhood job.*
Level 3: Severe	20-35	Toddler	*Minimal self-help skills* and independent behavior (toilet training, dressing self) School placement in handicapped or TMR program. Some are able to work in a sheltered workshop.
Level 4: Profound	Less than 20	Young infant	May require *total care;* may have CNS damage.

Nursing Process

ASSESSMENT
1. Developmental lags in motor and adaptive behaviors
2. Persistence of neonatal reflexes
3. Perceptual deficits
4. Level of functioning (Table 5-13)

ANALYSIS/NURSING DIAGNOSIS (see p. 435)

PLANNING, IMPLEMENTATION, AND EVALUATION (see General Nursing Plans, p. 435)

> **Goal** When hospitalized, the mentally retarded child will adapt to hospitalization, will maintain independence in ADL, will ingest adequate food and fluids.

Implementation
1. Adapt hospital routines to child's as much as possible.
2. Explain all procedures and treatments carefully, at level child can understand.
3. Maintain consistency to promote security within child's environment.
4. Encourage parent and family participation in care.
5. Assist with feeding as necessary; bring special cups and feeding utensils from home.
6. Be sure to follow through on what you tell child (e.g., if you say you will return at a certain time, be sure to do it).
7. Use positive reinforcement.

Evaluation
Child accepts staff members' explanations and cooperates in care; feeds and dresses self; takes prescribed diet and fluids.

⚕ ATTENTION DEFICIT DISORDER

1. Definition: syndrome of behaviorally related problems that include inattention and impulsivity; *DSM-IV classification differentiates attention deficit disorder (ADD) with and without hyperactivity; previously known as minimal brain dysfunction or hyperkinesis*
2. Causes: no definite pathophysiologic basis has been determined; possible causes include neurotransmitter imbalances, lead poisoning, allergies, and genetic factors
3. Incidence: 5% to 10% of school-age children, boys affected 4 to 6 times more frequently
4. Medical treatment
   a. Diagnosis: parent and teacher report of behavior, objective home and classroom observation, psychologic evaluation; results compared with *DSM-IV* criteria
   b. Treatment
      1. behavioral management
      2. medication: methylphenidate (Ritalin)
         a. dosage: 0.3 to 1.0 mg/kg/day adjusted according to child's behavior (begun on small dose)
         b. side effects: anorexia, upper abdominal pain, insomnia, growth suppression, tachycardia
         c. nursing implications
            ▪ administer with or after meals to minimize appetite suppression
            ▪ do not administer after 4 PM to minimize insomnia

Nursing Process

ASSESSMENT
1. Distractability
2. Impulsiveness
3. Emotional lability
4. Low frustration tolerance
5. High incidence of learning disabilities
6. Hyperactivity (may or may not be present)

ANALYSIS/NURSING DIAGNOSIS (see p. 435)

PLANNING, IMPLEMENTATION, AND EVALUATION

> **Goal** Child and parent will be prepared for home management.

Implementation
1. Help parents to
   a. Provide a highly structured environment with regular routines.
   b. Establish clear, simple rules and firm limits.
   c. Prevent overstimulation and fatigue in the child.
   d. Provide daily rest or quiet times.
   e. Reward any partially successful efforts at self-control.
   f. Encourage adherence to diet therapy.
2. Teach parents and child administration, action, and side effects of medication.
3. Reinforce importance of regular, routine administration of medications.
4. Refer for family or individual counseling as necessary.
5. Encourage parents to work closely with school personnel to minimize impact of ADD on learning.

Evaluation
Child continues to learn and progress in school; parents are satisfied with child's behavior pattern.

⚕ DOWN SYNDROME (TRISOMY 21)

1. Definition: extra chromosome 21 (trisomy 21), resulting from a failure of the chromosome to split during gametogenesis; mental capacity varies from level 1 (educable) to level 3 (severely retarded); one of the most common causes of mental retardation
2. Cause: associated with increased maternal or paternal age
3. Incidence: 1 in 600 to 650 live births
4. Medical treatment: diagnosis is usually based on clinical manifestations; chromosome studies may be done

Nursing Process

ASSESSMENT
1. Physical manifestations
   a. Small, round head; flat nose; protruding tongue; high, arched palate; low-set ears; fat roll at back of neck
   b. Slanted eyelids, Brushfield's spots (speckles in iris)
   c. Muscle hypotonia, hyperflexible joints
   d. Simian crease, short fingers, clinodactyly
   e. Congenital heart malformations in 40% of cases
   f. Weak respiratory accessory muscles
   g. Increased incidence of leukemia and GI anomalies
2. Mastery of development tasks
3. Intellectual functioning
4. Child's routine ADL

ANALYSIS/NURSING DIAGNOSIS (see p. 435)
PLANNING, IMPLEMENTATION, AND EVALUATION

Goal I Child will be free from respiratory infection.

Implementation
1. Teach parents (and child as appropriate) preventive health measures.
   a. Prevent exposure to individuals with URIs.
   b. Encourage optimal nutrition, adequate rest.
   c. Keep immunizations up-to-date.
2. Obtain medical care at onset of infection (may need antibiotics).

Evaluation
Child has no more than two URIs each year.

Goal 2 Child will ingest adequate food and fluids and will experience minimal feeding difficulties.

Implementation
1. Teach parents appropriate feeding techniques.
   a. Use bulb syringe to clear nasal passages before feeding.
   b. Use a long-handled infant spoon (rubber-coated) to place food to side and back of mouth.
2. Reassure parents that infant's tongue thrust does not mean dislike of food.
3. When hospitalized or in school, encourage foods from home if child not ingesting adequate amounts.
4. Adjust caloric requirements based on child's size and activity level to prevent child from becoming overweight.
5. Provide high-roughage foods and liberal fluids to prevent constipation.

Evaluation
Child's airway remains clear during feeding; child ingests food sufficient for growth; maintains weight within expected limits for height; remains free from constipation.

⚒ CEREBRAL PALSY

1. Definition: nonprogressive muscular impairment resulting in abnormal muscle tone and uncoordination; spastic type most common (upper motor neuron involvement), dyskinetic (athetoid) type second most common; may be mild to severe
2. Associated defects: mental retardation (may have normal or superior intelligence), seizures, minimal brain dysfunction; speech, hearing, oculomotor impairment
3. Incidence
   a. 25,000 babies with cerebral palsy born annually (5 per 1000 live births)
   b. Most common developmental disability of childhood
   c. Higher incidence in low-birth-weight babies or from pregnancies with complications that can result in cerebral anoxia (prenatal or perinatal)
4. Medical treatment
   a. Braces, ambulation devices (crutches, walker)
   b. Surgical correction of extremity deformities (especially lengthening of heel cord to improve stability and function)

   c. Medications: muscle relaxants, anticonvulsants, tranquilizers

Nursing Process
ASSESSMENT
1. Spasticity
   a. Hypertonicity of muscles (continuous reflexive contraction of muscles leading to tightening and shortening)
   b. Persistence of neonatal reflexes
   c. Scissoring
   d. Poor posturing
   e. Delayed gross and fine motor development
   f. Uneven muscle tone
   g. Intellectual functioning may be impaired
2. Dyskinesis (athetosis)
   a. Continuous uncontrollable, wormlike movements of arms, legs, torso, face, and tongue
      1. intensified by stress
      2. absent during sleep
   b. Drooling
   c. Poor speech articulation
ANALYSIS/NURSING DIAGNOSIS (see p. 435)
PLANNING, IMPLEMENTATION, AND EVALUATION

Goal I Child will ingest adequate nutrition.

Implementation
1. Provide adequate calories to meet additional energy demands of constant muscle activity (athetoid).
2. Feed slowly; provide calm, peaceful environment.
3. Modify feeding technique to deal with extrusion reflex.
4. Ensure adequate fluid intake.
5. Use special silverware and dishes as needed (e.g., padded spoon, nonskid dishes).
6. Teach importance of daily dental hygiene; routine dental care.

Evaluation
Child exhibits adequate growth; chews and swallows food adequately; is free from dental caries or gum problems.

Goal 2 Child will develop maximum mobility and self-help skills.

Implementation
1. Teach parents appropriate stretching and range-of-motion exercises.
2. Teach use of braces or splints, special support chair, or wheelchair as needed.
3. Encourage participation in programs of physical and occupational therapy, speech therapy as needed.
4. Avoid movement that triggers abnormal reflexes.
5. Teach self-help skills, beginning with simplest ones first; teach only one skill at a time until it is learned.
6. Provide needed adaptive devices (special utensils, Velcro fastenings).

Evaluation

Child is free from contractures; demonstrates maximum mobility (with assistance as needed); participates in self-care tasks (e.g., feeds self, dresses self).

Goal 3 Child will be free from skin breakdown.

Implementation

1. Reposition frequently and gently massage pressure points with lotion.
2. Check braces, splints for tightness and pressure; adjust as needed.
3. Use special equipment ("egg-crate" mattress, sheepskin).
4. Keep linens and clothes dry; if wet with urine or stool, change as soon as possible.

Evaluation

Child's skin is intact, free from pressure sores.

✺ HYDROCEPHALUS

1. Definition: excessive accumulation of cerebrospinal fluid (CSF) within the ventricles of the brain; three common types
   a. Excess secretion of CSF
   b. Obstructive (noncommunicating): results from an obstruction in the ventricular pathway
   c. Communicating: results when the CSF is not absorbed from the subarachnoid space
2. Causes: developmental malformation (congenital), tumors, infections, head injury
3. Treatment
   a. Diagnosis: lumbar puncture, ultrasound, computed tomography (CT), magnetic resonance imaging (MRI) (refer to Nursing Care of the Adult, diagnostic tests, p. 222)
   b. Surgical insertion of shunt to bypass obstruction or drain excess fluid
      1. ventriculoperitoneal (VP) shunt: lateral ventricle to peritoneal cavity
      2. atrioventricular (AV) shunt: lateral ventricle to right atrium of heart
      3. one-way valves are used in both cases to prevent backflow of blood or peritoneal secretions
   c. Extraventricular drainage system
   d. Rehospitalization is common for blocked or infected shunt or for lengthening of shunt as child grows

Nursing Process

ASSESSMENT

1. For signs and symptoms of increased intracranial pressure to prevent or minimize brain damage (Table 5-14)
2. Shiny scalp with dilated veins (congenital hydrocephalus)
3. Sunset eyes (congenital hydrocephalus)

ANALYSIS/NURSING DIAGNOSIS (see p. 435)
PLANNING, IMPLEMENTATION, AND EVALUATION

Goal 1 Child will maintain adequate nutrition and hydration.

Table 5-14 Signs and symptoms of increased intracranial pressure in infants and children*

Causes	Hydrocephalus
	Intracranial tumors
	Cerebral trauma
	Meningitis, encephalitis
Manifestations Infants	Bulging fontanels; wide suture lines
	High-pitched cry
	General irritability
	Vomiting, feeding difficulty (poor suck)
	Seizures
	Opisthotonos
	Rapid increase in head circumference (especially occipitofrontal diameter)
Older children after closure of fontanels	Headache
	Nausea, vomiting
	Change in level of consciousness
	Papilledema
	Diplopia
	Motor dysfunction (grasp, gait)
	Behavior changes, irritability
	Change in vital signs (elevated systolic BP, wide pulse pressure, decreased pulse and respirations)
	Seizures

*Review Nursing Care of the Adult, p 226, for content on head injury.

Implementation

1. Offer small, frequent feedings; do not overfeed.
2. Burp often.
3. After feeding, position on side with head elevated.
4. Provide rest period after feedings.
5. Assess for dehydration.

Evaluation

Child demonstrates adequate growth; has elastic skin turgor, moist mucous membranes.

Goal 2 Postoperatively, child will be free from complications.

Implementation

1. Measure infant's head circumference daily.
2. Position on unoperative side relative to appearance of fontanel: if fontanel normal, elevate head; if fontanel depressed, position child flat in bed.
3. Observe for signs of redness, skin breakdown on scalp; use sheepskin or water mattress. Check for signs of fluid leakage.
4. Turn at least q2h.
5. Do frequent neurologic checks (LOC, PERRLA). Check fontanel q2-4h. Sedation will mask signs of consciousness.
6. Observe for signs of infection along shunt tract (swelling, redness, bruising along shunt tract common for 24 to 48 hours after sugery).

7. *Pump shunt only with a physician's order, to maintain patency (usually done when shunt valve is a bubble type).*
8. Blood pressure monitoring.
9. Signs of infection (vital sign changes, irritability, poor feeding, vomiting).

Evaluation

Child's fontanels remain flat (no bulging or depression) with no further increase in head circumference; has no signs of infection or pneumonia (e.g., elevated temperature, increased pulse rate, reddened area around operative site); suffers no brain damage.

✲ SPINA BIFIDA

1. Definition: congenital defect involving incomplete formation of vertebrae, often accompanied by herniation of parts of the central nervous system
   a. Meningocele: herniation of sac containing spinal fluid and meninges
   b. Meningomyelocele: herniated sac containing CSF, meninges, and malformed portion of spinal cord and nerve roots (most serious type); sac may be covered by skin or by a thin, transparent tissue layer that tears easily and permits leakage of CSF
2. Motor and sensory impairment: relative to level and extent of defect; usually involves sensorimotor deficits of lower extremities, bowel and bladder dysfunction, associated orthopedic anomalies, and often hydrocephalus
3. Medical treatment
   a. Prenatal diagnosis: maternal serum levels of alpha-fetoprotein can be screened in all pregnancies at 16 to 18 weeks of gestation; amniocentesis is done when levels are 2 times normal or mother has a history of having a child with a neural tube defect; ultrasound useful for visualizing defect
   b. Surgical intervention to close defect within 24 to 48 hours to decrease chance of infection and minimize nerve damage

Nursing Process

ASSESSMENT

1. Condition of sac
2. Motor and sensory impairment: flaccid or spastic paralysis, response to painful stimuli, lower-extremity movement
3. Bladder and bowel function; dribbling of urine, leakage of stool
4. Associated orthopedic anomalies: clubfoot, congenital dislocated hip
5. Signs of infection (fever, irritability, lethargy)
6. Signs of increased intracranial pressure (Table 5-14), increased head circumference (especially after surgery)

ANALYSIS/NURSING DIAGNOSIS (see p. 435)
PLANNING, IMPLEMENTATION, AND EVALUATION

Goal I Child will be free from rupture of sac and infection; postoperatively, incision will heal without complications.

Implementation

1. Position on side or prone.
2. Use Bradford frame.
3. Protect sac with sponge doughnut when holding infant.
4. Apply moist, sterile dressings as ordered.
5. Observe for leakage of CSF from sac.
6. Observe for signs of meningitis (e.g., fever, irritability, bulging fontanel, nuchal rigidity).
7. Meticulously cleanse diaper area to prevent contamination of sac or postoperative wound site with urine or stool; check incision frequently for signs of infection.
8. Postoperatively, observe for signs of hydrocephalus or shunt malfunction; daily head circumference; neurologic checks.

Evaluation

Child is free from local or systemic infection (e.g., reddened skin around site, elevated temperature); has intact sac (preoperatively); has optimal wound healing postoperatively.

Goal 2 Child will maintain skin integrity (lifelong goal).

Implementation

1. Observe for reddened areas, breaks in skin.
2. Change position frequently.
3. Use sheepskin or water mattress.
4. Massage pressure areas to promote circulation.
5. Teach self-help skills concerning skin care.

Evaluation

Child's skin is intact, free from reddened areas or pressure sores.

Goal 3 Child will experience love and physical contact.

Implementation

1. Talk to infant (use face-to-face position).
2. Touch and stroke child.
3. Encourage parents to caress, stroke, and talk to infant (cannot be held preoperatively or early postoperatively) to promote parent-infant attachment.

Evaluation

Child experiences physical and voice contact from staff and parents and family; parents caress and talk to infant.

Goal 4 Child will gain optimal bowel and bladder function (long-term goal).

Implementation

1. Empty bladder manually by applying gentle downward pressure (Credé method), or catheterize as ordered.
2. Provide diet with adequate fluids (those that acidify urine such as apple and cranberry juice) and fiber (as child grows older).
3. Teach parent (and child when older) to care for
   a. Intermittent catheterizations (self-catheterization)
   b. Indwelling Foley catheter
   c. Ileal conduit

4. Administer urinary antiseptics, stool softeners as prescribed.

Evaluation

Child has adequate urinary output and an established bowel routine; is free from urinary tract infection.

Goal 5 Child will develop minimal lower extremity deformity.

Implementation

1. Provide passive ROM exercises.
2. Keep hips abducted using blanket rolls.
3. Provide physical therapy; fitting with braces (usually long leg braces) and crutches for ambulation as child grows older.

Evaluation

Child maintains full ROM of joints; has no contractures of hip or lower extremity.

SEIZURE DISORDERS

1. Definition: episode of uncontrolled electrical activity in the brain; neuronal discharges become excessive and irregular, resulting in loss of consciousness, convulsive body movements, or disturbances in sensations or behavior
2. Incidence: occur in 0.5% of all children; it has been estimated that 4% to 6% of all children will experience one or more seizures by the time they reach adolescence
3. Cause: possible causes include infection, tumors, trauma, acid-base imbalances, epilepsy, allergies, anoxia, and hypoglycemia
4. *Epilepsy: chronic brain dysfunction manifested by recurrent seizures; unknown etiology; higher incidence in children; may see status epilepticus: recurrent seizures occurring at such frequency that full consciousness is not regained between seizures.*
5. Types of seizures and manifestation
   a. Generalized seizures
      1. *grand mal:* sudden loss of consciousness followed by tonic phase (stiffening of body) and clonic phase (jerky movements of trunk and extremities); periods of depressed or apneic breathing may occur; child may fall asleep after the seizure or be confused and irritable
      2. *absence seizures;* child appears to be daydreaming; all verbal and motor behavior stops; may occur 10 or more times a day; usually lasts 10 to 30 seconds; child usually alert after the seizures; no memory of episode
      3. *akinetic:* child experiences a sudden loss of body tone accompanied by loss of consciousness; lasts a few seconds; resumes ADL afterwards
      4. *infantile spasms:* similar to a startle reflex; involves jerking of the head and clonic movements of the extremities; usually disappear by 2 to 3 years of age; may develop into more generalized seizures; usually accompanied by other problems (e.g., mental retardation)

   b. Partial seizures
      1. *jacksonian:* twitching begins at distal end of extremity, eventually involving entire extremity and possibly entire side of body; no loss of consciousness; not commonly seen in children
      2. *psychomotor:* characterized by altered state of consciousness (e.g., dreamlike); may chew, smack lips, mumble; lasts several minutes; child has no memory of behavior

   c. Febrile seizures: transient disorder usually the result of an extracranial infection (e.g., otitis media); peak incidence between 6 months and 3 years of age; resemble grand mal seizures
   d. Breath holding: usually benign; child begins to cry, holds breath, and experiences brief cyanosis with loss of consciousness; precipitating factors may be anger or frustration
6. Diagnosis: complete and accurate history and physical; thorough description of the seizure including onset, time of day, type of seizure, precipitating factors; EEG necessary for evaluating the seizure disorder
7. Medical treatment: anticonvulsants to elevate the child's excitability threshold and prevent seizures (Table 5-15)

Nursing Process

ASSESSMENT

1. History of seizure activity, recent episodes, management
   a. Preseizure behavior: aura, loss of consciousness
   b. Seizure activity: tonic/clonic phase; inappropriate behavior; fecal or urinary incontinence during the seizure
   c. Postseizure behavior: memory lapse, headache, instability, loss of consciousness, lethargy
   d. Obtain information from parents about differences in seizure activity over time and how medication has affected seizure activity
2. Use of anticonvulsant medications, side effects and effects on seizure outcome

ANALYSIS/NURSING DIAGNOSIS (see p. 435)

PLANNING, IMPLEMENTATION, AND EVALUATION

Goal 1 Child will maintain adequate respiratory function and be free from injuries during a seizure (primary concern with status epilepticus).

Implementation

1. Gently lower the standing or sitting child to the floor (supine position).
2. Maintain a patent airway by hyperextending the neck and pulling the jaw slightly forward; turn the head to the side to facilitate drainage of mucus and saliva.
3. Have O_2 and suction available (if possible).
4. *Do not place anything in the child's mouth; in the past it was believed that a padded tongue blade prevented the child from swallowing or biting tongue; simply turning the child's head to the side accomplishes the same effect and diminishes trauma.*
5. Do not restrain child.

Table 5-15 Medications used to treat seizure disorders

Drug	Route	Side effects	Nursing implications
Carbamazepine (Tegretol)	PO	Drowsiness Ataxia Vertigo Anorexia Aplastic anemia	Periodic CBC and liver enzymes. Avoid excessive sunlight because of photophobia. Administer with food.
Clonazepam (Klonopin)	PO	Nausea and vomiting Rash Nystagmus Drowsiness Anemia	Monitor behavioral changes. Frequent respiratory assessment because bronchial secretions are increased.
Diazepam (Valium)	IV push over 1-2 min; may repeat q15min × 2	Drowsiness Dry mouth Constipation Anorexia	Used for status epilepticus. Only inject 5 mg/min. Monitor BP (hypotension) and respirations (respiratory depression). Do not dilute with IV solutions.
Ethosuximide (Zarontin)	PO	Drowsiness Ataxia Blurred vision Anorexia GI upset	Monitor liver and kidney function. Administer with food.
Phenobarbital	PO	Nausea and vomiting Drowsiness Rash Irritability Mild ataxia	Monitor BP and respiration during IV administration. Paradoxic reaction in children. Taper medication when discontinuing.
Phenytoin (Dilantin)	PO, IV	Gingival hypertrophy Dermatitis Ataxia Drowsiness Nystagmus Bone marrow suppression	Meticulous oral hygiene. Administer with food to reduce GI upset. Monitor liver enzymes.
Primidone (Mysoline)	PO	Nausea and vomiting Drowsiness Ataxia Headache Gingival pain	Observe for folic acid deficiency. Taper medication when discontinuing. Monitor for hemorrhage in newborns whose mothers are taking this medication.
Valproic acid (Depakene)	PO	GI upset Nausea and vomiting Drowsiness Leukopenia; thrombocytopenia	Administer with meals. Potentiates phenytoin/phenobarbital. Monitor liver enzymes. Periodic CBC, bleeding time.

6. Remove any toys or dangerous objects that might injure the child during a seizure; pad side rails of bed if possible.
7. Loosen tight or restrictive clothing.
8. Observe the seizure carefully.
   a. Preseizure activity; aura, incontinence
   b. Seizure activity; include onset and initial focus of seizure, duration, change in respirations, progression of movement through body, and changes in neurologic status
   c. Postseizure activity: duration, status, and behavior
9. Administer anticonvulsant medication as ordered.
10. Monitor blood gases if possible.

Evaluation
Child has normal respiratory rate and normal color; is free from injuries; experiences cessation of seizure activity.

Goal 2 Child and family will learn how to cope with the long-term problems associated with seizure disorders.

Implementation
1. Encourage good health practices, including adequate sleep, good nutritional habits, and exercise.

2. Provide appropriate explanations concerning cause of seizure activity, actions of medications, importance of periodic reevaluation.
3. Teach the importance of adhering to medication routine, common side effects, importance of periodic blood and urine studies, behavior changes that may occur as a result of anticonvulsant medication.
4. Stress the importance of never discontinuing anticonvulsant medication abruptly.
5. Instruct family concerning care of child during a seizure.
6. Encourage child and family to discuss fears, anxieties concerning seizure disorder.
7. Inform child and family about situations that might precipitate seizure.
   a. Illness, fever, stress
   b. Occur more frequently during menses or as a result of alcohol ingestion
8. Ensure child wears a Medic Alert bracelet.
9. Provide information concerning vocational guidance and federal and state laws regarding limitations that might be imposed on the younger child or adolescent.
10. Provide information concerning support groups in the community.

Evaluation

Child functions independently regarding ADL; adheres to medical regimen; child and family discuss fears and anxieties concerning seizure disorder; become involved in support groups.

✖ MENINGITIS

1. Definition: a disorder caused by inflammation of the meninges of the brain and spinal cord; two basic types
   a. *Bacterial: H. influenzae, Streptococcus pneumoniae,* or *Neisseria meningitidis* (meningococcus)
   b. *Aseptic:* viruses, parasites, fungi
2. Cause: may be preceded by otitis media, tonsillitis, or other URI
3. Incidence: occurs more often in boys; peak incidence is late infancy and toddlerhood; *Haemophilus influenzae* b conjugate vaccine (HbCV) will protect child from meningitis caused by *H. influenzae* (recommended for all babies beginning at birth to 2 months)
4. Characteristics
   a. Generally determined by age of child
      1. newborn has nonspecific symptoms such as poor sucking and feeding, lethargy or irritability, apnea, weak cry, diarrhea, jaundice; tense anterior fontanel does not occur until late
      2. infant may have fever, poor feeding, nausea and vomiting, increased irritability, high-pitched cry, and seizures
      3. child or adolescent shows classic signs of fever, headache, nuchal rigidity, seizures, altered sensorium, projectile vomiting
   b. Petechial or purpural rash resulting from extravasation of red blood cells (RBCs) usually seen in meningococcal meningitis
   c. Long-term complications include bindness, deafness, mental retardation, hydrocephalus, cerebral palsy, and seizures

5. Medical treatment
   a. Diagnosis: lumbar puncture to examine CSF; usual findings:
      1. elevated WBC
      2. decreased glucose (compare with serum glucose)
      3. elevated protein
      4. positive results from CSF culture; blood culture may be elevated also
      5. spinal fluid pressure usually increases
   b. Medications
      1. antibiotics (large doses given IV)
      2. anticonvulsants
      3. antipyretics

Nursing Process
ASSESSMENT

1. Neurologic status (may see increased ICP [Table 5-14] secondary to cerebral edema resulting from inappropriate antidiuretic hormone (ADH) secretion)
   a. Neurologic check (LOC, PERRLA, motor activity, vital signs)
   b. Brudzinski's sign (pain on flexion of neck)
   c. Kernig's sign (pain on knee extension while lifting knee from a supine position)
   d. Opisthotonos
2. Meningeal irritation (e.g., high-pitched cry, nuchal rigidity, irritability)
3. Seizure activity (see p. 441)
4. Hydration (e.g., output, specific gravity, signs and symptoms of dehydration)
5. Skin (poor perfusion to extremities—change in skin temperature and color); check for rashes

ANALYSIS/NURSING DIAGNOSIS (see p. 435)
PLANNING, IMPLEMENTATION, AND EVALUATION

Goal 1 Others will be free from infecting organism; disease will not spread.

Implementation

1. Use standard precautions (with droplet precautions for at least 24 hours after antibiotics started).
2. Teach parents and others isolation procedures.
3. Assist with lumbar puncture to determine causative organism.
4. Administer antibiotics as soon as ordered; observe side effects.

Evaluation

Disease does not spread to others; family adheres to isolation procedures.

Goal 2 Child will remain free from neurologic complications and long-term sequelae.

Implementation

1. Implement seizure and safety precautions (e.g., bed's side rails up [padded], oxygen and suction available).
2. Perform frequent neurologic checks with vital signs.

3. Minimize environmental stimuli (lights, noise) and movement to lessen possibility of seizures.
4. Elevate head of bed slightly (to decrease intracranial pressure).
5. Administer anticonvulsants as ordered.
6. Monitor fluid intake to prevent dilutional hyponatremia (resulting from inappropriate ADH secretion).
7. Monitor for long-term sequelae: seizures, hydrocephalus, mental retardation, ataxia, hemiparesis, deafness.
8. Provide parental support and reassurance concerning recovery.

Evaluation
Child shows no signs of complications (e.g., seizure activity); resumes normal activities.

Goal 3 Child will maintain adequate hydration and nutrition.

Implementation
1. Maintain NPO during acute phase of illness.
2. Administer IV fluids as ordered; restrain as needed to maintain infusion site.
3. Carefully monitor I&O to prevent fluid overload (can increase intracranial pressure), specific gravity, weight.
4. Advance diet as tolerated as child recovers.

Evaluation
Child is adequately hydrated; is free from signs of fluid overload; maintains weight.

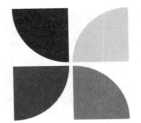

Oxygenation

OVERVIEW OF PHYSIOLOGY

1. Respiratory system (developmental differences)
   a. Chest configuration (AP diameter) changes from round to more flattened as child grows
   b. Steady increase in number and surface area of alveoli from birth to age 12; infants and young children have less alveolar surface for gas exchange
   c. Cricoid cartilage is at the level of the fourth cervical vertebra in infants and the fifth cervical vertebra in children (important when positioning children for resuscitation, intubation, or tracheostomy)
   d. Susceptible to respiratory obstruction and atelectasis because of narrow tracheal and bronchiolar pathways
   e. Susceptible to infections because of immature immune system and frequent contacts with infectious organisms
   f. In infancy, nasal passages are narrow and infants are obligatory nose breathers (important to remember when feeding infants—mucus accumulation and mucosal swelling may interfere with feeding)
   g. Diaphragmatic-abdominal breathing is normal at birth to age 6 to 7 years; abdominal distention from gas or fluid can impede diaphragmatic movement
2. Cardiovascular system (developmental differences)
   a. Changes during transition from fetal to postnatal circulation
      1. lungs inflate, resulting in increased pressure in left side of heart, decreased pulmonary vascular pressure
      2. foramen ovale closes
      3. ductus arteriosus closes
      4. obliteration of ductus venosus and umbilical vessels
   b. Blood pressure gradually increases, and pulse and respiratory rates gradually decrease as child grows
3. Hematologic system (developmental differences)
   a. All components necessary for normal hematologic functioning are present at birth except vitamin K, which is administered intramuscularly to the newborn (refer to Nursing Care of the Childbearing Family, p. 361); see Table 5-16 for normal values
   b. *All* bones are engaged in blood cell production until growth ceases in late adolescence

Application of the Nursing Process to the Child with Respiratory Problems

ASSESSMENT

1. Nursing history
   a. Any known breathing problems, respiratory allergies, activity intolerance (does child have problems keeping up with other children during play?), incidence of respiratory illnesses, medications, home management
   b. Environmental factors: dust, pollen, pets in home, or school environments; do parents or child smoke?
2. Clinical appraisal
   a. General appearance: color (pallor, cyanosis), respiratory effort (dyspnea, stridor, grunting, prolonged expirations), restlessness, irritability, fatigue, prostration, clubbing of fingers and toes
   b. Respiratory rate, depth, and character; presence of respiratory signs (cough: character, productive or nonproductive; rhinitis; retractions; nasal flaring)
   c. Fever
   d. Breath sounds: upper respiratory tract, all lobes of lungs; presence of wheezing, rales, or rhonchi
3. Diagnostic tests (refer to Nursing Care of the Adult, p. 123)

ANALYSIS/NURSING DIAGNOSIS

1. Safe, effective care environment
   a. Knowledge deficit
   b. Risk for infection
2. Physiologic integrity
   a. Ineffective breathing pattern
   b. Impaired gas exchange
   c. Ineffective airway clearance
3. Psychosocial integrity
   a. Anxiety
   b. Social isolation
4. Health promotion/maintenance
   a. Diversional activity deficit
   b. Altered growth and development

GENERAL NURSING PLANNING, IMPLEMENTATION, AND EVALUATION

Goal I Child will maintain adequate oxygenation and a patent airway.

Table 5-16 Hematology values in children

Hematocrit	35%-47%
Hemoglobin	10.5-16 g/dl
Red blood cell count (RBC)	3.9-5.1 million/mm³
White blood cell count (WBC)	5500-13,500/mm³ (between 2-13 years)
	5000-20,000/mm³ (under age 2)
Platelets	150,000-400,000/mm³
Arterial blood gases	
P_{O_2}	83-108 mm Hg (65-80 mm Hg newborn)
P_{CO_2}	35-45 mm Hg (27-40 mm Hg newborn)
pH	7.35-7.45 (7.27-7.47 newborn)

Implementation

1. Monitor respiratory status.
   a. Vital signs (respirations, pulse, and temperature)
   b. Skin and nail bed color, capillary refill, dyspnea, cough, nasal flaring, and retractions
   c. Adventitious lung sounds (e.g., pleural friction rub)
   d. Use of sternal and thoracic muscles
   e. Behavioral changes (restlessness, irritability, or disruptions in patterns)
2. Be alert for signs of airway obstruction.
   a. Rapidly rising heart rate and increased respiratory rate; diaphoresis
   b. Restlessness, anxiety, or agitation (indicate hypoxia)
   c. Increased stridor, retractions
   d. Pallor or cyanosis
3. Position to ease respiratory effort (semi- to high- Fowler's); loosen clothing to allow maximum chest expansion.
4. Avoid sedatives that depress respirations and cough reflex (e.g., narcotics).
5. Keep endotracheal tubes, laryngoscope, and tracheostomy tray at bedside for emergency use.
6. Never leave child unattended if in respiratory distress (changes in condition can occur rapidly).
7. Initiate CPR when necessary.
Infant (age 1 and younger):
   a. Position on back on a flat, firm surface (move child as a single unit).
   b. Clear airway of foreign matter and mucus.
   c. Open airway by placing head in a neutral position (sniff position), lift chin (avoid overextension).
   d. Look, listen, and feel for breaths.
   e. Give 2 breaths of 1 to 1½ seconds each, mouth to mouth and nose (small puffs of air)
   f. Check *brachial* pulse to assess circulation.
   g. Perform chest compressions if necessary with fingers
      1. location: one finger breadth below nipple line on sternum (lower third of sternum)
      2. compress with two fingers ½ to 1 inch at a rate of at least 100 compressions a minute; give 20 breaths per minute
      3. give 5 compressions to 1 breath
   h. Reassess after 10 cycles and every few minutes thereafter.

Child (age 1 to 8):
   i. Position on back on a flat, firm surface (move child as a single unit).
   j. Clear airway of foreign matter and mucus.
   k. Open airway and head tilt–chin lift maneuver (avoid overextension).
   l. Look, listen, and feel for breaths.
   m. Give two breaths of 1 to 1½ seconds each, mouth to mouth.
   n. Check *carotid* pulse to assess circulation.
   o. Perform chest compressions if necessary with heel of one hand.
      1. location: two finger breadths above costal-sternal notch in sternum (lower third of sternum)
      2. compress lower sternum with heel of one hand 1 to 1½ inches at a rate of 100 compressions each minute; give 20 breaths per minute
      3. give 5 compressions to 1 breath
   p. Reassess after 10 cycles and every few minutes thereafter.
8. Provide care for child with an endotracheal (ET) tube or tracheostomy.
   a. Perform ET tube/tracheostomy care and suctioning.
   b. Monitor blood gases, pulse oximetry.
   c. Restrain child as needed.
   d. Provide reassurance to child and parents.
   e. Change position q2h.
   f. Anticipate needs because child cannot verbalize.
   g. Inform child and parents of inability to speak.
   h. Devise alternate means of communication; reassure that voice will return when able to breathe normally again.

Evaluation

Child maintains a patent airway; exhibits signs of adequate oxygenation (normal skin color, quiet breathing, alert and oriented, clear lung sounds).

Goal 2 Child will be free from respiratory distress.

Implementation

1. Provide care for child under a hood or in mist tent with cool mist and O_2 as ordered (analyze O_2 level q4h and as needed).
   a. Plan care to minimize opening of tent or hood.
   b. Tuck sides of tent tightly to prevent loss of O_2 and mist.
   c. Monitor tent chamber temperature.
   d. Keep child as warm and dry as possible to prevent chilling (change clothing and bed linens frequently).
   e. Provide diversion and comfort measures to minimize child's fear and anxiety.
      1. reassure that child will not be left alone; encourage parent to stay with child (allow parent inside tent)
      2. provide favorite toy or object; inspect all toys for safety and suitability (no furry, electrical, or mechanical toys)
2. Assist with chest percussion, vibration, and postural drainage as needed; position child so gravity facilitates drainage from specific lobes.

Evaluation

Child cooperates with mist tent therapy; is free from respiratory distress.

Goal 3 Child will be adequately hydrated.

Implementation

1. Provide humidified atmosphere to help loosen secretions.
2. Ensure adequate fluid intake.
   a. Withhold oral fluids until respiratory distress subsides.
   b. Monitor IV fluids to prevent dehydration or fluid overload.
   c. Encourage oral fluids when respiratory distress subsides. Avoid cold liquids because they can trigger bronchospasm.
3. Monitor intake and output.

Evaluation

Child has elastic skin turgor, normal urine output, adequate fluid intake; is free from signs of dehydration or fluid overload.

Goal 4 Child will conserve energy and remain physically comfortable.

Implementation

1. Administer sedatives, analgesics as ordered (no narcotic sedatives, no cough suppressants).
2. Administer antipyretics, tepid sponge bath for fever.
3. Schedule treatments and nursing activities to allow uninterrupted periods for maximum rest and sleep.
4. Monitor child's response to care (feeding, chest physical therapy) to prevent tiring.
5. Provide quiet age-appropriate play activities.

Evaluation

Child conserves energy; cooperates with care and treatments; approximates normal rest and sleep patterns; engages in quiet play activities.

SELECTED HEALTH PROBLEMS RESULTING IN AN INTERFERENCE WITH RESPIRATION

✖ SUDDEN INFANT DEATH SYNDROME (CRIB DEATH)

1. Definition: sudden, unexpected death of an infant or young child, in which an adequate cause cannot be determined
2. Incidence: leading cause of death in children between the ages of 1 month and 1 year; higher incidence in boys, premature infants (especially with low birth weight), infants with CNS disturbances and respiratory disorders, multiple births, lower socioeconomic status

3. Etiology: unknown; evidence supports theory of relationship between periodic apnea and chronic hypoxemia
4. Peak occurrence: winter or early spring; between ages 2 and 4 months

Nursing Process
ASSESSMENT
1. Parents' knowledge of sudden infant death syndrome (SIDS)
2. Availability of support systems (e.g., family, friends, SIDS organization, or mental health center)
3. Apnea monitoring of high-risk infants (premature infants with pathologic apnea, siblings of two or more SIDS victims) or "near-miss" infants
   a. Parents' knowledge of and adjustment to home apnea monitoring
   b. Infant's apnea patterns

ANALYSIS/NURSING DIAGNOSIS (see p. 445)
PLANNING, IMPLEMENTATION, AND EVALUATION

Goal 1 Parents will receive information and support to help them adjust to loss.

Implementation

1. Explain that they are not responsible for infant's death (parents feel guilty).
2. Provide information about SIDS.
3. Allow expression of feelings; provide support as parents cope with loss, grief, and mourning.
4. Refer to local SIDS organization or support group: Foundation for Sudden Infant Death.
5. Refer to other community supports (e.g., church or community mental health centers).

Evaluation

Parents ventilate feelings about loss of infant; have a referral for counseling.

Goal 2 Parents will maintain and cope with home apnea monitoring.

Implementation

1. Teach parents mechanics of home monitoring equipment.
2. Teach parents infant CPR.
3. Provide emotional support to parents.
4. Help parents identify and use resources for relief (e.g., qualified sitters).

Evaluation

Parents demonstrate ability to implement home monitoring, demonstrate correct infant CPR, adjust to home apnea monitoring.

✖ ACUTE SPASMODIC LARYNGITIS (SPASMODIC CROUP); ACUTE EPIGLOTTITIS; ACUTE LARYNGOTRACHEOBRONCHITIS; BRONCHIOLITIS

(Refer to Table 5-17).

Table 5-17 Acute upper respiratory tract infections

	Acute spasmodic laryngitis (spasmodic croup)	Acute epiglottitis	Acute laryngotracheobronchitis (LTB)	Bronchiolitis
Definition	Acute spasm of larynx, resulting in partial upper airway obstruction	Severe inflammation of the epiglottis that progresses rapidly	Inflammation of larynx, to a lesser extent of trachea and bronchi, resulting in spasm and partial airway obstruction	Inflammation of the bronchioles with accumulation of mucus and exudate, resulting in lung hyperinflation, dyspnea, and cyanosis. Lower airway disease
Peak age of occurrence	3 months-3 years	1 to 8 years	3 months-8 years (most common form of croup)	2- to 12-month-olds (third-leading cause of death in this age group)
Cause	Viral	Bacterial (usually *H. influenzae*, type B)	Usually viral, but may be bacterial	Viral (especially RSV*)
Assessment	Sudden onset. Awakens with barklike, metallic cough. Hoarseness. Inspiratory stridor. Usually occurs at night. No fever. May be preceded by URI. Attack may recur for several nights	Sore throat. Inflamed, cherry-red epiglottis. Dysphagia, drooling. Muffled voice. Tripod posturing. Suprasternal and substernal retractions. High fever. Restlessness. Sudden onset, rapid progression	Preceded by URI. Slowly progressive. Harsh, brassy cough. Inspiratory stridor. Substernal and suprasternal retractions, rales, and rhonchi. Labored, prolonged expirations. Low-grade fever	Paroxysmal cough. Flaring nares. Intercostal and subcostal retractions. Rales with prolonged expirations, wheezing, grunting. Diminished breath sounds, areas of consolidation. Irritability, fatigue
Specific medications and treatment, additional nursing plan/ implementation (see also General Nursing Plans, p. 445)	Usually treated at home. Teach emergency home care: Steam inhalation. Cool-mist humidifier. Ensure adequate fluid intake (clear liquids). Prepare parents for possible recurrence for several nights	Emergency hospitalization: intubation or tracheostomy. IV antibiotics (ampicillin, chloramphenicol). Antipyretics. *Do not try to view child's throat* (may precipitate laryngospasm and death). Be alert for signs of airway obstruction	Hospitalization (intubation if needed). Humidity. Racemic epinephrine in severe cases. IV fluids until respiratory distress subsides	Home care; hospitalization in severe cases. Epinephrine or aminophylline in severe cases. Oxygen mist. Percussion, vibration, and postural drainage. If RSV, practice good hand washing. May use Ribavirin in high risk infants.

*Respiratory syncytial virus.

⊠ BRONCHOPULMONARY DYSPLASIA

1. Definition: an iatrogenic, chronic, obstructive pulmonary disease characterized by thickening of the alveolar walls and bronchiolar epithelium; most surviving infants recover by 1 year of age
2. Occurrence: primarily in low-birth-weight infants with insufficient levels of surfactant who have been mechanically ventilated with high concentrations of oxygen for prolonged periods of time
3. Medical treatment
   a. Prevention by using lowest pressures and lowest concentrations of inspired oxygen during mechanical ventilation
   b. Treatment: administer oxygen and prevent progression of the disease
   c. Medications: bronchodilators, diuretics (when complicated by congestive heart failure), antibiotics for respiratory infection

Nursing Process

ASSESSMENT (Refer also to General Nursing Goal 2, p. 446)
1. Respiratory distress
2. Ventilator dependence
3. Delayed growth and development
4. Signs of pulmonary hypertension and right-sided heart failure (e.g., fluid retention, rales, wheezing, and retractions)

ANALYSIS/NURSING DIAGNOSIS (see p. 445)

PLANNING, IMPLEMENTATION, AND EVALUATION (see General Nursing Plans, p. 445)

Table 5-18 Medications used to treat bronchial asthma

Drug	Administration	Nursing responsibilities
BRONCHODILATORS		
Beta-adrenergic agents		
Metaproterenol (Alupent)	Oral, inhalation	Side effects: nervousness, tremor, tachycardia, headache.
Albuterol (Proventil, Ventolin)	Oral, inhalation	Side effects: tremor, anxiety, nervousness, headache. Oral route recommended in small children.
Terbutaline (Brethine, Bricanyl)	Oral, inhalation, subcutaneously	Side effects: nervousness, tremor, headache, tachycardia, nausea. Use 1 cc syringe for accuracy.
Methylxanthines		
Theophylline	IV, oral	Use IV pump to regulate.
Aminophylline		Monitor vital signs, observe for tachycardia. Monitor blood levels (therapeutic level 10-20 mg/ml; toxicity > 20 mg/ml. Toxicity signs and symptoms: irritability, restlessness, vomiting, dysrhythmias, seizures.
ANTIINFLAMMATORY AGENTS		
Corticosteroids		
Hydrocortisone (Solucortef)	IV	IV form used for status asthmaticus.
Prednisone	Oral (shorter acting)	Antiinflammatory, reduces allergic response, enhances smooth muscle dilation of airway. Long-term oral steroids—risk of significant adverse effects. Inhaled steroids—few or no side effects.
Dexamethasone (Decadron, Azmacort)	Oral (longer acting)	
PROPHYLACTIC AGENTS		
Cromolyn sodium (Intal)	Inhalation	Prevents release of histamine. Used to prevent attacks. (Preventive only, not effective during acute attack.)

✳ BRONCHIAL ASTHMA (REACTIVE AIRWAY DISEASE)

1. Definition: an obstructive, reversible condition of the trachea and bronchial tissues; a complex health problem that involves biochemical, immunologic, endocrine, and psychologic factors leading to
   a. Edema of mucous membranes
   b. Congestion of airways with tenacious mucus
   c. Spasm of smooth muscle of bronchi and bronchioles causing narrowed airway and trapping of air in alveoli
2. Cause: believed to be an allergic hypersensitivity to foreign substances such as plant pollens, mold, dust, smoke, animal hair, or foods; other contributing factors are changes in environmental temperatures (especially cold air), emotional distress, fatigue, physical exertion, and infections
3. Medical treatment: acute asthma is a medical emergency
   a. Drug therapy is directed toward relieving bronchial spasm, obstruction, and edema (Table 5-18)
      1. bronchodilators
      2. corticosteroids
      3. no sedatives or cough suppressants
   b. Supportive measures
      1. cool, humidified environment
      2. IV fluids to ensure adequate hydration
      3. allergen control
   c. Status asthmaticus: continued severe respiratory distress in spite of medical intervention; child is in imminent danger of respiratory arrest and requires immediate hospitalization (to treat dehydration and acidosis and improve ventilation)
      1. NPO or sips of clear liquids
      2. IV fluids for hydration and medication administration
      3. sodium bicarbonate (IV) to correct acidosis
      4. humidified O_2
      5. mechanical ventilation in severe cases
      6. corticosteroids (hydrocortisone or methylprednisolone IV)
      7. aminophylline
      8. beta-adrenergics via nebulizer
   d. Long-term therapy includes removing the offending allergens, desensitization to allergens, normalization of respiratory function, and development of a personalized and effective therapeutic regimen

Nursing Process
ASSESSMENT
1. Prolonged expiratory wheezing
2. Hacking, paroxysmal, nonproductive coughing; cough then becomes rattling with thick, clear mucus
3. Deep-red lips; may progress to cyanosis
4. Anxious expression, restlessness
5. Child sits in upright position
6. Intercostal and suprasternal retractions (infants)
7. Coarse breath sounds

tions with sudden increase in
g may signal impending as-
;)
shoulders (chronic asthma)
ee p. 445)
ND EVALUATION

normal breathing pattern,
ay, and will liquefy and
...secretions.

Implementation

1. Monitor frequency, amount, and appearance of expectorated mucus.
2. Position in high Fowler's or in a chair; administer O_2 to relieve cyanosis and hypoxia (cyanosis appears in children with a Po_2 of less than 55 to 65 mm Hg).
3. Teach child to use diaphragm rather than just lungs, to pull in and expel deep breaths of air when first feeling a tightening sensation in chest.
4. Administer prescribed medications, including nebulizers; know the action, dose ranges, side effects, and contraindications for all medications administered.
5. Teach child and parents how to measure peak expiratory flow rate with peak flow meter to monitor condition.

Evaluation

Child resumes normal breathing pattern (no wheezing, rales, or cyanosis), maintains patent airway, liquefies and raises secretions.

Goal 2 Child will control anxiety during acute attacks.

Implementation

1. *Never leave child alone during an acute attack; if parental anxiety is too high, it is better for child if someone who is calm and supportive stays with child; work with parent until parent can be a calming influence.*
2. Hold child in an upright position and rock (as effective as bed rest if a relaxed, confident approach is used).
3. Reduce the level of nonproductive stimuli by keeping room quiet, with dimmed lighting; use touch, soft music, and controlled noise levels to induce relaxation and rest.
4. Teach child and parents panic control (i.e., teach to imagine how to stay calm [what works best] in stressful situations).

Evaluation

Child remains calm and copes with asthma attack.

Goal 3 Attacks will be prevented or minimized.

Implementation

1. Identify possible precipitating factors with child and family; teach child and parents to avoid stressful experiences, extremes of temperature, unnecessary fatigue, and exposure to infections.
2. Modify environment as indicated (no furry pets, damp dusting, nonallergenic pillows and bedding, elimination of allergenic foods with diet, air filters).

3. Assist with immune therapy (hyposensitization for allergens such as dust, molds, and pollens).
4. Administer prophylactic antibiotics during periods of high susceptibility (e.g., winter, pollen or flu season).
5. Guide parents in planning a total program that promotes rest, moderate exercise, appropriate activities (swimming, baseball, skiing), balanced nutrition, controlled levels of emotional stress.
6. Remind and urge child and parents to see physician regularly and at the first indication of a respiratory infection or attack.
7. Refer family to psychologic/mental health services when indicated.
8. Teach older children to assume responsibility for taking medications.

Evaluation

Child and parents describe the importance of good nutrition and rest in preventing respiratory infections; identify situations or agents that precipitate an asthmatic attack and conscientiously try to modify or avoid these; recognize signs of an impending attack (cough, wheezing, fever, nausea and vomiting, increased anxiety or tension) and the steps to take to minimize distress (position, rest, medications, fluids).

Application of the Nursing Process to the Child with Cardiovascular Dysfunction

ASSESSMENT

1. Nursing history
   a. Delayed growth patterns, physical and emotional
   b. Frequent respiratory infections
   c. Activity intolerance, weakness, fatigue
   d. Anorexia, weight loss, fatigue during feedings
   e. Chest pain, dyspnea, pallor or cyanosis, clubbing of fingers and toes
   f. Medications: parental knowledge of side effects
   g. Family and obstetric history
2. Clinical appraisal
   a. General appearance: pallor, cyanosis, clubbing of fingers and toes, cold extremities, mottling, edema, distended neck veins, and poor capillary refill
   b. Vital signs: apical pulse rate and character, presence of murmurs, gallops, friction rubs; blood pressure in upper and lower extremities; rate, depth, and character of respirations; rate, quality, and symmetry of peripheral pulses, especially of lower extremities
3. Diagnostic tests (refer to Nursing Care of the Adult, p. 123)
   a. Cardiac catheterization in infants and children: aids in diagnosis of congenital anomalies through direct visualization of chambers as well as detection of abnormalities in oxygen saturation, pressure, and cardiac output; femoral artery or vein may be used for catheter insertion (Table 5-19)
   b. Blood gas determination (Table 5-16), pulse oximetry
   c. Echocardiogram

ANALYSIS/NURSING DIAGNOSIS

1. Safe, effective care environment
   a. Risk for infection
   b. Sensory-perceptual alteration
2. Physiologic integrity
   a. Activity intolerance

Table 5-19 Cardiac catheterization in children: nursing considerations

Preprocedural	Postprocedural
Psychologic preparation (see Ill and Hospitalized Child for developmental considerations)	Maintain bed rest with frequent checks on vital signs until stable.
Explain in simple terms what child will experience and what it will feel like (e.g., skin prep: "cold"; catheter insertion: "pressure"; injection of contrast medium: "warm all over" [do not use the word "dye"]; darkness of room, and sounds of "picture-taking"); do not explain too far in advance of procedure.	Check dressing for bleeding, edema, and hematoma formation.
	Maintain sandbag or pressure dressing on operative site as ordered.
	Do not take blood pressure in affected extremity.
	Monitor skin color and warmth, especially distal to catheter insertion site.
Allow child to play with and manipulate equipment (e.g., gown and mask, syringes, sandbag).	Palpate brachial or pedal pulses distal to catheter insertion for presence, strength, and symmetry.
Arrange for child and parent to visit catheterization room the day before to see the equipment and meet staff.	Notify physician of any signs of complications (e.g., poor circulation, unstable vital signs, fever, and bleeding).
Physical preparation	Apply direct pressure 1 inch above insertion site if bleeding occurs.
NPO 4-6 hr before the procedure (give 5% DW orally as prescribed 2-3 hr before the procedure for infants with cyanotic heart disease and polycythemia); use pacifier for infants.	
Obtain baseline vital signs, including brachial and pedal pulses.	
Administer preoperative medications as ordered (child is not anesthetized).	

   b. Decreased cardiac output
   c. Impaired gas exchange
   d. Decreased tissue perfusion
3. Psychosocial integrity
   a. Anxiety
   b. Fear
4. Health promotion/maintenance
   a. Diversional activity deficit
   b. Ineffective family coping: compromised
   c. Altered family process

GENERAL NURSING PLANNING, IMPLEMENTATION, AND EVALUATION

Goal 1 Child will have adequate oxygenation and decreased workload on heart.

Implementation
1. Monitor vital signs frequently.
   a. Apical pulse 1 full minute while sleeping
   b. Peripheral pulses
   c. BP in all four extremities on initial assessment
   d. Respiratory status
   e. Body temperature
   f. Capillary refill
   g. Pulse oximetry
2. Schedule treatments and nursing care to prevent tiring and promote adequate rest and sleep.
3. Maintain bed rest as ordered.
4. Provide age-appropriate diversional activities to prevent boredom and help child maintain bed rest.
5. Avoid restrictive clothing and tight diapers.
6. Minimize crying and emotional distress (preoperatively).
   a. Encourage parent to room-in or visit frequently.
   b. Provide pacifier or favorite attachment object.
   c. Hold and cuddle child, anticipate needs (feeding, etc.)
7. Relieve anoxic spells (cyanotic heart disease).
   a. Place child in knee-chest (squatting) position.

   b. Administer O_2 as ordered.
   c. Administer sedatives and analgesics as ordered.
8. Avoid extremes of environmental temperature.

Evaluation
Child is free from signs of respiratory or cardiac distress (e.g., no dyspnea, tachycardia); cooperates with bed rest, rests comfortably, plays quietly.

Goal 2 Child will be free from infections.

Implementation
1. Protect child from exposure to others with respiratory infections.
2. Immunize child according to recommended schedule (see Table 5-3).
3. Observe for signs of endocarditis (fever, malaise, anorexia) and pneumonitis (dyspnea, tachycardia, fever).
4. Teach child and parents importance of antibiotic prophylaxis when prescribed (long-term therapy or short-term course for dental work, surgery, childbirth).

Evaluation
Child remains free from upper respiratory infections; is immunized on schedule; child and parents comply with antibiotic prophylaxis.

SELECTED HEALTH PROBLEMS RESULTING IN AN INTERFERENCE WITH CARDIAC FUNCTIONING

✖ CONGENITAL HEART DISEASE

1. Hemodynamics: related to three principles
   a. Pressure gradients: blood flows from higher pressure to lower; normally left side of heart is higher pressure

b. Resistance: the higher the resistance the less the flow; normally the systemic circulation has higher resistance than pulmonary circulation; larger vessels have less resistance than smaller, narrow ones

c. Quality of pumping action of heart affects the flow

2. Physical consequences of cardiac problems
   a. Increased workload of the heart (causes changes in systolic and diastolic pressures)
   b. Pulmonary hypertension (from increased pulmonary resistance)
   c. Inadequate systemic output from recirculated blood flow
   d. Cyanotic defects: no pure oxygenated blood in body, tissue hypoxia and hypoxemia, stimulates erythropoiesis, resulting in polycythemia

3. Cause: not known exactly; predisposing factors include
   a. Certain chromosome disorders (e.g., Down syndrome)
   b. Maternal and fetal infections (e.g., rubella in first trimester)
   c. Maternal alcoholism, undernutrition, diabetes, age over 40 years

4. Classification of defects: two different classification systems based on
   a. Physical characteristic of cyanosis: traditional classification that can be confusing and misleading
      1. acyanotic defects: blood flows from the arterial (left, oxygenated) side of the heart to the venous (right, unoxygenated) side; left-to-right shunt; there is no mixing of oxygenated and unoxygenated blood in systemic circulation; less serious defects
      2. cyanotic defects: those in which unoxygenated blood from the right side of the heart mixes with oxygenated blood on the left side, causing unoxygenated blood to be circulated throughout the body; right-to-left shunt; can result in cyanosis; severe defects
   b. Hemodynamic characteristics: more descriptive, practical, and frequently used classification
      1. increased pulmonary blood flow: defects that allow left-to-right shunting resulting in increased blood flow to the lungs and congestive heart failure
      2. obstructive defects: those that impede blood flow out of the ventricles
      3. decreased pulmonary blood flow: defects that cause right-to-left shunting or impede blood flow to the lungs
      4. mixed blood flow: oxygenated and unoxygenated blood is allowed to mix within the heart or great arteries

5. Specific defects (Fig. 5-2)
   a. *Atrial septal defect (ASD):* acyanotic; increased pulmonary blood flow
      1. flow of blood is from left atrium to right atrium (normal flow resistance)
      2. increased blood flow to right side of heart
      3. treatment: surgical closure or patch graft of defect; 99% survival rate

   b. *Ventricular septal defect (VSD):* acyanotic; increased pulmonary blood flow
      1. most common cardiac defect
      2. flow of blood is from left ventricle (higher pressure) to right ventricle, where oxygenated blood mixes with venous blood
      3. may cause right-ventricular hypertrophy and increased pulmonary-vascular resistance
      4. 50% close spontaneously within 1 to 3 years of age
      5. often associated with other cardiac defects (tetralogy of Fallot, transposition of great vessels, patent ductus arteriosus [PDA], pulmonic stenosis)
      6. infants with severe VSD may develop congestive heart failure
      7. treatment: surgical closure or patch graft of defect, survival rate 99%
      8. complications include conduction disturbances, congestive heart failure (CHF), or endocarditis

   c. *Patent ductus arteriosus (PDA):* acyanotic; increased pulmonary blood flow
      1. ductus arteriosus (normally open in fetus) fails to close: some blood is shunted by higher pressure in aorta to pulmonary artery
      2. leads to recirculation through lungs and return to left atrium and ventricle; effect is increased workload on left side of heart and increased pulmonary congestion
      3. pulse pressure is wide; left-ventricular hypertrophy and congestive heart failure may develop
      4. characteristic machinery-like murmur
      5. treatment: surgical ligation (closed-heart surgery) before 2 years of age; 99% survival rate
      6. in extremely ill newborns, medical closure of the ductus with the prostaglandin inhibitor indomethacin may be tried; most effective in premature newborns

   d. *Coarctation of the aorta:* acyanotic; obstructive
      1. narrowing of the aorta
      2. blood pressure higher in upper extremities
      3. bounding upper-extremity pulses, weak or absent femoral and popliteal pulses
      4. lower extremities may be cool, pale
      5. cramps (claudication)
      6. headaches, dizziness, epistaxis
      7. treatment: surgical resection and end-to-end anastomosis within first 2 years of life

   e. *pulmonic/aortic stenosis:* acyanotic; obstructive
      1. pulmonic stenosis interferes with flow of blood from right ventricle to pulmonary artery
      2. aortic stenosis interferes with blood flow from left ventricle to aorta
      3. both pulmonic and aortic stenosis
         a. may be asymptomatic
         b. are usually of the valves
         c. increased resistance can cause right ventricular hypertrophy with pulmonary stenosis, left ventricular hypertrophy with aortic stenosis
         d. aortic stenosis may result in sudden death after strenuous exercise or activity because of in-

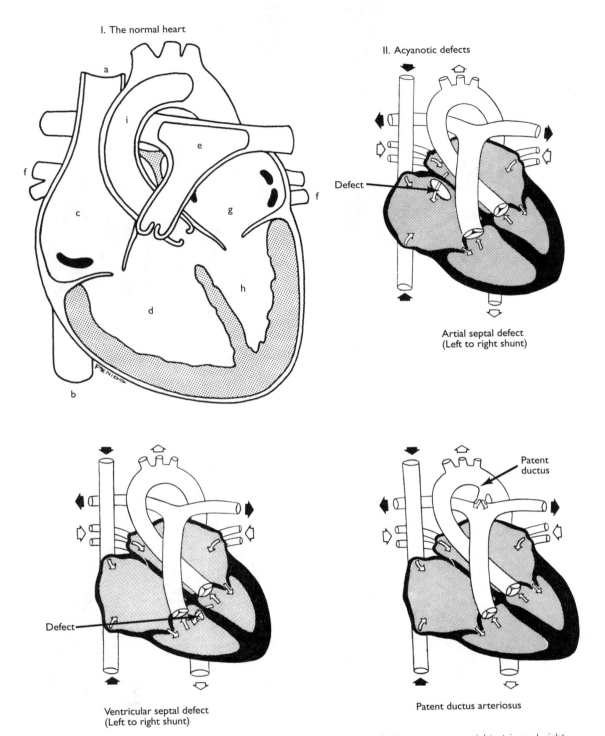

I. The normal heart

II. Acyanotic defects

Defect

Artial septal defect
(Left to right shunt)

Defect

Ventricular septal defect
(Left to right shunt)

Patent
ductus

Patent ductus arteriosus

Fig. 5-2 Normal and abnormal hearts. *a,* Superior vena cava; *b,* inferior vena cava; *c,* right atrium; *d,* right ventricle; *e,* pulmonary artery; *f,* pulmonary vein; *g,* left atrium; *h,* left ventricle; and *i,* aorta. (From *Nursing inservice aid #2, congenital heart abnormalities aid,* Columbus, Ohio, Ross Laboratories.)

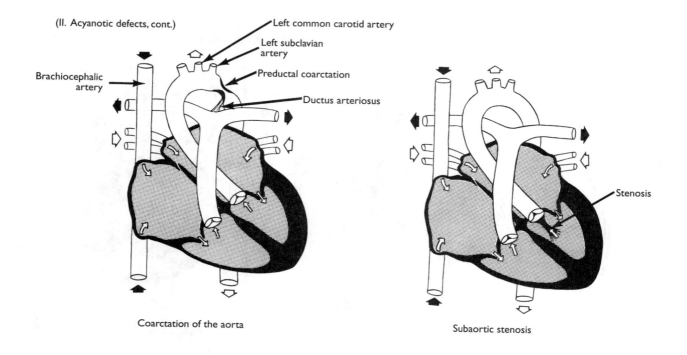

(II. Acyanotic defects, cont.)

Left common carotid artery

Left subclavian artery

Brachiocephalic artery

Preductal coarctation

Ductus arteriosus

Stenosis

Coarctation of the aorta

Subaortic stenosis

III. Cyanotic defects

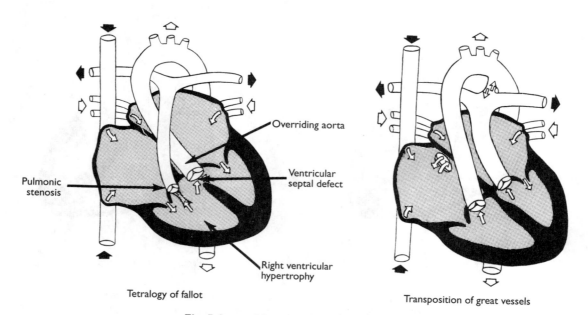

Overriding aorta

Ventricular septal defect

Pulmonic stenosis

Right ventricular hypertrophy

Tetralogy of fallot

Transposition of great vessels

Fig. 5-2, cont'd   For legend see previous page.

creased sudden oxygen demand and resultant myocardial ischemia

    4. treatment: valvotomy or valve replacement

  f. *tetralogy of Fallot:* cyanotic; decreased pulmonary blood flow

    1. most common cyanotic heart defect in children

    2. four (tetra) defects

      a. severe VSD

      b. severe pulmonic stenosis: right-to-left shunting of blood through ventricular septal defect because of pulmonic stenosis and increased pulmonary resistance; results in desaturated blood entering systemic circulation

      c. right ventricular hypertrophy

      d. overriding aorta: because the aorta overrides the septal defect, much of the systemic flow is venous and therefore unoxygenated

    3. treatment

      a. palliative surgical correction in infancy to increase pulmonary blood flow (Blalock-Taussig anastomosis of right or left subclavian artery and corresponding pulmonary artery)

      b. corrective surgical repair; closure of VSD (corrects overriding aorta) and pulmonary valvotomy or valve replacement; trend now for early primary repair

  g. *transposition of the great vessels:* cyanotic; mixed blood flow

    1. the aorta arises out of the right ventricle so that venous blood enters directly into the systemic circulation, bypassing the lungs; the pulmonary artery arises out of the left ventricle and goes through the lungs; once the foramen ovale and ductus arteriosus close, the situation is incompatible with life (unless ASD or VSD is present)

    2. treatment

      a. palliative surgical correction to prevent CHF and reduce pulmonary vascular resistance

        ▪ surgical creation of an ASD

        ▪ balloon atrial septostomy during cardiac catheterization to enlarge existing ASD

        ▪ pulmonary artery banding

      b. corrective surgical repair: creation of a new atrial septum that tunnels blood to the correct ventricle

6. Additional medical management: digoxin, potassium, diuretics (if in congestive heart failure), antibiotics

Nursing Process

ASSESSMENT: MAJOR MANIFESTATIONS

1. Congestive heart failure
  a. Tachycardia, tachypnea, dyspnea
  b. Diaphoresis
  c. Cold extremities, weak pulses, exercise intolerance
  d. Poor feeding, poor weight gain
  e. Edema, hepatomegaly
  f. Crackles, cough, respiratory infections

2. Hypoxemia
  a. Cyanosis
  b. Babies have difficulty eating because of inability to breathe and suck at same time

  c. Delayed physical growth because of chronic hypoxia

  d. Moderate to severe exercise intolerance

  e. Chest pain that becomes severe with O_2 demand

  f. Hypoxic spell may occur during periods of high O_2 demand (feeding, crying, or physical exertion during play)

    1. severe shortness of breath

    2. increased cyanosis and chest pain

    3. squats with arms thrown over knees, and knees on chest to relieve respiratory distress

  g. Chronic hypoxia causes erythropoietin to be released from kidneys to stimulate bone marrow to produce more red blood cells; also causes clubbing of fingers and toes

    1. Hgb may rise 20 to 30 g or more with a hematocrit as high as 60% to 80%

    2. increased RBC results in increased blood viscosity (polycythemia)

  h. Polycythemia and sluggish circulation may cause cerebral thrombosis (stroke) and paralysis, sometimes occurring at a very young age

3. Preoperative assessment
  a. Baseline vital signs, including apical pulse; existence and quality of peripheral pulses, especially of lower extremities; compare pulses; BP on all extremities
  b. Educational needs of child and parents for preoperative teaching and postoperative experience
  c. Laboratory values to assess potential problems

4. Postoperative assessment
  a. Respiratory status, chest tubes, chest-tube drainage, breath sounds
  b. Vital signs, including apical and femoral pulses, arterial and venous pressures, cardiac rhythm
  c. Hydration status and output
  d. Signs and symptoms of congestive heart failure
  e. Color of skin, mucous membranes, nail beds, and earlobes
  f. Level of discomfort and anxiety
  g. Surgical incisions (suture line)

ANALYSIS/NURSING DIAGNOSIS (see p. 450)
PLANNING, IMPLEMENTATION, AND EVALUATION

> **Goal I** Child will maintain adequate oxygenation and a patent airway.

Implementation

Preoperative and postoperative:

1. Count respirations and apical pulse for 1 full minute; BP frequently as needed.
2. Pin diapers loosely; use loose-fitting pajamas.
3. Feed slowly with frequent rest periods; burp frequently.
4. Position at 45-degree angle after feeding.
5. Suction nose and throat mucus if cough is inadequate.
6. Give O_2 as ordered and necessary.
7. Administer digoxin as prescribed.
  a. Give at regular intervals.
  b. Do not mix with other foods or fluids.
  c. Hold drug and notify physician if apical pulse rate is below 100 in infants, below 90 in toddlers, or be-

low 70 in older children or if significant change in pulse rate.
   d. Give 1 hour before or 2 hours after meals or feedings.
   e. Observe for signs of toxicity (bradycardia, nausea, anorexia, vomiting, disorientation).
8. Administer diuretics as prescribed.
   a. Monitor I&O closely.
   b. Ensure that fluid intake is within prescribed restrictions.
   c. Encourage high-potassium foods or administer prescribed potassium supplements.

Postoperative (palliative or corrective surgery):

9. Monitor constantly.
10. Take precautions in care of closed chest drainage (bottles below level of bed, no kinks in tubing, do not empty bottles, monitor fluid level and fluctuation in tube, character of drainage). Notify doctor if excessive fluid or blood.
11. Avoid elevating foot of bed (causes intestines to put pressure on diaphragm).
12. Administer O_2 as ordered.
13. Establish and follow coughing routine; allow crying postoperatively in infant and young child to facilitate lung expansion; use inspirometer (incentive spirometry) with older children.
14. When child has recovered from anesthesia, elevate head of bed to reduce pressure on diaphragm.
15. Use nasogastric suction to reduce gastric distension.
16. Be alert to signs of CHF, hypovolemic shock, pneumonia, hemothorax (dyspnea), atelectasis (dyspnea, increased pulse), cerebral thrombosis.

Evaluation

Child has normal skin color, a patent airway, breathes freely; no signs of complications.

Goal 2 Child will maintain adequate hydration and electrolyte balance.

Implementation

1. Encourage fluid intake within fluid restrictions for child; monitor I&O extremely *accurately (be especially alert to thoracotomy drainage, fluid used to administer IV medications or flush CVP and arterial lines).*
2. Monitor daily weights.
3. Check urine specific gravity and pH.
4. Be alert to early signs and symptoms of pulmonary edema, cardiac overload, and congestive heart failure (e.g., tachycardia, dyspnea, tachypnea, moist respirations, rales, rhonchi, sweating [in infants], edema).
5. Be aware that dehydration with cyanotic heart disease increases blood viscosity and therefore risk of thrombosis.
6. Observe for signs of hypokalemia (altered lab values, cardiac dysrhythmias).

Evaluation

Child has adequate I&O; no signs or symptoms of fluid or electrolyte imbalance, stroke, or congestive heart failure.

Goal 3 Child and parents will experience no more than moderate anxiety.

Implementation

1. Encourage child and parents to disclose their feelings about the surgery, hospitalization, and treatments (use projective techniques with child); answer their questions.
2. Prepare child and parents for treatments, surgical routine, and discharge; consider developmental age, environment, culture and ethnicity, timing needs, and ability to understand.
3. Help parents and others understand the importance of treating child as normally as possible (to provide for optimal emotional-social development and to avoid overprotecting and sheltering).

Evaluation

Child and parents describe realistic expectations about child's illness and hospitalization; establish and adhere to age-appropriate limits; demonstrate knowledge about procedures, medications.

Goal 4 Child and parents will be adequately prepared for discharge and home care.

Implementation

1. Encourage and support parents in their attempts to allow child age-appropriate independence and responsibilities.
2. Teach parents safe administration of medications, side effects, signs of complications, when to seek medical attention.
3. Refer parents to community health nursing agency for home follow-up if indicated.

Evaluation

Child gradually assumes self-care responsibilities and age-appropriate independence, including education level; parents state signs of complications and when to seek attention; administer medications correctly.

RHEUMATIC FEVER AND RHEUMATIC HEART DISEASE

1. Definition: an inflammatory disease caused by an immune response to group A beta-hemolytic streptococcal infection; affects collagen (connective) tissue such as heart, joints, central nervous system, and subcutaneous tissue
2. Occurrence: primarily affects school-age children; higher incidence in cold or humid climates, crowded living environments, and with strong family history of rheumatic fever
3. Medical treatment
   a. Antibiotics (penicillin or erythromycin)
      1. to eradicate any lingering infection
      2. for long-term prophylactic treatment
   b. Salicylates to control joint inflammation, fever, pain

Nursing Process

ASSESSMENT (REVISED JONES CRITERIA [AMERICAN HEART ASSOCIATION])

1. Major manifestations
   a. Carditis: mitral and aortic valves most commonly affected with symptoms of tachycardia, cardiomegaly, pericarditis, murmurs, congestive heart failure; carditis is the only manifestation that may cause permanent damage
   b. Painful migratory polyarthritis in large joints with manifestations of acute pain, warmth, redness, edema; permanent deformities do not follow
   c. Chorea (Saint Vitus' dance or Sydenham's chorea): purposeless, irregular movements of the extremities, muscular weakness, emotional lability, facial grimacing
      1. follows the acute febrile phase
      2. may last for months, but is self-limiting
      3. relieved by rest and sleep
   d. Erythema marginatum rheumaticum: macular rash with wavy, well-defined border on trunk
   e. Subcutaneous nodules: small, nontender swellings in groups over bony prominences
2. Minor manifestations
   a. Arthralgia
   b. Fever
   c. Nonspecific tests indicating inflammation
      1. elevated erythrocyte sedimentation rate (ESR)
      2. elevated C-reactive protein
      3. leukocytosis
   d. Anemia
   e. Prolonged PR and QT intervals on electrocardiogram (ECG)
3. Other
   a. Positive throat culture
   b. Elevated antistreptolysin (ASO) titer (indicates a preceding streptococcal infection)

ANALYSIS/NURSING DIAGNOSIS (see p. 450)

PLANNING, IMPLEMENTATION, AND EVALUATION

Goal 1 Child will be free from pain and will rest comfortably.

Implementation
1. Administer salicylates as ordered.
2. Use cradles to keep bed linens off painful joints.
3. Position joints on pillows; handle gently.
4. Encourage use of relaxation, distraction, and imagery as appropriate.

Evaluation
Child does not complain of pain, rests and sleeps comfortably.

Goal 2 Child with chorea will be protected from injury.

Implementation
1. Use side rails and pad sides of bed.
2. Provide understanding and emotional support; reassure child and family that chorea will resolve spontaneously.
3. Provide with alternative means to do written work (e.g., typewriter, personal computer, oral reports).
4. Assist child in self-care to promote independence and positive self-concept.

Evaluation
Child ambulates without falling, does not sustain injury.

Goal 3 Child and family will be prepared for home care and long-term management.

Implementation
1. Emphasize importance of compliance with long-term antibiotic therapy for prevention of serious heart damage.
   a. Teach daily oral antibiotic administration.
   b. Prepare child for monthly injections of penicillin if compliance with oral antibiotic therapy is poor.
   c. Stress seriousness of recurrence and need to seek medical care for subsequent infections.
2. Plan for continuation of schoolwork, realistic career goals.
3. Refer to community health nurse for follow-up as needed.
4. Instruct parents to take vital signs, administer medications, ensure restrictions.

Evaluation
Child returns to full activity with no residual cardiac involvement.

Application of the Nursing Process to the Child with Hematologic Problems

ASSESSMENT
1. Nursing history
   a. Dietary intake, especially dietary iron
   b. History of bleeding tendencies (easy bruising, gum bleeding, epistaxis), response to injury or trauma
   c. General symptoms: fatigue, irritability, anorexia, pain, or edema
   d. Recent stressful situations: exposure to temperature extremes, emotional stress
   e. Family history of hematologic disorders
   f. Current treatment, home management, general health
2. Clinical appraisal
   a. General appearance: pallor, lethargy, bruising, physical growth (overweight or underweight for age)
   b. Vital signs: tachycardia, tachypnea, hypotension
3. Diagnostic tests (refer to Nursing Care of the Adult, p. 116)

ANALYSIS/NURSING DIAGNOSIS
1. Safe, effective care environment
   a. Risk for injury
   b. Risk for infection
   c. Knowledge deficit
2. Physiologic integrity
   a. Impaired gas exchange
   b. Fatigue
   c. Altered cerebral tissue perfusion
3. Psychosocial integrity
   a. Anxiety

b. Altered role performance
c. Body-image disturbance
4. Health promotion/maintenance
   a. Ineffective family coping: compromised
   b. Diversional activity deficit
   c. Altered growth and development

GENERAL NURSING PLANNING, IMPLEMENTATION, AND EVALUATION

Goal 1 Child will be free from pain.

Implementation
1. Administer prescribed analgesics (no aspirin).
2. Handle and move child gently.
3. Provide bed rest with covers off affected areas.
4. Provide age-appropriate diversional activities.

Evaluation
Child is free from pain; rests comfortably.

Goal 2 Child will conserve energy.

Implementation
1. Schedule nursing care and treatment to prevent tiring and to provide uninterrupted periods of rest.
2. Provide quiet age-appropriate play activities.
3. Counsel parents concerning plan for activity and rest at home.

Evaluation
Child engages in activities of daily living without tiring, has age-appropriate rest and sleep periods.

SELECTED HEALTH PROBLEMS RESULTING IN AN INTERFERENCE WITH FORMED ELEMENTS OF THE BLOOD

�֎ IRON-DEFICIENCY ANEMIA

1. 1. Definition: a decrease in the number of erythrocytes, a decreased Hgb level (less than 10 g/dl), or both
2. Occurrence: most common nutritional disorder in United States, resulting in reduced oxygen-carrying capacity of blood; most common childhood anemia
   a. Primarily in children 6 to 24 months of age who have a diet low in iron; 16% of lower income children 6 to 24 months of age are anemic
   b. In premature infants (inadequate iron stores)
   c. In adolescent girls, with increased growth and menstruation
   d. In adolescent boys, with androgen-related increase in hemoglobin concentration
3. Cause: impaired production of red blood cells, resulting from deficient iron stores
   a. Inadequate dietary intake
   b. Impaired absorption
   c. Blood loss
   d. Excessive demand (prematurity, puberty, or pregnancy)

4. Medical treatment
   a. Oral iron supplements (ferrous iron), 10 to 15 mg/day for 3 months
   b. Parenteral iron therapy (iron dextran [Imferon]) IM or IV
   c. Blood transfusions with packed red cells (if Hgb is less than 4 g/dl)

Nursing Process
ASSESSMENT
1. Nutritional history (daily intake)
2. Pallor (porcelain-like skin)
3. Poor muscle development
4. May be overweight ("milk baby")
5. Exercise intolerance, lethargy
6. Susceptible to infection

ANALYSIS/NURSING DIAGNOSIS (see p. 457)

PLANNING, IMPLEMENTATION, AND EVALUATION

Goal Child will ingest diet and medications to maintain adequate Hgb level.

Implementation
1. Explain the necessity for a proper diet to parents of child.
   a. Provide adequate sources of iron, and teach parent and child what they are.
   b. For infants, give iron-fortified formula and cereal and iron supplements.
   c. For older children, give foods high in iron (e.g., meat, green leafy vegetables, and fruit).
   d. Give solids before milk.
2. Teach parents correct administration of oral iron preparations as ordered.
   a. Give ferrous sulfate (Fer-In-Sol) in three divided doses per day, between meals with citrus juice.
   b. Continue for 4 to 6 weeks after red blood cell count returns to normal.
   c. Liquid iron temporarily stains teeth (use straw or dropper to back of mouth; brush child's teeth).
   d. Oral iron causes stools to become dark green.
   e. Because iron ingested in large amounts may be fatal, teach parents to store iron out of reach of children.
3. If oral preparations are ineffective, administer parenteral iron as prescribed using IM Z-track method: painful and stains subcutaneous tissue; do not use deltoid; no more than 1 ml per site; use air bubble, do not massage over injection site, avoid tight clothing over injection site.
4. Limit milk intake to 1 quart per day or less.

Evaluation
Child takes diet and medications as ordered; child's Hgb level returns to normal.

✖ SICKLE CELL ANEMIA

1. 1. Definition: autosomal recessive defect (Fig. 5-3) found primarily in blacks, resulting in production of abnormal hemoglobin (hemoglobin S) and characterized by intermittent episodes of crisis
2. Occurrence: 8% of African Americans; 1 in 12 African Americans carries the sickle cell trait
   a. Sickle cell trait: heterozygous form (carrier); 1 in 12 black persons is a carrier

A. Autosomal dominant diseases

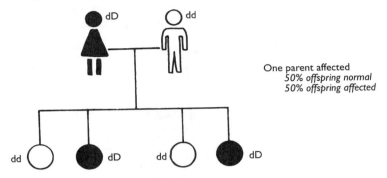

One parent affected
  50% offspring normal
  50% offspring affected

Key: d = normal gene; D = abnormal, *dominant* gene

Examples: Huntington's disease, osteogenesis imperfecta, neurofibromatosis

B. Autosomal recessive diseases

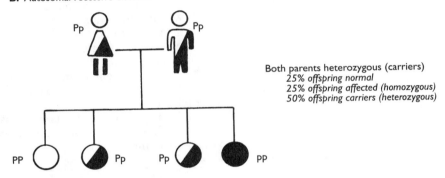

Both parents heterozygous (carriers)
  25% offspring normal
  25% offspring affected (homozygous)
  50% offspring carriers (heterozygous)

Key: P = normal gene; p = abnormal, *recessive gene*

Examples: phenylketonuria, cystic fibrosis, sickle cell disease, galactosemia, Tay-Sachs disease, thalassemia

C. Sex-linked recessive diseases (X-linked)

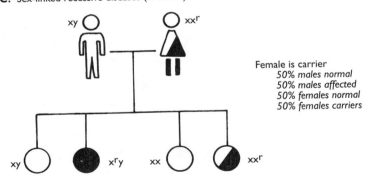

Female is carrier
  50% males normal
  50% males affected
  50% females normal
  50% females carriers

Key: xy = normal *male* sex chromosome pattern; xx = normal *female* sex chromosome pattern; r = sex-linked *recessive* gene

Examples: hemophilia, color blindness, agammaglobulinemia, G6PD deficiency, X-linked Duchenne's muscular dystrophy

Fig. 5-3   Common modes of genetic transmission.

b. Sickle cell disease: homozygous form (has the disease); may have vasoocclusive crisis; painful, acute occurrence usually precipitated by decreased O_2 tension, which causes cells to assume a sickle shape and blood to become viscous, obstruct blood vessels, and cause tissue ischemia, infarction, and necrosis
3. Cause: defective form of hemoglobin (hemoglobin S), inherited by autosomal recessive genetic transmission
4. Medical treatment: symptomatic treatment of crisis
   a. Bed rest to decrease O_2 expenditure
   b. Adequate hydration: oral and IV fluids to increase blood volume and mobilize sickled cells
   c. Electrolyte replacement (hypoxia causes metabolic acidosis)
   d. Relief of pain
      1. acetaminophen
      2. codeine
      3. morphine
      4. may use client-controlled analgesia
   e. Blood transfusions, for severe drop in hemoglobin (aplastic crisis)
   f. O_2 for severe hypoxia (on a short-term basis)
   g. Antibiotics to treat concurrent infection

Nursing Process
ASSESSMENT
1. Parents with sickle cell trait
2. Signs and symptoms (depend on organ involved); not evident until after 6 months of age
   a. Chronic hemolytic anemia
   b. Frequent infections, related to decreased ability of spleen to filter bacteria
   c. Organ deterioration (spleen, liver, kidney, heart, or CNS)
   d. Chronic pain: joints, abdomen, back
   e. Bone deterioration (osteoporosis, skeletal deformities) from increase in marrow
   f. Repeated episodes of pneumonia—may cause restrictive lung disease and pulmonary hypertension.
3. Manifestations of vasoocclusive crisis
   a. Severe abdominal pain: caused by organ hypoxia
   b. Hand-foot syndrome: swelling of hands and feet
   c. Fever: resulting from dehydration or possible concurrent infection
   d. Arthralgia

ANALYSIS/NURSING DIAGNOSIS (see p. 450)
PLANNING, IMPLEMENTATION, AND EVALUATION

Goal 1 Child's episodes of vasoocclusive crisis will be prevented or minimized.

Implementation
1. Teach crisis-prevention methods to child and parent.
   a. Avoid situations resulting in decreased O_2 concentration such as high altitudes, constrictive clothing, extreme physical exertion, and exposure to cold.
   b. Avoid emotional distress.
   c. Maintain adequate hydration (child should receive at least *minimum* daily fluid requirement: approximately 150 ml/kg/day).

d. Protect from infection.
   1. prevent exposure to persons with infections
   2. promote adequate nutrition
   3. obtain medical care at onset of infection (may need antibiotics)
   4. keep immunizations current, pneumoccocal vaccine

Evaluation
Parent and child adhere to plan for crisis prevention; child's crisis episodes are minimized.

Goal 2 Child will receive appropriate supportive care during crisis.

Implementation
1. Relieve pain.
   a. Administer analgesics.
   b. Handle gently.
   c. Use heating pad on painful areas.
   d. Encourage use of nonpharmacologic techniques (relaxation, distraction, etc.)
2. Monitor hydration and electrolyte status.
   a. Monitor I&O; offer liquids frequently.
   b. Regulate IV fluids, blood transfusion.
   c. Observe for fluid or electrolyte imbalance.
3. Assess for signs of infection; protect from exposure to infectious sources during crisis.

Evaluation
Child is relieved of pain during crisis; has no elevated temperature; has elastic skin turgor, moist mucous membranes, adequate fluid intake.

Goal 3 Parent and child at risk will receive screening and genetic counseling.

Implementation
1. Teach parent about screening and diagnostic techniques.
   a. Nonspecific screening tests for trait or disease: Sickledex
   b. Specific identification of trait and disease: Hgb electrophoresis ("protein fingerprinting") used if screening tests are positive
   c. Give information on available genetic counseling.

Evaluation
Parents receive screening and genetic counseling as indicated; demonstrate knowledge of transmission and implications for subsequent pregnancies.

✖ HEMOPHILIA

1. Definition, occurrence, and cause: hereditary coagulation defect, usually transmitted to affected male by female carrier through sex-linked recessive gene (Fig. 5-3), resulting in prolonged clotting time; most common type is hemophilia A, factor VIII deficiency; severity of the deficiency varies from mild to severe; 70% to 90% of hemophiliacs who received blood products before 1985 are HIV-positive; those diagnosed and treated since 1985 are at virtually no risk for developing HIV infection from blood products (see Table 5-9)

2. Medical treatment
   a. Replacement of factor VIII: transfusion of plasma or factor VIII concentrate to prevent bleeding episodes
   b. Additional treatment measures for more severe bleeding episodes
      1. immediate administration of factor VIII to control bleeding
      2. bed rest with covers off affected area to relieve pain; temporary immobilization of affected joints in a slightly flexed position with casts, splints, or traction
      3. physical therapy to prevent contractures, beginning 48 hours after bleeding stops
      4. pain relief with sedatives or narcotics
   c. Administration of DDAVP, a synthetic form of vasopressin, for treatment of mild hemophilia (DDAVP raises factor VIII activity)

Nursing Process

ASSESSMENT
1. Infant
   a. Umbilical-cord hemorrhage
   b. Hemorrhage after circumcision
   c. Family history of hemophilia
2. Any age
   a. Hemarthrosis (bleeding into a joint space) is the most frequent site of bleeding; may result in crippling bony deformities
   b. Epistaxis
   c. Spontaneous hematuria
   d. Hemorrhage after tooth extraction or minor falls and cuts
3. Diagnostic laboratory tests: only tests that measure clotting factors (e.g., PTT) are abnormal; platelet function tests (e.g., bleeding time) are normal

ANALYSIS/NURSING DIAGNOSIS (see p. 450)
PLANNING, IMPLEMENTATION, AND EVALUATION

Goal 1 Parent and child will receive education to *prevent* bleeding, provide safety measures; will know how to treat minor bleeding episodes.

Implementation
1. Prepare parents and child for home care and administration of factor VIII (where available).
   a. Teach about the disease.
   b. Teach venipuncture procedure and how to monitor the transfusion.
   c. Provide regular follow-up (family must be sufficiently motivated and stable to maintain a home-care program).
2. Teach local treatment measures for minor bleeding episodes.
   a. Apply direct pressure to site (10 to 15 minutes).
   b. Apply ice pack to promote vasoconstriction.
   c. Immobilize and elevate affected part.
3. Teach safe administration of medication.
   a. Give orally if possible.
   b. Avoid injections; if necessary, after injection apply pressure until bleeding stops.
4. Avoid medications that increase bleeding (aspirin, phenacetin, phenothiazines, indomethacin [Indocin]).
5. Institute dental precautions: soft toothbrush, Water Pik, good dental hygiene to avoid extractions.
6. Encourage appropriate toys, games, and sports.
   a. Soft toys for infants
   b. Quiet activities (e.g., reading, swimming)
   c. Avoid body-contact sports
   d. Careful handling of sharp objects
   e. Use of electric shavers (not razors)
7. Use protective devices for young child: padded crib, playpen, side rails, protective padding.
8. Teach to avoid overweight (causes strain on affected joints).
9. Teach to wear Medic Alert identification.
10. Inform appropriate school personnel.
11. Avoid stressful situations (they increase susceptibility to bleeding).
12. Seek emergency medical treatment in cases of uncontrolled bleeding.

Evaluation
Parent and child demonstrate ability to correctly manage home administration of factor VIII; state medication precautions, activities to avoid, and those that are permitted; parent provides appropriate protective devices at home; adequately cares for minor bleeding episodes (e.g., local pressure, ice pack); school personnel and friends are informed about child's condition and necessary restrictions or appropriate action during a bleeding episode.

Goal 2 Child and parents will receive emotional support.

Implementation
1. Encourage realistic career goals.
2. Allow child and family to discuss feelings and concerns about bleeding tendency and treatment, subsequent absences from school, reactions to peers, and parental protectiveness.
3. Encourage independence while maintaining safety.
4. Urge testing for HIV status.
5. Refer to the local chapter of the National Hemophilia Foundation.

Evaluation
Child seeks independence within reasonable limits; asks questions about reactions of school friends; adolescent seeks out appropriate job opportunities.

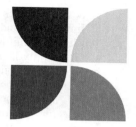

Nutrition and Metabolism

OVERVIEW OF PHYSIOLOGY

1. Fluid balance (developmental differences)
   a. Greater proportion of body water, especially in extracellular space, until 2 years of age (increases vulnerability to changes in body water)
   b. Three times greater water-turnover rate per unit of body weight in infants because of
      1. higher metabolic rate
      2. faster respiratory rate
      3. functional immaturity of kidneys that impairs ability to conserve water (increases infant's susceptibility to fluid volume deficit)
   c. Greater skin surface area in proportion to body weight (increases susceptibility to insensible water loss)
   d. Greater gastrointestinal surface area (leads to greater fluid loss from diarrhea)
2. Calculation of daily fluid requirements for infants and children
   a. Average daily fluid requirements are calculated according to child's weight in kilograms
      1. 100 ml/kg for the first 10 kg
      2. 50 ml/kg for the next 10 kg
      3. 20 ml/kg for each additional kg
   b. Example of calculation for a 25-kg child

	1000 ml (100 ml × 10 kg)
	500 ml (50 ml × 10 kg)
	100 ml (20 ml × 5 kg)
TOTAL	1600 ml per day

3. Digestive system (developmental differences)
   a. High rate of peristalsis (increases susceptibility to diarrhea)
   b. Immature cardiac sphincter that relaxes easily (predisposes to gastroesophageal reflux)
   c. Low production of intestinal antibodies until 6 or 7 months of age (increases susceptibility to infection)
   d. Increased permeability of intestines to whole proteins such as those found in cow's milk (increases susceptibility to allergies)
   e. Decreased levels of lactase in intestinal mucosa (predisposes to lactose intolerance and subsequent diarrhea)
   f. Immature liver (leads to an inability to conjugate water-soluble bilirubin in the newborn, resulting in physiologic jaundice; results in difficulties with drug metabolism)

4. Endocrine system (developmental differences)
   a. Functionally immature
   b. Blood glucose levels fluctuate (predisposes to hypoglycemia)
   c. Hormonal feedback mechanisms are not fully operational (leads to less ability to tolerate stresses and metabolic demands of illness)

Application of the Nursing Process to the Child with Problems of Nutrition and Metabolism

ASSESSMENT

1. Nursing history
   a. Dietary-intake history: type, amount, frequency, and tolerance
   b. Vomiting or diarrhea: onset, severity, duration, description, precipitating factors, and home management
   c. Infant/child behavior: irritability, lethargy, and change in disposition
   d. Other signs and symptoms of illness such as fever, respiratory infection, and abdominal pain
   e. Frequency and amount of voiding
   f. History of exposure to illness in family or community
   g. Family history of hereditary disorders: cystic fibrosis, phenylketonuria, diabetes mellitus, cleft lip and palate, or lactose intolerance
2. Clinical appraisal
   a. General appearance: color, cry, behavior
   b. Physical growth (refer to The Healthy Child, p. 402)
   c. Vital signs, presence of fever
   d. Nutrition and hydration status, including signs of dehydration
      1. mild dehydration: weight loss of up to 5%
         a. dry mucous membranes
         b. poor tear production
         c. decreased urine output with increased specific gravity (more than 1.030)
         d. pallor
         e. pulse normal or slightly increased
         f. normal blood pressure
      2. moderate dehydration: weight loss between 5% and 9%
         a. extremely dry mucous membranes
         b. poor skin turgor
         c. pale to gray skin color

d. oliguria (less than 1 ml/kg/hr)
e. tachycardia
f. slight increase in BP
3. severe dehydration: weight loss between 10% and 15%
   a. parched mucous membranes
   b. poor skin turgor
   c. marked oliguria
   d. gray to mottled skin color
   e. severe tachycardia
   f. decreased blood pressure
   g. sunken eyes and fontanel
   h. tetany and convulsions (late sign of electrolyte imbalance)
4. laboratory findings: elevated hematocrit and BUN
3. Diagnostic tests (refer to Nursing Care of the Adult, p. 158)

ANALYSIS/NURSING DIAGNOSIS

1. Safe, effective care environment
   a. Risk for infection
   b. Risk for injury
2. Physiologic integrity
   a. Fluid volume deficit
   b. Altered nutrition: less than body requirements
   c. Risk for aspiration
   d. Risk for impaired skin integrity
3. Psychosocial integrity
   a. Anxiety
   b. Self-esteem/body-image disturbance
   c. Fear
4. Health promotion/maintenance
   a. Altered family processes
   b. Altered growth and development
   c. Knowledge deficit

GENERAL NURSING PLANNING, IMPLEMENTATION, AND EVALUATION

> **Goal** Child will maintain fluid and electrolyte balance.

Implementation

1. Monitor for signs of electrolyte imbalance (refer to Nursing Care of the Adult, p. 188).
2. Administer fluids (PO, IV) as prescribed; usually includes sodium chloride and potassium replacement.
   a. Use infusion pump to maintain accurate rate.
   b. Restrain child as necessary to protect infusion site.
   c. Observe infusion site for infiltration or redness, and report promptly.
3. Provide pacifier if infant is NPO.
4. Administer electrolytes as prescribed (give potassium only when urinary output is adequate [i.e., 1 to 2 ml/kg/hr]).
5. Carefully monitor and record I&O (weigh diapers, indicate urine and stool output separately if possible).
6. Monitor response to therapy (improved skin color and turgor, moist mucous membranes, stable vital signs, urine output within normal limits, urine specific gravity within normal limits [e.g., 1.005 to 1.030]).

7. Weigh child daily before breakfast or every shift on same scale.
8. Administer antiemetics as ordered.
9. Gradually return to diet for age as tolerated.

Evaluation

Child regains and maintains fluid and electrolyte balance; shows no signs of dehydration or electrolyte or acid-base imbalance; returns to usual diet without recurrence of vomiting or diarrhea.

SELECTED HEALTH PROBLEMS RESULTING IN AN INTERFERENCE WITH NUTRITION AND METABOLISM

✖ VOMITING AND DIARRHEA

1. Although vomiting and diarrhea are usually symptoms of other underlying problems or diseases, they are often the primary diagnosis in infants because fluid and electrolyte imbalance can develop rapidly and become critical in a few hours.
2. Occurrence: these are common health problems in infancy; younger infants and children who are debilitated, and those who are exposed to unsanitary environmental conditions, are at greater risk of developing diarrhea.
3. Causes:
   a. Vomiting
      1. gastrointestinal infection
      2. allergy to formula, food, medications
      3. emotional upsets
      4. GI obstruction
      5. toxin ingestion
      6. increased intracranial pressure
      7. overfeeding
      8. diabetic ketoacidosis
      9. migraine headaches
      10. helminthic infestation
      11. appendicitis
      12. other infections (e.g., otitis media, meningitis, respiratory and urinary tract infections)
   b. Diarrhea (may be acute or chronic)
      1. infection
         a. viruses (e.g., rotavirus [self-limiting])
         b. parasites (e.g., *Giardia*)
         c. enteropathogenic organisms such as *Shigella, Salmonella, E. coli, Campylobacter*
      2. diet: formula or food allergy, high sugar or fat content, high bulk, overfeeding
      3. emotional upsets
      4. prolonged use of antibiotics (may destroy normal flora)
      5. intestinal malabsorption
      6. inflammatory bowel disease
      7. extraintestinal: hepatic, pancreatic, thyroid disorders
      8. ingestion of heavy metals such as lead and mercury
      9. parenteral infections

4. Medical treatment depends on severity of symptoms and degree of dehydration.
   a. Medical intervention
      1. bowel rest; IV or oral fluid and electrolyte replacement therapy (type and amount determined on basis of child's age and hydration status)
      2. antibiotic therapy for bacterial diarrhea
      3. antiemetics, usually by rectal suppository
      4. gradual reintroduction of solid foods
      5. diagnosis and treatment of extraintestinal cause
   b. Surgical intervention for GI obstruction

Nursing Process

ASSESSMENT
1. Feeding technique and formula preparation (amount, type, formula reconstitution, position of infant, and burping)
2. Type of vomiting or diarrhea
   a. Vomiting
      1. *forceful* vomiting: evacuation of stomach contents; usually caused by overdistention from formula or air
      2. *projectile* vomiting: stomach contents propelled 2 to 3 feet from infant; indicates GI obstruction or increased intracranial pressure
      3. *regurgitation:* "spitting up" milk after feeding; smells sour; usually associated with rumination or gastroesophageal reflux
   b. Diarrhea
      1. *mild:* weight loss of 5% or less; stools are loose, runny, usually brown or brownish yellow
      2. *severe:* explosive, green, watery stools, 10 to 12 per day; weight loss 10% or more
3. Character of vomitus or stool (ACCT)
   a. *Amount:* measure or estimate
   b. *Color/Consistency*
      1. vomitus
         a. undigested food, uncurdled milk
         b. sour milk curds
         c. bile stained (indicates lower GI tract obstruction)
         d. blood tinged or "coffee grounds"
      2. diarrhea
         a. color (brown, green, yellow)
         b. consistency (bulky, watery, runny, mucoid, bloody, seedy, or pasty)
   c. *Time*
      1. frequency
      2. precedents (feeding, stimulants, emotional upsets)
4. Diagnostic tests
   a. Stool pH and stool glucose with Clinitest
   b. Stool blood with guaiac or Hemoccult
   c. Stool sample for bacteria culture, ova, and parasites
5. Associated symptoms: anorexia, nausea, cramping, abdominal pain, fever, headache
6. Signs of dehydration
7. Change in acid-base balance
   a. Vomiting causes loss of HCl, which results in metabolic alkalosis
      1. compensation: kidneys conserve Na^+ and K^+, excrete HCO_3^-

2. lab findings: urine pH greater than 7; serum pH greater than 7.45
   b. Diarrhea causes loss of HCO_3^-, which results in metabolic acidosis
      1. compensation: respiratory hyperventilation (deep, rapid respirations)
      2. lab findings: urine pH less than 6; serum pH less than 7.35

ANALYSIS/NURSING DIAGNOSIS (see p. 463)
PLANNING, IMPLEMENTATION, AND EVALUATION

Goal 1 Child's close contacts will be free from signs of infection.

Implementation
1. Obtain stool culture to determine infecting organism.
2. Isolate infant; use good hand-washing technique; dispose of excreta and contaminated laundry appropriately.
3. Teach parents protective measures.
4. Administer antibiotics as ordered, observe for side effects.

Evaluation
Individuals involved with care of child (and other children in close proximity) show no signs of spread of infection.

Goal 2 Child (with diarrhea) will maintain skin integrity.

Implementation
1. Cleanse perineum and buttocks well after each stool.
2. Expose to heat lamp or air (buttocks must be free of ointment before exposing to heat lamp).
3. Apply ointment to protect skin.
4. Take axillary temperatures to avoid stimulating peristalsis.

Evaluation
Child is free from skin breakdown; heals excoriated areas.

Goal 3 Child will maintain comfort and safety.

Implementation
1. Position to prevent aspiration (on side or abdomen, or in infant seat).
2. Give mouth care after vomiting and while NPO.
3. If infant is NPO, offer pacifier to meet sucking needs.
4. Change soiled clothing and linen immediately.
5. Exercise restrained limbs.

Evaluation
Child is free from aspiration; rests and sleeps comfortably.

Goal 4 Child will resume diet for age without recurrence of vomiting or diarrhea.

Implementation
1. Begin clear liquids such as noncarbonated soft drinks, Gatorade, and half-strength flavored gelatin; use oral

rehydration solutions (e.g., Pedialyte, Lytren) for infants and young children.
2. Give liquids at room temperature (cold liquids stimulate bowel activity).
3. If vomiting, offer frequent, small amounts (5 to 15 ml depending on child's age) every 20 minutes; increase the amount and intervals between feedings slowly.
4. For diarrhea, offer large amounts of clear liquids at infrequent intervals.
5. Discourage use of Popsicles and Kool-Aid as sole source of fluid replacement because they lack electrolytes.
6. Limit apple juice (may cause diarrhea).
7. Discourage use of homemade electrolyte solutions.
8. If infant is breast-feeding, continue and supplement with clear liquids.
9. Add other liquids and solids gradually as tolerated.
10. Encourage bananas, applesauce, strained carrots, rice cereal, and toast for child with diarrhea.
11. Discourage foods with high fat content.
12. Add milk products last because temporary lactose intolerance is common after diarrhea.
13. Switch to soy formula for 1 to 3 weeks if necessary.

Evaluation
Child tolerates diet for age without recurrence of diarrhea or vomiting; gains weight or maintains present weight.

✖ NONORGANIC FAILURE TO THRIVE

1. Definition: A term used to describe infants and children who fail to gain weight as a result of psychosocial factors such as environmental deprivation; usually results from a disrupted relationship between child and primary caregiver
2. Medical treatment
   a. Comprehensive diagnostic testing to rule out organic failure to thrive, which results from physical causes (e.g., malabsorption syndrome, gastroesophageal reflux, cystic fibrosis, genitourinary or cardiac defects, and neurologic or endocrine disorders)
   b. Criteria used for diagnosis
      1. absence of organic disease
      2. weight below the 5th percentile with subsequent weight gain when nurtured
      3. developmental lags that improve with stimulation
      4. improvement in clinical signs of deprivation when nurtured
      5. disruption in psychosocial environment

Nursing Process
ASSESSMENT
1. Infant
   a. Growth retardation: height and weight below 5th percentile
   b. Developmental delay: social, motor, language, or cognitive
   c. Flat affect, withdrawn
   d. Feeding and elimination disorders
   e. Absence of stranger anxiety
   f. Avoids eye-to-eye contact
   g. Visually scans the environment
   h. Posture stiff or floppy

   i. Difficulty in feeding or eating (e.g., poor suck, anorexia, vomiting, rumination)
   j. Slow in smiling or socially responding to others
2. Parent
   a. Handles infant only when necessary
   b. Does not talk to, play with, or cuddle infant
   c. Bothered by infant's sounds and smells
   d. Holds infant away from body, no eye contact with infant
   e. Responds inappropriately and inconsistently to infant's cues
   f. Refers to infant as "bad" and "unloving"

ANALYSIS/NURSING DIAGNOSIS (see p. 463)
PLANNING, IMPLEMENTATION, AND EVALUATION

Goal I Infant will show evidence of weight gain.

Implementation
1. Calculate caloric requirements based on infant's weight: 115 kcal/kg/day for the first year of life.
2. Suggest dietary consultant.
3. Monitor I&O; describe frequency and precipitating events of any vomiting.
4. Obtain daily weights before breakfast on same scale, and weekly length and head circumferences.
5. Observe feeding patterns.
6. Observe parent-infant interactions around feeding. Feeding by staff may be necessary (consistent caregivers as much as possible).

Evaluation
Infant shows steady weight gain, ingests and retains appropriate amount of nutrients necessary to meet caloric requirements.

Goal 2 Infant will show progression in development while hospitalized.

Implementation
1. Use primary caregivers.
2. Hold, cuddle, talk to infant lovingly with reassurance to model for caregivers.
3. Monitor infant's response to care.
4. Provide age-appropriate developmental and sensory stimulation.

Evaluation
Infant responds appropriately to developmental stimulation and nurturing; maintains eye contact, smiles; allows self to be held closely; demonstrates interest in environment.

Goal 3 Parents will show positive interaction with infant.

Implementation
1. Welcome parents when visiting.
2. Encourage parent participation in care, teaching as appropriate.
3. Use anticipatory guidance regarding infant's capabilities, physical care, emotional needs (demonstrate by example).

4. Encourage parents to express feelings about infant and their parenting.
5. Urge parents to talk to infant; point out positive responses.
6. Identify stressors in family; refer to social services and family counseling as appropriate.
7. Praise parents' involvement with child.
8. Determine progress in parent-child relationship.
9. Maintain a nonjudgmental attitude.

Evaluation

Parents provide some care to infant; hold, cuddle, and talk to infant; express feelings about infant.

Goal 4 Parents will participate in follow-up care after discharge.

Implementation

1. Assess home environment.
2. Refer to community resources (e.g., public health nurse, parent support group) as needed.
3. Refer to agencies that can provide family counseling, financial assistance (e.g., WIC).
4. Review infant's regimen with parents (nutrition, elimination, stimulation, etc.).
5. Arrange for return visit for infant to physician/clinic.
6. Review developmental milestones and age-appropriate stimulation.

Evaluation

Parent keeps all appointments, including those with community resources and groups; infant continues weight gain and developmental progress.

✱ PYLORIC STENOSIS

1. Definition and occurrence: narrowing of the pylorus caused by hypertrophy of circular muscle fibers; more commonly affects firstborn white males, 2 weeks to 3 months of age
2. Medical treatment
   a. Medical intervention
      1. barium swallow to confirm diagnosis; abdominal ultrasound
      2. IV fluids to hydrate and correct metabolic alkalosis
      3. nasogastric tube to decompress stomach
   b. Surgical intervention: Fredet-Ramstedt procedure (pylorotomy); hypertrophied muscle is *split down to but not through* submucosa, permitting pylorus to expand (if mucosa is cut, gastric contents will leak into peritoneum, causing peritonitis)

Nursing Process

ASSESSMENT

1. Vomiting: amount, color, consistency, and time
2. Classic signs
   a. Projectile vomiting (not bile stained because obstruction is above the duodenum)
   b. Palpable, olive-size mass (usually in right upper quadrant)
   c. Observable left-to-right gastric peristaltic waves
3. Metabolic alkalosis, caused by the loss of HCl and K^+

4. Signs and symptoms of food and fluid loss
   a. Hunger after feeding
   b. Weight loss or failure to gain weight
   c. Dehydration
   d. Scanty, concentrated urine
   e. Progressive constipation

ANALYSIS/NURSING DIAGNOSIS (see p. 463)
PLANNING, IMPLEMENTATION, AND EVALUATION

Goal I Preoperatively, infant will regain and maintain fluid and electrolyte balance.

Implementation

1. Assess vital signs frequently.
2. Assess signs of dehydration.
3. Offer pacifier while NPO.
4. Follow correct principles of IV fluid and electrolyte administration.
5. Carefully monitor I&O and urine specific gravity.
6. Weigh infant daily or every shift if condition warrants.
7. Maintain nasogastric decompression as ordered.

Evaluation

Infant regains and maintains fluid and electrolyte balance; is free from signs of dehydration and metabolic alkalosis.

Goal 2 Postoperatively, infant will be free from vomiting and will ingest adequate nutrition.

Implementation

1. Initiate glucose water or electrolyte solutions 4 to 6 hours postoperatively and gradually advance to full-strength formula during second postoperative day.
2. Give small, frequent feedings; feed slowly.
3. Burp infant after every half ounce; position on right side in semi-Fowler's position after feeding.
4. Teach parent how to feed child; supervise as needed.
5. Handle gently and minimally after feeding.
6. Offer pacifier during period of restricted feeding.
7. Keep accurate I&O.

Evaluation

Infant ingests adequate caloric and fluid intake; has no vomiting, no signs of dehydration; gains or maintains present weight.

Goal 3 Postoperatively, infant will be free from infection.

Implementation

1. Observe operative site routinely for any drainage or signs of inflammation or infection.
2. Perform incision care and dressing change as ordered.
3. Assess for signs of peritonitis (e.g., abdominal distention, fever, rigid abdomen, increased irritability, tachycardia, decreased or absent bowel sounds, or rapid thoracic breathing).

Evaluation

Infant remains afebrile, has soft abdomen, exhibits no signs of discomfort.

✳ CELIAC DISEASE (GLUTEN ENTEROPATHY)

1. Definition: a disease of unknown etiology characterized by the permanent inability to tolerate gluten (one of the proteins found in wheat, rye, oats, and barley)
2. Occurrence: 1 in 4000 live births; second leading cause of malabsorption in children; positive familial tendency
3. Pathophysiology: the ingestion of gluten results in the inability to fully digest gliadin (a fraction of gluten); subsequently, there is an accumulation of the amino acid glutamine, which is toxic to the mucosal cells of the small intestine; this may lead to malabsorption of the following nutrients, causing various complications
   a. Fats: steatorrhea, malnutrition
   b. Proteins and carbohydrates: peripheral edema
   c. Vitamin D and calcium: osteomalacia, osteoporosis
   d. Vitamin K: bleeding
   e. Iron, folic acid, and vitamin B_{12}: anemia
4. Medical treatment
   a. Diagnosis
      1. positive fecal fat
      2. decreases in serum protein, prothrombin, folic acid, vitamin B_{12}, calcium
      3. anemia
      4. x-rays to determine bone age
      5. sweat test (to rule out cystic fibrosis)
      6. improvement of clinical signs and symptoms after withdrawal of gluten from diet
      7. bowel studies
      8. peroral jejunal biopsy (diagnosis is confirmed when atrophic changes are seen in the mucosal wall)
   b. Dietary management
      1. gluten-free diet (corn, rice, and millet are substituted for wheat, rye, oats, and barley)
      2. supplemental calories, vitamins, iron, and calcium
      3. parenteral alimentation if malnourished
   c. Management during celiac crisis (acute episode of profuse, watery diarrhea and vomiting that frequently leads to severe dehydration and metabolic acidosis; usually precipitated by gastrointestinal infection, dietary sources of gluten, and anticholinergic drugs)
      1. IV fluids and electrolytes
      2. albumin infusions (to prevent shock)
      3. nasogastric decompression
      4. corticosteroids (to decrease bowel inflammation)

Nursing Process

ASSESSMENT
1. Clinical manifestations (highly variable)
   a. Chronic diarrhea (usually begins late in the first year of life, several months after gluten-containing foods have been introduced)
   b. Failure to thrive
   c. Irritability
   d. Anorexia
   e. Vomiting
   f. Abdominal pain and distention
   g. Excessive appetite
   h. Rectal prolapse
   i. Peripheral edema
   j. Clubbing of fingers
   k. Wasting of muscles
   l. Excessive bruising
2. In celiac crisis
   a. Severe pale, bulky, foul-smelling stools
   b. Vomiting
   c. Signs of shock and metabolic acidosis
   d. Dependent edema

ANALYSIS/NURSING DIAGNOSIS (see p. 463)
PLANNING, IMPLEMENTATION, AND EVALUATION

Goal 1 Child will remain free from injury during intestinal biopsy.

Implementation
1. Prepare child and family for diagnostic procedure.
2. Assess bleeding times and platelet count.
3. Administer vitamin K prophylactically as ordered.
4. Assess frequently, following procedure for shock (early signs: tachycardia and signs of peripheral vasoconstriction; late signs: hypotension).

Evaluation
Child tolerates intestinal biopsy well, recovers free from signs of hemorrhage.

Goal 2 Child will adhere to nutritional management.

Implementation
1. Assess family's understanding of disease process and need for gluten-free diet.
2. Educate family regarding gluten-free foods; show parents how to read food labels (gluten is often listed as hydrolyzed vegetable protein or cereal fillers).
3. Encourage balanced diet (offer foods high in calories and protein such as pudding and milkshakes) and use of substitute foods; consult dietitian to help in meal planning.
4. Reinforce to family the need for lifelong dietary adherence.

Evaluation
Parents list elements of a gluten-free diet; child ingests only gluten-free, balanced meals.

Goal 3 Child will remain free from fluid and electrolyte imbalance during celiac crisis.

Implementation
1. Monitor vital signs frequently.
2. Assess for signs of shock and metabolic acidosis.
3. Keep accurate I&O.
4. Weigh child daily on same scale.
5. Maintain nasogastric decompression as ordered.
6. Administer corticosteroids, albumin, IV fluids, and electrolytes as ordered.
7. Test all stools and nasogastric drainage for occult blood.
8. Educate family regarding precipitating factors of celiac crisis.

Evaluation

Child recovers from celiac crisis free from complications; achieves homeostasis.

✳ CLEFT LIP AND PALATE

1. Definition
   a. *Cleft lip:* incomplete fusion of facial process; may be small notch in the upper lip (incomplete) or extend to nasal septum and dental ridge (complete); may be unilateral or bilateral
   b. *Cleft palate:* fissures in soft or hard palate and alveolar (dental) ridge; may be midline, unilateral, or bilateral
2. Occurrence
   a. Cleft lip (with or without cleft palate): 1 in 800 live births; higher in males, whites, and Asians
   b. Cleft palate: 1 in 2500, higher in females
3. Cause: often unknown, multifactorial inheritance, chromosomal abnormalities, maternal alcohol or drug ingestion, prenatal infection
4. Surgical treatment: cleft lip is usually repaired (by Z-plasty surgical technique) within the first few days to weeks of life if the infant is demonstrating steady weight gain and is free from infection; early correction is important for nutrition and cosmetic purposes; cleft palate repair may be delayed until 12 to 18 months of age to allow for bone growth and changes in contour of palate but may be done in first few months of life, depending on degree of involvement

Nursing Process

ASSESSMENT

1. Infant's ability to suck and and swallow (will depend on type and extent of defect)
2. Nutritional status
3. Parents' reaction to birth of an infant with a facial defect

ANALYSIS/NURSING DIAGNOSIS (see p. 463)
PLANNING, IMPLEMENTATION, AND EVALUATION

Goal 1 Preoperatively, child will maintain adequate nutrition and will not aspirate fluids.

Implementation

1. Feed slowly in upright position; use one of the following:
   a. Special nipple, soft nipple with large or cross-cut opening, lamb's nipple
   b. Asepto syringe (bulb syringe with rubber catheter tubing attached) or Breck feeder
   c. Cup for older infant with cleft palate
2. For infants with palate cleft be careful not to place nipple inside cleft.
3. Burp frequently.
4. Rinse mouth with water after feedings to keep lip/palate cleansed.
5. Teach parents how to feed and burp infant.
6. Teach parents use and care of palate prosthesis.

Evaluation

Child ingests adequate fluids and calories; is free from aspiration and lip/palate infections.

Goal 2 Postoperatively, child will maintain a patent airway.

Implementation

1. Observe for respiratory distress; assist in respiratory effort by positioning child to facilitate breathing; aspirate oral secretions *gently* from the sides of the mouth.
2. Cleft palate: place in mist tent.
3. Position infant to provide for drainage of mucus and to prevent trauma to suture lines.
   a. Cleft lip repair: on side or in infant seat
   b. Cleft palate repair: on side or abdomen
4. Keep oxygen and suction equipment at bedside; suction only if assessment reveals signs of airway obstruction.

Evaluation

Child has patent airway and adequate oxygenation; has no signs of respiratory distress.

Goal 3 Postoperatively, child will be free from trauma and infection of suture lines.

Implementation

1. Monitor vital signs including temperature every 4 hours.
2. Minimize crying by holding and soothing infant as needed. Do *not* use pacifiers. Provide adequate analgesia.
3. Put elbow restraints on child; remove *one at a time* q2h for ROM exercises.
4. Position as stated previously.
5. Maintain Logan bar (a metal-wire arch) on upper lip to decrease tension on suture line.
6. Cleanse suture lines after feeding with sterile swabs and solution (usually diluted hydrogen peroxide) as ordered to limit crusting and inflammation
   a. For cleft lip repair: *roll* applicator without rubbing
   b. For cleft palate repair: rinse mouth with sterile water after feeding
7. Apply antibiotic ointment to lip suture line as prescribed.
8. Encourage parents to stay with infant and participate in care.

Evaluation

Child has healing of suture lines without trauma and scarring associated with infection.

Goal 4 Postoperatively, child will ingest adequate nutrition.

Implementation

1. Feed with medicine dropper, Asepto syringe (cleft lip), or cup (cleft palate); no sucking, straws, or spoons to prevent trauma to suture line.
2. For children with cleft palate repair, give soft diet high in calories and protein (encourage milkshakes and pudding); avoid hard foods such as toast or cookies.

Evaluation

Child takes food and fluids (appropriate for age); is free from choking or aspiration.

Goal 5 Child and parents will be referred for ongoing, long-term intervention and promotion of optimum development.

Implementation

1. Teach parents signs of otitis media (fever, turning head to side, pulling at ear, discharge from ear, pain, or crying); encourage parents to seek medical treatment for upper respiratory infections.
2. Refer for regular evaluation of child's hearing, speech, and dental development.
3. Help parents to express feelings and concerns about defect and surgery.
4. Refer parents to community resources.
   a. Parent groups; local and state cleft-palate associations
   b. Crippled Children's Services or social services

Evaluation

Parents list early signs of ear infections and when to seek treatment; child has no permanent hearing loss; has age-appropriate language development, intelligible speech, and normal tooth alignment; parents and child receive community support (emotional, financial, and social).

✳ CONGENITAL HYPOTHYROIDISM

1. Definition: congenital condition in which the fetal thyroid fails to develop, resulting in inadequate levels of T_4 and other thyroid hormones in the fetus and newborn; also called cretinism; early diagnosis is essential to prevent mental retardation
2. Incidence: one of the most common endocrine problems of childhood; 1 in every 4000 live births; twice as common in females as in males; higher incidence in Down syndrome
3. Pathophysiology: thyroid hormones have a stimulating effect on metabolic rate, heart production, cardiac output, and growth of almost all tissues; lack of these hormones specifically affects brain, bone, and muscle growth in infants
4. Diagnosis
   a. Elevated serum thyroid-stimulating hormone (TSH) and decreased T_4 levels in early days of life; screening is mandatory in most states
   b. Decreased uptake of radioactive iodine by thyroid after oral administration of isotope
5. Causes
   a. Hypoplasia or aplasia of thyroid gland
   b. Pituitary dysfunction
   c. Unresponsiveness of tissue to existing thyroid hormones
   d. Autoimmune destruction of the thyroid (juvenile hypothyroidism)
6. Medical treatment: thyroid hormone replacement as soon as diagnosis is suspected
   a. Levothyroxine (Synthroid), 0.006 mg/kg/day or desiccated thyroid (Proloid), 4 mg/kg/day; adjusted according to clinical symptoms and T_4 level
      1. doses in children usually *higher* than adult doses
      2. given as a single dose in morning
      3. replacement is a lifelong necessity
   b. Side effects of excessive dosage: dyspnea, tachycardia, fever, irritability, tremors, diarrhea, weight loss, and sleep disturbance

Nursing Process
ASSESSMENT
1. Prolonged gestation and high birth weight
2. Signs of hypothyroidism usually appear after about 6 weeks of age.
3. Puffy face with coarse features
4. Wide fontanels and sutures
5. Flattened nasal bridge
6. Low anterior hairline
7. Described as "good, quiet baby"
8. Hoarse, weak cry
9. Lethargy and excessive sleeping, resulting in poor feeding
10. Poor abdominal muscle tone; constipation
11. Weak reflexes
12. Large, protruding tongue
13. Cold, mottled skin (hypothermia: 95°F or less)
14. Delayed cognitive and motor development
15. Delayed physical growth
16. Prolonged physiologic jaundice
17. Delayed passage of meconium
18. Respiratory distress
19. See also Hypothyroidism, p. 176

ANALYSIS/NURSING DIAGNOSIS (see p. 463)
PLANNING, IMPLEMENTATION, AND EVALUATION

Goal I Child's condition will be identified at the earliest possible stage.

Implementation

1. Screen all children before discharge from the hospital or within first week of life.
2. Be alert to earliest clinical manifestations and parental comments (e.g., "She is such a good baby, she hardly ever cries").
3. Educate and support parents during diagnostic tests.

Evaluation

Infant is diagnosed within first several weeks of life; replacement therapy begins.

Goal 2 Child will experience normal growth and development.

---

1. Provide information to family about condition.
2. Encourage expression of concerns about child's behavior and development.
3. If diagnosis is delayed, explore possible guilt feelings and discuss probability of mental retardation.

4. Teach parents about medication administration, side effects, need for lifelong administration.
    a. Do not change brands without physician knowledge because hormone content varies.
    b. Store in dry, dark place.
    c. Measure child's pulse daily before administration (indication of drug effectiveness).
    d. Teach importance of regular, consistent administration of medication.
    e. If a dose is missed, give twice the dose the next day.
    f. Look for signs of overdose (e.g., dyspnea, fever, diaphoresis, irritability, rapid pulse, and weight loss).
5. Teach parents how to measure pulse rate; consult physician if pulse is above normal range (Table 5-1).
6. Monitor child's growth and development periodically.
7. Refer family to community support groups if needed.

Evaluation

Child is alert, active; grows normally; development continues within normal range; parents and child assume self-care responsibilities.

✕ INSULIN-DEPENDENT DIABETES MELLITUS (IDD: TYPE I)

1. Definition: metabolic disease of unknown inheritance mechanism that results in insulin deficiency because of reduction in pancreatic islet cell mass or destruction of islets and consequent alterations of carbohydrate, fat, and protein metabolism; also results in long-term alterations in vascular, nervous, renal, and ocular systems; damage to other organ systems may be related to degree of control of diabetes (see Table 5-20 for comparison with adult-onset diabetes)
2. Theories of etiology
    a. Viral infection (e.g., mumps, coxsackievirus): stress of the illness may decrease glucose tolerance and precipitate onset of IDD
    b. Genetic inheritance
    c. Autoimmune disease (child produces antibodies that destroy the islet cells of the pancrease)
3. Pathophysiology: refer to Diabetes Mellitus, p. 179

4. Medical treatment
    a. Medication
        1. insulin therapy: human insulin usually recommended because of limited antigenicity, decreased dosage, increased solubility, and increased absorption
            a. dosage: 0.5 to 1 U/kg/day (usually in two divided doses)
            b. refer to Table 3-37, p. 180
        2. oral hypoglycemics: not used with children
    b. Meal plan: more flexible nutrition options than with adults; most commonly used are free (no concentrated sweets), exchange, and food pyramid (usually three meals and three snacks a day); prudent fat intake
5. Modifying factors
    a. Puberty
        1. onset complicates control by increasing insulin demands (growth is stimulated by gonadal steroids, which antagonize isulin action; larger doses of insulin usually needed)
        2. asociated growth significantly increases caloric needs
    b. Exercise
        1. reduces insulin requirements because glucose is catabolized without insulin during muscular activity
        2. increases risk of insulin shock if an extra snack is not provided before vigorous exercise
    c. Illness and emotional disturbance
        1. lessens ability to use glucose
        2. may increase insulin requirements because of decreased activity
    d. Alcohol and drug usage (common problem in adolescents)
        1. alcohol suppresses gluconeogenesis, which may precipitate hypoglycemia
        2. stimulant drugs (e.g., cocaine and amphetamines) increase metabolism and decrease appetite, which may result in hypoglycemia

Table 5-20   Comparison of type I (insulin-dependent) and type II (non–insulin-dependent) diabetes mellitus

	Type I	Type II
CHARACTERISTICS		
Age of onset	Usually less than 20 years (peaks: 5-7 years; puberty)	Usually over 35 years
Type of onset	Abrupt	Gradual
Nutritional status	Underweight	Overweight
Symptoms	Polydipsia, polyuria, polyphagia	May be none
Remission	Yes (honeymoon period)	No
Plasma insulin	Absent	Usually decreased
MANAGEMENT		
Medication	Insulin only	Oral hypoglycemics frequently used
Meal planning	Free or exchange	Exchange
Self-monitoring	Blood glucose monitoring preferred; when testing urine, use Clinitest; first-voided specimen acceptable	Blood glucose monitoring preferred; when testing urine use Tes-Tape or Clinitest on second voided specimen
Hypoglycemia	Oral sugars and glucagon (for severe reactions)	Oral sugars only

Nursing Process

ASSESSMENT

1. Initial
   a. Polydipsia, polyphagia, polyuria (bed-wetting): classic signs
   b. Weight loss
   c. Irritability, fatigue
   d. Abdominal discomfort
   e. May be mistaken for influenza, gastroenteritis
   f. Initial symptoms may follow physical or emotional stress (illness, injury, growth spurt, etc.)
   g. Frequent infections, slow-to-heal skin injuries
2. Often characterized by remission or honeymoon period
   a. Common in children with IDD
   b. Decreased amounts of insulin required
   c. Occurs once, lasting for a few weeks up to one year
3. Diabetic ketoacidosis (DKA): polydipsia, polyphagia, polyuria, dehydration with possible hypovolemic shock, nausea and vomiting, acetone breath, Kussmaul's respiration, flushed dry skin (children with DKA for the first time often show signs of abdominal pain and rigidity, which may mimic appendicitis); refer to Table 3-39, p. 183; DKA is presenting symptom in children 10% to 20% of the time
4. Hypoglycemia: irritability, trembling; apprehension; headache; hunger, blurred vision; mental confusion; sweating, pallor, seizures (more likely in infants and children); temper tantrums (common in toddlers)

ANALYSIS/NURSING DIAGNOSIS (see p. 463)
PLANNING, IMPLEMENTATION, AND EVALUATION

> **Goal** Child and parents will be prepared for home management.

Implementation

1. Teach blood glucose monitoring (preferred self-monitoring method).
   a. Finger-stick technique
   b. Importance of exact timing
   c. Variation among different products (use same product for consistency and accuracy)
   d. Importance of checking expiration dates
   e. Four measurements per day (before each meal and bedtime snack)
   f. Interpretation of results
   g. Importance of record keeping
2. Contact community resources for financial assistance as needed for blood glucose monitoring at home.
   a. Medicaid coverage in some states
   b. Local diabetes association
   c. Rentals available
   d. Private insurance
3. Demonstrate urine testing for glucose and acetone (to be done if blood glucose level is greater than 240 mg); two- to five-drop Clinitest preferred; first-voided specimens used because of difficulty in obtaining second-voided specimens in children.
4. Teach insulin administration.
   a. Knowledge of medication
   b. Proper mixing
   c. Injection technique
   d. Rotation of sites
   e. Use of insulin pump when indicated
5. Involve dietitian with nutrition planning; adjust meal plans for activity and growth with periodic reassessment at least every 6 months.
6. Teach management of hyperglycemia.
   a. Recognition of early signs and symptoms
   b. Importance of good control
   c. Food, activity, and insulin adjustment to improve control
7. Teach management of hypoglycemia: ingest a rapidly absorbed glucose-containing food or liquid, such as 4 oz of orange juice, 2 teaspoonfuls of honey, 5 or 6 Life Savers (chewed); for the unconscious child with a severe reaction, squeeze glucose gel or cake frosting between the child's cheek and gums and administer glucagon subcutaneously (raises blood glucose level by stimulating the release of glucose from glycogen stores in the liver).
8. Demonstrate foot care: same as adult except bare feet acceptable.
9. Prepare parents for developmental concerns with respect to management.
   a. For toddlers and preschoolers
      1. inform parents of major concerns (finger sticks and injections threaten body integrity; fears of loss of control and autonomy)
      2. encourage parents to offer choices when possible
      3. prepare parents for finicky eating habits and assist in meal planning
      4. teach parents how to recognize hypoglycemia and hyperglycemia
      5. encourage parents to involve child in creative play to allow expression of fears and emotions
   b. For school-age children
      1. inform school, teacher, and peers about symptoms/treatment
      2. arrange for child to participate in gym classes and sports, adjusting medication as needed
      3. anticipate nutrition needs of lunches, parties, and holidays
      4. feelings of being different
   c. For adolescents
      1. discuss feelings and concerns about future: career, marriage, and pregnancy
      2. acting-out behaviors (anticipate and prevent)
      3. onset of puberty, changes in body image
      4. discuss the effects of drugs, alcohol, and birth control pills on blood glucose levels
10. Teach self-management as appropriate.
    a. At 6 to 8 years: assisting with urine tests, injections, diet selection, and blood glucose measurement
    b. At 8 to 9 years: physical readiness; teach to do urine tests, injections, and blood glucose monitoring
    c. At 12 to 13 years and beyond: cognitive readiness; teach meal planning, how to maintain food, activity, and insulin balance
11. Develop an exercise program that allows for optimal growth and development.

12. Advise child and parents of need to obtain and wear medical-alert identification.

Evaluation

Child and parents incorporate necessary skills to daily routine; child does not have recurrent episodes of ketoacidosis or hypoglycemia; continues normal growth and development.

�֍ CYSTIC FIBROSIS

1. Definition: an inherited multisystem disorder characterized by widespread dysfunction of the exocrine glands (those whose secretions reach an epithelial surface, either directly or through a duct)
2. Cause and occurrence: autosomal recessive disorder (both parents are carriers: see Fig. 5-3); most common genetic defect in white children; approximately 1 in 2000 live births; 1 in 20 persons estimated to be a carrier
3. Pathophysiology: abnormal secretion of thick tenacious mucus by the exocrine glands causes obstruction and results in varying degress of pathology
   a. *Pulmonary effects:* depressed respiratory-cilia cells result in increased infection, bronchiole obstruction, and eventually pulmonary fibrosis; child ultimately develops chronic obstructive pulmonary disease; may progress to cor pulmonale; death can occur from respiratory infection or heart failure
   b. *Pancrease effects:* pancreatic fibrosis and eventual decrease of digestive enzymes (lipase, amylase, and trypsin) resulting in severe malnutrition and failure to thrive; steatorrhea: fatty, bulky, foul-smelling stools that float because of undigested fat cells; also can affect pancreatic endocrine functions, resulting in hyperglycemia, glucosuria, and ultimately requiring insulin replacement (occurs late in the disease process)
   c. *Salivary effects:* fibrosis and enlargement of glands caused by thickened secretions; elevated sodium and chloride in saliva
   d. *Sweat gland effects:* elevated sodium and chloride in sweat
   e. *Reproductive effects*
      1. males: inability to produce sperm; the semen is thickened and tenacious; it plugs the ducts in the testes, resulting in fibrosis; males are generally sterile but not impotent
      2. females: difficult to conceive because cervical plug cannot be penetrated by normal sperm
   f. *Hepatic effects:* bile secreted by the liver to emulsify fat in the duodenum is thickened (inspissated) and may plug liver ductules, resulting in biliary cirrhosis and jaundice; can lead to esophageal varices (in newborn and infant, condition may be misdiagnosed as biliary atresia)
4. Medical treatment
   a. Diagnostic testing
      1. prenatal diagnosis: DNA analysis of chorionic villi samples; DNA or enzyme analysis of amniotic fluid samples
      2. postnatal diagnosis: pilocarpine electrophoresis (sweat chloride test)
         a. normal sweat chloride values: less than 40 mEq/L
         b. suggestive of cystic fibrosis (CF): 40 to 60 mEq/L
         c. diagnostic of CF: greater than 60 mEq/L
   b. Medication
      1. pancreatic enzymes by mouth (Pancrease, Cotazym-S: preparations that resist destruction by stomach acids)
      2. fat-soluble vitamins A, D, E, and K in water-miscible form
      3. "high-dose" antibiotics for respiratory infections: penicillins, cephalosporins, and aminoglycosides (ticarcillin, piperacillin, tobramycin); NOTE: with aminoglycoside therapy, toxic effects include renal toxicity and ototoxicity
      4. stool softeners, when necessary, for constipation
      5. NaCl tablets added to diet in hot weather, during febrile illness, or strenuous activity; liberal dietary salt encouraged
      6. oral iron supplements
   c. Oxygen therapy, aerosols, nebulizers, bronchodilators
   d. Percussion, postural drainage, and breathing exercises
   e. Sweat chloride testing or gene-marker studies of other family members along with genetic counseling

Nursing Process
ASSESSMENT

1. Effects of mucous gland involvement
   a. Dry, paroxysmal cough
   b. Wheezing
   c. Barrel-shaped chest as child grows older
   d. Cyanosis and clubbing of child's fingers and toes as a result of hypoxia from chronic pulmonary disease
   e. Thick, mucoid, tenacious pulmonary secretions expectorated after chest physical therapy
   f. Because GI tract has a mucoid lining, newborn is at risk of meconium ileus (failure to pass meconium; impacted meconium causes bowel obstruction); older children are also at risk of bowel obstruction caused by fecal impactions
2. Effects of pancreatic involvement
   a. Abdominal distention
   b. Ravenous appetite
   c. Small stature
   d. Delayed puberty
   e. Decreased subcutaneous tissue
   f. Pale, transparent skin
   g. Easy fatigability
   h. Malaise
   i. Fatty, bulky, foul-smelling stools
   j. Rectal prolapse
3. Skin tastes "salty" when kissed

ANALYSIS/NURSING DIAGNOSIS (see p. 463)
PLANNING, IMPLEMENTATION, AND EVALUATION

Goal I Child will maintain effective airway clearance and remain free from pulmonary complications.

Implementation

1. Teach parents how to administer nebulizer treatment with prescribed solution and carry out percussion and

postural drainage at least twice daily, including on arising and at bedtime; discourage treatments immediately before or after meals.

a. Percussion and postural drainage are carried out before and after nebulizer treatment.

b. Nebulizer solution usually contains bronchodilators and saline; mucolytics rarely used.

2. Teach child and family correct administration of medications (antibiotics, bronchodilators, expectorants).

3. Teach child and family breathing exercises (done after postural drainage).

4. Encourage child to engage in physical activities (e.g., swimming, gymnastics, or baseball).

5. Teach child and family general health measures to prevent respiratory infections (e.g, immunizations on time avoid crowds and people with URIs, prevent chilling, no smoking in the home, provide proper nutrition).

6. Observe and record sputum amount, color, and consistency.

7. Review social implications of sputum by age.

a. Two-year-olds and under cannot expectorate.

b. Socially unacceptable for older children to spit, especially for teenager with beginning sexual identity and relationships.

c. Review with older children how to take care of bad breath.

d. If tetracycline given, warn that it stains teeth.

Evaluation

Child and parents implement daily pulmonary therapies; child is free from respiratory infections or they are detected and treated early and vigorously; maintains optimal ventilation.

Goal 2 Child will maintain adequate nutritional and electrolyte intake.

Implementation

1. Give pancreatic enzymes as ordered.

a. Dosage: individualized

b. Side effects: nausea, vomiting, and gastric irritation

c. Taken just before meals to assist digestion

d. Do not crush enteric-coated preparations

e. Capsules may be opened and sprinkled on food, especially with younger children

f. Mix with pureed fruit for infants; older children can swallow capsules

g. Antacid may be prescribed concurrently

h. Monitor I&O, appetite, quality of stools, and weight

2. Encourage intake of balanced nutrition high in protein and carbohydrate (use supplements such as Carnation Instant Breakfast or Sustacal); give snacks with high food value preceded by appropriate amounts of enzymes (these children have additional protein and caloric requirements); fats should be unsaturated.

3. Administer water-miscible vitamins daily.

4. Encourage child to assume responsibility for healthy food selection.

Evaluation

Child's nutritional intake is adequate to meet growth needs.

Goal 3 Child and parents will learn to cope with the chronicity of cystic fibrosis.

Implementation

1. Encourage and permit child and parents to express their feelings regarding diagnosis, its effects, and prognosis.

2. Discourage parents from overprotecting child and interfering with normal developmental processes.

3. Provide ongoing support and teaching as disease progresses.

4. Encourage child to assume age-appropriate responsiblity for care to increase feelings of self-control.

5. Provide positive reinforcement to enhance child's self-esteem.

6. Plan exercise program that allows for optimal growth and development.

7. Refer for genetic counseling: essential for persons with CF and all family members.

8. Support family in decision to seek genetic counseling.

9. Refer to community support groups and Cystic Fibrosis Foundation.

Evaluation

Child and parents verbalize their feelings about the disease, show adaptive behaviors, and seek genetic counseling and community support groups.

Elimination

OVERVIEW OF PHYSIOLOGY

1. Urinary elimination
   a. Kidney development is not complete until approximately 1 year of age
   b. Immature functioning of nephrons; poor filtration and absorption during first year of life; ability to concentrate urine increases gradually during first year of life
   c. Urinary bladder is an abdominal organ during infancy; as pelvic shape changes, the bladder gradually settles and becomes a pelvic organ
   d. Average daily urine output
      1. newborn: 150 to 300 ml
      2. infant: 400 to 500 ml
      3. 1 to 6 years: 500 to 700 ml
      4. 6 to 15 years: 700 to 1400 ml
2. Bowel elimination
   a. Large and small intestines serve as the major organs for detoxification during infancy while the liver and kidneys are maturing
   b. Development of digestive processes is complete by the early toddler years
3. Voluntary control of elimination
   a. Myelinization of the spinal cord is complete by 18 to 24 months of age, resulting in capacity for voluntary control of urinary and anal sphincters
   b. Bladder capacity increases (greater in girls than in boys) as voluntary control is achieved

Application of the Nursing Process to the Child with Elimination Problems

ASSESSMENT

1. Nursing history
   a. Voiding patterns: day and night; frequency; color, clarity, and estimated amount of urine output; recent changes or problems (e.g., nocturia, urgency, dysuria, or infections)
   b. Bowel elimination patterns: frequency, consistency, and color; recent changes or problems (e.g., diarrhea, constipation, or abdominal cramping)
   c. Alterations in elimination: neurogenic bowel and bladder, ostomy, enuresis, encopresis; problem management; medications (e.g., urinary antiseptics, laxatives, antidiarrheal drugs)
2. Clinical appraisal
   a. Observation of urine and stool elimination patterns
   b. Palpation and auscultation of abdomen and bladder

(normally nonpalpable), including bowel sounds (all quadrants) for at least 2 or 3 minutes per quadrant.
3. Diagnostic tests (refer to Nursing Care of the Adult, p. 186)

ANALYSIS/NURSING DIAGNOSIS

1. Safe, effective care environment
   a. Risk for infection
   b. Risk for impaired skin integrity
2. Physiologic integrity
   a. Activity intolerance
   b. Risk for fluid volume deficit/excess
   c. Constipation
   d. Bowel incontinence
   e. Altered urinary elimination
   f. Altered tissue perfusion
3. Psychosocial integrity
   a. Body-image disturbance
   b. Diversional activity deficit
4. Health promotion/maintenance
   a. Altered family processes
   b. Knowledge deficit

GENERAL NURSING PLANNING, IMPLEMENTATION, AND EVALUATION

See Selected Health Problems, following.

SELECTED HEALTH PROBLEMS RESULTING IN AN INTERFERENCE WITH URINARY OR BOWEL ELIMINATION

HYPOSPADIAS

1. Definition: congenital abnormality in which urethral opening is located behind the glans penis or lies on the ventral surface of penis; frequently associated with chordee, which results in a downward curve of penis
2. Treatment
   a. Surgical intervention required to provide normal function and appearance (usually two or three surgeries)
      1. urethroplasty: skin grafting to extend urethra and surgically construct a new urinary meatus
      2. surgical release of chordee
   b. Circumcision is contraindicated because foreskin may be needed for reconstructive surgery

Nursing Process

ASSESSMENT

1. Abnormal placement of urethral meatus
2. Abnormal urine stream
3. Associated problems
   a. Chordee
   b. Undescended testes

ANALYSIS/NURSING DIAGNOSIS (see p. 474)

PLANNING, IMPLEMENTATION, AND EVALUATION

> **Goal 1** Child will maintain integrity of surgical repair.

Implementation

1. Check dressing for evidence of bleeding and to ensure intact dressing.
2. Monitor function of urinary diversion apparatus (permits urine to bypass the operative site).
   a. Foley catheter
   b. Suprapubic tube
   c. Perineal urethrotomy
   d. Urethral stent
3. Check for adequate circulation to tip of penis.
4. Observe for difficulties after catheter removal.
   a. Inability to void
   b. Painful voiding (dysuria)
   c. Urinary tract infection
   d. Hematuria
   e. Urinary frequency
5. Prevent trauma to surgical site.

Evaluation

Child voids normally; maintains dry and intact surgical dressing and site.

> **Goal 2** Parents and child will experience minimal mutilation fears; will cope with altered body image.

Implementation

1. Identify defect in infancy to allow complete surgical repair before 5 to 6 years of age (most common age: 6 to 18 months).
2. Encourage child to express mutilation fears through play before surgery (if age appropriate).
3. Reinforce that surgery is to repair anomaly child was born with and is not punishment for sex play or masturbation.
4. Prepare parents and child for appearance after surgery.
5. Encourage child to examine surgical site after repair to minimize castration anxiety.
6. Encourage expression of parental concerns about child's future sexual functioning.

Evaluation

Parents and child discuss surgical outcome in positive terms; child expresses, through play, appropriate reasons for surgery.

URINARY TRACT INFECTION

1. Definition: bacteriuria with or without signs and symptoms of inflammation of the urinary bladder or kidneys, resulting in risk of renal damage; *E. coli* most common infecting organism
2. Incidence: 1% to 2% of the childhood population; girls have a 10 to 30 times greater risk than boys because of short female urethra close to vagina and anus (5% of girls have a urinary tract infection by age 18); peak age is 2 to 6 years
3. Predisposing factors
   a. Poor perineal hygiene, prolonged use of a single diaper (especially disposable diapers)
   b. Tight-fitting clothing (e.g., blue jeans)
   c. Ureteral reflux caused by congenital malposition of ureters
   d. Concurrent vaginitis or pinworms
   e. Neurogenic bladder
   f. Concentrated and alkaline urine
4. Treatment
   a. Antibiotic therapy: usually ampicillin, cefaclor (Ceclor), amoxicillin, or sulfonamides (e.g., Bactrim, Septra) for short, intensive treatment, 10 to 14 days
   b. Longer-term urinary antiseptic therapy: nitrofurantoin (Furadantin) or methenamine mandelate (Mandelamine) to maintain sterility of urine
   c. Surgical correction of congenital malposition of ureters (ureteral reimplantation) to correct reflux

Nursing Process

ASSESSMENT

1. Frequency, urgency, dysuria, dribbling, enuresis
2. Foul-smelling urine
3. Lower abdominal pain
4. Nausea, poor feeding, lethargy
5. Fever, chills, flank pain (all usually indicate an acute infection of the upper urinary tract)

ANALYSIS/NURSING DIAGNOSIS (see p. 474)

PLANNING, IMPLEMENTATION, AND EVALUATION

> **Goal 1** Child's urinary tract infection will be detected and treated early.

Implementation

1. Ensure that child receives annual routine urinalysis (especially girls, ages 2 to 6 years).
2. Provide age-appropriate preparation of child for intrusive diagnostic tests (usually done under general anesthesia).
3. Emphasize importance of full course of antibiotic therapy and continuing antiseptics even when child has no signs of infection.
4. Emphasize necessity of follow-up urine culture after antibiotic therapy completed.

Evaluation

Child is free from urinary tract infection; has no recurrence.

> **Goal 2** Child and parents will be knowledgeable about prevention of urinary tract infection.

Implementation
1. Teach good hygiene measures.
   a. Wipe front to back.
   b. Avoid bubble baths.
   c. Wear loose-fitting clothing and cotton panties.
2. Caution child not to "hold" urine, but to void as soon as urge is felt.
3. Teach child to empty bladder completely with each voiding.
4. Advise an increase in daily fluid intake, especially fluids that acidify urine (e.g., apple and cranberry juice).

Evaluation
Child is free from urinary tract infection; uses appropriate hygiene measures; empties bladder with each voiding; child's daily fluid intake is adequate.

✖ VESICOURETERAL REFLUX

1. Definition: retrograde flow of bladder urine into the ureters; increases the chance for infection
2. Causes
   a. Primary; results from congenitally abnormal insertion of the ureters into the bladder
   b. Secondary: occurs as a result of infection or a neurogenic bladder
3. Peak age: 46% of infants younger than 23 months with urinary tract infections and 9% of children 24 to 60 months of age with urinary tract infections exhibit vesicoureteral reflux (VUR)
4. Treatment
   a. Continuous, low-dose antibiotic therapy (nitrofurantoin and trimethoprim-sulfamethoxazole)
   b. Frequent urine cultures
   c. Surgical intervention (ureteral reimplantation is the procedure of choice)

Nursing Process

ASSESSMENT
1. Reflux of urine into kidneys
2. Chronic urinary tract infections
3. Associated problems
ANALYSIS/NURSING DIAGNOSIS (see p. 474)
PLANNING, IMPLEMENTATION, AND EVALUATION

> **Goal 1** Child will be free from infection.

Implementation
1. Monitor vital signs.
2. Encourage fluid intake.
3. Monitor urine cultures.
4. Continue to administer antibiotics as ordered.

Evaluation
Child is afebrile, has no complaints of dysuria.

> **Goal 2** Child will maintain integrity of surgical repair.

Implementation
1. Check dressing for intactness and evidence of bleeding.
2. Monitor function of urinary diversion apparatus (suprapubic catheter and left and right ureteral catheters or stent).
3. Monitor separate outputs from each catheter (suprapubic catheter will contain gross blood immediately after surgery).
4. Check bed, cradle, and four-point restraints if used to prevent trauma.
5. Hydrate with IV or oral fluids.
6. Administer postoperative antibiotics as ordered.
7. Observe for difficulties after catheter removal (removed separately beginning 5 to 10 days postoperatively).

Evaluation
The child has clean, dry wound; maintains patency of suprapubic catheter.

> **Goal 3** Child will not retain urine.

Implementation
1. Encourage child to void in a continuous stream and to empty bladder completely.
2. Observe and record amount, color, and frequency of each voided specimen.

Evaluation
Child empties bladder completely with each voiding.

> **Goal 4** Child and parents will understand methods to prevent problems.

Implementation
1. Teach child and family correct administration of antibiotics.
2. Teach regarding general health measures to prevent urinary tract infections (e.g., no bubble baths, empty bladder completely).

Evaluation
Child and parents list and follow measures to prevent further infections.

✖ NEPHRITIS

1. Definition: acute glomerulonephritis (AGN) is an immune complex disease that occurs as a reaction to group-A beta-hemolytic streptococci; causes inflammation and transient damage to the glomerulus; there is a latent period of 10 to 14 days between the streptococcal infection and the onset of symptoms (Table 5-21)
2. Incidence: peak age is 6 to 7 years; history of URI, scarlet fever, strep throat, or impetigo 1 to 3 weeks before the onset of symptoms; 2 times higher incidence in boys
3. Medical treatment
   a. Bed rest until hypertension and hematuria subside
   b. Medication
      1. antibiotics (penicillin) to eradicate streptococcal infection (indicated by an elevated anti-streptolysin-O [ASO] titer)
      2. antihypertensives and diuretics to control BP (diuretics are of limited value because they do not reach the distal tubules)
      3. digitalis (with congestive heart failure)
      4. anticonvulsants (with hypertensive encephalopathy)
   c. Diet
      1. fluid restriction for cardiac failure or anuria

Table 5-21 Comparison of nephrosis and nephritis

	Nephrosis	Nephritis/inflammatory
General information	Chronic condition	*Acute* condition
	Unknown cause	Caused by antigen-antibody response to group-A beta-hemolytic streptococci
Peak age	2-3 years (toddler)	6 years (school-age)
Medications	Prednisone	Antibiotic therapy; possibly antihypertensives and diuretics
Diet	High potassium	Low potassium until urine output normal
Assessment		
Edema	Massive	Moderate, usually facial and periorbital
Blood pressure	Normal	Elevated
Proteinuria	Massive	Moderate
Hematuria	Microscopic	Gross
Serum K$^+$	Normal	Elevated
Hypoproteinemia	Marked	Mild
Hyperlipidemia	Present	Absent

2. moderate sodium restriction
3. low potassium until urine output is normal
4. regular protein

Nursing Process

ASSESSMENT

1. Moderate edema
2. Elevated BP
3. Moderate proteinuria (rarely seen)
4. Gross hematuria
5. Elevated serum K$^+$
6. Mild hypoproteinemia
7. Elevated urine specific gravity
8. ASO titer

ANALYSIS/NURSING DIAGNOSIS (see p. 474)
PLANNING, IMPLEMENTATION, AND EVALUATION

Goal 1 Child will be free from infection and hematuria.

Implementation
1. Monitor temperature.
2. Keep child away from infected persons.
3. Administer antibiotics as ordered.
4. Teach parents administration, action, and side effects of medications.
5. Record frequency of urinary output; test each voided specimen for occult blood.
6. Measure I&O.
7. Restrict fluids if anuria is present.

Evaluation
Child has vital signs and lab values within normal ranges; has normal urine output.

Goal 2 Child will regain and maintain good nutrition within dietary limitations.

Implementation
1. Offer regular diet or low-protein and low-sodium diet if ordered.
2. Offer small, frequent, attractive meals with favorite foods that are allowed.

3. Restrict fluids if anuria is present.
4. Restrict high-potassium foods during oliguria.

Evaluation
Child ingests a diet adequate for age.

Goal 3 Child will maintain normal tissue perfusion.

Implementation
1. Monitor vital signs, especially BP.
2. Monitor urinary output.
3. Observe skin color.
4. Assess changes in edema by weighing daily.
5. Monitor arterial pulses.
6. Administer antihypertensives as ordered.
7. Keep environment calm.

Evaluation
Child is free from renal failure or cardiac decompensation; maintains BP within normal range.

Goal 4 Child and family will be prepared for home care.

Implementation
1. Let family verbalize concerns.
2. Refer to support groups as necessary.
3. Teach the family about
   a. Urine testing
   b. Side effects of drugs
   c. Diet therapies
4. Plan follow-up care.
5. Obtain throat cultures of each family member to check for streptococcal infections.

Evaluation
Child and family accurately describe discharge instructions in their own words.

✖ NEPHROSIS

1. Definition: a chronic condition characterized by glomerular membrane permeability to proteins, especially albumin; also called nephrotic syndrome (Table 5-21)
2. Causes
   a. Idiopathic (80% of cases)

b. Congenital
c. Drug toxicity
d. Sequelae of various diseases
3. Peak age: 2 to 5 years; 60% of those affected are boys
4. Medical treatment
   a. Activity as tolerated unless edematous, then bed rest
   b. Medication
      1. prednisone to reduce proteinuria and edema, induce remission, and produce diuresis
         a. dosage is 2 mg/kg/day until urine is free from protein
         b. side effects: immunosuppression, potassium loss, gastric ulcer, hypertension, growth failure, and Cushing's syndrome
         c. nursing implications
            ▪ taper dose gradually to avoid adrenal insufficiency
            ▪ administer with meals or milk to minimize gastric irritation
            ▪ monitor fluid balance
            ▪ protect from infection
      2. antibiotics to decrease risk of infection
      3. IV salt-poor albumin during acute phase
   c. Diet
      1. fluid and sodium restriction if edema present
      2. high protein, high potassium

Nursing Process
ASSESSMENT
1. Insidious weight gain
2. Severe edema
   a. Periorbital, facial
   b. Generalized: feet, scrotum/labia, ascites
3. Respiratory difficulty because of pleural effusion
4. Oliguria, increased urine specific gravity
5. Massive proteinuria
6. Marked hypoproteinemia
7. Hyperlipidemia
8. Irritability
9. Increased susceptibility to infection
10. Anorexia
11. Diarrhea
ANALYSIS/NURSING DIAGNOSIS (see p. 474)
PLANNING, IMPLEMENTATION, AND EVALUATION

Goal 1 Child will be free from infection and skin breakdown.

Implementation
1. Monitor vital signs and lab values.
2. Keep child away from infected persons.
3. Administer antibiotics as ordered.
4. Give medications by mouth if possible.
5. Teach parents administration, action, and side effects of medications.
6. Give meticulous skin care.
7. Support edematous organs (if needed, support scrotum with pillows or a rolled towel).
8. Change body position often.
9. Cleanse edematous eyelids with saline wipes.

10. Place in a semi-Fowler's position to facilitate breathing.
11. Handle gently with any movement.
Evaluation
Child has intact skin; has normal vital signs, lab values.

Goal 2 Child will conserve energy and play quiet activities suitable for age.

Implementation
1. Balance rest and activities; maintain bed rest with edema.
2. Provide quiet activities for age.
3. Observe for fatigue.
4. Explain reasons for bed rest.
Evaluation
Child tolerates play activities without fatigue.

Goal 3 Child will maintain fluid balance.

Implementation
1. Measure I&O; weigh diapers.
2. Weigh and measure abdominal girth daily.
3. Assess changes in edema each shift.
4. Limit fluids if necessary.
Evaluation
Child has no generalized edema or increased abdominal girth; maintains urine output, balanced I&O.

Goal 4 Child will maintain nutritional intake.

Implementation
1. Offer high-protein, high-carbohydrate, high-potassium diet.
2. Restrict sodium intake if edematous.
3. Serve small, frequent, attractive meals.
Evaluation
Child eats an adequate diet for age (within dietary restrictions).

Goal 5 Child will accept body changes.

Implementation
1. Provide feedback to child about body changes; reassure as needed.
2. Encourage child to verbalize feelings about body changes.
3. Teach child that changes are caused by medications and will diminish when medications are discontinued.
Evaluation
Child expresses feeling about body changes, capitalizes on positive aspects of self, looks forward to discontinuing medications.

Goal 6 Child and family will be prepared for home care.

Implementation
1. Let family verbalize concerns.
2. Refer to support groups as needed.
3. Teach about
    a. Urine testing
    b. Side effects of drugs
    c. Prevention of infection
    d. Diet therapies
4. Maintain follow-up contact with the family.

Evaluation
Child and family describe discharge instructions correctly.

✖ LOWER GASTROINTESTINAL TRACT OBSTRUCTION

1. Definitions
    a. *Intussusception:* telescoping of one portion of intestine into another, usually involving ileocecal valve, resulting in obstruction of blood supply with ischemia and death of telescoped portion; one of the most common causes of intestinal obstruction in infancy; most cases occur in previously healthy children under 2 years of age; 3 times more common in boys; higher incidence in children with cystic fibrosis and celiac disease
    b. *Hirschsprung's disease* (aganglionic megacolon): congenital absence of parasympathetic ganglia of distal colon and rectum, resulting in inadequate peristalsis; stool and flatus accumulate in colon proximal to defect, causing dilation and hypertrophy of bowel; usually diagnosed in neonatal period or early infancy; 4 times more common in boys; higher incidence in children with Down syndrome
2. Treatment
    a. *Intussusception*
        1. hydrostatic reduction with barium enema before bowel becomes necrotic
        2. surgical intervention (resection and anastomosis) if bowel necrosis has occurred
    b. *Hirschsprung's disease*
        1. barium enema to aid diagnosis
        2. rectal biopsy to confirm absence of ganglion cells
        3. resection of aganglionic portion of bowel, temporary colostomy of sigmoid or transverse colon to rest bowel and restore nutritional balance; abdominal-perineal pull-through anastomosis at approximately 1 year of age

Nursing Process

ASSESSMENT
1. *Intussusception:* acute, recurrent, episodic, severe, colicky, abdominal pain; "currant jelly" stools containing blood and mucus, caused by bowel gangrene (occurs about 12 hours after onset of abdominal pain); palpable sausage-shaped mass in right upper quadrant
2. *Hirschsprung's disease*
    a. Delayed passage of meconium in newborn; failure to thrive
    b. Chronic constipation
    c. Ribbonlike, foul-smelling stools
    d. Breath has foul odor
    e. Severe abdominal distention with shortness of breath

    f. At risk for enterocolitis, which increases risk of fatality
3. Both
    a. Bile-stained vomiting (the obstruction is below ampulla of Vater, which empties bile into duodenum)
    b. Abdominal distention

ANALYSIS/NURSING DIAGNOSIS (see p. 474)
PLANNING, IMPLEMENTATION, AND EVALUATION

> **Goal 1** Child will maintain adequate hydration and nutrition and regain normal elimination.

Implementation
1. Give IV fluids as ordered; hyperalimentation may be ordered for infants with Hirschsprung's disease.
2. Usually keep NPO; give mouth care, pacifier.
3. Keep accurate I&O; measure and record drainage (NG, colostomy); irrigate NG tube as ordered.
4. Assess bowel sounds frequently.
5. Take axillary temperature only.
6. Gradually reintroduce feedings and return to normal diet postoperatively after NG tube has been removed and bowel sounds have returned.

Evaluation
Child is adequately hydrated (elastic skin turgor, moist mucous membranes, etc.), has adequate caloric intake; returns to normal diet without complications (e.g., vomiting); is free from abdominal distention and establishes normal bowel elimination postoperatively.

> **Goal 2** Child with colostomy/ileostomy will have intact, functioning stoma without irritation or infection.

Implementation
1. Refer to Mechanical Obstruction of the Colon, p. 215.
2. Instruct child and parent about stoma care.
    a. Diaper only may be used in infants with sigmoid colostomy.
    b. Select appliance that fits child's size, activity level, and development.
    c. Use hypoallergenic supplies, because children's skin tends to be more sensitive; assess skin around stoma frequently; prevent breakdown.
    d. Encourage self-care.
        1. by 6 or 7 years, child should be able to remove and reapply pouch with assistance
        2. by 10 to 11 years, child should be able to assume all responsibility
3. Inspect stoma daily for redness, irritation, or breakdown.
4. Do not submerge colostomy in bath water.
5. Refer parents to local ostomy association for assistance and support.

Evaluation
Child has healthy, functioning stoma; becomes involved in developmentally appropriate self-care.

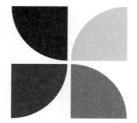

Mobility

OVERVIEW OF PHYSIOLOGY
1. Skeletal maturation
   a. Continued growth of bones and muscles throughout childhood
   b. Determined by accurate "bone age" through x-ray of ossification centers
   c. Correlates closely with other measures of physiologic maturity (e.g., onset of menarche) rather than with height or chronologic age
   d. Complete when epiphysis fuses completely with diaphysis, usually 18 to 21 years of age (earlier in girls than boys)
2. Differences in children's skeletal system compared with adults'
   a. Thick periosteum: stronger, more active osteogenic potential
   b. More plastic (pliable) bone: more porous, allows bending and buckling; this flexibility diffuses and absorbs a significant amount of the force of impact
   c. Rapid healing: decreases as child gets older (younger bones can be remolded more easily)
   d. Stiffness is unusual, even after lengthy immobilization
   e. Tendons and ligaments more flexible in children
   f. Injuries and treatments may be complicated by continuing growth of the child.

Application of the Nursing Process to the Child with an Interference with Mobility
ASSESSMENT
1. Nursing assessment
   a. Development of motor skills; delays, recent changes or interferences
   b. Signs and symptoms of current health problem; pain, altered structure or mobility
2. Clinical appraisal
   a. Muscle strength and symmetry
   b. Balance, gait, and posture
   c. Range of motion
   d. Obvious structural deformities or functional deficits
3. Radiologic tests of affected body part (refer to Nursing Care of the Adult, p. 246)

ANALYSIS/NURSING DIAGNOSIS
1. Physiologic integrity
   a. Risk for aspiration
   b. Impaired physical mobility
   c. Risk for altered peripheral tissue perfusion

2. Safe, effective care environment
   a. Risk for injury
   b. Knowledge deficit
   c. Risk for infection
3. Psychosocial integrity
   a. Body-image disturbance
   b. Social isolation
   c. Altered role performance
4. Health promotion/maintenance
   a. Altered growth and development
   b. Diversional activity deficit
   c. Bathing/hygiene self-care deficit

GENERAL NURSING PLANNING, IMPLEMENTATION, AND EVALUATION

Goal 1 Child's deformity will be detected and treated early.

Implementation
1. Screen child for skeletal deformity.
   a. In newborn period for congenital clubfoot and congenital hip dysplasia
   b. During preadolescence and adolescence for scoliosis
2. Refer child with possible deformity for immediate treatment.
3. Teach child and parents the importance of adhering to prescribed treatment plan to minimize or prevent serious, permanent deformity.
4. Stress importance of continued follow-up care to prevent recurrence.

Evaluation
Child's deformity is detected at an early age; parents initiate recommended treatment plan.

Goal 2 Child will maintain correct alignment of the affected body part during the period of treatment.

Implementation
1. Ensure that parents and child use braces and splints as prescribed.
2. For child in traction, ensure maintenance of effectiveness (Fig. 5-4; Tables 5-22 and 5-23).
   a. Maintain traction apparatus (elastic bandages, splints, rings, ropes, pulleys, and weights).
   b. Do not allow weights to rest on floor or bed.

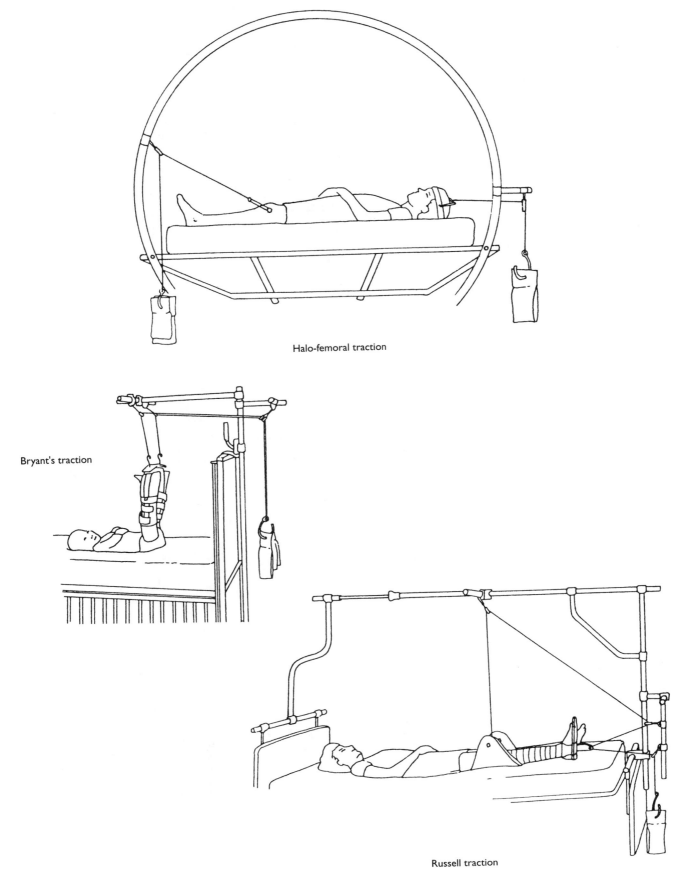

Halo-femoral traction

Bryant's traction

Russell traction

Fig. 5-4 Types of traction. (90° traction from Whaley L, Wong D: *Essentials of pediatric nursing,* ed 4, St Louis, 1991, Mosby.)

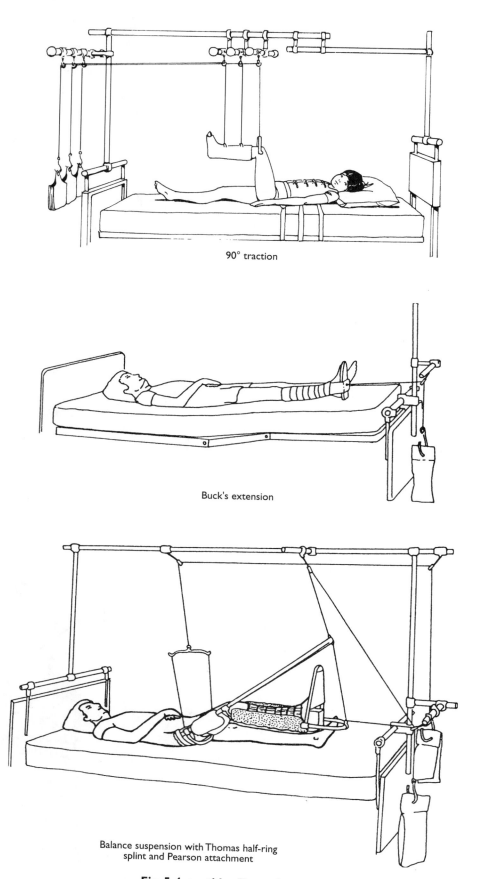

90° traction

Buck's extension

Balance suspension with Thomas half-ring
splint and Pearson attachment

Fig. 5-4, cont'd   Types of traction.

Table 5-22 Types of traction

GENERAL

Skin traction	Direct pull to skin surface and indirect pull to skeletal structures by means of adhesive strips or elastic bandage.
Skeletal traction	Direct pull to skeletal structures by means of pin, wire, or tongs inserted into bone distal to fracture.

SPECIFIC

Bryant's traction	Unidirectional, lower-extremity skin traction with child's hips flexed at 90-degree angle, knees extended, and legs and buttocks suspended (must weigh <26 lb).
Buck's extension	Skin traction to lower extremity with hips and legs extended. Used mostly when short-term traction is needed.
Russell traction	Two-directional, lower-extremity skin traction with padded knee sling; immobilizes hip and knee in flexed position. One pull line is longitudinal; the other is perpendicular to leg. Traction pull is twice the amount of weight applied.
Balance suspension with Thomas ring splint and Pearson attachment	Two-directional, skin or skeletal traction that suspends leg with hip slightly flexed; Thomas ring circles uppermost portion of the thigh while Pearson attachment supports lower part of leg. Alignment is maintained even when child lifts off bed.
Halo-femoral traction	Metal rings (halo) are attached to the skull and pins are inserted into distal femur also. Progressive traction is applied upward to the halo and downward to the distal end of the femur, increasing weights twice daily until alignment is achieved.

Table 5-23 Traction care

Purposes	Immobilize, realign fractures and reduce dislocations, stretch soft tissue, and reduce muscle spasm.
Types: Skin	Indirect pull to skeletal structure by means of direct pull to skin surface using adhesive or elastic bandage (example: Buck's traction).
Skeletal	Direct pull to skeletal structures by means of pins, wires, or tongs inserted into bone distal to the fracture or deformity (example: Halo-femoral traction).
Maintenance of dynamic traction	Weights swinging freely, body in correct alignment, maintenance of countertraction (body weight, shock blocks, feet not against foot of bed, ropes without obstruction through pulleys).
Nursing care	Understand the purpose of the traction, ensure adequate neurovascular function (check color, sensation, motor function, pulses, and especially presence of severe pain qh for 24 hours, then q4h), ensure skin integrity under adhesive and elastic bandage of skin traction, clean skin around skeletal pins and wires of skeletal traction.

c. Maintain correct body alignment (emphasis on shoulder, hip, and leg alignment).

d. Elevate head or foot of bed as needed to provide correct pull and countertraction.

e. Assess skin color, sensation, and movement of extremity every hour for the first 48 hours, then every 4 hours.

Table 5-24 Cast care

Purposes	Immobilization, realignment.
Types	Plaster or fiberglass; cylinder, cast brace, hip spica, other.
Nursing care	Ensure adequate neurovascular function (check color, sensation, motor function, pulses, and especially presence of severe pain qh for 24 hours, then q4h); observe for signs of infection under cast (fever, odor, drainage); observe for signs of bleeding under cast in postoperative period; protect skin around edges of cast by applying "petals" or soft, waterproof tape (Moleskin) (see Fig. 5-5); protect cast from soil of urine and stool; remove small toys from environment that can fit under cast and cause skin breakdown; change position as necessary; enhance drying of plaster cast by allowing for free air circulation to the plaster (use blankets on uncasted body parts); turn patient to ensure drying of all areas of cast; for hip spica care: give special attention to cleanliness by meticulous care with elimination to avoid soiling; do not use stabilizer bar for lifting.

3. Provide for care of child in cast (Table 5-24; see Nursing Care of the Adult, p. 248).

a. "Petal" cast edges of plaster cast (protects cast and skin); use waterproof adhesive tape petals (see Fig. 5-5).

b. Protect cast from being soiled with urine or stool (position child with buttocks lower than shoulders during toileting).

c. Use Bradford frame for smaller children.

d. Provide toys too large to fit down cast; make sure there are no removable small parts.

e. Stay with child during mealtimes and snacks.

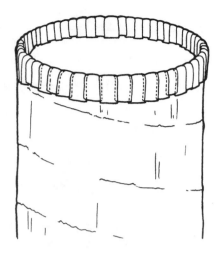

Fig. 5-5 Petaled cast edges.

f. Observe for signs of impaired circulation and infection (fever, lethargy, foul odor); do *not* rely on child to verbalize discomfort; change position frequently; do *not* use abduction-stabilizer bar on hip spica as a handle for turning child.
4. Provide exercise to maintain range of motion.

Evaluation

Child maintains correct alignment of affected body part; has permanent deformity prevented; parents provide appropriate care to child in cast, splint, or brace.

Goal 3 Child's skin integrity will be maintained during period of immobilization.

Implementation

1. Assess for areas of skin breakdown.
2. Change position frequently or encourage movement within limitations imposed by traction, cast, or brace to relieve pressure.
3. Check pin sites (skeletal traction) for bleeding, drainage, redness, edema, and signs of infection.
4. Clean pin insertion sites q8h.
5. Monitor neurovascular status of extremities (normal skin color, blanches easily, warm to touch; able to wiggle fingers and toes; peripheral pulses present). (See Tables 5-23 and 5-24.)
6. Provide meticulous skin care to areas near edges of cast or in contact with brace or traction apparatus.
7. Petal cast edges if necessary.

Evaluation

Child's skin is free from skin breakdown or infection.

Goal 4 Child's developmental progress will be maintained during immobilization.

Implementation

1. Provide age-appropriate stimulation and activity.
2. Encourage child to participate in own daily care and maintain control as much as possible.

3. Provide for child to maintain educational progress while immobilized (hospital teacher, homebound teacher, daily contact with regular teacher).
4. Arrange for and encourage interaction with peers and siblings (telephone at bedside).

Evaluation

Child maintains developmental and educational progress while immobilized; has no developmental delays; participates in own care.

SELECTED HEALTH PROBLEMS RESULTING IN AN INTERFERENCE WITH MOBILITY

❧ CONGENITAL CLUBFOOT

1. Definition: congenital deformity of the bones, muscles, tendons, and ligaments resulting in fixed inversion and platar flexion of the foot; may be unilateral or bilateral
2. Incidence: 1 in 1000; boys more often than girls, unilateral more frequent than bilateral
3. Medical treatment: serial casting; if unsuccessful: surgical correction

Nursing Process

See Application of Nursing Process: Analysis; General Nursing Planning, Implementation, and Evaluation.

Follow-up is essential because the deformity tends to reoccur over time.

ASSESSMENT

1. Differentiate true clubfoot from positional deformity.
   a. True clubfoot cannot be passively manipulated into an overcorrected position.
   b. Positional deformity can be passively corrected or overcorrected.

ANALYSIS/NURSING DIAGNOSIS (see p. 480)

PLANNING, IMPLEMENTATION, AND EVALUATION (see General Nursing Plans, p. 480)

❧ DISLOCATION OF THE HIP

1. Definition: head of the femur displaced from the acetabulum
   a. *Subluxation:* head of femur partially displaced but remains in contact with acetabulum
   b. *Complete dislocation of hip:* head of femur completely displaced
2. Incidence
   a. Developmental dislocation of the hip (DDH): occurs in infancy; more frequent in females; increased incidence in breech deliveries and among siblings of affected children
   b. Neurogenic dislocation of the hip: in the neurologically impaired (such as spina bifida, cerebral palsy)
3. Medical treatment: in the newborn, Pavlik harness; in older infants and children, traction, then open reduction and spica casting

Nursing Process
ASSESSMENT
1. *Infant*
   a. Limited abduction of affected hip
   b. Wide perineum
   c. Shortening of leg on affected side (Galeazzi's sign, Allis' sign)
   d. Asymmetry of thigh and gluteal folds
   e. Positive Ortolani's sign: clicking when leg abducted, caused by femoral head slipping over acetabulum (infant under 4 weeks of age)
   f. Barlow's sign: hand placed over knee, adduct leg past midline; abnormal movement is positive response
2. *Older child*
   a. Trendelenburg's sign: when child stands on affected leg, pelvis tilts downward on unaffected side instead of upward
   b. Limp on affected side
   c. Flattening of buttock on affected side

ANALYSIS/NURSING DIAGNOSIS (see p. 480)
PLANNING, IMPLEMENTATION, AND EVALUATION (see General Nursing Plans, p. 480)

🕸 LEGG-CALVÉ-PERTHES DISEASE
1. Definition: self-limiting avascular necrosis of the femoral head sometimes resulting in deformity of the hip joint
2. Incidence
   a. Onset between 3 and 11 years of age
   b. Four times more common in boys
   c. Usually unilateral; 15% bilateral
3. Treatment: controversial; may include non–weight-bearing traction; range-of-motion exercises; bracing in abduction; and perhaps osteotomy
   a. Bed rest and skin traction to the limb during the painful initial period
   b. Some weight bearing allowed after resolution of the initial stage of the disease; use of abduction braces, casts, or hip sling
   c. Full weight bearing if no new dense areas develop in femoral head in 2 months
   d. Surgical osteotomy of femur done if medical management is ineffective

Nursing Process
ASSESSMENT
Insidious onset of knee, thigh, or hip pain; stiffness; limited range of motion.
ANALYSIS/NURSING DIAGNOSIS (see p. 480)
PLANNING, IMPLEMENTATION, AND EVALUATION (see General Nursing Plans, p. 480)

🕸 SCOLIOSIS
1. Definition: lateral curvature and rotation of the spine
2. Incidence
   a. Affects 15% of children between ages 10 and 21
   b. Eight times more common in adolescent females
   c. 70% of cases are idiopathic (i.e., without apparent cause)
   d. May be associated with other disorders (spina bifida, cerebral palsy, muscular dystrophy, congenital abnormalities of the vertebral bodies)

3. Treatment
   a. Nonsurgical management techniques
      1. long-term monitoring
      2. bracing: two basic types
         a. Boston brace—underarm brace used for lumbar curves; made of molded plastic
         b. Milwaukee brace—an individually adapted steel-and-leather brace extending from chin to pelvis
   b. Surgical management techniques (curves greater than 40 degrees)
      1. Harrington instrumentation: metal rods implanted to hold vertebrae and bone fragments for permanent fusion
      2. Luque segmental instrumentation: flexible L-shaped metal rod fixed by wires to spinous processes; NOTE: child can get up and walk within a few days, and no postoperative immobilization is necessary
      3. Dwyer instrumentation: cable through cannulated screws that are fixed to each vertebra
      4. Cotrel-Dubousset procedure: bilateral segmental fixation using two knurled rods and multiple hooks

Nursing Process
ASSESSMENT
1. Screening of all children as newborns and especially during the school-age and adolescent years
2. Spinal curve may be obvious
3. Elevated shoulder or hip
4. Structural asymmetry (scapulae, waist, hips, shoulders, breasts)
5. Rib hump apparent when child bends at waist

ANALYSIS/NURSING DIAGNOSIS (see p. 480)
PLANNING, IMPLEMENTATION, AND EVALUATION

> **Goal** Adolescent and family will adjust to lengthy treatment regimen.

Implementation
1. Allow adolescent and parents to express feelings and concerns about long-term bracing or casting (6 months to 3 years for medical intervention).
2. Help adolescent cope with altered body image.
   a. Emphasize and enhance positive attributes (hair, makeup).
   b. Help with selection of attractive camouflage clothing.
   c. Encourage involvement in appropriate activities (choir, school clubs, etc.).
3. Demonstrate alternative ways of getting in and out of bed, dressing, and so on.
4. Advise standing at drafting table or easel for homework.
5. Teach application and removal of brace (must wear 23 hours per day; remove for 1 hour for hygiene or swimming).
6. Teach adolescent to wear T-shirt under brace.
7. Check for loosening of the brace; tighten the brace as necessary.

8. Keep brace clean: wash plastic with soap and water, clean leather with saddle soap.
9. Provide for needs of adolescent after surgical intervention (spinal fusion).
   a. Keep bed flat; log-roll q2h (varies with type of procedure).
   b. Assess circulatory and neurologic status of lower extremities.
   c. Administer analgesics for pain.
   d. Monitor incision sites for bleeding and signs of infection.
   e. Monitor respiratory status.
   f. Cough and deep breathe; use incentive spirometry.
   g. Monitor fluid and electrolyte status

Evaluation

Child adheres to treatment regimen; recovers from surgery free from complications and disability; adjusts to new body image.

MUSCULAR DYSTROPHY

1. Definition: a group of progressively degenerative inherited diseases of the connective tissue. Duchenne's muscular dystrophy is the most common of several forms of muscular dystrophy.
2. Incidence: Duchenne's muscular dystrophy occurs in 1 in 3000 male children; sex-linked recessive pattern of inheritance.
3. Treatment: range of motion, bracing, and surgery to maintain mobility and independence for as long as possible; maximize repiratory function; prevent obesity.

Nursing Process

ASSESSMENT

Monitor male children in families with history for delayed motor development; monitor weight gain, respiratory function, mobility, independence, and family coping abilities.

ANALYSIS/NURSING DIAGNOSIS

See Application of the Nursing Process, p. 480.

PLANNING, IMPLEMENTATION, AND EVALUATION

Implementation

1. Maintain optimum respiratory hygiene through use of incentive spirometry and other activities.
2. Minimize weight gain by anticipating and teaching dietary practices.

Evaluation

Condition is identified early and treated to reduce deformity and maintain independence for as long as possible; family is able to cope with child's long-term illness.

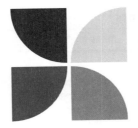

Cellular Aberration (Childhood Cancer)

See also Nursing Care of the Adult, p. 257.

OVERVIEW OF PHYSIOLOGY

1. Cancer: leading cause of death from disease between the ages of 3 and 15
   a. Leukemias and lymphomas account for more than 40% of childhood malignancies
   b. Brain tumors account for 20% of childhood cancers
   c. Embryonal tumors (e.g., Wilms' tumor and neuroblastoma) and sarcomas account for another 20% of childhood malignancies
   d. The survival rate for childhood cancer has dramatically increased in the last two decades, especially for acute lymphocytic leukemia
2. Differences in childhood cancers as compared with adult cancers
   a. Higher incidence of embryonal tumors
   b. Occur more frequently in rapidly growing tissues, such as bone marrow
   c. Higher rate of metastasis
3. Treatment
   a. Surgery: excision of all or part of solid tumors; may only be palliative if cancer has metastasized; most successful with localized and encapsulated tumors
   b. Chemotherapy: administration of antineoplastic drugs
      1. classification
         a. cell-cycle specific: destroys cells in specific phases of cell division
            ▪ most effective for rapidly growing cells
            ▪ least toxic
            ▪ examples: cytosine arabinoside, methotrexate
         b. cell-cycle nonspecific: destroys cells at any phase
            ▪ most effective for slow-growing, solid tumors
            ▪ examples: alkylating agents, hormones, antibiotics, nitrosoureas
         c. cytotoxic action (see Table 5-25 for specific drugs)
            ▪ alkylating agents: alkyl group; replaces hydrogen atom, causing cell to die
            ▪ antimetabolites: similar to essential elements needed for cell growth, but in altered form; prevent synthesis of DNA or RNA
            ▪ plant alkaloids: stop cell growth in metaphase
            ▪ antitumor antibiotics: interfere with cell division by reacting with DNA and RNA

            ▪ hormones, adrenocorticosteroids: depress mitosis of lymphoid cells; androgens and estrogens are used for breast and prostatic cancers, probably affecting growth regulation
            ▪ miscellaneous agents: enzymes, such as L-asparaginase, hydroxyurea, nitrosoureas; metals such as cisplatin
      2. combination chemotherapy: two or more drugs used simultaneously; each drug has a different effect on cell growth; increases effectiveness, decreases resistance of cancer cells to drugs
   c. Irradiation: frequently used in childhood cancers as an adjunct to surgery or chemotherapy; may be curative or palliative

Application of the Nursing Process to the Child with Cancer

ASSESSMENT

1. Nursing history (see Nursing Care of the Adult, p. 258)
2. Clinical appraisal: physical findings will vary according to the type of cancer
3. Diagnostic tests: same as for adult except that bone marrow aspiration is usually performed on the posterior iliac crest

ANALYSIS/NURSING DIAGNOSIS

1. Safe, effective care environment
   a. Risk for infection
   b. Risk for injury
   c. Impaired home maintenance management
2. Physiologic integrity
   a. Pain
   b. Diarrhea, constipation
   c. Fluid volume deficit
3. Psychosocial integrity
   a. Fear
   b. Social isolation
   c. Ineffective individual coping
4. Health promotion/maintenance
   a. Knowledge deficit
   b. Altered parenting
   c. Altered growth and development

GENERAL NURSING PLANNING, IMPLEMENTATION, AND EVALUATION

Goal I Child and family will be prepared for diagnostic tests.

Table 5-25 Commonly used chemotherapeutic agents

Drug	Uses	Side effects	Specific nursing concerns
ALKYLATING AGENTS			
Cyclophosphamide (Cytoxan)	Hodgkin's and other lymphomas Leukemias Neuroblastomas Retinoblastomas Multiple myeloma	Nausea and vomiting, occurring 2-6 hours after administration and lasting up to 48 hours Bone marrow depression (BMD) Alopecia	Chemical cystitis may result; force fluids, report burning or hematuria.
Mechlorethamine (nitrogen mustard, Mustargen)		Severe nausea and vomiting (½-8 hours later) BMD Alopecia Local phlebitis	Use immediately after reconstitution. Avoid vapors in eyes; if solution comes into contact with skin, flush with liberal amounts of water. Ensure IV is in place to prevent necrosis and sloughing.
Chlorambucil (Leukeran)		Mild nausea and vomiting, BMD, diarrhea Dermatitis	Side effects occur slowly and with high doses.
Cisplatin			Toxic to kidneys and ears; can cause anaphylaxis. Hydrate well before and during treatment with IVs and mannitol. Monitor renal function and audiograms.
ANTIMETABOLITES			
5-Fluorouracil (5-FU, Adrucil)	Acute lymphocytic leukemia; acute myelocytic leukemia; brain tumors; ovarian, breast, prostatic, testicular cancers	Mild to moderate nausea and vomiting Bone marrow depression Stomatitis Dermatitis Photosensitivity	Chronic nausea and vomiting with prolonged use. Check oral mucosa. If stomatitis and diarrhea are severe, stop drug.
Methotrexate (MTX)			Report signs of neurotoxicity immediately. Toxic to liver and kidney; avoid aspirin, sulfonamides, and tetracycline while on drug. Avoid vitamins containing folic acid. Leucovorin used as an antidote for high doses ("leucovorin rescue"). When outdoors, use sun screen.
6 Mercaptopurine (6-MP)	Allopurinol given concurrently increases drug's potency.		
Cytosine arabinoside (ara-C, Cytosar-U)			Crosses blood-brain barrier; may be hepatotoxic, monitor liver function.
PLANT ALKALOIDS			
Vincristine (Oncovin)	Acute lymphocytic leukemia, Hodgkin's disease, Wilms' tumor, sarcomas, breast cancer, testicular cancer	Minimal nausea and vomiting Alopecia Neurotoxicity	
Vinblastine (Velban) VP-16-213 (Etoposide, VePesid)		Neurotoxicity Fever SIADH	Monitor for neurotoxicity: reflexes, weakness, parasthesias, jaw pain, constipation. Check IV placement to prevent cellulitis. Headaches; less neurotoxic than vincristine.

Table 5-25 Commonly used chemotherapeutic agents—cont'd

Drug	Uses	Side effects	Specific nursing concerns
ANTITUMOR ANTIBIOTICS			
Bleomycin (Blenox-ane)	Sarcomas; neuroblastomas; head and neck tumors; testicular, ovarian, breast cancer		
Dacitnromycin (Cosme-gen, Actinomycin-D)		Mild nausea and vomiting Allergic reaction—fever, chills, anaphylaxis Pneumonitis Nausea and vomiting (2-5 hours later) BMD, immunosuppression Mucosal ulceration Alopecia	Should give test dose (SC) before therapeutic dose administered. Have emergency drugs at bedside. Used for Wilms' tumor; enhances effects of radiation (also increases toxicity). Extravasation can cause necrosis; maintain patent IV.
Doxorubicin hydro-chloride (Adriamy-cin)		Moderate nausea and vomiting Stomatitis BMD (7-14 days later)	Monitor for cardiac dysrrhythmias (cardio-toxicity is irreversible). Caution that urine turns red.
HORMONES			

Adrenocorticosteroids
  Prednisone
  Dexamethasone (Decadron)
	Leukemia, Hodgkin's disease, breast cancer, lymphomas, multiple myeloma, cerebral edema caused by brain metastasis	See Table 3-34	See Table 3-34

Androgens
  Testosterone (Ore-ton)
  Fluoxymesterone (Halotestin)
	Breast cancer in postmenopausal women	Fluid retention
		Nausea
		Masculinization
			Give low-sodium diet; provide psychologic support for masculinization effects.

Estrogens
  Diethylstilbestrol (DES)
  Ethinyl estradiol (Estinyl)
	Prostatic cancer, breast cancer that is estrogen-receptor positive in postmenopausal women	Fluid retention
		Feminization
		Gynecomastia in males
			Give low-sodium diet; provide psychologic support to males experiencing feminization.

Antiestrogens Tamoxifen (Nolva-dex)	Breast cancer; prostatic cancer	Hot flashes Generally mild nausea	
MISCELLANEOUS AGENTS			
Enzymes L-asparaginase (Els-par)	Leukemias, Hodgkin's disease		
Procarbazine (Matu-lane)		Severe nausea and vomiting; fever Liver dysfunction Anaphylaxis Nausea and vomiting (moderate) BMD Dermatitis Myalgia	Monitor BUN and serum ammonia levels. Observe for allergic reaction (have epinephrine 1:1000 at bedside). MAO inhibition sometimes occurs—all other drugs should be avoided unless medically approved.

Implementation
1. Provide age-appropriate explanation of procedure (what will happen, what it will feel like, what child is expected to do).
2. Give parents option of staying with child during procedure so they can provide needed emotional support to child.
3. Hold child firmly during procedure to facilitate needle insertion (e.g., bone marrow aspiration, lumbar puncture).
4. Reassure child throughout procedure.
5. After the procedure, provide child opportunities to express feelings (verbally, through therapeutic play).
6. Provide positive feedback to child concerning child's cooperation during the procedure.

Evaluation

Child copes with diagnostic procedures; cooperates with procedure; expresses feelings during and after procedure.

Goal 2 Child and family will be prepared for surgery (refer to The Ill and Hospitalized Child, p. 412).

Goal 3 Child and family will be prepared for chemotherapy.

Implementation

1. Explain benefits of chemotherapy, using terms the child and family can understand.
2. Reinforce physician's explanation of types of chemotherapy child will receive.
3. Explain side effects that may occur and identify measures that will help lessen side effects.
   a. Nausea and vomiting: administer antiemetics before chemotherapy; ensure adequate hydration
   b. Diarrhea: administer antispasmodics, adjust diet; monitor perianal skin condition
   c. Anorexia: monitor weight; provide soft diet; small, frequent feedings; favorite foods and liquids; give choices
   d. Stomatitis (see Goal 6)
   e. Alopecia: provide wig, scarf, or hat as desired; reassure that hair will grow back
   f. Fatigue: provide frequent rest periods, encourage quiet activities

Evaluation

Child and family list side effects; implement measures that minimize these effects and promote/enhance child's comfort.

Goal 4: Child and family will be prepared for radiation therapy.

Implementation

1. Reinforce reasons for and benefits of radiation.
2. Prepare for and manage side effects of radiation therapy.
   a. Nausea and vomiting: administer prescribed antiemetics as needed, bland diet, clear liquids
   b. Peeling skin: meticulous skin care; avoid direct exposure to sun; do not wash off skin markings (dark purple lines that define area to be irradiated)
   c. Risk of fracture: explain to child and family why child should avoid weight bearing; help plan to meet child's need for mobility through alternative means, such as crutches or stimulating activities while on bed rest
   d. Delays in physical development: discuss possible outcomes with parents and child (as appropriate) such as pathologic fractures, spinal deformities, growth retardation, sterility, delayed appearance of secondary sex characteristics, chromosomal damage

Evaluation

Child and family state reasons for radiation and knowledge of side effects that may occur.

Goal 5 Child will be free from infection.

Implementation

1. Maintain reverse isolation, or private room with strict hand washing if child is severely immunosuppressed.
2. Prevent contact with anyone with infection.
3. Have child rinse mouth regularly before meals, after meals, and q4h (removes debris as a source for growth of bacteria and fungi).
4. Administer antibiotics and observe for side effects.
5. Take measures to prevent skin breakdown.
6. Do not give immunizations until child's immune response is adequate.
7. Permit return to school when WBCs approach normal level (2000/mm^3).

Evaluation

Child remains free from infection; maintains skin integrity; child and family correctly assess immune response, risk factors, and modify lifestyle appropriately.

Goal 6 Child will receive care for ulcerations of mouth and rectal area.

Implementation

1. Provide meticulous oral hygiene before and after meals.
2. Offer mouthwash frequently; apply local anesthetic (viscous lidocaine [Xylocaine]) prn.
3. Encourage fluids, nonirritating foods (soft foods, cool drinks).
4. Avoid rectal temperatures and suppositories.
5. Encourage sitz baths; offer pericare after voiding or bowel movement.
6. Expose ulcerated anal area to air and heat.

Evaluation

Child is free from increased ulceration; experiences healing of lesions in mouth and rectum.

Goal 7 Child will ingest foods and fluids to meet nutritional needs.

Implementation

1. Rinse mouth before child eats.
2. Offer small, frequent meals.
3. Provide soft foods; permit favorite foods child tolerates.
4. Use nutritional supplements.

Evaluation

Child maintains appropriate nutrition and hydration status to meet developmental needs.

Goal 8 Child's pain will be relieved and comfort promoted.

Implementation

1. Administer nonnarcotic and narcotic analgesics as needed; consider "round-the-clock" dosing rather than prn.
2. Maintain comfortable body position, turning at least q2h and prn.
3. Teach child to focus on television, music, or friends when having pain.
4. Assess pain q2h using appropriate assessment tools.
5. Provide soothing skin care.

Evaluation

Child experiences relief of pain; child and family verbally identify and use available comfort measures.

> **Goal 9** Child's growth and development will be fostered throughout the course of illness and treatment.

Implementation

1. Refer to The Healthy Child, p. 402, for developmental needs appropriate to child's age.
2. Encourage child to participate in self-care to the extent possible.
3. Provide opportunities for child to exercise some control over daily routine (food choices, selection of play activities).
4. Maintain child's educational progress as much as possible.
5. Maintain child's contact with siblings and friends (through visiting, telephone calls, letters).

Evaluation

Child is free from significant developmental or educational delays; demonstrates age-appropriate skills and behaviors.

> **Goal 10** Child and family cope with the stresses of living with cancer and its treatment.

Implementation

1. Encourage parents and family to continue to provide care of child as much as desired and possible.
2. Encourage expressions of fear, feelings, and concerns about cancer and its treatment.
3. Refer to parent-support groups (Candlelighters, Compassionate Friends).
4. Assess child's understanding of diagnosis and prognosis (Table 5-26).
5. Help child express feelings through play and art.
6. Encourage family to treat child as normally as possible (i.e., age-appropriate limit setting and enforcement, avoid excessive gifts or privileges).
7. If child's condition becomes terminal, support family as they prepare for child's death; refer for home or hospice care, as appropriate and desired by family.

Evaluation

Child and family cope with child's illness and treatment; parents participate in community support groups as desired,

Table 5-26 Child's concept of death

INFANTS AND TODDLERS

React more to pain and to parents' responses and behaviors than to probability of death; cannot verbalize their understanding; only understand "alive," not "dead"; may persist in ritualistic activities.

PRESCHOOL

Death is a kind of sleep, temporary; believe their own illness is punishment; fear painful procedures and being separated from parents.

SCHOOL AGE

6-7 years old: personify death, such as God, devil, "bogeyman"; fear the mutilation of death.

9-10 years old: similar to adult concept; understand that death is eventually inevitable and irreversible; fear the unknown about death; need concrete explanations and a chance to share their fears and gain some control.

ADOLESCENTS

Have the most difficulty coping with death; have adult cognitive understanding, but death is a threat to their identity; fear the physical changes of terminal illness.

express their fears and feelings about child's illness and prognosis.

SELECTED HEALTH PROBLEMS RESULTING FROM CELLULAR ABERRATION

✠ LEUKEMIA

1. Definition: malignant neoplasm of unknown etiology that involves blood-forming organs and is characterized by abnormal overproduction of immature forms of any of the leukocytes; interferes with normal blood cell production, resulting in decreased erythrocytes, decreased platelets
   a. Types
      1. lymphocytic: predominance of stem cells, lymphoblasts, usually known as acute lymphocytic leukemia (ALL); 80% of childhood leukemias are of this type
      2. myelogenous: predominance of monocytes and immature granulocytes (more common in adults); 10% to 20% of childhood leukemias are myelogenous
   b. Pathophysiology: leukemic cells proliferate and deprive normal blood cells of nutrients needed for metabolism
      1. anemia results from decreased red blood cell production, blood loss
      2. immunosuppression occurs from large numbers of *immature* white blood cells or profound neutropenia

3. hemorrhage results from thrombocytopenia
4. leukemic invasion of other organ systems occurs (extramedullary disease)
   a. liver
   b. spleen
   c. lymph nodes
   d. CNS
   e. kidneys
   f. lungs
   g. gonads
5. hyperuricemia may result after the start of chemotherapy when large numbers of cells are rapidly destroyed
2. Incidence
   a. Most common childhood cancer
   b. Peak age of onset is 2 to 5 years; more frequent in males
   c. 80% of children with ALL who are treated in major research centers live 4 years or longer
3. Medical treatment
   a. Diagnostic measures
      1. bone marrow aspiration
      2. lumbar puncture
      3. frequent blood cell counts
   b. Chemotherapy—three phases
      1. remission induction: to reduce leukemia-cell population and attain remission, usually with corticosteroids and vincristine
      2. consolidation (sanctuary): usually begun after remission is achieved; may be done along with induction; prophylactic treatment of the CNS, usually with intrathecal use of methotrexate
      3. maintenance course: to maintain remission, usually with combination drugs
   c. Additional therapies
      1. radiation: irradiate cranium and spine as prophylaxis against CNS involvement
      2. bone marrow transplantation
4. Prognosis: disease is characterized by remissions and exacerbations; outlook varies according to type of cell involved, initial WBC, response to treatment, age at diagnosis, sex of the child, and extent of involvement

Nursing Process
ASSESSMENT
1. Bleeding tendencies
   a. Petechiae often the first sign, as a result of low platelet count
   b. Hemorrhage (nosebleeds, gingival bleeding; intracranial hemorrhage in advanced disease)
2. Anemia: fatigue, pallor
3. Neutropenia: immunosuppression leads to secondary infection and fever because cells are not capable of normal phagocytosis
4. Pain
   a. Abdomen: resulting from enlarged liver, spleen, lymph nodes, and other organs from cell infiltration
   b. Bones and joints
5. Anorexia and weight loss; ulcers of mucous membranes of GI tract

6. Vomiting and increased intracranial pressure from CNS involvement
7. Impaired kidney function
8. Emotional reaction, coping skills of parents, siblings, child, and significant extended-family members
9. Developmental and educational needs of child

ANALYSIS/NURSING DIAGNOSIS (see p. 487)

PLANNING, IMPLEMENTATION, AND EVALUATION

Goal 1 Child will be free from hemorrhage.

Implementation
1. Observe for epistaxis, gingival bleeding.
2. Handle gently.
3. Inspect skin and mucous membranes daily.
4. Keep lips and nostrils clean and lubricated.
5. Pad bed/crib to avoid trauma.
6. Monitor blood work.

Evaluation
Child is free from bruises and bleeding; has early signs of hemorrhage detected and reported.

Goal 2 Child will receive transfusions properly and safely.

Implementation
1. Administer blood products properly.
   a. Take baseline vital signs before transfusion.
   b. Check label with RN before transfusion for name, blood type, Rh, hospital number, and physician's name.
   c. Flush tubing with isotonic saline solution (hemolysis can occur if dextrose is in line).
   d. Administer blood at room temperature within 4 hours of refrigeration.
   e. Administer transfusion slowly to determine possible transfusion reaction, to prevent circulatory overload, and to protect small veins.
   f. Stay with child for first 15 minutes; have parent or other adult stay with young child throughout transfusion.
   g. Take vital signs q15min for first hour.
   h. Do not give IV medications while blood is infusing.
   i. Use blood filter.
2. Monitor intravenous transfusions.
   a. Whole blood/packed cells (cannot be continuously maintained on tranfusions because preservative in whole blood functions as anticoagulant)
   b. Platelets last 1 to 3 days; do not need to crossmatch for blood group or type, but doing so decreases chance of immunization to another platelet group; spontaneous hemorrhage can occur at platelet levels below 20,000/mm^3
   c. Leukocytes last 2 to 3 days; need compatible donors; febrile responses (with moderate to severe chills) are common; give antihistamines or antipyretics as ordered

3. Observe for complications and reactions to blood transfusions.
   a. Chills
   b. Fever (give antipyretic prn)
   c. Headache
   d. Apprehension (give sedatives prn)
   e. Pain in back, legs, or chest
   f. Hypotension (give IV fluids, vasopressors)
   g. Dyspnea (give O$_2$, bronchodilator [epinephrine] as ordered)
   h. Urticaria (give antihistamines prn)
4. Promptly manage a transfusion reaction.
   a. Stop the transfusion of blood.
   b. Monitor vital signs.
   c. Do not leave child alone.
   d. Run IV fluids to maintain patency of the IV line.

Table 5-27   Common solid-tumor cancers in children

Definition	Assessment	Medical treatment	Nursing planning/ implementation
BRAIN TUMORS			

Neoplasms in the cranium; most brain tumors in children are *infratentorial* (below the tentorium cerebelli), thus affecting the cerebellum and brain stem, making them less operable	Signs of increased ICP: see Table 5-14	Surgical excision to extent possible
		Irradiation
		Chemotherapy: methotrexate, vincristine
			Perform frequent neurologic checks.
			Institute seizure precautions.
			Postoperative care
			  Observe cranial dressing for drainage and record.
			  Reinforce but DO NOT CHANGE cranial dressing.
			  Position flat or on side with neck slightly extended.
			  Monitor fluid intake (IV, PO) carefully to prevent overload.
			  Avoid analgesics and sedatives that cause CNS depression.
			  Avoid coughing, straining, jarring movements.

NEUROBLASTOMA			
Malignant, embryonic abdominal tumor; most common in infancy	Abdominal mass that crosses midline Lymphadenopathy Urinary frequency or retention (pressure from tumor) Urine catecholamines (elevated)	Surgical excision and staging (to determine extent of other treatment and prognosis) Irradiation Chemotherapy	See General Nursing Plans, p. 487
WILMS' TUMOR			
Malignant, embryonic tumor of kidney, usually encapsulated until late stages; 90% survival rate if detected while encapsulated; peak age of occurrence—3 years; more common in boys; increased incidence in siblings or twin; usually unilateral	Palpable abdominal mass Abdominal distention Hypertension (excess renin secretion)	IV push Nephrectomy and adrenalectomy, staging (to determine treatment and prognosis) Irradiation Chemotherapy: actinomycin D, vincristine	Handle carefully; DO NOT PALPATE ABDOMEN. Monitor kidney function (e.g., I&O, urine specific gravity, BP).
OSTEOGENIC SARCOMA			
Primary bone tumor, usually affecting distal femur or proximal tibia; most common in adolescent males	Pain Localized swelling Limp or limited ROM	Amputation (above the knee or total hip disarticulation) Prophylactic lung irradiation Chemotherapy: doxorubicin, cisplatin, methotrexate with leucovorin rescue	Postoperative stump care (see Nursing Care of the Adult, p. 253). Support coping response in adjusting to loss of body part.

e. Notify physician.

f. Return untransfused blood to blood bank.

Evaluation

Child receives correct transfusion, is free from preventable complications (e.g., hemolysis); early signs of reaction (e.g., rash) are detected, and transfusion reaction is managed properly.

✖ SOLID TUMORS

General Information (Table 5-27)

Nursing Process (Table 5-27)

BIBLIOGRAPHY

General

Mott S, James S, Sperhac A: *Nursing care of children and families,* ed 2, Redwood City, Calif, 1990, Addison-Wesley.

Scipien GM et al: *Pediatric nursing care,* St Louis, 1990, Mosby.

Whaley L, Wong D: *Nursing care of infants and children,* ed 5, St Louis, 1995, Mosby.

The healthy child

American Academy of Pediatrics: *Report of the Committee on Infectious Diseases,* ed 22, Elk Grove Village, Ill, 1991.

Ball J, Bindler R: *Pediatric nursing,* Norwalk, Conn, 1995, Appleton & Lange.

Castiglia P, Petrini M: Selecting a developmental screening tool, *Pediatr Nurs* 11(1):8, 1994.

Jones NE: Childhood residential injuries, *MCN Am J Matern Child Nurs* 18(3):168, 1993.

Pineyard BJ: Assessment of infant growth, *J Pediatr Health Care* 6(5, part 2):302, 1992.

Pipes P: *Nutrition in infancy and childhood,* ed 5, St Louis, 1993, Mosby.

Poon CY: Childhood immunization: part 1, *J Pediatr Health Care* 6(6):370, 1992.

Report of the Committee on Infectious Diseases, ed 22, 1991, American Academy of Pediatrics.

Rimar J: *Haemophilus influenzae* type b polysaccharide, *MCN Am J Matern Child Nurs* 11:8, 1986.

Scipien GM, et al: *Pediatric nursing care,* St Louis, 1990, Mosby.

Sharts-Hopko NC: Current immunization guidelines, *Am J Matern Child Nurs MCN* 19:82, 1994.

Whaley L, Wong D: *Nursing care of infants and children,* ed 5, St Louis, 1995, Mosby.

The ill and hospitalized child

Castiglia PT, Harbin RE: *Child health care,* Philadelphia, 1994, Lippincott.

Gordin P: Assessing and managing agitation in a critically ill infant, *MCN Am J Matern Child Nurs* 15:26, 1990.

Jackson PL, Vessey JA: *Primary care of the child with a chronic condition,* St Louis, 1991, Mosby.

Knott C et al: Using the oucher: developmental approach to pain assessment in children, *Am J Matern Child Nurs MCN,* 19(6):314, 1994.

Landier W, Barrell M, Styffe E: How to administer blood components to children, *MCN Am J Matern Child Nurs* 12:178, 1987.

O'Brien S, Konsler G: Alleviating children's postoperative pain, *MCN Am J Matern Child Nurs* 13:183, 1988.

Reynolds E. Ramenofsky M: The emotional impact of trauma on toddlers, *MCN Am J Matern Child Nurs* 13:106, 1988.

Rimar J: Guidelines for the IV administration of medications used in pediatrics, *MCN Am J Matern Child Nurs* 12:322, 1987.

Rimar J: Recognizing shock syndromes in infants and children, *MCN Am J Matern Child Nurs* 13:32, 1988.

Sensation, perception, and protection

Crumrine P: A trio of pediatric neurologic emergencies, *Emerg Med* 25(2):103, 1993.

Dyer C, Roberts D: Thermal trauma, *Nurs Clin North Am* 25(1):85, 1990.

Gardner S: Pain and pain relief in the neonate, *MCN Am J Matern Child Nurs* 19(2):85, 1994.

Hurley A, Whelan E: Cognitive development and children's perception of pain, *Pediatr Nurs* 14:21, 1988.

Kachoyeanos M, Friedhoff M: Cognitive and behavioral strategies to reduce children's pain, *MCN Am J Matern Child Nurs* 18(1):14, 1993.

Knott C et al: Using the oucher developmental approach to apin assessment in children, *MCN Am J Matern Child Nurs* 19(6):314, 1994.

Lewis K, Bennett B, Schmeder N: The care of infants menaced by cocaine abuse, *MCN Am J Matern Child Nurs* 14(5):324, 1989.

Markiewicz T: Recognizing, treating, and preventing lead poisoning, *Am J. Nurs* 93(10):59, 1993.

Molinari F: Update on the treatment of pediculosis and scabies, *Pediatr Nurs* 18(6):600, 1992.

Morelli J: Pediatric poisonings: the 10 most toxic prescription drugs, *Am J Nurs* 93(7):27, 1993.

Mott S, James S, Sperhac A: *Nursing care of children and families,* ed 2, Redwood City, Calif, 1990, Addison-Wesley.

Paparone P: The summer scourge of Lyme disease, *Am J Nurs* 90(6):44, 1990.

Reynolds E: Controversies in caring for the child with a head injury, *MCN Am J Matern Child Nurs* 17(5):246, 1992.

Scheinblum S, Hammond M: The treatment of children with shunt infections: extraventricular drainage system care, *Pediatr Nurs* 16(2):139, 1990.

Scipien GM et al: *Pediatric nursing care,* St Louis, 1990, Mosby.

Selekman J: The guidelines for immunizations have changed . . . again! *Pediatr Nurs* 20(4):376, 1994.

Sharts-Hopko N: Current immunization guidelines, *MCN Am J Matern Child Nurs* 19(2):82, 1994.

Shiminski-Maher T, Disabato J: Current trends in the diagnosis and management of hydrocephalus in children, *J Pediatr Nurs* 9(2):74, 1994.

Thomson E, Cordero J: The new teratogens: accutane and other vitamin-A analogs, *MCN Am J Matern Child Nurs* 14(4): 244, 1989.

Vessey J et al: Caring for the child with Down syndrome, *J School Nurs* 9(1):20, 1993.

*Ward-Wimmer D: Nursing care of children with HIV infection, *Nursing Clin North Am* 23(4):719, 1988.

Yarber W, Parrillo A: Adolescents and sexually transmitted diseases, *J School Health* 62(7):331, 1992.

Oxygenation

Agamalian B: Pediatric cardiac catheterization, *J Pediatr Nurs* 1(2):73, 1986.

American Academy of Pediatrics, Committee on Infectious Diseases: Use of ribavirin in the treatment of RSV, *Pediatrics* 3:501, 1993.

American Heart Association: Guidelines for CPR and emergency cardiac care, *JAMA* 268(16):2171, 1992.

Cloutier M: Quick: what's the first-line therapy for acute asthma? *Contemp Pediatr* 10(3):76, 1993.

Fitzsimmons S: The changing epidemiology of cystic fibrosis, *J Pediatr* 122(1):1, 1993.

Filippell M, Rearick T: Respiratory syncytial virus, *Nurs Clin North Am* 28(3):651, 1993.

Freund B et al: Acute rheumatic fever revisited, *J Pediatr Nurs* 8:167, 1993.

Karsch AB: Assessment and management of status asthmaticus, *Pediatr Nurs* 20(3):217, 1994.

Nederhand K et al: Respiratory syncytial virus: a nursing perspective, *Pediatr Nurs* 15(4):342, 1989.

Jackson M: Tuberculosis in infants, children and adolescents: new dilemmas with an old disease, *Pediatr Nurs* 19(5):437, 1993.

Jury D: More on RSV and ribavirin, *Pediatr Nurs* 19(1):89, 1993.

Mott S, James S, Sperhac A: *Nursing care of children and families,* ed 2, Redwood City, Calif, 1990, Addison-Wesley.

Smith, J: Big differences in little people, *Am J Nurs* 88(4):458, 1988.

Wimberly TH, Parks BR: Iron preparations, it's elementary, my dear, *Pediatr Nurs* 17:274, 1991.

Zahr, LK: Assessment and management of the child with asthma, *Pediatr Nurs* 15(2):109, 1989.

Nutrition and metabolism

Bishop WP, Ulshen MH: Bacterial gastroenteritis, *Pediatr Clin North Am* 35(1):69, 1988.

Brink SJ: Pediatric adolescent and young-adult nutrition issues in IDDM, *Diabetes Care* 11:192, 1988.

Chase JP, Chase VC, Garg S: Self-care for the young diabetic—home but not alone, *Contemp Pediatr* 8:74, 1991.

Dibble SL, Savedra MC: Cystic fibrosis in adolescence: a new challenge, *Pediatr Nurs* 14(4):299, 1988.

Foster R, Hunsberger M, Anderson J: *Family-centered nursing care of children,* Philadelphia, 1989, Saunders.

Gavin JR III: Diabetes and exercise, *Am J Nurs* 88:178, 1988.

Grey M et al: Initial adaptation in children with newly diagnosed diabetes and healthy children, *Pediatr Nurs* 21(1):17, 1994.

Lipman TH: What causes diabetes? *MCN Am J Matern Child Nurs* 13(1):40, 1988.

Lipman TH et al: A developmental approach to diabetes in children: birth through preschool, *MCN Am J Matern Child Nurs* 14(4):255, 1989.

Lipman TH et al: A developmental approach to diabetes in children: school age–adolescence, *MCN Am J Matern Child Nurs* 14(5):330, 1989.

Meyer PA: Parental adaptation to cystic fibrosis, *J Pediatr Health Care* 2(1):20, 1988.

Savinetti-Rose B: Developmental issues in managing children with diabetes, *Pediatr Nurs* 20(1):11, 1994.

Vaughan V, Behrman R: *Nelson's textbook of pediatrics,* ed 13, Philadelphia, 1987, Saunders.

Wells PW, Meghdadpour S: Research yields new clues to cystic fibrosis, *MCN Am J Matern Child Nurs* 13(3):187, 1988.

Elimination

Betz C, Hunsberger M, Wright S: *Family centered nursing care of children,* ed 2, Philadelphia, 1994, Saunders.

Blackburn S: Renal function in the neonate, *J Perinat Neonat Nurs* 8(1):37, 1994.

Castiglia P, Harbin R: *Child health care,* Philadelphia, 1992, Lippincott.

Frost G: Hirschprung disease in infants and children, *Gastroenterol Nurs* 15(1):45, 1992.

Gilman C, Mooney K, Andrews M: Alterations of renal and urinary tract function in children. In McCance K, Huether S, editors: *Pathophysiology: the biologic basis for disease in adults and children,* St Louis, 1994, Mosby.

Hazinski M: *Nursing care of the critically ill child,* ed 2, St Louis, 1992, Mosby.

Ladebauche P: Intussusception in pediatric patients, *J Emerg Nurs* 18(3):275, 1992.

Mott S, James S, and Sperhac A: *Nursing care of children and families,* ed, 2 Redwood City, Calif, 1990, Addison-Wesley.

Sperhac AM: Abdominal pain in pediatric patients: assessment and management update, *J Emerg Nurs* 93, 1989.

Sugar E, Firlit C, Reisman M: Pediatric hypospadias surgery, *Pediatr Nurs* 19(6):585, 1993.

Welch V: The management of urologic disorders in the neonate, *J Perinat Neonat Nurs* 8(19):48, 1994.

Wilson D: Urinary tract infections in the pediatric patient, *Nurse Pract* 14(38):41, 1989.

Mobility

Brady M: The child with a limp, *J Pediatr Health Care* 7:226, 1993.

Butler AB, Salmond SW, Pellino TA: *Orthopedic nursing,* Philadelphia, 1994, Saunders.

Carlino HY: The child with an Ilizarov external fixator, *Pediatr Nurs* 17(4):355, 1991.

Cotton LA: Unit rod segnental spinal instrumentation for the treatment of neuromuscular scoliosis, *Orthop Nurs* 10(5):17, 1991.

Olson EV: The hazards of immobility, *Am J Nurs* 90:43, 1990.

Page-Goertz SS: Even children have arthritis, *J Pediatr Health Care* 5(1):18, 1989.

Staheli LT: *Fundamentals of pediatric orthopedics,* New York, 1992, Raven Press.

Cellular aberration (childhood cancer)

Austin J: Assessment of coping mechanisms used by parents and children with chronic illness, *MCN Am J Matern Child Nurs* 15:98, 1990.

Fernbach DJ, Hawkins EP, Pokorny WJ: Nephroblastoma and other renal tumors. In Fernbach DJ, Vietti TJ, editors: *Clinical pediatric oncology,* ed 4, St Louis, 1991, Mosby.

Galbraith L et al: Treatment for alteration in oral mucosa related to chemotherapy, *Pediatr Nurs* 17(3):233, 1991.

Hockenberry MJ, Coody DK, Bennett B: Childhood cancers, *Pediatr Nurs* 16:239, 1990.

Krulik T: *The child and family facing life threatening illness,* Philadelphia, 1988, Lippincott.

Lilley L: Side effects associated with pediatric chemotherapy: management and patient education issues, *Pediatr Nurs* 16:252, 1990.

Marcoux C, Fisher S, Wong D: Central venous access devices in children, *Pediatr Nurs* 16:123, 1990.

Meehan J: Pain control in the terminally ill child at home, *Issues Compr Pediatr Nurs* 12:187, 1989.

Young J, Eslinger P, Galloway M: Radiation treatment for the child with cancer, *Issues Compre Pediatr Nurs* 12:159, 1989.

*Highly recommended.

PAIN AND PAIN RELIEF IN THE NEONATE

The suffering of neonates can be avoided. Nurses must learn to recognize the symptoms of pain and advocate for effective treatment.

BY SANDRA L. GARDNER

In the past, neonates were not given anesthesia or analgesia for surgery because of the controversy over whether they felt pain or were physiologically stable enough to tolerate the effects of these drugs. It was believed that neonates have an immature central nervous system (CNS), with nonmyelinated pain fibers, and are thus incapable of perceiving pain. It was also believed that they have no memory of pain, and that pain cannot be assessed objectively in nonverbal patients. Moreover, it was thought that anesthetics and analgesics are dangerous when administered to neonates, and that neonates are safer without medication.

There is increasing evidence from recent research that neonates, including preterm infants, have a CNS that is far more mature than previously thought (1,2). Pain pathways are myelinated in the fetus during the second and third trimesters, and are completely myelinated by 30 to 37 weeks' gestation. Even thinly or nonmyelinated fibers carry pain stimuli. Incomplete myelination only implies slower transmission, offset in the neonate by the shorter distance the impulse must travel (2).

The infant's capacity for memory is also far greater than previously thought (1,3,4). Research has focused on measuring the infant's pain experience, and objective parameters have been developed to respond to the question of whether the neonate's responses are reflexive or a perception of pain. Local and systemic drugs now available, as well as new monitoring techniques and devices, enable neonates (including preterm infants) to be safely anesthetized and maintained in a stable condition (2).

Neonates, full-term and premature, exhibit physiologic, hormonal, metabolic, and behavioral responses to surgical procedures that are similar to, but more intense than, adult responses (2,3,5-7). Pain relief benefits the neonate by decreasing physiologic instability, hormonal and metabolic stress, and the behavioral reactions accompanying painful procedures (2,5,6,8). The Committee on Fetus and Newborn of the American Academy of Pediatrics has recommended the administration of local and systemic drugs for anesthesia or analgesia to neonates undergoing surgical procedures. It further states that any decision to withhold these drugs from infants is not to be based solely on the infant's age or perceived degree of cortical maturity, but rather on the same criteria used in older patients (1).

PREVENTION OF PAIN AND ITS INTENSIFICATION

Pain is produced with any surgical procedure, as a sequela to surgery, and with invasive procedures such as chest tube insertion and cutdowns. Since the myth that neonates do not feel pain has been proved incorrect, and since safe anesthetics and analgesics do exist, care providers need to anticipate and assess pain to provide prompt, safe, and adequate pain relief. Positive developmental and medical outcomes have been observed when very-low-birth-weight preterm infants are given individualized behavioral and environmental care that emphasizes the reduction of stress (9).

Some comfort measures may prevent the intensification of pain—guarding an abdominal incision by positioning, for example, will be less painful than four-point restraint. However, comfort measures, while helpful, may not relieve moderate to severe pain (10). In order to collect data about the neonate's pain, the nurse needs to review the history and evaluate signs, symptoms, and laboratory data.

History: The neonate's need for invasive procedures in the neonatal intensive care unit (NICU), surgery, and elsewhere necessitates the consideration of pain relief during and after the event. Agitation following invasive procedures or with medical problems, such as bronchopulmonary dysplasia, may also necessitate a combination of environmental interventions and sedative therapy (11-13).

Signs and Symptoms: It may be difficult to distinguish between pain and agitation. However, differentiation is absolutely necessary so that the correct interventions will be used. (To compare the two, see Indicators of Irritability/Agitation and Neonatal Pain Response.) If a pain behavior is interpreted as agitation, and the baby is treated with a sedative, the sedative will be ineffective and the baby may

Sandra L. Gardner, MS, PNP, is the director of Professional Outreach Consultation, a firm she owns in Aurora, Colorado. This article is adapted with permission from the section "Pain and Pain Relief," published in Handbook of Neonatal Intensive Care, *edited by G. B. Merenstein and S. L. Gardner, 3rd edition, 1993, St. Louis, Mosby-Year Book, pp. 496-502. It was also presented under the title "Correct Use of Sedatives and Analgesia in the Newborn," at the MCN Convention in Orlando, Florida, in March 1993.*

become more irritable and excessively sensitive to pain (13). Every agitated, irritable baby needs to be assessed for a locus of pain (for example, sepsis, hypoxia, uncomfortable position) and treated appropriately.

Assessment of neonatal pain is influenced by the attitudes, beliefs, and knowledge of care providers, the amount of time spent observing pain responses, the discrepancy between attitudes and practice, and prioritization of pain recognition and relief in the NICU (13-18). It is also complicated by the infant's state and level of neurodevelopment (7). The younger the gestational age, the more immature the central nervous system and the more difficult for the infant to communicate his internal experience of pain.

A more immature, fragile infant may manifest alterations in sleep-wake cycles and habituate to the overwhelming stimuli of the NICU, decreasing responsivity to external stimuli, and thus be unable to exhibit any behavioral responses to pain (9). Behavioral responses to pain may not be possible in the intubated baby, who cannot cry, the restrained baby, who cannot move, and the baby receiving neuromuscular blockers, such as pancuronium bromide.

When pain is repetitive or persists (immediately after the procedure or within hours or days), there is a decompensatory response resulting in hormonal and metabolic alterations. Because the "fight or flight" mechanism of the sympathetic nervous system is no longer able to compensate, an adaptation syndrome begins, with a return to baseline of physiologic parameters. The return of heart rate, respiration, and blood pressure to baseline parameters makes assessment of the infant for pain more difficult. It does not mean that the baby has "adjusted" to or no longer is experiencing pain (18). The nurse's responsibility is to understand that this phenomenon occurs and prevent its occurrence by use of timely and adequate pain relief. (For hormonal and metabolic changes, see Neonatal Pain Response.)

Laboratory Data: Serum glucose levels and reagent test strips are used to monitor for hyperglycemia, which may result in increased serum osmolality and increase the risk of intraventricular hemorrhage (IVH). Glucosuria,

---

INDICATORS OF IRRITABILITY/AGITATION

Physiologic
Increase in:
  Heart rate and blood pressure only with activity
  Oxygenation (TcPO$_2$ [transcutaneous partial pressure of oxygen]; PO$_2$ [partial pressure of oxygen]; SaO$_2$ [arterial saturation of oxygen])
  Respiratory rate and effort
Decrease in:
  Oxygenation (TcPO$_2$; PO$_2$; SaO$_2$) after prolonged agitation
  Heart rate (bradycardia)
  Respirations (apnea)
Alterations in color:
  Cyanosis, mottling, duskiness, pallor
Diaphoresis
Vomiting
Poor pattern of weight gain

Behavioral
Vocalizations:
  Whining cry
  Intense, urgent cry
  High-pitched cry
  Resumes fussiness when consolation ceases
Facial expressions:
  Frowning
  Worried facies
  Gaze aversion
  Closes eyes to tune out
Bodily movements:
  Random movements of head and body
  Hypertonic, rigid posturing; arching
  Hyperextended neck
  Flailing, thrashing, frantic activity of extremities during fuss/cry
  Decreased activity
  Tremulousness
States:
  Hyperalert—easily aroused from sleep; startles easily
  Rapid and frequent state changes to fuss/cry
  Sleep-wake cycles unpredictable
  Feeding difficulties
  Difficult to console, soothe
  High level of persistence
  Needs environmental structure to fall asleep; takes a long time to fall asleep
  Ineffective in self-consoling; requires vestibular stimulation or body containment to console; responds inconsistently to consolation
  Noncuddly

---

ketonuria, and proteinuria result in elevated specific gravity. Metabolic acidosis may result from increased serum levels of lactate, pyruvate, ketones, and nonesterified fatty acids.

COMFORT MEASURES AND MEDICATIONS

The judicious use of medications provides pain relief. (For a comprehensive list, see Analgesics and Sedatives for the Neonate.) Following a PRN schedule may result in peaks and valleys of pain relief because administra-

tion depends on the nurse's considering it necessary. Since analgesia is most effective if given *before* the peak of pain, a continuous intravenous infusion or regular schedule for administration precludes undue neonatal suffering (18).

Even though comfort measures alone do not relieve pain, their use reduces agitation, which indirectly reduces pain by promoting behavioral organization, relaxation, general comfort, and sleep (18,19). Nonnutritive sucking (on the baby's own fingers, hands,

NEONATAL PAIN RESPONSE

Compensatory Responses: Physiologic
Increase in:
  Heart rate
  Blood pressure
  Intracranial pressure
  Risk of intraventricular hemorrhage (IVH)
  Respiratory rate
  Mean airway pressure
  Muscle tension
  Carbon dioxide ($TcPco_2$ [transcutaneous partial pressure
    of oxygen]; Pco_2 [partial pressure of oxygen])
Decrease in:
  Depth of respirations (shallow)
  Oxygenation ($TcPo_2$; Po_2; Sao_2 [arterial saturation of
    oxygen]) that leads to apnea/bradycardia
Pallor or flushing
Diaphoresis/palmar sweating
Dilated pupils

Compensatory Responses: Behavioral
Vocalizations:
  Crying (higher pitched, tense, and harsh)
  Whimpering
  Moaning
Facial expressions:
  Grimacing
  Furrowing/bulging of the brow
  Quivering chin
  Eye squeeze
Bodily movements:
  General diffuse body activity

Limb withdrawal, swiping, thrashing
Changes in tone:
  Hypertonicity, rigidity, fist clenching
  Hypotonicity, flaccidity
  Touch aversion
States:
  Sleep-wake cycle changes—wakefulness
  Activity level changes: increased fussiness, irritability,
    listlessness, lethargy
Feeding difficulties
More difficult to comfort, soothe, quiet
Disrupts interactive ability with parents

Decompensatory Response: Hormonal/Metabolic
Increase in:
  Plasma renin activity
  Catecholamine levels (epinephrine and norepinephrine)
  Cortisol levels
  Nitrogen excretion
  Release of:
    Growth hormone
    Glucagon
    Aldosterone
  Serum levels of:
    Glucose
    Lactate
    Pyruvate
    Ketones
    Nonesterified fatty acids
Decrease in:
  Insulin secretion

or a pacifier) soothes by reducing the level of arousal and the duration of the cry while increasing the quiet-alert state (20,21).

Oral sucrose has been shown to calm distressed infants more quickly than a pacifier alone, enabling them to stay calm longer and spend more time in a quiet-alert state (22,23). Picking up, holding, and rocking provide tactile, soothing, vestibular stimulation and the soothing of rhythmic, repetitive movement.

Improper body position contributes to discomfort and pain. Containing extremities in a flexed position by holding, swaddling, or nesting, or providing the opportunity to grasp a finger or pacifier, decreases the gross motor movements that contribute to the infant's increased level of arousal (20). Therapeutic interventions by nurses include positions that support flexion, restraint of extremities in physiologic position, periodic release and exercise of extremities, gentle change in body position, and positioning to guard opera-

tive sites. Minimizing stimulation in the NICU environment enables the neonate who is agitated or in pain to use internal and external resources to organize his behavior and develop self-soothing strategies (9).

THE RAMIFICATIONS OF PAIN

The neonate's complex behavioral response to pain has both short- and long-term ramifications. Behavioral changes may disrupt parent-infant interaction and attachment, adaptation to the postnatal environment, and feeding behaviors (2). An alteration of brain development and maldevelopment of sensory systems can occur when distorted or inappropriate sensory input occurs during a critical period in development (24). Because of the neonate's memory, painful experiences increase his sensitivity to subsequent stressful medical encounters (4,25). These earliest experiences may affect the development of attitudes, fears, anxiety, conflicts, wishes, expectations, and patterns of interac-

tion with others (26). (Since it is beyond the scope of this article to discuss developmental impact in greater depth, the reader is encouraged to review the cited references, especially reference 9.)

Unanesthetized surgery and/or unrelieved pain caused by invasive procedures results in suffering that might itself be a risk to the life of the neonate (2,15). Release of stress hormones precipitates metabolic changes that lead to catabolism of the body's fat, carbohydrate, and protein reserves. Within physiologic limits, these changes may facilitate wound healing and recovery, but if severe and prolonged, they increase postoperative morbidity and mortality of the neonate (8,27,28). Maintaining metabolic homeostatis improves postoperative outcome by preventing protein wasting, electrolyte imbalance, impaired immune function, sepsis, metabolic acidosis, pulmonary and cardiac insuffciency, hypermetabolic state, and even death (6,8,16).

Analgesics and sedatives for the neonate

Drug	Dosage	Comments
ANALGESICS		Postsurgical incision pain is relieved by narcotic analgesia.
Narcotic Morphine	0.05-0.2 mg/kg/dose q 2-4 hours PRN IV, IM, or subcutaneous (SC). Continuous IV infusion: 10-15 µg/kg/hour.	Central nervous system (CNS) and respiratory depressant; peripheral vasodilation with hypovolemic infants; decreases intestinal motility; increases intracranial pressure; easily reversed with naloxone; slower onset but longer duration than fentanyl; withdrawal symptoms may occur.
Meperidine* (Demerol) *Not the drug of choice because of central nervous system (CNS) stimulation; use only if intolerant to all other drugs.	1-1.5 mg/kg/dose q 4 hours PRN IV, IM, SC, or PO.	Same as morphine; less respiratory depression with therapeutic dose; less likely to induce sleep/sedation than morphine or fentanyl. Active metabolite, normeperidine, may accumulate in tissues and cause CNS stimulation (e.g., tremors, muscle twitching, hyperactive reflexes, dilated pupils, seizures).
Fentanyl (Sublimaze)	1-2 µg/kg/dose q 4-6 hours PRN IV or SC. Continuous IV infusion: 2 µg/kg/hour. Anesthesia: 20-75 µg/kg/dose IV over 5 to 10 minutes.	Rapid onset of action; decreases motor activity; does not increase intracranial pressure; easily reversed with naloxone; short duration of action; may cause bradycardia, hypotension, apnea, seizures or rigidity if given too rapidly; withdrawal symptoms may occur.
Local Lidocaine (Xylocaine)	0.5-1 percent solution (to avoid systemic toxicity, volume should be <0.5 ml/kg of 1 percent lidocaine solution—5 mg/kg).	Local infiltration anesthesia for invasive procedures (e.g., circumcision, chest tube insertion/removal, cutdowns). Use solution without epinephrine to avoid vasoconstriction.
SEDATIVE/HYPNOTICS		Do not provide pain relief. Help reduce agitation precipitated by painful events.
Barbiturate		Frequently produces hyperalgesia and increased reaction to painful stimuli—contraindicated for neonates who have pain and also require sedation.
Phenobarbital	Loading: 10-20 mg/kg IV to maximum of 40 mg/kg. Maintenance: 5 to 7 mg/kg in 2 divided doses beginning 12 hours after last loading dose.	Prolonged sedation possible once therapeutic levels achieved (20-25 mg/cc); depresses CNS-motor and respiratory; slow onset of action; little or no pain relief; not easily reversed; withdrawal symptoms may occur; incompatible with other drugs in solution.
Nonbarbiturate Chloral hydrate	10-30 mg/kg/dose q 6 hours PRN PO to maximum daily dose of 50 mg/kg/day; per rectum (PR).	Gastric irritant—administer with or after feeding; paradoxical excitement; prolonged use associated with direct hyperbilirubinemia; not to be used for analgesia (29).
Benzodiazepine Diazepam (Valium)	0.02-0.3 mg/kg IV, IM, or PO q 6 to 8 hours.	Anti-anxiety agents; amnesiac. Do not dilute injection; may displace bilirubin; respiratory depression; hypotension; may cause agitation; induces sleep; relaxes muscles; withdrawal symptoms may occur; no analgesic effect.
Lorazepam (Ativan)	0.05-0.1 mg/kg/dose IV (give over ≥3 minutes) q 4 to 8 hours.	Respiratory depressant, partial airway obstruction, drowsiness. Respiratory depression potentiated when narcotics or barbituates also being given. Infuse slowly to avoid apnea, bradycardia, and hypotension.
Midazolam (Versed)	0.05-0.2 mg/kg/dose IV (give over ≥3 minutes) q 4 to 8 hours PRN. Continuous IV infusion: 0.2-6 µg/kg/min.	Same as above. Continuous IV infusion enables precise titration until sedative effect obtained; calms agitated infant on ventilator.

Modified from Bell S.G., and Ellis L.G. Use of fentanyl for sedation of mechanically ventilated neonates, Neonatal Network 6:28, 1987.

POTENTIAL COMPLICATIONS

Narcotic analgesics may produce respiratory depression severe enough to require mechanical ventilation. Naloxone (Narcan) (0.1 mg/kg IV or IM) is the specific antidote for narcotic potentiation or overdose. An ampule of neonatal naloxone must always be immediately available with the appropriate dose precalculated on the infant's emergency drug card.

Respiratory depression may produce hypoxemia. A pulse oximeter or transcutaneous oxygen monitor is standard postoperative equipment along with cardiorespiratory monitoring. If available, $TcPCO_2$ monitors (transcutaneous partial pressure of carbon dioxide) are also used to watch for hypercapnia. It is best to have all equipment necessary for assisted ventilation at the bedside.

Withdrawal symptoms (irritability, increased crying, ravenous sucking, vomiting, tremors, and jitteriness) may occur after the narcotic or sedative is discontinued. Minimal handling and a quiet, darkened environment help decrease external stimuli, and a pacifier, swaddling, and holding may provide comfort. To decrease the risk of withdrawal symptoms, a gradual extension of the time between doses or a gradual decrease in the size of the dose should be used.

PARENT TEACHING

Parents should be told before surgery about the anesthesia their infant will receive but often are not. The need for anesthesia and analgesia needs to be explained to parents, along with the physiologic and behavioral benefits of pain relief. The care provider's sensitivity to the neonate's pain and advocating for pain relief are comforting for parents (18). After surgery, comfort measures are ideally provided by parents, who may then actively participate in their infant's pain relief.

Neonates communicate both subjective and objective data about their painful experiences. They depend on the skilled observations, assessments, and interventions of care providers for prompt, safe, and effective relief. Nurses must ensure that they do not suffer unnecessarily.

One of the more sobering aspects of our acknowledgment of neonatal pain is the realization that we are the perpetrators and inflictors of pain on the most innocent and helpless of humankind. We must recognize this fact and deal cognitively, emotionally, and empathically with it, acknowledging that lifesaving care in an NICU is intrusive, noxious, and painful. From the infant's perspective, such care is indistinguishable from the pain of child abuse. Providing, and advocating for, effective pain relief are essential aspects of neonatal nursing care.

REFERENCES

1. American Academy of Pediatrics, Committee on Fetus and Newborn, Committee on Drugs, Section on Anesthesiology and Section on Surgery. Neonatal anesthesia. *Pediatrics* 80: 446, Sept. 1987.
2. Anand, K.J.S., and Hickey, P.R. Pain and its effect in the human neonate and fetus. *N. Engl. J. Med.* 317:1321-1329, Nov. 19, 1987.
3. Herzog, J.M. A neonatal intensive care syndrome: a pain complex involving neuroplasticity and psychic trauma. In *Frontiers of Infant Psychiatry,* edited by J. D. Call and others. New York, 1983, Basic Books, pp. 291-300.
4. Rovee-Collier, C., and Hayne, H. Reactuation of infant memory: implications for cognitive development. *Adv. Child Dev. Behav.* 10:185-238, 1987.
5. Anand, K.J.S., and Carr, D.B. The neuroanatomy, neurophysiology and neurochemistry of pain, stress and analgesia in newborns and children. *Pediatr. Clin. North Am.* 36:795-822, Aug. 1989.
6. Anand, K.J.S. Neonatal stress response to anesthesia and surgery. *Clin. Perinatol.* 17:207-214, Mar. 1990.
7. Grunau, R.V.E., and Craig, K.D. Pain expression in neonates: facial action and cry. *Pain* 28:395-410, Mar. 1987.
8. Anand, K.J.S., and Hickey, P.R. Halothane-morphine compared with high-dose sufentanil for anesthesia and post-operative analgesia in neonatal cardiac surgery. *N. Engl. J. Med.* 326:1-9, Jan. 2, 1992; Comment 326:55-56, Jan. 2, 1992.
9. Gardner, S.L., and others. The neonate and the environment: impact on development. In *Handbook of Neonatal Intensive Care,* 3rd ed., edited by G.B. Merenstein and S.L Gardner. St. Louis, Mosby-Year Book, 1993, pp. 564-608.
10. Marchette, L., and others. Pain reduction interventions during neonatal circumcision. *Nurs. Res.* 40:241-244, July-Aug. 1991; Comment 41:127, Mar-Apr. 1992.
11. Broome, M.E., and Tanzillo, H. Differentiating between pain and agitation in premature neonates. *J. Perinat. Neonatal Nurs.* 4:53-62, July 1990.
12. Budreau, G., and Kleiber, C. Clinical indicators of infant irritability. *Neonatal Netw.* 9:23-30, Feb. 1991.
13. Franck, L.S. A national survey of the assessment and treatment of pain and agitation in the neonatal intensive care unit. *J. Obstet. Gynecol. Neonatal Nurs.* 16:387-393, Nov.-Dec. 1987.
14. Butler, N.C. How to raise professional awareness of the need for adequate pain relief for infants. *Birth* 15:38-41, Mar. 1988.
15. Cunningham, N. Ethical perspectives on the perception and treatment of neonatal pain. *J. Perinat. Neonatal Nurs.* 4:75-83, July 1990.
16. Johnston, C.C., and Stevens, B. Pain assessment in newborns, *J. Perinat. Neonatal Nurs.* 4:41-52, July 1990.
17. Schecter, N.L. The undertreatment of pain in children. *Pediatr. Clin. North Am.* 36:781-794, Aug. 1989.
18. Shapiro, C. Pain in the neonate: assessment and intervention. *Neonatal Netw.* 8:7-21, Aug. 1989.
19. Gruenwald, P., and Becker, P. Developmental enhancement: implementing a program for the NICU. *Neonatal Netw.* 9:29-45, Mar. 1991.
20. Campos, R.G. Soothing pain-elicited distress in infants with swaddling and pacifiers. *Child Dev.* 60:781-792, Aug. 1989.
21. Field, T., and Goldson, E. Pacifying effects of non-nutritive sucking on term and preterm neonates during heelstick procedures. *Pediatrics* 74:1012-1015, Dec. 1984.
22. Blass, E.M., and Hoffmeyer, L.B. Sucrose as an analgesic for newborn infants. *Pediatrics* 87:215-218, Feb. 1991; Comments 88:655, Sept. 1991; 88:1287-1288, Dec. 1991.
23. Smith, B.A., and others. Orally-mediated sources of calming in 1-3 day old human infants. *Dev. Psychol.* 26:731, 1990.
24. Anders, T.F., and Zeanah, C.H. Early infant development from a biological point of view. In *Frontiers of Infant Psychiatry,* edited by J.D. Call and others. New York, Basic Books, 1983, pp. 55-69.
25. Fitzgerald, M., and others. Hyperalgesia in premature infants [letter]. *Lancet* 1:292, Feb. 6, 1988.
26. Tyson, P. Developmental lines and infant assessment. In *Frontiers of Infant Psychiatry,* edited by J.D. Call and others. New York, Basic Books, 1983, pp. 121-125.
27. Anand, K.J.S., and others. Randomized trial of fentanyl anaesthesia in preterm babies undergoing surgery: effects on

the stress response. *Lancet* 1:62-66, Jan. 10, 1987; Erratum 1:234, Jan. 24, 1987.

28. ———. Does halothane anesthesia decrease the metabolic and endocrine stress responses of newborn infants undergoing operation? *Br. Med. J.* (Clin. Res. Ed.) 296:668-672, Mar. 5, 1988.

29. Lambert, G.H., and others. Direct hyperbilirubinemia associated with chloral hydrate administration in the newborn. *Pediatrics* 86:277-281, Aug. 1990.

RESOURCES FOR PARENTS

American Association of Critical Care Nurses. *It's Critical That You Know . . . What You Should Do When Your Baby Is in the NICU. Aliso Viejo, CA: The Association, 1987.*

Butler, N.C. Questions parents and concerned professionals might ask of their local health care institutions, *Birth* 15:40, 1988.

PEDIATRIC POISONINGS: THE 10 MOST TOXIC PRESCRIPTION DRUGS

If your patient is taking certain medications, he should know how dangerous they can be to a child. Here's a rundown of 10 drugs that, in small hands, can be deadly.

BY JAMES MORELLI

oison control centers field thousands of calls every year about children who have swallowed toxic amounts of over-the-counter products. Acetaminophen poisoning in children under age six alone accounted for 57,377 calls in 1991. Children also often grab handfuls of chewable vitamins, and thus ingest dangerous levels of iron, or—more rarely since acetaminophen became more common—they overdose on aspirin.

Prescription drugs can be far more dangerous. It doesn't take very much at all—a few tablets, a couple of teaspoonfuls— of some highly potent prescription drugs to seriously, even fatally, poison a child.

The accident is sometimes due to look-alike containers, such as a topical solution dispensed in what look like cough syrup bottles, which confuses parents. Or, a drug may come in a bottle that isn't childproof. Often, the child thinks the drug is candy, since it's brightly colored, comes in many tiny pieces, and may even taste good.

The following 10 drugs (or, in some cases, drug classes) head the list of deadly prescription drugs. Some made the list because they're commonly prescribed for adults, but tiny doses in small children can be fatal. Others are

James Morelli, BS Pharmacy, is a registered pharmacist and poison information specialist at Georgia Poison Control Center, Atlanta.

on the list because, while prescribed for children, poisonings have occurred when the drugs were given at the wrong dose or by the wrong route.

Emergency department and ICU nurses, of course, need to be aware of their toxic effects and recommended treatments, but all nurses can help by warning adults who take or dispense these drugs about the threat to children.

1. CYCLIC ANTIDEPRESSANTS
Amitriptyline (Elavil), Desipramine (Norpramin), Imipramine (Tofranil)

Cyclic antidepressants are the great killers in the overdose world. Despite the drugs' relative antiquity, pediatric use of cyclic antidepressants is increasing: to control bedwetting, for example, and in attention deficit disorder, which means more opportunities for toxic exposures in children.

To children, the bright yellow, green, and blue tablets look like M&Ms. But 10 to 20 mg/kg of most cyclic antidepressants—a handful of, say, 25-mg Elavil tablets—will cause severe toxicity in a child. The first sign of poisoning may be extreme drowsiness. Within 20 to 30 minutes, the child may develop seizures and then lapse into coma. Deaths are linked to cardiac disturbances, and, in some cases, from intractable seizures.

Therapeutically, most cyclic antidepressants block the uptake of norepinephrine, a cardiostimulant. Mas-

sive blockade raises norepinephrine levels, resulting in massive stimulation, with tachycardia and other dysrhythmias possible. Anticholinergic effects raise blood pressure and alpha-receptor blocking effects lead mainly to postural hypotension, contributing to the cardiac instability.

Alkalinization of the blood with sodium bicarbonate protects the heart, probably by reducing the amount of unbound drug. Blood pH should be kept between 7.45 and 7.55. Phenytoin (15 mg/kg IV) also protects the heart and prevents seizures; lidocaine, or bretylium as a last resort, may also be used for dysrhythmia control.

Poison centers recommend cardiomonitoring all children with possible overdoses for at least six hours, and paying special attention to the QRS interval of the ECG. Widening of the QRS, especially if it's greater than 0.1 second, may indicate imminent dysrhythmias and seizures. All patients with symptoms of ECG changes must be admitted to ICU.

Patients with symptoms of overdose may benefit from intubation for airway protection and gastric lavage to remove any unabsorbed drug. Then, as long as the drug's anticholinergic effects have not caused paralytic ileus, the children can be given multiple doses of activated charcoal, usually 1 g/kg every four hours (for a maximum of 24 hours). The charcoal binds the cyclic antidepressant to prevent it from recirculating through the liver. A cathartic, such as sorbitol, may be given with the first dose of charcoal. Some poison control centers suggest adding sorbitol to every other dose, but it's not advisable to give repeated doses of sorbitol to children due to risk of excessive fluid and electrolyte loss.

Generally, patients are kept in intensive care until asymptomatic and dysrhythmia-free for 24 hours.

2. 4-AMINOQUINOLINES
Chloroquine (Aralen); Hydroxychloroquine (Plaquenil); Quinacrine (Atabrine)

Classified as antimalarials, some aminoquinolines (like Plaquenil) are prescribed for rheumatoid arthritis. As the population ages, these unusual remedies may show up more frequently in household medicine cabinets.

It's crucial to warn anyone who's taking this drug about its great threat to children: A tablet or two of 500-mg chloroquine phosphate can kill a child within an hour. The manufacturer of Plaquenil, Sanofi Winthrop, supplies red stickers warning consumers to keep the drug out of children's reach.

The aminoquinolines poison cardiac tissue directly, leading to vasodilation, hypotension, and shock. This massive breakdown in cardiac function happens quickly, and fatalities can occur within one to two hours after ingestion. If possible, poisoned children should immediately be intubated to preserve the airway, then lavaged and given a dose of activated charcoal to bind aminoquinoline residues. Ipecac syrup works too slowly to be useful in emergency treatment. It's not recommended unless the child is more than 20 minutes away from a hospital or definitive therapy.

Defibrillators, pacemakers, and mechanical ventilation may be needed in poisoned patients. Lidocaine may also be useful for dysrhythmias.

3. ANTIDIARRHEALS
Diphenoxylate with Atropine (Lomotil); Difenoxin (Motofen)

Few adults experience systemic effects from these tiny white tablets. Children, however, can slip into a coma after ingesting only a tablet or two. (Lomotil is also available as a tasty syrup.)

While most opioid ingestions cause rapid drowsiness and respiratory depression, the toxic effects of diphenoxylate (a meperidine derivative) are often delayed eight hours or longer, perhaps because atropine slows gastric motility. In fact, children have reportedly developed cardiopulmonary arrest 12 hours after swallowing Lomotil. Poison control centers recommend that all children who ingest diphenoxylate with atropine be observed in the ICU for 24 hours after decontamination. Be sure to instruct parents who elect to "watch" a child at home after to remain vigilant for the entire 24 hours.

In addition to shortness of breath or labored breathing, overdose is signaled by anticholinergic effects: Before drowsiness sets in, children may complain of feeling hot and thirsty and their pupils may dilate, signs of atropine poisoning.

Intravenous naloxone (Narcan) 0.4 to 2 mg reverses the respiratory depression and sedation seen with diphenoxylate. The dose may be repeated every two minutes until a patient improves, or until 10 mg has been given. Severely poisoned patients may require a continuous iv infusion of naloxone, after initial boluses.

Activated charcoal effectively binds opioids.

4. HYDROCODONE-BASED COUGH SYRUPS
Hycodan, Tussionex

Sweet, fruit-flavored, hydrocodone-based cough syrups present a temptation for youngsters.

Pediatricians sometimes prescribe small amounts of "low-strength" hydrocodone formulations for serious coughs. But a thin line divides therapeutic and toxic doses of these antitussives. As little as a teaspoonful or two (about 2.5 to 5 mg of hydrocodone, a derivative of codeine) can cause respiratory depression and severe drowsiness within an hour or two.

Naloxone reverses hydrocodone's depressive effects. Children often are given activated charcoal, as well.

INDIVIDUAL DRUGS

Besides the four drug classes just mentioned, the following individual drugs carry a high risk of toxicity in children:

INITIAL ASSESSMENT

Always begin with the basics. Many ingested drugs induce vomiting or depress the central nervous system. Be sure to check:
- airway, breathing, circulation
- vital signs
- level of consciousness and pupils
- perfusion

Ask the parents:
- the symptoms
- information about what was ingested—nature, time, amount; check the container if they brought it
- name and location of prescription medications they keep at home
- any prehospital treatment

Based on your assessment, stabilizing your patient's respiratory, cardiovascular, and neurological status is the priority. Once achieved, gastrointestinal decontamination can begin. Call the local poison control center to be sure you've covered all the bases. It's a valuable resource for information on clinical effects and treatment.

---

5. Propoxyphene (Darvon, Darvocet)

As few as four 65-mg capsules of propoxyphene can kill an average-sized two-year-old in an hour. Seizures complicate what otherwise presents as a classic opioid toxicity.

Naloxone reverses propoxyphene's respiratory depressant and sedative effects and, combined with oxygen, raises the seizure threshold. (Large doses may be required to counteract the respiratory effect.) Diazepam 0.1 to 0.3 mg/kg also controls propoxyphene seizures but increases sedation. Alternative antiseizure medications include phenytoin and phenobarbital. If administered early, activated charcoal extensively binds propoxyphene.

6. Ethchlorvynol (Placidyl)

Placidyl, one of the original sedative-hypnotics, is a dangerous dinosaur that was first marketed in the 1950s.

Rarely used anymore, ethchlorvynol capsules have a colorful, child-tempting appearance. They leave a minty smell on the breath. A single capsule can push a toddler into a deep, prolonged coma that reflects the drug's high liposolubility. The slow leaching of the drug from fat stores into systemic circulation can produce cyclic periods of sedation interspersed with periods of apparent recovery, followed by further coma. Be aware that flat EEG readings in a comatose child may be followed by recovery.

Two other effects mark ethchlorvynol overdose: severe hypotension and hypothermia. Should iv fluids fail to correct the drop in blood pressure, dopamine 2 to 5 µg/kg/minute can be used, or norepinephrine 0.1 to 0.2 µg/kg/minute. Charcoal may also be used. If the patient is both comatose and has a high blood level of the drug, resin hemoperfusion is the treatment of choice. If that's unavailable and treatment is begun within five hours, charcoal hemoperfusion may be substituted.

For hypothermia, wrap the child in warm blankets. Some may require warmed iv fluids and warm gastric lavage.

Naloxone doesn't relieve the respiratory and central nervous system depression seen with ethchlorvynol. These must be managed symptomatically.

7. Lindane (Kwell)

Used properly, lindane (1% solution prescribed for scabies and head and body lice) rarely causes systemic effects. But when applied liberally, frequently, or left on the skin for long periods (particularly on or near open cuts or sores), it can be absorbed and cause seizures.

More commonly, problems occur when the product is ingested. Pharmacists frequently repackage lindane products in the same brown glass bottles used for cough syrup. And, despite bright red "For External Use Only" stickers, parents sometimes give the product by mouth to infested children. As little as two teaspoonfuls of a lindane shampoo or lotion can poison a child.

Tremors and nervousness may mark the initial stages of lindane toxicity, but seizures can occur without warning. These signs of CNS stimulation are treated with pentobarbital, phenobarbital, or diazepam.

Avoid three things with oral lindane poisonings: ipecac, milk, and sympathomimetic amines. Ipecac may induce vomiting during a seizure. Milk and other fatty foods may increase the absorption of lindane. Sympathomimetic amines, such as phenylpropanolamine, pseudoephedrine, and metaproterenol—ingredients found in many common cold, allergy, and asthma medications—may irritate cardiac tissue and may cause dysrhythmias.

Most often, ingestions of lindane are treated with gastric lavage and activated charcoal.

8. Lithium Carbonate (Eskalith, Lithobid)

No one is quite sure how lithium stabilizes the mood swings of manic-depressives. One thing is known, though: A little lithium can change a life; a bit more can poison.

While lithium levels provide some benchmark for toxicity, they're unreliable predictors. Persistent, high lithium levels cause more severe toxicity than a high level due to an acute, accidental exposure. Nonetheless, lithium is highly toxic. A teaspoonful of lithium citrate syrup packs 300 mg of lithium, enough to poison a small child. Though the standard pediatric dose of syrup is 15 to 20 mg/kg day—which would give a 24-kg (53-lb) child 480 mg—that dose is divided over the course of the day. The danger is that parents can misunderstand and poison the child by giving an undivided dose or doubling doses when one is missed.

Nearly half of patients poisoned by lithium will present with gastrointestinal symptoms—nausea, vomiting, and diarrhea. They may be confused and lethargic. Dysrhythmias and hypotension may occur.

Lithium won't bind to activated charcoal and much of overdose therapy rests on replacing the body's sodium and water balance. Severe poisonings may require hemodialysis.

9. Glyburide/glipizide (DiaBeta, Micronase/Glucotrol)

Glyburide and glipizide are the twin terrors of the oral hypoglycemic world. Ingestions produce an intense, prolonged drop in blood glucose levels, sometimes after a single tablet.

The once-daily dosing (with nearly 24-hour duration of action) of these

drugs is a key factor in their toxicity. Their effects usually peak within a few hours, but symptoms of hypoglycemic poisoning—weakness, dizziness, lethargy, seizures, and coma—may be delayed for 12 hours or longer.

Begin with lavage to remove any unabsorbed drug, followed by a dose of activated charcoal to deactivate any remaining drug. If, after 24 hours, the child's blood glucose level is still low, give glucose as an antidote. For severe poisonings, 50 mL of 50% iv glucose solution should be given immediately, and an iv infusion of 10% glucose started. Glucose is preferred to glucagon, which takes nearly 20 minutes to work. Patients who respond to neither may benefit from diazoxide, which suppresses insulin secretion from the pancreas.

10. Clonidine (Catapres)

One of the more unusual antihypertensives, clonidine stimulates central alpha-receptors to lower blood pressure. This central action produces a toxicity similar to that of opioids, but compounded by severe hypotension, bradycardia, and sometimes dysrhythmias.

Children ingesting one or two 0.1- to 0.3-mg tablets of clonidine may become weak, pale, and lethargic within 30 minutes. Blood pressure may rise at first before dropping, and respiratory depression is likely.

Clonidine's quick onset precludes the use of ipecac syrup. Gastric lavage and activated charcoal are better choices. Clonidine's relationship to opioids allows for use of naloxone to reverse sedation and respiratory depression.

SELECTED REFERENCES

Ellenhorn, M.J., and Barceloux, D.G. *Medical Toxicology, Diagnosis and Treatment of Human Poisoning.* New York, Elsevier, 1987, p. 402.

Litovitz, T. L., and others. 1991 annual report of the American Association of Poison Control Centers National Data Collection System. *Am. J. Emerg. Med.* 10:452-505, Sept. 1992.

Physician's Desk Reference. 47th ed. Montvale, NJ, Medical Economics Data, 1993, pp. 2163, 2264, 2372.

Poisindex (software program). Denver, CO, Micromedex, Inc., 1993.

Thomas, D. O. *Quick Reference to Pediatric Emergency Nursing.* Gaithersburg, MD, Aspen, 1991, pp. 227-237.

CONTROVERSIES IN CARING FOR THE CHILD WITH A HEAD INJURY

Maintaining ventilation, oxygenation, and circulation is critical, but beyond these basics many approaches to care are controversial.

BY ELLEN A. REYNOLDS

Trauma is the leading killer of children, being responsible for between 40 and 60 percent of children's deaths each year. Nearly half of pediatric trauma cases involve head injury, which is a particularly lethal form of trauma. The mortality rate for pediatric trauma involving head injury is 26 times that of nonhead trauma (1). In addition, many head-injured children are left with significant disabilities. Many of these disabilities may not be apparent at hospital discharge, but show up months later as learning difficulties, behavioral changes, or emotional disturbances (2).

Thus, head injury is a common type of trauma in children that has nursing implications ranging from resuscitation needs to long-term care issues. Nursing care for the head-injured child tends to be complex, whether in the intensive care unit or on the acute care floor. Nowhere is the collaboration of medical and nursing care as important as it is in a child with a head injury. While many institutions have some type of "head injury protocol," the bases for various interventions are often unclear to nurses. In fact, many of the interventions for head trauma are controversial.

Ellen A. Reynolds, RN, CEN, MS, is a clinical research nurse specialist at Children's Hospital of Pittsburgh. This article is the basis for a talk presented at the MCN Convention in Atlanta in 1992.

CHILDREN ARE MORE VULNERABLE THAN ADULTS IN SOME RESPECTS, LESS SO IN OTHERS

Motor vehicle-related incidents are the most common cause of head injuries in children, and are associated with a high mortality rate. Falls are the next most common, and tend to be the least lethal mechanism. Ninety-seven percent of head trauma in children is blunt, although many urban centers are now reporting a higher than ever percentage of gunshot wounds to the head. Boys are more likely than girls to receive a head injury, and one-to-five-year-olds are the most common victims (1).

Certain aspects of child anatomy and physiology affect how young children are injured, how they manifest their injuries, and how they respond to various stressors and therapies. For example, infants and toddlers have large, heavy heads and underdeveloped neck muscles. This causes them to lead with their heads in impact situations, making them vulnerable to neck injuries as well as acceleration-deceleration brain injuries. Myelinization and other physiological processes in an infant's brain are incomplete (3). Young children have a pronounced vagal response that is manifested as bradycardia. This can compromise cardiac output in the young child. Children also have a tenuous fluid balance, which makes issues of fluid resuscitation and restriction even more complicated.

On the positive side, intracranial lesions are less common in children than adults. The open fontanelles and sutures in an infant's skull can accommodate expansion, affording some protection from an increase in intracranial pressure. While there is no clear-cut evidence, many experts feel that children suffering certain types of head injury tend to fare better than adults with the same type of injury—perhaps due to the plasticity or rapid growth state of the child's brain (4).

The concept of primary injury versus secondary injury is important since the category of injury determines the care. The primary injury occurs at the moment of impact—the bruising, laceration, or compression of the brain itself—and very few medical and nursing interventions are actually directed at the primary injury. The interventions are largely aimed at restoring equilibrium and preventing secondary injury, which is the sequelae of events triggered locally and systemically by the primary injury. These can range from compromised nutrient/waste exchange at the cellular level caused by ionic pump failure, to anoxia caused by respiratory failure.

Multiple trauma is common in children and may complicate treatment of any head injury. Hypotension resulting from a ruptured spleen, for example, can make attempts at cerebral resuscitation difficult or futile. Thus, the primary and secondary surveys, with careful attention to airway and circulation, are essential first steps in managing the child with head trauma.

505

KEY TO TREATMENT IS MAINTAINING BALANCE

The skull is normally a rigid structure that contains cerebrospinal fluid (CSF), blood, and brain tissue. These three volumes exist in equilibrium with each other and contribute to intracranial pressure (ICP). When the volume of one of these increases, another must decrease in order to maintain a stable ICP. This principle is referred to as the modified Monro-Kellie doctrine, and functions via the complex process of autoregulation. (See Concepts in Intracranial Dynamics.)

In head injury, three types of dysfunction may occur to alter this balance. Hyperemia, or an increase in blood flow, typically occurs in the head-injured child. Outflow of CSF may be compromised as a result of swelling related to injury. Intracranial lesions or edema may lead to increased brain volume. Thus, several or all three volumes may increase, leading to a net increase in ICP. As ICP rises, levels of consciousness, and respiratory rate and depth fall. The resulting hypoxia and hypercapnia lead to acidosis, which stimulates further increases in ICP. As this cycle perpetuates itself, autoregulation may be lost and ischemia may result.

The cerebral perfusion pressure (CPP), or the pumping pressure required to perfuse the brain, is the difference between the mean arterial pressure (MAP) and the ICP. Thus, if the MAP drops (as in shock), or if ICP rises, the CPP is decreased. In the early stages of increased ICP, the blood pressure often increases as the body attempts to compensate through the process of autoregulation. This is physiologically normal and can be a protective response. However, extreme or prolonged hypertension poses its own dangers, including worsening brain edema and damage to other organs.

The brain's responses to injury are still not clearly understood, and methods of treatment may not have the same effect in clinical care as they have in the laboratory. Thus, approaches to care are often controversial, and may vary among institutions. The objectives of neurosurgical and nursing management are similar: to maintain adequate ventilation, oxygenation, and circulation; to monitor and treat increased ICP; to minimize cerebral oxygen re-

---

CONCEPTS IN INTRACRANIAL DYNAMICS

The complex interrelationships among structures and processes in the brain are not fully understood. The concepts described here provide a brief review of intracranial pressure dynamics.

- **Brain swelling** can be the result of hyperemia (increased blood flow) or edema (excess fluid in brain tissue)
- **Intracranial pressure** (ICP) is a function of the volumes of brain tissue, blood, and cerebrospinal fluid. Its normal range is from 0 to 15 mm Hg.
- **Mean arterial pressure** (MAP) is the mean of the systolic and diastolic blood pressures, and reflects vascular tone as well as volume status. It is normally maintained by the process of *autoregulation*, which may be disrupted in head injury.
- **Cerebral perfusion pressure** (CPP) is the net pressure required to perfuse the brain. It can be represented by the equation CPP = MAP–ICP. In a normal healthy adult, the CPP is probably between 80 and 100 mm Hg (18). A normal value for children is not available, but since the CPP is based on mean arterial pressure, the normal value is probably somewhat lower for children than adults. The general recommendation for a head-injured patient has traditionally been to maintain the CPP above 50 mm Hg; however, in recent years new evidence has indicated that CPP should be maintained closer to 80 mm Hg to prevent ischemia (7).
- **Cerebral blood flow** (CBF) provides for the delivery of oxygen and necessary nutrients to the brain. Its value depends on cerebral perfusion pressure, blood viscosity, and the dimensions of the vascular bed.

---

quirements; and to provide support to the child and family during the recovery phases.

Ensuring Adequate Ventilation and Oxygenation. Carbon dioxide is a potent vasodilator that acts to maintain a high level of blood flow to the brain. As $PaCO_2$ drops, so does cerebral blood volume. The use of hyperventilation as therapy has been based on the premise that hyperemia is a significant component of increased ICP, and that decreasing the $PaCO_2$ will reverse acidosis in the brain and cerebrospinal fluid. Recent evidence suggests that the effects of hyperventilation on the pH of CSF are short-lived, and that prophylactic hyperventilation can actually retard recovery from head injury (5).

Although the reasons for this are unclear, it may be that hyperventilation reduces cerebral blood flow to ischemic levels or that prophylactic hyperventilation compromises the mechanisms available for volume regulation, leading to later increases in ICP.

Thus, while the elimination of CO_2 by hyperventilation can be helpful in limiting hyperemia and ICP spikes, an optimal maintenance $PaCO_2$ level must be found that will allow sufficient cerebral blood flow to prevent ischemia. A recently developed diagnostic tool,

xenon flow scan, identifies volume of blood flow to various parts of the brain. This information may then be correlated with the patient's $PaCO_2$ to determine his ventilation needs.

Optimal ventilation and oxygenation also depends on a healthy pulmonary system. Turning and positioning the child, chest physical therapy (PT), and suctioning are all necessary to prevent pulmonary complications, but are also associated with ICP spikes. Providing sedation and/or analgesia prior to such procedures is an important aspect of ICP control. Thorough preoxygenation prior to suctioning is required, and suctioning attempts are limited to 10 seconds. Lidocaine instilled into the endotracheal tube or given IV prior to suctioning blunts the cough reflex and can help to prevent ICP increases.

A recent nursing study demonstrated the efficacy of a protocol involving routine prophylactic chest PT with the head-injured patient in the Trendelenburg position. Although ICP was highest during chest PT in the Trendelenburg position, it declined to baseline more rapidly than when the horizontal position for chest PT was used (6). Proper neck alignment and sedation were important factors in avoiding ICP hypertension in this study. Careful consideration needs to

Advantages and disadvantages of various types of intracranial pressure monitoring

Type	Advantages	Disadvantages
Intracranial bolt	Provides direct measurement; useful if ventricles are small or collapsed; easy to insert	Requires closed skull, CSF can't be drained
Ventricular catheter	Provides direct measurement; can use to drain cerebral spinal fluid (CSF)	Very invasive; difficult to place if ventricles small or shifted; increased risk of infection
Epidural probe accuracy	Minimally invasive; fiberoptic system does not depend on patient position for accuracy	CSF can't be drained; fiber optic system requires special monitor

be given to findings such as these, which support the controlled use of interventions to prevent pulmonary complications.

Circulatory Support. Adequate fluid resuscitation is essential to successful cerebral outcome. Once fluids have been replaced, intake and output are monitored carefully to ensure a balance. Children with diabetes insipidus, a common complication of head injury, can lose a large volume of fluid in a short period of time. Such urine losses, as well as nasogastric losses, are replaced as needed. Pressors may be used to maintain adequate blood pressure. Positioning the child with the head of the bed elevated by 30 degrees or less enhances venous outflow from the head. However, the head of the bed cannot be elevated if the child is hemodynamically unstable, as cerebral perfusion will be compromised.

A recent study highlighted the importance of maintaining adequate cerebral perfusion (7). In that protocol, cerebral perfusion pressure was maintained at an average of 84 mm Hg by using volume expansion, flat positioning, and pressors as needed. Mannitol and CSF drainage were used as needed to decrease ICP. It was found that cerebral perfusion pressure could be artificially increased without inducing intracranial hypertension or negative systemic effects. This approach is based on enhancing the child's own physiological response, that is, increasing cerebral perfusion pressure when ICP is elevated.

Monitoring and Treatment of Increased ICP. Left untreated, persistent elevations in ICP can lead to focal ischemia, compression of brain structures, and ultimately herniation. Serial neurological exams are the most effective means of assessing changes in the child with a head injury. Level of consciousness is the most sensitive indicator of neurological status.

The nurse caring for the head-injured child needs to have solid knowledge of child development in order to assess for abnormalities. For example, it may be difficult to ascertain if a toddler who doesn't respond to verbal cues is unable or uncooperative. Also, the infant, toddler, or preschooler who doesn't fight or cry while blood work is being obtained is likely to have an altered level of consciousness.

In addition to following neurological status, intracranial pressure may be monitored directly using an intracranial bolt, a ventricular catheter, or an epidural probe system (see Types of Intracranial Pressure Monitoring). Each of these systems has advantages and disadvantages, but allows caregivers to monitor the effects of various stimuli and therapies (see Advantages and Disadvantages of Various Types of Intracranial Pressure Monitoring).

During the acute phase of management, fluid restriction may be employed to limit brain hyperemia and edema. Fluid restriction will also act to increase serum osmolality, thus enhancing fluid mobilization from brain tissue into the vascular space. Diuretics are often used in conjunction with fluid restriction. In the presence of an intact blood-brain barrier, mannitol acts to decrease edema by osmotic diuresis. It also decreases blood viscosity, lowering cerebral blood volume while maintaining cerebral blood flow (8). With osmotic diuretics, a temporary increase in cerebral blood flow may occur until the excess vascular fluid is cleared by the kidneys. Loop diuretics are often given alone or in conjunction with mannitol.

A current controversy in this area focuses on a study indicating that autoregulation may be intact in the majority of head-injured children (9). If this is the case, therapies such as fluid restriction and diuresis that potentially decrease systemic blood pressure could cause a corresponding increase in ICP and should be used with caution.

Environmental stimuli and routine nursing care measures are often the cause of ICP spikes in children with head injury. The environment is kept as quiet as possible, which can be difficult in a busy ICU. Dimming the lights and avoiding bedside discussion may help to decrease stimulation. However, nursing studies have shown that the presence of family, nonprocedural touch, and calm reassurances can help to decrease ICP, so observing the patient's responses may be the best guide to structuring stimulation (10).

Careful positioning, maintaining the head in a midline position, and avoiding lateral flexion can also help to limit ICP response. Acute hip flexion is also avoided (6).

An important aspect of controlling intracranial pressure is minimizing cerebral oxygen requirements. Fever and seizure activity can both increase metabolic demands on the brain and need to be aggressively managed. Febrile children may be given antipyretics or may be cooled by means of a cooling blanket. The medical approach to seizure prophylaxis varies among providers, but is most likely to be instituted in the child with penetrating injuries, severe cortical contusion, or recurrent seizures (3,11).

In the case of a moribund child, the presence of high blood levels of barbiturates will violate criteria for determining brain death. For this and other therapeutic reasons, phenytoin is generally the preferred anticonvulsant for children beyond infancy. Seizure medications can be sedating and may adversely affect cognitive and behavioral

Rancho Los Amigos scale of congnitive function

LEVEL	RECOVERY PHASE	APPROACH
I. No response		
II. Generalized response	Decreased response	Stimulation
III. Localized response		
IV. Agitated response	Agitated response	Structure
V. Confused, inappropriate, nonagitated	Confused response	Structure
VI. Confused, appropriate		
VII. Automatic approach	Automatic response	Community
VIII. Purposeful, appropriate		

The Rancho Los Amigos Scale of Cognitive Function identifies behavioral correlates of neurological recovery and can be used to guide care planning. Adapted from *Rehabilitation of the Head-Injured Adult—Comprehensive Management.* Downey, CA, Rancho Los Amigos Hospital, 1980, pp. 8-11.

functioning; recent studies indicate that the prophylactic effect lasts only about a week (12). These findings call into question the practice of long-term seizure prophylaxis.

Another controversial therapy for uncontrolled ICP is the use of barbiturate coma. In some studies, this treatment has been shown to directly decrease the brain's metabolic needs, but research on its success in improving outcome in children is inconclusive (13). The child in barbiturate coma requires complete ventilatory and circulatory support and monitoring. Neurologic status cannot be readily assessed due to the blunting or elimination of responses and reflexes.

In addition, continuous infusion of barbiturates is associated with complications, including arterial hypotension, liver failure, and immunosuppression (14). Because of the high risk and uncertain likelihood of success with this therapy, many use it only as a last-ditch effort in the child with uncontrollable ICP.

Routine sedation and analgesia also present a dilemma—the conflict between the need to promote comfort and relieve anxiety in the child versus the need to be able to assess for neurological changes. In most cases, a balance between the two can be met. Sedation can be provided prior to procedures and stimulation, and can be withheld prior to planned neurological evaluations. In addition, naloxone (Narcan) can be used to reverse the sedative effects of narcotics if evaluation is necessary. The role of the nurse in structuring the patient's daily schedule and providing nonpharmaceutical pain and anxiety relief measures is of key importance.

While steroids are still used with certain types of brain tumors to decrease edema, there is no clear evidence that the use of steroids following brain trauma is beneficial. Several studies point to the risks associated with this therapy (15,16).

Futuristic Approaches. The field of neurotrauma is filled with experimental modalities. Most traditional therapies act on the intact, or uninjured brain, and new directions of thought are aimed at limiting or reversing the effects of the injury itself. A current area of exploration is the use of pharmaceutical "scavengers" or "lazaroids" to neutralize the effects of complications that can occur during reperfusion of an injured tissue.

The processes that cause these complications include alterations in the calcium channel system, hydrolysis of cell membrane phospholipids, and formation of oxygen-derived free radicals. It is postulated that these processes can be interrupted by certain drugs, thus limiting further cell injury and death. The extent and clinical significance of reperfusion injury is still unclear. Studies in this realm are in early stages and have not yet established an effect on human outcome (8).

Other approaches propose the use of gangliosides and beta nerve growth factor to directly enhance neuronal regeneration. Based on the literature documenting brain recovery following cardiac arrest in cold water near-drowning, researchers are reexamining the usefulness of induced hypothermia—specifically, local cranial cooling's effect on limiting cell damage during reperfusion (8).

RECOVERY PHASE INVOLVES SUPPORT FOR BOTH CHILD AND FAMILY

The last area of challenge for the nurse caring for the child with a head injury is the management of the phases of recovery for both the child and the family. Discharge and rehabilitation planning, school needs, and home modifications are begun as soon as possible. Great strides are begun as soon as possible. Great studies have been made in the rehabilitation arena in recent years, and the principles of rehabilitative care can be incorporated into the initial nursing care plan.

The Rancho Los Amigos Scale of Cognitive Functioning is a useful tool for anticipating progress in brain recovery and for planning care during the different phases (17). For example, during the early phases, clinicians use aggressive stimulation to elicit any type of response from the child. This is modified to focus on selective stimulation as the child moves into more agitated phases. In addition, clinicians can help the parents to recognize characteristics of the various stages and thus be prepared for what may lie ahead.

Families are never prepared for the devastation of severe brain injury. Popular media tend to portray coma recovery as a quick, smooth process in which the child suddenly "wakes up," able to talk and ready to resume activities. In fact, the road to recovery is often painfully slow and filled with plateaus and valleys. Providing education and support to the entire injured family during this time is integral to their ability to accept the child's injury, deal with its implications for their lives, and move on to help the child achieve maximum functioning.

For the nurse caring for a child with

a head injury, these needs must be balanced with the complex physical care administered in the face of changing care modalities and technology. These interrelated complexities pose a significant challenge for the nurse designing and giving care to these youngsters.

REFERENCES

1. Lescohier, I., and DiScala, C. Causes and outcomes of blunt trauma in children, (US Dept. of Education NIDRR Grant #H133B80009-9). Boston, Tufts University School of Medicine, 1991 (Unpublished paper).
2. Ewing-Cobbs, L., and others. Neurobehavioral sequelae following head injury to children: Education implications. *J. Head Trauma Rehabil.,* 1(4):57-65, Dec. 1986.
3. Vernon-Levett, P. Head injuries in children. *Crit. Care Nurs. Clin. North Am.* 3:411-421, Sept. 1991.
4. Wagstyl, J., and others. Early prediction of outcome following head injury in children. *J. Pediatr. Surg.* 22:127-129, Feb. 1987.
5. Muizelaar, J.P., and others. Adverse effects of prolonged hyperventilation in patients with severe head injury: a randomized clinical trial. *J. Neurosurg.* 75:731-739, Nov. 1991.
6. Fontaine, D.K., and McQuillan, K. Positioning as a nursing therapy in trauma care. *Crit. Care Nurs. Clin. North Am.* 1:105-111, Mar. 1989.
7. Rosner, M.J., and Daughton, S. Cerebral perfusion pressure management in head injury. *J. Trauma* 30:933-940, Aug. 1990.
8. Kochanek P.M., and others. Hypoxic ischemic encephalopathy: pathobiology and therapy of the postresuscitation syndrome in children. In *Pediatric Critical Care Medicine,* ed. by B. Fuhrman and J. Zimmerman, St. Louis, Mosby Year Book, 1992, pp. 637-657.
9. Muizelaar, J.P., and others. Cerebral blood flow and metabolism in severely head-injured children. Part 2. Autoregulation. *J. Neurosurg.* 71:72-76, July 1989.
10. Farley, J.A. The comatose child. Analysis of factors affecting intracranial pressure. *Dimens. Crit. Care Nurs.* 9:216-222, July-Aug. 1990.
11. Wasco, J. To treat or not to treat? *Headlines* (New Medico Neurologic Rehabilitation System) Winter Issue, 1991, p. 20.
12. Ackerman, A.D. Current issues in the care of the head-injured child. *Curr. Opin. Pediatr.* 3:433-438, June 1991.
13. Pittman, T., and others. Efficacy of barbiturates in the treatment of resistant intracranial hypertension in severely head-injured children. *Pediatr. Neurosci.* 1989;15(1):13-17.
14. Dearden, N.M. Management of raised intracranial pressure after severe head injury. *Br. J. Hosp. Med.* 36:94-103, Aug. 1986.
15. Ford, E.G., and others. Steroid administration potentiates urinary nitrogen losses in head-injured children. *J. Trauma* 27:1074-1077, Sept. 1987.
16. Cooper, P.R., and others. Dexamethasone and severe head injury. A prospective double-blind study. *J. Neurosurg.* 51:307-316, Sept. 1979.
17. Reilly, A.N., and others. Head trauma in children: The stages to cognitive recovery. *MCN* 12:405-412, Dec. 1987.
18. Andrus, C. Intracranial pressure: dynamics and nursing management. *J. Neurosci. Nurs.* 23:85-91, Apr. 1991.

COGNITIVE AND BEHAVIORAL STRATEGIES TO REDUCE CHILDREN'S PAIN

The practical points of utilizing these strategies to reduce children's pain and stress.

BY MARY K. KACHOYEANOS AND MARGARET FRIEDHOFF

Despite a greater national awareness of the need for pain relief, children's pain continues to be undertreated. Moreover, even though children describe invasive procedures as the greatest source of distress and pain, they are inadequately prepared for procedures (1-3).

The negative physical and psychological consequences of pain are well documented. Patients in pain secrete higher levels of cortisol, have compromised immune systems, increased infections, and delayed wound healing (4).

Also, for their current and future mental health, helping children cope with pain is important. Adults who had traumatic experiences with needlesticks as children report a morbid fear of needles (5). Certain maladaptive behavior in adults has been attributed to traumatic experiences in childhood (5). Yet children who are helped to cope with painful procedures learn methods of self-control and mastery that can be applied in other stressful situations and future health care encounters (6).

The issue of pain control has prompted the development of federal guidelines, which address cognitive and behavioral strategies as well as analgesia (7). Imagery, distraction, relaxation, play, various tactile techniques, and other cognitive and behavioral strategies are known to be effective in managing a child's pain and distress from cancer and related therapies (8-11). Less reported is how to use these strategies to help other children deal with the pain and distress of hospitalization and procedures.

TYPES OF COGNITIVE STRATEGIES

The hypnotic technique, guided imagery, is a widely used cognitive strategy to minimize pain in children.

Through guided imagery, the child is helped to reach an altered state of consciousness in which she visualizes familiar or interesting images. Usually, children aged three and older are imaginative and able to participate in imagery experiences. The "pain switch' is an example of the use of guided imagery (12). Children are asked to imagine a pain switch, like a light switch; they may even give it a color. Then they mentally visualize turning the switch off in the area where pain is inflicted, such as in the thigh where intramuscular injections are given.

A creative method of using imagery is storytelling. Either the child develops the story or the child listens to a story (13). For example, during the changing of her colostomy dressings, Jane told a story about going to a picnic. She detailed the picnic setting, the kinds of food available, and the smells and tastes of the food.

A popular use of imagery combined with tactile sensation is the "magic glove." An imaginary glove is placed on the hand, finger by finger. The child is told the glove will help lessen the discomfort of a needlestick. Because children have vivid imaginations and few inhibitions, they are very receptive to the power of suggestion. An adaptation of the concept is the magic blanket, which can be used in areas where a glove might not be effective, such as the thigh, back, and hip.

Tactile transference is useful when areas on the body are not directly accessible to touch, such as during a spinal tap (12). Before the procedure, the nurse soothingly rubs the area on the child's back where the needle is to be inserted, at the same time stroking the child's hand. The child is told that when the spinal needle is inserted, the hand will be stroked, and the child will experience the same soothing sensations on her back.

To use emotive imagery, the nurse weaves the child's favorite superhero or fantasy image into the current clinical situation, to give a motivation for mastery (12). For example, the nurse might call upon one of the Ninja Turtles to help fight the pain impulses.

Distraction, either active or passive, is used to divert the child's attention from the intrusive procedure to other stimuli. In active distraction, the child is involved. For infants, a pacifier may help minimize the distress of heelsticks (14,15). For older children, blowing bubbles, counting the ceiling tiles or instruments in the examining room, or

Mary K. Kachoyeanos, RN, EdD, is nursing research coordinator at Children's Hospital of Wisconsin, Milwaukee, WI. Margaret Friedhoff, RN, MSN, is nursing instructor at Children's Hospital of Wisconsin. The authors would like to acknowledge the assistance of Julie Lathrope, RN, MSN, for reviewing the manuscript.

holding on tightly to the parent's hand are helpful (16).

In passive distraction, the child merely watches something distracting, such as a kaleidoscope. Dorthea Ross and Sheila Ross cite personal communication with orthodontists who report that children who watch television during orthodontic therapy appear almost oblivious to discomfort (16).

Music, being a captivating and inescapable stimulus, is a very effective distraction technique. Soft, low-pitched, instrumental music has been shown to reduce stress-related responses during orthodontic procedures and bone marrow aspirations (17-19).

Even comatose children respond to music. Music piped through earphones for children paralyzed with pancuronium bromide (Pavulon) was found to reduce their heart rate, blood pressure, and intracranial pressure (20).

Controlled breathing is often used in conjunction with other techniques or alone to encourage relaxation. The child is taught to take slow deep breaths in through the nose and slowly let the breath out through pursed lips. The process is repeated four to five times until the child is noticeably calm and quiet. Results may not be achieved on the first try. Encourage the child to practice between treatment sessions and try again during the next treatment. The nurse models the technique and encourages the child to use controlled breathing for future stressful encounters.

"Blowing the pain away," a form of controlled breathing, is very effective with young children. The child is taught to blow out, as hard as she can, at the first sensation of pain. Blowing out helps to change the meaning of the aversive stimulus by making the first sharp pain of the needle a signal for action. Concentrating on acting on the signal, the child is distracted from the thought of pain. Young children, who have confidence in magic, are especially receptive to this method (21). The element of magic in being able to blow out the pain heightens the credibility of the technique.

Relaxation techniques also work well for adolescents, especially those who have trouble getting to sleep. The child is taught to breathe in slowly and blow the tension out. The sounds of the ocean can be taped, and the child is encouraged to imagine the waves of the ocean as they roll in and out. The child may prefer the sounds of rain or a spring meadow. Most children enjoy picturing a favorite place. Since some children may fear certain images, such as a body of water, check with the child before using an image. Or have the child select her own image.

TYPES OF BEHAVIORAL STRATEGIES

Behavioral strategies help children work through anticipated and/or previously experienced pain. Modeling and the use of play are behavioral strategies that can be used singly or in combination with cognitive strategies.

Through modeling—either live or videotaped—children learn about the procedure and ways to master the experience. Another child is observed going through the experience and demonstrates behavior that helps to master the procedure. For example, a model child can be used to demonstrate how a cast is removed. The model child can be shown touching a cast cutter. The child sits still as the technician cuts and removes the cast. As children observe that the model child survives the experience without bodily harm, chances for these children's cooperation during the procedure increase. Behavioral rehearsal helps children learn about the impending experience by "pretending"—becoming familiar with, and preparing for, the painful event through playing.

Desensitization exposes the child to the anxiety-provoking experience in a hierarchical series through play. For example, the child who receives injections can be shown the syringe. Next, she is allowed to finger the equipment. Later, she can manipulate the equipment, use a needle, fill the syringe. Lastly, the child can give injections to a doll. By slowly helping the child to become accustomed to the equipment, fear and anxiety are reduced and the pain impulse is perceived as less intense (16).

HOW COGNITIVE AND BEHAVIORAL STRATEGIES WORK

The gate-control theory originated by Ronald Melzack and Patrick Wall is currently the most applicable theory to explain the perception and transmission of pain and how cognitive strategies work (22). They propose that mechanisms in the dorsal horn of the spinal cord act as a gate, and allow or prevent the flow of pain impulses from peripheral fibers to the central nervous system, depending on the extent to which the gate is opened.

A closed gate will inhibit transmission of impulses to the brain. Cells in the gelatinous substance of the spinal cord (the gating site) are thought to act on the signals transmitted by the large- and small-diameter fibers and modulate input before it is acted upon by the transmission cells.

The output in the transmission cells must reach a certain level before the message of pain can be transmitted to the brain. In addition, structures in the brain that control cognitive processes, such as attention, memory, and emotion, influence the gating mechanism and have an impact on the transmission cells and the consequent transmission of pain (23). Since emotions play a significant part in the perception of pain, cognitive and behavioral strategies help to minimize anxiety, thus reducing the amount of

---

BASIC PRINCIPLES OF COGNITIVE STRATEGIES

- The child must be willing to participate.
- The child must have energy to participate.
- The child must trust the coach.
- Ideally, the coach should not perform the painful procedure.
- The child's age will determine the most appropriate cognitive strategy to use.
- Several techniques may need to be used with the same child.
- Use parents to assist with cognitive strategies.
- The desired result may not occur on the first try.
- Allow sufficient time.
- When feasible, use cognitive strategies to supplement analgesia.

input into the transmission cells. Thus, the reduction of emotional and physical impulses also decreases the output of the transmission cells, which in turn inhibits pain impulses from reaching the central nervous system.

CREATING THE ENVIRONMENT

Before the situation of undertreated pediatric pain can change, nurses and physicians need to see it as an urgent problem, with cognitive and behavioral strategies as one solution. Educating staff in the use of cognitive strategies can be done by providing continuing education workshops. The target audiences are nurses, physicians, social workers, child life personnel, and physical and occupational therapists. Since phlebotomists perform most needlesticks, they should also be invited.

The idea is to train key people in each unit and department, who will act as mentors to their colleagues. These people may want to establish regular meetings to keep abreast of the use of the techniques and to share their successes, innovations in the techniques, and problems in instituting the various methods.

One of the best ways to demonstrate the power of the techniques is to apply a particular technique while a child is undergoing a procedure. A nurse who had scoffed at the use of these strategies was amazed when her colleague used the magic glove and gained full cooperation from an 11-year-old boy. The youngster previously had to be physically restrained to have a venipuncture. The formerly skeptical nurse currently uses the magic glove in her practice.

BASIC PRINCIPLES OF COGNITIVE PAIN CONTROL

In all cognitive strategies, certain principles apply (see Basic Principles of Cognitive Strategies). First of all, for the technique to be effective, the child must willingly participate (16). Second, learning cognitive strategies requires concentration and energy; seriously ill children are not always able to invest energy to learn *new* techniques. If the child declines to participate, her wishes should be respected (16). Those children who have previously mastered the techniques will of-

Age appropriate cognitive strategies*

AGE GROUP	TECHNIQUES
Infant	Pacifier, swaddling
	Tactile soothing
	Music, tapes (especially of the souffle sound of the fetal heart beat)
Toddler	Distraction (blowing bubbles, looking through a kaleidoscope, pop-up toys)
Preschooler	Emotive imagery (Superhero)
	Blowing pain away
	Behavioral rehearsal/desensitization
	Finding Waldo in the "Where's Waldo?" poster
	Looking through a kaleidoscope
	Magic glove or blanket
School Age	Magic glove
	Pain switch
	Blowing bubbles
	Behavioral rehearsal
Adolescent	Tactile transference
	Modeling
	Imagery

*Examples only—not a comprehensive list

ten use them, whatever their energy level.

Parent involvement and cooperation will further ensure success. By enlisting the parents in meeting the goals and involving them in the strategies, the nurse appears as an ally and the child's acceptance of the technique is more likely. Parents are also good predictors of how their child will respond (3).

For unexplained reasons, some children who have mastered a self-hypnosis technique—even those who have had great success—will start to use it less after a few months (16). For this reason, it is important to provide consistent contact with a professional (or parent) who can coach and support the child in practicing the technique regularly.

It is difficult to conduct the cognitive strategy and perform an intrusive procedure. Two nurses (or a nurse and a phlebotomist) can work as a team during the intrusive procedure. For example, the nurse can apply the magic glove, then the technician can insert the line. Cognitive strategies may not be right for all children. Certain children do worse with more information. Any additional information may overexcite them, making them less cooperative than if they were left to their own resources (24,25).

The child's age will often determine the most effective techniques (see Age Appropriate Cognitive Strategies). As the child develops cognitively, differ-

ent approaches to pain management may be more effective than others. The magical thinking of the preschooler makes techniques like storytelling and the magic glove very effective. The school-aged child likes to engage in emotive therapy and may enjoy calling upon his favorite hero to come and take the pain away. Adolescents' reliance on peers makes them especially receptive to modeling, and their need for control makes them especially open to behavioral rehearsal prior to any intrusive procedure.

There is no exact recipe; nor are the techniques always age-specific. For example, we have successfully used the magic glove with preschoolers, school-aged children, and adolescents. It may be necessary to experiment with a variety of cognitive and behavioral strategies until the desired result is obtained.

When arranging to use cognitive techniques, it is important to plan ahead. Warn the physician or lab technician that you plan to try a strategy, so they will be aware that you need a few extra minutes before they perform the procedure. When the other members of the health team see that using these techniques saves time and is more humane, they will enthusiastically cooperate with the plan.

In certain situations, like finger pokes, cognitive strategies can be used alone, but generally they are designed to augment analgesic medications. At no time should they replace analgesia.

When cognitive strategies are used in combination with analgesia, it is important to carefully monitor the child's vital signs. It has been our experience that in some children, blood pressure, heart rate, and SaO2 levels dropped to a point that it was necessary to temporarily discontinue the analgesic.

The scientific reason for this reaction is not clear. Richard Sternbach suggests that physiologic substrates, such as endorphins, account for the relief of pain when hypnosis is used (26). Others dispute this theory (27). Still, we have had several experiences where the dose of analgesia had to be reduced when used in combination with hypnosis. Therefore, we strongly encourage monitoring the vital signs of the child in case the analgesia dosage needs to be altered.

CASE HISTORIES: OUR EXPERIENCE

Ideally, each child is aided through invasive procedures from the beginning of the illness. In reality, this doesn't happen very often. Most hospitalized children have had previous traumatic experiences, the memories of which intensify the child's reactions to current therapies.

Sara, aged six, had been hospitalized at four years of age for treatment of a renal infection and diagnostic workup, which revealed a malformed kidney. To arrive at the diagnosis, Sara was subjected to multiple procedures: urinary catheterizations, I.V.P., kidney biopsy, and numerous needlesticks. Now, when faced with a needlestick, Sara responded by kicking and scratching. Given the psychological vulnerability of a preschooler, Sara's current intense reaction is not surprising.

When a renal scan was scheduled, Sara was referred by a pediatrician to the nurse clinical specialist for behavior rehearsal and relaxation therapy. Sara was seen twice in the two weeks prior to the renal scan. During the first visit we took a history from Sara's mother, who could not tell us much about Sara's coping styles. We also interviewed Sara herself, who had one renal scan already and could describe it. However, she could not describe anything she thought would make the procedure less frightening.

Given the history of responses, we took a multifaceted approach. We used behavioral rehearsal, in the form of doll play, to explain the procedure and to suggest ways in which the doll might cope with the procedure. We also went through a series of steps to desensitize Sara to the needlesticks. First, the nurse fingered the equipment, then gave the doll an injection while Sara watched.

Sara was invited to do the same. She was surprisingly adept at withdrawing fluid from the vial, manipulating the syringe, and administering the injections. She then carefully applied a Band-Aid. When asked, "What can the doll do to make this less scary?" Sara mimicked one of the suggestions previously offered, that of finding a secret place to think about.

During the second visit, she asked to play with the doll, repeated the procedure, and seemed less frenzied. The nurse offered other suggestions for control during the procedure, such as deep breathing and blowing bubbles.

On the morning of the procedure, the nurse met Sara and her parents in the waiting area of the Radiology Department. Sara was obviously agitated, dashing around the waiting room. Offered a bottle of blow bubbles, she was quickly engaged in blowing bubbles and enlisted other children in the activity. When the radiology technician came to escort her to the procedure room, Sara began to cry and asked that her daddy accompany her. She grasped his hand and the nurse's hand and went without further protest to the procedure room.

Once on the table she began to cry again and resist as the therapist started to insert the IV. She was asked to hold her father's hand and blow. Sara did not blow, but did hold her father's hand. The nurse immobilized her arm and the therapist quickly inserted the IV. Previously it had taken several people to restrain her for the procedure.

We used imagery during the procedure by asking her to tell a story. She did so by recounting an episode that she had engaged in with her sister. Sara was able to lie still during the following 15 minutes when the x-rays were taken. She was praised for the good job she'd done and seemed genuinely pleased with herself.

For children who are resistant or unable to engage in imagery, such as toddlers, distraction is extremely effective, as we found with three-year-old **Vickie,** who was hospitalized with severe otitis media. Vickie's inner ear canals were encrusted with dried exudate. They needed daily suctioning to allow the instilled medication to reach the target site, but the severe swelling of the external tissues of the ears made any contact especially painful. During the first treatment Vickie was as upset at being restrained as with the actual procedure.

Upon returning to her room, Vickie's cheeks were flushed and tear-stained, her IV in disarray. After the primary nurse obtained an account of the experience, she was determined that the child not be subjected to a replay of the distressing experience. The nurse planned to accompany Vickie to the next treatment and did so, armed with a bottle of blow-bubble solution. During a 10-minute wait for the physician, the nurse blew bubbles for her little patient's delight.

When the physician arrived, he grabbed a sheet, ready to restrain Vickie. The nurse asked that he not do so, stating that the bubbles were distracting her and, if necessary, she would restrain the child herself. Since the physician was willing to try anything that would prevent a repeat of the previous day's experience, he acquiesced.

The nurse helped Vickie to assume the position for the examination and continued to blow bubbles and encouraged her to blow them back. Vickie quickly got into the game. The procedure was half over when Vickie's mother entered the room, expecting to find a screaming, kicking Vickie. To her amazement her little one was blowing bubbles, lying still—the only restraint the nurse's reassuring hand on Vickie's thigh—as the physician probed the ear. The nurse turned over the bubble game to Vickie's mom while she repositioned Vickie to gain access to the other ear. The game went on as the physician completed the procedure with only a minor grimace from Vickie.

We use a magic blanket for children who receive intramuscular (IM) injections. **Billy,** four-years-old, requires biweekly intramuscular injections. At first, a magic blanket was placed over the anterior aspect of the thigh. His mother reported his response to the IM was more controlled than previously. At the next clinic visit, when the nurse offered to use a magic glove on his leg, Billy said, "No, use the blanket."

At the subsequent visit he produced his own very tattered and torn blanket. The blanket was laid over the thigh a few minutes before the injection was given. Then Billy turned a corner of the blanket back and, without a murmur, allowed the nurse to disinfect the area and administer the injection.

In preparation for his weekly IM injections, five-year-old **Wayne** imagines pain switches. He says he sees a red pain switch when pain is impending. Then he mentally turns the switch off. He knows the switch is off, because it turns black.

With **Latoya,** we tried imagery to augment the effect of analgesia. Latoya, a 13-year-old girl in sickle cell crisis, was receiving IV morphine but was so agitated that the morphine was ineffective. We asked her to imagine a safe place. Latoya readily responded to the imagery experience and quickly relaxed. However, at this point, her blood pressure dropped critically low and the morphine was stopped. Again, caution should be used when combining cognitive and behavioral strategies with medication. The dose of medication may need to be altered.

Music can also enhance the effect of analgesia, but in our experience, children respond best to music of their choice. **Jameel,** an eight-year-old who suffered burns over 40 percent of his body, responded best to the music of the rock star Michael Jackson, Jameel's hero. He found listening to the hit song, "Beat It," during painful burn débridement greatly enhanced the effects of pain-relieving drugs. In another instance, three-year-old **Frankie** liked to sing "Baby Balooga" at the top of his lungs when he had an IV inserted.

Children in emergency situations are particularly receptive to cognitive strategies. The stress of the emergency appears to cause children to move into an altered state of awareness and motivates them to ameliorate their discomfort [28]. Our emergency room nurses find that encouraging children to visualize how their favorite superhero would cope is particularly useful during stitching of lacerations.

A SENSE OF CONTROL

During the course of normal growth and development, children strive to be in control of their bodies and the world around them. Illness and accompanying diagnostic and therapeutic procedures place an additional burden on children's ability to cope. Providing children with cognitive strategies helps to lessen their discomfort and allows them some control in the medical procedure. Mastering a difficult situation not only reduces the child's anxiety, but raises her self-esteem.

The use of cognitive and behavioral strategies also suggests areas for further nursing research. Most of the research in this area has been conducted in oncology and by people in disciplines outside of nursing. Marion Broome has suggested that research should compare the effect of hypnosis on behavioral and physical responses to pain; such a study is contemplated [29,30].

In today's cost-conscious health care setting, cognitive and behavioral strategies are a wise choice—they cost nothing to implement and actually save staff time. But much more important, these strategies work! Children do not have to suffer needlessly. Such techniques do require a commitment on the part of caregivers. Nevertheless, practicing nurses can provide a pain-controlled environment for children, and gain much satisfaction in the process.

REFERENCES

1. Fowler-Kerry, S. Adolescent oncology survivors' recollection of pain. In *Pediatric Pain,* ed. by D. C. Tyler and E. Krane. (Advances in Pain Research and Therapy Series) New York, Raven Press, 1990, Vol. 15, pp. 365-371.
2. Weekes, D.P., and Savedra, M.C. Adolescent cancer: coping with treatment-related pain. *J. Pediatr. Nurs.* 3:318-328, Oct. 1988.
3. Schechter, N.L., and others. Individual differences in children's response to pain: Role of temperament and parental characteristics. *Pediatrics* 82:171-177, Feb. 1991.
4. Bonica, J. *The Management of Pain.* Vol. 1 2d ed. Philadelphia, Lea & Febiger, 1990, pp. 175-178.
5. Terr, L.C. Childhood trauma: an outline and overview. *Am. J. Psychiatry* 148:10-20, Jan. 1991.
6. Kohen, D.P., and others. The use of relaxation-mental imagery (self-hypnosis) in the management of 505 pediatric behavioral encounters. *J. Dev. Behav. Pediatr.* 5:21-25, Feb. 1984.
7. Agency for Health Policy and Research. *Acute Pain Management: Operative or Medical Procedures and Trauma.* (AHCPR Pub. No. 92-0032). Washington D.C., U.S. Government Printing Office, 1992, pp. 37-55.
8. Hilgard, J.R., and LeBaron, S. Relief of anxiety and pain in children and adolescents with cancer: quantitative measures and clinical observations. *Int. J. Clin. Exp. Hypn.* 30:417-442, Oct. 1982.
9. Jay, S.M. and others. Behavioral management of children's distress during painful medical procedures. *Behav. Res. Ther.* 23(5):513-520, 1985.
10. Valente, S.M. Using hypnosis with children for pain management. *Oncol. Nurs. Forum* 18:699-704, May-June 1991.
11. Zeltzer, L.K., and others. A randomized, controlled study of behavioral intervention for chemotherapy distress in children with cancer. *Pediatrics* 88:34-42, July 1991.
12. Kuttner, L. (1986) *No Fears—No Tears: Children With Cancer Coping with Pain.* (30 minute-videotape and manual). Vancouver, Canadian Cancer Society, 1986 (955 W. Broadway, Vancouver, BC VSZ 3X8, Canada).
13. Kuttner, L. Favorite stories: a hypnotic pain-reduction technique for children in acute pain. *Am. J. Clin. Hypn.* 30:289-295, Apr. 1988.
14. Campos, R.G. Soothing pain-elicited distress in infants with swaddling and pacifiers. *Child Dev.* 60:781-792, Aug. 1989.
15. Field, T. and Goldson, E. Pacifying effects of nonnutritive sucking on term and preterm neonates during heelstick procedures. *Pediatrics* 74:1012-1015, Dec. 1984.
16. Ross, D.M., and Ross, S.A. *Childhood Pain, Current Issues Research and Management.* Baltimore, Urban and Schwarzenberg, 1988, pp. 211-250.
17. Cook, J.D. Therapeutic use of music: a literature review. *Nurs. Forum* 20(3):252-266, 1981.
18. McGrath, P.J., and Vair, C. Psychological aspects of pain management of the burned child. *Children's Health Care* 13:15-19, Summer, 1984.
19. Ryan, E. The effect of musical distortion on pain in hospitalized school-aged children. In *Key Aspects of Comfort, Management of Pain, Fatigue and Nausea,* ed. by S.G. Funk and others. New York, Springer, 1989, pp. 101-107.
20. Wincek, J. *The Effects of Auditory Control on the Physiologic Responses*

of Brain Injured Children. Milwaukee, Medical College of Wisconsin, 1986 p. 63. (Unpublished Master's Thesis).

21. Fraiberg, S. *The Magic Years.* New York, Scribner, 1981, pp. 126-132 (Originally published 1959).

22. Melczak, R., and Wall, P.D. Pain mechanism: a new theory. *Science* 150:971, Nov. 1965.

23. Savedra, M., and others. Pain management. In *Nursing Intervention for Infants and Children,* ed. by M. Craft and J. Denehy. Philadelphia, W.B. Saunders Co., 1990, pp. 304-325.

24. Cohen, F., and Lazurus, R.W. Active coping process, coping disposition and recovery from surgery. *Psychol. Rep.* 45:867-873, 1979.

25. Harris, G., and Rollman, G.B. Cognitive techniques for controlling pain: generality and individual differences. In *Proceedings of the Fourth World Congress on Pain, Seattle,* ed. by H.L. Fields and others. (Advances in Pain Research and Therapy Vol. 9) New York: Raven Press, 1985.

26. Sternbach, R.A. On Strategies for identifying neurochemical correlates of hypnotic analgesia: a brief communication. *Int. J. Clin. Exp. Hypn.* 30:251-256, July 1982.

27. Barber, J., and Mayer, D. An investigation of the efficacy and neural mechanism of a hypnotic analgesia procedure in experimental and clinical dental pain. *Pain* 4:41-48, Oct. 1977.

28. Olness, K. Hypnotherapy: a cyberphysiologic strategy in pain management. *Pediatr. Clin. North Am.* 36:876-877, Aug. 1989.

29. Broome, M.E., and others. Pain interventions with children: a meta-analysis of research. *Nurs. Res.* 38: 154-158, May-June 1989.

30. Kachoyeanos, M., and others. *EMLA Versus Imagery for Children's Distress During Venipuncture,* 1992 (Unpublished).

Contents

Chapter 6

Practice Tests

The questions and answers in this section have been organized to simulate the stand-alone format of the questions on the computerized NCLEX-RN exam.

The 300 questions have been divided into four practice tests. Each exam tests your nursing knowledge regarding care of the adult, the child, the childbearing family, and the client with psychosocial problems.

INSTRUCTIONS FOR TAKING THE TEST

1. Review the information in Chapter One: Preparing for the NCLEX-RN.
2. Time yourself, allowing 1½ hours per test.
3. Read each question carefully, and select *one* best answer to each question.
4. Do not leave questions blank because you will not be able to return to questions on the computerized NCLEX-RN.

5. Score your exam using the answer key. Count any questions left unanswered as incorrect.
6. Review the questions you answered incorrectly and restudy that specific material.

At the end of each answer and accompanying rationale, you will find information regarding the assignment of each question into the section of this book covering the content, nursing process, and client need categories. These decisions were made after consultation with the section coordinators and are based on the NCLEX-RN Test Plan published by the National Council of State Boards of Nursing. You may use this information to determine if your incorrect answers reflect a weakness in a particular area. Remember, however, that NCLEX-RN is testing your abilities *to apply the steps of the nursing process,* not your ability to identify a category for an individual question.

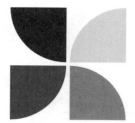

Practice Test 1

1. A young woman is being admitted for treatment of primary Cushing's disease. You will complete her admission assessment. You would expect her to exhibit which of the following signs and symptoms?
   ① Stretch marks on her hips and thighs
   ② Taut, dry skin
   ③ Thin, pale appearance
   ④ Protruding eyes

2. Lesley Morton calls the child and adolescent mental health center and expresses concern about her 15-year-old daughter, Margaret. She informs the nurse that her daughter is overly worried about gaining weight and exercising, although she looks healthy and has not lost weight. These behaviors indicate which of the following?
   ① Anxiety
   ② Anorexia
   ③ Chemical dependency
   ④ Bulimia

3. A multipara who attended childbirth classes with her husband has been successfully working toward an unmedicated delivery since admission to a birthing room when dilation was 4 cm. To best assist them during the second stage of labor, the nurse should
   ① Inform the couple about progress toward delivery and all procedures.
   ② Restrain the client's hands so that she will not contaminate the sterile field.
   ③ Do a nonsterile cleansing prep of the vulvular and perineal area.
   ④ Encourage strong pushing between contractions.

4. A 13-year-old boy is brought to the emergency department by his camp leader. During a summer overnight camp-out, the boy's kerosene lamp overturned and ignited his sleeping bag. The boy's shirt sleeve caught fire when he tried to put out the fire. He has second-degree burns of his right hand and forearm. Immediate care of the burn wound should include
   ① Immersing the hand and forearm in cool water.
   ② Applying ice packs to the injury.
   ③ Pulling adherent charred clothing from the burn wounds.
   ④ Covering the burn with cortisone cream.

5. If a client develops the syndrome of inappropriate antidiuretic hormone (SIADH), it will be critical for the nurse to
   ① Force fluids and monitor urine output carefully.
   ② Restrict fluids and monitor the serum sodium levels carefully.
   ③ Restrict the level of sodium in the diet and maintain accurate I&O.
   ④ Follow the urine specific gravity and monitor the serum potassium levels carefully.

6. The nurse is giving discharge instructions to the parents of a child hospitalized for second-degree burns. In teaching them how to change the child's dressing, which instruction should the nurse include in the teaching plan?
   ① The silver sulfadiazine cream will be painful when first applied to the burn.
   ② The child should return to the laboratory each day to have his blood pH monitored.
   ③ Old cream should be removed by soaking the wound in warm, soapy water.
   ④ The silver sulfadiazine cream may cause a change in color of adjacent healthy skin.

7. Ms. Harmony Jones underwent transsphenoidal hypophysectomy surgery today for treatment of a pituitary adenoma. Her "moustache" dressing is wet, and you observe a halo effect around the wet area of the drainage as you change the dressing. Which nursing diagnosis would take priority at this time?
   ① Risk for fluid volume deficit
   ② Risk for infection
   ③ Risk for injury
   ④ Risk for ineffective airway clearance

8. Mrs. Morley is scheduled to go on her first overnight pass with her husband. Before leaving she asks the nurse to tell her husband that she can't stay overnight and that she must return before lunch. The most appropriate nursing response is which of the following?
   ① "Most people are anxious about their first overnight pass. You will feel more comfortable when you get home."
   ② "I am unwilling to lie to your husband. Just tell him you don't want to go."
   ③ "If you are worried about how you will do on this pass, wait until you get home before you decide whether or not you want to stay overnight."
   ④ "Your husband and the staff will be very disappointed if you don't go on the pass."

9. After cleansing and debridement of a second-degree burn, the physician decides to apply silver sulfadiazine (Silvadene) and cover the wound with a bulky gauze dressing. The primary advantage of the closed method used to treat the burn is that it
   ① Protects the wound from further injury.
   ② Minimizes fluid loss from the burn surface.
   ③ Alleviates pain caused by exposure of the wound to air.
   ④ Prevents contractures of the hand and wrist.

10. A client has just been diagnosed with hepatitis A and is extremely distressed about the diagnosis, saying "I just can't imagine where I could have gotten something like this." Which of the following factors in the client's history is most likely to have contributed to this diagnosis?
    ① Receiving blood after a major surgery
    ② A recent severe viral illness
    ③ A beach party with clams and oysters on the half shell
    ④ A 20-year history of social drinking

11. The nurse is aware of hospital policy regarding suspected or actual child abuse. All of the following measures are appropriate nursing actions except:
    ① Document physical assessment, including bruises (their location, size, and color).
    ② Chart a description of parent-child interactions.
    ③ Delineate staff's impression of parent-child relationship.
    ④ Report to local child protective services.

12. A 13-year-old child is admitted to the pediatric unit with second-degree burns to 30% of his body. The child's immunization history indicates that he has received all childhood immunizations according to the recommended schedule. At this time, tetanus prophylaxis for the child should include
    ① Tetanus toxoid.
    ② Tetanus immune globulin.
    ③ Tetanus toxoid and tetanus immune globin.
    ④ No additional protection.

13. A laboring woman ambulates with her husband after hospital admission. Which of the following would warrant return to bed and evaluation of her condition?
    ① Contractions that are intense and last 60 seconds
    ② Progressive sacral discomfort during contractions
    ③ Warm flushed skin
    ④ A desire to defecate at the peak of contractions

14. A postoperative neck surgery client begins to experience respiratory distress. A check of the surgical dressing reveals it to be tight about the patient's neck with a small amount of bloody drainage. What should the nurse do?
    ① Administer oxygen at 2 L via nasal prongs.
    ② Reinforce the dressing and notify the doctor.
    ③ Loosen the dressing and notify the doctor.
    ④ Place the client in low Fowler's position and notify the doctor.

15. A family member suspected of child abuse is questioned about means of disciplining. The person comments aggressively by saying "Any child who disobeys should be punished. That's what's wrong with our so-ciety, not enough discipline! I don't do any more to my child than the next parent." The nurse recognizes this response as which of the following?
    ① Exaggerating the truth to avoid getting into trouble
    ② Being honest and protecting someone else who abused the child
    ③ Not recognizing that the behavior is abusive
    ④ Doing what any parent would do when a child is disobedient

16. A 10-year-old girl is recovering from first- and second-degree burns over 40% of her body that she received when she was playing with fireworks. She has been advanced to a regular diet. Which of the following foods should the nurse encourage the child to eat most often to promote healing?
    ① Meats, citrus fruits, and milk
    ② Vegetables, cheese, and yogurt
    ③ Breads, cereals, and pastas
    ④ Milkshakes, salads, and soups

17. Ten-year-old Jessica Linsson is brought to the emergency department by her grandmother. She has numerous burned areas over her entire body and a fractured left arm. Her grandmother reports that she was out riding her bike and fell in the street. She reports that the child disobeyed her and left the house without permission. The child refuses to talk to the nurse and grandmother and stares at the wall. The nurse suspects child abuse. All of the following contribute to the nurse's suspicions except:
    ① The physical presentation is inconsistent with the grandmother's story.
    ② The child is described as being disobedient.
    ③ There is a lack of warmth between the child and grandmother.
    ④ The child's disobedience suggests that discipline is appropriate.

18. Which of the following observations would be the most reliable guide to assess progress of a primigravida in labor?
    ① Contractions that are getting more intense
    ② Breathing that is becoming more rapid
    ③ Cervix that is progressively dilating
    ④ Vaginal discharge that is increasing

19. The school nurse observes that a 13-year-old student has mild acne and that the lesions are especially noticeable on his forehead and chin. When asked if he would like some suggestions to help clear up the lesions, the boy nods. The nurse should suggest that the boy
    ① Use a commercial sunlamp for 5 minutes daily.
    ② Wear an absorbent headband during exercise or hot weather.
    ③ Purchase an over-the-counter product that contains benzoyl peroxide.
    ④ Avoid chocolate, fried foods, and iodized salt.

20. The nurse is performing a well-child assessment of a 5-year-old boy. Part of the assessment includes vision screening using the Snellen E chart for visual acuity. The child's results are 20/30 vision in both eyes. Which action should the nurse take?
    ① Rescreen the child immediately.
    ② Rescreen the child in 2 weeks.

③ Refer the child to an ophthalmologist for a complete eye exam.

④ Explain to the child and his mother that his vision is normal.

21. A client goes out on an afternoon pass with his wife. During dinner the client is observed sitting alone away from other clients. What is the most appropriate nursing response?
① Tell him that he looks preoccupied.
② Allow him to sit alone because of the long day.
③ Discourage him from staying out so long.
④ Point out that he is quiet this evening.

22. In early labor, the fetal heart tones (FHT) are auscultated at regular intervals. The most appropriate time to listen to FHT is
① During contractions.
② Between contractions.
③ Soon after contractions.
④ During and soon after contractions.

23. The nurse frequently assesses the voice and ability to speak of a client who had a thyroidectomy. What is the nurse evaluating?
① Changes in level of consciousness
② Recovery from anesthesia
③ Injury to the parathyroid gland
④ Spasm or edema of vocal chords

24. A postpartum client comments, "I hope this is our last baby because we can't afford any more." The nurse's best response would be which of the following?
① "Discuss this with your physician at your postpartum checkup."
② "You need not worry until you stop breast-feeding."
③ "Let's talk about birth-control methods."
④ "Perhaps the social worker can help you."

25. Clint Jeston, a 14-year-old, was admitted to an acute psychiatric unit several weeks ago. His stay over this period has been extremely disorderly. He has difficulty interacting with his peers and staff during group activities. He becomes angry easily, and his behavior is disruptive. Which of the following best describes Clint's behavior?
① He is avoiding group activities because he is shy.
② He is intimidated by the group.
③ He is angry at a group member.
④ He is annoyed by the group leader.

26. While conducting preschool vision screening, the nurse assesses visual acuity. The nurse should also screen the children for which of the following?
① Strabismus
② Diplopia
③ Papilledema
④ Pupil reactivity

27. Which of the following demonstrates positive evidence of progress both in the child who has been abused and the abusing parent?
① Sleeping and eating patterns and other activities of daily living return to normal along with an absence of thoughts of abuse in both the child and parent.
② A lack of parent-child conflict.
③ When the child becomes frustrated, the parent uses other learned nonabusive options.

④ The parent develops activities that decrease the time of parent-child interactions.

28. A 5-year-old's height is at the 50th percentile. His weight is at the 90th percentile. A nutritional history reveals that the child's diet is high in carbohydrates and fats. The nurse helps the mother develop a plan to ensure that her child gets the nutrients he needs without overeating. This diet should provide approximately how many calories per day?
① 1200
② 1700
③ 2400
④ 2800

29. Postoperative care of the client after thyroidectomy includes which of the following actions?
① Keep the head of the bed flat to prevent neck flexion.
② Avoid coughing and deep breathing to prevent injury to the suture line.
③ Restrict ambulation until the suture line is healed.
④ Check the back of the neck and upper part of the back when assessing the dressing.

30. A 5-year-old boy returns to the clinic for a follow-up visit 6 months after an assessment of overweight (weight 90th percentile, height 50th percentile). Which of the following best indicates that the child is making satisfactory progress with his nutritional plan?
① The child has lost 5 pounds.
② The child's daily intake has been 300 calories less than recommended.
③ The child's weight is now in the 75th percentile.
④ The child has stopped craving junk food.

31. On the morning after delivery, a woman complains that excessive perspiring kept her awake all night. She is worried that there is a problem. Select an appropriate response to the client.
① "IV fluids administered during labor sometimes cause sweating."
② "Maybe you drank too much fluid during the day."
③ "Fluids that were retained during pregnancy are normally lost in this manner."
④ "You may be experiencing signs of infection."

32. All of the following nursing measures promote sleep in the client with bipolar disorder, manic type, *except:*
① Engage in a quiet activity.
② Offer a warm bedtime drink.
③ Provide Lorazepam for sleep.
④ Provide a piece of chocolate cake and tea.

33. A client in the emergency department complains of severe, sharp, deep lumbar pain radiating to his right side. An IVP reveals a kidney stone in the right ureter at the bifurcation of the iliac vessel. Upon his admission to the hospital, which of the following goals would take initial priority in this client's nursing care?
① Client will decrease risk of future kidney stones.
② Client will be prepared for possible urinary tract surgery.
③ Client will be free from discomfort of kidney stones.
④ Client will have fluid intake of 3 to 5 L per day.

34. Treatment of an otherwise healthy 5-year-old who is overweight would best include
   ① A planned program of activity and exercise.
   ② A daily appetite suppressant.
   ③ Large doses of supplemental vitamins.
   ④ Withholding all sweets.

35. A 31-year-old gravida 5 para 4 delivered a 9-pound, 10-ounce baby after a 20-hour labor. Based on the data, this woman is at risk for which of the following?
   ① Thrombophlebitis
   ② Postpartal hemorrhage
   ③ Puerperal infection
   ④ Urinary retention

36. The nurse is giving discharge instructions to the mother of a 5-year-old girl hospitalized for acute lymphoblastic leukemia. The mother tells the nurse that her daughter is supposed to receive a DPT and TOPV booster before she starts kindergarten this year and asks when she should take her to the health department to receive these. Which response by the nurse is accurate?
   ① "We can give it before she leaves the hospital."
   ② "Wait until a week or so before she starts school."
   ③ "When her white blood cell count returns to a normal level the immunizations may be given."
   ④ "Because of her diagnosis, she won't ever be able to be immunized again."

37. Which intervention would be a priority in discharge teaching for a client with a kidney infection?
   ① Drink at least 3 to 4 L of fluid per day.
   ② Take sitz baths 3 to 4 times per day for urethral burning.
   ③ Void immediately after sexual intercourse.
   ④ Avoid exposure to persons with upper respiratory infections.

38. A client with an elated mood tells the nursing staff that he is too busy for lunch. He also explains that he is scheduled to meet with the president later in the day. What is the most appropriate nursing response?
   ① "Your physician has not written an order for you to leave the unit."
   ② "When you are through, come to dinner."
   ③ "It is time to eat now and I will go with you and help."
   ④ "If you refuse to eat now, we will put you in seclusion."

39. Carol Perez, 21 years old, is in acute renal failure after a large loss of blood from injuries she received in a car accident. Her 24-hour urine output is 275 ml. Her serum BUN is 60 mg/100 ml and her serum creatinine is 2.5 mg/dl. Mrs. Perez fails to respond to therapy to correct her acute renal failure. She goes into chronic renal failure, with the prospect of having to start dialysis or have a kidney transplant. Which of the following indicators would you expect to see in Mrs. Perez as the renal failure becomes more severe?
   ① Anemia
   ② Hypokalemia
   ③ Diaphoresis
   ④ Hypotension

40. A 12-year-old boy with Hodgkin's disease is receiving radiation therapy. The boy's father says he has heard that there are serious side effects, and asks the nurse what these are. Which of the following is not a side effect of radiation therapy?
   ① Delays in physical development
   ② Susceptibility to bone fractures
   ③ Early onset of secondary sex characteristics
   ④ Possible damage to chromosomes

41. A 3-year-old girl hospitalized with a diagnosis of acute lymphocytic leukemia is crying softly and says she is "hurting." The child's pulse rate is elevated. Which of the following protocols would be most effective when administering the child's pain medication?
   ① Give when she becomes restless and is unable to sleep.
   ② Give on a preventive schedule after assessing her pain responses.
   ③ Give when the child or her parents request it be given.
   ④ Give every 3 to 4 hours around the clock.

42. After discharge, the physician wants the client to maintain his urine in a more acidic state by eating an acid-ash diet. Which food would you teach the client can be unrestricted in his diet?
   ① Milk
   ② Carrots
   ③ Grape Nuts cereal
   ④ Dried apricots

43. An appropriate response to a client who professes to seeing creatures from Mirkee is which of the following?
   ① Acknowledge that the client has seen the creatures, but you have not seen them.
   ② Help the client understand the underlying symbolism of the creatures.
   ③ Encourage the client to call if the creatures return.
   ④ Avoid responding to the statement and switch to another topic.

44. During the active phase of labor, a client, gravida 2, para 0, begins to complain of dizziness, tingling in her fingers, and numbness in her lips. The nurse caring for her should
   ① Have her breathe into a paper bag.
   ② Help her assume a left lateral position in bed.
   ③ Administer O_2 at 6 to 8 L per nasal cannula.
   ④ Notify the physician immediately.

45. A mother brings her 5-year-old son to the pediatrician's office for a complete health appraisal before he enters kindergarten next month. The nurse should focus part of the assessment on the child's achievement of psychosocial tasks. At this age, he should be trying to accomplish a sense of which of the following?
   ① Autonomy
   ② Identity
   ③ Mastery
   ④ Initiative

46. The nurse evaluates a 5-year-old's readiness to attend kindergarten. The child should be able to
   ① Tie his shoelaces.
   ② Count to 20.
   ③ Tell time on a clock.
   ④ Print his name.

47. A client is placed on a regimen of a sulfonamide antibiotic (Bactrim). As a nurse, you know which of the following statements to be true concerning this drug?
    ① It is metabolized by the liver and excreted through the bile.
    ② It produces a false-negative glucose on urine tests.
    ③ It is more soluble in acidic urine.
    ④ It can crystalize in the urine if fluid intake is insufficient.

48. During a conversation with a client with schizophrenia, the client remarks that "creatures from Mirkee recently left my room." The creatures from Mirkee represent which of the following?
    ① An adverse drug reaction, specifically extrapyramidal adverse effect
    ② An illusion
    ③ A symbol of the client's retreat from reality
    ④ An example of projection

49. A client will receive a spinal anesthetic for cesarean birth. As she discusses the surgery, she asks the nurse about the possibility of postanesthesia headaches. An appropriate response is
    ① "Headaches should not be a problem."
    ② "Medication is available to counteract headaches and is given as needed."
    ③ "If there is an allergy to the agent used, headaches may occur."
    ④ "This problem may be prevented by keeping the bed flat."

50. A client with a history of schizophrenia has been taking thioridazine (Mellaril) as ordered for a number of years. Her physician has recently prescribed antibiotics for a physical condition. What is the *most appropriate* nursing intervention?
    ① Formulate a psychoeducational program that addresses the basis of the client's problems, the effect on physical and mental processes, and changes arising from the physical problem.
    ② Provide instructions on taking the medication, and encourage the client to demonstrate the process several times to the nurse.
    ③ Strongly encourage hospitalization until the medication is completed.
    ④ Ask for a home health nurse to come in and administer the medications.

51. Which of the following behaviors would indicate to the nurse that a 5-year-old child is adequately prepared for bone marrow aspiration? The child
    ① Explains that her healthy blood cells are sick and need special medicine.
    ② Tells her mom that she likes her nurse and wants to play after the test.
    ③ Willingly allows the nurse to take her to the treatment room.
    ④ Tells her dolls that she has to have a needle in her hip to test her blood.

52. In teaching parents how to administer levothyroxine (Synthroid) to their infant with congenital hypothyroidism, the nurse should provide which instruction?
    ① The medication should be given until symptoms subside, then be gradually discontinued.
    ② The child can be expected to lose some weight as he adjusts to the medication.
    ③ The medication should be administered as a single morning dose.
    ④ Constipation may develop, indicating toxicity.

53. An intravenous pyelogram (IVP) is ordered. Which action would be the most important for the nurse to do before the IVP?
    ① Give a cathartic and enemas to cleanse the bowel.
    ② Instruct the client to be NPO after midnight.
    ③ Identify by history any client allergies to medicine or foods.
    ④ Teach the client that x-rays will be taken at multiple intervals.

54. Janice Carter is in the 37th week of pregnancy. Her husband calls the physician to report that his wife awakened in the middle of the night, lying in a pool of bright-red blood. The onset of third-trimester painless bleeding is usually a sign of potential
    ① Abruptio placentae.
    ② Placenta previa.
    ③ Incomplete abortion.
    ④ Ectopic pregnancy.

55. Primary needs of a client with schizophrenia are best described in which of the following statements?
    ① Assign a different staff member daily to decrease dependency.
    ② Assign the same staff as often as possible to foster trust.
    ③ Assign one staff member to stay with client constantly to promote closeness.
    ④ Daily assignments have little relevancy to the care of this client.

56. A 3-month-old boy is seen in the pediatric clinic for well baby care. During this visit, the physician diagnoses congenital hypothyroidism. When explaining the diagnosis to the parents, the nurse should describe which findings as characteristic of congenital hypothyroidism?
    ① Hyperirritability and prominent nasal bridge
    ② Tachycardia and small oral cavity
    ③ Constant hunger and runny stools
    ④ Inactivity and mottled skin

57. Jo Ellen Baxter, a 50-year-old with a diagnosis of chronic, undifferentiated schizophrenia, is hospitalized on a surgical unit for an appendectomy. The day after surgery, Mrs. Baxter tells the nurse that she feels creatures eating away at her abdomen. What is the first thing the nurse needs to do?
    ① Request an increase in her phenothiazine to control the psychosis.
    ② Talk with her more often to help control her stress level.
    ③ Assess for possible abdominal pains.
    ④ Request an order for benztropine (Cogentin) to control her extrapyramidal symptoms.

58. A chemotherapeutic regimen of vincristine and prednisone has been initiated for a child with acute lymphoblastic leukemia. The nurse should report which of the following reactions to the physician?
    ① Petechiae appear on the child's chest and face.
    ② The child vomits two times after breakfast.

③ The child complains of tingling in her fingers and toes.

④ The child develops small ulcerations on her lips.

59. When a client is discharged, he and his wife are referred to the Visiting Nurse Association. The client and his wife will more readily accept aid from this organization if which of the following is noted?

① The need they think they have for such help

② The enthusiasm of the nurse who plans their care

③ The availability of the help

④ The willingness of the client to accept the help

60. A child is receiving a unit of packed cells intravenously. Which intravenous solution would be appropriate to use to flush the tubing before initiating the transfusion?

① Lactated Ringer's solution

② 5% dextrose in water

③ 5% dextrose in one-fourth normal saline

④ Hyperalimentation solution

61. The most important blood test of kidney filtration is which of the following?

① Glucose

② Electrolytes

③ Creatinine

④ BUN

62. After a motorcycle accident, Tony, a 33-year-old construction worker, is admitted to the emergency department for treatment of a fractured pelvis and right clavicle. He was drinking and rear-ended a car. His blood alcohol level is elevated, but he contests that he is in severe pain and has a low tolerance to pain. Additionally, he requests several pain pills. Which is the most appropriate *initial* nursing response to this client?

① "Do you have any nonprescribed medication with you?"

② "Do not take any medication except what we give you for comfort."

③ "Do you routinely need medication to get through the day?"

④ "I need a verbal contract from you that says that you will take only the medications prescribed at this time. Any other drug can interfere with your anesthetic tonight."

63. A client is admitted to the labor room with possible placenta previa. Which of the following is contraindicated during the admission assessment?

① Vaginal examination

② X-ray pelvimetry

③ Type and crossmatch

④ Perineal prep

64. The nurse is planning care for a 13-month-old boy scheduled for surgery for transposition of the great vessels. Which activity would be most appropriate for the child preoperatively?

① A play stethoscope

② A push-pull toy

③ A shape sorter

④ A toy trumpet

65. The basis of withdrawal symptoms from psychoactive agents involves all of the following *except*:

① Physiologic dependence

② Noticeable tolerance

③ Decreased consumption

④ Cessation of use

66. A laboring woman is worried about her 2-year-old twins at home. Her spouse asks the nurse if he should remain or return home to check on the children and their teenage sitter. Which response indicates an understanding of their feelings at this time?

① "You would feel more secure if you checked on your family."

② "Your wife is well cared for here. You may go home for a while."

③ "You really belong here now. Call home and check on the children."

④ "Why not ask your wife what she feels would be best for her?"

67. While waiting for a suitable transplant kidney to be identified, a client has to begin dialysis. An arteriovenous (AV) fistula is created for hemodialysis. As a nurse, you understand that one major complication you must observe for after an AV fistula is

① Rejection of the silastic cannula connecting the artery and vein.

② Accidental dislodgment of the cannula with resulting hemorrhage.

③ Thrombosis of the artery and vein site.

④ Cardiac irritation caused by the cannula's insertion.

68. In the pediatric cardiology clinic a nurse observes a 2-year-old child with severe cyanotic heart disease playing in the waiting room. The child starts to investigate the contents of his mother's purse. When his mother takes her purse away from him, the child begins to cry, then screams, stomps his feet, and starts to gasp. Which action should the nurse take?

① Allow the child's mother to handle the situation.

② Distract the child with one of his favorite toys.

③ Advise the mother to "be as easy as possible on him" until after his heart defect is repaired.

④ Hold the child in a squatting position.

69. An IV of 1000 ml of 5% dextrose in saline is ordered. The solution is to infuse in 6 hours. Drop factor is 10. At what rate should the IV infuse?

① 2.7 drops per minute

② 3.7 drops per minute

③ 27 drops per minute

④ 37 drops per minute

70. In planning a client's diet, which of the following food sources would be the best source of high-biologic-value protein?

① Bananas

② Asparagus

③ Eggs

④ Mushrooms

71. Which of the following ego-defense mechanisms is a basic priority in the care of clients who have alcoholism?

① Dependency

② Denial

③ Suspiciousness

④ Projection

72. A newborn infant has a meningomyelocele. She is being transferred directly from the delivery room to a spe-

cial care unit. The nurse should place the infant in which position?

① Semi-Fowler's
② Supine
③ On her side
④ Prone

73. The nurse is caring for an infant with meningomyelocele in the newborn intensive care unit. The parents have consented to surgical closure of the defect. Before surgery, the defect should be

① Covered with dry, sterile dressings.
② Left open to the air.
③ Covered with sterile saline soaks.
④ Covered with gauze impregnated with petroleum jelly.

74. Which of the following is least effective in treating families of clients who use alcohol or other drugs?

① Genetic predisposition and other neurobiologic factors
② History of alcoholism as a generational disorder
③ Maladaptive coping behaviors among various family members
④ The degree of intimacy and distance within family structure

75. A 2-year-old child with tetralogy of Fallot is awaiting palliative surgery. The surgeon plans to anastomose the child's left subclavian artery to the pulmonary artery. The child's mother asks the nurse to explain the reason for this temporary palliative surgery. The nurse should give which of the following responses?

① "The surgery will increase the amount of blood that flows through the child's lungs so that his body gets more oxygen."
② "This procedure will change the direction of blood flow in his heart so his skin color will be less blue."
③ "The pressure on the heart chamber that pumps blood to the body will be relieved."
④ "The surgery will allow the child to grow and develop like a normal child."

Answers to this test begin on p. 545.

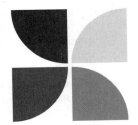

Practice Test 2

76. A 76-year-old client with a right modified radical mastectomy has just returned from surgery. In addition to assessing her vital signs, the nurse should assess for symptoms of hemorrhage by
① Asking her if her back feels wet.
② Assessing her level of consciousness.
③ Testing her stools for occult blood.
④ Visually checking under her back for drainage.

77. The primary potential problem for a woman in the third trimester of pregnancy with a history of cardiac disease is
① Premature delivery.
② Cardiac decompensation.
③ Dehydration.
④ Infection.

78. The *most critical* nursing care during the detoxification stage of alcoholism is
① Addressing manipulative behaviors used to gain access to alcohol.
② Knowing that alcoholism has depleted certain B-complex vitamins and replacing them.
③ Reporting a potassium level of 2.5 mEq/L.
④ To encourage socialization and improve social skills.

79. A 3-year-old girl's mother brings her to the emergency room because the child ate "half a bottle of acetaminophen tablets 15 minutes ago." The nurse ascertains that the bottle originally contained 100 tablets. The nurse's first action should be what?
① Have the child drink an 8 oz glass of milk.
② Give the child 30 ml of syrup of ipecac followed by a glass of water.
③ Insert a nasogastric tube and administer activated charcoal.
④ Obtain a brief history of events leading up to the ingestion from the mother.

80. Nursing assessment of the access site to the AV fistula would best include
① Taking blood pressures in the affected arm to monitor the presence of good circulation.
② Making sure the color of the blood in the fistula is bright cranberry-red.
③ Checking skin temperatures and pulses proximal to the fistula to assess circulation.
④ Palpating the access site for a thrill to assess circulation.

81. During a morning visit with the client in a chemical dependence program, the client states "I can't do anything right, my cocaine use has really messed up my life." An appropriate nursing response to this client's remarks is
① "What have you done that is so wrong?"
② "Yes, it's time you stopped smoking crack."
③ "Is this your first time in this stage of treatment?"
④ "It sounds like you are feeling guilty about using cocaine."

82. Which of the following is a correct analysis of problems associated with pregnancy-induced hypertension?
① Risk of recurrence affects future childbearing.
② Altered tissue perfusion leads to permanent maternal injury.
③ Homeotasis returns immediately after delivery.
④ Potential problems exist for 24 to 48 hours after childbirth.

83. A 14-month-old boy is scheduled for palliative surgery for tetralogy of Fallot. His mother is staying in his hospital room until he is taken to surgery. When reviewing the child's preoperative lab reports, the nurse should be most concerned about which value?
① White blood cell count 14,000/mm^3
② Hematocrit 52%
③ Serum pH 7.33
④ Platelets 220,000/mm^3

84. After surgery, the physician has ordered a 4-year-old child's ventriculoperitoneal shunt to be pumped four times every shift. When preparing the child for this procedure, the nurse should
① Explain to the child how it will feel when the shunt is pumped.
② Tell the child why the shunt has to be pumped.
③ Remind the child to be brave so she will get well soon.
④ Ask the child to close her eyes and relax so it will be over quickly.

85. A pregnant woman is hospitalized with severe pregnancy-induced hypertension in the third trimester. In evaluating her response to IV magnesium sulfate therapy, which effect is expected?
① Muscle cramps
② Hyperreflexia
③ Polyuria
④ Central nervous system depression

86. Caring for clients misusing alcohol and other drugs continues to challenge complex nursing skills. Of the following nursing orders, which is *inappropriate* for

the care of the client with alcohol and other drug problems?

① Maintain clear, firm, and consistent limits.

② Delineate acceptable and unacceptable behaviors and consequences.

③ Develop measures to ensure that all staff members provide consistent responses to client's behavior.

④ Demonstrate a high level of sympathy and concern for the client's problems.

87. A 76-year-old client with a right modified radical mastectomy has received discharge teaching. The discharge teaching has been effective if the client has

① Demonstrated incision care.

② Adapted to altered body image.

③ Completed the grieving process.

④ Received a Jobst pressure machine for home use.

88. The school nurse assesses a 6-year-old boy after a fall from the monkey bars. The child's teacher reports that she heard a loud "thunk" as his head hit the ground. The child entered the nurse's office crying loudly and asking for his mother. Which of the following findings is the most reliable indicator of a change in the child's intracranial pressure?

① Change in sensorium

② Tachycardia

③ Nausea and vomiting

④ Pulmonary rales

89. The nurse prepares to administer acetylcysteine (Mucomyst) as an antidote to acetaminophen. To make the drug more palatable the nurse should mix the drug with what fluid?

① Water

② Orange juice

③ Milk

④ Flavored milkshake

90. Which plan would best meet the learning needs in discharge planning for a 76-year-old woman?

① Provide written materials for her to read during the day.

② Offer brief, frequent, one-to-one sessions.

③ Teach her during a single session, taking a sufficient amount of time to provide complete factual material.

④ Have her join a group session with peers; use charts, several speakers, and handouts.

91. The best outcome of intervention to control aggressive and angry behavior occurs when it is implemented at which of the following times?

① Before initial frustration and anxiety culminate in aggression

② After cessation of aggressive behavior or act

③ During the aggressive incident

④ Shortly after the starting anxiety

92. When discussing concerns and discomforts with a woman in the third trimester of pregnancy, the nurse is aware that occasional dreams about labor are

① Common in women treated for infertility.

② Unique to the primigravida.

③ A sign of psychosocial problems.

④ Usual in the third trimester.

93. In caring for a child after accidental ingestion of acetaminophen, which laboratory values should the nurse monitor most closely for changes in the child's health status?

① Hemoglobin and hematocrit

② White blood cell count and differential

③ Blood gases (Po_2, Pco_2, and pH)

④ Serum transaminase levels (ALT and AST)

94. When preparing to administer a DTP booster to a toddler, the nurse should

① Allow the child to play with a syringe for a few minutes.

② Talk in a soothing tone to the child while her mother holds her firmly in her lap, and proceed quickly.

③ Explain to the child that she must "get a shot so you won't get sick."

④ Secure the assistance of at least one other nurse to help restrain the child.

95. While waiting for the AV-fistula site to mature for hemodialysis, a client is maintained using peritoneal dialysis. During peritoneal dialysis, the nurse notes a retention of 600 ml of dialysate fluid after draining the peritoneal cavity. The best initial response of the nurse would be to

① Infuse an additional 1400 ml of fresh dialysate and continue with dialysis.

② Have the client turn from side to side to help localize fluid to promote drainage.

③ Check vital signs to assess whether a fluid overload is occurring.

④ Notify the physician of the fluid retention.

96. The purpose of an ultrasound in the twelfth week of an uncomplicated pregnancy is to

① Measure biparietal diameters.

② Identify potential problems.

③ Confirm fetal viability.

④ Assess placental function.

97. Confidentiality is a client's right. When a client expresses concerns of privacy and confidentiality, it is important to know that provisions exist to address these concerns. Which of the following does *not* pertain to the client's interests?

① Phones are accessible to clients that allow them not to be overheard by others.

② The client's records are not accessible to the public.

③ Client data cannot be released without the client's authorization.

④ Specific client information should be kept in a separate chart and is not part of the hospital records.

98. A 2-year-old boy returns to the pediatric unit after insertion of a ventriculoperitoneal shunt. The nurse should plan for the child to be placed in what position in the early postoperative period?

① Semi-Fowler's on the operative side

② Semi-Fowler's on the unoperative side

③ Flat on the operative side

④ Flat on the unoperative side

99. A 5-year-old girl has been admitted with a diagnosis of noncommunicating hydrocephalus secondary to postmeningitis adhesions. What was probably the earliest manifestation of increased intracranial pressure that the child exhibited?
① Early-morning headache
② Clumsy gait
③ Projectile vomiting
④ Papilledema

100. While performing a nursing assessment on a 2-year-old Korean girl, the nurse finds that the child's weight and length are both below the 5th percentile. A nutritional history reveals that the child's caloric and nutrient intake is consistent with recommended guidelines. Which of the following interpretations is most valid?
① Growth norms are based on American children, who tend to be larger on the average.
② The child's parents may not have been truthful concerning her intake.
③ A hormone deficiency may be causing a growth lag.
④ The child may not be getting adequate activity and exercise.

101. Which of the following would be most effective in supporting an optimal level of function for the client who is confused?
① Maintain the client's daily routine as often as possible.
② Involve the client in all unit activities to increase socialization.
③ Establish a one-to-one nurse-client relationship to assist the client in understanding limitations.
④ Follow the unit's routines at all times.

102. To gain the trust and cooperation of a 2-year-old child during a physical assessment, the nurse should first
① Offer the child a toy to play with.
② Pick up the child and hug her warmly.
③ Use a puppet to "talk" to the child.
④ Establish a positive interaction with the child's parents.

103. A 16-year-old boy with hemophilia is admitted for hemarthrosis. While he is on bed rest, which activity should the nurse *not* include as part of the nursing care plan?
① Reading the daily newspaper
② Playing Nerf basketball with his older brother
③ Watching his favorite football team on television
④ Playing chess with his father

104. Shortly after a visit with his son, the client complains that his son has not been by in several days. Additionally, he expresses fear that something has happened to his son. Which is the most therapeutic nursing response?
① "Sounds like you don't think your son will return."
② "He is a good son and I am certain he will return."
③ "You are very confused, he just left your room."
④ "Your son was here and had dinner with you."

105. A newborn appears pink and active, but slight grunting on expiration is noted when he is scored using the Silverman-Anderson scale. What additional assessments are indicated?
① Heart rate
② Chest movements
③ Blood gases
④ Color

106. After a recent visit with his wife, Mr. Prallok states that his wife of 55 years is severely confused and does not remember or recognize him despite attempts to orient her. Additionally, he states that he is unsure if he should come back because she does not remember him anyway. The most appropriate nursing response to Mr. Prallok is which of the following?
① "Your visits are important, please come back tomorrow."
② "Are there others who can visit your wife?"
③ "If your wife wants to talk to you she will call."
④ "We will keep her busy on the unit and she will not miss you."

107. A 56-year-old client is diagnosed with ovarian cancer. She is likely to have which manifestation?
① Peau d'orange changes
② Constipation
③ Postcoital bleeding
④ Increased appetite

108. A nursing student tells the nurse she has a cousin with hemophilia and wants to know how the disease is inherited. The nurse explains that a female is usually the carrier of the disease, and when she marries a male who is free of the disease, the risk to their offspring for *each* pregnancy is
① 100% chance that a female baby will be a carrier.
② 100% chance that a male baby will have the disease.
③ 50% chance that a male baby will have hemophilia.
④ 50% chance that a female baby will have hemophilia.

109. Which of the following would best indicate increased intracranial pressure?
① BP change from 110/80 mm Hg to 140/50 mm Hg
② Pulse change from 78 per minute to 92 per minute
③ Respirations change from 16 per minute to 26 per minute
④ Change in level of consciousness from stupor to drowsy and restless

110. The nurse plans to obtain a nursing history from a 10-year-old child with AIDS. No direct body contact with the child will be necessary during this time. Because the child has AIDS, the nurse should take which precautions?
① Wear a mask only.
② Wear a mask and gown.
③ Wear a mask, gown, and gloves.
④ No special precautions are needed.

111. Mrs. Rankins, who is confused, discourages her son from visiting because he refuses to let her live with him. The son seeks out the nurse and lets him know that he is unsure of what to do. He further contends that his mother is angry and that he feels frustrated because he cannot keep her home because of her con-

fusion. The most sensible nursing response to this client is which of the following?

① "Your mother will be okay in several days, this is not unusual."

② "She will do fine after she gets a daily routine."

③ "It sounds like you are feeling guilty for leaving your mother here."

④ "This is a stressful time for you and your mother."

112. A 16-year-old boy has hemophilia. He has recently been diagnosed with acquired immunodeficiency syndrome (AIDS) resulting from contaminated blood products. The child is currently free from infectious disease. He has been hospitalized for hemarthrosis of his left elbow. He is complaining of severe elbow pain. In addition to placing the child on bed rest, the nurse should

① Apply a heating pad to his left elbow.

② Give him 10 grains aspirin PO.

③ Gently perform passive range-of-motion exercises to the left elbow.

④ Elevate and immobilize the left elbow in a flexed position.

113. When educating a client about continuous ambulatory peritoneal dialysis (CAPD), the top priority is to teach

① Sterile technique to help prevent peritonitis.

② To maintain a more liberal protein diet.

③ To maintain a daily written record of blood pressure and weight.

④ To continue regular medical and nursing follow-up.

114. The client with Alzheimer's disease is likely to have which of the following behaviors?

① Inattentiveness and inability to learn new information.

② Equal impairment of recall of both recent and long-past events.

③ Slight difficulty adapting to environmental changes.

④ Expanded interest in activities of daily living.

115. What is the optimal bed position for the client with congestive heart failure?

① Position of comfort, to relax the client.

② Semirecumbent, to ease dyspnea and metabolic demands of the heart.

③ Sims, to decrease danger of pulmonary edema.

④ Dorsal recumbent, to decrease edema formation in the extremities.

116. A child with Down syndrome can benefit from a comprehensive preschool stimulation program. The primary goal of such a program is which of the following?

① The child's muscle tone will improve.

② The child will achieve an optimal developmental level.

③ The child's family will be involved in his care.

④ The child will be ready to enter first grade at age 6.

117. Respirations of the client with congestive heart failure are usually of which kind?

① Rapid and shallow

② Deep and stertorous

③ Rapid and wheezing

④ Biot's respirations

118. Which of the following childhood problems poses the most serious threat to health for a child with Down syndrome?

① Conjunctivitis

② Milk allergy

③ Chickenpox

④ Bronchitis

119. A newborn has an initial axillary temperature of 96° F. If the infant is cold stressed and is not warmed immediately, the nurse would initially observe which of the following?

① Shivering

② Cyanosis

③ Respiratory rate increase

④ Irritability

120. Parents bring their 3-month-old infant to the pediatric clinic 1 month after surgical repair of a cleft lip. What is the most crucial indicator of successful treatment of the defect?

① The suture line is clean and well healed.

② The parents say they are "thrilled with how he looks now."

③ The infant is making cooing and babbling sounds.

④ The infant is now sleeping through the night.

121. Maintaining reality orientation is a major treatment goal for the cognitively impaired client. Which of the following interventions will facilitate reality orientation?

① Call the client by name and identify yourself during each interaction.

② Make the television available and encourage the client to watch it as often as possible.

③ Provide an array of activities daily.

④ Avoid assigning the same staff and ensure staff rotation.

122. When tourniquets are applied to extremities to relieve the symptoms of pulmonary edema, one tourniquet should be rotated, in order, on a regular basis. How often is it rotated?

① Every 5 minutes

② Every 10 minutes

③ Every 15 minutes

④ Every 20 minutes

123. A 3-year-old boy has Down syndrome. During a routine clinic visit, the boy's mother tells the nurse that her husband is being transferred to another city. She is concerned about the effect this move will have on her child. Which of the following suggestions should receive the highest priority when discussing the move with the child's mother?

① Adhere to the child's daily routine as much as possible during and after the move.

② Include the child in all the family discussions concerning the move.

③ Have the child stay with relatives until the move is complete.

④ Enroll the child in a special day-care program as soon as possible.

124. An adult client is admitted to the coronary care unit (CCU). His ECG indicates an anterior myocardial infarction. To assess the client's cardiac status, the nurse should monitor

① ECG changes, serum enzymes, and leg cramps.
② ECG changes, serum enzymes, and chest pain.
③ ST-segment changes, serum creatinine, and chest pain.
④ T-wave changes, serum electrolytes, and blood urea nitrogen.

125. A mother of a child with Down syndrome is concerned about her child's weight. "He is so much smaller than other children his age." The nurse's response should be based on the knowledge that
① The child needs more fluid and calories than the average child of the same age.
② The height and weight of children with Down syndrome is usually below chronologic norms.
③ The mother should discuss this concern with the pediatrician.
④ The child's growth will "catch up" in a few years.

126. The mother of an infant with cleft lip asks the nurse, "Why do you think this happened to my baby?" The nurse should reply
① "Cleft lip probably runs in your family."
② "Sometimes it's hard to know why these things happen."
③ "Did you have any infections or take any drugs while you were pregnant?"
④ "What thoughts do you have about why it happened?"

127. The nurse is caring for an infant who underwent surgical repair of a cleft lip yesterday. Oral feedings of 4 to 6 oz of infant formula every 4 or 5 hours are to be resumed. The nurse should teach the mother to feed her infant using what method?
① A bottle with a soft nipple
② A small paper cup
③ A syringe with catheter tubing
④ Nasogastric gavage

128. Mrs. Irving's daughter reports that her mother has lost 12 pounds over the past 2 or 3 months. Of the following, which promises the *most appropriate* nursing action to ensure adequate nutrition?
① Insist and feed the client when the client refuses to complete the meal.
② Provide the client with six small servings during the day.
③ Inform the client that she will be tube fed if she continues to refuse food.
④ Assess the client's eating patterns and weight and develop an individualized plan of care.

129. While being monitored for a ventricular dysrhythmia, an adult client in CCU goes into cardiac arrest. Which of these actions should the nurse take **first**?
① Check his carotid pulse.
② Put him on a hard surface.
③ Open his airway.
④ Start chest compression.

130. A 2-month-old infant was born with a unilateral complete cleft lip. It is 12 hours after surgical repair of the lip. His mother is staying in his hospital room. The infant is acting fussy and starts to cry softly. The nurse should
① Encourage the mother to hold and rock the infant.
② Give the infant his pacifier and rub his back.

③ Sedate the infant with 2.5 mg of diphenhydramine hydrochloride (Benadryl) elixir.
④ Allow the infant to cry to facilitate lung inflation.

131. An adult client is scheduled to have a cardiac catheterization in the morning. The nurse should inform the client that during the procedure the client will be
① Heavily sedated and moved by the doctor.
② Under general anesthesia and unconscious.
③ Not sedated, and told to remain still.
④ Mildly sedated, and asked to change position.

132. The nurse completes a health history from a couple with a history of infertility. What are the two assessment possibilities?
① Testicular biopsy and culdoscopy
② Laparoscopy and hormonal studies
③ Huhner test and thyroid screening
④ Semen analysis and cervical mucus observation

133. The nurse has just finished talking with the mother of a 2-year-old about accident prevention. Which of the following statements by the mother suggests that the nurse's teaching was *not* effective?
① "I can simply close the doors to the bathroom and basement in order to keep my child out."
② "It's very important that my daughter not think of medicine as candy."
③ "I've put the poison control center phone number by all the phones in the house."
④ "You know, no matter how hard I try I just can't monitor everything she does."

134. Select an appropriate goal for the client in the first trimester of pregnancy.
① Mother will adhere to regular clinic visit schedule.
② Father will participate in each prenatal class.
③ Couple will practice exercises each day.
④ Mother will rest for 30 minutes daily.

135. The information gathered from a left cardiac catheterization will include all except which of the following?
① Patency of the coronary arteries
② Status of collateral circulation
③ Patency of the pulmonary artery
④ Perfusion of the myocardium

136. Mrs. Onie Irving is an 85-year-old woman whose husband, Walter, died 3 years ago. Mrs. Irving constantly tries to leave the extended care facility, stating, "Walter is waiting for me at home. I must go to him now!" The most therapeutic nursing response is which of the following?
① "He is aware that you cannot come to him now; have a seat."
② "You know you retired 15 years ago and Mr. Irving is dead."
③ "We cannot let you leave now, you must stay."
④ "Your husband died 3 years ago, I know you miss him. Tell me about him."

137. A nurse makes a home visit to a mother of three girls, aged 3 months, 3 years, and 12 years. Which finding during a nursing assessment presents the greatest cause for concern?
① The 3-month-old infant is taking 28 oz of formula daily and 2 Tbsp. of cereal and pureed fruit twice daily.

② The 3-year-old wets the bed two or three times a week.

③ Mrs. Davis says she is "always exhausted."

④ The 12-year-old has been spending increasing amounts of time in her room talking on the telephone and playing video games.

138. Which of the following statements made by a couple after participation in Lamaze childbirth preparation classes indicates learning has occurred?

① "We'll continue to practice the breathing and relaxation techniques."

② "Our bonding as a couple will help us bond to the baby."

③ "This method will help us avoid all pain medications."

④ "The presence of the father ensures success."

139. During the oliguric phase of acute renal failure, which of the following would be an appropriate nursing intervention?

① Increase dietary sodium and potassium.

② Restrict fluid to 1500 ml daily.

③ Weigh client three times weekly.

④ Provide a low-protein, high-carbohydrate diet.

140. On admission to the hospital, a client with the diagnosis of parkinsonism reports that he is taking the medication levodopa. The nurse knows that one side effect of this drug that should be monitored and included in the care plan is

① Hypertension.

② Increased appetite.

③ Euphoria.

④ Orthostatic hypotension.

141. The nurse assesses a 4-month-old infant's development. Which of the following behaviors should be present?

① Bears some weight on his legs

② Imitates speech sounds

③ Sits with minimal support

④ Uses a thumb-finger grasp

142. A physician prescribes clomiphene citrate (Clomid) for a woman with a history of infertility. She should be informed that a side effect of this medication may be

① Uterine fibroids.

② Multiple gestation.

③ Hypertension.

④ Transitory depression.

143. A client having a spinal anesthetic is at greatest risk for which of the following complications?

① Respiratory paralysis

② Permanent motor dysfunction

③ Paralytic ileus

④ Hypotension

144. A patient has vaginal bleeding in the tenth week of pregnancy. When bleeding stops and the hCG levels remain elevated, discharge planning should include which of the following instructions?

① "Call the doctor if you experience abdominal pain or cramping."

② "Notify the doctor if you are nauseated or vomit."

③ "If you are very tired, call and make an appointment."

④ "Report any signs of urinary frequency."

145. Some clients experiencing confusion wander into other client's rooms or out into the street. One of the most effective deterrents to wandering is which of the following?

① Escort the client when wandering is noted and guide the client back to the room or day area.

② Question the client and provide an explanation for not remaining in the room or street.

③ Restrict the client to her room because of persistent wandering.

④ Restrain the client in her chair so that she remains confined and safe.

146. Preparation of the client's skin before applying Buck's extension traction should include which of the following?

① Surgical preparation of the area where pins will be inserted

② Close shaving of the leg with a safety razor

③ Washing and drying of the skin

④ Application of talc to the area

147. Which of the following behaviors could indicate potential problems with early attachment by a first-day postpartum mother?

① She complains of episiotomy pain while sitting with the infant.

② The woman appears discouraged with early breast-feeding attempts.

③ She makes little attempt to touch or speak to the newborn.

④ The mother often naps when the newborn is quiet.

148. A mother tells the nurse that she is concerned about her 3-week-old infant's "throwing up; he does it every time he eats." What would be the nurse's best first response to further clarify this potential problem?

① "About how much does he throw up each time, and what does it look like?"

② "Are you burping him after every ounce?"

③ "Perhaps you aren't diluting his formula correctly. Let's check."

④ "Is he taking formula with iron?"

149. Persistent confusion in the elderly client admitted to a long-term care facility is most like caused by which of the following?

① Frustration and anger at the family

② Increased personal space

③ Continued cortical deterioration

④ Unfamiliar environment

150. Your patient with hepatitis A has extensive jaundice and is experiencing severe pruritis. Which intervention would be appropriate?

① Administering sedative medications every 4 hours

② Encouraging frequent warm showers or long tub baths

③ Encouraging the use of light cotton clothing

④ Obtaining a dehumidifier for the room

Answers to this test begin on p. 550.

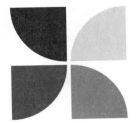

Practice Test 3

151. An infant looks directly at her mother while breast-feeding and seems to react to the voices of both parents. The mother asks the nurse if their daughter can see and hear. Which of the following responses is most accurate?
   ① "We think that the newborn can see light and hear loud sounds."
   ② "Research has shown that close-up vision and hearing are present."
   ③ "The newborn only appears to respond to sensory stimuli."
   ④ "It is impossible to determine this in the first days of life."

152. A client is admitted to the hospital for a kidney transplant. Which of the following interventions would do the most to help prevent transplant rejection?
   ① Transfusion of 4 units of typed and crossmatched blood
   ② Administration of prophylactic antibiotics
   ③ Hemodialysis until the transplant begins to function
   ④ Administration of immunosuppressive drugs

153. The mother of a child with acute glomerulonephritis asks the nurse if her child will "probably end up on one of those kidney machines." The nurse's reply should be based on the knowledge that the kidneys will most likely
   ① Return to normal functioning.
   ② Develop acute failure, requiring dialysis.
   ③ Develop chronic failure, necessitating a kidney transplant.
   ④ Have numerous recurrences of the infection.

154. Mr. Jefferson was brought to the emergency room vomiting blood. Esophageal varices were found to be the cause, and a Sengstaken-Blakemore tube was inserted. Which observation would lead the nurse to conclude that this intervention was effective?
   ① The client is relaxed and has stable vital signs.
   ② A sample of stomach aspirate tests guaiac-negative.
   ③ The client is able to swallow liquids without discomfort.
   ④ There is no increase in the client's abdominal girth.

155. The nurse makes a home visit to a 7-year-old child with acute glomerulonephritis. Which of the following meals reported by the child's mother indicates that she does not fully understand the child's dietary restrictions?
   ① Fried chicken, mashed potatoes, green beans, and apple juice
   ② Broiled fish, macaroni salad, applesauce, and grape juice
   ③ Scrambled eggs, bacon, muffin with jelly, and orange juice
   ④ Grilled cheese sandwich, carrots, fruit cocktail, and milk

156. Which of the following interventions, if implemented, would be the most likely to help a client avoid disequilibrium syndrome from hemodialysis?
   ① Withhold antihypertensive medications.
   ② Dialyze for a short time.
   ③ Dialyze in a sitting position.
   ④ Withhold protein from the diet.

157. Mrs. Lily becomes more confused after being admitted to a long-term care facility. Her confusion can be minimized by which of the following nursing actions?
   ① Helping the client with all activities of daily living.
   ② Assessing the client's normal routine and following it as much as possible.
   ③ Limiting visitors during the initial 2 weeks of admission until the client is used to the facility.
   ④ Waiting for the confusion to resolve; confusion is to be expected during the initial period and will abate after the client gets used to the facility.

158. While assessing an infant, the nurse notes nose breathing and occasional sneezing. What is the correct analysis of these data?
   ① There may be a respiratory problem.
   ② Further assessment is indicated.
   ③ The environment may be cold.
   ④ These are normal responses.

159. The physician orders a screening test to assess a client for glaucoma. That test is a(n)
   ① Myringotomy.
   ② Funduscopy.
   ③ Tonometry.
   ④ Iridectomy.

160. A 7-year-old girl had acute poststreptococcal nephritis. The nurse makes a home visit to monitor the child's response to treatment. Which of the following

531

is necessary for the nurse to include when evaluating this client?
① Blood pressure measurement
② Auscultation of breath sounds
③ Urine test for glucose and acetone
④ Abdominal circumference measurements

161. On an infant's admission to the newborn nursery, a gestational assessment is performed. Which of the following observations indicates that the newborn is probably full term?
① Apgar scores of 9 and 10 at 1 and 5 minutes
② Good reflex responses
③ Many sole creases present
④ Birth weight at 50th percentile

162. The underlying neurobiology of cognitive impairment that is caused by dementia and that follows altered intellectual functioning is which of the following?
① Impaired ability to manage anxiety
② Disorientation to time and place
③ Mood swings
④ Perceptual disturbances (e.g., paranoia)

163. A male, 68 years old, is diagnosed with idiopathic parkinsonism. He is likely to have which manifestations?
① Intentional tremors
② Hyperkinesia
③ Propulsive gait
④ Loss of sensation in both feet

164. You are performing preoperative teaching for a client who will undergo laparascopic cholecystectomy today. You should prepare the client for which common problem after the surgery?
① Severe nausea and possible vomiting for about 6 hours postoperative
② Pain that radiates to the shoulder region
③ Lethargy and extreme fatigue
④ Severe anorexia

165. A 31-year-old married man with two children has been diagnosed with leukemia, and the disease has been treated with drug therapy for 2½ years. The client has been admitted to the hospital with pneumonia and has been placed in protective isolation. He has told the nurses that he knows he is going to die, but that is all he has said about it. He talks about his disease in clinical terms to the nurses, never about his own experiences. One day he comments to his primary nurse, "I am so worried." The best response from the nurse is
① "It must frighten you to know you are dying."
② "It must make you very uncomfortable."
③ "Have you shared these feelings with your family?"
④ "Tell me exactly what things are worrying you."

166. The nurse can best help the dying client cope with death by which of the following?
① Use distraction by switching to another subject that does not focus on the client's disease.
② Encourage the client to reach out to loved ones and spend more time with them.
③ Listen to the client and encourage a life review of important events.
④ Encourage the client to spend more time sleeping and resting.

167. Mrs. Rosa Perez has had several episodes of acute cholecystitis, and her physician recommends a cholecystectomy. She asks whether she will be able to have the "belly button" surgery like several of her friends. Which factor would be a contraindication for this surgical approach?
① Ultrasound showing the presence of gallstones in the common bile duct
② Being 20 pounds overweight
③ Having chronic osteoarthritis
④ Working as a waitress (requires a lot of heavy lifting)

168. An 11-year-old girl is hospitalized with rheumatic fever with carditis and polyarthritis. She also has Sydenham's chorea. Which of the following is true concerning rheumatic fever?
① It is usually associated with glomerulonephritis.
② Symptoms disappear shortly after the fever abates and the temperature returns to normal.
③ The child should resume normal activities as soon as she feels well.
④ It usually follows a streptococcal infection.

169. In planning nursing care for a child with rheumatic fever, the nurse notes that the child is on bed rest. What is the rationale for this?
① To help ease the pain of the arthritis that accompanies the disease
② To minimize the effects of the carditis
③ So other children will not see the child's choreiform movements
④ To help alleviate the febrile effects of the disease

170. A client with a terminal illness tells the nurse not to let the family know of the impending death. What is the most effective response to this request?
① "They would not want to worry about upsetting you."
② "Sounds like you are concerned about them worrying."
③ "This is stressful to you. Let's talk about something more pleasant."
④ Sit and wait a minute without speaking.

171. A father asks you about laboratory charges for PKU screening and questions the need for the test. The nurse understands that PKU testing is valuable because
① It identifies newborns with chromosomal abnormalities.
② Routine screening tests meet state laws.
③ A rare metabolic disorder can be detected.
④ Autoimmune adaptation is evaluated.

172. A client with insulin-dependent diabetes mellitus comes in for a routine follow-up visit. Diabetic teaching is reinforced at each visit, and the emphasis of this visit is hygiene and foot care. Which statement or observation would indicate that the client needs further teaching on this topic?
① The nails are trimmed straight across.
② The client reports that she bathes and inspects her feet daily.
③ The client uses lotion to counteract dry areas on her heels.

④ The client is wearing attractive sandals and is not wearing stockings.

173. A 9-year-old girl is hospitalized with acute glomerulonephritis. Which of the following is likely to be the major psychologic stressor of this child during her illness and hospitalization?
① Fear of painful procedures
② Separation from her family
③ Activity restriction
④ Worry about possible outcomes

174. A posttrauma male patient has a mean blood pressure of 90. He is on nitroprusside drip and epinephrine drip with orders to keep blood pressure at a mean of 80. What is the action of the nitroprusside?
① Increased afterload
② Increased cardiac output
③ Decreased preload
④ Increased preload

175. What is the primary goal of therapy for a client in shock?
① Maintain adequate blood pressure.
② Improve tissue perfusion.
③ Maintain adequate vascular tone.
④ Improve kidney function.

176. During rooming-in, a client is taught many aspects of newborn care. Before discharge, she is observed feeding and handling the baby. Which of the following actions best indicates that she learned how to provide safe infant care?
① The infant is placed on her right side after the feeding.
② Breast-feeding is managed comfortably and effectively.
③ The diaper area is cleansed after passage of a stool.
④ The mother handles the baby gently while dressing her.

177. After ascertaining that an infant is experiencing normal newborn regurgitation, the nurse reassures his mother that newborns often experience this problem based on what knowledge?
① The newborn's stomach capacity is small.
② It takes some time for the newborn to adjust to the formula's richness.
③ The lining of the newborn's stomach is easily irritated.
④ The cardiac sphincter between the esophagus and stomach is not fully matured.

178. Which is most effective in helping families cope with the imminent death of a loved one?
① Help family members stay at the same level of grief.
② Encourage them to express their feelings and thoughts to the nurse.
③ Tell them to spend as much time at the hospital as possible even if just sitting in the waiting room.
④ Recommend crying, but not in front of the client.

179. A 90-year-old female client with a knee replacement expresses concern over her impending discharge. What would be the most effective intervention for the client?

① Ask what concerns her.
② Discuss the possibility of placing her in a nursing home.
③ Teach her about hazards in her environment.
④ Have the social worker make a visit to the client's home.

180. Which of the following children should the nurse select as a roommate for a 12-year-old girl with rheumatic fever?
① A 7-year-old girl who also has rheumatic fever.
② A 10-year-old girl with insulin-dependent diabetes.
③ A 13-year-old girl with sickle cell vasoocclusive crisis.
④ A 12-year-old girl with fever of unknown origin.

181. An adult male is admitted to a neurologic unit with a skull fracture he sustained in an auto accident. One of the goals of care for him is to prevent increased intracranial pressure. Which of the following signs indicates increased intracranial pressure?
① Increased pulse rate and increased blood pressure
② Increased pulse rate and decreased blood pressure
③ Decreased pulse rate and increased blood pressure
④ Decreased pulse rate and decreased blood pressure

182. Which of the following activities is most appropriate for a 12-year-old girl hospitalized with rheumatic fever with carditis and polyarthritis?
① Listening to tapes and the radio
② Watching television
③ Playing ping-pong in the game room
④ Crocheting a small afghan

183. When a client has kidney surgery, there is a high thoracic incision. The most appropriate outcome criterion to evaluate the status of the pulmonary system in this client would be
① Client is free from temperature elevation greater than 38.5°C.
② Client's breath sounds are clear.
③ Client's P_{O_2} is greater than 60 mm Hg.
④ Client shows no signs of cyanosis.

184. A severely depressed client ignores the nurse, who attempts to engage the client in conversation. The client walks away without responding. What is the most therapeutic nursing response?
① Avoid further pursuit of the client.
② Continue attempts to engage the client.
③ Confront the client's socially isolative behavior.
④ Ask another staff member to monitor the client.

185. Which maternal behavior is commonly observed during the "taking-in" phase?
① Asking about birth control measures
② Requesting information on infant development
③ Reliving and retelling labor/birth events
④ Experiencing mild transient depression

186. Blood tests of a child with rheumatic fever show the following results. Which is the most indicative of an improvement in her condition?
① Positive C-reactive protein
② White blood cell count of 11,000
③ Decreased erythrocyte sedimentation rate (ESR)
④ Elevated antistreptolysin O (ASO) titer

187. At a clinic visit, a postpartum client is discouraged about breast-feeding. She says, "Neither the baby nor I seem to be successful at breast-feeding. Maybe it's because I'm so small." The nurse's response should be based on understanding that
    ① Hormone levels may vary in individual women.
    ② Desire to breast-feed affects milk production.
    ③ Primiparas are usually apprehensive about feeding.
    ④ Breast size is not a factor in volume of milk produced.

188. An adult victim of cardiac arrest receives cardiopulmonary resuscitation. Which of the following observations would *best* indicate that the CPR is effective?
    ① Palpable carotid pulse
    ② Dilated pupils
    ③ Easily blanched nail beds
    ④ Normal skin color

189. When preparing a 12-year-old for cardiac catheterization, the nurse should take into account which of the following?
    ① Concrete explanations and experiences will be most meaningful.
    ② The child is likely to misinterpret the procedure as punishment for previous misbehavior.
    ③ The child should be given a full verbal explanation of the procedure using correct medical terminology.
    ④ The child should be allowed to make all decisions concerning her care.

190. Which statement by a new father indicates that he has a realistic understanding of newborn behavior?
    ① "I hope we can get him on a schedule of two naps and a full night's sleep."
    ② "I don't want him to be spoiled, so he'll learn quickly not to cry for attention."
    ③ "If we can get him on a schedule for feedings, he'll nurse better."
    ④ "It looks like the next weeks will be mostly feeding, changing, and caring for baby."

191. An adult client is suffering from shock postoperatively. The nurse should assess the person for signs and symptoms of adequate tissue perfusion. The *least* reliable indicator of tissue perfusion is
    ① Urinary output.
    ② Skin color.
    ③ Blood pressure.
    ④ Level of consciousness.

192. A 2-year-old is hospitalized for 4 days with a diagnosis of laryngotracheobronchitis. The child's parents visit every evening but are unable to stay with her overnight. Which behavior is this child most likely to demonstrate when separating from her parents?
    ① Readily seeks comfort from the nurse
    ② Sucks her thumb, whines, and curls up in a corner of her crib
    ③ Cries loudly and tries to cling to her parents
    ④ Waves and blows them a kiss

193. During a home visit the nurse notices that the TV is on, but the client is not watching it. This client is severely depressed and socially isolative. What is the most therapeutic approach to engaging the client in conversation?
    ① "What is going on today?"
    ② "Is the TV show interesting?"
    ③ "How are you doing today?"
    ④ "I noticed that you are not watching TV."

194. A client experiencing severe depression has recently been promoted and will soon receive a significant advance if he continues to do well. How does this information contribute to depression?
    ① Depression often accompanies success.
    ② Ideas of grandeur represent an aspect of depression.
    ③ Decreased feelings of worthlessness parallel the promotion.
    ④ The promotion will give him a purpose.

195. A postpartum patient asks if breast-feeding will change the shape of her breast. Which of the following is an appropriate response?
    ① "Yes, the shape of your breast may be affected if the baby is allowed to nurse too vigorously."
    ② "Breast-feeding does not affect the shape of the breast. However, wearing a proper breast support is important."
    ③ "If you breast-feed for more than 6 months, the shape of the breast will change."
    ④ "Breast-feeding may change the shape of the breast; however, this shouldn't be the most important consideration."

196. After chest percussion and postural drainage, which finding indicates that the treatment has not been entirely effective?
    ① Inspiratory stridor
    ② Crackles and wheezes
    ③ Suprasternal retractions
    ④ Harsh metallic cough

197. A client with congestive heart failure is given digitalis. Which finding indicates the earliest manifestation of digitalis toxicity?
    ① Hypokalemia
    ② Tachycardia
    ③ Nausea and vomiting
    ④ Gynecomastia

198. A client who is receiving Coumadin comes to a walk-in clinic. He has blood in his stool and reports that he has had several episodes of epistaxis. Because of these findings, which drug should the nurse have available?
    ① Ascorbic acid
    ② Vitamin K
    ③ Protamine sulfate
    ④ Calcium chloride

199. Which of the following nursing assessments suggests bladder distention 6 hours after delivery?
    ① Poor abdominal muscle tone
    ② Lochia rubra with stringy clots
    ③ Hard, contracted uterus
    ④ Uterus soft to the right of midline

200. Chest percussion and postural drainage are prescribed 4 times a day for a child with cystic fibrosis. When should the nurse plan to carry out the chest therapy?

① Just before the child eats and at bedtime.

② Halfway between mealtimes and at bedtime.

③ Upon arising and 1 hour after meals.

④ During intervals between the child's naps.

201. A 47-year-old male is admitted with an acute myocardial infarct. He is cold and clammy and has severe substernal chest pain with dyspnea. Because of these findings, which of these medical orders should the nurse carry out **first?**

① Apply a light blanket.

② Administer oxygen.

③ Place the client in a semi-Fowler's position.

④ Administer morphine by slow IV push.

202. What is the most reasonable interpretation of a client's regression before discharge from a program?

① The discharge is premature.

② The client has experienced increased attachment and dependency on nursing staff.

③ This is a common response to discharge.

④ The client needs reassurance that the nurse cares.

203. Which of the following tasks frequently would be contraindicated in the first trimester of pregnancy for a woman employed in an animal hospital?

① Operating a computer to prepare weekly statements.

② Preparing the surgical suite for minor procedures.

③ Handling rabies and distemper vaccines and syringes.

④ Administering antibiotic ear drops to small animals.

204. A toddler is in a mist tent with compressed air. Nursing care should include which measure?

① Explain to her why she must stay in the tent.

② Restrict her fluid intake to no more than 32 oz a day.

③ Administer a cough suppressant to control her cough.

④ Change her wet bed linens frequently.

205. A client with hypercholesterolemia is advised to eliminate foods high in cholesterol from his diet. This means he should avoid eggs and

① Liver.

② Yogurt.

③ Chicken.

④ Corn oil.

206. When taking a history from a pregnant client, the nurse finds out that her family has a kitten at home. Which teaching would be most appropriate at this time?

① "Realize that the kitten may be jealous of your infant."

② "Ask your husband if he will care for the litter box."

③ "Check to see if you and your husband have any allergies."

④ "Be sure to keep the animal indoors at all times."

207. The antidepressant sertraline (Zoloft) has been ordered for the client in a home health care setting. Which of the following questions *most* represents an understanding of safe administration of this medication?

① "When was your last meal?"

② "How long have you been off phenelzine (Nardil)?"

③ "How long have you been depressed?"

④ "When was your last dose of lithium?"

208. A child has an IV of 500 ml of 5% dextrose in 0.25% normal saline ordered to infuse over 8 hours. The nurse should set the microdrip regulator to infuse at a rate of how many drops per minute?

① 21

② 30

③ 63

④ 125

209. With left-sided congestive heart failure, which of the following symptoms is most expected?

① Nocturnal dyspnea

② Sacral edema

③ Oliguria

④ Anorexia

210. A pregnant client in the tenth week of pregnancy comes to the clinic complaining of vague flulike symptoms. Which of the following statements made by the client indicates that she has learned what was taught at the early antepartal visits?

① "I know I shouldn't take any over-the-counter remedies now."

② "I feel so tired all the time; I must need the rest."

③ "I urinate frequently, so I probably am drinking too many fluids."

④ "Between the morning sickness and the flu, I'll be happy to lose weight."

211. Developmentally, a 22-month-old should exhibit which of the following behaviors?

① Dress and undress herself without help.

② Share her toys with other children.

③ Speak in 5- to 6-word sentences.

④ Feed herself well with a spoon.

212. Which of the following persons is at greatest risk of suicide?

① The depressed woman who has had a recent stillbirth.

② The elderly man whose wife has recently been diagnosed with Alzheimer's disease.

③ The adolescent girl who recently broke up with her boyfriend.

④ The adolescent boy whose best friend was severely injured in a motor vehicle accident in which he was the driver.

213. Edema caused by right-sided congestive heart failure tends to be which of the following?

① Painful

② Dependent

③ Periorbital

④ Nonpitting

214. After a left cardiac catheterization, in what position will a client be placed?

① Supine with affected leg extended

② Supine with affected leg flexed

③ Side lying with both legs flexed

④ The position of most comfort

215. A pregnant woman with a history of two term births,

now healthy adolescents, and a 36-week fetal loss is determined to be
① T3, P0, A0, L2.
② T2, P1, A0, L2.
③ T2, P0, A1, L2.
④ T3, P0, A1, L2.

216. In the immediate postoperative period after a total laryngectomy, a client requires frequent suctioning of the tracheostomy tube and nasopharynx to maintain a patent airway and remove secretions. When suctioning the nurse would
① Use a clean setup each time.
② Apply constant suction.
③ Suction the tracheostomy tube, then the nasopharynx.
④ Lubricate the catheter with petroleum jelly.

217. A 22-month-old girl is admitted to the pediatric unit with acute laryngotracheobronchitis. When a nursing history is taken, the mother tells the nurse that her child is toilet trained. Which additional information is the most important for the nurse to ascertain?
① The age at which toilet training began
② The child's toilet habits and routine at home
③ The mother's understanding of the possibility of regression in her child's toileting habits while she is hospitalized
④ The child's willingness to accept help from the nursing staff with her toileting needs

218. Immediately after a laryngectomy, a nasogastric tube is used to provide fluids and nutrients for the client. The purpose of this treatment is to
① Prevent pain while swallowing.
② Prevent contamination of the suture line.
③ Decrease need for swallowing.
④ Prevent aspiration.

219. A client with depression is actively participating in treatment by interacting with staff and other clients. She states that she looks forward to going on pass with her family. She confidently states that she feels good about her life. What is the most therapeutic nursing response?
① "Are you planning to harm yourself?"
② "Slow down and take one day at a time."
③ "What other plans do you have?"
④ "It's good to see you taking an interest in people again."

220. Sam Baker, age 21, is admitted with a spinal cord injury from a diving accident. Shortly after admission, he develops bradycardia and hypotension. His skin is warm and dry. You suspect he is experiencing which of the following?
① Spinal shock
② Autonomic dysreflexia
③ Hypoxia
④ Infection

221. Which of the following is a correctly identified sign of pregnancy?
① Amenorrhea: probable
② Chadwick's sign: probable
③ Urine human chorionic gonadotropin (hCG): positive
④ Nausea and vomiting: presumptive

222. When a toddler is discharged after a brief hospitalization, which instruction to the parents is *not* appropriate?
① The child may show some regression in her behavior for a few weeks.
② The child should not be separated from her parents for lengthy periods until she feels secure again.
③ The child should be allowed to sleep with her parents for a few nights until she readjusts to being home.
④ The parents should reinstate limits that were in effect before her hospitalization.

223. Screening a population for tuberculosis with tuberculin skin testing is an example of
① Primary health promotion.
② Secondary health promotion.
③ Tertiary health promotion.
④ Primary prevention.

224. Histamine (H_2) receptor antagonist drugs are the mainstay of management for peptic ulcers. What is their major action?
① Increase gastric motility and emptying
② Neutralize acid in the stomach and duodenum
③ Reduce the production of gastric secretions
④ Coat and protect the mucosa of the stomach and duodenum

225. Selective serotonin reuptake inhibitors (SSRIs) are new-generation antidepressants. Which of the following indicates an understanding of possible adverse reactions of this type of medication?
① The SSRI should be taken at bedtime to encourage rest.
② The SSRI should be taken on an empty stomach to promote absorption.
③ The SSRI should be taken with food to reduce gastrointestinal disturbances.
④ The SSRI should not be taken for more than 6 months because it is addictive.

Answers to this test begin on p. 555.

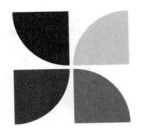

226. Because of normal physiologic changes, CBC results in the sixth month of pregnancy are expected to show
① An increase in the hematocrit.
② A decrease in the hematocrit.
③ An increase in the hemoglobin to meet the requirements of the fetus.
④ No change in the blood levels because the body will maintain homeostasis.

227. When planning care for the hospitalized toddler whose mother cannot room-in, which nursing action would be most appropriate?
① Encourage the mother to leave an article of her clothing.
② Assign the toddler a roommate close in age to keep him or her company.
③ Inform the mother that toddlers handle separation easily.
④ Suggest that mother limit visits to reduce the toddler's separation anxiety.

228. Your client has a subtotal gastric resection today (Billroth II) for treatment of a recurrent duodenal ulcer. Which postop order would you question?
① Monitor vital signs q4h.
② Attach the Salem sump to low suction.
③ Irrigate the NG tube with normal saline q2h and reposition as needed.
④ Accurately record all NG tube drainage as output.

229. The client is discharged on the antidepressant trazodone hydrochloride (Desyrel). Pertinent discharge information regarding this medication should include which of the following?
① It is addictive and should not be taken for more than several months.
② The benefits of sedation can be gained by taking it at bedtime.
③ Foods such as wines, aged cheese, chocolates, and over-the-counter cold preparations should be avoided.
④ It may cause hypertension, and the client's blood pressure should be closely monitored.

230. A woman 10 weeks pregnant finds herself questioning whether she can adapt to having a new baby with two preschoolers. The nurse's response is
① "Perhaps you should explore the possibility of terminating the pregnancy."
② "It's normal to feel ambivalent. Let's talk about it."

③ "Once you feel the life within you, these feelings will subside."
④ "I can arrange an appointment for counseling if you wish."

231. A 7-month-old infant has a congenitally dislocated right hip. The nurse should expect to note which finding when assessing this infant?
① Easily abducted right hip
② Lengthening of the right leg
③ Severe pain on hip movement
④ Widening of the perineum

232. One year after gastric resection, a client is diagnosed with pernicious anemia. The most appropriate treatment for this problem is
① Diet modification with iron-rich foods.
② Monthly vitamin B_{12} injections.
③ Daily multivitamin supplements.
④ Oral replacement of intrinsic factor.

233. The severely depressed client eats little at mealtime. Which of the following is the most accurate explanation for decreased appetite in the depressed client?
① It is an adverse reaction to antidepressants.
② Hospital food is unappetizing.
③ This is a manipulative, attention-seeking behavior.
④ It represents a symptom of depression.

234. Which instruction concerning diet should be given to a client with a duodenal ulcer?
① Following a strict bland diet is essential to the early healing stages for an ulcer.
② A regular diet may be used, but the client should limit intake of fat.
③ No specific diet restrictions are necessary, but the client should avoid any foods or seasonings that cause pain.
④ The client may follow his own food preferences but should be sure to increase the use of milk between meals.

235. At a first prenatal visit, the woman reports she had bladder infections during past pregnancies. Which of the following statements is true?
① Many women have a hereditary predisposition to bladder infection in pregnancy.
② Pregnancy predisposes a woman to bladder infections because of dilation of the ureters and decreased bladder tone.
③ Although bladder infections occur frequently in pregnancy, they are of little consequence.

④ Clients are generally placed on prophylactic anti-biotics when such a history exists.

236. Twenty-four hours before surgery for repair of meningomyelocele, a newborn develops a fever. She is fussy, irritable, and refuses her formula. Which of the following nursing measures should the nurse carry out first?
① Examine the meningomyelocele sac.
② Contact the physician.
③ Place the infant in strict isolation.
④ Ask the mother to feed the infant.

237. An adult client has active tuberculosis. Which of these actions best prevents the transfer of the tuberculosis organism?
① Having the client cover his nose and mouth with a tissue when he coughs or sneezes
② Instructing the family in effective hand washing
③ Having the client's laundry disinfected after use
④ Having the client's dishes sterilized after use

238. Which of the following would be a correct use of the drug misoprostol (Cytotec) in the management of peptic ulcer disease?
① Taken prn whenever gastric acidity or pain is present
② Taken one-half hour before meals and at bedtime
③ Taken when ibuprofen or other nonsteroidal anti-inflammatory drug (NSAID) is to be used long term for the management of arthritis
④ Taken to eradicate colonization by *H. pylori* bacteria

239. Your client with trauma suddenly begins to vomit bright-red blood. Which position should the client be placed in?
① Semi-Fowler's to high Fowler's position to support ventilation of the lungs
② Head elevated 30 to 45 degrees and turned to the side to prevent aspiration
③ Flat in bed to support blood pressure
④ Reverse Trendelenberg to support blood return to the heart and prevent shock

240. The initial priority in caring for clients with severe depression is which of the following?
① Foster self-esteem.
② Initiate a therapeutic relationship.
③ Encourage expression of feelings.
④ Safeguard against suicidal gestures.

241. In caring for an infant postoperatively after meningomyelocele repair, which nursing action should receive the highest priority?
① Maintain her legs in abduction.
② Measure her head circumference daily.
③ Provide tactile and verbal stimulation.
④ Change her position frequently.

242. You are caring for a client after insertion of a total hip prosthesis. Which action would you be sure to include in your nursing care plan?
① Maintain abduction of the legs through the use of an abductor splint or pillows
② Empty and reconstitute the hemovac every 12 hours

③ Ambulate the client, full weight bearing, within 8 hours after surgery
④ Administer Ativan for pain relief

243. Two months after gastric resection, a client is readmitted with complaints of dizziness, sweating, and tachycardia after meals. The client has lost 15 pounds since surgery. Which strategy is most likely to be effective in controlling the symptoms?
① Eat small meals that are low in simple carbohydrates.
② Eat meals that consist primarily of easily digested carbohydrates.
③ Drink at least two glasses of water with each meal.
④ Remain active and upright for at least 1 hour after meals.

244. A pregnant woman who dislikes milk may meet her needs for calcium by eating
① Nuts and sardines.
② Yogurt and cheese.
③ Meat and leafy vegetables.
④ Custard and dried fruits.

245. An infant diagnosed with meningitis is receiving ampicillin, 75 mg IV every 6 hours. When reconstituted with sterile saline, the vial contains 125 mg/1.2 ml. The nurse should administer what amount of the solution for the correct dose?
① 0.60 ml
② 0.72 ml
③ 0.84 ml
④ 1.00 ml

246. Which statement indicates that a 16-year-old diabetic rotates injection sites appropriately?
① "I can use each site only once every 4 to 6 weeks."
② "I can give myself my insulin with either hand."
③ "I alternate daily between sites on my thighs and upper arms."
④ "I can use sites on my arms, thighs, stomach, and buttocks for injections."

247. In the immediate postoperative period after a laminectomy, a client complains of a severe headache, numbness, and tingling in the feet bilaterally. What is the nurse's first action?
① Notify the physician at once.
② Medicate the client for the discomfort.
③ Explain that this is normal.
④ Compare this numbness and tingling with preoperative neurologic assessment data.

248. A client with insulin-dependent diabetes gives herself 29 units of NPH insulin and 6 units of regular insulin each day. She gives the insulin in two separate injections. What is the most accurate evaluation of this method?
① This is the only safe method because NPH should never be mixed with any other form of insulin.
② This is the preferred method because it prevents mistakes in dosage.
③ There are no real advantages or disadvantages to administering the insulin in one or two injections.
④ Accurately mixing the two insulins in one injection means that injection sites can be used less frequently.

249. When the nurse informs the depressed client that he will be seen in therapy on a regular basis, the client remarks, "Why do you want to see me?" The most appropriate nursing response is which of the following?
① You are certainly worth the time and effort.
② You were assigned to me.
③ Your feelings need to be explored.
④ You need help in dealing with your problems.

250. A client in the sixteenth week of pregnancy phones to report symptoms of frequency and burning on urination. Which of the following statements made by a woman in the sixteenth week of pregnancy indicates that she understood antepartal teaching?
① "I realize the frequency is due to pressure of the uterus on the bladder."
② "I have noticed mild symptoms for the last 10 days."
③ "I called immediately. I understand this problem may need treatment."
④ "I refilled my prescription for antibiotics from last year."

251. The physician has prescribed phenytoin (Dilantin) elixir, 20 mg PO bid, for an infant with seizures. The drug comes in a concentration of 30 mg/4 ml. The nurse should administer what amount?
① 0.67 ml
② 1.5 ml
③ 2.6 ml
④ 3.0 ml

252. Judy Rogers is a 25-year-old insulin-dependent diabetic. Her insulin routine has been 22 units of NPH plus 5 units of regular insulin daily. She takes her insulin each morning at 7. Which piece of subjective data obtained on the nurse's admission assessment indicates a potentially serious problem with Mrs. Rogers self-care management?
① "I'm not getting as much sleep as I used to. My child seems to wake up at least once every night."
② "I've been promoted at work, but the new job has more responsibility."
③ "I can't seem to find the time for morning blood glucose checks anymore."
④ "I'm careful about never skipping meals, but I frequently have to eat breakfast at our 10 AM coffee break."

253. The labor-room nurse is monitoring the induction of labor for a primigravida, who has failed to progress in labor over 24 hours. In evaluating the action of the medication oxytocin (Pitocin), which of the following indicates an adverse effect?
① A contraction lasting over 120 seconds
② A decrease in blood pressure
③ Urinary output of 100 ml per hour
④ Increasing intensity of contractions

254. Josie Morgan, a 34-year-old woman, was admitted several days ago for severe depression. She mentions to the nurse, "I cannot do anything right. I cannot go on like this." What is the most appropriate nursing response?
① "What a negative opinion you have of yourself."
② "It is difficult to listen to your self-deprecating remarks."
③ "What led you to believe that you cannot go on like this?"
④ "I don't think you give yourself enough credit."

255. Alda Clark is a 75-year-old widow who maintains her own residence. While cleaning the snow off her walk, she slips and falls. The nurse notices that Mrs. Clark is unable to move her left leg. The first priority is to
① Extend her leg into a normal position.
② Try to reduce the fracture.
③ Elevate the extremity.
④ Treat her as if a fracture has occurred.

256. Which potential problem presents the most serious threat to long-term management of an infant with meningomyelocele?
① Flexion contractures of the hips
② Frequent colds
③ Constipation
④ Recurrent urinary tract infection

257. The nurse suspects that a patient has a fractured left hip because of which manifestation?
① Edema around the site
② Internal rotation of the left hip
③ Abduction of the left hip
④ Shortened right leg

258. The community health nurse makes a home visit to a single mother with a 2½-year-old daughter and a 3-week-old son. The family lives on public assistance and receives food stamps. The infant's formula is supplied by the WIC program. The nurse would best initiate the visit with which remark?
① "You look tired. Are you getting enough sleep?"
② "Your little girl seems to like her new brother."
③ "Tell me what a typical day is like for you."
④ "Are you having any trouble meeting your expenses?"

259. A client reports a history of osteoarthritis for years. The client takes 600 mg of aspirin q4h to relieve the pain. Side effects of aspirin are indicated by which assessment finding?
① Urinary retention
② Bradycardia
③ Tinnitus
④ Diplopia

260. A 10-year-old boy has been admitted to the orthopedic unit for casting and traction of a fractured femur. Which of the following is most likely to be a major concern for this child during his hospitalization?
① Placement in unfamiliar surroundings
② Fear of painful treatments
③ Absence from school and social activities
④ Worry over restricted mobility

261. An infertile couple express their frustration with time-consuming diagnostic tests. Which of the following statements by the nurse is the most appropriate?
① "I know you want a family, but these tests take time."
② "Your doctor is a very competent infertility specialist."

③ "It is hard when you don't know which one of you is at fault."

④ "Feeling frustration is understandable; let's discuss it."

262. A client is in active labor. She expresses concern about her ability to behave as she would wish during the remainder of labor. Which of these nursing interventions would be most supportive?
① Acknowledge that responses are often influenced by culture.
② Inform her that medication is available if she needs it.
③ Instruct the client in relaxation and breathing exercises.
④ Reassure her that she is accepted regardless of behavior.

263. After a total thyroidectomy, what should the nurse teach the client?
① Take thyroid medication daily for the rest of life.
② Thyroid medication will be prescribed for 1 to 2 years.
③ Restrict intake of seafood, iodized salt, and green vegetables.
④ Take iodine solution daily for the rest of life.

264. Herbert McKay, an accountant for a large firm, has recurring thoughts that his coworker is stealing his clients. He has installed an elaborate security system in his computer, and he spends long hours after work checking for signs of theft. He isolates himself from social gatherings because he fears someone is getting into his computer. Which is the most appropriate description of his delusions?
① Grandiose
② Persecutory
③ Reference of ideas
④ Religiosity

265. Treatment of parathyroid hormone deficiency can be expected to include
① Thyroid preparations
② Digitalis
③ Calcium gluconate
④ High-phosphorus diet

266. A 10-year-old girl has had insulin-dependent diabetes mellitus (IDDM) since age 5. She is seen with her father in the diabetics' clinic for a routine follow-up. Which statement made to the nurse indicates that the child has achieved developmentally appropriate self-management of her diabetes?
① "My mom does my urine tests most of the time."
② "I give my injections, but Dad checks to be sure I do it right."
③ "I'm not allowed to help with my finger sticks yet."
④ "I decide what I want to eat and when."

267. Beginning plans for the client who has suspicious behavior generally involves which of the following?
① Encourage the client to initiate relationships and activities.
② Establish a one-to-one nurse-client relationship.
③ Encourage the client to engage in competitive sports.

④ Encourage the client to participate in a stress-reduction group.

268. Thirty minutes after delivery the following data are collected. The fundus firm, 1 inch below the umbilicus; lochia rubra; client complains of thirst; slight tremors of lower extremities. Analysis of these data suggests
① Impending shock.
② Circulatory overload.
③ Subinvolution.
④ Normal postpartum adaptation.

269. The best indication of improvement in the client experiencing paranoia is which of the following?
① The client talks about the nature of delusions in group.
② The client maintains personal hygiene and grooming.
③ The client clearly speaks of attempts to protect his clientele.
④ The client expresses feelings of anxiety to the nurse.

270. An adult female with right lobar pneumonia suddenly develops right-sided chest pain and increased dyspnea. A portable chest x-ray shows she has suffered a spontaneous pneumothorax. Which item should the nurse know in order to answer the client's questions?
① The pneumothorax was caused by a disruption in the integrity of the pleura.
② A rib has fractured and is causing changes in the thoracic pressure.
③ Air has collected in the mediastinal space.
④ The pneumothorax was caused by the accumulation of pus in the lung parenchyma.

271. A 50-year-old client who has been a heavy smoker for 20 years is admitted to the hospital with emphysema and right lower-lobe pneumonia. Which activity is most likely to have precipitated his emphysema flare-up?
① He wore a new linen suit 2 days ago.
② He smoked more cigarettes than usual 3 days ago.
③ He went bowling last week.
④ He has had a cold for the past week.

272. A 12-year-old girl with insulin-dependent diabetes mellitus (IDDM) tells the nurse, "I'm on our school's soccer team now. We just started practice, and we sure do a lot of running." What changes in the control of her diabetes should be expected as a result?
① Decreased insulin requirements
② Increased insulin requirements
③ Decreased risk of insulin shock
④ Increased risk of ketoacidosis

273. A 45-year-old male client with COPD tells the nurse he realizes proper nutrition is important for his future health, but he doesn't have much of an appetite. Which of these responses by the nurse would be most helpful?
① Eat three large meals a day that are high in calories.
② Eat three large meals a day that are high in protein.

③ Eat six small meals a day that are high in calories.

④ Eat six small meals a day that are high in protein.

274. During a daily session with the nurse, a client who has participated appropriately becomes restless, jumps up, and begins screaming. What is the most appropriate nursing response?

① Tell the client to stay in the room while the nurse gets a prn medication.

② Warn the client that if the behavior continues the session will end.

③ Walk around the room with the client.

④ Remain seated and quiet while observing the client.

275. Two hours after vaginal delivery, a client complains of severe perineal pain. Which nursing action is a priority?

① Administer prescribed pain medication.

② Initiate sitz baths.

③ Inspect the perineum.

④ Teach perineal muscle exercises.

276. An adult client with a pneumothorax has a chest tube connected to a Pleur-Evac. The client wants to know why there are intermittent "bubbles" in the water-seal chamber. Which answer by the nurse would be the best response to this client's question?

① "Perhaps you should ask your doctor to explain your treatment."

② "It indicates that the system is working correctly."

③ "You don't have to worry about the Pleur-Evac. We'll make sure it is functioning correctly."

④ "It indicates that your lung has not fully reexpanded."

277. As a 12-year-old girl with insulin-dependent diabetes mellitus (IDDM) enters early adolescence, it is most important that the nurse prepare the child and her family for which occurrence?

① A rapid gain in weight

② Changes in diet and insulin requirements

③ The need to limit physical activity

④ A switch to oral hypoglycemics

278. A 49-year-old female client with an acute pneumothorax is to have a chest tube inserted. The client asks how this tube will help her breathe with greater ease. Which explanation by the nurse is least likely to be correct?

① The chest tube will evacuate air from the pleural space.

② The chest tube will reestablish atmospheric pressure in the pleural space.

③ The chest tube will allow the affected lung to reexpand.

④ The chest tube will aid in reestablishing negative pressure in the pleural space.

279. A client with paranoia abruptly leaves a group therapy session and remarks to the nurse, "They don't know how to run a group. They're nuts. I refuse to attend these meetings." What is the most suitable nursing response?

① Establish a one-to-one nurse-client relationship before putting the client back into the group.

② Point out the benefits of participating in the group.

③ Maintain that the client must go back into the group immediately.

④ Excuse the client from today's group and tell him that he must attend tomorrow.

280. Which of the following tests provides the best information on fetal development?

① Urine estriol

② Amniocentesis

③ Ultrasound

④ Nonstress test

281. Each of the following nursing actions is significant in forming a one-to-one nurse-client relationship with a client who is suspicious except:

① Open and sincere communication.

② Clearly defined shared expectations.

③ Dispute the reality of delusions.

④ Keep promises regarding appointments.

282. Propranalol (Inderal) may be prescribed to a client with symptoms of Graves' disease to

① Control the associated problem of hypertension.

② Block the synthesis of thyroid hormone.

③ Control common symptoms such as palpitations, tachycardia, and chest pain.

④ Improve appetite and digestion.

283. The best way to prevent nosocomial infections is to

① Put the client in isolation.

② Use strict hand washing.

③ Meet with the staff members to instruct them individually.

④ Inform the family of needed restrictions.

284. A 6-year-old boy is admitted to the hospital in diabetic ketoacidosis. Which manifestations should the nurse expect to observe?

① Seizures and trembling

② Pallor and sweating

③ Vomiting and dry mucous membranes

④ Hunger and diplopia

285. Mr. Pylant discusses his delusions openly. He approaches the nurse and says, "See that lady in the red dress next to the door? She is here to pick me up for a date." What is the most appropriate nursing approach?

① Engage the client in unit activities.

② Listen attentively and ask the client to elaborate on the date.

③ Tell the client that no one is going to take him on a date.

④ Inform the client that you already know about his date.

286. A pregnant couple is told that the fetus suffers from intrauterine growth retardation. After the physician explains what this means, the woman cries and tells the nurse, "I don't think I can cope with a retarded baby." Which response is most appropriate?

① "Perhaps you were not listening to the doctor's explanation."

② "Are there other retarded children in either family?"

③ "There are many resources available to help you."

④ "Let's talk about what the doctor said to us all."

287. A client with a newly formed ileal conduit has received discharge instructions on the need for meticulous skin care. Which statement by the client indicates an understanding of the priority for the teaching session?
    ① "I know the drainage contains enzymes that irritate the skin."
    ② "I believe there will be continuous flow."
    ③ "Sometimes there may be mucous strings in the drainage."
    ④ "The bag needs to be placed and sealed correctly."

288. Which of the following is a *serious* side effect of Carbamazepine (tegretol)?
    ① Aplastic anemia
    ② Hypoglycemia
    ③ Hypothyroidism
    ④ Urinary obstruction

289. A 28-year-old woman has an enlarged thyroid and symptoms of hyperthyroidism. Typical symptoms would include
    ① Fatigue, weight gain, dry skin, and cold intolerance.
    ② Decreased pulse rate, slurred speech, constipation, and cold intolerance.
    ③ Nervousness, weight loss, tachycardia, and heat intolerance.
    ④ Abdominal pain, diarrhea, and heat intolerance.

290. A 5-pound infant is delivered vaginally at 39 weeks of gestation. Apgar scores are 9 and 10 at 1 and 5 minutes. The newborn appears active, wide-eyed, and alert. There was slight meconium staining of the placenta and cord. What analysis is justified?
    ① The baby may have suffered chronic hypoxia.
    ② It appears that the baby's condition is normal.
    ③ Assessments indicate good adaptation.
    ④ This child may have been somewhat premature.

291. Mr. Murray has been recently diagnosed with bipolar disorder, manic type. He has been on carbamazepine (Tegretol) for several days, and his blood level is 5 μg/ml. The appropriate nursing action includes which of the following?
    ① Call the physician because the level is too high.
    ② Administer the medication because the range is within normal parameters.
    ③ Call the physician because the level is too low.
    ④ Call the physician because Tegretol is not used to treat this disorder.

292. When is the best time for a client to start speech therapy after a laryngectomy?
    ① When the client leaves the hospital
    ② When the esophageal suture line is healed
    ③ Three months after surgery
    ④ When the client regains her strength

293. When Edward Barden, a 37-year-old construction worker, is admitted to the nursing unit, he tells you that he has pain radiating down his right leg. Which item is *not* appropriate to include in the assessment?
    ① Activities that occur before the pain
    ② What relieves the pain
    ③ How he carries out activities of daily living
    ④ How he got to the hospital

294. The nurse notes that an infant occasionally cries, then appears to quiet himself and fall asleep. What is the best explanation of this behavior?
    ① The baby's needs have not been met.
    ② This is normal, expected behavior.
    ③ The central nervous system may be immature.
    ④ The newborn is able to comfort himself.

295. A mother reports that her daughter's appetite has not changed, but she spends a lot of time in the bathroom after meals. The daughter denies problems at this time. An *initial* nursing response to the mother would be which of the following?
    ① "She is acting like a normal teenager, stuffing down food and going to her room."
    ② "I think she is anorexic."
    ③ "It sounds like you believe she has an eating disorder."
    ④ "She might be experiencing an anxiety disorder."

296. A client is scheduled for a myelogram. Which nursing care consideration is best included in the postprocedure care?
    ① Keep the client in bed for 6 to 8 hours.
    ② Allow the client to go to the bathroom as soon as he gets back to his room in order to excrete the dye.
    ③ Limit fluids.
    ④ Provide heavy sedation for his spinal headache.

297. The nurse makes a home visit to the family of a 4-month-old infant girl with a congenitally dislocated hip. The infant has been fitted with a von Rosen splint. In evaluating the effectiveness of teaching the parents how to care for the child during the treatment period, which outcome demonstrated by the parents indicates they understand the seriousness of the defect?
    ① Her parents apply and remove the splint correctly.
    ② The parents keep the infant in the splint at all times except when she is being bathed.
    ③ The parents change the infant's position at least every 2 hours.
    ④ The parents provide age-appropriate sensorimotor activities and stimulation for the infant.

298. A client relates fears that her newborn might choke. The nurse would provide which of the following instructions about choking episodes?
    ① Place the infant face down with head lower than the trunk and deliver sharp blows between the shoulders.
    ② Grasp the infant with two hands, place in a supine position, and apply chest thrusts.
    ③ Position the infant with head lower than trunk and milk the trachea to facilitate mucus drainage.
    ④ Place your mouth over the infant's nose and mouth to create a seal; administer two slow breaths.

299. The initial goal of treatment of clients with bulimia who are abusing laxatives and diet pills is which of the following?
    ① Aid the client in understanding reasons for these behaviors.
    ② Help the client accept self and body.

③ Maintain adequate nutritional intake and retention of food and fluids.

④ Help the client develop reasonable anticipation of dieting.

300. What does the nurse include in the preoperative teaching for a laminectomy patient?

① Postop "log-rolling"

② Getting out of bed the third postoperative day

③ Activities to be avoided after discharge

④ Use of a turning frame

Answers to this test begin on p. 560.

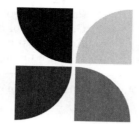

Answers and Rationales

KEY TO ABBREVIATIONS

Three abbreviations follow the rationales. The first abbreviation refers to the section in this book where discussion of the topic may be found. The second abbreviation refers to the step of the nursing process that the question addresses. The third abbreviation refers to the appropriate client need category.

Review Section

P = Psychosocial and Mental Health Problems
  I = Introduction
  T = Therapeutic Use of Self
  L = Loss and Death and Dying
  A = Anxious Behavior
  D = Delerium, Dementia, and Amnestic and Other Cognitive Disorders
  E = Elated-Depressive Behavior
  P = Personality Disorders and Other Maladaptive Behaviors
  S = Schizophrenia and Other Psychotic Disorders
  U = Substance Use Disorders
A = Adult
  H = Healthy Adult
  S = Surgery
  O = Oxygenation
  NM = Nutrition and Metabolism
  E = Elimination
  SP = Sensation and Perception
  M = Mobility
  CA = Cellular Aberration

CBF = Childbearing Family
  W = Women's Health Care
  A = Antepartal Care
  I = Intrapartal Care
  P = Postpartal Care
  N = Newborn Care
C = Child
  H = Healthy Child
  I = Ill and Hospitalized Child
  SPP = Sensation, Perception, Protection
  O = Oxygenation
  NM = Nutrition and Metabolism
  E = Elimination
  M = Mobility
  CA = Cellular Aberration

NURSING PROCESS CATEGORY

AS = Assessment
AN = Analysis
PL = Planning
IM = Implementation
EV = Evaluation

CLIENT NEED CATEGORY

E = Safe, Effective Care Environment
PS = Physiologic Integrity
PC = Psychosocial Integrity
H = Health Promotion/Maintenance

The correct answer option is listed after the question number.

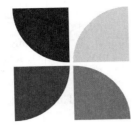

Answers and Rationales: Practice Test 1

Key to abbreviations may be found on p. 544.

1. no. 1. Cushing's disease produces a syndrome of cortisol excess, which causes the classic symptom pattern of weight gain; truncal obesity; moon face; cervicodorsal fat pad; thin, fragile skin with easy bruising; stretch marks on the breasts, hips, thighs, and abdomen; hypertension; and unstable mood. A-NM, AS, PS

2. no. 4. Lesley is showing the classic signs of bulimia: healthy appearance, normal weight, furtive trips to the bathroom after meals. These signs differentiate it from anorexia. Options no. 1, no. 2, and no. 3 are wrong for the symptoms presented. P-P, AN, PC

3. no. 1. Identification of progress maintains effort during the hard work of birth. Option 2 is not warranted, especially with an unmedicated client. A cleansing prep should be done using sterile technique. Pushing should be encouraged with contractions. CBF-I, IM, H, PS

4. no. 1. Emergency care of a burn wound such as this involves dousing or immersing the injury in cool water to prevent further thermal damage. Ice packs or ice water can cause further damage to the injured tissue and are contraindicated. Adherent clothing should never be pulled from a burn injury because of the possibility of damaging remaining tissue. Covering the burn with any kind of substance (cream, margarine, ointments) can trap heat and also cause further damage and increase the risk of infection. C-SPP, IM, E

5. no. 2. SIADH is a frequent temporary problem after neurologic surgery or trauma. It can usually be managed conservatively through fluid restriction while the body makes the necessary fluid adjustments. Serum sodium levels must be monitored carefully, however, to prevent the development of potentially life-threatening imbalances. A-NM, IM, PS

6. no. 3. Removal of old cream is essential in keeping the wound clean and ensuring that newly applied cream is effective in reducing the chance of bacterial contamination. The wound should be cleansed with warm sudsy water (using a soap such as Ivory flakes or Dreft, *not* a detergent). Silver sulfadiazine (Silvadene) is not painful when applied and does not interfere with acid-base or electrolyte balance. Silver nitrate, not Silvadene, may cause skin discoloration when used to treat burn wounds. C-SPP, PL, E

7. no. 2. A muscle plug is placed to fill the defect in the dura mater created by the surgery. If the seal is not tight cerebrospinal fluid can leak into the dressing or down the back of the throat causing frequent swallowing and a sense of postnasal drip. The CSF creates a halo effect on gauze as it dries. Fresh drainage will also test positive for glucose. The risk of infection in the form of meningitis is extremely high, and the physician must be notified immediately to begin antibiotic coverage. A-NM, AN, PS

8. no. 3. Reflects the concerns of the client while allowing the client to make decisions. P-T, IM, PC

9. no. 2. The major advantage of the closed method is to minimize fluid lost from the burn surface by applying gentle pressure to the burn wound. Use of silver sulfadiazine (Silvadene) will also reduce the possibility of wound infection. Although the dressing will protect the wound and reduce pain, these are not the primary reasons for using this method. Wrapping the wound will partially immobilize the hand and wrist and therefore may increase the possibility of contracture. C-SPP, IM, PS

10. no. 3. Hepatitis A (HAV) is usually transmitted through contaminated food or water. Routine viral illness does not increase the risk of contracting hepatitis, nor does social drinking. Hepatitis B (HBV) is transmitted through the blood, but it is rare for HBA to be contracted in that way. A-NM, AN, PS

11. no. 3. The nurse documents behaviors and factual information, which may become evidence. Ideas about what might have happened are not the hospital staff's responsibility to report. Accurate documentation and reporting is required and in the best interest of parent and child. P-P, IM, E

12. no. 1. Because the wound is not tetanus prone (i.e., does not involve muscle tissue, is not contaminated with saliva or excrement, and is less than 24 hours old) and he has received a full series of primary immunizations with his last booster less than 10 years ago (between 4 and 6 years of age) but more than 5 years ago, he needs tetanus toxoid (given in the form of Td). Tetanus immune globulin (passive immunity) is indicated only if the previous immunization history is unknown or uncertain or the burn wound is tetanus prone (i.e., burn wounds that involve muscle tissue or are highly contaminated). C-SPP, IM, H

13. no. 4. This symptom is related to transition and progression into the second stage of labor. The other options do not warrant further evaluation as long as the client is comfortably ambulating. CBF-I, AS, E

14. no. 3. Respiratory distress and a tightening neck dressing may indicate hemorrhage into tissues or increasing

edema in the neck area. Loosening the dressing to prevent further tracheal compression should be the nurse's first action. Reinforcement of the dressing would only increase tracheal compression. High Fowler's position alone will not decrease swelling; the dressing must also be loosened. A-O, IM, PS

15. no. 3. Some abusive parents do not see their behavior as inappropriate. They may have been abused as children and so raise their children as they were raised. None of the behaviors in no. 1, no. 2, and no. 4 are characteristics of abusive parent's actions. P-P, AN, PC

16. no. 1. The burn-injured client needs large amounts of protein and vitamin C for wound healing. Meats and milk are high in protein, and citrus fruits are high in vitamin C. C-SPP, PL, PS

17. no. 4. Although a symptom of child abuse is that the child exhibits behavior not appropriate to age, playing with a bike is appropriate for a 10-year-old. Options no. 1, no. 2, and no. 3 are classic behaviors found in abusive relationships. P-P, AS, PC

18. no. 3. Cervical dilation is the most reliable index of the progress of labor. Other options may or may not indicate true progress. Option no. 1 is possible with hypertonic dysfunction, option no. 2 could be related to anxiety, and option no. 4 can occur at any time and may not relate to progress. CBF-I, AS, PS

19. no. 3. Acne is caused by sebum blocking skin pores and is most effectively treated by adequate daily cleansing, followed by application of antiacne product that contains benzoyl peroxide, a peeling and drying agent. Use of a headband during exercise or hot weather can cause secretions to be retained, with further blockage of skin pores. There is no evidence that chocolate, iodine, or greasy foods contribute to acne. Use of ultraviolet light should be reserved for severe cases of acne and done under the supervision of a physician. C-SPP, PL, PS

20. no. 4. These results are normal; 20/20 or 20/30 vision is considered within normal limits at this age, because visual acuity may not be fully developed. C-H, AN, H

21. no. 4. Use open-ended communications to which the client may respond without being judgmental or uninterested. P-T, IM, PC

22. no. 4. To assess for late decelerations, it is necessary to listen during and soon after contractions. Early fetal distress would be completely missed if option no. 2 were followed. CBF-I, AS, PS

23. no. 4. Increasing hoarseness after a thyroidectomy may indicate injury to the recurrent laryngeal nerve or swelling in the area of the glottis. Parathyroid injury will be evidenced by muscular tingling or twitching. A-NM, EV, PS

24. no. 3. This is the best option and is an appropriate way to initiate teaching. Breast-feeding is not a means of contraception unless it is exclusive. Delaying a discussion until the checkup may lead to another pregnancy. CBF-P, IM, PC

25. no. 2. He is probably indicating his discomfort with the group. Perhaps projection is the main defense used in this situation. There is no evidence that Clint is shy or that he is angry with any one group member; likewise, there is no evidence that the therapist annoys him. P-T, AN, PC

26. no. 1. Strabismus is a common health problem that must be detected early to prevent amblyopia. The other options are used to assess neurologic status. C-H, AS, H

27. no. 3. This indicates learning alternatives to anger and harmful punishment, which are significant aspects of nursing interventions for the abusive parents. No. 1 does not indicate changes in behavior patterns when frustrated or angry. No. 2 is a positive change, but, again, does not indicate constructive coping during frustration. No. 4 indicates avoidance rather than successful coping. P-P, EV, PC

28. no. 2. Recommended caloric intake at this age is approximately 1700 calories per day. C-H, IM, H

29. no. 4. Hemorrhage is a serious complication after thyroidectomy. Because of gravity, drainage may not be visible along the suture line on the anterior neck dressing, but rather at the back of the neck and upper part of the back. The preferred position for the client after a thyroidectomy is semi-Fowler's with good neck support. Turning, coughing, and deep breathing as well as early ambulation can be accomplished while the head and neck are supported in a neutral position. A-NM, IM, PS

30. no. 3. Because of the slowing of the child's weight gain, his weight is now only one standard deviation from his height. Weight loss and caloric restriction are not desired outcomes. The child may not be craving junk food, but this option does not give enough information to evaluate his progress (e.g., he may not be eating junk food, but his caloric intake may be as high as previously if he is substituting other foods). C-NM, EV, PS

31. no. 3. Fluid shifts during the postpartal period cause a normal diaphoresis and diuresis. Intake is related to urinary output, but options no. 1 and no. 2 are not accurate. Although hormones dramatically affect adaptation after delivery, this symptom alone does not suggest infection. CBF-P, IM, H

32. no. 4. This would stimulate the client, not sedate him. Activities that decrease stimuli may help counteract insomnia. Rest and sleep are vital for the manic client because hyperactivity may lead to dangerous exhaustion. P-E, IM, E

33. no. 3. All of these goals are worthwhile and will need to be met before discharge; however, because of the severity of the renal colic, option no. 3 must be the first priority. Only then can the client respond to teaching and begin taking increased fluids. Morphine may have to be given for the pain, depending on the severity. IV fluids may have to be started to increase intake initially. A-E, PL, PS

34. no. 1. A carefully planned program of diet and exercise that meets the child's continued needs for growth is essential. Focus should be on slowing weight gain to allow height to catch up over a period of several months, rather than trying to have the child lose weight. Appetite suppressants are without merit in the treatment of childhood overweight and obesity. Large doses of vitamins are unnecessary if the child is eating a well-balanced diet, and they may actually be harmful to the child. Withholding all sweets is unrealistic and may lead to cheating. The child should be helped to change his eating habits with the recognition that an occasional sweet treat is acceptable. C-NM, PL, PS

35. no. 2. The uterine muscle may contract poorly as a result of overdistention from a large baby and several past pregnancies. Rapid labor may delay involution as well. The other complications may occur, but they are not specific in this case. CBF-P, AN, PS

36. no. 3. Immunosuppression is a contraindication for giving immunizations. Immunizing a child who is immunosuppressed can lead to overwhelming infection and death. As soon as the child's white blood cell count is normal, the DPT and TOPV boosters may be given because the child's immune system can respond normally. C-CA, IM, E

37. no. 1. A high urine output helps flush out bacteria from the urinary tract and maintain a low urine osmolarity. Encourage clients to void every 2 to 3 hours during the day and 1 to 2 times during the night. Sitz baths are helpful during an acute episode but are not a priority of discharge planning. Voiding after intercourse is recommended for women who have repeated urinary tract infections. Avoidance of exposure to respiratory infections would be highly desirable if the client was showing signs and symptoms of renal failure. A-E, IM, H

38. no. 3. A client in the manic phase of bipolar disorder tends to disregard physical needs and needs clear, concise, firm, and explicit directions to meet these needs. Option no. 1 evades the issue of taking care of physical needs. Option no. 2 is too passive, and left alone the client will not come. Option no. 4 is premature and punitive. P-E, IM, PC

39. no. 1. Anemia occurs in chronic renal disease because renal erythropoietin production is decreased and the bone marrow is depressed by the increasing uremia. Because of the decreased ability of the kidneys to excrete waste products and maintain normal fluid and electrolyte balance, hyperkalemia and hypertension develop. The stimulation of the renin-angiotensin mechanism also contributes to the hypertension. The skin becomes dry because the sweat glands atrophy. A-E, AS, PS

40. no. 3. Radiation therapy may cause delayed onset of puberty, delays in physical growth, pathologic bone fractures, and chromosomal damage because of its effects on normal cells. C-CA, AN, PS

41. no. 2. Pain control is best achieved on a preventive schedule after assessing the period that a particular dosage is effective for the child and the child's general pain responses. This prevents fluctuation in pain threshold levels. Waiting until the child becomes restless and unable to sleep will lessen the effectiveness of analgesics when given. Pain medications should not be given more often than every 3 to 4 hours, but giving them that often around the clock may not be necessary for a particular child. C-I, IM, E

42. no. 3. Whole grains are unrestricted in an acid-ash diet. Carrots and dried apricots are not allowed and only 1 pint of milk is allowed daily. A-E, IM, H

43. no. 1. This statement acknowledges the importance of the hallucination for the client without undermining her need for the symptom; it also does not indicate that the nurse regards the hallucination content as real. Interpretation is not usually a part of nursing practice. Option no. 3 supports her hallucination. Option no. 4 is not sensitive to the client's needs. P-S, IM, PC

44. no. 1. Symptoms reported are associated with hyperventilation. Resolution occurs through rebreathing CO_2. Options 2 and 3 are not physiologically related interventions. Option 4 is inappropriate because no medical problem exists. CBF-I, IM, PS

45. no. 4. The psychosocial task at this age is accomplishing a sense of initiative. Autonomy is the toddler's major task, and identity is the adolescent's. Mastery is important throughout childhood but is most characteristic of the school-age child. C-H, AS, PC

46. no. 2. The average 5-year-old can count to 20, recite the alphabet, and recognize most colors. It is not until about age 6 that children can print their names. At age 7, children can tell clock time and tie their shoelaces. C-H, AS, H

47. no. 4. Sulfonamides dissolve well in urine and are excreted unchanged in the urine; therefore they are excellent for treating urinary tract infections. However, if fluid intake is not sufficient, the drug can crystalize, resulting in renal toxicity. While on the drug regimen, intake should be sufficient to maintain a urine output of at least 1 L per day. Sulfonamides are metabolized by the liver and excreted through the kidneys, may produce a false-positive glucose on urine tests, and are more soluble in alkaline urine. A-E, AS, PS

48. no. 3. The creatures are part of her hallucinatory world into which she withdraws at times. Hallucinations as described are not usually associated with extrapyramidal reactions, nor is hallucinatory activity viewed as phobic or as flight of ideas. P-S, AN, PC

49. no. 4. The bed will be kept flat for 8 to 12 hours after use of spinal anesthetic to minimize the possibility of headaches. Although it is true that medication is available, the chief focus of teaching is on position. CBF-P, IM, H

50. no. 2. Lengthy explanations will be too confusing. Rather, tell and show her how to take the drugs and she will probably be as reliable with them as she has been with phenothiazines. It is better for the client to remain in her usual environment than to hospitalize her for the needs described. Reliable self-administration is better than forced dependency. P-S, IM, H

51. no. 4. Option no. 1 indicates some understanding of the disease, but not the bone marrow procedure. No. 2 and no. 3 reflect adaptation to hospitalization. No. 4 indicates that the child comprehends what will happen to her during the procedure. C-I, EV, PC

52. no. 3. Thyroid replacement should be given as a single morning dose throughout the child's lifetime. Diarrhea, tachycardia, and weight loss indicate toxicity. C-NM, IM, E

53. no. 3. The dye used for an IVP is iodine based and can cause a severe allergic reaction (anaphylaxis) in sensitive individuals. Food allergies to shellfish can indicate an iodine allergy, because shellfish are high in iodine content. The other options should be done, but because of the possible danger to the client, the allergy history takes priority. A-E, EV, E

54. no. 2. Low implantation of the placenta causes painless bleeding in the third trimester. Abruptio placentae often is accompanied by pain or tenderness. Ectopic pregnancy and abortion occur earlier in pregnancy. CBF-A, AN, PS

55. no. 2. Sameness will increase trust but intimacy will frighten the client and cause her to withdraw more into herself. A wide variety of caretakers will only increase confusion and reduce trust. Option no. 3 has advantages but may be overpowering to this client. P-S, IM, PC

56. no. 4. The infant with congenital hypothyroidism is inactive (often described as a good, quiet baby) and undemanding. The disease is also characterized by mottling of the skin, constipation, a large protruding tongue, and a flattened nasal bridge. C-NM, AS, PS

57. no. 3. Physical complaints of clients, such as those with chronic schizophrenia who might incorporate pain into their delusional *system*, must be assessed. P-S, IM, E Option no. 1 may be needed, but only after assessment of the behavior is completed. Although talking is important, the abdominal pains take priority. The symptom described is not an extrapyramidal reaction. P-S, IM, E

58. no. 3. Petechiae result from the leukemic process. Vomiting and stomatitis are expected side effects of chemotherapy. Vincristine causes neurotoxic responses, such as numbness and tingling, jaw pain, and constipation, which should be reported because they may indicate toxicity. C-CA, AN, E

59. no. 1. The willingness to accept professional help depends on the need as the client and family see it. All the other factors are important also, but first the client and family must want the service. P-T, AN, H

60. no. 1. When administering blood products, only saline solutions or solutions that do not contain any dextrose or glucose should be used. Dextrose and glucose solutions (hyperalimentation solutions contain hypertonic glucose concentrations) will cause hemolysis of the blood cells. C-CA, IM, PS

61. no. 3. This is a specific measurement to determine kidney function, primarily glomerular filtration. Creatinine is produced at a constant rate; it is not reabsorbed and is only minimally secreted. BUN is less reliable because urea, after being filtered, is reabsorbed back into renal tubular cells. Additionally, urea production varies according to liver function and protein intake and breakdown. The test for serum glucose is used to screen for disorders of metabolism. Electrolyte studies are not specific to kidney filtration. A-E, PL, PS

62. no. 3. This response encourages the client to discuss his feelings and can provide important clues to what is troubling him or what has been difficult for him. P-T, IM, E

63. no. 1. A vaginal examination is contraindicated for this client because it might stimulate contractions and increase the risk of placental delivery. The other options if ordered may be safely done. CBF-A, IM, E

64. no. 3. The shape sorter is age appropriate (toddlers are

interested in how things fit together, such as how different shapes fit into their respective slots) and is a quiet activity. A priority goal preoperatively is to minimize the workload of the heart. The push-pull toy and the toy trumpet will increase the oxygen demands and therefore the cardiac workload. A play stethoscope is too advanced for this child (it is an appropriate toy for a preschooler). C-H, IM, H

65. no. 4. Even diminished intake can lead to withdrawal symptoms. Cessation is not a prerequisite to their occurrence. P-U, AN, PC

66. no. 4. Because the mother is worried, her feelings should be considered. The nurse appropriately suggests shared decision making. CBF-I, IM, PC

67. no. 3. An AV fistula is an *internal* access created by a side-to-side or end-to-end anastomosis of an adjacent vein and artery. This results in an enlarged vein because of the high pressure in the artery. The resulting vessel provides an easy access for venipuncture. Thrombosis at this site can be a major complication. Rejection does not occur, because no foreign material is involved. Dislodgment is not a problem, because the fistula is internal. (An AV *shunt* is external.) Cardiac irritation is a problem with subclavian catheters used for temporary access for hemodialysis. A-E, AS, PS

68. no. 4. Gasping indicates that this child is at risk for having an anoxic spell and should be placed in a knee-chest (squatting) position to increase the blood flow to his heart, lungs, and brain. Although options no. 1 and no. 2 are appropriate responses for handling a toddler's temper tantrums, in this instance, this child's physiologic needs take priority over his developmental needs. Encouraging the mother to set few limits is not in the child's best interests developmentally. C-O, IM, E

69. no. 3. With a drop factor of 10 drops per milliliter, the desired rate is 27 drops per minute. CBF-I, IM, PS

70. no. 3. Milk, meats, fish, and eggs are considered the best sources of high-biologic-value protein. Some vegetables have essential amino acids but are not consistently the best sources. In contrast, fruits are poor sources of high-biologic-value protein. A-H, PL, E

71. no. 2. The alcoholic client's denial of problems is evidenced by recognition that something is wrong, but denying that medical, emotional, or social problems are related to the consumption of alcohol. No. 1 and no. 4 may be seen, but are not the priority for developing nursing care. Once the problem of denial is addressed, dependency and projection will decrease. No. 3, paranoia, is not a defense mechanism. P-U, AN, PC

72. no. 4. The infant must be kept in the prone position to reduce tension on and prevent trauma to the sac. The supine and semi-Fowler's position would place tension on the sac. The side-lying position is difficult to maintain in a newborn. C-SPP, IM, E

73. no. 3. Before surgical closure of the sac, it is important to prevent drying of the sac so the fragile tissue does not tear and allow cerebrospinal fluid to leak, increasing the risk of meningitis. Sterile saline soaks help prevent drying. Dry, sterile dressings or leaving the sac open to the air is advocated only if surgery is to be delayed. Petroleum jelly gauze is contraindicated in either case. C-SPP, IM, E

74. no. 1. Although genetic factors and chronic disease effects are important, options no. 2 through no. 4 are important areas to explore and focus on in the family-therapy sessions. P-U, AN, PC

75. no. 1. The purpose of palliative surgery for the child with tetralogy of Fallot is to increase the pulmonary blood flow, which increases the amount of oxygenated blood to the tissues. The procedure will not affect the intracardiac shunting of blood from right to left or provide enough oxygen to his tissues to allow for normal development. In tetralogy of Fallot, the pressure is increased in the right ventricle (not the left) because of the pulmonary stenosis. C-O, IM, PS

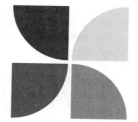

Answers and Rationales: Practice Test 2

Key to abbreviations may be found on p. 544.

76. no. 4. Drainage is drawn to the back of the dressing by gravity. A client may have significant amounts of bloody drainage while the upper portion of the dressing remains dry and intact. This drainage may be undetected unless the back and bed linen are visually inspected for drainage. In no. 1, a client may not be able to detect and feel drainage on the back because of receiving pain medications and a decreased number of nerve endings that innervate the back. In no. 2, changes in level of consciousness may be caused by a number of physiologic problems such as receiving pain medication. This client would need to lose a significant amount of blood before a change in level of consciousness would occur. In no. 3, there is no indication to test stools for blood. A-S, A, PS

77. no. 2. This is a period of maximum cardiac output, and, as a result, cardiac decompensation may occur. The other potential problems are not necessarily associated with cardiac disease. CBF-A, AN, PS

78. no. 3. In the detoxification stage of alcoholism the body chemistry changes can be rapid and severe. Sodium-potassium level changes are especially vulnerable because of vomiting and fluid shifts. The heart, already burdened by the process of detoxification, is especially sensitive to low potassium levels. Option no. 1 is important, but not as dangerous a problem. No. 2 is true but is not an immediate concern. No. 4 is a priority at a later stage. P-U, PL, PS

79. no. 2. Use of syrup of ipecac in age-appropriate dosage and with an alert client is the safest, most effective emergency treatment of accidental ingestion of all substances *except* hydrocarbons or caustics. The priority goal is to empty the potentially toxic acetaminophen from the stomach. Having the child drink milk may cause more rapid absorption of the tablets. Gastric lavage with administration of activated charcoal should be carried out *after* gastric emptying. Option no. 4 would waste valuable time and allow greater amounts of the acetaminophen to be absorbed. The history may be obtained during or immediately after administration of the syrup of ipecac. C-SPP, IM, E

80. no. 4. The presence of a bruit and a thrill indicates good circulation. Skin temperatures and pulses should be assessed *distal* to the fistula. Blood pressure and venipunctures should never be done in the affected limb in order to help promote the longevity of the fis-

tula. Because an AV fistula is *internal,* it is not possible to assess the color of the blood. A-E, AS, E

81. no. 4. The client must do his own evaluating as to his readiness to change direction. The nurse serves best by helping him clarify his thoughts and feelings. No. 2 is judgmental and insensitive. The timing belongs to the client. No. 3 is inconsequential in light of the client's remarks. No. 1 might be appropriate, but no. 4 is geared more to the feeling level of the statement. P-U, IM, PC

82. no. 4. Maternal blood pressure, reflexes, and level of consciousness must be closely monitored. Effects of pregnancy-induced hypertension may continue for 1 to 2 days postpartum before homeotasis is restored. There is generally low risk of recurrence unless hypertension is chronic. With proper management, the woman recovers fully from pathophysiologic changes. CBF-P, AN, PS

83. no. 2. The child with cyanotic heart disease is prone to polycythemia (an increase in circulating red blood cells), which leads to a rise in hematocrit. Normal hematocrit values for a child are 32% to 47%. All other values are within normal limits. C-O, AN, PS

84. no. 1. Four-year-olds are in the preoperational stage of cognitive development and are most concerned about what sensations they will feel when facing an unfamiliar experience. The 4-year-old would have difficulty understanding why the shunt must be pumped and, in any event, why is not as important as what or how. Options no. 3 and no. 4 do not actively involve the child in the experience or give her any sense of control and will probably increase her fear and lessen her cooperation. C-I, IM, PC

85. no. 4. Magnesium sulfate is a central nervous system depressant. The client must be closely observed for profound symptoms such as diminished respiratory rate. Muscle cramps indicate toxic effects of the drug; hyperstimulation of reflexes may indicate impending seizure. Anuria is sometimes observed in such a client. CBF-A, EV, E

86. no. 4. Too much sympathy and empathy reinforces the client's view of himself as a victim of alcohol, drugs, or other people. The client will not accept responsibility for himself, nor will he be able to break through his denial, if a high level of sympathy and empathy is given. The client would then manipulate his nurse and avoid dealing with his problems. Options no. 1, no.

2, and no. 3 are critical to setting the stage for the client to work on his problems. The client must internalize limits. P-U, IM, E

87. no. 1. Before discharge, clients should be able to do a return demonstration of incisional care. No. 2, adapting to altered body image, takes several months. No. 3, completing the grieving process, can take an older adult several months to over a year. It is unrealistic to expect that the client will adapt to altered body image or complete the grieving process by the time of discharge from the hospital. No. 4, a Jobst pressure machine, is used only when all other methods of preventing lymphedema have failed. Based on this scenario, there is no indication that this client needs to have a Jobst pressure machine at home. A-CA, EV, E

88. no. 1. The primary indicator of changing intracranial pressure is a change in sensorium or level of consciousness. C-SPP, EV, PS

89. no. 2. Orange juice will help disguise the taste of acetylcysteine (Mucomyst), whereas water will not. Milk products may interfere with the absorption of the Mucomyst and are therefore not recommended. C-SPP, IM, E

90. no. 2. This best allows the nurse to assess understanding of material and provides an opportunity to adapt to the elderly client's concentration span. Option no. 1 is not best with this age group because those in this group may have trouble with written content or may not be motivated to read. No. 3 and no. 4 may overtax the client and do not allow feelings about the surgery and diagnosis to be expressed. Note the teaching that is described as "complete factual." Option no. 4 is more appropriate with 20- to 30-year-olds. A-H, IM, H

91. no. 1. Anger is cyclic. Once the client works out his anger and frustration in an aggressive act, he feels guilty and needs to justify and explain his behavior. His anxiety is temporarily decreased, but he experiences a decrease in self-esteem, which further increases the anxiety and can result in more acting-out behavior. The best intervention is to stop the anger cycle before it begins. Options no. 2, no. 3, and no. 4 reflect the later aspects of the anger cycle when intervention is more difficult. P-P, IM, PC

92. no. 4. These fears and dreams are common, especially in the last trimester. There is no higher incidence with infertility or in a first pregnancy. CBF-A, AN, PC

93. no. 4. Acetaminophen is potentially toxic to the liver. Serum transaminase (AST and ALT) levels should be closely monitored every 24 hours for 3 to 5 days after the ingestion to detect hepatic damage. Acetaminophen toxicity is not reflected by any of the other laboratory findings listed. C-SPP, AN, PS

94. no. 2. It is best to have a parent assist with holding the child during a briefly painful procedure, such as an immunization, if possible. Proceeding quickly is the desirable approach with a child this age for a procedure that will be over quickly. Prolonged explanations only increase the child's anxiety and, in this child's case, would not be understood because she does not speak English. She may be given the needle-

less syringe to play with *after* the injection. C-I, IM, PC

95. no. 2. Any fluid retention greater than 300 ml must be assessed before continuing with dialysis. As an initial response, turning the client from side to side may help drain the remaining dialysate, thereby eliminating the need for contacting the physician. Vital signs must be monitored at frequent intervals throughout the dialysis. A-E, IM, PS

96. no. 3. At this time in pregnancy, when the client has a history of bleeding, the test is performed to confirm fetal viability. Biparietal diameters are a useful assessment between 18 and 24 weeks of gestation. Neither option no. 2 nor no. 4 is accurate. CBF-A, AS, PS

97. no. 4. The law does deal with the confidentiality concerns of clients. Limiting the documentation of staff is in violation of the portion of most state laws that indicates the record must contain specific data. Options no. 1, no. 2, and no. 3 address laws protecting client confidentiality. P-I, AN, PC

98. no. 4. Positioning the client flat on the unoperative side will prevent pressure on the shunt valve and allow for gradual drainage of the spinal fluid. The other positions would place additional pressure on the shunt. C-SPP, PL, E

99. no. 1. Early morning headaches are frequently the earliest sign of increased intracranial pressure. The other manifestations are later signs of increased ICP. C-SPP, AS, PS

100. no. 1. Asian children are shorter and weigh less, on the average, than American children, on whom growth norms are usually based. Even though the graphs have been revised recently to be more representative of children from varying backgrounds, the nurse should always consider the child's family heritage when evaluating variances from normal. No information has been provided to support any of the other options. C-H, AN, PC

101. no. 1. Decreasing the number of adjustments needed in a new environment lessens confusion. Do not overstimulate or confront clients with deficits. Provide for individualization of care instead of rigid routines. P-D, PL, PC

102. no. 4. At this age, it is best to allow the child to make the first move. Establishing interaction with the parents gives the child time to size up the nurse and see that her parents demonstrate trust in the nurse. The other nursing actions may be perceived by the child as direct threats because of her developmental level. C-H, IM, PS

103. no. 2. Playing Nerf basketball would be contraindicated for this patient because it would require him to move his elbow, which should remain immobilized while he is on bed rest to prevent further bleeding. The other activities are age appropriate and acceptable for his treatment plan. C-H, IM, E

104. no. 4. Provide concrete information that reinforces reality without emphasizing the client's deficits. Probing for feelings increases confusion and argumentativeness in these clients. P-D, IM, PC

105. no. 2. All are important assessments of respiratory

function, but only breathing movements are scored as part of the Silverman-Andersen scale. CBF-N, AN, E

106. no. 1. Assist with feelings and client situations so family members will not withdraw from the client. Encourage regular visits. Options no. 2, no. 3, and no. 4 tend to separate family and client rather than enhance their feelings at this difficult time. P-D, IM, H

107. no. 2. Changes in bowel function may be one of the first symptoms of ovarian cancer. Clients often associate this with advancing age and tend to treat it with over-the-counter laxatives rather than reporting it. No. 1 is a sign of breast cancer. No. 3 is a sign of cervical cancer. No. 4 is incorrect; clients with ovarian cancer report anorexia. A-CA, AS, PS

108. no. 3. When a female carrier of hemophilia has children fathered by a male who is free of the disease, the risk to their offspring *(with each pregnancy)* is as follows: half the males will have hemophilia (XrY), half the males will be normal (XY), half the females will be carriers of the hemophilia gene (XrX), and half the females will be normal (XX). C-O, AS, PS

109. no. 1. A widening pulse pressure is characteristic of increasing intracranial pressure; also, pulse rate decreases, respirations decrease, and level of consciousness decreases. A-SP, AS, PS

110. no. 4. AIDS is transmitted in body secretions such as urine, stools, blood, and saliva. As long as the nurse does not have direct body contact with the patient, no special precautions are needed. C-SPP, IM, E

111. no. 4. Help family members explore their feelings. Maintaining family contact is necessary for orientation and self-identity. Reassurance will not help family members deal with feelings or the situation. There is insufficient evidence to justify an inference of guilt. P-T, IM, PC

112. no. 4. During a bleeding episode involving a joint, the joint should be elevated and immobilized in a flexed position to minimize further bleeding and decrease pain. Heat will cause vasodilation and aggravate the bleeding episode. Ice packs, which promote vasoconstriction, should be applied to the elbow instead. Aspirin is contraindicated for the child with hemophilia because it interferes with platelet function. Another analgesic would be necessary. Range-of-motion exercises may cause further trauma to the joint during a bleeding episode. C-O, AN, E

113. no. 1. The most common recurring problem with peritoneal dialysis is peritonitis; therefore education on proper techniques to help decrease its occurrence should take priority. All other listed interventions are also important and should be included in the teaching. A-E, IM, H

114. no. 1. Decreased ability to learn because of decreased attention span is a characteristic of Alzheimer's disease. Recent and remote memory changes are variable. As memory changes occur, the person will have more difficulty adapting to change and attending to usual activities of daily living. P-D, AS, PC

115. no. 2. The client with congestive heart failure can breathe with more ease in a Fowler's or semi-Fowler's position. Maximal lung expansion is permitted be-

cause there is full expansion of the rib cage and there is less upward pressure from the abdominal organs on the diaphragm. In option no. 1, position of comfort may be appropriate; however, the second part ("to relax the client") incorrect. A-O, IM, PS

116. no. 2. The priority goal of caring for a child with any form of retardation is to promote optimal development. Options no. 1 and no. 3 are important goals, but are not as crucial as the broader goal of maximizing development. No. 4 may be unrealistic because of the mental retardation that accompanies Down syndrome. C-SPP, PL, H

117. no. 1. Respirations in congestive heart failure are rapid and shallow because of pulmonary circulatory congestion. Deep, stertorous, wheezing, or Biot's respirations are not characteristic of congestive heart failure. A-O, AS, PS

118. no. 4. Respiratory infections are common in children with Down syndrome and account for high morbidity. The hypotonicity of the chest and abdominal muscles is a major predisposing factor to respiratory infections. C-SPP, AN, H

119. no. 3. Cold stress increases metabolic efforts; respiratory distress can result. Irritability is not usually related to cold stress. Cyanosis is a late change. A newborn does not shiver to maintain body temperature. CBF-N, AS, PS

120. no. 1. The goal of surgical repair of cleft lip is to achieve primary closure of the defect to ensure adequate nutrition through normal sucking and to minimize scarring for cosmetic reasons. A clean, well-healed suture line indicates that the infant has the capacity to suck and that he will have minimal scarring. Although it is important for the parent-infant relationship that the parents are pleased with the repair, the infant's physiologic needs are more crucial when evaluating treatment outcomes. Options no. 3 and no. 4 illustrate typical development progress for a 3-month-old and do not provide direct evidence of goal achievement. C-NM, EV, H

121. no. 1. Identify yourself to avoid misidentification and call the client by name to reinforce her sense of identity. Option no. 2 would decrease her interaction with others, possibly increasing confusion. Options no. 3 and no. 4 provide an inappropriate degree of stimulation. P-D, IM, PC

122. no. 3. Rotation every 15 minutes ensures that the venous return of a single extremity is occluded for no more than 45 minutes. Shorter or longer periods of venous occlusion are not recommended. A-O, IM, E

123. no. 1. Maintaining consistency in the child's environment is the single most effective way to promote a sense of security and continuity during the move. No. 2 is unrealistic in view of the child's age and limitations. No. 3 and no. 4 may increase his fear by adding more change in his life. C-I, PL, PC

124. no. 2. ECG changes, serum enzymes, and chest pain best indicate cardiac status after a myocardial infarction. All of these will show definitive changes as the infarction process evolves. Leg cramps and changes in serum electrolytes, creatinine, and blood urea ni-

trogen are not indicators of post–myocardial infarction cardiac status but rather renal function or the effect of medications. A-O, AS, PS

125. no. 2. Children with Down syndrome are smaller than healthy children the same age and will continue to be as they grow older. No data suggest that fluid and caloric intake is inadequate. Referring this mother's concern to the pediatrician is inappropriate because it is within the scope of nursing practice. C-SPP, AN, H

126. no. 4. This reply allows the nurse to ascertain what the mother believes to be the cause of her infant's defect and what specific concerns or unanswered questions about the cause she may have. The nurse can then further validate the mother's concerns before responding with information or appropriate supportive comments. Although cleft lip is known to be transmitted multifactorially, thus increasing the possibility of occurrence in families with a history of defect, option no. 1 has not been validated and is not responsive to the mother's concern. Option no. 2 ignores the mother's feelings in the situation. Teratogens, such as viruses or drugs, may also cause cleft lip, but option no. 3 is worded as a closed question and does not address the mother's question. C-NM, IM, PC

127. no. 3. A syringe fitted with soft catheter tubing will allow the mother to feed him adequate amounts of formula to the side and back of his mouth and prevent the infant from sucking, which may injure the lip repair. The infant should not be allowed to suck from a nipple in the postoperative period because of possible damage created by tension on the suture line. The infant is too young to be able to drink from a cup; additionally, placement of the cup to his lips may stimulate his suck reflex or directly irritate the suture line. There is no reason to institute nasogastric feedings when a less invasive method, effective in providing adequate nutrition, is available. C-NM, IM, E

128. no. 2. Provide smaller meals that require less attention to complete. The other choices would decrease independence, threaten the client, or allow the problem to continue. P-D, IM, E

129. no. 3. The first step in a cardiac arrest is to ensure that the client has an open airway. The second priority is to establish breathing. The third priority is to establish cardiac function. A-O, IM, PS

130. no. 1. Sucking and crying are contraindicated postoperatively in infants who have had a cleft lip repair because of potential damage to the repair. Sedation with diphenhydramine hydrochloride (Benadryl) is indicated only if the infant becomes restless or agitated and is unable to be calmed by other measures such as holding, stroking, or rocking. Allowing the mother to hold and rock the infant also involves her directly in his care and thus increases her sense of control. C-NM, IM, E

131. no. 4. During a cardiac catheterization, the client may be asked to make verbal responses, change position, cough, and deep breathe. In order to do this, the client is only mildly sedated. A-O, IM, E

132. no. 4. Although the other tests may be performed later, they are involved or invasive. Semen analysis is a simple assessment. Cervical mucus consistency changes during the menstrual cycle and gives clues to ovulation. CBF-W, IM, PC

133. no. 1. Usually by 2 years, the toddler can turn knobs and open doors; simply closing the door is not enough; the door should be locked and all harmful substances placed in a locked cabinet. Parents should be told that medicine should not be treated as candy, the Poison Control Center number should be easily accessible, and no matter how hard they try they cannot watch their children all the time. Accidents will happen. C-H, EV, H

134. no. 1. The priority goal for any pregnant client is compliance with regular prenatal care. CBF-A, PL, H

135. no. 3. A left-sided cardiac catheterization will show coronary artery patency and perfusion of the myocardium. A left-sided cardiac catheterization will not demonstrate any pathologic condition in the right side of the heart or the pulmonary artery. A-O, AS, E

136. no. 4. This provides reality orientation without degrading or arguing with the client. Inaccurate information confuses the client further. Option no. 2 does not tell the client where she is now, and verbal constraints may confuse the client. P-D, IM, E

137. no. 3. Although tiredness is a common complaint of mothers of small children, the mother's feeling "exhausted" may indicate anemia or poor coping. This should be further investigated. Although the infant does not need solids at his age, her caloric intake is within recommended ranges. Bed-wetting is not considered unusual in 3-year-old children, and she may still be adjusting to her new sister. The homemade toys provide appropriate developmental stimulation for children. C-H, AN, H

138. no. 1. The focus of Lamaze classes is the practice of breathing, relaxation, and conditioned responses for use during labor. It is positive that bonding and support were noted, but these are not criteria for evaluation of learning. Requests for analgesics during labor do not influence successful delivery outcome for Lamaze couples. CBF-A, EV, PC

139. no. 4. Nitrogenous waste products from protein metabolism result in an elevation of BUN; therefore a low-protein diet is needed. The protein given should be of high biologic value (i.e., contain all essential amino acids). A high-carbohydrate diet will help reverse gluconeogenesis. The client should be weighed daily. Intake is calculated on urine output plus 500 to 1000 ml of insensible water loss every 24 hours. The potassium is already elevated; therefore the diet should be restrictive of potassium and may even require the administration of ion-exchange resins such as sodium polystyrene sulfonate (Kayexalate). A-E, IM, PS

140. no. 4. This is a common side effect of levodopa. Rather than euphoria, depression is a second common side effect of this drug. Option no. 2 is incorrect. Most parkinsonian clients have a decreased appetite. A-SP, AN, PS

141. no. 1. The 4-month-old infant should be bearing some weight on his legs when held upright. Inability to do

so may indicate a neuromotor delay. The other skills are too advanced for this infant's age. C-H, AS, H

142. no. 2. Clomiphine citrate (Clomid), a drug frequently prescribed to correct infertility, increases the risk of ovarian cysts and multiple births. None of the other choices is correct. CBF-W, IM, E

143. no. 4. Spinal anesthesia results in vasodilation and pooling of blood with a resultant decrease in effective circulatory volume. Respiratory paralysis could occur if the anesthetic is given improperly, but it is not a potential complication. The anesthetic agent is injected below the level of the spinal cord, so spinal cord injury is not a complication. Paralytic ileus is a complication of surgery but is due to factors other than spinal anesthesia. A-S, AN, PS

144. no. 1. If the client experiences contractions, cramping, or more bleeding, she may be experiencing a miscarriage. The other symptoms listed are common in the first trimester and need not be reported. CBF-A, IM, PS

145. no. 1. Personal attention and assistance for client's safety will enhance feelings of security. Confinement and restraints increase feelings of hopelessness and inadequacy, which may lead to increased confusion. These clients will not be able to explain their behavior, and requests for such explanations may increase argumentativeness. P-D, IM, PC

146. no. 3. Washing and drying of the skin aids in securing the traction. Buck's traction does not involve the insertion of pins. Healthy skin (i.e., without abrasions) tolerates skin traction well. C-M, IM, E

147. no. 3. Talking to the infant in the first 24 hours is part of early bonding. Because this is the first day, she may need more time to get acquainted with the newborn. It is normal to feel discouraged with initial feeding; this is not likely to indicate attachment problems. CBF-P, AN, H

148. no. 1. The nurse's first response should be to clarify and validate the problem by gathering additional information. Option no. 2 might be asked as the nurse proceeds to narrow the scope of the cause. no. 3 is likely to make the parent feel defensive, and no. 4 is irrelevant because research does not implicate iron as a cause of regurgitation or vomiting. C-H, AS, E

149. no. 4. Admission to a care facility often exacerbates symptoms because of the new environment. Although options no. 1, no. 2, and no. 3 are important considerations, it is unlikely that they produced the confusion as it is described in this situation. P-D, AN, PC

150. no. 3. The pruritus associated with hepatitis can be severe, and clients can cause a significant amount of skin damage with scratching. Appropriate interventions include cool temperatures, skin lotions, cold packs, keeping the nails short, light cotton clothing, and the possible use of antihistamines. Sedative medications should be avoided because they require liver action to break down. Warm water opens the pores and frequently exacerbates pruritus, which is also worsened if the environment lacks humidity. A-NM, IM, PS

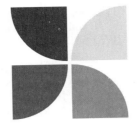

Answers and Rationales: Practice Test 3

Key to abbreviations may be found on p. 544.

151. no. 2. Studies indicate that sensory development at birth is good. This response is more specific than option no. 1. CBF-N, IM, H

152. no. 4. The main defense against transplant rejection is immunosuppressive drugs (e.g., azathioprine [Imuran], prednisone). This therapy is begun before surgery and continues after surgery. It is important for the client not to discontinue this drug therapy unless instructed to do so by a physician, and then the reduction is done slowly over an extended time. Immunosuppressive drugs increase the client's susceptibility to infection. A-E, IM, E

153. no. 1. Fewer than one quarter of the children with poststreptococcal nephritis develop chronic renal failure. Recurrences are rare. With proper treatment, these children return to normal renal functioning within 3 to 4 weeks. C-E, EV, PS

154. no. 2. The Sengstaken-Blakemore tube is used to provide tamponade for the bleeding vessels in the esophagus. If it has been successful in stopping the bleeding, stomach contents will not test positive for blood. The client is not able to swallow at all while the tube is in place and inflated, and the client will require assistance to expectorate his secretions. Active bleeding may stimulate abdominal cramping and diarrhea, but an increase in abdominal girth would not be expected. A-NM, EV, PS

155. no. 3. The child with poststreptococcal nephritis needs a diet with normal protein, moderate sodium restriction, and low potassium. This meal is high in sodium (bacon) and high in potassium (orange juice) and therefore indicates the mother does not clearly understand the diet or the importance of the restrictions. C-E, AN, PS

156. no. 2. Disequilibrium syndrome is believed by some to be caused by too rapid or excess fluid removal from the circulatory system. Dialysis for a short time (2 to 4 hours) and at a reduced rate of blood flow is effective in decreasing occurrence and severity. A-E, IM, E

157. no. 2. A familiar, established routine decreases confusion and the demands on the client's coping mechanisms. Efforts should be made to minimize further dependence. No. 3 would lead to increased feelings of isolation. Waiting will not lessen the confusion. P-D, IM, E

158. no. 4. These are normal responses. CBF-N, AN, PS

159. no. 3. Tonometry is the measurement of intraocular pressure. A myringotomy is an opening into the tympanic membrane. Funduscopy is a procedure to observe the tissue in the cavity of a body of any organ (e.g., the eye or uterus). An iridectomy is the removal of the iris of the eye. A-SP, AS, H

160. no. 1. Elevated blood pressure is one of the primary manifestations of poststreptococcal nephritis and should be monitored on a regular basis. Return of the blood pressure to normal indicates that the disease process is resolving. The edema associated with this disease affects the face and extremities, not the abdomen, so it is not necessary to measure abdominal girth. The urine should be checked for specific gravity, protein, and blood. Although assessment of breath sounds is an important part of evaluating general health status, it is not essential in this case. C-E, EV, PS

161. no. 3. This is the only assessment that refers to gestational age. Apgar scores measure immediate adaptations to extrauterine life; birth weight is not necessarily related to length of gestation; reflexes may be good in some infants who were born before term. CBF-N, AN, PS

162. no. 2. This is the only symptom listed that is indicative of a problem with intellectual function. Options no. 1, no. 3, and no. 4 indicate changes in emotional and psychologic functioning. P-D, AS, PC

163. no. 3. With bradykinesia (not hyperkinesia) and muscle rigidity, the client with Parkinson's disease is unable to lift his feet; hence he shuffles and propels forward with such momentum that he often is unable to control body movement. Parkinsonian clients manifest nonintentional or resting tremors. Option no. 4 is not a manifestation of parkinsonism. A-SP, AS, PS

164. no. 2. The laparascopic cholecystectomy has proved to be an excellent alternative to traditional surgical approaches. Hospitalization has been reduced to 1 day, and clients make rapid recoveries without experiencing anorexia or nausea and vomiting. Clients resume their normal activities promptly and may be vulnerable to fatigue, but increased rest should reverse the fatigue promptly. The most common complaint involves pain that radiates to the shoulder area and is the result of irritation of nerves by the carbon dioxide gas use to increase visualization of the abdomen. The pain usually responds quickly to mild analgesics and the use of a heating pad to the shoulder. A-NM, PL, PS

165. no. 2. This response acknowledges empathy and encourages further expression of feeling. No. 1 is too confrontive, too fast. No. 3 cuts off communication of feelings between client and nurse. No. 4 is too demanding of information and cuts off spontaneous discussion of feelings by the client. P-L, IM, PC

166. no. 3. Terminally ill clients need to review their lives to explore the meaning their lives have had. No. 1 and no. 4 reinforce denial and nonacceptance of the inevitable. Withdrawal from relationships normally occurs among the terminally ill. P-L, IM, PC

167. no. 1. The laser cholecystectomy can be used in most routine cases of cholecystitis and is not affected by the presence of chronic illnesses such as arthritis or mild obesity. It cuts recovery time and causes less tissue trauma so it is of benefit to persons who need to return to stressful occupations. The procedure cannot be used, however, when stones are located down in the common bile duct and would not be reached with laparascopic removal of the gallbladder. Abdominal cholecystectomy would be necessary. A-NM, AN, PS

168. no. 4. Two possible sequelae of a streptococcal infection are rheumatic fever and glomerulonephritis, but the two do not necessarily occur in conjunction with each other. C-O, AS, PS

169. no. 2. The major sequela of rheumatic fever is heart damage, particularly scarring of the mitral valve. Bed rest is recommended for the client with carditis to minimize metabolic needs and ease the workload of the heart. C-O, PL, E

170. no. 2. Verbalize implied feelings, give the client permission to discuss feelings, and help the client work through the denial stage. Options no. 1 and no. 3 cut off communication. Silent support is important but is not appropriate when the client is demonstrating a need to talk and is asking for information. P-L, IM, H

171. no. 3. Although state laws do require PKU screening, the most appropriate response gives the major purpose of the test. The PKU test is specific for an inherited metabolic disorder rather than for vague chromosomal abnormalities. CBF-N, AS, H

172. no. 4. Foot care is extremely important for diabetics. The feet must be carefully cleansed and inspected daily, and the nails should be kept short and trimmed straight across. Lotion can be used on dry areas such as the heels, but the feet and toes should not be oversoftened because they are more vulnerable to skin breakdown. Diabetics should always wear socks or stockings with their shoes, should avoid going barefoot, and should avoid open-toed shoes that expose the feet to injury. A-NM, EV, H

173. no. 3. All are potential stressors, but the school-age child is especially vulnerable to the loss of control that results from decreased and restricted mobility. The 9-year-old is old enough to understand and accept explanations of possible outcomes, reasons for hospitalization, and procedures such as venipuncture, but in addition is likely to be easily frustrated by bed rest requirements. C-I, PL, PS

174. no. 3. Nipride causes vasodilation, which decreases both preload and after load. A-O, AN, PS

175. no. 2. All are goals of shock treatment, but tissue perfusion must be improved to prevent irreversible damage and death of tissues. If tissue perfusion improves, the other goals will be accomplished secondarily. A-O, PL, PS

176. no. 1. A newborn should be positioned on the right side after feeding to prevent aspiration of milk or mucus. The other behaviors are appropriate, but do not evaluate *safe* care. CBF-N, EV, E

177. no. 4. The young infant's cardiac sphincter is not yet fully matured and as a result often relaxes, allowing regurgitation of stomach contents. Although the newborn's stomach capacity is small, it is not the size per se, but the weak cardiac sphincter that precipitates spitting up. There is no scientific basis to support options no. 2 or no. 3. CBF-N, AN, PS

178. no. 2. Verbal expression of grief facilitates mourning. Option no. 1 is too controlling and does not permit individual needs of family members in dealing with their grief. No. 3 discourages family members from taking care of themselves and could impede the family grieving process. No. 4 does not facilitate the family's communication about the grieving process. P-L, IM, PC

179. no. 1. Additional information is needed from the client regarding her concerns. The other choices *may* be appropriate, but clarification regarding the clients' concerns is needed first. P-T, IM, PO

180. no. 2. The 7-year-old is somewhat young to be the best choice, even though she has the same health problem. Because the patient has carditis and had a recent streptococcal infection, she should not be placed with the child with sickle cell vasoocclusive crisis, which may be aggravated by exposure to a potential source of infection. The 12-year-old with fever of unknown origin may also have a concurrent infection to which the patient should not be exposed. The 10-year-old with diabetes is the best choice because she is close enough in age, has no infectious condition, and, like the patient, has a chronic illness. C-O, PL, H

181. no. 3. Intracranial pressure rises as a result of tissue injury, edema, and hypoxia. Blood pressure increases in response to the hypoxic stimulation of the vasomotor center. Pulse rate slows as blood pressure increases. A-SP, AS, PS

182. no. 4. The child is on bed rest with bathroom privileges and cannot go to the playroom. Listening to records and watching television are passive activities. Crocheting requires minimal exertion, does not involve the large joints (which may be painful), and also fosters feelings of accomplishment. C-I, IM, E

183. no. 2. Atelectasis is the major pulmonary risk for this client. Clear breath sounds are the best indicator of an adequately functioning pulmonary system in the client. Temperature elevation is not an early sign of atelectasis and, if present, might signify many other problems. A lowering of the P_{O_2} may not occur early in atelectasis, and cyanosis is a late sign of hypoxia. A-E, EV, PS

184. no. 2. Stay with her to demonstrate caring. Encourage her to talk, but do not push or confront her. Options no. 1 and no. 4 may be interpreted by the client as a lack of caring. In this initial, early phase, confrontation might be destructive to the relationship. P-T, IM, PC

185. no. 3. There is a need during the taking-in phase to integrate the experience of labor and delivery into reality. An interest in birth control measures or infant development usually follows in 2 or 3 days during "taking hold." Mild depression is usually present 3 to 10 days postpartum. CBF-P, AN, PL

186. no. 3. A decreasing ESR indicates a decrease in the body's inflammatory response. The WBC is slightly elevated; a positive C-reactive protein indicates continued inflammation; the elevated ASO titer indicates a recent streptococcal infection. C-O, EV, PS

187. no. 4. Breast size is not a factor in volume of milk produced. This mother needs support and teaching. CBF-P, IM, H

188. no. 1. A palpable carotid pulsation with each chest compression would be the best indicator of adequate CPR. It is a better indicator of effective CPR than skin color. Easily blanched nail beds and dilated pupils indicate inadequate perfusion. A-O, EV, PS

189. no. 3. A 12-year-old is able to cognitively understand full explanations using correct terminology. Such explanations also consider her emotional needs and foster feelings of control. However, although she should be included in making decisions that affect her, she is not legally able to give consent for or refuse necessary care. Concrete thinking and misunderstanding of the causes of illness characterize the younger child. C-H, AN, PS

190. no. 4. The newborn sleeps more than 20 hours daily, nurses every 2 to 3 hours, urinates often, and has frequent stools. New parents will find their lives dramatically changed. The newborn will feed on demand in the first weeks, and parents cannot schedule naps or feedings. The father's comment on crying indicates a lack of understanding of the newborn's need to communicate and need for love. CBF-N, EV, H

191. no. 2. Options 1, 3, and 4 are reliable indicators of vital tissue perfusion. Alteration in skin color is the least reliable. Skin color may be altered by changes in vasomotor tone and gives little indication of the status of the perfusion of vital tissue (cerebral, renal, cardiovascular). A-O, AS, PS

192. no. 3. Protest behavior most characterizes the toddler's separation from parents. Despair or detachment behavior is unlikely to appear when hospitalization is short, especially when parents visit daily. C-I, AS, PS

193. no. 3. Encourage the client to talk by using general, open-ended question. Option no. 1 is too vague and option no. 4 does not encourage the client to talk. The TV is not the concern. P-T, IM, PC

194. no. 1. Success can cause depression in some persons because of a fear of failure, which will lead to a loss of self-esteem. The promotion will increase stress and responsibility. Option no. 2 is not correct because

there is no indication of delusions, and no. 3 may lead to argument over worth. P-E, AN, PC

195. no. 2. The shape of the breast will not be changed by breast-feeding. The bra will prevent breakdown of breast musculature and provide comfort. CBF-P, IM, E

196. no. 2. Chest therapy is carried out to keep the lower airway passage clear and to facilitate drainage of lower airway secretions. Inspiratory stridor, suprasternal retractions, and a harsh metallic cough indicate upper airway involvement and are not used to evaluate the effectiveness of chest percussion and drainage. The presence of crackles and wheezes indicates that the lower airway passages are still congested, and therefore the treatment has not been completely effective. C-O, EV, PS

197. no. 3. Early digitalis toxicity is manifested by gastrointestinal upset. Severe toxicity is characterized by tachycardia. Hypokalemia potentiates the effects of digitalis but is not a toxic effect. Gynecomastia is an uncommon side effect. A-O, AS, PS

198. no. 2. Bleeding indicates excessive anticoagulation by Coumadin. Vitamin K is the antidote for *oral* anticoagulants such as Coumadin. Protamine sulfate is the antidote for heparin. Neither ascorbic acid nor calcium chloride acts as an antidote against an anticoagulant drug. A-O, AN, E

199. no. 4. A full bladder displaces the uterus and prevents contraction. Suggest that the client void and reassess fundus and lochia. CBF-P, AN, E

200. no. 1. Chest therapy in a child with a respiratory infection should be carried out just before mealtimes so the airway is cleared and the child will be able to eat without tiring. Chest therapy should also be done at bedtime to facilitate sleep by helping the child breathe more easily. Chest therapy after meals may cause vomiting. Trying to schedule the treatment around nap times is inefficient and too unpredictable. C-O, PL, E

201. no. 4. Relief of acute chest pain is the priority goal for a client with a myocardial infarction. All the interventions may be carried out, but relief of pain is first. A-O, IM, PS

202. no. 3. Clients often become anxious near discharge and reexperience symptoms they may not have shown for some time. There have been no data given to indicate that the client is not ready for discharge or is overly dependent. P-A, AN, E

203. no. 3. This is a task that poses potential danger to a pregnant woman in the first trimester. There would appear to be no risks with the other tasks. CBF-A, AN, H

204. no. 4. Bed linens should be changed frequently to prevent chilling and promote comfort. Cough suppressants are contraindicated, and children with croup need a liberal fluid intake because of the possibility of dehydration secondary to increased sensible fluid loss. The child is too young to comprehend an explanation of why she must stay in the tent. C-O, IM, E

205. no. 1. Organ meats are high in cholesterol. Chicken and yogurt are low in cholesterol. Vegetable oils such as corn oil have no cholesterol. A-O, AN, H

206. no. 2. There is danger of contracting toxoplasmosis from handling cat litter, so this is an essential aspect of teaching. CBF-A, IM, H

207. no. 2. Severe drug interactions exist between SSRIs (e.g., Zoloft) and MAOIs. The client must be off the MAOI at least several weeks before starting Zoloft (up to 5 weeks for Prozac). No. 1, taking the medication with meals, is important, but not as significant as determining the last dose of Nardil. No. 3 is insignificant at this point because obviously the client is depressed. No. 4, lithium can be taken with some antidepressants. P-E, AN, E, PS

208. no. 3. When a microdrip is used for an intravenous infusion, the number of milliliters per hour is equal to the number of drops per minute. Therefore the nurse should divide the total amount of 500 ml by 8 hours to determine the amount per hour to be infused. This amount equals 63 ml per hour; therefore the microdrip regulator should be set at 63 drops per minute. C-H, IM, E

209. no. 1. Left-sided congestive heart failure causes pulmonary congestion and symptoms. Oliguria, although present in both right-sided and left-sided congestive heart failure, is not an initial or most expected finding. Sacral edema and anorexia occur with right-sided congestive heart failure. A-O, AS, PS

210. no. 1. This response indicates that she has learned *essential* content of antepartal teaching. Rest is always important, but first-trimester fatigue is related to hormone changes. The pregnant woman should drink six to eight glasses of fluids daily. Weight should be maintained in early pregnancy to provide for fetal growth. CBF-A, EV, H

211. no. 4. Dressing without supervision, sharing with other children, and using complete sentences are characteristics of preschoolers, not toddlers. The child should have learned to use a spoon well by 18 months of age. C-H, AS, H

212. no. 2. The elderly male whose wife has a debilitating illness is more at risk for suicide. The clients in options no. 1, 3, and 4 may also be at risk at some point, but elderly men experiencing major losses pose the highest risk of suicide. P-L, AN, PC, E

213. no. 2. Because of gravity, dependent edema occurs in right-sided congestive heart failure. Cardiac failure edema is also painless and pitting. It does not involve the face. A-O, AS, PS

214. no. 1. During a left-sided cardiac catheterization, the catheter is introduced into the femoral artery of the leg. After catheterization, the client is cautioned to keep the affected leg extended (not flexed) to avoid any increase in pressure at the inguinal puncture site. A-O, PL, PS

215. no. 2. This item requires correct identification of terms used in a TPAL chart; analysis of data in the history leads to the only correct response. T = term births (two pregnancies carried to 40 weeks of gestation); P = premature births (the stillborn delivered at 36 weeks of gestation is considered a premature birth); A = abortion history (the client has no history of abortions because all pregnancies extended beyond 20 weeks); L = number of living children (two living children). CBF-A, AS, H

216. no. 3. A tracheostomy tube enters directly into the trachea. It should be suctioned first with sterile equipment to prevent lower airway infections. The nose requires clean technique and can be suctioned with the same catheter after the trachea is suctioned. Intermittent, not constant, suction is used. Only a sterile, water-soluble lubricant is used for the catheter. Oil-based lubricants, such as petroleum jelly, can cause pneumonia if aspirated into the lower airway. A-O, IM, E

217. no. 2. Although all these pieces of information may be important and may be ascertained at some point during the child's hospital stay, the nurse must know the child's usual patterns in order to develop an appropriate care plan to meet her toileting needs. C-I, AS, H

218. no. 2. The NG tube is used immediately postoperatively, primarily to prevent food and fluid from contaminating the pharyngeal and esophageal suture line during healing. Swallowing may be reduced, but it is not the primary reason for using the NG tube. Aspiration is not possible unless a fistula forms between the pharynx and larynx later in the postoperative recovery. A-O, PL, E

219. no. 3. Further assessment is necessary to decide whether the client is suicidal or making realistic plans and steps to become more involved with her environment. No. 1 is a possibility, but the nurse needs more information before asking this direct question. No. 2 and no. 4 do not encourage further exploration of the client's actions and feelings and pose a barrier to talking about her plans. P-E, IM, PC

220. no. 1. These manifestations are characteristic of spinal shock, which typically develops 30 to 60 minutes after a spinal cord injury. With spinal shock, suppression of the reflexes below the level of injury results in loss of temperature control, vasomotor tone, and sweating. Autonomic dysreflexia is the exaggerated reflex response to stimuli (e.g., distended bladder) characterized by hypertension, severe headache, bradycardia, and profuse sweating. Autonomic dysreflexia occurs only with spinal cord injuries above T-6 and rarely occurs until spinal shock has subsided. Hypoxia and infection are not characterized by these signs. A-S, AN, PS

221. no. 4. Morning sickness is correctly classified as a "presumptive sign." Amenorrhea and Chadwick's sign are also presumptive signs of pregnancy. Urine positive for hCG is a probable sign of pregnancy (95% to 98% accuracy). CBF-A, AN, PS

222. no. 3. Allowing the child to sleep with her parents may increase her insecurity and reinforces dependency (not autonomy) because this was not part of her routine before hospitalization. C-H, PL, PS

223. no. 2. The goal of tuberculin skin testing is the early diagnosis and treatment of tuberculosis (i.e., secondary health promotion). Primary health promotion and primary prevention aim at preventing the occurrence

of a disease. Tertiary health promotion has a focus on restoration and rehabilitation. A-H, AS, H

224. no. 3. Histamine receptor antagonists work directly to reduce gastric acid secretion. Metoclopramide (Reglan) increases the rate of gastric emptying, antacids neutralize gastric acid, and Carafate coats and protects the mucosa of the stomach. A-NM, EV, PS

225. no. 3. Selective serotonin reuptake inhibitors tend to cause gastrointestinal disturbances. Taking them with food reduces this side effect. No. 1 is incorrect because these agents usually increase insomnia and interfere with sleep. No. 2 is incorrect. No. 4 is incorrect because these agents are not addictive. P-E, AN, PC

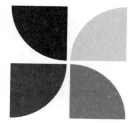

Answers and Rationales: Practice Test 4

Key to abbreviations may be found on p. 544.

226. no. 2. There is an increase in both plasma and cells during pregnancy. However, the increase in plasma is greater than the increase in red blood cells. This results in a hemodilution of blood, causing a fall in the hematocrit. This is referred to as the normal physiologic anemia of pregnancy. CBF-A, AS, PS

227. no. 1. Of all the age groups, toddlers handle separation and hospitalization most poorly. If a mother cannot room-in, the next best thing is an article of clothing to remind the child of the mother. C-I, PL, PS

228. no. 3. The suture line must be protected after gastric surgery. Therefore the NG tube is not routinely irrigated or repositioned. Routine vital sign monitoring and output measurements are performed. Salem sump tubes are used to prevent distention of the stomach wall and thus tension on the suture line. A-NM, EV, E

229. no. 2. The most common side effect of trazodone hydrochloride (Desyrel) is sedation. Antidepressants are not addicting. No. 3 and no. 4 are common for MAO inhibitors. P-E, IM, H

230. no. 2. Ambivalence is a normal psychologic reaction during the first trimester. In communicating therapeutically, it is important to relate to the client that such feelings are frequently experienced. The nurse should allow the client to ventilate her feelings regarding this. The other options do not encourage the client to share feelings; rather, they immediately suggest an alternative or focus on long-term changes. CBF-A, IM, PC

231. no. 4. The findings of congenital dislocated hip include *limited abduction* of the affected hip, *shortening* of the leg on the affected side, and widening of the perineum caused by the head of the femur slipping out of the acetabulum. The infant rarely experiences pain in the affected hip. C-M, AS, PS

232. no. 2. The parietal cells of the fundus of the stomach secrete intrinsic factor which is essential for the absorption of vitamin B_{12} in the intestine. Its loss gradually produces pernicious anemia. The anemia does not respond to diet changes or oral vitamin therapy. No oral form of intrinsic factor exists. Vitamin B_{12} must be administered by injection to reverse the anemia. A-NM, IM, PS

233. no. 4. Anorexia is a common occurrence in depressed clients, but it is not a common side effect of antidepressants. Hospital food usually meets client needs.

There has been no indication that the client desires staff attention. P-E, AN, PC

234. no. 3. Treatment of a peptic ulcer does not require any particular diet restrictions. Bland diets are not necessary and do not aid in healing. Fat intake is not related to ulcer healing and milk has been found to increase gastric acid secretions. Clients should avoid any food item or seasoning that causes pain. A-NM, IM, H

235. no. 2. Increasing progesterone levels during pregnancy result in smooth-muscle relaxation, leading to dilation of the ureters (especially the right ureter) and decreased bladder tone. Urinary stasis is thus created, contributing to bladder infections. Bladder infection during pregnancy can lead to serious complications for both mother and fetus. If an infection occurs, antibiotics may be prescribed. However, using such medication preventively is never suggested because of the teratogenic potential. CBF-A, IM, H

236. no. 1. An elevated temperature accompanied by behavioral changes may be an early sign of infection. Any leak, abrasion, or tear of the meningomyelocele sac would further support the possibility of infection (e.g., meningitis). Assess the sac before notifying the physician. Isolation precautions should be instituted to protect the other babies and would be appropriate once the sac has been assessed. Although the mother might help calm the infant, it is not appropriate until the nursing assessment is complete. C-SPP, AN, E

237. no. 1. Tuberculosis is usually transmitted by the inhalation of airborne particles (droplet nuclei containing *M. tuberculosis*) from a person with active disease. Covering the mouth and nose of the infected person with a tissue best prevents the transmission of the tuberculosis organism. Hand washing removes the tubercle bacilli from the hands but is not the best way to prevent the transmission of airborne organisms. No special laundry or dishwashing techniques are needed. A-O, IM, E

238. no. 3. Misoprostol cannot be used to treat active peptic ulcer disease. Its only use is in prevention. The drug supports prostaglandin synthesis and helps protect the mucous layer of the stomach and duodenum from breakdown by the action of NSAIDs. The drug is recommended for all high-risk clients (elderly females) who will need long-term NSAID administration. A-NM, EV, H

239. no. 2. Aspiration of vomited blood is a serious risk for the client. The head should be elevated, but the client also needs to be turned to the side to facilitate removal of the vomited blood. Because 85% of GI bleeds spontaneously stop, the concern for the airway takes priority over concerns for shock, at least in the initial interventions. No data are given to suggest assessment findings of shock. A-NM, IM, PS

240. no. 4. From 50% to 80% of all suicides are committed by depressed persons. Although options no. 1, no. 2, and no. 3 are good objectives of care, they are not the first priority at this time. P-T, PL, PC

241. no. 2. Although all of these nursing actions would be appropriate, measuring head circumference daily is essential. Hydrocephalus is a common complication of meningomyelocele. The primary sign of hydrocephalus in infants is head enlargement. Any change in the size of the infant's head can be assessed by taking daily measurements. C-SPP, IM, E

242. no. 1. The client, after insertion of a total hip prosthesis, must be positioned with the legs abducted at all times. This prevents the slippage of the prosthesis out of position. The hemovac is reconstituted every 8 hours or when half full. The client is not ambulated with full weight bearing on the affected leg for several months. Ativan does not relieve pain. A-M, PL, PS

243. no. 1. The symptoms of dumping syndrome are related to the rapid movement and absorption of food and nutrients from the stomach to the duodenum. Clients are encouraged to eat small meals, drink liquids only between meals, lie on their left side after eating, and avoid easily digested carbohydrates or high-CHO diets. The malabsorption can become severe. A-NM, IM, PS

244. no. 2. Cheese and yogurt are both good substitutes for milk. Other sources of calcium include some fish, including sardines, ice cream, and dried beans. Although leafy vegetables and grains contain calcium, recent research indicates that it is poorly absorbed. CBF-A, IM, H

245. no. 2. The equation should be set up with 125 mg per 1.2 ml = 75 mg per X ml. Thus $125X = 1.2$ multiplied by 75, which becomes $125X = 90.90$ divided by 125 = 0.72. Therefore the nurse should administer 0.72 ml as the correct dose. C-I, IM, PS

246. no. 1. No injection site should be used more than once a month. Although the other statements are all correct to some degree, this statement tells you the exact, correct information about "rotating injection sites." A-NM, EV, E

247. no. 4. Postoperative numbness and tingling should be compared with the client's preoperative neurologic assessment data. If the client had no numbness and tingling preoperatively, or if numbness and tingling are more severe, the nurse notifies the physician. Sensory manifestations may be due to inflammatory changes and will be temporary. However, new findings always must be assessed further. A-M, EV, E

248. no. 4. NPH and regular insulin may be mixed. Accurately and consistently drawing up insulin, whether mixed or not, is the key to preventing mistakes in dos-

age. There is no need for two injections, and this gives the client more sites for rotation, decreasing the incidence of lipohypertrophy. A-NM, EV, E

249. no. 3. This option focuses on the client's needs without challenging the client. Option no. 1 reassures the client of his worth but does not provide information necessary to set the tone for the nurse-client relationship. No. 2 presents factual information but does not focus on client needs or the purpose of the nurse-client relationship. No. 4 challenges the client and does not focus on needs. P-T, IM, PC

250. no. 3. This reflects an understanding of potential risks. Although bladder pressure causes frequency in the first and third trimesters, burning is never expected. Because the remaining options indicate delayed or self-treatment, they are incorrect. CBF-A, EV, E

251. no. 3. The equation is set up with 30 mg per 4 ml = 20 mg per X ml. Thus $30X = 20$ multiplied by 4, which becomes $30X = 80.80$ divided by 30 = 2.6. Therefore the nurse should administer 2.6 ml as the correct dose. C-I, IM, PS

252. no. 4. This is a potentially serious problem because she takes her insulin at 7 AM but does not eat until 10 AM. Regular insulin's onset is within 1 hour from the time injected S.Q., and it peaks in 2 to 4 hours. A-NM, AS, E

253. no. 1. If contractions exceed 90 seconds in duration, there is a danger of a ruptured uterus. Adverse blood pressure changes with oxytocin (Pitocin) are seen in hypertension. A desired effect is increased strength and frequency of contractions. CBF-I, AN, E

254. no. 3. This is the only response that recognizes and acknowledges the client's perception of her situation and that encourages her to explore it with the nurse. This response is therapeutic and conveys respect for the client's point of view and a desire to help her learn to cope with her problems. It promotes a relationship of trust. Option no. 1 is slightly sarcastic and option no. 2 makes a listening relationship contingent on the client's behavior. Option no. 4 contradicts the client's ideas. P-T, IM, PC

255. no. 4. The diagnosis has not been confirmed; you only suspect a fractured hip. You should never attempt to reduce a fracture or extend or elevate the extremity. You may cause more damage. A-M, AN, PS

256. no. 4. Renal problems present a major threat to the life of the child with spina bifida as well as to her self-image and willingness to become involved with activities and individuals outside the home. The other areas may become problematic, but they are generally not life threatening. C-SPP, AN, PS

257. no. 3. Fractured hips are indicated by abduction of the affected extremity and movement away from the main axis of the body. There is also external rotation of the hip, and the leg is shortened. It is difficult to assess edema at this point. A-M, AS, PS

258. no. 3. This opening statement allows the nurse to gain an overall perspective of family functioning, yet is specific enough to focus the response (as opposed to, "Tell me how you are doing"). The other choices focus narrowly on one aspect, which might be appro-

priate as the visit proceeds, but are haphazard initial questions. Also, two of them (no. 1 and no. 4) require only a "yes" or "no" response and thus do not encourage disclosure by the client. P-T, AS, PC

259. no. 3. Doses of aspirin sufficient to relieve pain may cause tinnitus. The other side effects listed are not characteristic of aspirin side effects. A-M, AS, PS

260. no. 3. The school-age child is developmentally concerned with a sense of industry, which is accomplished through peer interactions and school activities. Fear of painful procedures characterizes preschoolers. The school-age child has little difficulty adjusting to new environments. The child's activity should not be restricted; therefore, restricted mobility will not be a concern. C-I, AS, PC

261. no. 4. This response indicates understanding of common feelings about infertility and is considered therapeutic communication because it encourages further discussion. Although options no. 1 and no. 2 are true, neither is helpful. Option no. 3 blocks communication by introducing the concept of blame. P-T, IM, PC

262. no. 4. Acceptance is needed in time of stress, as the woman seeks to maintain control. CBF-I, IM, E

263. no. 1. After total removal of the thyroid gland, the client must take thyroid medication daily for the rest of life to supply the hormones essential for maintaining body metabolism. Because the thyroid hormones themselves are taken, dietary iodine is no longer needed to support their synthesis within the body. Dietary iodine need not be advised or restricted. A-NM, IM, H

264. no. 2. Delusions of persecution are defined as false beliefs that one has been singled out for harassment. Delusions in this situation do not relate to ideas of superiority (no. 1) or focus on the self (no. 3) or on religious ideation (no. 4). P-S, AN, PC

265. no. 3. The treatment of choice, both on an emergency and long-term basis, is the administration of calcium gluconate. Thyroid preparations have no influence on parathyroid functioning. Digitalis is a cardiotonic and requires normal levels of calcium to produce desired effects. Because phosphate levels increase in hypoparathyroid conditions, high dietary phosphorus would be contraindicated. A-NM, PL, PS

266. no. 2. The 10-year-old should be involved in all aspects of managing her diabetes, but she still requires supervision and support by an adult. Options no. 1 and no. 3 indicate overinvolvement of the parents, and option no. 4 indicates that the parents are not providing adequate supervision. A 10-year-old is not yet capable of full self-management. C-I, EV, PC

267. no. 2. Interventions would begin with one-to-one activities. Socialization is increased gradually. The client will need assistance in developing a relationship. Participation in demanding group activities may seem threatening. P-S, PL, E

268. no. 4. These are normal adaptations. CBF-P, AN, PS

269. no. 4. The goal for a suspicious client is to recognize and express the anxiety that causes the delusion. No disruption of work or self-care abilities has been in-

dicated. Discussion of delusions would indicate no change. P-S, EV, PC

270. no. 1. The pneumothorax was caused by a disruption in the integrity of the pleura, which allowed air from the lung to enter the pleural (not mediastinal) space. A *pneumo*thorax involves *air,* not pus, in the pleural space. In this case, there was no rib involvement. A-O, AS, PS

271. no. 4. Respiratory infections, such as colds or flu, are the most common cause of exacerbations of emphysema, a chronic obstructive pulmonary disease (COPD). Clients with COPD should be instructed to seek early treatment for any respiratory infection. A-O, AS, E

272. no. 1. Exercise reduces insulin requirements because glucose can be used without insulin during periods of muscular activity. There is an increased risk of insulin shock if nutrition is not modified to reflect changes in caloric requirements during exercise. The risk of hyperglycemia is lowered as a result of exercise. C-NM, AN, PS

273. no. 3. Clients with COPD may be unable to tolerate eating large meals; they might tolerate small, frequent meals better. Also, their need for calories is increased as a result of the increased energy expended by the work of breathing. A-O, IM, PS

274. no. 3. It communicates interest and willingness to stay with the client during difficult moments without increasing his agitation, being judgmental, or taking away the client's control. P-T, IM, PC

275. no. 3. Such pain may be associated with the development of a hematoma. Assessment should precede intervention. Comfort measures may follow. CBF-P, PL, E

276. no. 4. Correct information allays anxiety. Option no. 4 is more accurate and specific than no. 2. The removal of air from the pleural space is facilitated when intrathoracic pressure is increased with exhalation, coughing, or sneezing. During these activities, bubbles are seen in the water-seal chamber of the Pleur-Evac. When the lung is reexpanded, this intermittent bubbling will cease. (*Continuous* bubbling may indicate an air leak.) Options no. 1 and 3 do not answer the client's question. A-O, AS, PC.

277. no. 2. The effect of changes in puberty on dietary and insulin management should be anticipated and discussed with the preadolescent and her family. Rapid weight gain is unexpected in adolescents with IDD, and they cannot be maintained on oral hypoglycemics at any point in their lives. Physical activity should be encouraged. C-NM, PL, PS

278. no. 2. The primary purpose of chest tube drainage is to reestablish *negative* (subatmospheric) pressure in the pleural space by the removal of air and fluid. This allows the lung to reexpand. Atmospheric or supraatmospheric pressure in the pleural space causes the lung to collapse. A-O, AS, E

279. no. 1. Involve the suspicious client in group activity and relationships gradually. Begin by developing a one-to-one relationship; then involve others slowly.

Options no. 2, no. 3, and no. 4 do not allow for this gradual involvement. P-S, IM, PC

280. no. 3. An ultrasound examination would provide information on the fetal development. Estriol and non-stress tests indicate placental-fetal well-being, and the amniocentesis may provide a variety of information, from genetic information to the extent of lung development. CBF-A, AS, PS

281. no. 3. Do not argue with the client about delusions. Consistency and clarity will enhance development of trust and are crucial in developing a relationship. P-T, IM, PC

282. no. 3. Clients with Graves' disease frequently experience catecholamine-related symptoms such as palpitations, tachycardia, and chest pain. The administration of a beta blocker such as propranolol (Inderal) effectively blocks these symptoms and increases the client's sense of well-being. It does not directly affect the client's thyroid overactivity, however. A-NM, E, PS

283. no. 2. The other responses have nothing to do with prevention of nosocomial infections. Nosocomial infections are those infections acquired during hospitalization. Commonly these are tracked to the lack of hand washing by health care providers between clients or before procedures. A-S, IM, E

284. no. 3. Ketoacidosis is manifested by nausea, vomiting, acetone breath, flushing, dry skin and mucous membranes, and dehydration. The other manifestations are commonly seen with hypoglycemia. C-NM, AS, PS

285. no. 1. Maintain a focus on reality without demeaning the client or becoming involved in arguments. Options no. 2 and no. 3 may lead to an argument. Option no. 4 shows a condescending attitude by the nurse and is not therapeutic. P-S, IM, PC

286. no. 4. This best meets the couple's needs. Apparently they have misunderstood the physician's explanation. Time to discuss feelings should be provided. CBF-A, IM, PC

287. no. 4. The discharge instructions are focused on skin care. Option 1 is incorrect information for an ileal conduit. Options 2 and 3 are correct statements; however, they are not focused on skin care. A-E, EV, H

288. no. 1. Aplastic anemia is a serious side effect of Tegretol. Options 2, 3, and 4 are not side effects of Tegretol. P-E, AS, PS

289. no. 3. Options no. 1 and no. 2 suggest hypofunction of the thyroid gland. The symptoms listed in option no. 4 are not, as a group, specific for thyroid dysfunction. A-NM, AS, PS

290. no. 1. The signs indicate hypoxia. Meconium staining can be associated with distress. Although the Apgar score is normal, the deprivation of nutrients and oxygen in utero causes retarded intrauterine growth. CBF-N, AN, PS

291. no. 3. This level is too low. The therapeutic range of Tegretol is 7 to 12 μg. Options no. 1 and no. 2 are not appropriate. Option no. 4 is incorrect because Tegretol is an effective antimanic agent. P-E, AN, PS

292. no. 2. Speech rehabilitation can be started as soon as the esophageal suture line has healed. Time of healing is determined on an individual basis. A-O, IM, PS

293. no. 4. The mode of transportation to the hospital is not significant as part of the initial assessment. The other assessments listed are pertinent to the client's admitting complaint. A-M, AS, E

294. no. 2. The newborn has the ability to self-console and go into a quiet sleep state. CBF-N, AN, PC

295. no. 3. From the signs described, it is evident she suspects her daughter has an eating problem. But the lack of weight loss does not seem to fit with what she knows, so she's not sure. Option no. 3 verbalizes the implied question the mother seems to be asking as well as gets to the point of her daughter having an eating disorder, which the symptoms support. Options no. 1 and no. 2 are wrong because the daughter has typical symptoms of bulimia. Option no. 4 may be true, but the central problem is the eating disorder, bulimia. P-P, IM, PC

296. no. 1. Bed rest is necessary for 6 to 8 hours to prevent a spinal headache. Although the client may need to void, he cannot get out of bed. Fluids are to be encouraged for rehydration and replacement of cerebrospinal fluid and to minimize headache after the lumbar puncture. Only mild sedation is required for a spinal headache. If a water dye was used, the head of the bed is elevated at least 20 degrees after the procedure to prevent the dye from coming into contact with the meninges and causing irritation. If an oil dye was used, the bed may be kept flat. A-M, IM, E

297. no. 2. All of these outcomes are desirable, but the parents' compliance with keeping the infant in her splint at all times except bath time is the most crucial indicator that they understand the possible consequences of not adhering to the treatment plan. C-M, EV, H

298. no. 1. A choking infant requires immediate attention to clear the airway. Option no. 2 can be carried out after clearing the airway. Option no. 3, milking the trachea, may cause trauma. Option no. 4 is contraindicated with choking. CBF-N, IM, E.

299. no. 3. Initially the client will show some of the physical effects of use of laxatives. Options no. 1, no. 2, and no. 4 are also good objectives of care, but they are secondary to stabilizing her food retention and intake. P-P, PL, PC

300. no. 1. Postoperatively, the client is turned as a unit (i.e., log-rolled). A turning frame is used if the client has a fusion. The client will be out of bed on the first or second postoperative day. Activities to be avoided after discharge would be included in discharge instructions. A-M, IM, E

Appendix A

Approved Nursing Diagnoses from the North American Nursing Diagnosis Association, 1994

Activity intolerance
Activity intolerance, risk for
Adaptive capacity, decreased: intracranial
Adjustment, impaired
Airway clearance, ineffective
Anxiety
Aspiration, risk for
Body image disturbance
Body temperature, altered, risk for
Bowel incontinence
Breastfeeding, effective
Breastfeeding, ineffective
Breathing pattern, ineffective
Cardiac output, decreased
Caregiver role strain
Caregiver role strain, risk for
Communication, impaired verbal
Community coping, potential for enhanced
Community coping, ineffective
Confusion, acute
Confusion, chronic
Constipation
Constipation, colonic
Constipation, perceived
Coping, defensive
Coping, family: potential for growth
Coping, ineffective family: compromised
Coping, ineffective family: disabling
Coping, ineffective individual
Decisional conflict (specify)
Denial, ineffective
Diarrhea
Disuse syndrome, risk for
Diversional activity deficit
Dysreflexia
Energy field disturbance
Environmental interpretation syndrome: impaired
Family processes, altered
Family processes, altered: alcoholism
Fatigue
Fear
Fluid volume deficit (1)
Fluid volume deficit (2)
Fluid volume deficit, risk for
Fluid volume excess

Gas exchange, impaired
Grieving, anticipatory
Grieving, dysfunctional
Growth and development, altered
Health maintenance, altered
Health-seeking behaviors (specify)
Home maintenance management, impaired
Hopelessness
Hyperthermia
Hypothermia
Incontinence, functional
Incontinence, reflex
Incontinence, stress
Incontinence, total
Incontinence, urge
Infant behavior, disorganized
Infant behavior, disorganized, risk for
Infant behavior, organized: potential for enhanced
Infant feeding pattern, ineffective
Infection, risk for
Injury, perioperative positioning: risk for
Injury, risk for
Knowledge deficit (specify)
Loneliness, risk for
Management of therapeutic regimen, community: ineffective
Management of therapeutic regimen, families: ineffective
Management of therapeutic regimen, individuals: effective
Management of therapeutic regimen, individuals: ineffective
Memory, impaired
Mobility, impaired physical
Noncompliance (specify)
Nutrition, altered: less than body requirements
Nutrition, altered: more than body requirements
Nutrition, altered: risk for more than body requirements
Oral mucous membranes, altered
Pain
Pain, chronic
Parent/infant/child attachment, altered, risk for
Parental role conflict
Parenting, altered
Parenting, altered, risk for
Peripheral neurovascular dysfunction, risk for
Personal identity disturbance

Poisoning, risk for
Posttrauma response
Powerlessness
Protection, altered
Rape-trauma syndrome
Rape-trauma syndrome: compound reaction
Rape-trauma syndrome: silent reaction
Relocation stress syndrome
Role performance, altered
Self-care deficit, bathing/hygiene
Self-care deficit, dressing/grooming
Self-care deficit, feeding
Self-care deficit, toileting
Self-esteem, chronic low
Self-esteem, disturbance
Self-esteem, situational low
Self-mutilation, risk for
Sensory/perceptual alterations (specify) (visual, auditory, kinesthetic, gustatory, tactile, olfactory)
Sexual dysfunction
Sexuality patterns, altered

Skin integrity, impaired
Skin integrity, impaired, risk for
Sleep pattern disturbance
Social interaction, impaired
Social isolation
Spiritual distress (distress of the human spirit)
Spiritual well-being, potential for enhanced
Suffocation, risk for
Swallowing, impaired
Thermoregulation, ineffective
Thought processes, altered
Tissue integrity, impaired
Tissue perfusion, altered (specify type) (renal, cerebral, cardiopulmonary, gastrointestinal, peripheral)
Trauma, risk for
Unilateral neglect
Urinary elimination, altered
Urinary retention
Ventilation, inability to sustain spontaneous
Ventilatory weaning process, dysfunctional
Violence, risk for: self-directed or directed at others

Appendix B
Common Laboratory Values—Adult*

	Conventional	SI units
HEMATOLOGIC TESTS		
Hematocrit	Male: 42%-52%	0.42-0.52
	Female: 37%-47%	0.37-0.47
Hemoglobin	Male: 14-18 g/dl	8.1-11.2 mmol/L
	Female: 12-16 g/dl	7.4-9.9 mmol/L
Red blood cells	Male: 4.7-6.1 million/mm^3	4.7-6.1 × 10^{12}/L
	Female: 4.2-5.4 million/mm^3	
White blood cells	5000-10,000/mm^3	5-10 × 10^9/L
Platelets	150,000-400,000/mm^3	150-400 × 10^9/L
Erythrocyte sedimentation rate	Male: 0-15 mm/hr	
	Female: 0-20 mm/hr	
Prothrombin time	11.0-12.5 seconds	11.0-12.5 seconds
Partial thromboplastin time	30-40 seconds	30-40 seconds
BLOOD CHEMISTRY TESTS		
Acid phosphatase†	0.10-0.63 U/ml	28-175 nmol/sec/L
Alkaline phosphatase†	30-85 ImU/ml	
Albumin	3.5-4.5 g/dl	35-55 g/L
ALT (SGPT)†	5-35 IU/L	5-35 U/L
Ammonia	15-110 μg/dl	47-65 μmol/L
Amylase†	56-190 IU/L	25-125 U/L
AST (SGOT)†	5-40 IU/L	5-40 U/L
Bilirubin	Direct: 0.1-0.3 mg/dl	1.7-5.1 μmol/L
	Total: 0.1-1.0 mg/dl	5.1-17 μmol/L
Calcium	9.0-10.5 mg/dl	2.25-2.75 mmol/L
CO_2	23-30 mEq/L	21-30 mmol/L
Chloride	90-110 mEq/L	98-106 mmol/L
Cholesterol	150-200 mg/dl	3.90-6.50 mmol/L
Creatine phosphokinase (CPK)†	5-75 mU/ml	12-80 U/L
Creatinine	0.7-1.5 mg/dl	<133 μmol/L
Globulin	2.3-3.4 g/dl	20-35 g/L
Glucose	70-115 mg/dl	3.89-6.38 mmol/L
Iron	60-190 μg/dl	13-31 μmol/L
Iron-binding capacity	250-420 μg/dl	45-73 μmol/L

Modified from Pagana KD, Pagana TJ: *Mosby's diagnostic and test reference*, St. Louis, 1992, Mosby.
*Normal value ranges will vary from laboratory to laboratory.
†Enzyme value ranges may vary widely from laboratory to laboratory. Any actual client result must be compared with laboratory standards for accurate evaluation.

	Conventional	SI units
BLOOD CHEMISTRY TESTS—cont'd		
Lactic dehydrogenase (LDH)†	90-200 ImU/ml	0.4-1.7 μmol/sec/L
Lipase†	Up to 1.5 U/ml	0.4-17 U/L
Lithium	0.8-1.4 mEq/L‡	
O_2 saturation	95%-100%	0.95-1.00
P_{CO_2}	35-45 mm Hg	
pH	7.35-7.45	7.35-7.45
P_{O_2}	80-100 mm Hg	
Potassium	3.5-5.0 mEq/L	3.5-5.0 mmol/L
Protein	6-8 g/dl	55-80 g/L
Sodium	136-145 mEq/L	136-145 mmol/L
Triglycerides	Male: 40-160 mg/dl	0.4-1.6 g/L
	Female: 35-135 mg/dl	0.35-1.35 g/L
Urea nitrogen	10-20 mg/dl	3.6-7.1 mmol/L
Uric acid	Male: 2.1-8.5 mg/dl	0.15-0.48 mmol/L
	Female: 2.0-6.6 mg/dl	0.09-0.36 mmol/L
URINE TESTS		
pH	4.6-8.0 (average 6.0)	
Specific gravity	1.010-1.025	
Odor	Aromatic	
Color	Amber-yellow	
Appearance	Clear	
Glucose	Negative	
Protein	<8 mg/dl	
Hemoglobin	Negative	
Acetone	Negative	

†Enzyme values ranges may vary widely from laboratory to laboratory. Any actual client result must be compared with laboratory standards for accurate evaluation.

‡Therapeutic level

Appendix C
State and Territorial Boards of Nursing

Alabama State Nurses Association
360 North Hull St.
Montgomery, Alabama 36104-3658
(334) 262-8321
FAX (334) 262-8578

Alaska Nurses Association
237 East Third Ave.
Anchorage, Alaska 99501
(907)274-082/264-1706
FAX (907) 272-0292

Arizona Nurses Association
1850 East Southern Ave., Ste. 1
Tempe, Arizona 85282
(602) 831-0404
FAX (602) 839-4780

Arkansas Nurses Association
117 South Cedar St.
Little Rock, Arkansas 72205
(501) 664-5853
FAX (501) 664-5859

ANA/California
P.O. Box 225
3010 Wilshire Blvd.
Los Angeles, California 90010
(213) 486-6555
FAX (213) 486-6565

Colorado Nurses Association
5453 East Evans Place
Denver, Colorado 80222
(303) 757-7483, ext. 13
FAX (303) 757-2679

Connecticut Nurses Association
Meritech Business Park
377 Research Parkway, Ste. 2D
Meriden, Connecticut 06450
(203) 238-1207
FAX (203) 238-3437

Delaware Nurses Association
2634 Capitol Trail, Ste. A
Newark, Delaware 19711
(302) 368-2333
FAX (302) 366-1775

District of Columbia
Nurses Association
5100 Wisconsin Ave. NW, Ste. 306
Washington, DC 20016
(202) 244-2705
FAX (202) 362-8285

Florida Nurses Association
PO Box 536985
Orlando, Florida 32853-6985
(407) 896-3261
FAX (407) 896-9042

Georgia Nurses Association
1362 West Peachtree St. NW
Atlanta, Georgia 30339
(404) 876-4624
FAX (404) 876-4621

Guam Nurses Association
PO Box CG
Agana, Guam 96910
011 (671) 477-NURS

Hawaii Nurses Association
677 Ala Moana Boulevard, Ste. 301
Honolulu, Hawaii 96813
(808) 521-8361
FAX (808) 524-2760

Idaho Nurses Association
200 North 4th St., Ste. 20
Boise, Idaho 83702-6001
(208) 345-0500
FAX (208) 345-1163

Illinois Nurses Association
300 South Wacker Dr., Ste. 2200
Chicago, Illinois 60606
(312) 360-2300
FAX (312) 360-9380

Indiana State Nurses Association
2915 North High School Rd.
Indianapolis, Indiana 46224
(317) 299-4575
FAX (317) 297-3525

Iowa Nurses Association
1501 42nd St., Ste. 471
West Des Moines, Iowa 50266
(515) 225-0495
FAX (515) 225-2201

Kansas State Nurses Association
700 SW Jackson, Ste. 601
Topeka, Kansas 66603
(913) 233-8638
FAX (913) 233-5222

Kentucky Nurses Association
1400 South First St.
PO Box 2616
Louisville, Kentucky 40201
(502) 637-2546/2547
FAX (502) 637-8236

Louisiana State Nurses Association
712 Transcontinental Dr.
Metairie, Louisiana 70001
(504) 889-1030
FAX (504) 888-1158

Maine State Nurses Association
PO Box 2240/295 Water St.
Augusta, Maine 04338-2240
(207) 622-1057
FAX (207) 623-4072

Maryland Nurses Association
849 International Dr.
Airport Square 21, Ste. 255
Linthicum, Maryland 21090
(410) 859-3000
FAX (410) 859-3001

Massachusetts Nurses Association
340 Turnpike St.
Canton, Massachusetts 02021
(617) 821-4625
FAX (617) 821-4445

Michigan Nurses Association
2310 Jolly Oak Rd.
Okemos, Michigan 48864-4599
(517) 349-5640
FAX (517) 349-5818

Minnesota Nurses Association
1295 Bandana Blvd. North, Ste. 140
Saint Paul, Minnesota 55108-5115
(612) 646-4807, (800) 536-4662
FAX (612) 647-5301, ext. 82

Mississippi Nurses Association
135 Bounds St., Ste. 100
Jackson, Mississippi 39206
(601) 982-9182
FAX (601) 982-9183

Missouri Nurses Association
1904 Bubba Lane
Box 105228
Jefferson City, Missouri 65110
(314) 636-4623
FAX (314) 636-9576

Montana Nurses Association
104 Broadway, Ste. G-2
PO Box 5718
Helena, Montana 59601
(406) 442-6710
FAX (406) 442-6738

Nebraska Nurses Association
1430 South St., Ste. 202
Lincoln, Nebraska 68502-2446
(402) 475-3859
FAX (402) 475-3961

Nevada Nurses Association
3660 Baker Lane, Ste. 104
Reno, Nevada 89509
(702) 825-3555
FAX (702) 825-3555

New Hampshire Nurses Association
48 West St.
Concord, New Hampshire 03301
(603) 225-3783
FAX (603) 226-4550

New Jersey State
Nurses Association
320 West State St.
Trenton, New Jersey 08618
(609) 392-4884
FAX (609) 396-2330

New Mexico Nurses Association
909 Virginia NE, Ste. 101
Albuquerque, New Mexico 87108
(505) 268-7744
FAX (505) 260-1919

New York State Nurses Association
46 Cornell Rd.
Latham, New York 12110
(518) 782-9400
FAX (518) 782-9530

North Carolina Nurses Association
103 Enterprise St.
Box 12025
Raleigh, North Carolina 27605
(919) 821-4250
FAX (919) 829-5807

North Dakota Nurses Association
549 Airport Rd.
Bismarck, North Dakota 58504-6107
(701) 223-1385
FAX (701) 223-0575

Ohio Nurses Association
4000 East Main St.
Columbus, Ohio 43213-2950
(614) 237-5414
FAX (614) 237-6074

Oklahoma Nurses Association
6414 North Santa Fe, Ste. A
Oklahoma City, Oklahoma 73116
(405) 840-3476
FAX (405) 840-3013

Oregon Nurses Association
9600 SW Oak, Ste. 550
Portland, Oregon 97223
(503) 293-0011
FAX (503) 293-0013

Pennsylvania Nurses Association
2578 Interstate Dr.
PO Box 68525
Harrisburg, Pennsylvania
17106-8525
(717) 657-1222
FAX (717) 657-3796

Rhode Island State
Nurses Association
550 South Water St., Unit 540B
Providence, Rhode Island
02903-4334
(401) 421-9703
FAX (401) 421-6793

South Carolina Nurses Association
1821 Gadsden St.
Columbia, South Carolina 29201
(803) 252-4781
FAX (803) 779-3870

South Dakota Nurses Association
1505 South Minnesota Ave., Ste. 6
Sioux Falls, South Dakota 57105
(605) 338-1401

Tennessee Nurses Association
545 Mainstream Dr., Ste. 405
Nashville, Tennessee 37228-1201
(615) 254-0350
FAX (615) 254-0303

Texas Nurses Association
7600 Burnet Rd., Ste. 440
Austin, Texas 78757-1292
FAX (512) 452-0648

Utah Nurses Association
455 East 400 South, Ste. 402
Salt Lake City, Utah 84111
(801) 322-3439
FAX (801) 322-3430

Vermont State Nurses Association
Box 26 Champlain Mill, 1 Main St.
Winooski, Vermont 05404-2230
(802) 655-7123
FAX (802) 655-7187

Virgin Islands State
Nurses Association
Box 583
St. Croix, US Virgin Islands
00820-4355
(809) 773-2323, ext. 119/116
FAX (809) 776-0610

Washington State
Nurse Association
2505 Second Ave. Ste. 500
Seattle, Washington 98121
(206) 443-9762
FAX (206) 728-2074

West Virginia Nurses Association
2003 Quarrier St.
Charleston, West Virginia
25311-4911
(304) 342-1169
FAX (304) 345-1538

Wisconsin Nurses Association
6117 Monona Dr.
Madison, Wisconsin 53716
(608) 221-0383
FAX (608) 221-2788

Wyoming Nurses Association
Majestic Building, Room 305
1603 Capitol Ave.
Cheyenne, Wyoming 82001
(307) 635-3955
FAX (307) 635-3965

Canadian Provincial Registered Nurses Associations

Alberta

Alberta Association of Registered Nurses
11620—168th Street
Edmonton, Alberta
T5M 4A6
(403) 451-0043

British Columbia

Registered Nurses Association of British Columbia
2855 Arbutus Street
Vancouver, British Columbia
V6Y 3Y8
(604) 736-7331

Manitoba

Manitoba Association of Registered Nurses
647 Broadway Avenue
Winnipeg, Manitoba
R3C 0X2
(204) 774-3477

New Brunswick

Nurses Association of New Brunswick
231 Saunders Street
Fredericton, New Brunswick
E3B 1N6
(506) 458-8731

Newfoundland

Association of Registered Nurses of Newfoundland
55 Military Road
P.O. Box 6116
St. John's, Newfoundland
A1C 5X8
(709) 753-6040

Northwest Territories

Northwest Territories Registered Nurses Association
P.O. Box 2757
Yellowknife, Northwest Territories
X1A 2R1
(403) 873-2745

Nova Scotia

Registered Nurses Association of Nova Scotia
6035 Coburg Road
Halifax, Nova Scotia
B3H 1Y8
(902) 423-6156

Ontario

College of Nurses of Ontario
101 Davenport Road
Toronto, Ontario
M5R 3P1
(416) 928-0900

Prince Edward Island

Association of Nurses of Prince Edward Island
P.O. Box 1838
Charlottetown, Prince Edward Island
C1A 7N5
(902) 892-6322

Québec

Ordre des infirmières et infirmiers du Québec
4200 ouest, boulevard Dorchester
Montréal (Quebec)
H3Z 1V4
(514) 935-2501

Saskatchewan

Saskatchewan Registered Nurses Association
2066 Retallack Street
Regina, Saskatchewan
S4T 2K2
(306) 757-4643

Yukon

Yukon Nurses Society
P.O. Box 5371
Whitehorse, Yukon
Y1A 4Z2
(403) 667-4062

Appendix D

Information for Foreign Nurse Graduates Who Wish to Practice in the United States

Nursing practice in the United States is regulated by each state through its Nurse Practice Act and the State Board of Nursing (or State Board of Nurse Examiners). These licensing laws and appointed boards establish the qualifications for obtaining a license in the state and the grounds for denying a license to an applicant or suspending a nurse's license. Of particular significance is the board's role in defining the scope of nursing practice in a particular state. Qualifications for obtaining a license generally include:

- graduation from an accredited nursing education program
- a satisfactory score on the National Council Licensure Examination (NCLEX) or Canadian Nursing Association Testing Service (CNATS)
- submission of a completed application form with specified fee

Foreign nurse graduates must also obtain an H1 visa, which is a temporary working visa granted to individuals who are not seeking permanent residency in the United States. To obtain an H1 visa, a foreign nurse graduate must have a certificate issued by the U.S. Commission on Graduates of Foreign Nursing Schools (CGFNS). This requirement also applies to Canadian nurses who want to obtain a license in Indiana, Montana, South Dakota, and Washington state. The CGFNS certificate is awarded for successful scores on an examination. This multiple-choice examination is intended to screen foreign nurse graduates and evaluate their understanding of written English and medical terminology, as well as their basic nursing knowledge. The CGFNS examination is given twice a year in sites throughout the world. To take this examination, the foreign nurse graduate must submit a completed application form and a filing fee 3 months before the examination is held (i.e., January 1 for the April exam and July 1 for the October exam). The CGFNS address is 3624 Market St., Philadelphia, PA 19104.

After obtaining a CGFNS certificate, the employing hospital will file for an H1 visa on behalf of the foreign nurse. The Bureau of Immigration and Naturalization Service returns the visa to the hospital, which will send it to the nearest U.S. embassy for delivery to the nurse. Because this visa restricts the holder to working at only one hospital in the United States, a new H1 visa must be obtained if the nurse wishes to work in another hospital or health care facility. Before coming to the United States, the nurse should write to the appropriate State Board for information about obtaining a license and for an application to take the NCLEX at the next available opportunity. The foreign nurse graduate may then move to the United States and practice nursing, usually with some restrictions, until the next NCLEX examination is given. Although the NCLEX examination is identical throughout the states, each state grants a license (that is, the designation "Registered Nurse") based on the individual's score.

The NCLEX is a 2-day-long, multiple-choice examination that evaluates a nurse's ability to systematically analyze and conceptualize nursing care using the scientific method of problem solving commonly called the "nursing process." Successfully obtaining a minimum score on the examination enables the recipient to obtain a license to practice nursing in that state. Generally, once a license is obtained in one state, other states will recognize that license and grant their state license by endorsement. A nurse who wishes to relocate or move to another state (remember that a new H1 visa is required) should contact the State Board of Nursing of the prospective employer's state before the anticipated move to inquire about obtaining a license by endorsement. Requirements for licensure by endorsement vary and may change periodically, so it is important to obtain the most current information from the individual State Board of Nursing.

The H1 visa may be extended annually for a total of 5 years. A resident alien who wishes to remain in the United States beyond this period must apply for permanent residency.

A WORD FOR CANADIAN NURSES

Like the United States, each Canadian province has its own nurse practice act and laws that vary slightly from province to province. All provinces, except Prince Edward Island and Ontario, require nurses to join the provincial nursing association to obtain a license. The provincial nursing association requires successful completion of the CNATS. Several U.S. states also accept the CNATS, thus exempting those Canadians who wish to practice in those states from taking the NCLEX. Those states include:

Alabama	Idaho	Ohio
Alaska	Kentucky	Pennsylvania
Arizona	Maine	Rhode Island
Arkansas	Mississippi	Tennessee
California	Missouri	Utah
Delaware	New Mexico	Wisconsin
Georgia	North Dakota	

Appendix E
Commonly Used Abbreviations

NOTE: Abbreviations in common use can vary widely from place to place. Each institution's list of acceptable abbreviations is the best authority for its records.

° C	degrees Centigrade
° F	degrees Fahrenheit
μg	microgram
μm	micrometer
ʒ	dram
@	at
aa	of each
ABG	arterial blood gas
ac	before meals
ad lib	freely as desired
ADL	activities of daily living
AFB	acid-fast bacilli (e.g., *M. tuberculosis*)
Ag	silver, antigen
AIDS	acquired immunodeficiency syndrome
ALS	amyotrophic lateral sclerosis
AM	morning
ama	against medical advice
AMI	acute myocardial infarction
amp	ampule
AP	anterior posterior
ARC	AIDS-related complex
ARDS	adult respiratory distress syndrome
AS	aortic stenosis
ASD	atrial septal defect
Ba	barium
BCG	bacille Calmette-Guérin vaccine for TB
BE	barium enema
bid	two times a day
BM, bm	bowel movement
BMR	basal metabolic rate
BP	blood pressure
BPH	benign prostatic hypertrophy
BRP	bathroom privileges
BSA	body surface area
BUN	blood urea nitrogen
c̄	with
c/o	complains of
Ca	calcium, cancer, carcinoma
CAD	coronary artery disease
cap	capsule
CAT	computed axial tomography
cath.	catheter, catheterize
CBC	complete blood count
CBR	complete bed rest
CC	chief complaint
cc	cubic centimeter
CCU	coronary care unit, critical care unit
CDC	Centers for Disease Control and Prevention
CEA	carcinoembryonic antigen
CFT	complement-fixation test

cg	centigram
CHF	congestive heart failure
CHO	carbohydrate
Cl	chlorine
cm	centimeter
cm³	cubic centimeter
CNS	central nervous system
CO	carbon monoxide or cardiac output
CO₂	carbon dioxide
COPD	chronic obstructive pulmonary disease
CPK	creatine phosphokinase
CPR	cardiopulmonary resuscitation
cps	cycle per second, unit of frequency
C&S	culture and sensitivity
CSF	cerebrospinal fluid
CT	computed tomography
CVA	cerebrovascular accident, costovertebral angle
CVP	central venous pressure
D&C	dilatation and curettage
D5W	5% dextrose in water
db, dB	decibels
dc	discontinue
DIC	disseminated intravascular coagulation
diff	differential blood count
dil	dilute
DJD	degenerative joint disease
dl	deciliter
DM	diastolic murmur
DNR	do not resuscitate
DOE	dyspnea on exertion
DSA	digital subtraction angiography
dx, Dx	diagnosis
EBV	Epstein-Barr virus
ECF	extracellular fluid
ECG	electrocardiogram
ECT	electroconvulsive therapy
EDC	estimated date of confinement
EDD	estimated date of delivery
EEG	electroencephalogram
EKG	electrocardiogram
elix	elixer
EMG	electromyogram
ENG	electronystagmography
ER	emergency room
ERG	electroretinogram
ESR	erythrocyte sedimentation rate
ESRD	end-stage renal disease
EST	electroshock therapy
f ʒ	fluid ounce
FANA	fluorescent antinuclear antibody test
Fe	iron
FEV	forced expiratory volume
FHR	fetal heart rate
FRC	functional residual capacity
FUO	fever of unknown origin

Fx, fx	fracture, fractional urine test		MICU	medical intensive care unit
g, gm, Gm	gram		ml	milliliter
Gc, GC	gonococcus		mm	millimeter
GCS	Glasgow Coma Scale		mm³	cubic millimeter
GI	gastrointestinal		mm Hg	millimeters of mercury
gr	grain		MRI	magnetic resonance imaging
grav I, II, III, etc	pregnancy one, two, three, etc		MS	multiple sclerosis
			MW	molecular weight
gtt, gt	drop, drops		N	nitrogen
GTT	glucose tolerance test		Na	sodium
GU	genitourinary		NICU	neonatal intensive care unit
GYN, Gyn	gynecological		NIDDM	non–insulin-dependent diabetes mellitus
H₂O	water		NIH	National Institutes of Health
h	hour		nm	nanometer
H⁺	hydrogen ion		NMR	nuclear magnetic resonance
h/o	history of		NPO	nothing by mouth
H&P	history and physical examination		NS	normal saline
HAV	hepatitis A virus		NSAID	nonsteroidal anti-inflammatory drug
Hb	hemoglobin		O₂	oxygen
HBAg	hepatitis B antigen		OD	right eye; optical density; overdose
HBV	hepatitis B virus		OL	left eye
Hct, HCT	hematocrit		OOB	out of bed
Hg	mercury		ORIF	open reduction and internal fixation
Hgb	hemoglobin		OS	left eye
HIV	human immunodeficiency (AIDS) virus		OT	occupational therapy
HLA	human lymphocyte antigen		OTC	over-the-counter
hs	at bedtime		oz, ℥	ounce
HSV	herpes simplex virus		P&A	percussion and auscultation
HZ	hertz, unit of frequency, equal to one cycle/second		Paco₂	partial pressure of carbon dioxide (arterial blood)
I&O	intake and output		Pao₂	partial pressure of oxygen (arterial blood)
IC	inspiratory capacity		para I, II, etc	unipara, bipara, etc
ICP	intracranial pressure		PAT	paroxysmal atrial tachycardia
ICU	intensive care unit		pc	after meals
IDDM	insulin-dependent diabetes mellitus		PCA	patient-controlled analgesia
IE	immunoelectrophoresis		PCG	phonocardiogram
Ig	immunoglobulin		Pco₂	partial pressure of carbon dioxide
IgA, etc	immunoglobulin A, etc		PCP	pulmonary capillary pressure, phencyclidine
IM	intramuscular		PTCA	percutaneous transluminal coronary angioplasty
IOP	intraocular pressure		PCV	packed cell volume
IPPB	intermittent positive pressure breathing		PCWP	pulmonary capillary wedge pressure
IV	intravenous		PD	interpupillary distance; postural drainage
IVP	intravenous push; intravenous pyelogram		PE	pulmonary embolism, physical examination
IVU	intravenous urogram		PEEP	positive end expiratory pressure
JRA	juvenile rheumatoid arthritis		PEG	pneumoencephalography
K	potassium		per	through, by way of
kg	kilogram		PERRLA	pupils equal, round, and reactive to light and accommodation
KUB	kidney, ureters, and bladder (radiograph)			
KVO	keep vein open		PET	positron emission tomography
L	liter		PG	prostaglandin
L&A	light and accommodation		pH	hydrogen ion concentration (acidity and alkalinity)
LBBB	left bundle branch block		PID	pelvic inflammatory disease
LE	lupus erythematosus		PKU	phenylketonuria
LGV	lymphogranuloma venereum		PM	postmortem
LLL	left lower lobe		PM	evening
LLQ	left lower quadrant		PMS	premenstrual syndrome
LMP	last menstrual period		PND	paroxysmal nocturnal dyspnea, postnasal drip
LNMP	last normal menstrual period		Po₂	partial pressure of oxygen
LOC	level of consciousness		PO, po	orally
LP	lumbar puncture		PPD	purified protein derivative
LUL	left upper lobe		ppm	parts per million
LUQ	left upper quadrant		prn	when required, as often as necessary
LVH	left ventricular hypertrophy		PT	physical therapy; prothrombin time
m	meter		PTT	partial thromboplastin time
m, min, ℳ	minim		PUO	pyrexia of unknown origin
MAP	mean arterial pressure		PVC	premature ventricular contraction
mgc	microgram		q	every
MCH	mean corpuscular hemoglobin		q2h	every 2 hours
MCHC	mean corpuscular hemoglobin concentration		q3h	every 3 hours
MCV	mean cell volume, mean corpuscular volume		q4h	every 4 hours
MDR-TB	multidrug-resistant tuberculosis		qd	every day
mg	milligram		qh	every hour
Mg	magnesium		qid	four times a day
MG	myasthenia gravis		qn	every night
MI	myocardial infarction		qod	every other day

qns	quantity not sufficient
R/O	rule out
RA	rheumatoid arthritis
RBBB	right bundle branch block
RBC	red blood cell; red blood count
RDA	recommended daily (dietary) allowance
RDS	respiratory distress syndrome
Rh+	positive Rh factor
Rh−	negative Rh factor
RHD	rheumatic heart disease
RLL	right lower lobe
RLQ	right lower quadrant
RML	right middle lobe
ROM	range of motion
ROS	review of systems
RS	Reiter's syndrome
RSV	Rous sarcoma virus
RUL	right upper lobe
RUQ	right upper quadrant
Rx	take; treatment
$\bar{s}$	without
SB	sternal border
SC	subcutaneous
SCI	spinal cord injury
sib.	sibling
SICU	surgical intensive care unit
SIDS	sudden infant death syndrome
Sig	write on label
SLE	systemic lupus erythematosus
sol	solution, dissolved
sos	if necessary
sp. gr., SG, s.g.,	specific gravity
SQ, subq	subcutaneous
SR	sedimentation rate
ss	half
SSS	sick sinus syndrome, specific soluble substance, short-stay surgery
stat	immediately

STD	sexually transmitted disease
STS	serological test for syphilis
susp	suspension
T_3	triiodothyronine
T_4	tetraiodothyronine
T&A	tonsillectomy and adenoidectomy
TAB	typhoid and paratyphoid A and B
TAH	total abdominal hysterectomy
TAT	tetanus antitoxin; thematic apperception test
TB, TBC	tuberculosis
TBG	thyroxin-binding globulin
TG	triglyceride
TIA	transient ischemic attack
TIBC	total iron-binding capacity
tid	three times a day
TKO	to keep open
TLC	total lung capacity; thin-layer chromatography
TPN	total parenteral nutrition
TPR	temperature, pulse, and respirations
tr, tinct	tincture
TST	triple sugar iron test
UIBC	unsaturated iron-binding capacity
URI	upper respiratory infection
UTI	urinary tract infection
V&T	volume and tension
VC	vital capacity
VD	venereal disease
VDA	visual discriminatory acuity
VDH	valvular disease of the heart
VDRL	Venereal Disease Research Laboratory (test for syphilis)
VS	vital signs
VSD	ventricular septal defect
V_T	tidal volume
W/V	weight/volume
WBC	white blood cell; white blood count
WNL	within normal limits
WR	Wasserman reaction

Index

f following number indicates figure or illustration; t following page number indicates table.